Brief Contents

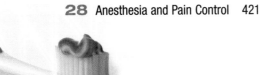

PEARSON'S COMPREHENSIVE
DENTAL ASSISTING

LORI TYLER, MS, Editor

Authors of This Text

Charity Butler, CDA, EFDA
Lead Dental Assistant
Kind Kids in Need of Dentistry, Denver, CO

Angela McGrady, BS, MBA
Former Dental Assistant Instructor
PIMA Medical Institute, Colorado Springs, CO

Ellen Nuss, CDA, RDA
Dental Assisting Instructor
Concorde Career College, Aurora, CO

Angela Osborn, D.D.S.
General Dentist
Solo Practice, Lone Tree, CO

With Contributions by:

Kathy Chitti, CDA, EFDA, AAS
Instructional Specialist
KCTCS Bluegrass CTC, Prestonsburg, KY

Sherri Cooper, CMA, BA
Instructor
College America, Denver, CO

Vickie Hawkins Hash, RDH, BSDH
Dental Hygiene Faculty
Wytheville Community College, Wytheville, VA

Brandy Hoffman-Freeman, CDPMA, CDA, RDA, EFDA
Director of Education
Georgian Institute, GA

Martha L. McCaslin, CDA, BSBM
Dental Assisting Program Director
Dona Ana Community College, Las Cruces, NM

Roxanne Medinger, CDA, RDA, B.S.H.S
President Elect
New Jersey Dental Assistants Association, Shamong, NJ

Cynthia Meekins, CDA, RDA, EDDA
Director for Dental Assisting Program
Concorde Career College, Aurora, CO

Aamna Nayyar, DDS
Director Dental Department
Santa Fe Community College, Santa Fe, NM

Tonya Robinson, CDA, RDA, EFDA
Dental Instructor
Denver Public Schools, Denver, CO

Rita Sheaves, BSDH, RDH, MSEd
Assistant Professor
Wytheville Community College, Wytheville, VA

Brenda Stevens, CDA
Dental Assisting Program Director
Emily Griffith Opportunity School, Denver, CO

Eleanor D. Vanable, CDA, RDH, BS, MA, EdD
Lecturer, Department of Dental Health
Community College of Rhode Island, Harrisville, RI

Brenda Weiman, CDA
Dental Office Business Administrator
Dr. Angela Osborn, Lone Tree, CO

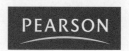

Upper Saddle River, New Jersey 07458

Library of Congress Cataloging-in-Publication Data

Tyler, Lori.
  Comprehensive dental assisting / Lori Tyler.
      p. ; cm.
  Includes bibliographical references and index.
  ISBN-13: 978-0-13-174419-6
  ISBN-10: 0-13-174419-4
 1. Dental assistants. 2. Dentistry. I. Title.
  [DNLM: 1. Dental Assistants. WU 90 T982c 2009]
  RK60.5.T95 2009
  617.6.'0223—dc22   2008021657

Publisher: Julie Levin Alexander
Publisher's Assistant: Regina Bruno
Executive Editor: Joan Gill
Associate Editor: Bronwen Glowacki
Editorial Assistant: Mary Ellen Ruitenberg
Development Editor: Lori Tyler
Director of Marketing: Karen Allman
Senior Marketing Manager: Harper Coles
Marketing Coordinator: Michael Sirinides
Marketing Assistant: Lauren Castellano
Managing Editor, Production: Pat Walsh
Production Liaison: Yagnesh Jani
Production Editor: Heather Willison, S4Carlisle Publishing Services
Media Project Manager: Steven Hartner
Media Editor: Amy Peltier
Manufacturing Manager: Ilene Sanford
Manufacturing Buyer: Pat Brown
Composition: S4Carlisle Publishing Services
Printer/Binder: R.R. Donnelley/Willard
Interior and Cover Designer: Laura Gardner
Cover Printer: Phoenix Color Corp.

Pearson Education Ltd., London
Pearson Education Singapore, Pte. Ltd
Pearson Education Canada, Inc.
Pearson Education–Japan
Pearson Education Australia PTY, Limited

Pearson Education North Asia, Ltd., Hong Kong
Pearson Educación de Mexico, S.A. de C.V.
Pearson Education Malaysia, Pte. Ltd.
Pearson Education, Upper Saddle River, New Jersey

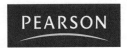

10 9 8 7 6 5 4 3 2 1
ISBN-13: 978-0-13-174419-6
ISBN: 0-13-174419-4

Contents

Pearson's Comprehensive Dental Assisting

Introduction

Dental assistants are a vital part of the delivery of oral health care. Dental assistants work with the dental team to ensure that dental patients receive the highest level of professional care related to their oral health. The dental assistant's responsibilities vary depending on the state in which a dental assistant is employed and the size of the dental practice.

The story of this book began about four years ago when Pearson was asked again and again by instructors "What do you have in Dental Assisting?" In response, we went back to Dental Assisting Instructors to ask them, "What do you and your students want and need in a Dental Assisting textbook and how can we best provide that material?" The answer is here in this complete learning package.

Pearson's Comprehensive Dental Assisting is all about ensuring that you will be a successful student and dental assistant. To help ensure this success, a focus is placed on learning both technical and people skills. This comprehensive textbook helps you learn the right skills for becoming the very best and most effective Dental Assistant by presenting a step-by-step, competency based approach that covers all the facets of the dental assisting profession. People skills are covered throughout the text as various areas related to cultural and lifespan considerations are discussed.

This text was developed and organized with both the needs of the instructor and student in mind. Attention was paid to ensure that the information flowed smoothly and that the topics were presented simply for students to be able to grasp the concepts.

Various authors participated in the development of this textbook. In addition to the numerous years of experience they all have in the field of dentistry, many of the authors offer their expertise as educators. Teaching students how to become a professional, well-trained dental assistant was the goal of this textbook. The authors' style is engaging and straightforward. Difficult concepts are presented clearly and simply to ensure understanding. Procedures are presented with step-by-step instructions. Throughout the text, students are provided critical thinking questions that challenge students to think about various aspects of being a dental assistant.

To be prepared to take certification exams, students must accomplish various learning objectives. A list of these objectives is provided at the beginning of each chapter in the section titled *"Preparing for Certification Exams."* *Learning Objectives* listed at the beginning of each chapter provide a list of competencies that the student must demonstrate after completing each chapter. *Key terms* are terms critical for students to understand. These terms are listed and defined at the beginning of each chapter. The first time each key term is mentioned in the chapter, the terms are placed in bold. Throughout each chapter *Critical Thinking Questions* are asked at various points within the narrative. These questions provide an opportunity for students to further think through the material being learned.

At the end of each chapter a *Check Your Understanding* test is provided. These questions represent the type of questions that would be asked on certification exams. The format of multiple choice matches the format used in certification exams. Other learning aids found throughout the textbook include hundreds of color photos and photo sequences; hundreds of full color, detailed drawings; easy to understand charts and tables; step-by-step procedures; and clear, informative guidelines.

Special features are placed throughout the chapters. These include segments on Dental Assistant Professional Tips, Cultural and Life Span Considerations, Patient Education, Legal and Ethical Issues, Preparing for Externship, and Professionalism. These features have been praised by reviewers of the text as valuable tools that further assist the dental assistant student in learning more about the profession of dental assisting.

Special Features

Dental Assistant Professional Tip

Utilizing the topics covered in the chapter a brief example or scenario has been provided that describes how the information will be used on the job. The focus of these tips is on being a professional in the field of dentistry and the success that will occur with the knowledge gained from the materials presented in the text.

Internet Activities

Internet activities are suggested in each chapter. These activities expand the students' understanding of the material by providing them an opportunity to perform further research on the Internet.

Web References

Web references are provided at the end of each chapter. These references relate to the topics presented in the chapter and offer an opportunity for students and faculty to further research the subjects discussed.

Reviewer comment regarding this feature:

"Internet Activities and Web References are good for the teacher to be able to use. Information literacy is a big thing in college and this will help the teacher out when making assignments."

Patient Education or Legal and Ethical Issue

In each chapter a patient education or legal and ethical issue is presented. The patient education scenarios help students consider their role as a dental assistant in providing patient education. Issues such as patient confidentiality are presented in the legal and ethical feature. With the presentation of these issues students can further their understanding of the legal and ethical issues faced in the field of dental assisting.

Cultural Considerations

The cultural considerations feature addresses the dental assistant's encounters with people of different cultural backgrounds. Brief tips, advice, or general guidelines on how to deal with a specific cultural or communication issue are presented in this feature.

Life Span Considerations

This feature highlights how the dental assistant deals with people of all different ages, with a major focus on older and pediatric patients.

Preparing for Externship

The preparing for externship feature deals with topics and issues relating to students' participation in an externship program as a capstone to their training. Pertinent issues are addressed including student responsibilities, caring attitude, enthusiasm, grooming/dress, interpersonal skills with patients and colleagues, language skills, poise under pressure, preceptor role, etc.

Professionalism

The focus of this feature is on issues important to being successful as a dental assistant. Issues discussed include grooming/dress, interpersonal skills, ethical standards, language skills, punctuality, dependability, and the need for a caring attitude.

Ancillary Materials

The **Instructor's Manual and Instructor's Resource CD-ROM** is available both in print and online at www.prenhall.com. The *Instructor's Manual and CD* contains the following for each chapter:

- Chapter Spotlight
- Lesson Overviews
- Learning Activities
- Pre- and Posttest
- Discussion Questions
- Lecture Notes
- PowerPoint Slides
- Image Bank of every image in the text for use in PowerPoint Slides
- TestGen—with more than 5,000 questions

The **Student Workbook**
The *Student Workbook* contains the following for each chapter:

- Chapter outline
- Short summary of the chapter
- Learning activities/study aids
- Terminology review
- Critical thinking questions
- Chapter review test
- Weighted competency checklists

Student CD-ROM is in the back of every textbook and includes:

- Dental charting activities
- Tray set-up activities
- Dental billing activities
- Scheduling activities
- Radiography exercises
- Quizzes
- Audio glossary
- Games and other learning activities

The Companion Website online at www.prenhall.com/tyler includes:

- Games and learning activities
- Quizzes
- Key terminology
- Audio glossary

Acknowledgments

The Reviewers of This Text

The authors would like to extend appreciation to the following reviewers for providing valuable feedback throughout the review process:

Lynnea Adams, CDA, BA
Associate Professor and Program Coordinator
New Hampshire Technical Institute, Concord, NH

Emily Addison, CDA, BS
Director of Dental Assisting
Pear River Community College, Hattiesburg, MS

Barbara Bennett, CDA, RDH, MS
*Department Chair, Dental Hygiene and Dental
    Assisting Programs Co-Division Director, Allied
    Health Division*
Texas State Technical College, Harlingen, TX

Karen Betts, CDA, RDA
Associate Academic Dean
Concorde Career College, San Diego, CA

Patricia Bradshaw, RDH, BSDH, MS
Coordinator of Health Professions
Lord Fairfax Community College, Middletown, VA

Tonja Bowcut, CDA, AAS
Dental Assisting Program Director/Assistant Professor
College of Southern Idaho, Twin Falls, ID

Roderic Caron Jr., DMD
Supervising Dentist/Professor
New Hampshire Technical Institute, Concord, NH

Kathy Chitti, CDA, EFDA
Instructional Specialist
Big Sandy Community and Technical College,
    Prestonsburg, KY

Dawn Conley, RDH, MEd
Assistant Professor
Camden County College, Blackwood, NJ

Susan Cutler, CDA, BA
Director of Dental Assisting
Martin Community College, Williamston, NC

DeAnna Davis, CDA, RDA, MEd
Dental Assisting Program Director
Pulaski Technical College, North Little Rock, AR

Michelle Davis, CDA, RDA, BSBM
Dental Assisting Program Director
Bryman College, Alhambra, CA

Jan DeBell, CDA, BS
Dental Assisting Instructor
Front Range Community College, Fort Collins, CO

Che' Evans, CDA, QDA, DRT
Dental Assisting Instructor
Medix School-Towson, Towson, MD

Ann Gallerie, RDA
Technical Assistant and Dental Assistant Instructor
Hudson Valley Community College, Troy, NY

Jacquelyn Goodman, CDA
Dental Assisting Director
Tri-State Business Institute, Erie, PA

Gabriele Hamm, CDPMA, NYSLCDA
Dental Assisting Instructor
Hudson Valley Community College, Troy, NY

Patti Harris, RDA, BS
Dental Assisting Instructor
Career Centers of Texas, Fort Worth, TX

Jan Hills, RDH, MA
Chair, Dental Hygiene Program
Iowa Western Community College, Creighton, IA

Anastasia Holler, DMD
Dental Instructor
Pima Community College, Tucson, AZ

Barbara Jarrett, CDA, RDH
Program Coordinator
Trident Technical College, Hanahan, SC

Debra Jennings, DMD
Faculty, Dental Services
Trident Technical College, Charleston, SC

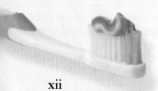

Linda Kihs, CDA, EFDA, MADAA
Instructor
Linn Benton Community College, Albany, OR

Stella Lovato, CDA, RDA, MS, MAEd
Department Chairperson Allied Health
*   Program Coordinator Dental Assisting*
San Antonio College, San Antonio, TX

Lesa McCabe, CDA
Dental Assisting Instructor
Cape Fear Community College, Wilmington, NC

Glenda Miller, CDA, EDA, BS
Dental Assisting Professor
Florida Community College, Jacksonville, FL

Melynn Moore, RDA
Dental Assisting Instructor
Career Centers of Texas, Fort Worth, TX

Cynthia Perry-Knittel
Dental Assisting Program Manager
Ohio Institute of Health Careers, Elyria, OH

Kori Preble, CDA, BS
Dental Programs Clinic Manager
Middlesex Community College, Lowell, MA

Juanita Robinson, CDA, EFDA, LDH, MSEd
Program Director
Indiana University Northwest, Gary, IN

Dana Scott, CDA, CDPMA, RDA, BSOE
Dentist Aide Program Director
Amarillo College, Amarillo, TX

Rita Sheaves, BSDH, RDH, MSEd
Adjunct Faculty
Wytheville Community College, Wytheville, VA

Dorothy Smith, CDA, EFDA, BA
Dental Assisting Program Director
Atlanta Technical College, Atlanta, GA

Crystal Stuhr, CDA
Dental Assisting Instructor
Southeast Community College, Lincoln, NE

Kelly Svanda, CDA
Dental Assisting Instructor
Southeast Community College, Lincoln, NE

Sherie Tynes-Deitz, RDH
Dental Assisting Program Director
YTI Career Institute, Lancaster, PA

Marilyn Westerhoff, CDA, BS
Professor Emeritus
Elgin Community College, Elgin, IL

Jannette Whisenhunt, PhD
Department Chair Dental Education
Forsyth Technical Community College,
    Winston-Salem, NC

A special thanks goes to Cynthia Meekins, Ellen Nuss, Dr. Angela Osborn, and Dr. Scott Greenhaugh who voluntarily offered significant amount of support and hours ensuring that this textbook is a successful and useful tool to dental assisting instructors and students.

Successful Connections

PEARSON'S COMPREHENSIVE
DENTAL ASSISTING

This book connects skills in the classroom and skills on the job, by helping dental assistant students achieve success in school and in their careers.

With Pearson's Comprehensive Dental Assisting, students learn what to do and how to do it. Strong integration of tips, hints, and guidelines helps students overcome common difficulties in performing various dental assisting tasks and problems related to interpersonal skills.

Skills in the Classroom
- Presentation of objectives necessary for students to become prepared for taking certification exams
- Internet Activities
- Web References
- Open design makes using the text easy and clear to the student

Skills on the Job
- Dental Professionalism Tip
- Legal and Ethical Issues
- Cultural Considerations
- Life Span Considerations
- Professionalism
- Patient Education
- Preparing for Externship

Chapter Opener Features . . .

Learning Objectives
The learning objectives help guide the students in understanding the important topics discussed in the chapter.

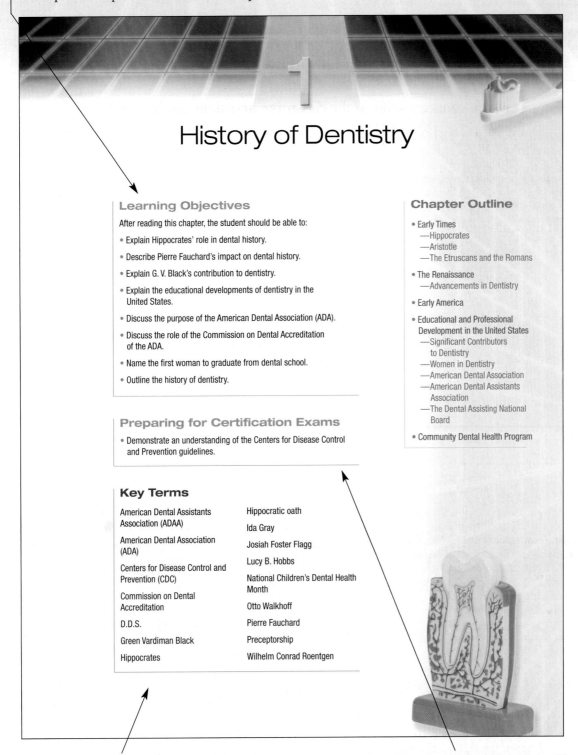

1

History of Dentistry

Learning Objectives

After reading this chapter, the student should be able to:

- Explain Hippocrates' role in dental history.
- Describe Pierre Fauchard's impact on dental history.
- Explain G. V. Black's contribution to dentistry.
- Explain the educational developments of dentistry in the United States.
- Discuss the purpose of the American Dental Association (ADA).
- Discuss the role of the Commission on Dental Accreditation of the ADA.
- Name the first woman to graduate from dental school.
- Outline the history of dentistry.

Preparing for Certification Exams

- Demonstrate an understanding of the Centers for Disease Control and Prevention guidelines.

Key Terms

American Dental Assistants Association (ADAA)

American Dental Association (ADA)

Centers for Disease Control and Prevention (CDC)

Commission on Dental Accreditation

D.D.S.

Green Vardiman Black

Hippocrates

Hippocratic oath

Ida Gray

Josiah Foster Flagg

Lucy B. Hobbs

National Children's Dental Health Month

Otto Walkhoff

Pierre Fauchard

Preceptorship

Wilhelm Conrad Roentgen

Chapter Outline

- Early Times
  - —Hippocrates
  - —Aristotle
  - —The Etruscans and the Romans
- The Renaissance
  - —Advancements in Dentistry
- Early America
- Educational and Professional Development in the United States
  - —Significant Contributors to Dentistry
  - —Women in Dentistry
  - —American Dental Association
  - —American Dental Assistants Association
  - —The Dental Assisting National Board
- Community Dental Health Program

List of Key Terms
The list of key terms represents the most significant key terms discussed in the chapter. These terms are critical for students to master in order to be a successful dental assistant.

Preparing for Certification Exams
These objectives are different from the learning objectives in that these are focused on the skills students must learn to be prepared in taking dental assistant certification exams.

Additional Features

These features provide students the opportunity to review concepts relevant to the dental assistant's success as a professional in the field of dentistry.

Legal and Ethical Issues

A patient may take a variety of prescription drugs. Medications can sometimes affect or cause changes in the oral tissues. If a patient is taking a medication for a condition with which the dental assistant is unfamiliar, the *Physicians' Desk Reference* (PDR) can be a useful reference tool. The PDR provides rapid access to a variety of drug information. It provides information on generic and brand names of drugs, drug class, drug actions, drug side effects, and drug interactions. The PDR has a picture section of medicines where medication can be identified by sight if the name is unknown. This is a valuable tool and a good reference for the latest information on drugs. It is updated and published each year for health care professionals.

Legal and Ethical Issues

Various legal and ethical issues must be understood by the dental assistant. This special feature addresses the complex topics in a practical and relevant manner, assisting the student in understanding and applying these concepts.

Professionalism

Professionalism is one of the most important keys to career success. These featured highlights help students understand the importance of always exhibiting professional behaviors as a dental assistant.

Professionalism

The American Dental Association helps set and approve standards and guidelines for each state dental society. These guidelines and bylaws will help you maintain your professionalism as a dental assistant. Chapter 2 discusses the specific responsibilities and professionalism of each dental team member.

Cultural Considerations

In many dental practices the English language is not the first language of many patients. Compiling a list of available translators for communications between the dentist and non–English-speaking patients will provide quality of care necessary in patient treatment as well as good risk management. Providing multilingual patient information forms makes it easier for patients to provide accurate and complete information.

Cultural Considerations

The world is full of diversity. As a dental assistant it is important to recognize and have the skills and sensitivity to deal with a variety of different types of people. The Cultural Considerations provide students the opportunity to consider various issues as they relate to individuals with diverse cultures.

Life Span Considerations

Life Span Considerations help students develop the skills required as a dental assistant to relate to people of all ages.

Life Span Considerations

Technology in dentistry is making treatment much more comfortable and faster for patients. Doctors are discovering the use of more comfortable laser treatments as opposed to the use of less comfortable intraoral drills. Recently there have been the trials of non–anesthetic-based treatments for patients who have a fear of needles. Studies to increase the life span of restorative materials continue to grow.

Patient Education

The dental assistant has a unique opportunity to educate each patient at every visit. Recent studies by microbiologists suggest that brushing teeth and using dental floss may help prevent heart disease. Reducing inflammation caused by gingivitis and periodontal disease can also reduce the inflammation that leads to atherosclerosis, which is thickening of the walls of the arteries due to a buildup of cholesterol.

Patient Education

The Patient Education features provide hints and important tips on how dental assistants can share information with patients in a professional and complete manner.

Preparing for Externship

As part of their educational experience, students may be required to participate in an externship program. Preparing for Externship discusses topics and issues students may encounter while on externship.

Preparing for Externship

As you prepare to work in your first dental office, it is important to understand the origins of dentistry to appreciate how far dentistry has advanced and gain a further appreciation regarding what might be possible for the future. The externship offers a unique opportunity to learn much about the dental field. During this time, act like a sponge and soak up as much information as possible. Do not just rely on the experience of the dental office. Spend time researching your field online or in the library. Go to websites such as the American Dental Association's site, which contains useful information that will not only serve you in your career but can be utilized as a tool to provide further assistance to those you work with and to your patients.

Dental Assistant PROFESSIONAL TIP

Knowing dental history may not directly help you on the job, but it does expand your knowledge so you can further your growth in the dental career field. Note that the ADA is the main source of information for the dental team. If you are planning an oral hygiene presentation to an elementary class, for instance, the ADA has lesson plans, handouts, and oral health instruction information that can be extremely useful for your presentation.

Dental Assistant/Professional Tip

This feature focuses on addressing important issues that the dental assistant must have knowledge in and how this knowledge will be used as a dental health professional.

Additional Features (continued)

Check Your Understanding

The Check Your Understanding section at the end of each chapter provides the students an opportunity to build confidence in demonstrating their knowledge in the material covered in the chapter. These questions represent the types of questions that may be asked on a certification exam.

● CHECK YOUR UNDERSTANDING

1. Who was the "chief of the toothers and the physicians"?
   a. Hesi-Re
   b. Hippocrates
   c. Pierre Fauchard
   d. Aristotle

2. What is the meaning of the Hippocratic oath?
   a. to provide dental treatment to everyone
   b. to do no harm
   c. to cure dental disease
   d. to extract teeth

3. Who is known as the "father of modern dentistry"?
   a. Aristotle
   b. G. V. Black
   c. Pierre Fauchard
   d. Hippocrates

4. Who was one of George Washington's dentists?
   a. John Greenwood
   b. Robert Woofendale
   c. John Baker
   d. Both a and c

5. Which dentist is recognized for his invention of the dental chair?
   a. Isaac Greenwood
   b. Josiah Foster Flagg
   c. Chapin Harris
   d. Pierre Fauchard

6. Preceptorship is defined as
   a. studying and training with someone already in the field.
   b. studying at a formal college.
   c. reading a book on the subject.
   d. observing a dentist.

7. The acronym D.D.S. stands for
   a. dental doctor of surgery.
   b. doctorate degree in surgery.
   c. doctor of dental surgery.
   d. doctorate of dental surgery.

8. When was the American Dental Association formed?
   a. 1859
   b. 1869
   c. 1879
   d. 1866

9. Who was the first woman to graduate from dental school?
   a. Ida Gray
   b. Chapin Harris
   c. Lucy B. Hobbs
   d. Irene Newman

10. Who was the first person to x-ray teeth?
    a. Wilhelm C. Roentgen
    b. Otto Walkhoff
    c. Edmund Kells
    d. Horace Wells

Internet Activities

Knowing how to use the computer to find information on the World Wide Web is an important tool for any professional. The Internet Activities feature helps students build their confidence in using the computer and conducting research on the Internet on topics related to their dental assisting profession.

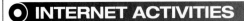

INTERNET ACTIVITIES

- Using the Internet, research the history behind the toothbrush, toothpaste, and dental floss. How do the original versions of these items differ from those available today? How are they similar?

- Search the ADA website for information on National Children's Dental Health Month and learn more about this fun month.

Web References

Students can use the Web References feature to learn more about the topics discussed in the chapter.

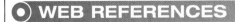

WEB REFERENCES

- American Dental Association www.ada.org
- British Dental Journal www.nature.com/bdj/journal/v199/n8/full/4812913a.html
- Centers for Disease Control and Prevention www.cdc.gov
- National Museum of Dentistry www.dentalmuseum.org
- Oral Health America www.oralhealthamerica.org

History of Dentistry

Learning Objectives

After reading this chapter, the student should be able to:

- Explain Hippocrates' role in dental history.
- Describe Pierre Fauchard's impact on dental history.
- Explain G. V. Black's contribution to dentistry.
- Explain the educational developments of dentistry in the United States.
- Discuss the purpose of the American Dental Association (ADA).
- Discuss the role of the Commission on Dental Accreditation of the ADA.
- Name the first woman to graduate from dental school.
- Outline the history of dentistry.

Preparing for Certification Exams

- Demonstrate an understanding of the Centers for Disease Control and Prevention guidelines.

Key Terms

American Dental Assistants Association (ADAA)

American Dental Association (ADA)

Centers for Disease Control and Prevention (CDC)

Commission on Dental Accreditation

D.D.S.

Green Vardiman Black

Hippocrates

Hippocratic oath

Ida Gray

Josiah Foster Flagg

Lucy B. Hobbs

National Children's Dental Health Month

Otto Walkhoff

Pierre Fauchard

Preceptorship

Wilhelm Conrad Roentgen

Chapter Outline

- Early Times
  - Hippocrates
  - Aristotle
  - The Etruscans and the Romans

- The Renaissance
  - Advancements in Dentistry

- Early America

- Educational and Professional Development in the United States
  - Significant Contributors to Dentistry
  - Women in Dentistry
  - American Dental Association
  - American Dental Assistants Association
  - The Dental Assisting National Board

- Community Dental Health Program

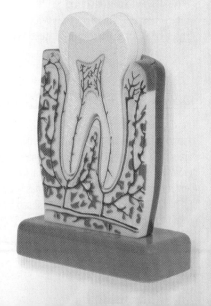

Oral health problems have plagued society since the beginning of time. Understanding how oral diseases affected early society has helped dentists over time discover ways to perform more humane treatments. Dentistry has evolved from being a very primitive practice to one that now involves sophisticated technology. In addition, the development of professional organizations for dentistry has assisted in advancing the field of dentistry. As the field has advanced, the need for well-trained, skilled professionals has increased. This chapter provides the dental assistant with an introduction to the field of dentistry and helps dental assistants gain an appreciation of the advancements made in their chosen career.

Early Times

In studying early society, ancient remains have proven that tooth ailments such as decay and impacted or missing teeth were common. As early as 5000 BCE, people thought "toothworms" caused tooth pain. This folklore was believable because people thought demons lived in the body. The belief was that if an individual had a toothache, the individual must have upset the demons and deserved the pain. It is now thought that the "worms" were either the appearance of the pulp or maggots from rotting food. Other evidence of dentistry during early society includes these examples:

- The Chinese used acupuncture around 2700 BCE to treat pain associated with tooth decay.
- The Babylonians used sticks called chewing sticks to clean teeth. This practice was one of the earliest recordings of dental hygiene. These sticks were chewed until

Dental Assistant   PROFESSIONAL TIP

Knowing dental history may not directly help you on the job, but it does expand your knowledge so you can further your growth in the dental career field. Note that the ADA is the main source of information for the dental team. If you are planning an oral hygiene presentation to an elementary class, for instance, the ADA has lesson plans, handouts, and oral health instruction information that can be extremely useful for your presentation.

the ends were soft and brush-like. Then the brush was used to remove debris from between the teeth.

Around 2600 BCE a man by the name of Hesi-Re, an Egyptian scribe, is referenced as the first "dentist," known as "chief of the toothers and the physicians." Evidence of dentistry during this time has been traced back to some Egyptian remains that contained a bridge constructed of gold bands and a calf's tooth. In Egypt during this time, it has been reported that the Pharaohs and others were afflicted with teeth ailments. It is thought that these teeth disorders resulted from chewing the coarse grain used to make bread. Through the examination of ancient remains, evidence of jaw surgery that took place in Egypt has been discovered. In addition, procedures such as drilling two holes just below the root of a molar to treat an abscess and splinting of teeth are evident.

Table 1-1 lists some of the important highlights in dental history.

Why is the Hippocratic oath important to us today?

Hippocrates

Around the fifth century, **Hippocrates,** known as the "father of medicine," began to teach a civilized approach to medicine (Figure 1.1). He rejected the notion that spirits or demons caused illness and embraced medicine as a science. Hippocrates taught that magic and medicine should be separate. He felt that fluids in the body such as phlegm, yellow bile, black bile, and blood caused disease or led to good health. His writings included patient confidentiality and documentation of treatment to be passed down to other physicians. This information was later described and recorded in the Hippocratic oath.

The **Hippocratic oath** stems from Hippocrates' early approach to medicine and is a code of ethics that guides those in the medical and dental fields. The Hippocratic oath essentially means "do no harm." Hippocrates helped to advance the field of dentistry by emphasizing the importance of healthy teeth. Many of his writings described the illnesses of the teeth and gums. He believed that decay was caused by corrosive foods and dirt trapped in the teeth and recommended the use of rinses to remove the debris. Hippocrates invented dental instruments such as extraction forceps. These forceps helped the advancement of the dental field.

In spite of Hippocrates' logical approach to medicine, "majic" was still thought of as the way to treat a variety of ailments. Some extreme examples of the use of magic include the belief that women with halitosis (bad breath) should take the head of a hare and three mice with intestines removed and grind these together to make a powder. This powder would then be mixed with chalk and rubbed onto the teeth with unwashed wool. A concoction suggested for toothaches was for patients to

TABLE 1-1 Highlights of Dental History

3000–525 BCE	The earliest known dentist was Hesi-Re, who was known as the "chief of the toothers and the physicians."
700–510 BCE	This was the Etruscan period, in which fixed and removable bridgework was constructed.
460–370 BCE	Hippocrates, considered the founder of medicine, recorded information on teeth and is the first to recognize teeth *in utero,* humoral pathology.
384–322 BCE	Aristotle is the first to study comparative anatomy of the teeth.
30 CE	Celsus is the first to mention filling teeth with lint or lead.
130–201 CE	Galen is the first to mention the nerves of the teeth.
249 CE	St. Apollonia, the patron saint of dentistry, has her teeth extracted in Alexandria.
1308–1745 CE	The Guild of Barber-Surgeons is founded.
1452–1519 CE	Leonardo da Vinci presents the earliest accurate drawings of teeth.
1498 CE	The Chinese invent the modern toothbrush.
1542 CE	Ambroise Pare, a military surgeon, mentions transplantation and filling of teeth and ligation of teeth with gold wire.
1683 CE	Antony Van Leeuwenhoek uses a primitive microscope to view bacteria.
1728 CE	Pierre Fauchard writes "Le Chirurgien Dentiste."
1763 CE	John Baker is the earliest qualified dentist to practice in America.
1790 CE	Josiah Flagg constructs the first dental chair.
1790–1859 CE	Dental floss is invented by a New Orleans dentist named Levi Spear Parmly.
1794 CE	John Greenwood constructs dentures for George Washington.
1840 CE	Horace Hayden and Chapin Harris establish the world's first dental school, the Baltimore College of Dental Surgery. The school merges with the University of Maryland School of Dentistry in 1923.
1844 CE	Horace Wells discovers nitrous oxide anesthesia.
1848 CE	Waldo Hanchett patents the dental chair.
1872 CE	The first toothpick manufacturing machine is developed and patented by Silas Noble and J. P. Cooley.
1885 CE	H. N. Wadsworth is credited as the first American to receive a toothbrush patent.
1891 CE	G. V. Black develops "Extension for Prevention" and cavity classifications.
1895 CE	Roentgen discovers the x-ray.
1948 CE	The Dental Assisting National Board is established.

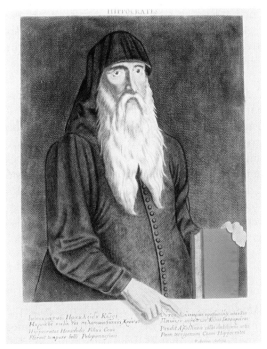

FIGURE 1.1
Hippocrates.

grind mice, mix the grinds with marble, and put the grinds on the ailing tooth. A mouthwash remedy made with dog teeth boiled in wine was another idea. Although these suggestions were popular at the time, there is no evidence that these remedies were successful in addressing the issues.

Aristotle

During the time of Aristotle various beliefs about teeth existed. Aristotle, a Greek philosopher, wrote a study on comparative anatomy. He concluded that teeth were animal instead of human. He explored how blood was supplied to teeth and, like Hippocrates, discussed the tooth extraction process. Another example of Aristotle's beliefs can be seen in his writings, which contained misinformation about the number of teeth men and women have. Aristotle purported that men had 32 teeth and women had only 30 teeth. Today we know this not to be the case. Aristotle's writings continue to demonstrate that during this early time in history individuals had an interest in dentistry.

The Etruscans and the Romans

Between 100 and 400 BCE, the Etruscans in Italy contributed to the restorative art of dentistry. A bridge from this era has bands made of gold that fastened to natural teeth and artificial teeth that were made of calves' teeth. The Etruscans also made the first dentures. Over time the Romans conquered the Etruscans; as a result the cities came under Roman rule and the Etruscan people were absorbed into the community as Romans. The Romans actually learned the field of dentistry from the Etruscans.

Some famous Romans specialized in dentistry. Celsus (50 CE) believed that deterioration of the body caused dental decay. He recommended hot water, mustard seed, and narcotics for tooth pain. It is believed that Celsus performed the first filling using lint and lead. This was done to give the tooth strength and keep the crown from cracking during extraction. Archigenes (100 CE) believed that dental disease resulted from an infection inside the tooth. He treated afflicted teeth by cutting holes into them to drain the pus. Galen (200 CE) categorized teeth into central incisors, cuspids, and molars. He also was said to be the first to recognize that teeth have nerves.

The Renaissance

The Middle Ages, most commonly referred to as the time between 500 and 1500 CE, saw dentistry and medicine being practiced by monks, who were typically the most educated people at the time. In 1210 CE, France established the Guild of Barbers. The barbers were split into two groups: the educated group, who performed dental surgeries, and the lay group, who performed routine dental services such as shaving and tooth extraction. Other individuals known as tooth-drawers were tradesmen who specialized in extracting teeth (Figure 1.2). These individuals usually traveled from town to town and pulled teeth at markets or fairs. Tooth-drawers were thought of as quacks who tried to make the public believe they were educated and skilled although this was not the case.

Advancements in Dentistry

Advancements in dentistry during the Middle Ages included the development in China of a "silver paste" to fill cavities. This advancement occurred in 700 CE and the

> ### Cultural Considerations
>
> The American Dental Association website provides a variety of resources for public use. If you have a patient whose second language is English, it is important to ensure that your communications with that patient will be understood. To help with your non–English-speaking patients, you will want to become familiar with the information provided on the ADA website. If possible, either print out the materials or suggest to patients who seek further information to conduct a search for more information at the ADA site (www.ada.org). Never assume that your patients are computer literate. Individuals may be afraid to tell you that they do not have computer skills. Be sure to offer assistance in accessing the information they are seeking.

material today is known as amalgam. In 1723, **Pierre Fauchard,** known as the "father of modern dentistry" (Figure 1.3), published *The Surgeon Dentist, A Treatise on Teeth* in which he describes a comprehensive system of dentistry. He is credited for writing the first comprehensive book on dentistry called *Surgeon Dentist.*

Fauchard held a variety of beliefs about dentistry. Fauchard felt that sugar was bad for the teeth and should be limited in the diet. He recommended that teeth be filled with lead or gold, after the removal of decay, to strengthen them. Fauchard also believed that if a tooth was knocked out it should be reimplanted. Fauchard was

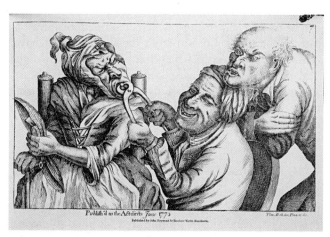

FIGURE 1.2
Tooth-drawers extracting a tooth.

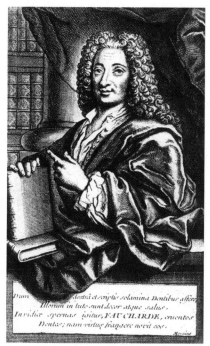

FIGURE 1.3
Pierre Fauchard, the "father of modern dentistry."

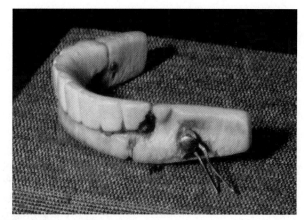

FIGURE 1.4
George Washington's lower dentures.
Courtesy of the Samuel D. Harris National Museum of Dentistry, Baltimore, MD

the first to determine that a patient should be seated in a comfortable position on a chair and that the dentist should stand behind the patient so as not to block any available light. He prescribed oil of cloves and cinnamon for pulpitis (inflamed pulp of tooth). Today oil of cloves is still used in sedative filling materials.

In his writings Fauchard recommended that his patients rinse with their own urine to combat decay, which he discovered was not toothworms, as believed in earlier times, but dirt, decay, and muck. Because Fauchard was such a highly regarded dentist, his teachings were used for more than 100 years. For instance, the practice of rinsing with baby urine was a suggested treatment for periodontal disease until the early 1900s.

Why was Pierre Fauchard considered the "father of modern dentistry"?

Early America

In early colonial America, a blacksmith or barber performed most of the dental work. The famous American revolutionary Paul Revere was one of those part-time dentists. He performed procedures such as fillings and cleanings and constructed bridges and dentures.

Trained dentists began arriving to the colonies from England. One such person was Robert Woofendale, who marketed his abilities to perform a variety of different dental procedures. A dentist named John Baker arrived in America around 1763, shortly after Woofendale's arrival, and practiced in the Boston area. He later became one of George Washington's dentists.

The first native-born dentist in colonial America was Isaac Greenwood. Later, John Greenwood, Isaac's son, became another dentist of George Washington's. John Greenwood is credited with constructing an upper denture for George Washington that was made out of a sheet of gold with ivory riveted into it. Washington's lower dentures were carved from a single piece of hippopotamus tusk (Figure 1.4). Many dentures were made for Washington, and none of them were made of wood as legend leads us to believe. George Washington had the various dentures because they would stain when he drank

wine, prompting Greenwood to recommend that Washington remove his dentures when drinking wine!

Other notable individuals during this time include Josiah Foster Flagg and Robert Tanner Freeman. **Josiah Foster Flagg** is most recognized for his invention of the dental chair. Robert Tanner Freeman was the first African American to graduate with a formal dental education. He graduated from Harvard University School of Dental Medicine in 1869.

What differences might there be between the dentures used today and those used in the past?

Educational and Professional Development in the United States

Throughout early history the profession of dentistry was obtained through **preceptorship,** the study and hands-on training of someone already in the field. Dental schools and colleges did not exist until the 1800s when a dentist named Chapin A. Harris began advocating a more formal education for dentists. He began with a library of many publications including his own, *The Dental Art: A Practical Treatise on Dental Surgery* and *The American Journal of Dental Science.* Thanks to Harris and other dental pioneers, the Baltimore College of Dental Surgery was founded on March 6, 1840, and began to award **doctor of dental surgery (D.D.S.)** degrees. This college is now called the University of Maryland School of Dentistry, and it houses the National Museum of Dentistry (Figure 1.5). Today the museum has many artifacts and exhibits so visitors can learn about the history and the future of dentistry.

Significant Contributors to Dentistry

One dental pioneer who advocated an independent dental profession was a dentist named **Green Vardiman Black,** or G. V. Black (Figure 1.6). He earned the title of the "grand old man of dentistry" because of his many contributions to the field. Black taught in dental schools and was responsible for the standardization of cavity preparations.

In 1844 another American dentist played a key role in dental history. Horace Wells discovered a way to use nitrous oxide gas to relieve the pain of extractions on his patients. Other individuals who contributed to advancements in dentistry include the following individuals:

- An intern named Karl Koller first used local anesthetics for dentistry in 1884 to numb the gingiva. He ini-

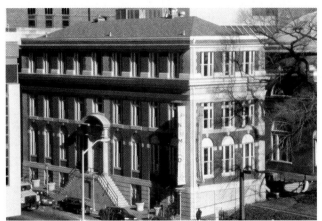

FIGURE 1.5
The National Museum of Dentistry, Baltimore, Maryland.
Courtesy of the Samuel D. Harris National Museum of Dentistry, Baltimore, MD

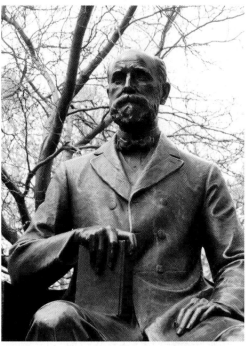

FIGURE 1.6
Green Vardiman Black, the "grand old man of dentistry."
Photo by Falke Bruinsma, http://photos.innersource.com

tially used cocaine, which was a popular painkiller, to anesthetize the eye.

- William S. Halstead, a surgeon, demonstrated the use of anesthetic to block a nerve on the mandible.

- **Wilhelm Conrad Roentgen,** a German physicist, is credited with the 1895 discovery of radiation usage (Figure 1.7). His research involved the use of certain rays to develop photographic films. He did not know exactly what the rays were so he called them x-rays. When these films were exposed to radiation, a picture or shadow appeared. In fact, Roentgen tested this unknown ray on his wife's hand. It took 25 minutes to expose the bones in her hand (Figure 1.8).

- **Otto Walkhoff,** a dentist and medical doctor in Braunschweig (Brunswick), Germany, took a dental radiograph on January 14, 1896. This was only 14 days after the publication of the experimental results of the discovery of x-rays by Roentgen. Walkhoff made the first dental radiograph by placing an unexposed photographic glass plate wrapped in black paper in his own mouth and covering it with a rubber dam. He lay on the floor and submitted himself to 25 minutes of x-ray exposure.

- An American dentist named C. Edmund Kells also experimented with the use of x-rays. He held film plates in hundreds of patients' mouths while exposing them to radiation. As a result, he lost his hand to cancer and ultimately the suffering led to suicide. This unfortunate event did lead to some safety changes in the use of radiation. Kells was also known for hiring the first "lady in attendance." During that time it was

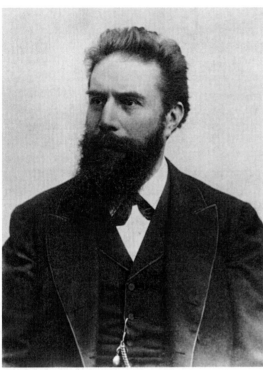

FIGURE 1.7
Wilhelm Roentgen.

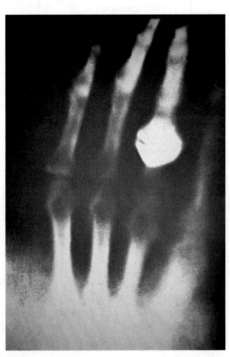

FIGURE 1.8
X-ray of Roentgen's wife's hand.

improper for women patients to visit the dentist alone. However, having a "lady in attendance" present made it possible for women to receive dental care without an escort. In the 1930s educational guidelines were formed to begin formal training for dental assistants (Figure 1.9).

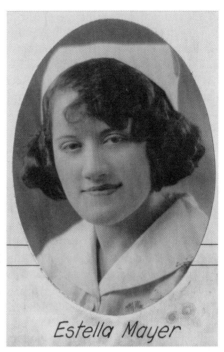

Estella Mayer

FIGURE 1.9
A dental assistant in 1923.
Courtesy of the Galter Health Sciences Library, Special Collections, Northwestern University, Chicago, IL

Women in Dentistry

Women played a small role in practicing dentistry, mostly through preceptorship with family members. In 1859, Emeline Jones was the first woman to have a regular dental practice in the United States. **Lucy B. Hobbs** practiced dentistry with her husband, but felt the need for a formal education. After a lot of determination she was finally accepted and graduated from the Ohio College of Dental Surgery in Cincinnati in 1866. In 1890, **Ida Gray** became the first African American woman to graduate with a dental degree from the University of Michigan School of Dentistry. Around 1885, Malvina Cueria became the first female dental assistant. Irene Newman became the first dental hygienist in 1906.

What do you think it would be like to be a dental assistant in 1930? How has dental assisting advanced since the 1930s?

American Dental Association

Due to the work of the dental pioneers just discussed and others, the dental field continued to advance and in 1859 twenty-six dentists formed the **American Dental Association (ADA)**. Regional organizations formed over time, and in 1897, the Southern Dental Association merged with the American Dental Association, resulting in a national organization. Today, each state has its own organization with bylaws approved by the ADA. The

ADA is an educational source for the public and dental professionals such as dentists, assistants, and hygienists. The ADA's large reference library contains approximately 33,000 books and 17,500 journals.

The ADA's **Commission on Dental Accreditation** evaluates and provides accreditation for dental assistant and hygiene programs as well as programs for dentists in the United States.

American Dental Assistants Association

The first society for dental assistants was formed in Nebraska in 1917. In 1921, Juliette Southard formed a dental assistant society in New York City. By 1923, Juliette Southard and other women began researching the idea of forming an association just for dental assistants. The idea was discussed in 1923 at the ADA meeting in Cleveland. By 1924 bylaws and a constitution were presented and the **American Dental Assistants Association** (**ADAA**) officially became incorporated on March 17, 1925, in Illinois.

The Dental Assisting National Board

In 1948 the Dental Assisting National Board (DANB) was established. DANB is a credentialing and certification organization for dental assistants. DANB identifies quality dental assistants for the public by measuring and promoting skills. By the 1950s education programs for dental assistants were in existence throughout the United States.

What obstacles do you think the first female dentist faced?

Community Dental Health Program

Not only does the American Dental Association promote education for dental professionals, but for the public as well. The ADA has long monitored and promoted the safety and effectiveness of dental health products. Consumers across the country recognize the ADA's seal of acceptance on dental products such as toothpaste, toothbrushes, and mouth rinses (Figure 1.10).

One of the most popular public dental health activities initiated by the ADA is the observance of Children's Dental Health Month. It began as a single day of observance on February 8, 1949, and turned into a weeklong celebration in 1955. In 1981 it evolved into a monthlong celebration known as **National Children's Dental Health Month.**

The **Centers for Disease Control and Prevention** (**CDC**) is a government organization that plays a role in community public health in the area of water fluoridation. Water fluoridation is one of the most cost-effective means of ensuring the community receives fluoride. Because fluoride is added to some public water supplies, everyone benefits from this cost-effective method of dental disease prevention.

A variety of other organizations advocate improving oral health for all individuals. One such organization is called *Oral Health America*. This is an independent organization that is dedicated to improving oral health for all

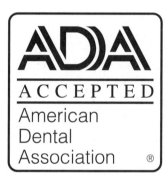

FIGURE 1.10
The ADA's seal of acceptance.
Courtesy of the American Dental Association

Life Span Considerations

Consider your elderly patients who may have experienced dental care without all of the technological advances we have today. If you know some of the history of dentistry and the future of dentistry, you may be able to educate them and calm some of their dental fears. For example, your patient may not be comfortable receiving restorations because of the pain of receiving the anesthetic and the sound of the "drill." You can explain to such a patient how restorative dentistry has advanced from early times to the use of many techniques that minimize the pain the person may experience.

Preparing for Externship

As you prepare to work in your first dental office, it is important to understand the origins of dentistry to appreciate how far dentistry has advanced and gain a further appreciation regarding what might be possible for the future. The externship offers a unique opportunity to learn much about the dental field. During this time, act like a sponge and soak up as much information as possible. Do not just rely on the experience of the dental office. Spend time researching your field online or in the library. Go to websites such as the American Dental Association's site, which contains useful information that will not only serve you in your career but can be utilized as a tool to provide further assistance to those you work with and to your patients.

Americans. Additional programs offered to improve oral health include the National Sealant Alliance. This program pledges to provide sealants (a type of dental material applied to one or more teeth to help prevent dental caries) to 225,000 children by 2010. The National Spit Tobacco Education Program is a program that provides education about the dangers of spit tobacco.

As a dental assistant, becoming involved with community dental health is a natural progression in one's professional career. Dental professionals can become involved in the community by contacting these organizations, providing dental health presentations at schools, and working with the dental employer to ensure that dental patients receive education in oral health.

Why have a National Children's Dental Health Month?

SUMMARY

The history of the dental profession is important for dental assistants to learn. In order for the profession to grow, individuals in the dental field must learn from the past and look toward the future. Dental professionals must strive to continue the educational path established by the pioneers of dentistry.

Many significant advances in dentistry continue to occur: (1) the use of lasers for removing decay often without anesthetics and aiding in cosmetic dentistry; (2) digital radiology, which often results in less radiation exposure and is more convenient; (3) dental implants to replace missing teeth; (4) porcelain veneers to hide gray or chipped teeth; (5) dental spas, where patients are provided shoulder and neck massages, paraffin wax dip for hands, and aromatherapy to ensure that the dental experience is less frightening and more enjoyable; and (6) the discovery that stem cells from human exfoliated deciduous teeth contain supplies of stem cells that can develop into tooth-generating cells. This discovery is very promising for restoring tissues and teeth destroyed by gingivitis and periodontitis. It is an exciting time to be a part of this great profession.

KEY TERMS

- **American Dental Assistants Association (ADAA):** Professional organization that represents the profession of dental assisting. p. 8
- **American Dental Association (ADA):** Professional organization that represents the profession of dentists in the United States. p. 7
- **Centers for Disease Control and Prevention (CDC):** Federal agency that makes recommendations on health and safety issues. p. 8
- **Commission on Dental Accreditation:** Evaluates and provides accreditation for programs for dentists, dental assistants, and dental hygienists in the United States. p. 8
- **D.D.S.:** Doctor of Dental Surgery degree. p. 6
- **Green Vardiman Black:** Referred to as the "grand old man of dentistry." Black was responsible for the standardization of cavity preparations. p. 6
- **Hippocrates:** The "father of medicine." p. 2
- **Hippocratic oath:** An obligation to refrain from wrongdoing and to treat patients to the best of one's ability. p. 2

- **Ida Gray:** The first African American woman to graduate with a dental degree. p. 7
- **Josiah Foster Flagg:** Man who invented the dental chair. p. 5
- **Lucy B. Hobbs:** First woman to graduate from dental school. p. 7
- **National Children's Dental Health Month:** Initiated by the ADA to observe children's dental health; occurs during the month of February each year. p. 8
- **Otto Walkhoff:** German dentist credited with taking the first x-rays of teeth in 1896. p. 6
- **Pierre Fauchard:** Known as the "father of modern dentistry." p. 4
- **Preceptorship:** Studying and training for a field under the guidance of a professional already practicing in the field. p. 6
- **Wilhelm Conrad Roentgen:** German physicist who discovered radiographs (x-rays) in 1895. p. 6

CHECK YOUR UNDERSTANDING

1. Who was the "chief of the toothers and the physicians"?
   a. Hesi-Re
   b. Hippocrates
   c. Pierre Fauchard
   d. Aristotle

2. What is the meaning of the Hippocratic oath?
   a. to provide dental treatment to everyone
   b. to do no harm
   c. to cure dental disease
   d. to extract teeth

3. Who is known as the "father of modern dentistry"?
   a. Aristotle
   b. G. V. Black
   c. Pierre Fauchard
   d. Hippocrates

4. Who was one of George Washington's dentists?
   a. John Greenwood
   b. Robert Woofendale
   c. John Baker
   d. Both a and c

5. Which dentist is recognized for his invention of the dental chair?
   a. Isaac Greenwood
   b. Josiah Foster Flagg
   c. Chapin Harris
   d. Pierre Fauchard

6. Preceptorship is defined as
   a. studying and training with someone already in the field.
   b. studying at a formal college.
   c. reading a book on the subject.
   d. observing a dentist.

7. The acronym D.D.S. stands for
   a. dental doctor of surgery.
   b. doctorate degree in surgery.
   c. doctor of dental surgery.
   d. doctorate of dental surgery.

8. When was the American Dental Association formed?
   a. 1859
   b. 1869
   c. 1879
   d. 1866

9. Who was the first woman to graduate from dental school?
   a. Ida Gray
   b. Chapin Harris
   c. Lucy B. Hobbs
   d. Irene Newman

10. Who was the first person to x-ray teeth?
    a. Wilhelm C. Roentgen
    b. Otto Walkhoff
    c. Edmund Kells
    d. Horace Wells

INTERNET ACTIVITIES

- Using the Internet, research the history behind the toothbrush, toothpaste, and dental floss. How do the original versions of these items differ from those available today? How are they similar?

- Search the ADA website for information on National Children's Dental Health Month and learn more about this fun month.

WEB REFERENCES

- American Dental Association   www.ada.org
- British Dental Journal   www.nature.com/bdj/journal/v199/n8/full/4812913a.html
- Centers for Disease Control and Prevention   www.cdc.gov
- National Museum of Dentistry   www.dentalmuseum.org
- Oral Health America   www.oralhealthamerica.org

2

The Dental Team

Learning Objectives

After reading this chapter, the student should be able to:

- Describe the responsibilities and characteristics of dental assistants.
- Discuss how to receive credentialing as a dental assistant.
- Define the steps for becoming a dentist.
- Explain the responsibilities of dental hygienists.
- List the training requirements for dental laboratory technicians.
- Compare team support staff positions and their role in office functions.

Preparing for Certification Exams

- Apply effective communication techniques with a variety of patients.
- Demonstrate knowledge of ethics/jurisprudence/patient confidentiality.

Chapter Outline

- Dental Assistant
  —Responsibilities of a Dental Assistant
  —Characteristics of a Professional Dental Assistant
  —Credentialing, Professional Growth, and Development
  —Expanded Function Dental Assistant

- Dentist

- Dental Specialist

- Registered Dental Hygienist

- Dental Laboratory Technician

- Support Staff in the Dental Office

Key Terms

American Medical Technologists (AMT)

Dental Assisting National Board (DANB)

Doctor of Dental Medicine (D.M.D.)

Doctor of Dental Surgery (D.D.S.)

Endodontist

Oral and maxillofacial surgeon

Oral pathologist

Orthodontist

Periodontist

Prosthodontist

Public health dental official

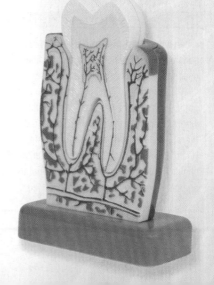

The profession of dentistry is composed of a variety of professionals who are trained to perform various responsibilities. The dental assistant performs a vital role in assisting the dentist. Other members of the dental team include individuals trained in performing administrative duties, clinical duties, or both. Some individuals choose to specialize in practices such as pediatrics or oral surgery. As a member of the dental team, it is important to be familiar with the responsibilities held by dental team members and to understand the training involved for the various positions held by those individuals.

What are the duties of the dental assistant?

Dental Assistant

The history of dental assistants started in the 1880s. At this time all dental assistants were women and were known as "ladies in attendance." Over the years more males have joined the profession of dental assisting. Newer technology has allowed for more patients to be seen each day, and extra responsibilities have been placed on the dental assistant. These added responsibilities provide the dentist the time needed to address the needs of each patient.

Responsibilities of a Dental Assistant

The responsibilities of the dental assistant are often confused with the responsibilities of the dental hygienist. There are significant differences in these two professions.

Dental Assistant PROFESSIONAL TIP

When working with outside salespeople, remember that all patient personal information should be kept confidential. Full names are never used when discussing a patient's case.

The office will typically choose to use last names only or the patient's first name with last name initial. Do not leave patient charts where a sales representative or other patient may have easy access to them. This is a violation of patient confidentiality as set forth in the Health Insurance Portability and Accountability Act. Patient charts should be kept in a secure filing cabinet that must be accessed with a combination or key lock.

In many cases the dental assistant, also called DA or dental auxiliary, is the first to see the patient in the operatory prior to seeing the dentist or hygienist. Dental assistants have many duties that sometimes go unnoticed. These duties are critical to ensuring that the practice runs smoothly. The dental assistant's responsibilities will vary depending on the dental practice laws in the state in which the DA works. To find the legal requirements for your state, contact the state's dental board of examiners.

Duties of the dental assistant can include the following:

- Operatory setup and disassembly after each patient
- Operatory disinfection and instrument sterilization after each patient
- Seating and dismissal of patients
- Exposing, developing, and mounting of dental radiographs
- Instructing patients on home care techniques and dental products
- Making alginate impressions and pouring diagnostic casts
- Maintaining inventory and ordering of supplies
- Documenting patient medical histories
- Front-office practice management
- Laboratory procedures such as making custom trays and temporaries
- Comforting patients during procedures
- Taking vital signs
- Assisting the dentist during procedures
- Coronal polishing
- Sterilizing instruments
- Placing sealants
- Charting patient information
- Applying topical fluorides
- Applying fluoride varnishes

The dental assistant's responsibility can involve either or both clinical and administrative duties. Those dental assistants who are directly involved in patient care are often called *chairside assistants* (Figure 2.1). The skill of working chairside with a dentist is called *four-handed dentistry*. For some procedures more than one assistant is

Legal and Ethical Issues

Keep in mind that even though dental assistants are usually taught to coronal polish or expose radiographs in school, most states require certification to practice these skills. The DA who works in a state that does not require either a CDA or RDA must still obtain coronal polish and radiographic certification. These are considered dental assistant expanded functions.

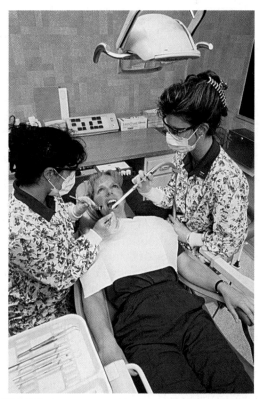

FIGURE 2.1
The chairside assistant.

required to assist. When a dentist uses two assistants, the skill is referred to as *six-handed dentistry*. This second assistant may help with mixing materials, passing instruments, holding the patient's tongue, or suction.

The second individual may be referred to as the *circulating assistant*. Circulating assistants provide help to the front desk, hygienist, chairside assistant, and dentist. Responsibilities of circulating assistants include performing lab work, sterilizing and disinfecting rooms and instruments, answering phones, filing charts, scheduling patients, charting, taking and processing x-rays, ordering supplies, and maintaining dental equipment.

Administrative duties assigned to the dental assistant vary depending on the dental office. The dental assistant may have the responsibility for sterilization procedures, including the management of biohazardous waste. This individual may also be given the responsibility of opening and closing the office each day. This task can entail turning on the air compressor or x-ray processor to ensure that certain temperatures and pressures are maintained. Dental material supply ordering is another essential task typically assigned to the dental assistant. Ensuring that supplies are present is critical to a practice's success.

What type of attire is appropriate for the office?

Characteristics of a Professional Dental Assistant

Professionalism must be upheld in every aspect of being a dental assistant, including the way we speak, what we wear, how we respond to other people, and our knowledge of the field. The DA's appearance can greatly impact whether a patient takes the DA seriously and listens to the DA's advice. The following list contains items that can influence a patient's first impression of the dental assistant and other team members:

- Personal hygiene
- Work uniform
- Makeup and fingernails
- Hair
- Jewelry, tattoos, and visible piercings
- Facial expressions and attitude

As a dental assistant it is important to practice good oral hygiene habits. Having good oral hygiene as an assistant lends credibility to any recommendations the DA may make to a patient. If the DA has visible gingival (gum) problems or extreme yellowing of teeth, this type of image can negatively impact what the dental assistant is saying to his patients.

Good oral hygiene habits include everyday brushing and flossing. These are the most important tasks one can do to ensure a clean mouth. Brushing with dentifrice (toothpaste) helps to keep away stain and odor. This should be performed approximately two to three times per day. The morning is the most important brush of the day. It removes bacteria that have accumulated during the night. For breath odor control between brushings, a sugar-free breath mint is suggested. Because assistants work in close proximity with patients and staff, fresh breath is important. Cigarette smoke produces an offensive odor that stays in the clothes, hair, and mouth. Tobacco creates an odor that emanates from the mouth and lungs, and no mint can hide that odor.

Not only is oral hygiene important but hygiene in general is of significant importance. Bathing should be done each day. Application of fragrance-free deodorant is recommended to reduce the possibility of bad body odor. The wearing of colognes or perfumes on the job should be avoided. Many patients are allergy sensitive to perfumes or colognes or they do not enjoy scents.

The employer will decide what constitutes a work-approved uniform. Some facilities prefer the dental assistant to wear scrubs. In many cases wearing scrubs underneath a laboratory coat would be considered appropriate attire. Every office has a uniform policy that needs to be followed. It is not appropriate for employees to show up in jeans and/or a t-shirt unless the dentist has said otherwise. Some dental assistants arrive at the office in street clothes and then change into the approved office uniform. Uniforms approved by the Occupational Safety and Health Administration (OSHA) include scrubs, a three-quarter length or full-length fluid-repellent lab coat with button or snap top collar and cuffs that roll back to prevent materials from reaching tissue on the arms of team members, an aerosol filtration mask that filters 95% or higher bacterial filtration efficiency (BFE), goggles with side shields, and white vinyl or leather shoes.

Makeup should be kept to a minimum. The following should be avoided: red lipstick, brightly colored fingernail polish, heavy eye shadow or blush, and thickly applied mascara. Fingernails should be cut to one-eighth of an inch. Longer nails are harder to clean and promote the growth of bacteria underneath the nail bed. Long nails also increase the chance of puncturing personal protective equipment (PPE), which could be a health hazard to both the employee and the patient. Fingernail polish should be clear or neutral. Acrylic nails are typically not acceptable. Hair needs to be neat and cleaned regularly. If hair is long it should be worn pulled back above the collar. If long hair is allowed to hang, it can get in the way during patient care and could possibly become entangled in rotating equipment, causing harm or serious injury to the dental professional or the patient. During surgical procedures the assistant is usually required to wear a hair net to prevent the contamination of the surgical site.

Jewelry should be kept simple. Large-stoned rings or rings on multiple fingers should be removed before work. Facial jewelry of any type is considered intolerable and should be removed before work. Examples of these include eyebrow rings, tongue rings, nose rings, cheek rings, and lip rings. Single piercings on the ears can be worn, and stud earrings are the suggested style. Long earrings should not be worn. Many people, both male and female, are wearing tattoo artistry. Most dental offices enforce the rule that tattoos must not be visible, meaning that tattoos must be covered during work hours.

Greeting patients cheerfully and with enthusiasm is important. A positive attitude can be contagious. The dental assistant can set the tone for how patients will feel about their appointment. When stress runs high in the office, keep a positive attitude with a smile. Take initiative, set an example, help coworkers as much as possible, and be reliable with shift hours and completing tasks. Stay away from gossip that can occur among coworkers. Office gossip only breeds bigger problems, creates an unpleasant working environment, and is unprofessional.

In the field of dentistry the dental assistant will hear, smell, and see things that are sometimes unusual and may be unpleasant. When this occurs it is important that the dental assistant not respond either verbally or nonverbally. Part of the reason for this is to show respect to patients. Keep in mind that dental patients come to the office with various beliefs and practices. Patient differences should be honored and each should be treated with respect.

Cultural Considerations

The clothing a DA selects to wear can significantly impact a patient's opinion regarding the presence of—or lack of—professionalism. Depending on a patient's age or culture, the DA's clothing can be offensive if it is unprofessional. While treating patients the dental assistant should wear the required personal protective equipment (PPE), which includes a lab coat, face mask, gloves, and protective eyewear. PPE is worn to prevent contamination between operator and patients. Clothing under the DA's lab coat should be professionally appropriate, such as scrubs. If street clothing is worn under the lab coat, items such as see-through blouses, low-cut V-neck shirts, and short skirts should be avoided. Flat comfortable shoes should complete the outfit. Individuals in positions such as that of administrative assistant, supply salesperson, office manager, or equipment technician usually dress in business casual attire in the dental office.

Why should a dental assistant become certified?

Credentialing, Professional Growth, and Development

Credentialing requirements for dental assistants are dependent on the state in which the DA practices. In some states dental assistants are required to be certified; in others they must be registered. To become certified the dental assistant must pass a national certification exam. Various organizations offer certification exams. The **Dental Assisting National Board (DANB)** offers such an exam. The registration exam can be taken through the **American Medical Technologists (AMT)** association. On passing the DANB exam, the applicant becomes a certified dental assistant (CDA). On completion of the AMT exam, the applicant becomes a registered dental assistant (RDA). The CDA is recognized nationally, whereas the RDA is recognized by some states.

Dental Assisting National Board

Several states require dental assistants to pass the DANB exam in order to practice as CDAs. The DANB exam is offered three times a year for two consecutive days. Applicants may also choose to take a computerized exam. DANB has three eligibility pathways from which the applicant can choose. Each pathway requires a current cardiopulmonary resuscitation (CPR) card.

The DANB exam is four hours long and is divided into three separate parts. If one particular portion of the test is not successfully passed, the applicant can pay and reregister to take that portion of the exam. The first portion of the test consists of 120 questions on chairside procedures, oral health management, office emergencies, dental materials, records management, and office procedures. The second portion of the test focuses strictly on x-ray information. There are 100 questions on this portion covering processing of radiographs, mounting, and safety for the operator and patient. The last section tests the dental assistant's knowledge of infection control issues such as cross-contamination, sterilization and disinfection, environmental asepsis, and occupational safety. There are 100 multiple-choice questions in this section.

Once an individual passes the CDA exam, she becomes a certified dental assistant. This certification is good for one full year. To keep a certification current, the dental assistant must complete 12 credit hours of continuing education. To fulfill continuing education credits, applicants can do volunteer work in the community, purchase at-home video courses and books, attend seminars, or take dental-related courses.

American Medical Technologists

The American Medical Technologists exam is very similar to the DANB. States that do not recognize the DANB exam will usually require that the AMT exam be taken for state registration. Administration of the AMT exam started in the early 1970s and was originally focused only on registration for medical assistants, but is now offered to many other medical professionals such as phlebotomy technicians, medical assistants, laboratory technicians, and allied health instructors. Applicants must be 18 years old. Participants must have attended and graduated from an accredited dental assisting school with three years of full-time work experience in a dental office. Verification from the employer must be documented, and a current CPR certification from the American Heart Association or Red Cross must be completed before the individual is allowed to take the exam.

Although some states do not require dental assistants to be either certified or registered, graduates of dental programs are strongly urged to obtain these credentials. Having credentials can make a difference in your chances of gaining employment. Maintaining your credentialing will let your employer know you are dedicated to your career and that you are willing to stay current on new dental materials and procedures. Salary increases are not guaranteed, but employers will often increase salaries based on personal goals accomplished and the employee's credentials.

Expanded Function Dental Assistant

The duties of the *expanded function dental assistant* (EFDA) or *expanded duties dental assistant* (EDDA) are covered by the dental practice act for each state. Therefore, the credential cannot be carried from state to state. Salary is determined solely by the employer. There are assisting positions that will encourage pay raises with additional responsibilities (Figure 2.2). A dental assistant who is trained as an EFDA or EDDA will command a salary that can range anywhere from $17 to $33 per hour.

To obtain these credentials, the DA must take additional continuing education courses as determined by each state. There are also DANB and AMT exams specifically designed to ensure national board recognition for expanded functions. When an applicant passes the exam, the applicant receives a certificate from the state in which the exam is taken. Expanded functions are recognized in

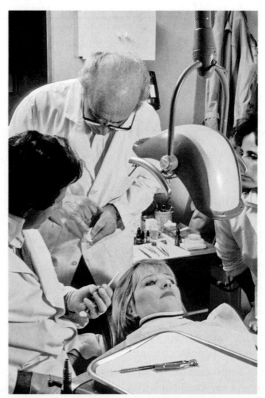

FIGURE 2.2
The dentist and dental assistant working side by side.

many states and may allow the DA to perform many of the following expanded functions:

- Packing gingival retraction cords
- Taking final impressions
- Packing and carving amalgam restorations
- Placing and finishing composite restorations
- Coronal polishing
- Placing and removing dental dams
- Placing and removing Tofflemire/matrix bands
- Applying varnishes, bases, and liners
- Removing sutures
- Placing and adjusting sealants
- Placing and removing provisional crowns
- Applying topical fluoride or topical anesthetic

Dentist

The dentist is licensed to perform various dental procedures on patients, provide patient education on oral hygiene, and monitor patient home care. Dentist responsibilities include evaluation of oral health status and screening for pathology; placement of restorations, crowns, bridges, and veneers; fabrication of full and partial denture appliances; tooth extractions; dental implants; writing prescriptions; and staff and office management. Those entering the field of dentistry either become degreed as a **doctor of dental medicine (D.M.D.)** or as a **doctor of dental surgery (D.D.S.).** The degree is determined by the school at which the individual attends. Seven to nine years is the average time spent on completing all degree requirements.

Which specialist performs root canal therapy?

Dental Specialist

On graduation from dental school, some dentists choose to further their education in a dental specialty. Specializing in a specific field of dentistry takes about two to three years of additional education. Several different specialties are available:

- A pediatric dentist specializes in oral care for children. The pediatric dentist treats children from birth through adolescence. Pediatric oral care includes restorations, crowns, space maintainers, orthodontic appliances, pulpotomies/pulpectomies, and extractions.
- An **oral and maxillofacial surgeon** treats the entire head and neck region. Specialties include extractions of third molars (wisdom teeth), which is a very common procedure for oral surgeons; reconstruction of the facial bones or mandible caused by genetic deformities or injuries;

and treatment of pathology. Oral and maxillofacial surgeons are often referred to as oral surgeons.

- An **endodontist** treats the pupal tissues, which is the blood and nerve supply for teeth. Dentists refer patients who need endodontic therapy (root canals) to an endodontist.
- A **prosthodontist** fabricates prosthetic appliances for dental patients to maximize masticular function and improve occlusion due to missing teeth. Some appliances that a prosthodontist fabricates are crowns, bridges, veneers, inlays/onlays, implants and dentures (full and partial), and snore/night guards.
- A **periodontist** handles any conditions concerning the supporting structures of the teeth and prevention of gingival disease with treatment. Periodontists perform gingival grafting surgeries, crown lengthening procedures, implant surgeries, and a number of hygiene procedures to decrease tooth loss.
- A **public health dental official** works for organizations that offer oral health care on county, state, and national levels. Public health dental officials provide oral hygiene education to the general public/community.
- An **orthodontist** deals with the correction of malocclusion by realignment of the teeth and also deals with temporomandibular joint dysfunction.
- An **oral pathologist** performs any testing that must be done on tissue that originates from the oral cavity to confirm the detection of disease.
- Although not specialists, *general practitioners* are allowed to perform any of the above-stated tasks, depending on the task's complexity and the dentist's desires/strengths. Some refer many procedures; others like to do almost all procedures themselves and only refer the most problematic and complex cases.
- Oral and maxillofacial radiology was added to the list of specialties in 1999. The oral and maxillofacial radiologist is usually a dentist who is a specialist in performing, understanding, and interpreting diagnostic imaging of facial, neck, and oral structures.

How do the responsibilities of a dental assistant and a dental hygienist differ?

Life Span Considerations

Technology in dentistry is making treatment much more comfortable and faster for patients. Doctors are discovering the use of more comfortable laser treatments as opposed to the use of less comfortable intraoral drills. Recently there have been the trials of non–anesthetic-based treatments for patients who have a fear of needles. Studies to increase the life span of restorative materials continue to grow.

Registered Dental Hygienist

The registered dental hygienist (RDH) plays a key role in the dental office providing oral hygiene care for patients (Figure 2.3). Dental hygienists are in high demand, and it is a growing field in the United States. A dental hygienist works independent from the dentist, which allows for a flexible work schedule. In the past this field was predominantly a female career. In recent years more males have entered the field. The hygienist has several responsibilities, including the following:

- Instructing patients on home care techniques and dental products
- Scaling/removing calculus
- Exposing, processing, and mounting intraoral and extraoral radiographs
- Coronal polishing
- Sterilizing instruments
- Placing sealants
- Charting patient information
- Scheduling recall patients
- Making alginate impressions (in some states)
- Applications of topical fluorides and other medicinal agents

About two to four years are required for an individual to complete a degree in dental hygiene. After completion of a state and an American Dental Association (ADA) accredited program in dental hygiene, the hygienist must successfully pass the National Dental Hygiene Board examination and a regional or state clinical examination in order to obtain state licensure, which allows the dental hygienist the opportunity to practice dental hygiene in a variety of settings within the state. The American Dental Hygienists Association or local state dental examiners board provides information on education or licensure.

Dental Laboratory Technician

The certified dental laboratory technician (CDT) (Figure 2.4) provides all fabricated prosthetic appliances made for patients. Common prescription orders that a CDT will fill for the dentist include these:

- Crowns/bridges
- Implants
- Palatal expanders and orthodontic appliances
- Space maintainers
- Veneers/inlays/onlays
- Night guards and snore guards
- Full and partial dentures

For an order to be placed, the doctor writes a prescription documenting exactly what needs to be made for the patient, the due date for delivery, the shade and material used, and the tooth number. A doctor's signature and license number are required and are generally included on the prescription form.

A laboratory technician should have in-depth knowledge of specific oral anatomy shapes and dimensions to be able to fabricate the prosthetic device to resemble natural tooth and oral structures.

In order to be a CDT you must complete three separate examinations within a four-year period. There are five examination subjects to choose from, including crown and bridge, partial denture, full denture, ceramics, and orthodontics. Each involves a written and practical element. The average pay for a lab technician is $6 to $12 an hour, depending on the state in which one works.

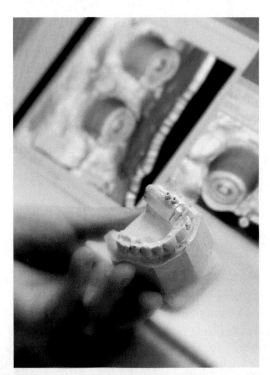

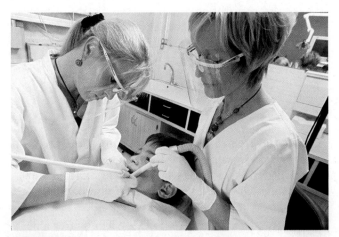

FIGURE 2.3
Hygienist performing dental work on a child's teeth.

FIGURE 2.4
Dental technician examining a plaster cast with dental implants.

Support Staff in the Dental Office

The support staff may consist of an office manager, administrative assistant, dental aide (sterilization technician/hygiene assistant), equipment technician, and dental supply salesperson. These team members are important to the business of the dental practice. Without their expertise the practice would not flow smoothly.

The front-office staff handles scheduling and finances for the office. The office manager and administrative assistant work together to carefully schedule patients for their dental needs. The office manager, also known as the business assistant, handles crucial bookkeeping paperwork that must be processed to insurance companies and employee payroll checks.

The administrative assistant keeps track of all front-office supplies. This individual schedules patients and puts together a yearly schedule. Administrative assistants ensure that all necessary health history information is documented in the patient's chart before the patient is seen by the doctor. The assistants also keep track of special appointments or dates the doctor may have on the office schedule. A specialized certification through DANB is offered for office managers or dental assistants who would like to become certified dental practice management administrators.

Dental aides provide assistance to the dental practice by performing tasks such as sterilizing instruments, pouring diagnostic casts, mounting radiographs (x-rays), charting oral conditions, and seating/dismissing patients.

The job of the dental aide is similar to that of the dental assistant, but these individuals do not perform all-encompassing intraoral work.

Equipment technicians are hired by the dental office to deliver, install, and repair dental equipment. To keep the dental office running efficiently, it is critical to keep all equipment in good running condition. Broken equipment can significantly impact office production. No production means zero income. Keeping a log of when equipment should be serviced is important. Most major dental equipment should be checked quarterly.

The dental supply salesperson assists the dental office in dealing with supply orders. This individual's knowledge regarding the dentist's likes and dislikes is helpful in determining what new products the office may want to try and when bargains are available. Problems with orders can be handled expertly by the supply salesperson.

Preparing for Externship

When preparing to use classroom skills at the externship site, be open to exploring other positions in the office. One advantage of exploring other positions is that it allows the DA to be cross-trained in various aspects of the dental office, making the DA more valuable to employers. Another advantage is that the DA may discover aspects of other positions that might be of future interest.

SUMMARY

As a member of the dental team, it is important for the dental assistant to be familiar not only with the dental assistant's role but also with the roles of the other dental team members. The members of the dental team include the dentist, the dental hygienist, the dental assistant, and the office administrator. The type of practice is dependent on the specialty of the dentist. Most dental practices are general dental practices, although some dentists choose to specialize in specific areas of dentistry such as endodontics or orthodontics. The dental assistant is typically the individual who assists the dentist in patient pro-

cedures. Depending on the state where the dental assistant works, the DA may be required to become certified. Certification can be acquired through the Dental Assisting National Board. Once an individual has successfully completed the DANB exam, the individual becomes a certified dental assistant (CDA). Some states require dental assistants to be registered. The dental assistant who passes the registration exam offered by the American Medical Technologists association becomes a registered dental assistant.

KEY TERMS

- **American Medical Technologists (AMT):** An organization of medical professionals that administers certification tests in order to become registered.   p. 14
- **Dental Assisting National Board (DANB):** Provides a nationally recognized test for front-office professionals or chairside assistants to become certified in their profession.   p. 14

- **Doctor of Dental Medicine (D.M.D.):** The degree a person receives on graduation from dental school; awarded to individuals who complete clinical hours of training in dentistry and successfully complete board examinations.   p. 16
- **Doctor of Dental Surgery (D.D.S.):** The degree a person receives on graduation from dental school; awarded to individuals who complete clinical hours

KEY TERMS (continued)

of training in dentistry and successfully complete board examinations. This degree is the same as the D.M.D degree. The degree awarded is determined by the university.   p. 16

- **Endodontist:** A dentist who specializes in the diagnoses and treatment of dental pulp diseases.   p. 16
- **Oral and maxillofacial surgeon:** A dentist who specializes in the treatment of the entire facial structure due to injury or disease.   p. 16
- **Oral pathologist:** A dentist who specializes in examining tissue samples to provide proper diagnosis and treatment of biopsy results.   p. 16
- **Orthodontist:** A dentist who corrects malocclusions by realignment of the teeth and/or joints.   p. 16

- **Periodontist:** A dentist who specializes in the treatment of the surrounding structures that support the teeth due to injury or disease.   p. 16
- **Prosthodontist:** A dentist who specializes in the fabrication of prosthetic dental devices for tooth replacement.   p. 16
- **Public health dental official:** Provides dental health care on county, state, and national levels by providing education and demonstration of proper oral hygiene instruction to elementary schools, high schools, businesses and the general population/community.   p. 16

CHECK YOUR UNDERSTANDING

1. A sterilization technician is another title for
   a. dental assistant.
   b. dental hygienist.
   c. dental aide.
   d. lab technician.

2. The DANB exams are based on
   a. radiography.
   b. sterilization/disinfection.
   c. dental chairside skills.
   d. all of the above.

3. Which staff member keeps track of office supplies and bookkeeping?
   a. dental hygienist
   b. dental assistant
   c. dentist
   d. office manager

4. DANB and AMT memberships must be renewed
   a. every 10 years.
   b. every year.
   c. every 3 years.
   d. every 5 years.

5. This dental specialist will treat malocclusion by realignment of the teeth or joints.
   a. orthodontist
   b. periodontist
   c. endodontist
   d. prosthodontist

6. Expanded function dental assistants are not allowed to
   a. make impressions.
   b. process radiographs.
   c. place gingival retraction cords.
   d. scale.

7. The acronym for a doctor of dental surgery is
   a. D.O.D.
   b. D.D.S.
   c. D.S.D.
   d. A.D.D.

8. When writing out lab slips, which item is not on the prescription?
   a. shade
   b. sex
   c. birth date
   d. name

9. This dental specialty deals with the treatment of children from birth to age 17.
   a. pediatric dentist
   b. oral surgeon
   c. prosthodontist
   d. dental public health official

10. This skill is not a dental hygienist's responsibility.
    a. coronal polishing
    b. delivery of oral hygiene instruction
    c. extracting teeth
    d. periodontal probing

INTERNET ACTIVITY

- Go to www.danb.org/ and find out more about your state's requirements for becoming a certified dental assistant.

WEB REFERENCES

- American Dental Association education information   www.ada.org/public/careers/team/index.asp
- Bureau of Labor Statistics Occupational Outlook Handbook   www.bls.gov/oco/ocos097.htm
- California Committee on Dental Auxiliaries licensing information   www.comda.ca.gov/licensing.html
- California Committee on Dental Auxiliaries examination information   www.comda.ca.gov/exam_rdh.html

3

Dental Ethics and Law

Learning Objectives

After reading this chapter, the student should be able to:

- Identify the basic principles of ethics.
- Explain the American Dental Association's Code of Ethics.
- Discuss the purpose of a state dental practice act.
- Compare and contrast the terms *direct supervision* and *general supervision*.
- Discuss the difference between the terms *legal* and *ethical*.
- Define the terms *negligence* and *malpractice*.
- Differentiate between written and implied consent.
- Explain the requirements for releasing a patient record.
- Demonstrate how to make corrections on a patient's record.

Preparing for Certification Exams

- Demonstrate knowledge of ethics and jurisprudence.

Key Terms

Abandonment

Civil law

Criminal law

Dental jurisprudence

Dental practice act

Due care

Expanded function

Express contract

Health Insurance Portability and Accountability Act (HIPAA)

Implied contract

Informed consent

Informed refusal

Malpractice

Negligence

Reciprocity

Res gestae

Res ipsa loquitur

Respondeat superior

Risk management

Tort

Written consent

Chapter Outline

- Ethical Principles in Dentistry
  —Autonomy
  —Nonmaleficence
  —Beneficence
  —Justice
  —Veracity
- Professional Code of Ethics
- State Dental Practice Act
- Dental Jurisprudence
  —Criminal and Civil Law
  —Contracts
  —Negligence and Malpractice
  —Tort Law
- Risk Management
- Confidentiality
  —Health Insurance Portability and Accountability Act
- Dentist–Patient Relationship
  —Abandonment
- The Patient Record

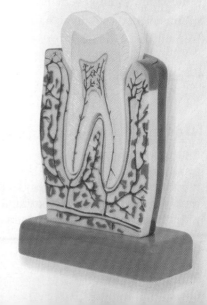

On a daily basis the dental health care team is required to maintain ethical and legal principles in which **dental jurisprudence,** the governing laws in the science of dentistry, is critical at all times. **Dental practice acts** provide legal restrictions, as set forth by each state's legislative body, that describe the statutes regarding performance guidelines of licensed and nonlicensed dental health care professionals. By understanding the dental practice act, the law, moral responsibilities, and ethics, the dental team will be successful in maintaining good risk management and aid in the prevention of costly lawsuits for the dental practice.

Ethical Principles in Dentistry

Ethics deals with moral judgments and behaviors, right versus wrong, good versus evil. In the dental field ethical behavior is defined by a code known as the American Dental Association Principle of Ethics. Unlike the law, which rarely changes, ethics are constantly changing. One's ethics are learned through various means including personal values (right from wrong), education (study, don't cheat), religion (golden rule: "Do unto others as you would have them do unto you"), parents ("How would you like it if that happened to you?"), and learning from others' behaviors.

Ethical principles help guide the dental team's actions as it makes decisions about patient care. Basic principles used in the health care profession by providers to recognize, explain, and rationalize moral and ethical choices include the following:

- Autonomy ("self-governance")
- Nonmaleficence ("do no harm")
- Beneficence ("do good")
- Justice ("fairness")
- Veracity ("truthfulness")

Dental Assistant   PROFESSIONAL TIP

It is important for the dental assistant to understand the state dental practice act regarding the practice of dental assisting in his or her state. Dental practice requirements and regulations for dental assisting can vary greatly from state to state. It is very important for dental assistants to understand the laws and regulations for the state in which they practice.

Legal and Ethical Issues

Ethically, we ask ourselves "What *should* I do?" Legally, we ask "What *must* I do?" Legal questions are very specific; we know what is right or wrong and the minimum standard of behavior is all that is required. Ethics are not as specific; we question our principles, and set a high standard on behavior. For instance, there may be times when the dental assistant witnesses or may be instructed to perform actions that may violate ethical standards.

Ethical dilemmas can be handled by making a few simple decisions. First, distinguish the alternatives and establish what is at risk, categorize your options, and then decide on a plan of action. Decisions will need to be made on the part of the dental assistant. Should the DA remain at the practice under these conditions or should she seek other employment? Ethically, the dental assistant would not want to participate in substandard care or practice unlawful dentistry that may harm the patient. If the dental assistant decides not to make any choice, how will it affect her employment history? The dental assistant is the only one who can ethically answer these questions with regard to her own decisions about how to handle a situation.

The American Dental Assistants Association's Principles of Ethics and Code of Conduct can be viewed by visiting the following website: www.dentalassistant.org.

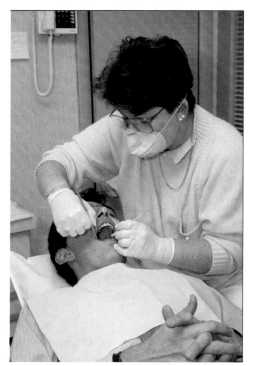

FIGURE 3.1
Expanded functions.

Autonomy

The autonomy principle expresses the concept that the dental team has a duty to treat the patient according to the patient's desires, within the bounds of accepted treatment, and to protect the patient's confidentiality. Under this principle, the dental team's primary obligations include involving patients in treatment decisions in a meaningful way, with due consideration being given to the patient's needs, desires, and abilities, and safeguarding the patient's privacy.

Nonmaleficence

The principle of nonmaleficence means that the dental team has a duty to protect the patient from harm. The dental team's primary obligations include keeping knowledge and skills current, knowing one's own limitations and when to refer to a specialist or other professional, and knowing when and under what circumstances delegation of patient care to auxiliaries is appropriate according to the dental practice act of the team's specific state.

Beneficence

The beneficence principle expresses the concept that the dental team has a duty to promote the patient's welfare. The dental team's primary obligation is service to the patient and the public-at-large. The most important aspect of this obligation is the competent and timely delivery of dental care.

Justice

The principle of justice means that the dental team has a duty to be fair in their dealings with patients. The dental team's primary obligations include dealing with people justly and delivering dental care without prejudice.

Veracity

Under the principle of veracity the dental team has a duty to be honest and trustworthy in their dealings with people. The dental team's primary obligations include respecting the position of trust inherent in the dentist–patient relationship, communicating truthfully and without deception, and maintaining intellectual integrity. The concept of veracity must also be reflected in dental practice advertising. Truthfulness in the ads designed by the staff for media such as the newspaper and Yellow Pages is critical for the overall reputation of the practice.

The five principles of ethics just discussed are summarized in Table 3-1.

How does a dental assistant establish patient trust within the dental office?

Professional Code of Ethics

Many professions, such as the dental, medical, and legal professions, have written codes of ethics. In fact, the American Dental Assistants Association (ADAA) publishes a guide for the professional dental assistant.

The high standard of care provided to dental patients is based both on the code of ethics set forth by the profession of dentistry as well as the laws that have been established to govern this profession. A common question that might be asked when addressing an ethical situation would be "What should I do?" This is different from the question "What must I do?" which would refer to something being decided by a set law.

TABLE 3-1 Basic Ethical Principles

Principle of Ethics	Code of Conduct	Example
Autonomy (self-governance)	Patient involvement	The dental team should inform the patient of the proposed treatment and any reasonable alternatives in a manner that allows the patient to become involved in treatment decisions.
Nonmaleficence (do no harm)	Education	All credentialed dental team members are obligated to keep their knowledge and skills current.
Beneficence (do good)	Service to community	Dental teams are obligated to continue their learning and go to continuing education meetings to keep abreast of new developments in dentistry.
Justice (fairness)	Patient selection	Although dental teams may exercise reasonable discretion in selecting patients for their practices, dentists shall not refuse to accept patients into their practice or deny dental service to patients because of the patient's race, creed, color, sex, or national origin.
Veracity (truthfulness)	Standard of care	Dental teams shall not represent the care being rendered to their patients in a false or misleading manner.

Courtesy of the American Dental Assistants Association

State Dental Practice Act

Each state's board of dentistry is an administrative board responsible for supervising, enforcing, and ensuring adherence to the dental practice act of its specific state. The Board of Dental Examiners usually consists of dentists, public consumers, and dental auxiliaries appointed by the governor of the state. Each state imposes regulations and legal rules that act as the professional standards for dental practice through the state dental practice act. This act regulates all areas of dentistry and provides protection for both those in the dental profession and their patients.

The credentialing of dental personnel varies from state to state according to the state's dental practice act. Dentists and dental hygienists must be licensed in the states in which they practice. **Reciprocity** allows an individual to transfer licensure, with the same rights, from one state to another without having to retake licensure exams. The purpose of licensing dentists and regulating the duties performed by dental auxiliaries is to protect the public from unqualified or incompetent practitioners.

It is important to remain educated about the state regulations where you are employed. For instance, some states require dental assistants to perform certain tasks under the direct supervision of the dentist; other duties, however, may be performed under just general supervision. Disregarding these requirements could lead to performing a duty illegally.

Expanded functions are duties performed by qualified dental auxiliaries who have increased training, have additional education, or have registered with their state according to specific regulations set forth in the state's dental practice act. (See Figure 3.1, page 22.) Depending on the state, the rules may indicate that certain dental auxiliary duties are subject to direct supervision. Direct supervision requires the dentist to be physically present in the dental office while procedures are being performed, and work must be examined once procedures are completed. Under general supervision, the dental auxiliary

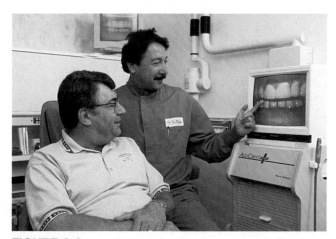

FIGURE 3.2
The dentist–patient relationship.

may perform procedures under the dentist's instructions, but the dentist does not have to be physically present. *Respondeat superior,* a Latin term defined as "the master answers," means that the employer is responsible for all employee actions.

Dental Jurisprudence

Dental *laws* point out what the dental assistant *must* do—that is, a minimum standard of behavior. Dental *ethics* refers to what the dental assistant *should* do—that is, a highest standard of behavior. Dental jurisprudence is written by the state dental board, and the statutes (laws) and regulations are very precise.

How would you explain the difference between ethics and jurisprudence?

Criminal and Civil Law

There are two types of laws, criminal law and civil law. **Criminal law** involves a state or government action against individuals who perform illegal procedures or violate laws. Such lawsuits can result in disciplinary action, fines, and/or imprisonment. Individuals in a criminal case can be charged with an infraction, a misdemeanor, or a felony. **Civil law** refers to noncriminal legal actions that a patient may pursue against a dentist that may result in a compensation lawsuit for pain, suffering, and loss of wages resulting from a dental treatment or dentist's actions (Figure 3.2).

Contracts

Express contracts are verbal or written words that are agreed on in an established contract. Such a contract specifies what each party will do. In contrast to a verbal or written contract, an **implied contract**, also called **implied consent**, is an agreement that is implied based on the patient's actions. Dentists usually treat their patients under implied contracts. For example, when a patient comes to the dental office for the dentist to treat a toothache, the patient implies that he wants treatment (Figure 3.2).

Negligence and Malpractice

Failure to take **due care** can result in either a negligence or malpractice lawsuit. Due care can be defined as what any reasonable or prudent dental care professional would do under similar circumstances. Dental malpractice and **negligence** can occur due to a variety of circumstances:

- Failure to properly detect an oral disease or malformation
- Improper utilization of dental or surgical utensils
- Installation of defective or inferior dental products
- Personal injury to oral cavity or surrounding bone and tissue
- Wrongful death due to dental procedures or anesthetic

Another example of malpractice is when a dentist performs unnecessary procedures on a patient purely for financial gain. Intentionally processing an inaccurate insurance claim on which unnecessary diagnosis and exams have been listed for the sole purpose of collecting higher insurance reimbursements is known as fraud.

Malpractice, also known as professional negligence or incorrect or negligent treatment by a professional, occurs when the four elements of malpractice are present. These are known as the "four D's":

- Duty (relationship)
- Derelict (negligence)
- Direct cause (injury)
- Damage (loss)

For example, the dentist directs the dental assistant to administer nitrous oxide to a dental patient (duty: relationship) who then becomes ill from oversedation of the nitrous gases (direct cause: injury), preventing the patient from returning to work that day (damage: loss). The dentist was aware that the dental practice act clearly states that nitrous oxide is not to be administered by unlicensed personnel (derelict: negligence).

An act of omission occurs when a reasonable person does *not* do something that a similar person or peer in the same situation would do under the same circumstances. For example, if a dentist does not diagnose decay in posterior teeth at contacts because she did not take diagnostic x-rays that would have aided in the diagnosis of decay, leading to treatment that could have prevented now deeper decay that has resulted in possible root canal treatment, then an act of omission has occurred.

Tort Law

A **tort** is an act, which may be intentional or unintentional, that has caused harm to another person. Note that harm must result from the act. For example, consider this scenario: when recording which tooth needs to be extracted, the dental assistant (DA) writes down the wrong tooth number. If, prior to the dental extraction, the dentist reviews the dental radiographs and history with the patient and corrects the appropriate tooth number before extracting it, no harm has occurred and, therefore, no tort. However, if the dentist had extracted the wrong tooth because of the incorrectly written number, harm would have occurred, resulting in a tort. Tort law regulates which acts are considered torts and what remedies, if any, will be applied.

Sometimes in malpractice cases the evidence is so clear that the doctrine of *res ipsa loquitur* ("the act speaks for itself" in Latin) is implemented. A classic example of *res ipsa loquitur* arises when a root canal file breaks and is left inside a root following root canal treatment, and the patient is not informed. Typically, dental documentation will not state "dentist broke root canal file in patient's tooth root canal and did not inform

patient"; furthermore, if not documented, there may be no recorded proof of how or why the negligence occurred. The proof would not be evident until the patient began to experience discomfort, leading to a radiograph that would reveal the broken file. In this situation the evidence produced from the x-ray showing that the file is inside the root would "speak for itself" and fall under the doctrine of *res ipsa loquitur*. The dentist who performed the root canal and left the broken file inside the root could be charged with malpractice.

Who can be held responsible for the result of a negligent act in the dental office?

Risk Management

The prevention of lawsuits is part of **risk management**. Various tasks performed in a dental office are done to help minimize legal risks to the dental practice. The dental team needs to be constantly aware of and cautious about risk management so that unnecessary errors can be avoided. Tasks involved in preventing lawsuits include keeping accurate and complete patient records, gaining written authorizations and informed consent for treatment prior to performing procedures on patients, and practicing and maintaining due care. Good patient rapport and communications are key in risk prevention. When a dental assistant is working with a patient, the dental assistant must constantly guard against making flippant or inappropriate remarks regarding a patient. Inappropriate remarks can be used as evidence should litigation occur. Statements made at the time of an alleged negligent act are admissible in court as evidence under the *res gestae* doctrine.

Informed consent is the procedure of fully informing a patient about the choices the patient has regarding his dental care and addressing any concerns he may have. Complete informed consent includes a discussion of the following elements:

- The nature of the diagnosis/procedure
- The cost of and healing time for the proposed treatment
- Reasonable options

Cultural Considerations

In many dental practices the English language is not the first language of many patients. Compiling a list of available translators for communications between the dentist and non–English-speaking patients will provide quality of care necessary in patient treatment as well as good risk management. Providing multilingual patient information forms makes it easier for patients to provide accurate and complete information.

Professionalism

Res gestae is a statement or words made at the time of an alleged negligent act that are admissible in court as evidence. These same statements or words can also cause undue anxiety to the patient. When excellent communication occurs between the dental team and the patient, good dental–patient rapport is established. This is a key element in reducing lawsuits in dentistry.

- The risks and benefits to each alternative
- Evaluation of patient understanding

Written consent is the preferred method for documenting the patient's awareness of the diagnosis, required treatment, treatment options, and what might occur if the condition is left untreated. Written informed consent is mandatory in a variety of circumstances including these:

- When new drugs will be used
- When experimental or clinical testing is involved
- When photographs are used that identify a patient
- When general anesthesia is being used
- Anytime treatment will take more than one year

Informed refusal occurs when the patient refuses treatment after he has been fully educated regarding the consequences of not receiving the treatment. Accepting informed refusal from a patient does not release the dentist from providing due care. For instance, sometimes patients refuse radiographs. When this occurs the dentist has the right to refer the patient to another dental provider for the patient's continued care. If the dentist chooses to continue the patient's treatment without the radiographs, the dentist may require the patient to sign a written and dated informed refusal form. This form is then filed in the patient's file.

When a patient presents an unusual condition or case that is beyond the scope of the dentist's expertise, the dentist typically refers the patient to a provider who can properly perform the required specialized services. When referring a patient, proper documentation placed in the patient's file is important and should include:

- A description of the problem requiring referral
- The reason for the referral
- The name of the specialist to whom the patient is being referred, as well as the referring dentist's name
- The patient's acceptance of the referral

Patients also have a responsibility regarding their treatment outcome. Contributory negligence occurs when a patient's actions or lack thereof negatively affect the treatment outcome. The patient's record needs to include documentation of broken appointments, last minute cancellations, rescheduled appointments, along with any information about the patient's lack of attention to her personal dental care that may have resulted in a decline in the progress of the treatment outcome.

What are the various consent requirements in the dental office? What are some good risk management procedures for a dental practice?

Confidentiality

Invasion of a patient's privacy occurs when information is disclosed that should remain confidential. Invasion of privacy is a type of tort and can occur when patient information is shared inappropriately (verbally or in writing) with the wrong individual. Dental teams must take precautions to protect patient information.

A patient's health information is protected through the **Health Insurance Portability and Accountability Act (HIPAA)**. Protected health information (PHI) includes any information that can be used in some manner to identify the person, such as a patient's Social Security number, zip code, or birth date. It is very important to keep this information protected and private, and dental practices are legally required to comply with the standards set by HIPAA. (See Chapter 52 for more information on confidentiality in the dental office.)

Health Insurance Portability and Accountability Act

HIPAA was enacted in 1996. The compliance deadline for dental offices was April 14, 2003. Under HIPAA, protection of patient health information was established for transactions regarding claims and remittances, eligibility inquiries, and claims status. HIPAA privacy laws require that appropriate administrative, technical, and physical safeguards be maintained to ensure the integrity and confidentiality of patient health information. HIPAA security rules identify steps to take to secure PHI that is in an electronic format. Equally as important are guidelines that establish the rights of patients concerning their personal health information. The rules help the dental office ensure that processes are in place to protect the patient information covered by HIPAA privacy rules.

Federal HIPAA privacy requirements consist of three categories:

- Privacy standards
- Patients' rights
- Administrative requirements

Privacy standards require that as of April 14, 2003, dental offices provide a copy of the office's Notice of Privacy Procedure to each patient when he or she first visits the practice. Under HIPAA, the policy states that patients have rights regarding their own PHI. These rights include the right to:

- Access and obtain copies of their PHI
- Amend PHI in their records
- Be notified of nonroutine and nonauthorized disclosure
- Have confidential communications with their care providers
- File complaints to the practice and/or the Secretary of Health and Human Services

To meet the administrative requirement, policies, procedures, and documentation must be created. Every office must have in place a HIPAA privacy contact person with whom patients may file complaints concerning their PHI. Each office must also provide training in privacy and safeguarding of PHI. Other administrative requirements include the establishment of a complaint system and a system on how to mitigate a complaint if a breach of privacy does occur. When business associates are involved with dental practices, agreements protecting PHI must be contracted and documented within the HIPAA policy manuals.

Compromised PHI penalties handed down from the Health and Human Services Office of Civil Rights can include fines up to $250,000 and 10 years imprisonment. It is important that dental offices stay compliant with changes to HIPAA. Updates through the American Dental Association can be checked at www.osap.org.

Dentist–Patient Relationship

When establishing a relationship with a dental patient, the dentist and his dental team must practice a standard of care or due care. The standard of care that patients expect when they enter a dentist office includes:

- Access to a qualified licensed dentist who is knowledgeable and skillful in his or her field of practice

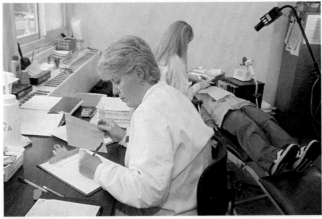

FIGURE 3.3
The patient file.

- Use of standard materials and appropriate drugs for the patient's treatment
- Care and treatment that is completed successfully within a given period of time
- Fees that are similar to those of other dental offices in the area
- Accurate and clear instructions as needed

When a patient enters into a contract with a dental office, the patient agrees to provide the dentist with accurate patient information and health history, follow the special directions during treatment and with regard to medications, keep their scheduled appointments, and pay for services as set forth in practice terms.

Abandonment

Withdrawing from patient care without reasonable notice or failing to provide a referral for completion of dental treatment is illegal and is known as **abandonment.** Dentists cannot terminate contracts with patients without reasonable notice. Dentists can decide not to treat a patient initially. If, however, the dentist has treated the patient, then terminating a patient must be done in writing and usually with 30 days' notice to give the patient a reasonable length of time to establish treatment with another dentist. It may also be considered abandonment if, for example, a dentist leaves the area for a weekend without giving patients of record who have recently had emergency treatment instructions on who to contact regarding emergency care while the dentist is unreachable.

What type of information should be contained in the patient's record?

The Patient Record

The patient record is a legal document (Figure 3.3). The dentist and the dental team are responsible for maintaining accurate, up-to-date records within the dental chart, known as the dental record. The treating dentist is the owner of the original patient record. The patient may request a copy of his or her patient record and radiographs to be sent to other dental providers directly as long as a signed disclosure from the patient noting the provider's name and address where the records are being sent is kept in the original patient record. HIPAA regulations give patients the right to review their patient charts and request copies of their records and radiographs.

Information in the patient record includes chart notes, exam records, radiographs, informed consent forms, medical histories, copies of diagnostic tests, prescriptions, diagnoses, treatment plans and acceptance records, and copies of referrals and communications pertaining to the patient's care. (See Chapter 5 for more information about the patient's record.) Financial records are not kept in the patient chart.

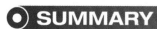

Life Span Considerations

Documentation requirements for minor children are the same as for adult patients. However, obtaining information and permission for treatment requires the presence of a parent or legal guardian. Sometimes obtaining information is difficult due to the fact that a grandparent or family friend may bring in the child for a dental appointment. Obtaining informed consent for dental treatment in the absence of the legal guardian is critical prior to dental procedures being performed. Disclosure on who may have rights to the minor child's information and treatment decisions must be documented.

a patient chart, individuals should always sign their entries and notes. If entries are made electronically, attention must still be paid to ensure accurate placement of dates and information. If an error is made in a manual record, the error should be corrected by drawing a single line through the incorrect entry, placing your initials beside the deleted entry, and then making an accurate entry. Do not erase, scribble through, or otherwise cover up entries in patient charts.

Dental radiographs (x-rays) are a legal component of the dental record. All radiographs should be clearly labeled with the patient's name, date of radiograph, and dentist's name.

Although the future of the electronic record is certain, many health care and dental facilities still use paper records. Regardless of which format is used for the patient record, any information that is entered into a patient's record should be dated and entered clearly and accurately. Information written into the paper record should be done in ink. When manually entering data into

Preparing for Externship

To be successful on one's externship it is important to be familiar with how the dental office functions. At the start of your externship be sure to ask to review the office's procedures on issues related to record-keeping and privacy safeguards.

SUMMARY

Every day dental assistants are expected to perform procedures that require good judgment and protect the dental office both ethically and legally while providing the best care to the patient. It is important as a dental assistant to know the state dental practice act requirements for the state in which you are employed. Dental health care is a rapidly changing field and all dental assistants must understand the laws that affect their profession and how to apply ethical principles to the requirements of their jobs.

KEY TERMS

- **Abandonment:** Withdrawing care from a patient without reasonable notice or without providing a referral for completion of dental treatment. p. 27
- **Civil law:** Noncriminal legal action that a patient may pursue against a dentist that may result in a compensation lawsuit for pain, suffering, and loss of wages resulting from a dental treatment or dentist's actions. p. 24
- **Criminal law:** Involves a state or government action against individuals who perform nonlegal procedures or violate laws. Such lawsuits can result in disciplinary action, fines, and/or imprisonment. p. 24
- **Dental jurisprudence:** The governing laws in the science of dentistry. p. 22
- **Dental practice act:** Legal restrictions set forth by each state legislative body that describe the statutes regarding performance guidelines for licensed and nonlicensed dental health care professionals. p. 22

- **Due care:** The actions any reasonable or prudent dental care professional would perform under similar circumstances. p. 24
- **Expanded function:** Advanced task that requires increased skill and training performed by a dental auxiliary when delegated by a dentist in accordance with the governing state dental practice act. p. 24
- **Express contract:** Verbal or written words that are agreed on in an established contract. p. 24
- **Health Insurance Portability and Accountability Act (HIPAA):** An act passed by Congress to address the security and privacy of health data. p. 26
- **Implied contract:** A contract that is implemented by the patient's actions, not verbally or written. Also known as implied consent. p. 24
- **Informed consent:** The procedure of fully informing a patient about the choices the patient has regarding his/her dental care. p. 25

KEY TERMS (continued)

- **Informed refusal:** Occurs when the patient refuses treatment after he/she has been fully educated regarding the consequences of not receiving the treatment.   p. 26
- **Malpractice:** Incorrect or negligent treatment by a professional.   p. 25
- **Negligence:** Failure to use a standard of care that a reasonable person would apply under related situations.   p. 24
- **Reciprocity:** Allows an individual to transfer licensure, with the same rights, from one state to another without having to retake licensure exams.   p. 24
- *Res gestae:* Statements made at the time of an alleged negligent act that are admissible in court as evidence.   p. 25

- *Res ipsa loquitur:* "The act speaks for itself" (Latin). The cause is obvious.   p. 25
- *Respondeat superior:* "The master answers" (Latin). The employer is responsible for all employee actions.   p. 24
- **Risk management:** Actions implemented to minimize legal risks to the dental practice.   p. 25
- **Tort:** Intentional or unintentional act that causes harm.   p. 25
- **Written consent:** A written document signed by the patient that provides consent to receive treatment.   p. 26

CHECK YOUR UNDERSTANDING

1. Knowledge of intentional misrepresentation of facts is called
   a. fraud.
   b. slander.
   c. felony.
   d. libel.

2. Keeping patient record information private is an act of
   a. screening.
   b. negligence.
   c. legality.
   d. confidentiality.

3. A law set forth by the legislature is a
   a. licensure.
   b. statute.
   c. tort.
   d. restriction.

4. If an erroneous entry is made in a patient clinical record, which of the following is true?
   a. Rewrite the correct entry just above the incorrect entry.
   b. Circle the incorrect entry and write the correct entry with red ink.
   c. Draw one line through the middle of the incorrect entry, enter initials, and write the correct entry on the next line below.
   d. Erase or cover up the incorrect entry and write in the correct entry.

5. Radiographs and a patient's original dental record are the lone ownership of the
   a. patient.
   b. treating dentist.
   c. state dental examiner.
   d. depends on the state dental practice act.

6. Which type of supervision means that the dentist must be in the office, authorize treatment, and examine the completed procedure prior to dismissing the patient?
   a. personal
   b. indirect
   c. general
   d. direct

7. Which of the following is the science of law as it applies to dentistry?
   a. dental jurisprudence
   b. malpractice
   c. ethics
   d. due care

8. Which of the following would refer to the control and restrictions that govern the practice of dentistry within each state?
   a. a state's board of dentistry
   b. a state's dental practice act
   c. the ADA Code of Ethics
   d. a state's department of public health

9. What does HIPAA stand for?
   a. Health Insurance and Personal Authorization Act
   b. Health Insurance Portability and Accountability Act
   c. Health and Individual Personal Accounts Act
   d. Health and Individual Privacy on Accounts Act

10. Which of the following should be obtained if a patient denies the dentist permission to provide necessary treatment?
    a. informed consent
    b. implied consent
    c. referral to specialist
    d. informed refusal

INTERNET ACTIVITY

- Go to www.crest.com and register as a dental professional under New Member. Once registered, select "Practice Management" and then "Communications Skills." Choose the lesson titled "The Health History." Review and learn legal and ethical issues surrounding the importance of a health history for a patient record. Also pay particular attention to the advice on communicating with patients.

WEB REFERENCES

- ADAA Ethics and Code of Conduct   www.dentalassistant.org
- HIPAA information   www.hipaaadvisory.com

General Anatomy and Physiology

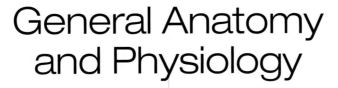

Learning Objectives

After reading this chapter, the student should be able to:

- Define the differences between anatomy and physiology.
- Identify locations of body planes and directions, body systems, body cavities, and body regions.
- List the components of a cell and their functions.
- Name the four types of tissues in the human body.
- Explain how each of the 11 body systems functions.
- Discuss diseases, conditions, and disorders of the 11 body systems.

Preparing for Certification Exams

- Identify systems and diseases of the human body.

Key Terms

Appendicular	Myelin sheath
Articulation	Myocardium
Atria	Nucleus
Axial	Organelle
Cancellous bone	Osteoblast
Cartilage	Osteoclast
Compact bone	Parietal
Endocardium	Pericardium
Epiglottis	Periosteum
Epithelial	Ventricle
Hemostasis	Visceral
Homeostasis	

Chapter Outline

- Planes and Body Directions
- Structural Units
  - Cells
  - Tissues
  - Organs
  - Body Systems
- Body Cavities
- Body Regions
- Introduction to Major Body Systems
- Skeletal System
  - Function of the Skeletal System
  - Divisions of the Skeletal System
  - Composition of Bones
  - Types of Joints
  - Diseases and Disorders of the Skeletal System
- Muscular System
  - Function of the Muscular System
  - Characteristics of Muscles
  - Diseases and Disorders of the Muscular System
- Cardiovascular System
  - Circulatory System
  - Diseases and Disorders of the Circulatory System
- Lymphatic System
  - Structure of the Lymphatic System
  - Diseases and Disorders of the Lymphatic System
- Nervous System
  - Structure of the Nervous System
  - Diseases and Disorders of the Nervous System
- Respiratory System
  - Structure of the Respiratory System
  - Diseases and Disorders of the Respiratory System
- Digestive System
  - Function of the Digestive System
  - Structure of the Digestive System
  - Diseases and Disorders of the Digestive System
- Endocrine System
  - Structure of the Endocrine System
  - Diseases and Disorders of the Endocrine System
- Urinary System
  - Structure of the Urinary System
  - Diseases and Disorders of the Urinary System
- Integumentary System
  - Structure of the Integumentary System
  - Diseases and Disorders of the Integumentary System
- Reproductive System
  - Structure of the Male Reproductive System
  - Diseases and Disorders of the Male Reproductive System
  - Structure of the Female Reproductive System
  - Diseases and Disorders of the Female Reproductive System
- The Interaction of the Eleven Systems of the Body

The quality of health care delivered to dental patients is greatly dependent on the knowledge the dental team has regarding the functions and structures of the human body. Dental assistants must understand both the anatomy of the body, which is the body structure, and the physiology that deals with the functions of the body structures. In addition to providing a detailed study of anatomy and physiology, this chapter introduces the dental assistant to the basic medical terminology needed to communicate effectively with dental patients and other medical personnel.

Planes and Body Directions

Communication between health care professionals is important for the overall health of the patient. The medical and dental communities use a specific language when discussing the human body. When discussing the *anatomic position* of the human body, the reference is understood to mean that the body is standing erect, face forward, feet together, and arms hanging to the sides with palms forward (Figure 4.1). With this image in mind, body planes and directional terms are more clearly understood.

A plane is an imaginary line, like the plane of the goal line in football. The players do not have to touch the line,

---

Dental Assistant   PROFESSIONAL TIP

Before educating the dental patient about dental procedures, try experiencing as much of the procedure as you can from the patient's point of view. For example, wear a type of splint for a period of time such as those worn by a patient with temporomandibular joint disorder. When you can relate to the experience, explaining the procedure to the patient will be much easier.

---

but they must make the ball cross the plane. Anatomically, three planes are used to divide the body (Figure 4.2):

1. *Midsagittal plane* (also known as the sagittal or median plane): This plane divides the body into left and right equal sides.
2. *Horizontal plane* (also known as the axial or transverse plane): This plane divides the body into upper and lower sections.
3. *Coronal plane* (also known as the frontal plane): This plane divides the body into front and back.

Directional terms describe the positions of structures relative to other structures or locations in the body. They are usually described in pairs, as shown in Figure 4.3 and listed in Table 4-1. The *superior* direction is toward the head of the body or above another part. An example would be the eyebrows, which are superior to the eyes. *Inferior* is away from the head or below another part. For example, the foot is inferior to the knee. *Anterior* is toward the front, such as the lips are anterior to the teeth. *Posterior* is toward the back. For example, the shoulder blades are located on the posterior side of the body. *Ventral* is on the front. As an example, the ribs are ventral to internal organs. Other directional terms include the following:

- *Dorsal:* on the back. Example: the dorsal fin of the shark.
- *Medial:* toward the midline of the body. Example: the mouth is medial to the ears.
- *Lateral:* on the side or away from the midline of the body. Example: the thumb is located laterally on the hand.
- *Proximal:* toward or nearest the trunk of the body or the point of attachment. Example: the knee is proximal to the ankle.
- *Distal:* away from or farthest from the trunk or the point or attachment. Example: the hand is located distally to the forearm.

Correct and consistent use of directional terms allows the dental assistant to identify locations during clinical situations.

Life Span Considerations

The geriatric patient in the dental practice may require some special comfort considerations in several areas of patient care techniques, especially during longer dental appointments. Attention to things such as permitting extra time for dental appointments so the patient does not feel rushed, dental chair positioning to help reduce back and/or neck pain, and mouth props for jaw resting during longer procedures can assist the patient in having a positive dental experience.

Understanding the body systems and the disabilities of medically compromised patients can affect how patients are handled in the dental practice and allows the dental assistant to help create a visit that is more efficient for the dental team yet maintains the comfort of the patient. Many geriatric patients can tolerate early morning appointments better than later appointments.

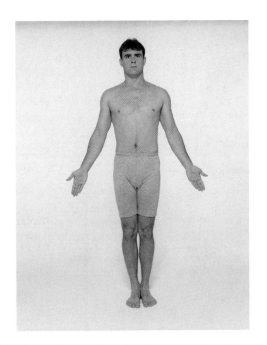

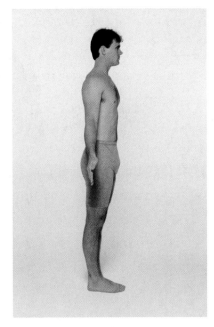

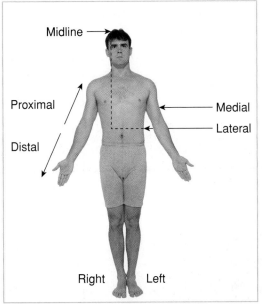

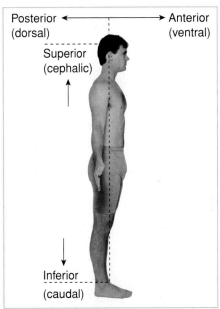

FIGURE 4.1
Directional anatomic terms.

Structural Units

The study of the human body's anatomy can be quite complex. To simplify the information, it is helpful to think of the body in layers. The structuring is made up of four main components: cells, tissues, organs or glands, and systems (Figure 4.4). The cell is the basic functioning unit, and all other layers are based on the smallest of the components. Cells work together to make tissue, tissues work together to make organs and glands, and organs and glands work together to make systems.

Cells

To understand the anatomy of the body it is important to understand the basic cell structure. This is the simplest component of the human body. Human life begins with one cell. Tissues and organs unite to form the body system. **Homeostasis**, a term literally meaning "under the same control," occurs when all of the body systems and their cells, tissues, and organs perform together to maintain harmony in the body.

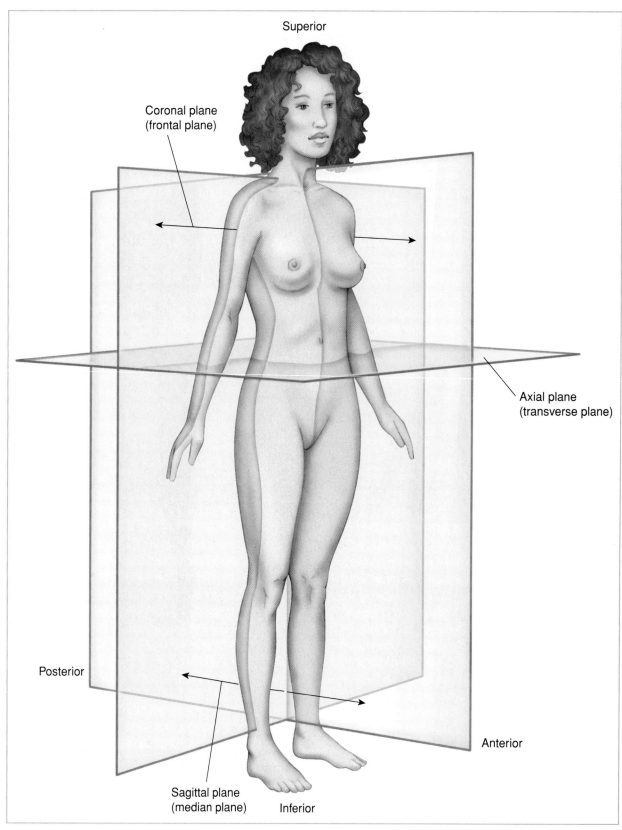

Superior

Coronal plane
(frontal plane)

Axial plane
(transverse plane)

Posterior

Anterior

Sagittal plane
(median plane)

Inferior

FIGURE 4.2
Planes of the body.

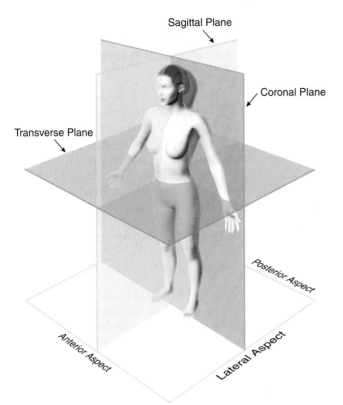

Sagittal Plane

Coronal Plane

Transverse Plane

Posterior Aspect

Anterior Aspect

Lateral Aspect

FIGURE 4.3
Anatomic positions and body planes.

TABLE 4-1 Directional Terms for Anatomy and Physiology

Term	Definition
Superficial	Close to the surface
Deep	Farther from the surface
Ventral	Belly side or front
Dorsal	Back of the body or back of the organ
Anterior	Front or situated in the front
Posterior	Back or situated in the back
Cephalic	Toward the head
Caudal	Toward the tail
Superior	Above or uppermost
Inferior	Below or lowermost
Lateral	Toward the side
Medial	Toward the middle or midline
Proximal	Nearer to the point of attachment
Distal	Farther from the point of attachment

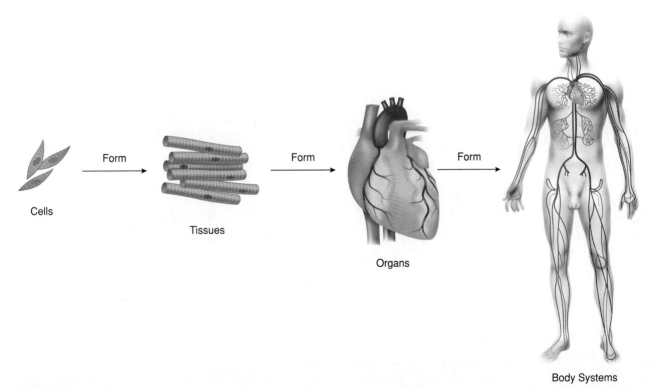

Cells   Form →   Tissues   Form →   Organs   Form →   Body Systems

FIGURE 4.4
Cells are the foundation of structural units to the human body.

Cells are the basic functioning units of the body (Figure 4.5). They are microscopic structures that carry genetic information and are the very foundation of life. All cells have certain similarities and certain differences in appearance, structure, and function. Genes (determined by heredity) control each cell. Each cell carries identical genes unique to the individual. These genes are the blueprints that shape and form the body.

In the reproductive process, cells divide in a process known as *mitosis*. The cell continually divides until the adult human body is complete. The overall structure of a cell is much like that of an egg in that it is enclosed and has a thicker center designated as the processing center. The basic components of a cell are the cell membrane, **nucleus**, and cytoplasm.

Cell Membrane

On the outside of each cell there is a permeable membrane. This membrane, which encircles the cell, has two main functions. One function is to help maintain the cell's form and separate the cell's substance from the immediate environment. The second function of the cell membrane is seen in its chemical and physical properties. Permeability means the membrane recognizes other cells and acts like a gateway with those other cells. These gateways allow substances such as nutrients (oxygen) to enter the cell and waste products (carbon dioxide) to leave. This chemical process is called *diffusion*.

Nucleus

The **nucleus** is the "little brain" of the cell. The nucleus influences growth, repair, and reproduction in the cell. All cells have at least one nucleus during some point in the cell's existence. Some cells have multiple nuclei and others lose the nucleus in maturity. Every cell nucleus contains chromosomes, which are structures that contain DNA (deoxyribonucleic acid) and RNA (ribonucleic acid). These two chemicals contain all of a human being's genetic information.

Cytoplasm

Cytoplasm is a watery gelatin fluid inside of the cell that is thick enough to hold the different components of the cell. These components are called **organelles** and they have specific purposes to complete the function of the cell. Organelles produce, modify, store, and transport proteins, and dispose of waste. Some organelles have reproductive functions and others are necessary for the production of energy.

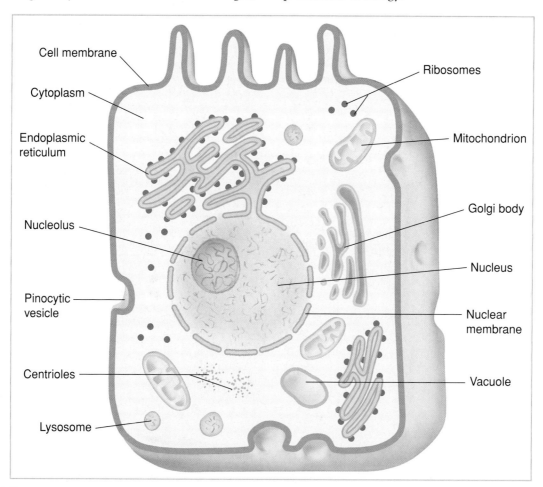

FIGURE 4.5
Parts and structures of a cell.

Tissues

Cells working together become tissue. Tissues are formed when a collection of cells with common features and characteristics group together to perform the same functions for the body. The four primary tissue types are as follows (Figure 4.6):

1. *Epithelial:* covering tissue
2. *Muscle:* contracting tissue
3. *Connective:* supporting tissue
4. *Nerve:* conducting tissue

Epithelial Tissue

Epithelial tissue consists of tightly packed cells that form continuous sheets to serve as a lining over the external and internal body surfaces. The external epithelial tissue covers the exposed surfaces of the body, such as the skin, eyes, and lips. The internal epithelial tissue covers internal body surfaces such as the cavities, passageways, tracts, and vessels of the body in addition to the interior of the body. The lining keeps the body's organs separate and protected. Specialized epithelial tissues allow for the production of secretions such as sweat and mucus, and the production of nails, hair, and melanin for pigmentation.

Muscle Tissue

Muscle tissue is a specialized tissue that allows for movement and has the ability to lengthen and shorten. The myofilaments, or muscle fibers, are drawn together, resulting in contraction of the muscle. Once relaxation occurs between the myofilaments, the muscle relaxes. Striated or skeletal muscles are the most obvious muscle type because they are voluntary. They attach to bone and react to a conscious desire to move. They are composed of bundles of long, thin, cylindrical fibers that are arranged parallel to each other.

Smooth muscles produce involuntary movements such as breathing and digestion. Smooth muscle tissue makes up the internal organs such as the stomach and diaphragm. The contractions of each cell result in a shortening or thickening in particular tissue (e.g., during digestion). The heart muscle is made of cardiac muscle tissue. Cardiac tissue resembles the striated muscle tissue, but it conducts electricity, it lacks elasticity, and its movement is involuntary.

Connective Tissue

The body has several types of connective tissue. Connective tissue adds support and structure to the body, usually providing a fundamental connection of tissues. Some examples of connective tissue include the inner layers of skin, tendons, ligaments, cartilage, bone, and fat tissue.

Nerve Tissue

Nerve tissue has the ability to produce and direct electrical signals in the body. These electrical messages are directed by nerve tissue in the brain and transmitted down the spinal cord to the body. Nerve tissues carry messages from all areas of the body to the brain and are responsible for coordinating and controlling the body's activities. Nerves are primarily found in the brain, spinal cord, and sensory organs.

Organs

Organs are the next level of organization in the body. An organ is formed when at least two different types of tissues work together to perform a function. Organs are contained within body cavities. The primary cavities are the dorsal and ventral cavities. The dorsal cavities are in the back of the body and house the brain and spinal column. The ventral cavity is located in the front and contains the organs of digestion, circulation, breathing, and reproduction. There are many different organs in the body, including the liver, kidneys, heart, and skin.

The skin is the largest organ in the human body. The skin is made up of three layers: the epidermis, dermis, and subcutaneous layer. The epidermis is the outermost layer of skin. It consists of epithelial tissue and provides a protective barrier. The dermis, a layer of connective tissue, lies just under the epidermis. Besides providing support for the skin, the dermis has other purposes:

• Provides blood vessels that nourish skin cells
• Contains nerve tissue that allows sensation via the skin
• Contains muscle tissue that reacts to stimuli, for example, getting "goosebumps" when you get cold or frightened
• Contains hair and the hair root, sweat glands, and oil glands

The subcutaneous layer lies beneath the dermis and consists primarily of a type of connective tissue called adipose tissue. The adipose tissue is known as fat and it helps protect the skin from extreme temperatures and provides a cushion for the skin.

Body Systems

A body system is two or more organs working together to provide a major function. For example, the circulatory system is composed of various organs, which transport nutrients, oxygen, hormones, and wastes through the body. Organs of the circulatory system are the heart, blood vessels, and blood. Each organ has a specific job,

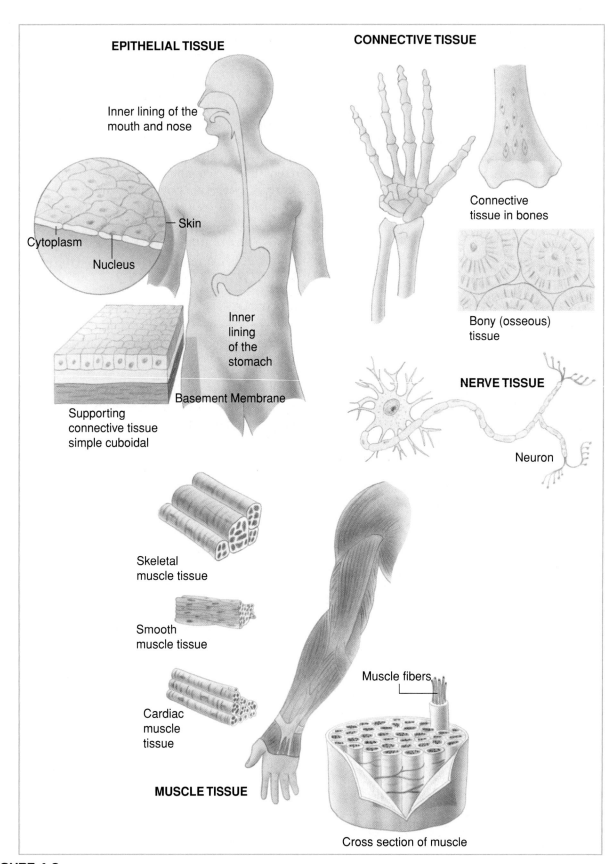

EPITHELIAL TISSUE

Inner lining of the mouth and nose

Cytoplasm

Nucleus

Skin

Inner lining of the stomach

Basement Membrane

Supporting connective tissue simple cuboidal

CONNECTIVE TISSUE

Connective tissue in bones

Bony (osseous) tissue

NERVE TISSUE

Neuron

Skeletal muscle tissue

Smooth muscle tissue

Cardiac muscle tissue

Muscle fibers

Cross section of muscle

MUSCLE TISSUE

FIGURE 4.6
Types of tissue found in the human body.

but as a collective group they function together to ensure that the body system remains healthy.

Body Cavities

The body has a series of spaces, hollow cavities or compartments that hold different organ systems (Figure 4.7). The two main body cavities are called the ventral and dorsal cavities. The ventral, the larger cavity, is located in the front

Preparing for Externship

It is interesting to witness the manifestations of decreased health care in the oral cavity. Be sure to ask how other body systems and their unique contributions to the overall health of the patient show in dental care. Pay careful attention to the patient intake forms and observe common characteristics among medical diseases.

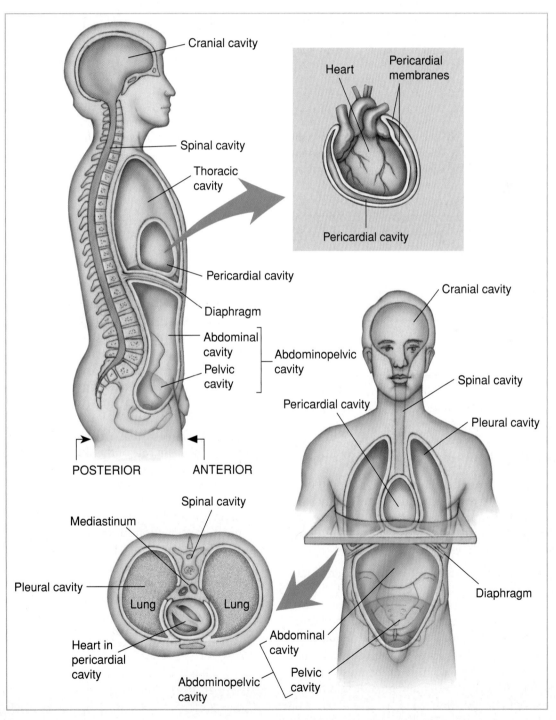

FIGURE 4.7
Cavities of the human body.

of the body, and is subdivided into two parts: the thoracic and the abdominopelvic cavities. The upper ventral thoracic (or chest) cavity contains the heart, lungs, trachea, esophagus, large blood vessels, and nerves. The lower part of the ventral or abdominopelvic cavity can be further divided into two portions: the abdominal portion and the pelvic portion. The abdominal cavity contains most of the intestines, liver, gallbladder, spleen, and stomach. The pelvic cavity contains most of the small and large intestines, urinary bladder, internal reproductive organs, and the rectum.

The dorsal cavity, the smaller of the two main cavities, is located in the back of the body, and can be divided into two portions: the upper portion, or the cranial cavity, which houses the brain, and the spinal cavity, which houses the spinal cord.

Body Regions

The human body is divided into two major regions, the **axial** and the **appendicular**. The axial region involves the head, neck, and trunk. The appendicular region consists of the extremities, arms, and legs. The abdominal area of the body is also divided into quadrants by the crossing of two imaginary lines. The quadrants are referred to as the left and right upper quadrants and the left and right lower quadrants.

Sometimes the abdominal area is divided by the crossing of four imaginary lines, as in a pound sign or tic-tac-toe pattern. The region in the middle located by the belly button or navel is called the umbilicus region. To the immediate right and left of the center region are the right and left lumbar regions. The region above the umbilicus region is called the epigastric region, and below the umbilicus region is the hypogastric region. The lowest right and left regions are called the inguinal or iliac region, and the uppermost right and left regions are the hypochondriac regions.

Introduction to Major Body Systems

An organ system is composed of two or more different organs. The major systems within the human body each have a specific function; however, their ability to work together supports life. The 11 major organ systems in the human body are as follows:

1. *Skeletal system:* Consists of 206 bones in the adult and includes cartilage, tendons, and ligaments. The main roles of the skeletal system are to provide a framework for the body; to protect, support, and shape internal organs; to store minerals; and to produce blood cells.
2. *Muscular system:* Consists of skeletal, smooth, and cardiac muscles. The main role of the muscular system is to hold the body erect and provide movement. It also produces body heat.
3. *Cardiovascular system:* Consists of the heart, blood vessels, and blood. The main role of the circulatory system is to transport nutrients, oxygen, hormones, and wastes throughout the body.
4. *Lymphatic/immune system:* Consists of the lymph, lymph nodes and vessels, white blood cells, spleen, tonsils, and lymphocytes. The main role of the immune system is to defend the body against disease. The lymphatic system also removes fat and excess fluids from the blood.
5. *Nervous system:* Consists of the brain, spinal cord, and peripheral nerves. The main roles of the nervous system are to receive stimuli and transmit electrical signals and messages to the brain.
6. *Respiratory system:* Consists of the nose, sinuses, larynx, epiglottis, trachea, and lungs, including lung structures such as the bronchus, bronchioles, and alveoli. The main role of the respiratory system is to provide oxygen to the cells. Oxygen is absorbed from the atmosphere into the body (inhaled), and carbon dioxide is expelled from the body (exhaled).
7. *Digestive system:* Consists of the oral cavity, esophagus, pharynx, stomach, and the small and large intestines. Accessory organs to the digestive system are the pancreas, liver, and gallbladder. The main roles of the digestive system are to digest food, absorb nutrients, and eliminate solid waste.
8. *Endocrine system:* Consists of the thymus, gonads, pituitary, thyroid, pancreas, and adrenal glands. The main role of the endocrine system is to assist the body in maintaining homeostasis by controlling growth, stimulating sexual development, producing insulin, and regulating water balance.
9. *Urinary or excretory system:* Consists of the kidneys, ureters, bladder, and urethra. The main role of the urinary system is to maintain the amount of fluid in the body by filtering wastes, toxins, and excess water and nutrients from the bloodstream.
10. *Integumentary system:* Consists of the skin, hair, and nails. The main role of the skin is protection. It is the largest organ and covers more area than any other organ. The skin provides the first line of defense against disease, absorbs essential vitamins, helps maintain fluid balance in the body, and aids in temperature regulation for the body.
11. *Reproductive system:* In the female, consists of the ovaries, oviducts, fallopian tubes, uterus, vagina, and mammary glands; and in the male, the testes, seminal vesicles, prostate, and penis. The main role of the reproductive system is to produce cells that allow reproduction. In the male, sperm are created to inseminate the egg cells or ova produced in the female.

Where do body systems overlap? Think about the overlapping in purpose and in structures.

Skeletal System

The skeletal system is made up of 206 bones that provide a framework for attached muscles (Figure 4.8). It plays a crucial role in movement and in supporting the brain and spinal cord. The skeletal system is the body's major framework and supports and protects the major organs.

Function of the Skeletal System

The skeletal system has five major functions:

1. Providing a framework for the body.
2. Aiding in movement of the body in conjunction with muscles that are attached to the skeletal bones.
3. Protecting internal organs. For example, the ribs protect the heart and other organs within the thoracic cavity.
4. Producing blood cells. The process of *hematopoiesis*, the term for the production of blood cells, occurs in the bone marrow housed within the long bones. On average, 2.6 million red blood cells are produced each second by the bone marrow.
5. Storing minerals such as calcium and phosphorus, which are essential for the proper functioning of muscles and nerves and for blood clotting.

Divisions of the Skeletal System

The skull, face, spine, sternum, and rib cage form the axial skeleton and consist of 80 of the 206 bones that compose the framework of the head and trunk of the body. The upper extremities, shoulder areas, the arms and hands, lower extremities, the hip area, and the legs and feet make up the appendicular skeleton, which consists of 126 of the 206 bones in the body.

A child has 240 bones at birth because several bone groups have not yet fused together and are counted separately. The best example of this phenomenon is the baby's soft spot on top of the head, called the fontanelles. As the baby grows, the soft spot disappears because the bones have grown together.

Composition of Bones

The bones in the body are placed into one of the following five categories:

1. Irregular bones vary in shape, size, and surface traits. These include the bones of the spinal column and the skull.
2. Short bones are small and cube shaped and are found in the wrists and ankles.
3. Flat bones are recognized by their broad surfaces that protect the organs and serve as attachment areas for muscles. Examples include the ribs, cranial bones, and the shoulder blades.

4. Long bones are longer and wider than short bones and are located in the upper and lower extremities. The inside of the bone is made of three primary tissue layers: periosteum, compact bone (hard bone), and cancellous bone (spongy bone) (Figure 4.9). The femur or thigh bone is the largest, strongest long bone in the body.
5. Sesamoid bones are small floating bones found near joints. The largest, most well-known sesamoid bone is the kneecap (also called the patella).

The Primary Tissue Layers

The **periosteum** is a double layer of tissue that covers the compact bone. The outer layer is thin, white connective tissue that houses nerves and blood cells. It provides a venue for nutrients, bone growth, and repair and also removes waste. The importance of the periosteum is in the inner or lower layer of loose connective tissue, which is responsible for bone-forming cells called **osteoblasts**. Osteoblasts form immature bone cells that mature to make way for new bone cells. The periosteum also serves as a place for the muscles system to insert and fasten to the bone. Its primary responsibility is the repair and maintenance of the bones in the skeletal system.

Patient Education

Common conditions specific to dental anatomy and physiology include temporomandibular joint (TMJ) disorders. TMJ pain is often described as a dull aching pain in the jaw joint, with referred pain, including the ear. Some people still have problems using their jaws without experiencing the pain associated with TMJ. Other symptoms can include trismus, being unable to open the mouth comfortably; clicking, popping, or grating sounds in the jaw joint; locking of the jaw when attempting to open the mouth; headaches; and neck, shoulder, and back pain. It is important to remember that some discomfort in the jaw joint or chewing muscles is common and is not always a cause for concern.

Most TMJ problems get better without treatment; in fact, the problems often go away on their own over the course of a few weeks to months. However, anytime pain is severe and lasts more than a few weeks, care should be sought. Treatments vary according to severity of damage that has occurred to the joint. Some home care, such as eating soft foods, alternating ice or moist heat, and avoiding extreme jaw movements (e.g., wide yawning, loud yelling or singing, and gum chewing), are useful in easing symptoms. Therapies include occlusal splint or bite guards to prevent wear and tear on the joint. Improving the alignment of the upper and lower teeth and surgical options are available for advanced cases.

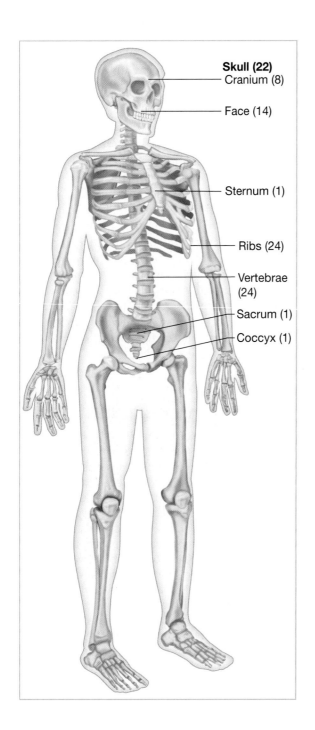

Skull (22)
Cranium (8)
Face (14)

Sternum (1)

Ribs (24)

Vertebrae (24)

Sacrum (1)

Coccyx (1)

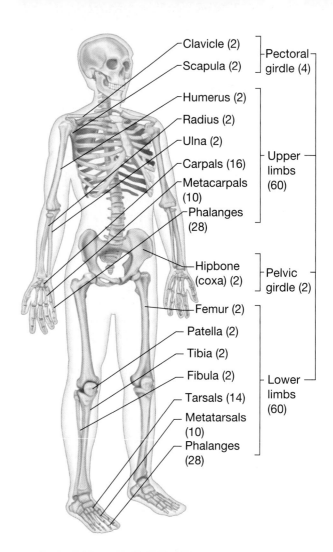

Clavicle (2)
Scapula (2)
— Pectoral girdle (4)

Humerus (2)
Radius (2)
Ulna (2)
Carpals (16)
Metacarpals (10)
Phalanges (28)
— Upper limbs (60)

Hipbone (coxa) (2)
— Pelvic girdle (2)

Femur (2)
Patella (2)
Tibia (2)
Fibula (2)
Tarsals (14)
Metatarsals (10)
Phalanges (28)
— Lower limbs (60)

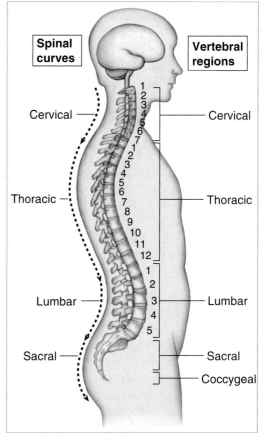

Spinal curves

Vertebral regions

Cervical

Thoracic

Lumbar

Sacral

Cervical

Thoracic

Lumbar

Sacral

Coccygeal

1 2 3 4 5 6 7
1 2 3 4 5 6 7 8 9 10 11 12
1 2 3 4 5

FIGURE 4.8
The skeletal system including divisions and spinal sections.

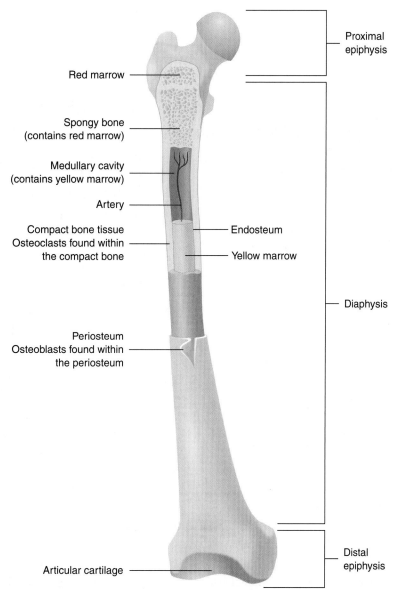

Red marrow

Spongy bone
(contains red marrow)

Medullary cavity
(contains yellow marrow)

Artery

Compact bone tissue
Osteoclasts found within
the compact bone

Periosteum
Osteoblasts found within
the periosteum

Articular cartilage

Proximal
epiphysis

Endosteum

Yellow marrow

Diaphysis

Distal
epiphysis

FIGURE 4.9
Composition and other features of bones.

Compact bone tissue or cortical bone is also known as hard bone due to its density and strength. It forms the main shaft (diaphysis) of long bones and comprises the outer layer of other bones. **Osteoclasts** are found in compact bone. These cells are responsible for destroying bone by dissolving or reabsorbing calcium when bone is stressed or damaged as in a break.

Cancellous bone, or spongy bone, is less dense and is lighter in weight than compact bone. A meshwork of trabeculae strengthens the bone. Trabeculae (plural for trabecula) have a sponge-like or web-like appearance on radiographs that are formed by interlaced bony spicules located in the hollow center of the surrounding compact bone in long bones and in the outside layer of other bones. Located within the cancellous bone tissue of long bones is the bone marrow. There are two types: red bone and yellow bone marrow. Yellow bone marrow stores fat.

Red bone marrow produces blood cells including the red blood cells, which carry oxygen.

How do the two types of bone complement each other? How do the two types of bone differ from each other?

Types of Joints

A joint is where two or more bones of the skeleton meet (Figure 4.10). A joint is also called an **articulation**. Joints can be classified according to the type and amount of movement they provide. The following are the three basic types of joints:

1. Immovable or synarthrotic joints are fibrous and connect bones without allowing any movement.

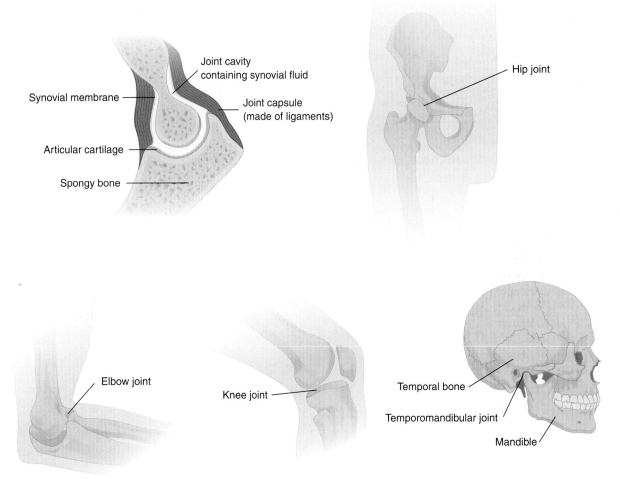

FIGURE 4.10
Skeletal joints.

These joints are held together by a thin layer of strong connective tissue. No movement occurs between the bones involved, for instance, the sutures of the skull and the teeth.

2. Slightly movable or diarthrotic joints are cartilaginous joints and are made of connective tissue attached to the bones by **cartilage**. These joints allow slight motion, such as in the spine or ribs.

3. Freely movable or amphiarthrotic joints are synovial joints that allow relatively free movement between the bones that meet. This type of joint is the most common in the body. Some synovial joints are lined with a fibrous sac referred to as bursa sacks and are filled with synovial fluid. This fluid helps lubricate and protect the bones. The six types of synovial joints are named by their movements:

- *Hinge:* Hinge joints allow extension and retraction of an appendage. An example is the knee.
- *Saddle:* Saddle joints allow movement back and forth and up and down; they do not, however, allow for rotation like a ball-and-socket joint. An example is the fingers.

- *Ball-and-socket:* Ball-and-socket joints allow for a rotating motion in most directions. An example is the hip.
- *Ellipsoid:* Ellipsoid joints are much like the ball-and-socket joint except that the motion is more limited than with a ball-and-socket joint. The wrist is an example of an ellipsoid joint.
- *Pivot:* A pivot joint allows for rotation around a fixed point. An example is found in the neck.
- *Gliding:* A gliding joint allows bones to slide past each other with a limited amount of movement. An example of this type of joint is found inside the wrist.

Diseases and Disorders of the Skeletal System

As with any body system, the skeletal system can be affected by disease and disorder. The more common ones are listed here:

- *Arthritis:* inflammation of one or more joints. Arthritis is often a sign that other diseases are present in the body. These diseases include osteoarthritis, rheumatoid arthritis, and gout. Signs and symptoms are pain, redness, swelling, and heat. Motion at the joint is usually restricted in arthritis.

- *Gout:* arthritis due to excessive uric acids and salts called urates, which accumulate, causing uric acid crystals to accumulate in the joints. Usually the big toe up to the ankle is affected. The signs and symptoms include swelling, redness, heat, and pain. Gout can lead to kidney damage and stones due to the excess urates.

- *Osteoporosis:* a loss of bone tissue. Osteoporosis is common in elderly Caucasian and Asian women who are of slight build. It is caused by demineralization in the bones. Signs and symptoms include a thinning of the bone, which causes the bones to become brittle and more conducive to fracture. The disease can lead to decreased height and increased back pain.

- *Fractures:* breaks of the bone and/or cartilage. Fractures can be caused by stress or injury to the bones. Signs and symptoms are dependent on the severity of the fracture. Severe fractures can involve severe pain, swelling, and potential disfigurement. Fractures of a more simple nature are characterized by pain and swelling. Fractures are categorized according to the type of break.

- *Osteomyelitis:* an infection to the bone tissue caused by fungi or bacteria. Signs and symptoms include a severe throbbing pain over the affected area, and fever is also common.

What other disorders can you think of that might develop in the skeletal system?

Muscular System

Approximately 40% to 45% of a human's body weight is composed of muscle mass. There are three types of muscles: striated, smooth, and cardiac. Each muscle is named for its appearance and/or its function. Movement is the primary function of the muscles. The body has more than 600 individual muscles. Some of the main muscles are shown in Figure 4.11.

Function of the Muscular System

The functions of the muscular system include movement, posture, joint stability, and the production of heat. The muscles hold the body erect; that is, they maintain a person's posture. A person with poor posture has weak muscle activity. Many of the joints are surrounded by muscle, thus providing stability to that joint. Nearly 85% of body heat is a result of muscle contraction. Whenever a person gets cold, goosebumps, technically known as *cutis anserina,* are produced by the contraction of the muscles in the skin.

Voluntary movement is only possible in conjunction with the skeletal system. Skeletal muscles are attached to bones by strong fibers called tendons. The muscles contract and tendons hold the muscle to the bone to allow for movement. The muscle origin is the location where the muscle attaches to the bone originally, and it is fixed or nonmovable. The attachment to the bone where the muscle ends is called the muscle insertion point. The muscle attachment at this end is more movable than at the origin.

Some muscles move by coordination of antagonistic muscle pairs. This requires the one muscle to work while the other rests, and then as the working muscle rests, the resting muscle goes to work. One set of muscles contracts or shortens, while another set of muscles is responsible for relaxing or expanding. A good example of antagonistic muscle pairs is the biceps and the triceps. If the biceps are flexed, then the triceps relax, but if the biceps are relaxed, the triceps contract. It is the fundamental action of joints, bones, and skeletal muscles working together that creates obvious movements such as walking and running. Any conscious movement is a result of skeletal muscles, including the more subtle movements such as raising the eyebrows, batting the eyes, and sighing. Some muscles move only when instructed such as the arms and legs; others move involuntarily. The nervous system and hormones automatically regulate or control involuntary muscles such as the heart, stomach, and intestines.

Characteristics of Muscles

The muscles are made of groups of cells that work together to form fibers. Fibers are very small—about the width of a hair. There are more than a trillion fibers in the body, and each one has its own blood supply and can support more than 1,000 times its own weight. Other specialized connective layers known as fascia protect the fibers. The fascia covers, separates, and supports muscle fibers. The ability of a muscle to react to stimuli is called excitability. Extensibility is the term for the muscle as it stretches. Muscle tone is the tension maintained within the muscle. A muscle that has contracted is short and thicker, whereas a muscle that is relaxed is longer and thinner.

Diseases and Disorders of the Muscular System

The muscular system can be affected by a variety of diseases and disorders, some of which are simple and others are life threatening:

- *Sprains and strains:* Strains occur when a muscle or tendon is overstretched or overused. Sprains are strains that involve the surrounding tissues such as ligaments. Signs and symptoms are pain, swelling, and tenderness around the area affected and can result in possible muscle spasms and restriction of motion. Treatment is remembered by use of the acronym RICE: rest, ice, compression, and elevation.

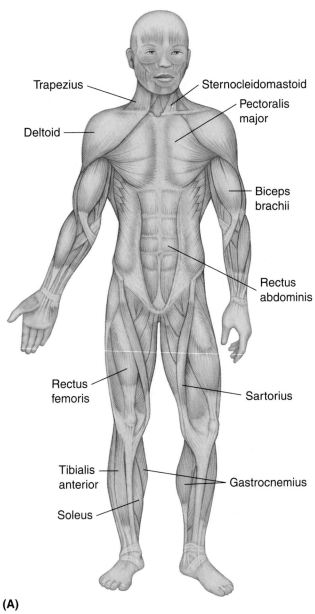

(A)

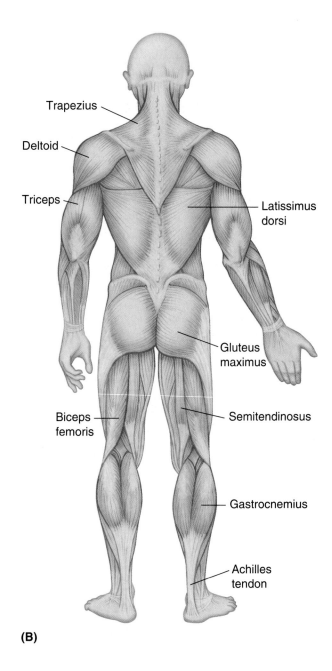

(B)

FIGURE 4.11
The muscular system.

- *Muscular dystrophy:* Muscular dystrophy is a genetic disorder a person is born with that affects the muscles. Over time the muscles break down and, in essence, become useless. The most common form usually strikes children. Signs and symptoms are the inability to walk, shriveling of the muscles, and weakness.
- *Myasthenia gravis:* This is an autoimmune disorder that affects the muscles, making them weak and sore. Signs and symptoms include weakness in the facial muscles or in the muscles of the throat.
- *Fibromyalgia:* Fibromyalgia is a pain disorder involving the muscle fibers and the surrounding soft tissue near a joint. Signs and symptoms are deep throbbing alternating with sharp shooting pains and/or a feeling

of intense burning from the inside. Multiple muscle groups are usually involved.

How is one's posture affected by the muscles?

Cardiovascular System

The cardiovascular system involves a circulatory process, which includes the veins, arteries, heart, and blood (Figure 4.12). The major function of the cardiovascular system is to circulate blood, carrying oxygen into the body and filtering and eliminating the waste product called carbon dioxide.

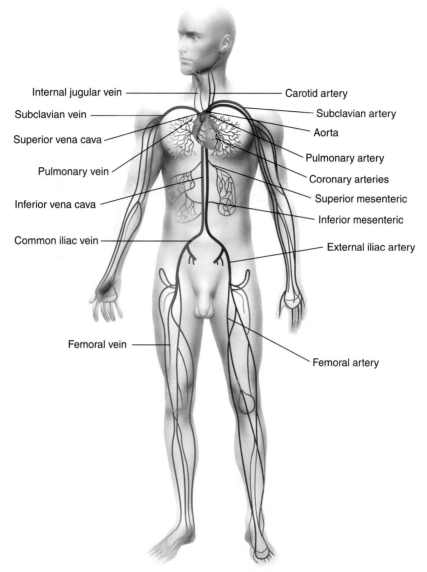

Internal jugular vein — Carotid artery
Subclavian vein — Subclavian artery
Superior vena cava — Aorta
Pulmonary vein — Pulmonary artery
Inferior vena cava — Coronary arteries
Common iliac vein — Superior mesenteric
Inferior mesenteric
External iliac artery
Femoral vein — Femoral artery

FIGURE 4.12
Cardiovascular system including the heart, arteries, and veins.

Circulatory System

The circulatory system is made up of the heart, blood, blood vessels, lymph, and lymph vessels. The circulatory system is the body's transportation system. The heart is the pump that keeps the blood moving throughout the body. Blood carries oxygen and nutrients to every part of the body. Blood also picks up the waste products for delivery to the filtering stations and ultimately for disposal. The blood vessels include the arteries, veins, and capillaries. Capillaries are the only vessels small enough to allow for the exchange of chemicals, such as gases, nutrients, and waste products. The lymph vessels meet the blood vessels at the capillary bed so that the blood can carry lymphocytes (lymph cells that fight infection). Arteries are the larger vessels that carry blood away from the heart. Most of them carry oxygen-rich blood. All veins return blood to the heart, and most of them carry deoxygenated blood.

The circulatory system is divided into two types of circulation: pulmonary and systemic. Systemic circulation is the exchange of blood between the heart and the body. According to the American Heart Association, if all of the blood vessels of an average-size child were lined up, they would measure about 60,000 miles long. For an adult the blood vessels would measure about 100,000 miles long.

The blood leaves the heart from the largest artery, the aorta. As it moves away from the heart, blood is channeled into smaller arteries called arterioles to be taken ultimately to the capillaries throughout the body. The oxygen and nutrients are dropped off and the wastes are picked up. The blood is then channeled into smaller veins called venules that lead to the larger vessels known as veins. The largest veins are the ones nearest to the heart, called the vena cavae. The blood is then channeled into the heart for pulmonary circulation, which can be thought of as the refreshing station. Arteries are imbedded deeper into the body for protection. They pulsate in order to move the blood more efficiently. The term *pulse* refers to the pulsation of the arteries. The pulse can be felt most commonly in the wrist, neck, upper arm, and thigh.

Veins are more superficial. They do not pulsate but they have valves that are designed to prevent backflow. Both veins and arteries have several layers of tissue that make up the vessel. Food products enter the blood from the digestive organs into the portal vein. Waste products are filtered through the liver and kidneys. All systems ultimately return to the right side of the heart via the inferior and superior vena cavae.

Heart

Pulmonary circulation is the exchange of blood between the heart and the lungs. The heart is a muscle about the size of a clenched fist that contracts and relaxes (Figure 4.13). It consists of four chambers, two on the top called **atria** and two on the bottom called **ventricles**. The chambers are separated in the middle by a thick layer of tissue known as the septum, which divides the heart into right and left halves. The chambers are identified by the side of the heart on which they are located. The atria are smaller than the ventricles and contract to push the blood through the heart valves into the ventricles located just inferior.

The heart repeats a cycle of contraction and relaxation at about 60 to 100 beats per minute. The structure of the heart allows the blood that contains mostly carbon dioxide to be separated from the blood that carries mostly oxygen. The heart keeps the blood flowing. The strength of the heart is measured by taking one's blood pressure. This test determines the amount of force exerted on the walls of the arteries. The heart also responds to increased or decreased needs of the body for blood supply, so whenever a body is excited or in motion, the heart can respond by pumping more blood. Likewise, whenever the body is relaxed, the heart can also slow itself and preserve the energy it takes for the heart cycle to be complete.

The heart is composed of three layers: the pericardium, the myocardium, and the endocardium. The **pericardium** surrounds the outside of the heart by enclosing the heart in a double-walled membranous sac. The **visceral** or inside pericardium of the heart sac is identical to the **parietal** or outside pericardium of the heart wall. Fluids are contained within these layers to help avoid friction while the heart beats. The **myocardium** is a thick layer of tough cardiac muscle that is responsible for the contraction and relaxation of the heart. The **endocardium** is a thin layer of tissue lining inside the heart. The heart is surrounded by coronary arteries that have the sole purpose of supplying the heart with oxygen and nutri-

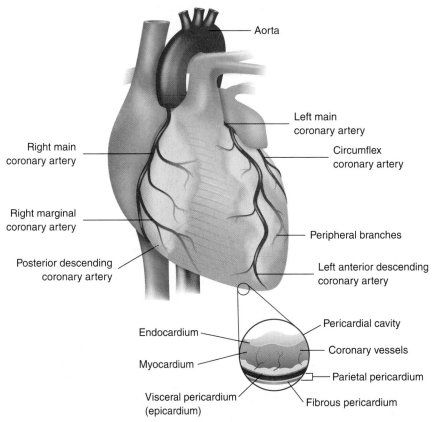

FIGURE 4.13
The heart showing the coronary arteries and a look at the layers of the heart.

tion. It is this network of blood vessels that supplies the myocardium.

Blood flows through the heart in a continuous but consistent manner. The heart carries oxygen and nutrients that are distributed to every cell. The blood also picks up wastes such as carbon dioxide. As the blood full of wastes returns to the heart, it is carried through the vena cavae and dumped into the right atrium, which fills with the blood. The heart beats and the right atrium squeezes shut, forcing the blood to move downward through the tricuspid valve into the right ventricle. The right ventricle fills and the heart beats, again forcing the blood into the pulmonary artery through the pulmonary semilunar valve.

The blood is pushed through the pulmonary artery into the lungs where carbon dioxide and oxygen are exchanged within the capillaries of the lungs. The blood comes back to the heart through the pulmonary vein and is deposited into the left atrium. The atrium fills and the heart beats, forcing the blood through the bicuspid or mitral valve and into the left ventricle. The heart beats again and the blood leaves through the aortic semilunar valve going into the aorta. The aorta carries the blood out to the rest of the body.

The heartbeat is regulated by the electrical impulses received from the brain. The impulse is received at the sinoatrial (SA) node, a thickened area of nervous tissue near the right atrium. This impulse starts atrial contractions and sends the impulse to be received in the atrioventricular (AV) node, located atop the left ventricle. The impulse is then sent to the bundle of His. The bundle of His is a length of nervous fibers that runs the lower half of the septum. These fibers are more superficial than the SA and AV nodes. As the fibers reach the bottom of the pointed end of the heart, called the apex, the bundle of His splits into right and left bundle branches. The electrical impulse is carried to the smallest of the electrical fibers, called Purkinje fibers. These fibers are very small and surround the heart. Because the current has nowhere to go, the ends of the fibers send an electrical shock that triggers the muscle to react with a contraction. The heart sounds are actually due to the closing of the heart valves, not from any muscular action. Cardiac output refers to the amount of blood released by the heart in one minute.

The circulating blood is often referred to as the river of life. It has several functions: continuous transportation of all nutrients, gases, waste products, and hormones; regulation of the pH balance; regulation of body fluids; and regulation of body temperature. Blood also carries elements, such as white blood cells, lymphocytes, and clotting agents, that are key to the body's immune response. Blood is composed of solids and liquids. Water makes up 90% of the blood contents. About half of that is plasma, which is a clear yellowish colored fluid. It contains many different substances such as proteins, glucose, salts, vitamins, hormones, and antibodies.

The solid portion of blood is referred to as the formed elements such as the red blood cells, white blood

cells, and platelets. Red blood cells are small biconcave disks, meaning they are sunken in the middle on both sides to have the appearance of something like this:)(. They carry the oxygen via a protein and iron substance called hemoglobin that binds oxygen to the red blood cell, also called the erythrocyte. A mature erythrocyte does not have a nucleus. The blood has far more erythrocytes than any of the other formed elements.

White blood cells, also called leukocytes, are larger than red blood cells and have very clearly defined nuclei. They are fewer in number than red blood cells. Their purpose is to seek out and destroy any pathogens, that is, disease-producing microorganisms. Each type of white blood cell assists the body in resisting these foreign substances on an individual basis. White blood cells are colorless and are categorized according to the appearance of grains on the cell. They are granulocytes or agranulocytes, white blood cells with a grainy appearance and white blood cells without a grainy appearance, respectively. Some leukocytes produce antibodies, others detoxify foreign substances, and still others perform by ingesting certain bacteria.

White blood cells travel throughout the circulatory system to sites where they are needed. Types of white bloods cells include:

- Eosinophils
- Basophils
- Monocytes
- Segmented neutrophils
- Nonsegmented neutrophils

Thrombocytes are commonly referred to as platelets and are necessary for blood clotting. They contain the clotting factors such as fibrin and fibrinogen. The process by which the body controls bleeding is called **hemostasis.**

The blood type of a human is determined by detecting the kind of antigen located on the outer rim of the red blood cell. An antigen is a foreign substance found in the blood. These red blood cell antigens are categorized into the four types of blood: A, B, AB, and O. This way of categorizing these antigens is known as the ABO system. Blood types are established before birth and are determined by the genes inherited from an individual's biological parents.

The ABO system is used mostly for blood transfusions. Correct blood typing or cross-matching is vital to ensure that patients who require blood transfusions receive blood compatible with their own blood type. The body will attack a red blood cell antigen if it is different than what is already present. The consequences of introducing a foreign blood type into the body can be serious—even fatal.

Another antigen identified is the Rh factor. The Rh factor is an antigen that is located along the edges of the red blood cell. If a pregnant woman is Rh negative (Rh−), she does not have the antigen on her red blood cells. If the baby she is carrying has the Rh factor on its cells (Rh positive or Rh+), the mother's body will prepare to defend the body against tissues that it considers foreign. Usually a first baby is born without problems, but a second baby carrying the Rh factor will not survive the attack of the mother's immune system. In these cases, the mother is given an immunoglobulin called RhoGAM to prevent the mother's response to the foreign antigen.

Diseases and Disorders of the Circulatory System

Cardiovascular disease can affect the heart or the blood vessels. Some types of cardiovascular disease are hereditary; others are a result of natural processes such as aging or a result of unhealthy lifestyles, including smoking, obesity, and poor diet and exercise habits.

- *Coronary artery disease:* This is the leading cause of heart attacks. It occurs when blood flow to the arteries is blocked from the heart muscle. If the coronary arteries cannot serve the heart, the tissue dies, which can cause severe structural damage to the heart. It can lead to myocardial infarction, commonly known as a heart attack. The blockage is usually plaque, a sticky substance that adheres to the artery walls and then accumulates. This plaque also stiffens the walls of the artery, causing a condition known as atherosclerosis. Arteriosclerosis is hardening of the arteries without plaque as seen in the vessels of the elderly. Angina pectoris is the name given to chest pains that are due to a lack of oxygen. Signs and symptoms are pain in the chest, back, jaw, and down the arm, shortness of breath, and diaphoresis or sweating. An ashen or gray color along with anxiety are common. Coronary artery disease may be a preventable disease that can be avoided with proper care such as eating a healthy diet, exercising regularly, and abstaining from smoking—unless the disease was inherited, in which case treatment may not help.

  Heart failure occurs when the heart is unable to pump a sufficient amount of blood to the body. This does not mean that the heart has stopped or is no longer pumping blood at all. It simply means that the heart has become less effective in pumping and that the organs are not receiving enough blood. Signs and symptoms include shortness of breath, fluid retention, and fatigue. Heart failure may develop suddenly or over many years. It may occur because of other cardiovascular diseases that have damaged or weakened the heart, such as hypertension or high blood pressure, congenital problems such as atrial septal defects or ventricular septal defects, lung disease, or valve disorders such as a prolapsed mitral valve.

- *Pericardial disease:* This disease, also called pericarditis, includes inflammation of the pericardium, as well as fluid accumulation around the pericardium, which results in constriction of the heart. Both of these signs

can occur alone or together. The causes of pericardial disease can include the presence of a bacteria or virus. For this reason, many dentists will prescribe a proactive treatment of antibiotics to patients who report a history of heart problems. However, the American Heart Association has learned from research that prophylactic antibiotics may not be necessary, but that good oral hygiene is always good for the dental patient with a heart condition. Certain heart conditions still require prophylactic antibiotic therapy, but good hygiene is recommended for all. Signs and symptoms are joint pain, shortness of breath, weight loss, enlarged spleen, high fever, heart murmurs, blood clots, and/or fatigue.

- *Endocarditis:* This disease is characterized by an inflammation of the endocardium of the heart. Like pericarditis, bacteria, virus, or cancer usually cause endocarditis. Signs and symptoms are increased body temperature, joint pain, shortness of breath, fatigue, an enlarged spleen, and blood clots.

- *Hemophilia:* Hemophilia is called the free bleeding disease. It is an inherited disease in which the blood fails to clot. This inability can lead to serious—possibly fatal—outcomes. Some cardiovascular medications known as blood thinners can have the same effect as hemophilia. Be sure you note whether a patient is taking any of these types of medications. Patients with hemophilia are not treated in the dental office; they are usually treated at the hospital instead.

What additional factors not mentioned here can you think of that would contribute to a healthy heart?

Lymphatic System

The lymphatic system performs three main functions for the body: It drains and filters the lymph and also fights infection. As the blood moves throughout the body, a clear fluid oozes out into the body tissues starting at the capillary bed (Figure 4.14). The fluid is called *lymph,* Greek for a pure, clear stream. The lymph

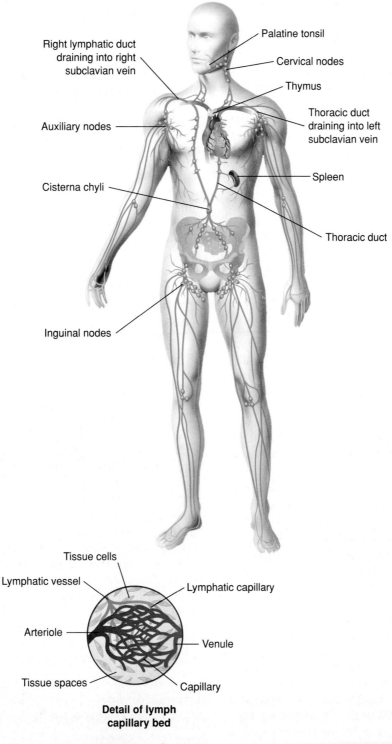

Palatine tonsil

Right lymphatic duct draining into right subclavian vein

Cervical nodes

Thymus

Thoracic duct draining into left subclavian vein

Auxiliary nodes

Spleen

Cisterna chyli

Thoracic duct

Inguinal nodes

Tissue cells

Lymphatic vessel

Lymphatic capillary

Arteriole

Venule

Tissue spaces

Capillary

Detail of lymph capillary bed

FIGURE 4.14
Lymphatic system with a close-up of the capillary bed.

drains into the lymph vessels and then is passed through the lymph vessels to the base of the neck, where it is drained back into the bloodstream. This circulation of fluid through the body is continuous, much like the circulation of the blood in the circulatory system except that there is no pump. The vessels move the lymph by way of rhythmic wavelike contractions and relaxation called peristalsis.

Structure of the Lymphatic System

Part of the lymphatic system includes thin pipes or vessels that run throughout the body. These tubes are called lymph vessels (also known as lymphatic vessels). The lymph vessels reach throughout all parts of the body in a network much like that of the arteries and veins. The lymph contains a high number of white blood cells and lymphocytes, also known as lymph cells. The cells have phagocytic properties or the ability to engulf other cells. The cells latch onto the antigens that get into the bloodstream, and the foreign substance is carried to the lymph nodes for further filtering. The major lymph nodes are located in the armpit area, the groin area, and down the sides of the neck. Other less significant lymph nodes are located in the abdomen, pelvis, and chest regions.

The lymphatic system also includes the spleen, thymus, tonsils, and adenoids.

- The spleen is under the ribs between the stomach and diaphragm on the left side of the body. It produces lymphocytes and monocytes, a type of white blood cell, and works to filter out all of the old red blood cells. The red blood cells are destroyed and replaced by new red blood cells made from the bone marrow. The spleen also assists in maintaining a balance between cells and plasma in the blood.
- The thymus is a small gland under the breast bone near the heart, beneath the sternum and just below the thyroid. It is usually most active in teenagers and begins to atrophy after puberty. The thymus is important in the development of the immune system and helps to produce white blood cells. It also provides a place for T cells, a type of lymphocyte, to mature.
- The tonsils are glands located in the back of the throat. (Refer to Chapter 5 for more information on the tonsils.) There are three types: the palatine tonsils, which are located on each side of the throat; the lingual tonsil, located on the base of the tongue; and the pharyngeal tonsils, known as the adenoids, which are at the back of the nose. The adenoids are also called the nasopharyngeal tonsils. The main purpose of the tonsils is to protect the digestive system and the lungs from bacteria and viruses.

Diseases and Disorders of the Lymphatic System

After a person has recovered from a disease, the lymphatic system aids the immune system to remember the identity of the antigen so the body can respond quickly to any future similar threat.

The following are some diseases and disorders of the lymphatic system:

- *Lymphoma:* Lymphoma refers to a broad category of cancers of the lymphatic system. Two common types of lymphoma are Hodgkin's disease and non-Hodgkin's lymphoma. Lymphoma causes enlargement of the lymph nodes. Signs and symptoms include lymph node swelling, reduced energy and fatigue, weight loss, itching, fever, and night sweats.
- *Leukemia:* Leukemia is a proliferation of white blood cells, with a swelling of the glands. Signs and symptoms include enlarged spleen, liver, and lymphatic glands, diarrhea, swelling, reduced energy, and weight loss.
- *Infectious mononucleosis:* This disease is commonly called the "kissing disease." It is a viral infection most often seen in young adults that gets into the system by contact with the Epstein-Barr virus. It lives in the body until the conditions are correct for mononucleosis to surface. It is spread by direct contact. Symptoms usually begin to appear four to seven weeks after contact with the virus. Signs and symptoms include constant and extreme fatigue, fever, sore throat, decreased appetite, swollen lymph nodes, headaches, sore muscles, skin rashes, and abdominal pain.
- *Allergies:* These are hypersensitivities to certain materials. Allergies occur when the molecules known as antibodies and antigens become sensitive to foreign materials. This sensitivity leads the body to react to them like it would react to a bacteria or other invader. Some allergic reactions, known as anaphylaxis, can be so severe as to cause a life-threatening situation. Signs and symptoms range from minor runny noses, rashes, itchy, watery eyes, to complete allergic reactions of swollen airways and trouble breathing.
- *Inflammation:* This is the reaction that occurs whenever the immune system goes to work. As the cells that fight infection gather to take on the invader, blood fills the area, causing swelling, heat, and redness. Inflammation occurs also in the event of an injury, such as a sprained ankle, where there is usually no infection, just inflammation. A person can have inflammation without infection, but infection always leads to inflammation. The signs and symptoms of inflammation are redness, heat, swelling, and pain.

Why is it important for dental assistants to understand the function of the lymphatic system?

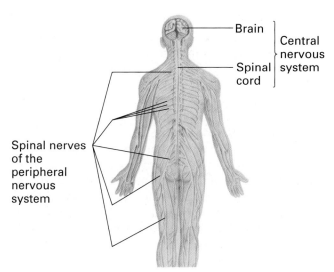

FIGURE 4.15
The nervous system.

Nervous System

The brain, the spinal cord, and all of the nerves comprise the nervous system (Figure 4.15). This system initiates muscles to contract, stimulates glands to secrete, and standardizes other systems within the body. The nervous system permits sensation to be perceived, such as pain, pressure, and touch. These nerve impulses trigger the muscles and organs to begin their processes, and they are responsible for the body's response to the environment.

Structure of the Nervous System

The nervous system is divided into three sections: the central nervous system, the peripheral nervous system, and the autonomic nervous system. The central nervous system (CNS) consists of the brain and spinal cord. Signals are sent and received by nerve impulses along the spinal column that provide information from the sensory data for the brain and relay the brain's response about things seen, heard, smelled, tasted, and felt (the five senses).

The peripheral nervous system (PNS) includes 12 pairs of craniospinal nerves that branch off the brain and 31 pairs of nerves that branch off the spinal cord. The PNS is a continuation of the nerve impulses that originate in the CNS to ultimately trigger the muscles and glands.

The autonomic nervous system (ANS) automatically regulates the involuntary actions required for vital functioning of the body, such as the heartbeat and digestion. Another function of the ANS is to stimulate a response to physical danger or to emergency. This response is known as the "fight-or-flight" response. The ANS releases a series of hormones, such as adrenalin and norepinephrine, to ensure that the body can protect itself if necessary.

The neuron is the basic functioning unit of the nervous system (Figure 4.16). The nervous system operates according to the principles of electricity, which requires a circuit. Neurons serve as conduits, or paths of electrical conduction, which are linked together. The neuron is shaped like a tree with a linked tail. The tree-like projections are called dendrites, and they receive impulses as they begin to pass through a cell. The impulse is routed

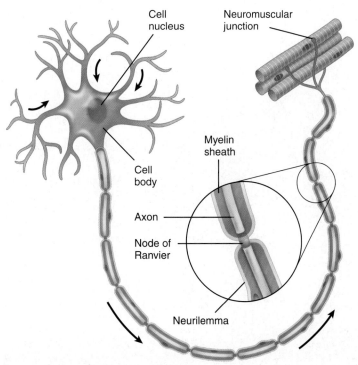

FIGURE 4.16
The neuron with a close-up of the axon structure.

through the nucleus of the cell, processed, and sent out of the neuron via a linked tail called the axon. It is encased in a layer of protective tissue called the **myelin sheath**. If a neuron has a myelin sheath, it is considered white matter. The neurons in the brain do not have myelin sheaths and are called gray matter. At the end of the axon is a small gap, called the synapse. The synapse is filled with fluids that allow for the conduction of electricity.

There are generally three types of neurons: motor neurons, sensory neurons, and associative neurons. They are characterized by their purpose. Sensory neurons carry messages from all over the body, like the skin (a sensory organ), toward the brain and spinal cord. Motor neurons carry messages away from the brain and spinal cord toward the muscles and glands of the body, giving directions to the body to act. Associative neurons (also called connecting neurons) send messages between motor neurons and sensory neurons.

The Brain

The bones of the skull protect the brain, a small organ covered with grooves and cracks. The five main parts of the brain are the cerebrum, the cerebellum, the brainstem, the pituitary gland, and the diencephalon (Figure 4.17).

The largest part of the brain is the cerebrum. The cerebrum is the part of the brain dedicated to higher thought such as reasoning, learning, and creative activity. The cerebrum makes up 85% of the brain's weight. The cerebrum has two halves, one on either side of the head. The pituitary gland is about the size of a pea and is located in the cerebrum. Its major function is to produce and release hormones. The cerebellum, a much smaller part of the brain, is located at the back of the brain, below the cerebrum. It is a very important part of the brain in that it controls fine-movement coordination, balance, and equilibrium and also helps to maintain muscle tone.

Another brain part is the brainstem. It is located beneath the cerebrum, just in front of the cerebellum. It serves as a connection from the brain to the spinal cord. The brainstem is responsible for life-sustaining activities such as breathing air, circulating blood, and digesting food.

The diencephalon is composed of the thalamus and the hypothalamus. The thalamus assists in the control of motor activity and also receives auditory and visual sensory signals. The hypothalamus is responsible for the maintenance of the body's temperature, among other physical functions. If the body is too hot, the hypothalamus signals the production of sweat for cooling. If the body is too cold, the hypothalamus triggers the processes for shivering and making goosebumps to provide warmth. Both mechanisms are attempts to get the body's temperature back to normal.

The Spinal Cord

The brain and spinal cord are considered to be two separate organs. The spinal cord is a thick bundle of nerves that serves as the main pathway for information connecting the brain and peripheral nervous system. The brain communicates with the rest of the body through the spinal cord and the nerves. Ring-shaped bones called vertebrae protect the spinal cord, allowing for a pair of spinal nerves to lead out from each segment of the spinal cord. Each spinal nerve is connected to the spinal cord by a dorsal root and a ventral root. Nerves then divide many times as they depart the spinal cord so that they may reach all parts of the body. The spinal cord runs down a tunnel created by aligned holes in the spinal column. The spinal cord is made up of 31 segments of bone. Each segment has a layer of protection, as does the skull, called the meninges. The meninges have three layers of protective fibers called the pia mater, the arachnoid, and the dura mater. They serve to further protect the most vital organs of the body: the brain and the spinal cord.

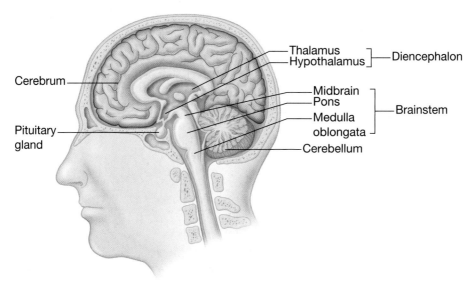

FIGURE 4.17
The structures of the brain.

Cranial Nerves

The cranial nerves send impulses from the brain to control the movements made in the face, forehead, and eyes. As shown in Table 4-2, these nerves are identified by name and are numbered using Roman numerals in sequential order starting from the front surface of the brain moving to the back. The sensory and motor nerves are key in the cranial nerves.

Diseases and Disorders of the Nervous System

Nervous disorders can present a variety of obstacles for the dental assistant. Uncontrollable shaking and incapable muscles are just a few of the signs and symptoms of nervous conditions. The tremors and uncontrolled movements can present a challenge to the dental assistant who prefers the patient remain still. Some patients with behavior problems may also engage in activities that make it difficult or impossible to perform certain routine dental tasks. Common disorders of the nervous system that are seen in dentistry are presented in Table 4-3.

How does the nervous system interact with other body systems?

Respiratory System

The respiratory system has the life-sustaining responsibility of bringing oxygen into the body (Figure 4.18). This task is accomplished by the processes of inhalation (bringing oxygen from the air into the body) and exhalation (releasing carbon dioxide from the body). *Respiration* is the term for a full cycle of inhalation and exhalation. The air is brought into the lungs through the nose or mouth by a contraction of the diaphragm. The air proceeds down a long tube called the trachea and into smaller passageways that lead to the blood. Once the air comes in contact with blood, the oxygen is absorbed through the walls of the capillaries and is carried to all parts of the body. As the oxygen is absorbed into the blood, the waste matter or carbon dioxide is transferred to the air and exhaled out of the lungs when air is exhaled.

Structure of the Respiratory System

The sinuses are hollow spaces in the skull just above the nasal cavity. (See Chapter 5 for information on the anatomy of the sinuses.) Small openings connect them to the nasal cavity. The sinuses serve to help regulate the temperature and humidity of air breathed in, to lighten the bone structure in the skull, and to give tone to the voice. The nasal cavity, which is known as the nose, is the main path by which outside air gets into the respiratory system. The nasal cavity is divided into a right and left passageway. Hairs, called cilia, exist in the nasal cavity as part of the air-cleansing system. As air is inhaled through the nose, small specks of debris are trapped by the cilia. The body expels the dirt by way of sneezing and blowing the nose. A mucous lining surrounds the nasal cavity and the lungs. The tissue that covers the wall of the nasal cavity contains many blood vessels to keep a constant flow of heat to warm the inhaled air. The mucus assists in warming and moisturizing the air before it enters the lungs. In human beings, air also enters through the mouth, known as the oral cavity.

TABLE 4-2 Cranial Nerves and Their Functions

Nerve Name	Function
I. Olfactory nerve	Leads from nasal receptors to the brain; provides sense of smell.
II. Optic nerves	Leads from the retina and some eye muscles to the brain; allows for vision.
III. Oculomotor nerves	Consists of two components with distinct functions: responsible for allowing the eyes to focus and for the accommodation of light through the lens. It is also responsible for reflexes of the eyes.
IV. Trochlear nerves	Allows for the precise movement of each eye in visual tracking or to work together fixating on an object.
V. Trigeminal nerves	Divides into three branches and controls the activity of the respective areas: • Ophthalmic branches lead to the eyes and the forehead. • Maxillary branches lead to the upper jaw. • Mandibular branches lead to the lower jaw.
VI. Abducens nerves	Controls the voluntary lateral (side-to-side) movement of the eye.
VII. Facial nerves	Has four components with distinct functions: to control facial expression muscles, salivary glands, lacrimal glands, and taste sensory in the front part of the tongue.
VIII. Acoustic nerves	Each divides into two branches: • Cochlear branches facilitate the sense of hearing. • Vestibular branches facilitate the sense of balance.

TABLE 4-3 Examples of Diseases and Disorders of the Nervous System and Their Signs and Symptoms

Diseases and Disorders	Signs and Symptoms
Alzheimer's disease (AD): progressive degenerative disease type of dementia involving parts of the brain that control thought, memory, and language	Loss of memory may include asking the same questions repeatedly; becoming lost in familiar places; being unable to follow directions; being disoriented about time, people, and places; and neglecting personal safety, hygiene, and nutrition. People with dementia lose their abilities at different rates. Disoriented and/or confused
Bell's palsy: condition in which one side of the face becomes paralyzed, usually temporary	Twitching, weakness, or partial to full paralysis of the face
Brain tumors: can be categorized into one of two groups: cancerous (malignant) or noncancerous (benign)	Headaches, seizures, cognitive or personality changes, eye weakness, nausea or vomiting, speech disturbances, or memory loss
Cerebrovascular accident: also known as a stroke; occurs when the blood supply to the brain is interrupted, resulting in brain cells lacking oxygen, which can cause some cells to die and leave other cells damaged	Weakness, paralysis or numbness of the arm and leg, unable to speak, hard to swallow, or loses consciousness
Epilepsy: seizure disorder	Varies from just staring off, being forgetful (called a petit mal seizure) to the body going rigid and exhibiting jerking motions (called a grand mal seizure)
Head injuries: trauma to the head or skull	Depending on the force of the injury and location, bleeding, pressure, and swelling can lead to other serious to fatal nervous system disorders
Migraine headaches: severe to disabling headache	Flashes of light, blind spots, nausea, vomiting, and extreme sensitivity to light and sound
Multiple sclerosis (MS): inflammatory disease in which the body loses the ability to transmit signals from the brain and spinal cord to other parts of the body	Loss of sensory, motor, and coordination skills
Parkinson's disease: degenerative neurologic disease in which the production of dopamine, a vital chemical that allows smooth, coordinated functioning of the body's muscles and movement, is discontinued	Tremor (shaking), slowness of movement, rigidity (stiffness), and difficulty balancing
Trigeminal neuralgia (tic douloureux): neurologic disorder of the fifth cranial trigeminal nerve that causes attacks of pain to one side of the face	Episodes of intense, stabbing, electric shock-like pain in the areas of the face, lips, eyes, nose, scalp, forehead, upper jaw, and lower jaw

The pharynx, commonly called the throat, is divided into three parts:

- Nasopharynx
- Oropharynx
- Laryngopharynx

The nasopharynx is located above the soft palate of the roof of the mouth just behind the nose. A narrow tube, called the Eustachian tube, extends from the middle ear into the nasopharynx. The Eustachian tube allows for the equalization of pressure between the inside of the skull and the outside atmosphere. The oropharynx is the visible part of the throat as seen through the mouth. It extends from the soft palate to the epiglottis, which covers the trachea or windpipe. The laryngopharynx contains the vocal cords, which are located near the Adam's apple. The vocal cords are lengths of tissue that are stretched by muscular contractions. As air moves across the vocal cords, the vibrations form sounds.

The adenoids are thick patches of lymph tissue located toward the top of the pharynx. The function of the adenoids is to assist the body in rejecting unfamiliar material, including germs. The adenoids produce lymphocytes to fight any pathogens. The tonsils are lymph nodes in the wall of the pharynx that serve to filter the inhaled air. Although the tonsils and the adenoids are an important part of the germ-fighting system of the body, they can be removed when infected.

The throat or pharynx channels incoming air from the nose or mouth. Air is pulled downward into the trachea, also known as the windpipe, where it enters the upper respiratory tract. Cartilage rings that can be easily felt protect the trachea. The **epiglottis** is a flap of tissue

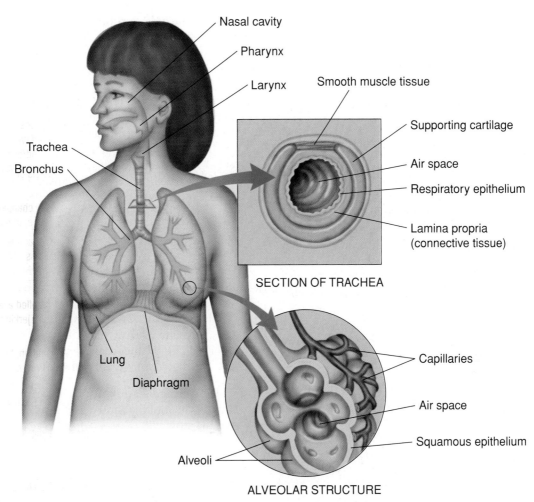

FIGURE 4.18
Structures of the respiratory system with expanded views of the trachea and alveolar structure.

located deep within the pharynx that protects the entrance to the trachea. It covers the opening to the trachea and prevents food and drink from entering the windpipe. Substances that are swallowed for digestive purposes should go into the esophagus, a tube that lies behind the trachea and leads to the stomach.

The bottom of the trachea splits into two branches called bronchi. Each branch extends into both lungs. The bronchi narrow to smaller passageways once in the lungs called bronchioles. The function of the bronchial tree is to spread the air from the trachea over a very wide area as quickly as possible. These smaller branches or bronchioles open into little air sacs called alveoli. The alveoli contain the capillaries where the oxygen can be extracted from the air. The capillaries are imbedded in the walls of the alveoli. The sac-like alveoli give the lungs increased surface area for the absorption of oxygen from the air. The blood in the capillaries carries the waste products, which are exchanged and then breathed out. To exit the body, the air travels the same passageways as when it was inhaled except in reverse.

The lungs, in general, provide the breath of life. They are always working, taking in oxygen and releasing carbon dioxide. Oxygen is required for all body processes. The pleura are two membranes that surround each of the lungs to separate the lungs from the chest wall. The bronchial tubes are lined with small hairs, or cilia, to aid in cleaning incoming air. The cilia also provide a fluid motion of movement that helps carry mucus upward and out into the throat, where it is either coughed up or swallowed. The mucus catches much of the dust, germs, and other unwanted matter that is then expelled.

The diaphragm is the strong muscle under your chest that separates the chest cavity from the abdomen. The diaphragm contracts, causing air to be pulled into the trachea and down the breathing passageways. Exhalation occurs as a result of the relaxation of the diaphragm. Chest muscles are also instrumental in the breathing process because they pull the ribs up and out, allowing the lungs to expand upon inhalation. The chest muscles allow for exhalation by pulling the ribs and consequently pushing air out.

Diseases and Disorders of the Respiratory System

Diseases of the respiratory system can be classified into four general areas:

- Obstructive diseases
- Restrictive diseases
- Vascular diseases
- Infectious, environmental, and other diseases

Obstructive diseases include emphysema and bronchitis. Emphysema is characterized by loss of elasticity or a stretching out of the alveoli and destruction of the capillaries. The small airways collapse during expiration, making it difficult to breathe out. Signs and symptoms include shortness of breath on exertion. Bronchitis is an inflammation of the bronchi of the lungs. It is a common disease that strikes habitual tobacco smokers, persons with chronic allergies, and drug abusers. Individuals who are exposed to high levels of pollution can also develop bronchitis. Like many disorders, bronchitis can be acute (short term) or chronic (long lasting). Signs and symptoms are a productive cough, fatigue, mild fever, and/or mild chest pains.

Restrictive diseases are ones that affect the airway by reducing its capacity. Sarcoidosis is a disorder of the immune system characterized by small inflammatory nodules. Common symptoms include complaints of fatigue regardless of any amount of sleep, an associated lack of energy, aches and pains, dry eyes, blurry vision, shortness of breath, a dry hacking cough, and skin lesions. Another example of a restrictive disease is asthma. Asthma is characterized by restricted airways due to inflammation of the bronchial tree.

Vascular diseases include pulmonary edema and pulmonary embolism. Pulmonary edema is swelling and/or an accumulation of fluid in the lungs. The accumulated fluids can lead to impaired gas exchange and respiratory failure. Signs and symptoms include difficulty breathing, coughing up blood, excessive sweating, anxiety, and pale skin. Pulmonary edema can be fatal if untreated. Pulmonary embolism occurs when a blood clot becomes dislodged from its site of formation, travels through the bloodstream, and lodges itself in the lungs. Signs and symptoms include difficulty breathing and pain during breathing. An untreated pulmonary embolism can result in death.

Infectious, environmental, and other diseases of the respiratory system include pneumonia, tuberculosis, and lung cancer. Tuberculosis is an important respiratory disease for the dental assistant to be aware of because it is caused by airborne bacteria. The dental assistant must take all necessary precautions to protect him- or herself from coming into contact with the bacteria.

Digestive System

The digestive system is divided into the alimentary canal and the accessory organs (Figure 4.19). Each of these divisions includes a complex series of organs and glands that are used to process food. In order for food to be processed, the body must break it down into smaller molecules. Most of the digestive organs such as the stomach and intestines are tube-like and hold the food as it makes its way through the body. The digestive system is essentially a long, twisting tube that runs from the mouth to the anus. It is referred to as the gastrointestinal (GI) tract or alimentary canal. The remainder of the digestive system is located outside of the GI tract and is collectively referred to as the accessory organs. The accessory organs include the liver, the gallbladder, and pancreas, which primarily produce or store digestive chemicals.

Function of the Digestive System

The function of the digestive system is to ingest and process nutrition into molecules that can be absorbed and used by the body. The digestive system's organs work together to break down the chemical components of food into nutrients. These nutrients are then carried and absorbed into the bloodstream to generate energy for each cell. The digestive system breaks down food in two ways:

- Mechanical digestion, which occurs through the chewing in the mouth, known as mastication, and churning in the stomach
- Chemical digestion, which occurs in the mouth, stomach, and small intestines

Through the basic actions of the digestive system, the process of ingestion, digestion, movement, absorption, and elimination occurs under involuntary control. The digestive process begins in the mouth when the teeth bite off, chew, and grind the food. The saliva is produced by the salivary glands located under the jaw, under the tongue, and just anterior to the ears. Saliva contains an enzyme called ptyalin that begins the chemical breakdown of carbohydrates. The tongue moves the food around, mixing the saliva and pushing the food toward the proper teeth.

Food, before being swallowed, is a lump of partially ground food called a bolus. After the bolus is swallowed, it enters the esophagus. The esophagus is a long muscular tube that runs from the back of the pharynx to the stomach. The muscles move the food down the esophagus via rhythmic, wave-like muscular contractions called peristalsis to force food from the throat into the stomach.

The stomach is a large, flexible, sac-like organ that churns the food and mixes the bolus with a very strong gastric acid. In the stomach, the bolus becomes a thin watery liquid called chyme. The chyme leaves the stomach and enters the duodenum, the first part of the small intestine. The second part of the small intestine is called the jejunum, and the final part of the small intestine is called the ileum. The small intestine's purpose is absorption. Finger-like projections called villi extend from the walls of the small intestines and are embedded with capillaries. These capillaries are thrust into the stream of chyme mixed with

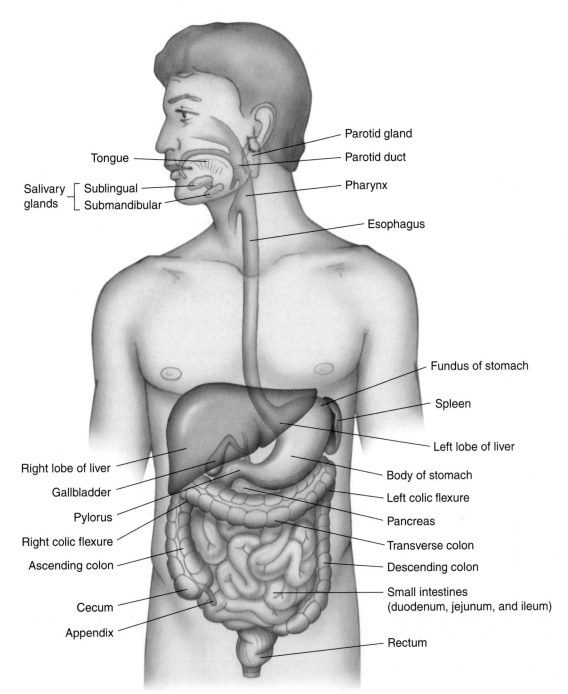

FIGURE 4.19
The major structures of the digestive system.

pancreatic enzymes. The capillaries absorb the nutrients for distribution throughout the circulatory system.

After passing through the small intestine, the chyme passes into the large intestine. In the large intestine, the chyme is dried as some of the water and electrolytes are removed from the food. Many microbes in the large intestine help in the digestion process but would be deadly outside of the digestive tract. The first part of the large intestine is called the cecum. It is a rounded pouch with the appendix affixed to the upper right section of

the cecum. It has no known purpose but can cause severe, sometimes fatal problems. Food proceeds from the cecum upward into the ascending colon. The transverse colon carries fecal matter across the abdomen, following down the left side of the body in the descending colon. The colon rounds out in a slight "S" formation called the sigmoid colon. The sigmoid colon leads to the rectum, where fecal matter is stored until released through the anal canal and out the anus. The large intestines absorb excess water from chyme so it can be used by the body.

Structure of the Digestive System

The major structures of the digestive system that assist in the function of the digestive system include the mouth, esophagus, stomach, small intestine, large intestine, appendix, rectum, anal canal, and anus.

The accessory organs of the digestive system are outlying organs that contribute to the digestive process by completing their own specific functions. These accessory organs are the liver, gallbladder, pancreas, and the structures of the oral cavity, which include the teeth, tongue, and salivary glands. The liver is the second largest organ (skin is the largest). It is located on the left side of the abdominal cavity, above and in front of the stomach. It is the chemical center of the body because it filters toxins from the blood, makes protein, produces cholesterol, and makes bile, which breaks down fats and some blood proteins.

The gallbladder is a small, sac-like organ situated near the duodenum toward the center of the abdominal cavity; it stores and releases bile. The pancreas is an oblong organ situated on the right side of the abdominal cavity just below the stomach and above the intestines. The pancreas produces enzymes that aid in the digestion of carbohydrates, fats, and proteins in the small intestine. The pancreas also serves an important function for the endocrine system.

Diseases and Disorders of the Digestive System

Various diseases and disorders affect the digestive system, including peritonitis, diverticulitis, hemorrhoids, and ulcers. Of most importance to the dental assistant are those digestive diseases that affect the oral cavity, such as bulimia, anorexia, and xerostomia.

Bulimia is a condition commonly seen in young women. The bulimic person will eat large amounts of food and then induce vomiting to purge the food. As the stomach acids come into repeated contact with the teeth, it causes a breakdown of the enamel (called erosion), increased decay, and xerostomia. In contrast the anorexic will severely limit her intake of food, which leads to xerostomia. Xerostomia is the condition of having a dry mouth. Other diseases and disorders, medications, and dehydration can also lead to xerostomia. For a more comprehensive list of diseases and disorders of the digestive system see Table 4-4.

In your own words how would you describe the digestive process?

Endocrine System

The endocrine system is composed of a series of glands (Figure 4.20).

The glands of the endocrine system secrete hormones that impact almost every cell, organ, and major function of the body. The endocrine system regulates mood, growth and development, tissue function, and metabolism. It also stimulates sexual development and triggers the body to respond to any threat to survival, via the fight-or-flight response. Hormones are chemical messengers that circulate through the bloodstream to affect distant organs. The various glands associated with the endocrine system react in response to the hormonal messages sent from the brain by way of the pituitary gland. Those hormones affect the glands that control the body's metabolism and its growth and development.

Other hormones released from the pituitary gland help protect the body in stressful situations, and yet others stim-

TABLE 4-4 Examples of Diseases and Disorders of the Digestive System and Their Signs and Symptoms

Diseases and Disorders	Signs and Symptoms
Hemorrhoids: condition in which the veins around the anus or lower rectum are swollen and inflamed	Pain, itching, and burning in and around rectum during defecation, sometimes with bleeding
Bulimia: condition in which individuals intentionally "purge" or vomit after eating	Serious dental problems caused by hydrochloric acid from the stomach that can lead to breakdown of the enamel of the teeth
Gastroesophageal reflux (GERD): condition in which esophageal mucosa is exposed to gastric contents that back flow into the esophagus	Most common symptom is heartburn, but patients may have other symptoms; at times it can be difficult to swallow
Hepatitis: currently, five kinds (A, B, C, D, and E) of hepatitis viruses have been identified that cause liver disease; the three main types are A, B, and C	Signs and symptoms vary; jaundice, fever, cold and chills, irritability depending on which type of viral liver disease is contracted
Crohn's disease: chronic inflammatory disease of the intestines that causes ulcerations and breaks in the lining of the small and large intestines, but can affect the digestive system anywhere from the mouth to the anus	Abdominal pain, diarrhea, and weight loss; less common symptoms include poor appetite, fever, night sweats, rectal pain, and rectal bleeding

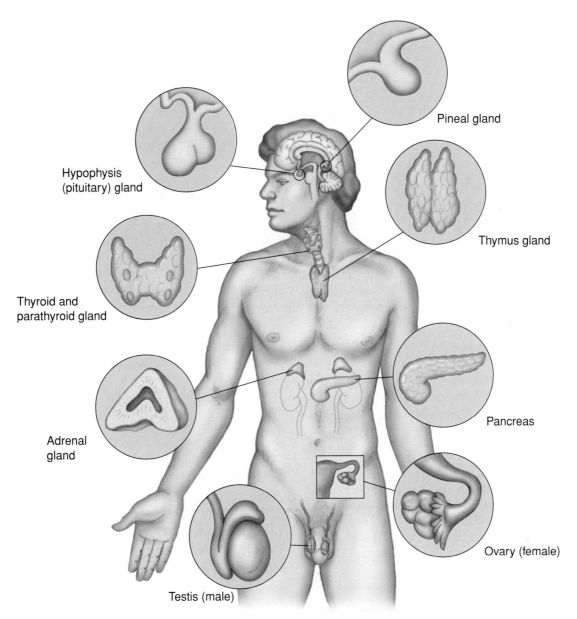

FIGURE 4.20
Primary glands of the endocrine system.

ulate sexual development and reproduction. Hormones are responsible for regulating the balance of water in the body and the body's utilization of calcium. One of the most critical functions of the body is the production of insulin, which aids in the transport of glucose in the cells.

Structure of the Endocrine System

Endocrine glands release more than 20 major hormones directly into the bloodstream. The major glands that make up the human endocrine system are the pituitary, the thyroid, the parathyroid glands, the adrenals, the pineal body, and the reproductive glands, which include the ovaries in females and the testes in males. Table 4-5 provides examples of the endocrine glands, their hormones, and their purpose.

The pituitary gland is sometimes called the "master" gland of the endocrine system, because it controls the functions of the other endocrine glands. The pituitary gland is very small, no larger than a pea, and is located at the base of the brain. The gland is attached to the hypothalamus (a part of the brain that affects the pituitary gland) by nerve fibers. The pituitary gland itself consists of three sections: the anterior lobe, the intermediate lobe, and the posterior lobe.

Each lobe of the pituitary gland produces certain hormones. The anterior lobe produces:

- Growth hormone (GH)
- Prolactin (PR) to stimulate the breast to release milk after giving birth
- Adrenocorticotropic hormone (ACTH) to stimulate the adrenal glands

TABLE 4-5 Examples of Endocrine Glands and Their Hormones and Purpose

Name of Endocrine Gland	Hormones	Purpose
Thyroid gland; located in the front of the neck	Secretes thyroid hormone	Regulates the body's overall metabolism
Parathyroid gland (4); located behind the thyroid	Secretes parathyroid hormone	Have absolute control over calcium levels throughout the body
Adrenal glands (2); located on the top of each kidney	Inner part secretes adrenaline; outer part secretes aldosterone and cortisol	Maintain salt levels in the blood, maintain blood pressure, help control kidney function, control overall fluid concentrations in the body
Pancreas (neuroendocrine gland); located deep in the abdomen behind the stomach; primarily a digestive organ	Contains extremely important endocrine cells that secrete insulin, glucagon, somatostatin, and others	Controls blood sugar and overall glucose metabolism; helps control other endocrine cells of the digestive tract
Pituitary gland; located at the base of the brain	Secretes thyroid-stimulating hormone, follicle-stimulating hormone, adrenocorticotropic hormone, and others	Controls the activity of many other endocrine glands such as thyroid, ovaries, and adrenal glands

- Thyroid-stimulating hormone (TSH) to stimulate the thyroid gland
- Follicle-stimulating hormone (FSH) to stimulate the ovaries and testes
- Luteinizing hormone (LH) to stimulate the ovaries or testes

The intermediate lobe produces a melanocyte-stimulating hormone that regulates skin pigmentation. The posterior lobe produces two key hormones: ADH and oxytocin. ADH (antidiuretic hormone) is released to increase absorption of water into the blood by the kidneys, and oxytocin is released to contract the uterus during childbirth and stimulates milk production during pregnancy and thereafter.

The pineal gland is shaped like a pinecone and is located in the middle of the brain. It secretes melatonin, a hormone that helps regulate the wake/sleep cycle. The pineal gland shrinks during puberty. The thymus gland plays a role in the body's immune system allowing for the maturity and screening of the T cells. The thymus also shrinks during puberty.

Other structures in the endocrine system include the reproductive glands. Male gonads, or testes, secrete hormones called testosterone. Testosterone regulates body changes associated with male sexual development including enlargement of the penis, the growth spurt that occurs during puberty, and the appearance of other male secondary sex characteristics such as deepening of the voice, growth of facial and pubic hair, and the increase in muscle growth and strength. Testosterone is also required for the production of sperm by the testes.

In the female, the ovaries produce eggs and secrete estrogen. Estrogen is required for the development of female sexual features such as breast growth, the accumulation of body fat around the hips and thighs, and the growth spurt that occurs during puberty.

The pancreas produces hormones associated with the digestive system: insulin and glucagons. These hormones work together to maintain a steady level of glucose, or sugar, in the blood, which keeps the body supplied and sustained with fuel for energy. Although the endocrine glands are the body's main hormone producers, some nonendocrine organs, such as the brain, heart, lungs, kidneys, liver, thymus, skin, and placenta, also produce and release hormones.

Diseases and Disorders of the Endocrine System

Hormones must be balanced in the blood; too much or too little can be detrimental to the function of the body. For example, if the pituitary gland produces too much growth hormone, a child may grow excessively tall. If it produces too little, a child may be abnormally short. Many endocrine disorders are easily treatable by either stopping or slowing the release of hormones or by replacing the insufficient hormones. Diseases of the endocrine system are somewhat common and include conditions such as diabetes, thyroid disease, and the following diseases:

- *Hyperthyroidism:* Occurs when too much thyroid hormone is present.
- *Hypothyroidism:* Occurs when not enough thyroid hormone is present.
- *Thyroiditis:* An inflammatory process that occurs within the thyroid gland. Can present with a number of symptoms such as fever and pain. It can also appear as subtle findings of hypothyroidism or hyperthyroidism.
- *Cushing's syndrome:* Can be caused by excessive amounts of synthetic corticosteroid drugs (such as prednisone) used to treat autoimmune diseases such as lupus. Cushing's disease occurs when a tumor in the pituitary

gland produces excessive amounts of corticotropin and stimulates the adrenals to overproduce corticosteroids.

• *Type 1 and type 2 diabetes:* Due to either a decreased or increased production of insulin.

Urinary System

The urinary system is also known as the excretory system because it filters waste, toxins, and excess water or nutrients from the circulatory system. It helps regulate the chemical composition of body fluids. The system serves to help retain the proper amounts of water, salts, and nutrients as well. Components of this system include the kidneys, the ureters, the bladder, the urethra, and the urethral meatus (Figure 4.21).

Structure of the Urinary System

According to the National Institute of Diabetes and Digestive and Kidney Diseases, "Every day, the kidneys process about 200 quarts of blood to sift out about 2 quarts of waste products and extra water." During circulation, blood passes through the kidneys in order to deposit used and unwanted water, minerals, and a nitrogen-

rich molecule called urea. The kidneys filter the wastes from the blood, carrying the blood through the capillary system of the nephron, the basic functioning unit of the kidney where urine is produced. Billions of nephrons are located in the cortex or outer layer of the kidney.

As urine is produced, it trickles to the floor of the kidney called the renal pelvis. The urine pools there and then spills over into the ureters. Urine is then transported to the bladder by a rhythmic motion made by the squeezing of the muscles that cause the urine to be moved through the ureters. The bladder holds urine until it is eliminated through the urethra. The bladder can hold up to 1000 mL of urine. A person feels the urge to urinate at about 250 mL, and the daily average output of urine is about 1500 mL. The urethra carries the urine from the bladder to the outside of the body. In women it is about two inches long; in men, about six to eight inches long. In men the urethra carries urine and semen.

In addition to removing wastes, the kidneys release three important hormones: erythropoietin, which stimulates bone marrow to reproduce red blood cells; renin, which regulates blood pressure; and calcitriol (vitamin D), which helps maintain calcium for bones and homeostasis in the body.

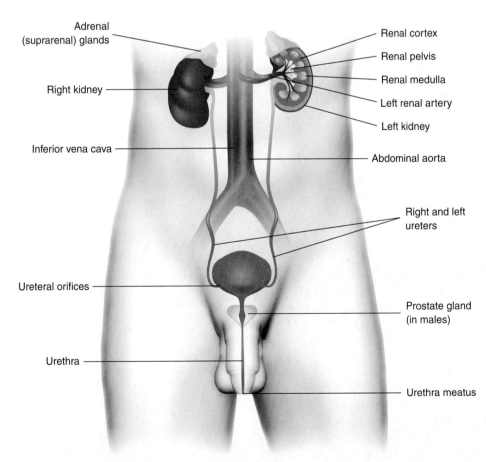

FIGURE 4.21
The major structures of the urinary system.

TABLE 4-6 Example of Disorders of the Urinary System and Their Signs and Symptoms

Disorders	Signs and Symptoms
Incontinence: inability to control urination; bladder pressure intensifies	Unable to control urine output during coughing, sneezing, laughing, or when any pressure is put on the bladder. Can be a symptom of many diseases or infections
Cystitis: inflammation in the bladder	Pain when urinating, feeling of urgency, fever, and sometimes lower back pain
Renal failure: loss of kidney function	Rapid retention of body fluids and inability to remove wastes or filter poisons from the body

Diseases and Disorders of the Urinary System

If kidneys are diseased and not working properly, the buildup of waste in the body system will eventually lead to death. Diseases of the urinary system include bladder and kidney infections, and the presence of stones in the kidney. Table 4-6 lists three common disorders of the urinary system.

Integumentary System

The integumentary system consists of the skin, hair, and nails. This system serves as a barrier to guard the body from the outside environment and keep the body intact. Additional functions are to retain body fluids, defend against disease, eliminate waste products, and regulate body temperature. The skin is the human body's largest organ. The skin contains several types of sensory receptors through which sensations such as pressure, hot and cold temperatures, and pain can be felt. One of the most important purposes of the integumentary system is to protect the body.

Fingerprints are the pattern of ridges on the skin of an individual's fingertips and thumbs. They are formed by dermal tissue and are unique to each individual. The patterns found in one's fingerprints never change.

Structure of the Integumentary System

The skin is composed of three main layers, the epidermis, the dermis, and the subcutaneous layer (Figure 4.22). The epidermis is the outermost layer of the skin and is composed of many sheets of flattened, scaly **epithelial** cells. These epithelial cells create a thin outer layer of skin. This thin outer layer has no blood supply and consists of dead cells. As new cells are pushed to the surface, the older cells begin to die and then fall off. The epidermis contains cells that produce melanin, a dark brown pigment that

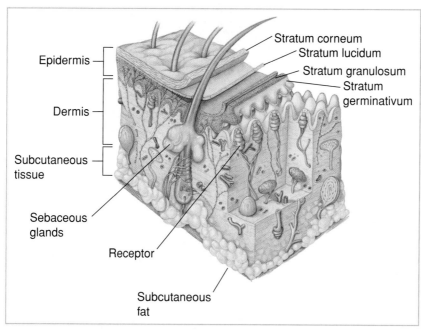

FIGURE 4.22
Structures of the skin with associated glands.

acts to keep the skin color consistent even as the cells die and slough off. Both light- and dark-skinned people have the same amount of melanocytes. The difference in skin color is caused by the amount of melanin the melanocytes produce and distribute. The amount of melanin produced in skin depends on heredity and the amount of exposure the skin has to ultraviolet radiation or tanning. Melanin is important for protection. Light-skinned people need to minimize exposure to the sun and protect themselves from its ultraviolet radiation. However some exposure to the sun is required for the absorption of vitamin D.

The dermis is the thickest layer of inner skin composed of living cells. It provides bulk for the skin. The dermis lies beneath the epidermis and contains a source of blood vessels, nerve receptors, oil and sweat glands, sensory organs, smooth muscles, and hair follicles.

The dermis helps to control the body's temperature. When an individual is cold and needs to conserve heat, the blood vessels in the dermis narrow or tighten. When the body is too warm, the skin allows for the release of sweat that cools the body.

Beneath the dermis is the subcutaneous fat layer consisting of fat and loose connective tissue. The subcutaneous fat insulates the body from heat loss and cushions the underlying organs. The subcutaneous fat layer is also known as the hypodermis.

Skin Appendages

The skin has a number of appendages, including the hair, nails, and glands. The dermis contains three major types of glands in the skin: sebaceous glands, sudoriferous glands, and the apocrine sweat glands. The sebaceous glands (oil glands) produce an oily secretion that spreads along the surface of the skin, keeping the epidermis flexible and waterproof. Sebaceous glands are connected to hair follicles by tiny ducts that provide the surface of the skin and the shafts of hair with a coating of protective oils. The oil prevents excess water loss and provides lubrication and softening to the skin and hair. The sebaceous glands become active during puberty and less active with age. These glands are found all over the body except for the palms of the hands and the soles of the feet.

Sudoriferous glands and apocrine glands are sweat glands. Sudoriferous glands are spread throughout the body. This type of gland senses core temperature directly and with input from temperature receptors from the skin the sweat output is determined according to the temperature. The sudoriferous glands are also known as the eccrine sweat glands and are activated in response to stress. The sweat glands release sweat at the surface of the epidermis. The apocrine sweat glands are the largest sweat glands and are located under the arms, around the nipples, and in the genital region. Sweat, which contains salt and water, incorporates a bacterial action causing secretions to break down, helping the body to cool. The main cause of sweat odor is bacteria.

The integumentary system supports the excretory system in the removal of waste. Skin, hair, and nails make up the system by removing wastes and transporting them to the surface level of the body. The skin protects the body and provides removal of dead cells and sweat, which are composed of waste products.

The body's hair and nails are a gathering of dead epidermal cells. As cells die and need to be removed, the hair and nails grow. A hair follicle is part of the skin that grows hair by packing old cells together. The thicker the hair, the more sebaceous glands exist. Hair grows from a hair follicle on all areas of the body's skin, regardless of sex or race, except in the palms of hands and the soles of feet. Hair projects from the skin and grows from follicles found in the dermis. Hair serves to provide insulation from the cold and heat.

Some people seem to have less body and facial hair than others; however, the total number of follicles is comparatively even. Older people tend to develop gray hair due to a loss of pigment. Gray or white hair along with hair loss is considered to be a sign of the normal aging process.

As with hair, nails are composed of dead epidermal cells. The nail is made up of a root and a body. The nail root or matrix grows from an area of rapidly dividing cells. The root of the nail is located at the end or tip of the fingers and toes. During cell division, cells produce a tough, strong platelike nail that covers and protects the tips of the fingers and toes. The nails rest on a bed of tissue filled with blood vessels, giving the nails a pinkish color. The body of the nail is the visible portion seen growing from the skin out through the cuticle. The free edge hangs over the end of the finger, and the white crescent shape at the base of the nail is called the lunula.

Diseases and Disorders of the Integumentary System

Many disorders can occur in the integumentary system. These include basal cell carcinoma (BCC), acne, blisters, and athlete's foot. BCC is a skin cancer of the outer layer of skin where basal cells are located. It is the most common type of skin cancer and is highly curable when detected early. The early warning signs of BCC are listed in Table 4-7.

Squamous cell carcinoma (SCC) is the second most common type of skin cancer. Squamous cells are flat, scaly cells on the surface of the skin and are malignant. Cure rates are increased upon early detection. Table 4-8 lists warning signs for SCC.

Acne, a disorder of the hair follicles, occurs when the skin becomes clogged and infected. If the ducts of oil glands become clogged with too much oily secretions, dead cells, and bacteria, acne will result. Symptoms of acne include comedones (blackheads) and pustules (whiteheads) on the face, chest, and back.

TABLE 4-7 The Five Warning Signs of Basal Cell Carcinoma

A **reddish patch** or irritated area, frequently occurring on the chest, shoulders, arms, or legs. Sometimes the patch crusts. It may also itch or hurt. At other times, it persists with no noticeable discomfort.

An **open sore** that bleeds, oozes, or crusts and remains open for three or more weeks. A persistent, nonhealing sore is a very common sign of an early basal cell carcinoma.

A **pink growth** with a slightly elevated rolled border and a crusted indentation in the center. As the growth slowly enlarges, tiny blood vessels may develop on the surface.

A **scar-like area** that is white, yellow, or waxy, and often has poorly defined borders. The skin itself appears shiny and taut. This warning sign can indicate the presence of an aggressive tumor.

A **shiny bump**, or nodule, that is pearly or translucent and is often pink, red, or white. The bump can also be tan, black, or brown, especially in dark-haired people, and can be confused with a mole.

TABLE 4-8 Warning Signs of Squamous Cell Carcinoma

A **persistent, scaly red patch** with irregular borders that sometimes crusts or bleeds.

An **elevated growth** with a central depression that occasionally bleeds. A growth of this type may rapidly increase in size.

An **open sore** that bleeds and crusts and persists for weeks.

A **wart-like growth** that crusts and occasionally bleeds.

A decrease in the production of oil to the skin and hair is the reason the skin becomes very dry and loses elasticity, resulting in wrinkles of the skin.

Sometimes when friction damage occurs to the soft skin tissue layers, the epidermis separates from the dermis and tissue fluid can collect causing a blister. An example of when this might occur is when an individual is breaking in a new pair of shoes. If the skin is continuously subjected to pressure, the skin will reproduce replacement cells rapidly, creating a thicker epidermis called a callus.

Athlete's foot, a common fungus infection, can cause soreness and pain in the foot. Symptoms of athlete's foot include itchy, sore skin on the toes, with scaling, cracking, inflammation, and blisters. If the blisters break, raw patches of tissue may be exposed. If the infection spreads, itching and burning may increase.

There are few threats more serious to the skin than burns. Burns are injuries to tissues caused by intense heat, electricity, or chemicals. When skin is burned and cells are destroyed, the body readily loses its precious supply of fluids as well as its first line of defense in the immune system. Infection of the dead tissue by bacteria and viruses occurs one to two days after the skin has been burned. Infection is the leading cause of death in burn victims.

Burns are classified according to their severity or depth:

- First-degree burns occur when only the epidermis is damaged. The burned area is painful. The outer skin is reddened and some swelling may occur. Although first-degree burns may cause discomfort, these minor burns are usually not serious and heal within a few days. Sunburns are usually first-degree burns.

- Second-degree burns occur when the epidermis and the upper region of the dermis are damaged. The burned area is red, painful, and may have a wet, shiny appearance because of exposed tissue. Blisters may form with a second-degree burn. If the blisters are not broken and care is taken to prevent infection, the burned skin may regenerate or grow again without permanent scars. Second-degree burns take longer to heal than first-degree burns.

- Third-degree burns occur when the entire depth of skin is destroyed. Because nerve endings have been destroyed, the burned area has no sensitivity. The area may be blackened or gray-white in color. Muscle tissue and bone underneath may be damaged. In these serious to critical burns, regeneration of the skin is not possible. Third-degree burns take weeks to heal and will leave permanent scarring.

Melanoma is a malignancy of the skin in which the cells that give the skin its color become cancerous. Melanoma occurs most frequently in light-skinned people. It is usually found in adults, though occasionally melanoma may develop in children and adolescents. Melanoma is most often associated with too much exposure to the sun. Half of all melanomas are thought to arise from a noncancerous form such as a mole. Symptoms include increase in size, changes in color, lack of symmetry, indistinct borders, itching, and possibly ulceration and bleeding of the skin area.

Why is the skin so important?

Reproductive System

The major function of the reproductive system is to ensure survival of the human species. The reproductive system, unlike the other body systems, is not essential to the body's survival. An individual may live a long, healthy, and happy life without producing children. The reproductive system has four functions:

- To produce hormones
- To produce egg and sperm cells
- To transport and sustain these cells
- To nurture developing offspring

The male and female reproductive systems have the same function but operate in completely different manners. The idea is that the male contribution meets the female contribution to reproduce another individual. In the first six weeks after fertilization, the male and female embryos are identical in appearance. Sometime around the seventh week of development major changes occur. These changes include the development of testes, the primary reproductive organ in males, where male hormones and sperm are produced, or the development of ovaries, the primary reproductive organ for females. The tissue of the embryo responds to these hormones by developing into the male reproductive organs or developing into the female reproductive organs.

During infancy and childhood, the testes and ovaries produce small amounts of sex hormones. These hormones aid in the development of the other reproductive organs. Active reproductive cells are not capable in either the male or female until puberty. Puberty is the period of time at which the sexual growth and maturation of the reproductive systems become fully functional and the male and female reproductive organs are fully developed. The age of onset of puberty varies among individuals, although it usually occurs anytime from 9 to 15 years of age in females and about one year later for males.

Structure of the Male Reproductive System

Unlike the female, whose sex organs are located entirely within the pelvis, the male has reproductive organs called genitals that are both inside and outside the pelvis (Figure 4.23). The male genitals include:

- The external genitalia consisting of the penis and scrotum.
- The urethra, the common passageway for semen and urine.

- The testes or male gonads. The primary functions of the gonads are to produce and store sperm. The production of testosterone is secondary to the purpose of the production of sperm. The testes are held within the scrotum, which keeps the glands away from body heat, allowing a cooler temperature for the production of sperm. Other organs in the male reproductive system prepare sperm for the possible fertilization of an egg.
- Accessory glands contribute to the nutrition, secretion, and release of sperm as the sperm travel along the pathway from the testes to the urethra. The secretions of the accessory glands constitute most of the volume of the semen that the male eventually ejaculates.

Diseases and Disorders of the Male Reproductive System

The male reproductive system can be very susceptible to diseases and disorders. If any of the passageways are blocked or discontinued, the reproductive system will not be effective. Some diseases, such as cancer and the mumps, attack the cells of the reproductive system. Other diseases are of an accidental nature as in injury or in sexually transmitted diseases. Diseases and disordes of this system include:

- *Testicular trauma:* Because the testes require a cooler temperature, the testicles are held at a vulnerable position. Even a mild injury to the testicles can cause severe pain, bruising, or swelling. Most testicular injuries occur when the testicles are struck, hit, kicked, or crushed, usually during sports or due to other trauma.
- *Varicocele:* A varicocele is a varicose vein in the testicles. It is a painful and possibly dangerous situation, especially if the vein bursts. Varicoceles commonly develop while a boy is going through puberty.

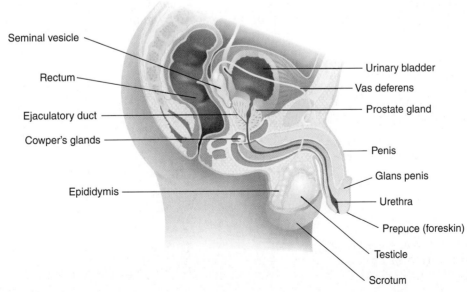

FIGURE 4.23
The male reproductive system.

- *Testicular cancer:* The most common cancer in men younger than 40 is testicular cancer. It occurs when cells in the testicle divide abnormally and form a tumor. Testicular cancer often spreads to other parts of the body like the prostate, lungs, and lymph nodes. Early detection can result in improved cure rates.
- *Sexually transmitted diseases (STDs):* STDs that can affect men include human immunodeficiency virus/ acquired immunodeficiency syndrome (HIV/AIDS), human papillomavirus (HPV, or genital warts), syphilis, chlamydia, gonorrhea, genital herpes, and hepatitis B. Some are bacterial infections and others are viral or fungal. They are spread from one person to another mainly through sexual activities.

Structure of the Female Reproductive System

The female reproductive system has two main functions: to present the female eggs for possible fertilization and to prepare for the fertilized egg to grow into the embryo. The reproductive structure enables fertilization to occur and then accommodates and nourishes a developing baby.

The female reproductive system is shown in Figure 4.24. At the top of the uterus are two ovaries that store all female eggs. The fallopian tubes are thin, narrow passageways that lead from the ovaries to the uterus. If fertilization by sperm occurs, it usually occurs in the outer third of the fallopian tube. The egg, whether fertilized or not, moves down the fallopian tube to the top part of the uterus. This part is called the fundus. If the egg is fertilized, it will cling to the inner lining of the uterus called the endometrium. The regular menstrual cycle should stop so that the egg is nourished properly. If the egg is not fertilized, it is passed from the body with the uterine tissue that is excreted during menstruation. The end of the uterus is marked by the cervix, which serves as a gatekeeper for the uterus. The cervix connects to the vagina, a hollow muscular sac that leads to the outside of the body. The genitalia, or vulva, is composed of the mons pubis, the clitoris, the labia, the urinary opening, and the vagina.

Diseases and Disorders of the Female Reproductive System

Because the female reproductive system is very complicated and relies on an intricate hormonal matrix, the system is open to a series of diseases and disorders. Many of the problems associated with this system are related to the structure and function of the parts. Sexually transmitted microorganisms cause some of the diseases. Diseases and disordes of this system include:

- *Vulvovaginitis:* This disorder is an inflammation of the vulva and vagina. Irritating substances such as laundry soaps, bubble baths, or poor personal hygiene may cause vulvovaginitis. Symptoms include redness, itching, and vaginal discharge.
- *Ectopic pregnancy:* This type of pregnancy occurs when a fertilized egg implants itself anywhere outside the uterus. It is an occurrence most commonly found in the fallopian tube. If a female has this condition, she can develop severe abdominal pain and must be seen by a doctor immediately. Surgery may be necessary.
- *Endometriosis:* This disorder occurs when tissue that makes up the inner lining is found outside of the uterus. The endometrium starts to grow outside the uterus such as in the ovaries, fallopian tubes, or other parts of the pelvic cavity. It can cause abnormal bleeding, painful periods, and general pelvic pain.
- *Sexually transmitted diseases:* STDs that affect women include infections and diseases such as pelvic inflammatory disease (PID), HIV/AIDS, HPV (genital warts), syphilis, chlamydia, gonorrhea, and genital herpes. Most are spread from one person to another by sexual intercourse.
- *Toxic shock syndrome:* This uncommon illness is caused by toxins released into the body during a type

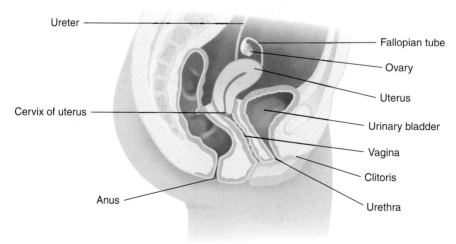

FIGURE 4.24
The female reproductive system.

of bacterial infection that is more likely to develop if a tampon is left in too long. It can produce high fever, diarrhea, vomiting, and shock. Death can occur.

Many types of menstrual problems can affect females. Some of the more common conditions include dysmenorrhea (painful periods), menorrhagia (very heavy periods with excessive bleeding), and oligomenorrhea (missed or infrequent periods, without pregnancy).

The Interaction of the Eleven Systems of the Body

Each major system within the human body has specific functions that are interconnected and must work together to maintain body functions. Consider what would happen if the muscle system did not have the support of the skeletal system. Alternatively, think of how swallowing would occur if the digestive system did not have the muscle system helping it to contract and relax. What if the urinary system was not filtering poisons and then removing the waste from our bodies—how long would life be sustained without that balance?

Most functions within the body occur without thought or involuntarily, relying on all the body systems to continually support each other. The interaction of all the body systems working together to maintain harmony is homeostasis. Homeostasis is the key to preventing a breakdown in health and ensuring a long life.

● SUMMARY

The health of one's body is often taken for granted. In learning and understanding the body systems, the dental assistant can assist patients in developing habits that sustain a healthy life. Within the dental office, dental assistants who are aware of overall health issues can contribute and take the precautions necessary to ensure more pleasant dental visits for those patients with medical concerns. Recognizing key factors that can influence the health of dental patients enables the dental assistant to distinguish abnormalities that may be exhibited by the patient.

● KEY TERMS

- **Appendicular:** Region of the body pertaining to the arms and legs. p. 40
- **Articulation:** Where two or more bones meet or form a junction; joints. p. 43
- **Atria:** Upper chambers of the heart. p. 48
- **Axial:** Portion of the body pertaining to the head, neck, and trunk. p. 40
- **Cancellous bone:** Lightweight bone (sponge-like) located in the interior area of the bones. p. 43
- **Cartilage:** Tough nonvascular, flexible, connective tissue. p. 44
- **Compact bone:** Hard and dense layer of bone. p. 43
- **Endocardium:** Thin lining inside the heart. p. 48
- **Epiglottis:** Elastic cartilage covered with mucous membrane that forms a part of the larynx; its function is to close off the larynx during swallowing. p. 56
- **Epithelial:** Tissue consisting of tightly packed cells that form a covering over external and internal body surfaces. p. 64
- **Hemostasis:** The process by which the body controls bleeding. p. 49
- **Homeostasis:** The process of all body functions performing together to maintain harmony in the body. p. 33

- **Myelin sheath:** Protective, insulated covering that surrounds some nerves. p. 54
- **Myocardium:** Middle layer (muscular wall) of the heart. p. 48
- **Nucleus:** Control center portion of a cell that is responsible for growth, repair, and reproduction of cells. p. 36
- **Organelle:** Special component of a cell that performs a particular function for the cell. p. 36
- **Osteoblast:** Cells responsible for forming bone. p. 41
- **Osteoclast:** Cells responsible for destroying bone. p. 43
- **Parietal:** Pertaining to the walls of a body cavity. p. 48
- **Pericardium:** Fibrous (double-walled) sac that surrounds the heart. p. 48
- **Periosteum:** Tough, fibrous lining that covers the compact coronal bone. p. 41
- **Ventricle:** Lower chamber of each half of the heart. p. 48
- **Visceral:** Pertaining to the internal organs or the covering of the internal organs. p. 48

CHECK YOUR UNDERSTANDING

1. When referring to the "anatomic position," the body is said to be in which position?
   a. standing erect with face forward, feet together, arms hanging to the sides, and palms forward
   b. standing erect with face forward, feet apart, arms hanging to the sides, and palms down
   c. standing erect with face forward, feet together, knees slightly bent, and arms hanging behind the back
   d. standing erect with face looking to either side, feet together, arms hanging to the sides, and palms facing up

2. Which of the following is an example of dorsal location?
   a. The nose is in front the ears.
   b. The spine is on the back side of the body.
   c. The pinky finger is located at the outside side of the hand.
   d. The knee is above the ankle.

3. Homeostasis occurs when all the body systems, cells, tissues, and organs
   a. vary by appearance, structure, and function.
   b. build into specialized groups of cells that form tissues, and tissue grouped together form into organs.
   c. perform together to maintain harmony in the body.
   d. are the blueprints that shape and form the body.

4. The nucleus is the _____ for the cell.
   a. waste storage
   b. control center
   c. energy source
   d. starting point

5. Striated or skeletal muscles create _____ movement.
   a. involuntary
   b. uncontrollable
   c. partial
   d. voluntary

6. The main role of the circulatory system is to
   a. transport nutrients, oxygen, hormones, and wastes through the body.
   b. hold the body erect and provide movement, production of body heat, and a means of communication.
   c. absorb oxygen from the atmosphere into the body (inhale) and expel carbon dioxide from the body (exhale).
   d. receive stimulation, transmit electrical signals and messages, and coordinate the body's activities.

7. Which bone is known as spongy bone?
   a. cortical bone
   b. cancellous bone
   c. crustiform bone
   d. alveolar bone

8. Muscle origins are the places where
   a. muscles begin.
   b. muscles end.
   c. muscles originate.
   d. muscles insert.

9. The hardest substance in the human body is
   a. bone.
   b. cartilage.
   c. cementum.
   d. enamel.

10. What two tissues of the human body can identify and are unique to an individual?
   a. hair and skin
   b. blood type and fingerprints
   c. saliva and tissue
   d. sweat and body fluids

INTERNET ACTIVITIES

- Go to Human Anatomy Online at www.innerbody.com/htm/body.html and choose "Begin your tour by choosing a system...." Enjoy the visual learning and ability to interact with all body systems.
- Visit www.kidinfo.com/Health/Human_Body.html to find more educational information regarding the human body systems.
- Go to www.tvdsb.on.ca/Westmin/science/sbi3a1/digest/digdiag.htm and view an interactive diagram of the digestive system.

WEB REFERENCES

- American Cancer Society   www.cancer.org
- American Heart Association   www.americanheart.org
- Anatomy of the Brain   www.biology.about.com/library/organs/brain/blcerebellum.htm
- Hypothalamus Gland   www.heumann.org/body.of.knowledge/k1/hypothalamus.html
- The Hypothalamus Gland   www.ask.com
- Muscular Dystrophy Association education information   www.mdausa.org/publications
- National Kidney Foundation   www.kidney.org

5

Head and Neck Anatomy

Chapter Outline

- Regions of the Head
- Bones of the Skull
  —Cranial Bones
  —Facial Bones
  —Temporomandibular Joint
- Muscles of the Face and Oral Cavity
  —Muscles of Mastication
  —Muscles of Facial Expression
  —Muscles of the Neck
  —Muscles of the Floor of the Mouth
  —Muscles of the Tongue
- Structure and Function of the Salivary Glands and Ducts
  —Parotid Gland
  —Sublingual Gland
  —Submandibular Gland
  —Disorders of Salivary Glands
- Sinuses
- Lymph Nodes of the Face and Neck
- Nerves of the Face and Neck
- Circulatory System of the Face and Neck
  —Arteries of the Face
  —Veins of the Face

Learning Objectives

After reading this chapter, the student should be able to:

- Identify major structures of the cranium and face.
- Describe landmarks of the maxilla and mandible.
- Differentiate the parts of the temporomandibular joint and their functions.
- Discuss muscles of mastication, facial expression, the floor of the mouth, and the tongue.
- Describe the major salivary glands and saliva ducts and list the paranasal sinuses.
- Name major nerves and blood vessels of the face and neck.
- Recognize and note any abnormal findings in the head and neck region.

Preparing for Certification Exams

- Identify intraoral anatomy.

Key Terms

Alveolar process	Maxilla
Articulate	Maxillary tuberosity
Bruxism	Mentalis
Cancellous bone	Origin
Crepitus	Saliva
Foramina	Sialolith
Glenoid fossa	Sinuses
Insertion	Suture
Mandible	Temporomandibular joint
Masseter	Xerostomia
Mastication	Zygomatic

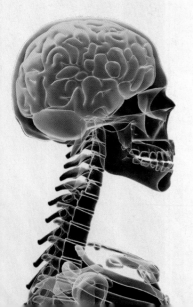

Anatomy is the study of the structure of organisms, and physiology is the study of the function of organisms. It is important for the dental assistant to understand head and neck anatomy in order to recognize when an abnormal condition exists so the dentist may be alerted. Anatomic structures of the head and neck include the bones of the skull and the temporomandibular joints, the muscles of the face and oral cavity, salivary glands and ducts, sinuses, lymph nodes, nerves, and arteries and veins.

Regions of the Head

The regions of the head are named according to the corresponding landmarks (Figure 5.1). The various anatomic regions of the head include the following:

- Frontal
- Parietal
- Temporal
- Occipital
- Mastoid
- Facial
- Oral
- Nasal
- Orbital
- Mental
- Zygomatic
- Buccal
- Submandibular

The frontal region corresponds to the frontal bone and is located at the forehead. The sides of the head include the parietal region, which spans the outline of the parietal bone, and the temporal region, which outlines the temporal bone. The occipital region is located at the

Preparing for Externship

Often subjects such as anatomy can be quite challenging. This information though is critical for dental assistants to learn and understand. If this area of your studies has been challenging, utilize the externship experience to continue learning. Ask a lot of questions during the externship experience. The externship supervisor and dentist are there to assist you in your learning process. Look, listen, and learn!

Dental Assistant PROFESSIONAL TIP

When the dental assistant is performing oral evacuation and tissue retraction with the high-volume evacuator during intraoral procedures, knowledge of oral soft tissues, the tongue, and cheek muscles is valuable to ensure the best possible patient comfort. (See Chapter 26 for information on evacuators.) Familiarity with the nerves, arteries, and veins of the face is valuable for the dental assistant to understand during local anesthesia procedures in order to place topical anesthetic in the correct location. (See Chapter 28 for more on anesthesia.)

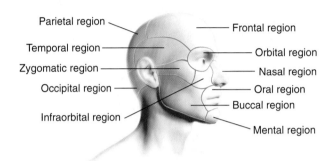

FIGURE 5.1
Regions of the head.

base of the skull. Either side of the head has a mastoid region, which corresponds to the outline of the mastoid process and is a projection of the temporal bone. The facial bones compose the facial region. The area of the head around the mouth is the oral region, and the nasal region includes the nose. The orbital region is the area around the eye, and the chin is called the mental region. The **zygomatic** region corresponds to the cheekbone, and below that is the buccal region. The submandibular region includes the submandibular salivary gland, the mylohyoid muscle, and the hyoglossus muscle.

How many bones make up the skull? Why do you think humans have sutures on the bones of the head?

Bones of the Skull

The bones of the skull consist of the bones of the cranium and the bones of the face. Twenty-two bones make up the skull, 8 cranial bones and 14 facial bones. Within many bones are openings, called foramen (plural: **foramina**) through which nerves and blood vessels pass.

Cranial Bones

The cranium houses and protects the brain. The cranial bones are one frontal, two parietal, two temporal, one sphenoid, one occipital, and one ethmoid. See Table 5-1 and Figure 5.2 for more details about the cranial bones.

TABLE 5-1 Cranial Bones

Name of Bone	Position	Articulates with
One frontal bone	Forehead	Parietal bones
Two parietal bones	Each side of the skull	Occipital, frontal, temporal, sphenoid
Two temporal bones	Sides and base of skull	Parietal, occipital, sphenoid, zygomatic, mandible
One ethmoid bone	Eye orbits and above nose	Sphenoid, lacrimal, vomer, inferior turbinate
One sphenoid bone	Sides of skull, behind and across nose and eyes	All cranial bones
One occipital bone	Back and base of cranium	Temporal, parietal, sphenoid

Frontal Bone

The frontal bone forms the anterior portion of the skull (that portion toward the front of the body), including the forehead, part of the nasal cavity, the main portion of the roof of the eye orbits, and the nose. The frontal bone is connected to both parietal bones by the coronal **suture**, which is an immovable union between two bones, and contains air spaces for the frontal sinuses. Sutures allow the bones of the head to be temporarily compressed in order to go through the birth canal. They also allow the skull to grow.

Parietal Bones

There are two parietal bones, one on each side of the head. They form the sides and roof of the skull and are joined at the midline by the sagittal suture. The parietal bones **articulate**, or join, the occipital, the frontal, the temporal, and the sphenoid bones.

Temporal Bones

At the sides and base of the skull are the temporal bones. Projecting from the anterior portion of each temporal bone is the zygomatic process, which meets the zygomatic bone or cheekbone. The lower portion of this fan-shaped bone includes a depression, called the **glenoid fossa**, which is a shallow depression that articulates, or joins with, the mandible. A raised portion of the temporal bone, just in front of the glenoid fossa, is called the articular eminence. The opening for the outer ear (called the external auditory meatus), the mastoid, and the styloid processes are also situated within the temporal bone.

Sphenoid Bone

The sphenoid bone, also called the butterfly bone, articulates with all of the other cranial bones to bind them together. It is shaped similar to a butterfly with its wings extended. It forms the anterior portion of the base of the skull and the floors and sides of the eye orbits. The sphenoid bone is divided into a central portion or body with two greater and two lesser wings extending outward on each side, and two pterygoid processes, which project beneath. In Greek, *sphenoid* means "wedge shaped" and *pterygoid* means "wing shaped." The greater wings of the sphenoid bone form the sides of the skull and are

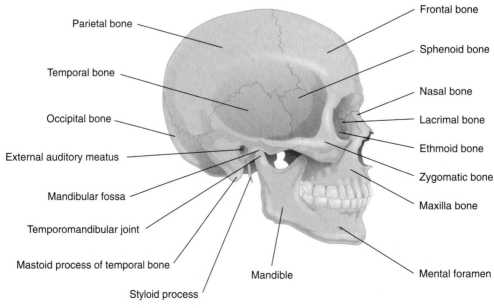

FIGURE 5.2
Bones of the cranium.

located anterior to the temporal bones. Descending from each side of the greater wings are the pterygoid processes. The lateral pterygoid plate projects posterolaterally from the pterygoid process and provides attachment points for the lateral and medial pterygoid muscles. The medial pterygoid plate projects posteriorly from the pterygoid process.

Ethmoid Bone

The ethmoid bone is a light, spongy bone situated between the two orbits of the eyes. It forms the bony wall of the nasal septum and encases the ethmoid sinuses. It articulates with several bones including the sphenoid, lacrimal, inferior turbinate, and the vomer.

Occipital Bone

The occipital bone is situated at the back and base of the cranium, or posterior, which is a term used to designate toward the back of the body. A large opening, the foramen magnum, allows the spinal cord to pass through this bone and into the brain. The occipital bone articulates with the interior of the sphenoid bone and the parietal and temporal bones on each side of the skull.

What is the longest and strongest bone of the face?

Facial Bones

The bones of the face consist of 13 stationary bones and a mobile mandible (Table 5-2 and Figure 5.3). They form the basic shape of the face and provide attachment for facial muscles.

Nasal Bones

The nasal bones are small oblong bones that are fused at the midline and form the bridge of the nose. They articulate with the frontal, ethmoid, and maxillary bones.

Maxilla

The second largest bone of the face is the **maxilla**, which is made up of two portions joined by a median suture. It forms the upper jaw, and contains pyramid-shaped cavities called the maxillary sinuses. The maxilla includes the zygomatic, frontal, and palatine bones and alveolar processes. The **alveolar process** is the thickest and most spongy part of the maxillary bone and contains sockets for the teeth. As mentioned in Chapter 4, spongy bone is also called **cancellous bone**, which is more porous than dense bone. Cancellous bone is permeated by many blood vessels and nerves enclosed in membranous periosteum. The most posterior portion of the maxillary alveolar bone, behind the molars, is a rounded projection of bone, called the **maxillary tuberosity**. The maxilla articulates with the ethmoid, lacrimal, inferior turbinate, zygomatic, and palatine bones. It also contains the infraorbital foramina and assists in forming the roof of the mouth, the floor and lateral walls of the nose, and the floor of the orbits.

Lacrimal Bones

The smallest and most fragile bones of the face are the lacrimal bones. They are very thin; situated at the front part of the inner wall of the eye orbit, anterior to the ethmoid bones; and contain tear ducts.

Zygomatic Bones

The zygomatic, or malar bone, is a paired bone, with one on each side of the human skull. Three major processes articulate (join) with the bones that surround it. The frontal process articulates with the frontal bone. The temporal process articulates with the zygomatic process of the temporal bone, and together these two processes assist in forming the zygomatic arch, which serves as the attachment point for the masseter muscle. The temporal muscle runs beneath the arch and also assists the mandible in chewing. The maxillary process of the zygomatic bone articulates with the zygomatic portion of the maxilla.

TABLE 5-2 Facial Bones

Name of Bone	Position	Articulates with
Two nasal bones	Bridge of nose	Frontal, ethmoid, maxilla
Two maxillary bones	Upper jaw	Ethmoid, lacrimal, inferior turbinate, zygomatic, palatine
Two lacrimal bones	Front part of inner wall of eye orbit	Frontal, ethmoid, maxilla, inferior turbinate
Two zygomatic bones	Cheek	Maxilla, sphenoid, ethmoid, inferior turbinate, vomer, temporal bone
Two palatine bones	Roof of mouth	Maxilla, sphenoid, ethmoid, inferior turbinate, vomer
Two inferior turbinates	Outer wall of nasal fossa	Maxilla, ethmoid, lacrimal, palatine
One vomer bone	On the nasal septum	Ethmoid, sphenoid, maxilla, palatine
One mandible	Lower jaw	Temporal bone

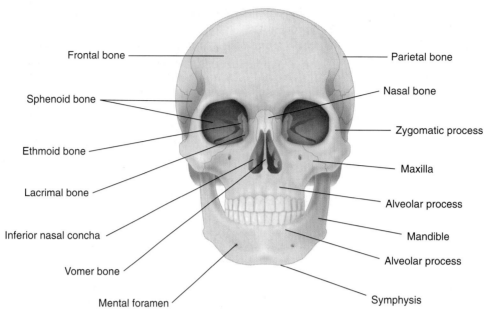

FIGURE 5.3
Bones of the face.

Palatine Bones

The palatine bones consist of a horizontal and vertical plate. The horizontal plate forms the hard palate, and contains the median palatine suture, the transverse palatine suture, and several foramina (Figure 5.4).

The vertical plate is a thin oblong form that rises up behind the nose to meet the orbits of the eyes. The palatine bones articulate with the maxillary, sphenoid, ethmoid, inferior turbinate, and vomer bones.

Inferior Turbinate

Each side of the outer wall of the nasal fossa has a thin layer of curled bone called the inferior turbinate, also known as the inferior nasal concha. These bones provide support for mucous membranes.

Vomer Bone

The vomer is a single bone, situated vertically at the back of the nasal fossa, and forms part of the septum or partition of the nose.

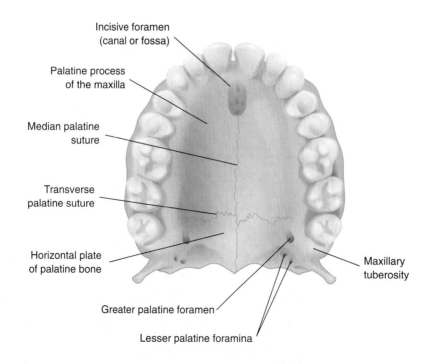

FIGURE 5.4
Palatal bones.

Mandible

- The word *mandible* is derived from the Latin word *mandere*, meaning "to chew."
- The word *mental* is derived from the Latin word *mentum*, meaning "chin."

The **mandible** is the longest and strongest bone of the face and holds the teeth of the lower jaw (Figure 5.5). The mandible is thick, dense, compact bone that lacks the porosity of the maxilla. It is a U-shaped bone that has a horizontal portion, the body, and a vertical portion, the ramus (plural: rami).

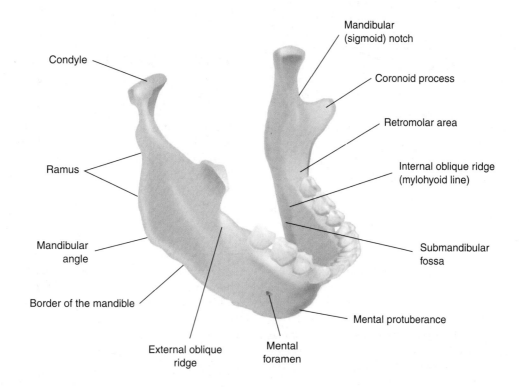

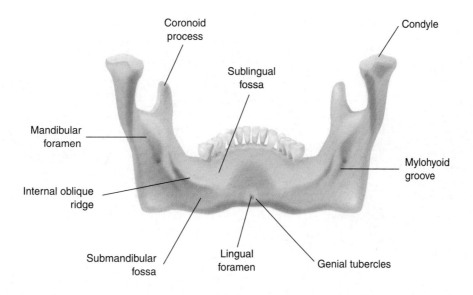

Lingual view

FIGURE 5.5
Landmarks of the mandible.

Patient Education

The dental assistant is often instrumental in assisting patients to understand their conditions. The Internet is full of valuable information. To assist a patient with temporomandibular joint dysfunction (TMD) and to understand how the mandible functions and how headaches increase with overuse of muscles of the head and neck as well as the various treatments the dentist can provide to aid in TMD management, have the patient visit the following website: www. tmjfriends.com/articles/pain.html.

The external surface of the body of the mandible includes the symphysis at the midline of the chin, a mental foramen on each side, the external oblique ridge, the border of the mandible, and the alveolar process. The posterior portion of the alveolar process on the mandible is called the retromolar area. External portions of the ramus consist of the angle of the mandible on the lower portion, the coronoid process on the anterior, and the condyloid process (also called the condyle) on the posterior portion. The coronoid and condyloid processes are separated by the mandibular (sigmoid) notch. The condyloid process extends to form rounded condyles, which articulate with the glenoid fossa of the temporal bones to form the **temporomandibular joint** or TMJ. The TMJ is an encapsulated joint between the temporal bone of the skull and the condyle of the mandible.

Internal surfaces of the mandible include an irregular eminence, or projection of bone, called genial tubercles,

the internal oblique ridge, mandibular foramen, and the internal oblique ridge (also called the mylohyoid ridge).

Hyoid Bone

The hyoid bone is a U-shaped bone that is suspended in the neck and attached to the neck by muscles of the tongue (Figure 5.6). It supports the tongue and provides attachment for numerous muscles.

Temporomandibular Joint

The temporomandibular joint, or TMJ, is formed by the union of the condyle of the mandible with the glenoid fossa and the articular eminence of the temporal bone (Figure 5.7). It is located in front of each ear. Ligaments surrounding the joint form a loose capsule.

As with other joints, synovial fluids enclosed within membranes provide nutrition and lubricate the TMJ. A meniscus, or disc made up of cartilage, separates the bony parts of the fossa and condyle, allowing the mandible to slide easily. The mandible moves at this joint by hinge and glide actions where the head of the condyle rotates, allowing movement up and down, side to side (lateral or excursion), and forward (protrusion) and backward (retrusion) (Figure 5.8). This gives the mandible the mobility needed for biting, chewing, and swallowing food and for speaking. This joint functions through extensive combined actions of several groups of muscles that bring the mandibular arch against the maxillary arch.

Problems with the TMJ are known as temporomandibular joint dysfunction (TMD). The symptoms may be mild or severe and include **bruxism** (grinding of

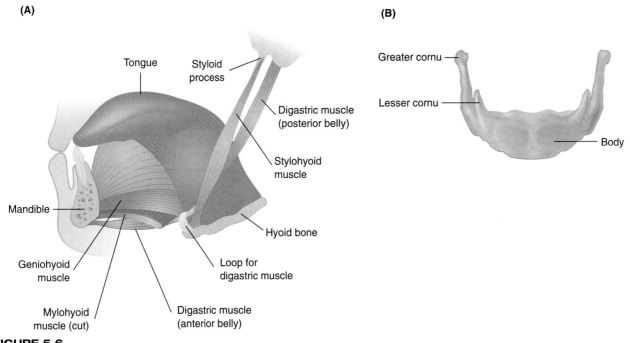

(A)

Tongue
Styloid process
Digastric muscle (posterior belly)
Stylohyoid muscle
Hyoid bone
Mandible
Geniohyoid muscle
Loop for digastric muscle
Mylohyoid muscle (cut)
Digastric muscle (anterior belly)

(B)

Greater cornu
Lesser cornu
Body

FIGURE 5.6
(a) Hyoid bone and muscles of floor of mouth. (b) Hyoid bone.

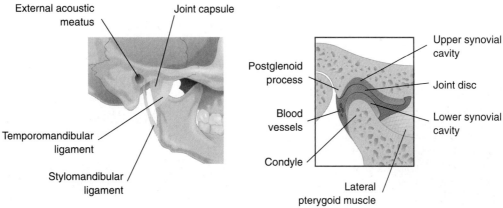

FIGURE 5.7
The temporomandibular joint.

the teeth), muscle soreness, headaches, popping noises, and **crepitus**, which is a crackling or grinding sound. The meniscus may also become perforated through trauma, the muscles can spasm, the joint may become displaced forward, the bone of the condyle can wear down over time, and inflammation of the joint or arthritis can occur. The dental assistant should report to the dentist any patient complaints that include irregular jaw movements, headaches, jaw pain, or joint sounds.

Which bone binds all other cranium bones together? Why is the maxilla bone cancellous while the mandible is denser?

Muscles of the Face and Oral Cavity

The muscles of the body shorten or contract in order to provide movement. They are connected with the bones, cartilage, and skin through fibrous ligaments. As discussed in Chapter 4, the point at which the end of a muscle is attached to a fixed structure is called the **origin** and its **insertion** is the movable point toward which the muscle is directed. Some muscles are spindle shaped; others form flat sheets of bands. Muscles may be attached directly to the periosteum of the bones, or may be attached through means of tough cords of connective tissue known as tendons.

Muscles of the body can be divided into three distinct groups: voluntary, involuntary, and cardiac. Voluntary muscles are attached to the skeleton and move bones at the joints. These muscles contract when an individual makes a conscious decision to move the muscle. Involuntary muscles are found in the walls of the body's internal organs. Their contraction is not under an individual's conscious control. Cardiac muscles are found only in the walls of the heart. Cardiac muscles contract to allow the heart to pump blood through it.

Head muscles fall into three primary groups: the muscles of mastication, muscles of facial expression, and neck muscles. Muscles of the oral cavity include those that aid in swallowing and speech, and muscles that function to control and support the tongue.

Muscles of Mastication

Mastication is the process of chewing food and mixing it with saliva in preparation for swallowing and digestion. This process involves the skull and mandible, their articulation, or joining together at the TMJ, and four sets of muscles. Jaw movements in mastication include elevation, side-to-side motion, protrusion, and retrusion (front-to-back movement). The four pairs of muscles that move the mandible and provide the primary focus of mastication are the temporalis, masseter, and the lateral and medial pterygoid muscles (Table 5-3 and Figure 5.9).

Temporalis

The temporalis or temporal is a large fan-shaped muscle that is attached to the temporal fossa on the side of the skull and connects to the coronoid process of the mandible. It functions to close the jaw as well as to pull the mandible forward.

Masseter

The **masseter** is a thick powerful muscle of mastication that closes the jaw during chewing. It starts at the zygomatic arch and inserts at the lateral surface on the ramus of the mandible.

Lateral and Medial Pterygoid

The lateral pterygoid, also known as the external pterygoid, originates from the greater wing of the sphenoid bone and the pterygoid plate of bone. It inserts onto the condyle of the mandible, and its purpose is to protrude the jaw and open the mouth. The medial pterygoid, also called the internal pterygoid, pulls the mandible upward and forward. It closes the mouth to aid in chewing. The medial pterygoid originates from the pterygoid plate and inserts onto the ramus and angle of the mandible.

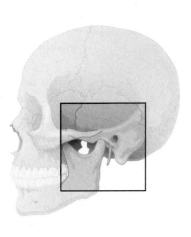

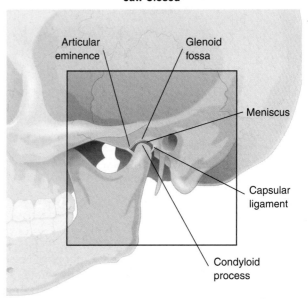

Jaw Closed

Articular eminence

Glenoid fossa

Meniscus

Capsular ligament

Condyloid process

Jaw Open—hinge action

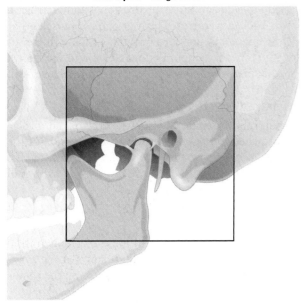

Jaw Wide Open—glide-and-hinge action

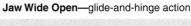

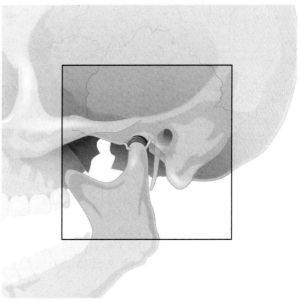

FIGURE 5.8
TMJ hinge and glide function.

Muscles of Facial Expression

The muscles of the face permit facial expression and therefore contribute to nonverbal communication. The main muscles of facial expression are the frontalis, orbicularis oris, buccinator, and the zygomatic muscles (Figure 5.10).

Unlike other skeletal muscles which attach to bones, the facial muscles attach to other muscles or skin. The frontalis muscle runs vertically along the forehead and raises and lowers the eyebrows. Surrounding the mouth is the orbicularis oris muscle. It is sometimes known as the kissing muscle because it closes the mouth and puckers the lips when it contracts. The thin, flat muscle that forms the walls of the cheek is the buccinator. The buccinator muscle contracts to compress the cheeks and lips in

TABLE 5-3 Muscles of Mastication

Muscle	Function	Origin	Insertion
Temporalis	Closes jaw and pulls mandible forward and backward (retrude)	Temporal bone	Coronoid process and ramus of mandible
Masseter	Closes jaw and retrudes mandible	Zygomatic arch	Ramus and angle of mandible
Lateral pterygoid	Protrudes jaw and opens mouth	Sphenoid bone and pterygoid plate	Condyle of mandible and TMJ capsule
Medial pterygoid	Pulls mandible upward and forward, and closes mouth	Pterygoid plate, palatine bone, and maxillary tuberosity	Ramus and angle of mandible

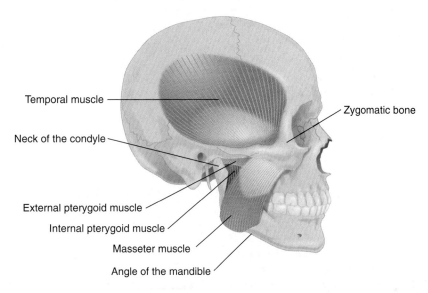

FIGURE 5.9
Muscles of mastication.

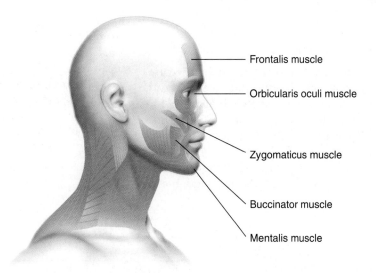

FIGURE 5.10
Muscles of facial expression.

order to keep food in contact with the teeth. The zygomatic muscle retracts and pulls the corners of the lips upward, outward, and backward. Located at the tip of the chin is the **mentalis** muscle, which protrudes the lower lip and wrinkles the skin. Table 5-4 summarizes these major muscles of facial expression.

Assorted other muscles contribute to facial expression. The zygomaticus major draws the upper lip backward,

TABLE 5-4 Muscles of Facial Expression

Muscle	Function	Origin	Insertion
Frontalis	Raises and lowers eyebrows	Frontal bone	Skin above eyes
Orbicularis oris	Puckers lips	Maxilla, mandible, lips, and buccinator	Mucous membrane and lip muscles
Buccinator	Compresses cheeks and lips	Maxilla and mandible	Orbicularis oris
Zygomatic	Pulls corner of lips up, back, and outward	Zygomatic bone	Orbicularis oris
Mentalis	Pushes lower lip up	Midline of mandible	Skin of chin

Cultural Considerations

Facial expressions are understood across all cultures. When dental team members are masked, the patient can still see the team member's eyes and the muscles surrounding them. Negative and positive emotions can be conveyed to patients without the dental assistant even being aware that it is happening. The dental assistant needs to remain positive and sensitive to what his or her facial expressions are conveying at all times.

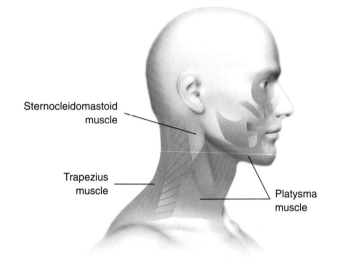

FIGURE 5.11
Muscles of the neck.

upward, and outward. The zygomatic minor draws the upper lip up and out. The depressor anguli oris depresses the angle of the mouth. The depressor labii inferioris draws the lower lip down and somewhat laterally. The levator anguli oris elevates the angle of the mouth, and the levator labii superioris elevates and extends the upper lip.

Muscles of the Neck

The largest and primary neck muscles of importance are the sternocleidomastoid, the platysma, and the trapezius muscles, as listed in Table 5-5 and shown in Figure 5.11. The sternocleidomastoid, also called the SCM, runs along the side of the neck and tilts the head to the right and left. The SCM is attached to the sternum bone in the chest and inserts at the mastoid process of the temporal bone and the anterior portion of the occipital bone.

Extending from both sides of the neck to the jaw muscles around the mouth is a wide layer of muscle called the platysma, which assists in depressing the mandible and the lower lip. The trapezius is a large flat triangular muscle at the back of the shoulder with parts leading to the neck and spine.

Which muscles help in chewing? Which muscles contribute to a smile? Which muscles aid in a kiss?

TABLE 5-5 Muscles of the Neck

Muscle	Function	Origin	Insertion
Sternocleidomastoid	Rotates head right and left	Sternum and clavicle bones	Mastoid process of temporal bone and anterior of occipital
Platysma	Depresses mandible and lower lip	Skin on chest	Mandible and lower part of face
Trapezius	Moves the head to one side or backward	Occipital bone and spine	Shoulder and clavicle bones

Muscles of the Floor of the Mouth

Four muscles support the tongue and suspend the hyoid bone within the neck: the digastric, stylohyoid, mylohyoid, and geniohyoid. (Table 5-6). These muscles, along with the muscles of the tongue, are important in the act of swallowing.

The digastric muscle depresses the mandible and elevates the hyoid bone, the stylohyoid muscle draws the hyoid bone upward and backward, and the mylohyoid forms the floor of the mouth. The geniohyoid muscles are short narrow muscles that contact each other at the midline of the mandible and reinforce the floor of the mouth. These groups of muscles function to elevate and draw the hyoid bone forward, depress the mandible, and shorten the floor of the mouth, which widens the pharynx for receiving food during the important process of swallowing.

Muscles of the Tongue

• The word parts *gloss, glossa,* and *glossal* mean "relating to the tongue."

The tongue functions to provide us with speech, mastication, and help in swallowing food. Movements of the tongue are numerous and complicated. The complex arrangement of the muscular fibers of the tongue and the various directions in which they run allow this organ to form the various positions needed for pronouncing different sounds. As mentioned earlier, mastication is the act of bringing the teeth together in order to grind food. The act of swallowing, or deglutition, is the process by which masticated food is moved from the mouth to the stomach for digestion.

The four primary muscles of the tongue are the genioglossus, the hyoglossus, the styloglossus, and the palatoglossus (Table 5-7 and Figure 5.12). The genioglossus muscles function to protrude the tongue forward as well as to move it to opposite sides of the mouth. This action aids in speech and articulation of words. It also helps form a channel for fluids to pass through into the throat. The hyoglossus depresses the tongue and draws down its sides. The styloglossus is shorter and smaller and functions to bring the tongue upward and backward in the mouth. The palatoglossus brings the tongue upward during the act of swallowing, where it touches the soft palate at the back of the mouth.

Structure and Function of the Salivary Glands and Ducts

Saliva is important for the process of digesting food. Saliva is normally tasteless, clear, and odorless. The average amount secreted daily by a person is 1 to 1.5 liters or 4 to 6 cups. Included in this fluid are enzymes, proteins, and some amino acids. Saliva initiates the digestion process by acting as a solvent and moistening food to aid in chewing and swallowing. The enzyme

TABLE 5-6 Muscles of the Floor of the Mouth

Muscle	Function	Origin	Insertion
Digastric	Depresses mandible and elevates hyoid bone	Mandible and temporal bone	Tendon of hyoid bone
Stylohyoid	Elevates and retracts hyoid bone	Styloid process of temporal bone	Hyoid bone
Mylohyoid	Elevates hyoid bone and tongue and depresses mandible	Mandible	Hyoid bone
Geniohyoid	Elevates hyoid and tongue and depresses mandible	Mandible	Hyoid bone

TABLE 5-7 Muscles of the Tongue

Muscle	Function	Origin	Insertion
Genioglossus	Protrudes and depresses tongue	Mental symphysis at midline of chin	Base of tongue and hyoid bone
Hyoglossus	Depresses down sides and retracts tongue	Hyoid bone	Intrinsic tongue muscles
Styloglossus	Brings tongue upward and backward	Styloid process	Side of tongue
Palatoglossus	Brings tongue upward during swallowing	Soft palate	Side of tongue

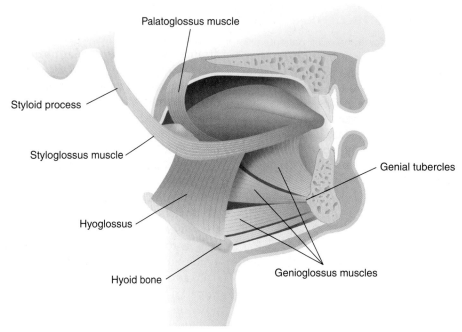

FIGURE 5.12
Muscles of the tongue.

ptyalin is a salivary enzyme that begins breaking down food starches in the mouth.

The three major pairs of salivary glands in the oral cavity that secrete saliva are the parotid, sublingual, and submandibular glands (Figure 5.13). In addition to these major salivary glands, several smaller glands also secrete saliva. Salivary glands release two types of liquid. One type of gland secretes a ropy fluid that contains mucin and is therefore called mucous, while the other secretes a thinner (serous), more watery fluid. Saliva is also important in remineralizing enamel broken down by bacterial by-products and is a component in the formation of dental plaque.

Parotid Gland

The parotid gland is the largest salivary gland and is located below the ear. Stensen's duct conveys saliva from the parotid gland into the mouth at the inner surface of the cheek opposite the second molar of the upper jaw. The parotid gland produces about 50% of daytime saliva and produces serous secretions only.

Sublingual Gland

Found under the tongue, in the anterior region of the floor of the mouth, is the sublingual gland. It lies on the mylohyoid muscle and provides saliva via Bartholin's duct. It is the smallest salivary gland and is shaped somewhat like an almond. The sublingual gland produces mucous secretions.

Submandibular Gland

The submandibular gland is found below the mandible in the mouth, farther back from the sublingual gland. It is slightly larger than the sublingual gland and produces the most saliva volume. It forms a tube that opens into Wharton's duct, which conveys saliva into the oral cavity. The submandibular gland produces both serous and mucous secretory products.

What is xerostomia and what are some of its causes? Why would it be difficult for a patient with xerostomia to wear a denture?

Disorders of Salivary Glands

When the flow of saliva is insufficient or almost nonexistent, the mouth feels extremely dry. This condition is called dry mouth or **xerostomia**. It is a common disorder affecting the salivary glands. Certain diseases and disorders can cause the salivary glands to malfunction and thus decrease saliva production; they include Parkinson's disease, diabetes, depression, and HIV infection. Some drugs can decrease saliva production as well, such as certain antidepressants, antihistamines, and diuretics. The salivary glands often malfunction after a person has had chemotherapy or head and neck radiation for the treatment of cancer. Dry mouth due to radiation is usually permanent, especially if the radiation dose is high; xerostomia due to chemotherapy, however, is usually temporary.

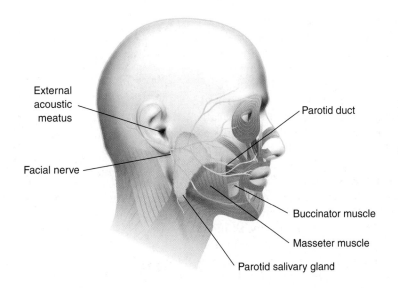

(A)

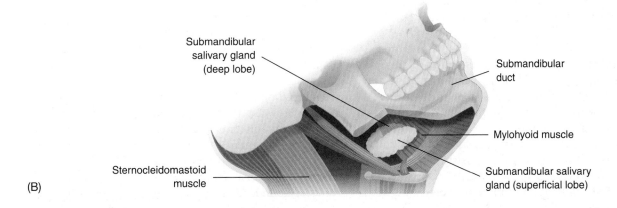

(B)

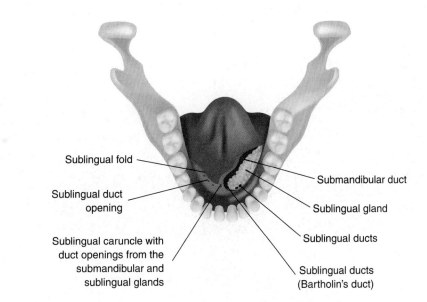

(C)

FIGURE 5.13

(a) Parotid salivary glands. (b) Submandibular salivary glands. (c) Sublingual salivary glands.

Not all cases of dry mouth are caused by salivary gland malfunction. The mouth may also dry somewhat as a person ages, although this is probably due to the greater likelihood of taking medications that cause dry mouth than to the aging process itself. Because saliva offers considerable natural protection against tooth decay, an inadequate amount of saliva leads to more caries—especially on the roots of teeth. Dry mouth, if severe, can also lead to difficulty with digestion, speaking, and swallowing.

Saliva lubricates the oral cavity and aids a denture in adhering to tissues properly via suction. Without saliva, oral tissues will become chafed and irritated and especially uncomfortable for those patients who wear dentures. A thorough medical history listing medications taken is necessary to aid in diagnosis of this condition. Patients should be advised to avoid smoking and drinking alcohol, to drink lots of water, to soak dentures overnight, to lubricate the lips, and to discuss with the dentist other options to stimulate saliva (sialogogue). Commercial products are available that may help patients with this problem.

Another disorder that occurs in salivary glands is salivary stones. Occasionally an object will show up on a patient's radiograph that is caused by mineralization and calcification processes. A calcified stone in the ducts of salivary glands is called a **sialolith**. The duct may be blocked creating discomfort and problems for the patient, but most are insignificant and do not cause harm. If the sialolith causes pain or persistent swelling for the patient, it will need to be removed. Occasionally, removal of the salivary gland itself is necessary. Stones usually occur in the submandibular glands, less frequently in the parotid gland, and rarely in the sublingual and minor salivary glands.

Name of Sinus	Location in the Skull
Maxillary	Anterior—within the maxillary bone
Frontal	Anterior—within the frontal bone on each side of midline above the bridge of the nose
Ethmoid	Posterior—within the ethmoid bone
Sphenoid	Posterior—occupy body of sphenoid bone on both sides

TABLE 5-8 Major Paranasal Sinuses

Sinuses

The nose is the organ of smell and a main passageway for air into and out of the lungs. The nose warms, moistens, and filters air before it enters the lungs. The bones of the face around the nose contain hollow spaces called paranasal sinuses. There are four groups of paranasal sinuses: the maxillary, ethmoid, frontal, and sphenoid sinuses (Table 5-8 and Figure 5.14). They are located on each side of the nose (maxillary), behind and in between the eyes (ethmoid), in the forehead (frontal), and one much farther back in the head (sphenoid). Sinuses reduce the weight of facial bones while maintaining bone strength and shape. The air-filled spaces of the nose and sinuses also add resonance, or full deep sound, to the voice. They are lined with mucus and very fine hair-like projections called cilia, which move secretions through tiny holes that provide drainage.

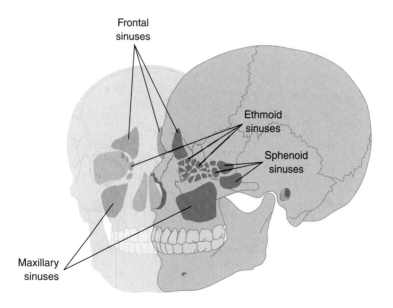

FIGURE 5.14
Major paranasal sinuses.

Lymph Nodes of the Face and Neck

The lymphatic system is closely related to the circulatory system. It is a network of lymph capillaries and larger vessels that empty into the bloodstream. Like the circulatory system that supplies blood, the network of lymph vessels supports almost every cell in the body. The lymph nodes serve as a series of cleaning filters. Lymph slowly circulates in a one-way direction toward the thoracic duct through body movements and breathing. The thoracic duct is the main lymph duct of the body. It returns cleansed and enriched lymph to the blood supply.

The lymphatic system has several important functions:

- Removes excess fluid and dissolves substances that leak from the capillaries
- Transports fats from the small intestine to the bloodstream
- Defends the body by exposing bacteria and viruses to white blood cells

The linings of the digestive and respiratory systems in the head and neck include patches of connective tissue that contain large numbers of lymphocytes. The largest of these patches is the tonsils in the back of the throat. Large lymph vessels are interrupted periodically by kidney bean–shaped structures called lymph nodes. Lymph fluid is forced through the nodes, which are lined with masses of macrophages. Lymphocytes are also produced in the lymph nodes. Both macrophages and lymphocytes recognize and destroy foreign particles such as bacteria and viruses. Painful swelling of lymph nodes accompanies certain diseases. Palpation of lymph nodes in the head and neck is part of an extraoral examination.

Lymph nodes the dentist will palpate include:

- Nodes that lie on either side of the neck
- Tonsillar areas below the angle of the mandible
- Along the underside of the jaw
- Underneath the chin

Infected lymph nodes tend to be firm, tender, enlarged, and warm. Following infection the lymph nodes occasionally remain enlarged. Enlargement of lymph nodes is frequently associated with upper airway infections, systemic infections, and oral cancer.

Nerves of the Face and Neck

The brain controls all functions of the body via the nervous system. The nervous system is a network of nerves and nerve cells that relay messages back and forth from different parts of the body. It does this through thread-like nerves that branch out to every organ. The majority of nerves connect with the brain via the spinal cord, but cranial nerves emerge from the brainstem instead of the spinal cord. Cranial nerves are found on each side of the head and neck. They control the sensory and muscle functions of the eyes, nose, tongue, face, and throat. There are 12 cranial nerves: olfactory, optic, oculomotor, trochlear, trigeminal, abducens, facial, vestibulocochlear, glossopharyngeal, vagus, spinal accessory, and hypoglossal.

As discussed in Chapter 4, basic functioning of the nervous system depends on tiny cells called neurons that have specialized functions. Sensory neurons take information from the eyes, ears, nose, tongue, and skin to the brain. Motor neurons carry messages away from the brain and back to the rest of the body. With the help of nerves, the body is able to carry out voluntary and involuntary actions, that is, conscious and unconscious decisions, respectively. These activities occur almost instantly through electrochemical impulses. An electrochemical impulse is a process that uses chemicals to create an electrical impulse. When a nerve impulse (electrical signal) travels across a neuron to the junction (synapse) between a neuron and another cell, it causes the release of neurotransmitters. Neurotransmitters are chemicals that carry the nerve signal across the synapse to another neuron.

The facial nerve carries signals that provide for the sensation of taste on the anterior two-thirds of the tongue, sensation on the skin of the external meatus, taste from the palate, muscles producing facial expression, the pterygopalatine, and the submandibular and sublingual glands.

The primary nerve of concern to the dental assistant is the trigeminal nerve. This nerve gets its name because it has three branches: the ophthalmic, maxillary, and mandibular. The ophthalmic branches to the lacrimal, frontal, and nasociliary nerves. The maxillary branch of the trigeminal nerve includes the zygomatic, infraorbital, posterior superior alveolar, pterygopalatine, and sphenopalatine nerves.

From the ophthalmic, maxillary, and mandibular branches, other nerves branch off and stimulate areas on the face and neck. The infraorbital nerve branches into the middle superior alveolar and the anterior superior alveolar nerve. The middle superior alveolar nerve stimulates the maxillary (premolars) bicuspids, the mesial buccal roots of the maxillary first molar, and the sinus mucosa. The anterior superior alveolar innervates (or stimulates) the lateral and central incisors, canines (cuspids), buccal gingiva, and the maxillary sinus. The posterior superior alveolar branches off from the maxillary nerve and stimulates the following:

- Buccal gingiva
- Maxillary sinus
- Cheeks
- Maxillary second and third molars
- Maxillary first molars except the mesiobuccal root of the first molar, which receives its nerve supply from both the posterior superior alveolar and the middle superior alveolar

The pterygopalatine nerve has five branches which supply the pharynx, hard palate, lingual gingiva of the maxillary molars, premolars (bicuspids), and the canines (cuspids) (Figure 5.15).

The mandibular branch of the trigeminal nerve subdivides into anterior and posterior divisions (Figure 5.16). The anterior division serves the temporal, masseter, and lateral and medial pterygoid muscles and also branches into the buccal nerve, which innervates the skin and mucosa of the cheeks and gingiva. The posterior division of the mandibular nerve branch serves the auriculotemporal, lingual, and inferior alveolar nerves. The auriculotemporal nerve innervates the parotid gland, TMJ, external auditory meatus, eardrum, and temporal skin. The lingual nerve serves the anterior two-thirds of the tongue. The inferior alveolar nerve serves all mandibular teeth, the lower lip, and the mandibular gingiva.

The mylohyoid nerve is derived from the inferior alveolar nerve just before it enters the mandibular foramen. It supplies the mylohyoid and the anterior belly of the digastric muscles. The mental nerve emerges from the larger branch of the inferior superior alveolar and innervates the chin and lower lip, while a smaller incisive branch innervates the mandibular anterior teeth and labial gingiva.

What is the nerve of primary concern to the dental assistant and why?

Circulatory System of the Face and Neck

Arteries convey blood from the heart to all structures of the body and carry oxygenated blood away from the heart. The artery supplying the head and neck is the common carotid artery. It rises upward in the neck and divides into two branches: the external and internal carotid arteries. All veins, except the pulmonary vein, receive deoxygenated blood and return it to the heart. The pulmonary vein returns oxygenated blood to the heart. The circulatory system of the head and neck can allow the spread of infection from teeth and associated oral tissues. Pathogens can travel in the veins and drain the infection into other tissues and organs. The spread of dental infection by way of the blood system can create serious complications in other parts of the body. The arteries of the face and neck are shown in Figure 5.17.

Arteries of the Face

The external carotid artery supplies the surface parts of the head and face while the internal carotid artery supplies blood to the brain and eyes. The external carotid artery has eight branches that are named according to the areas they supply. They are the ascending pharyngeal, superior thyroid, lingual, facial, occipital, posterior auricular, superficial temporal, and maxillary.

The lingual artery rises from the external artery and provides circulation to the hyoid muscles, tissues on floor of the mouth, the tongue, gingival tissues, soft palate, and tonsils.

The facial artery rises above the lingual artery, passing upward and forward of the mandible, across the cheek, and continuing upward along the side of the nose until it terminates at the inner corner of the eye. It has six branches, which supply the pharynx muscles, soft palate, tonsils, posterior portion of the tongue, submandibular and sublingual salivary glands, and muscles of the face and neck, ear, nose, and eyelids.

The maxillary artery is the largest branch of the external carotid artery and rises behind the ramus of the

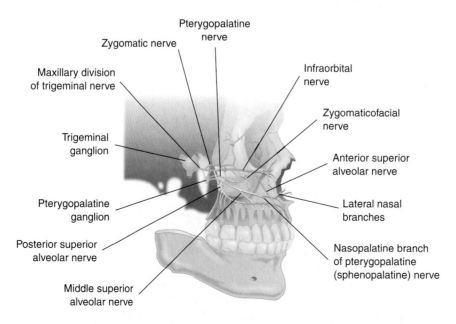

FIGURE 5.15
Nerves of the maxilla.

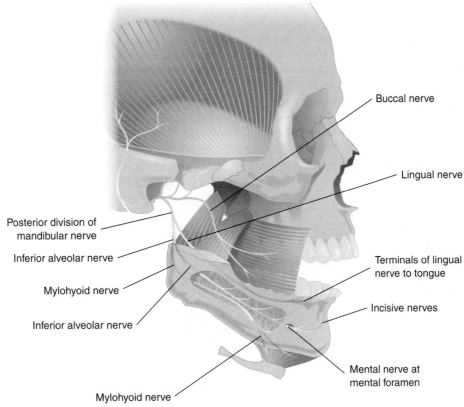

Buccal nerve

Lingual nerve

Posterior division of
mandibular nerve

Inferior alveolar nerve

Mylohyoid nerve

Inferior alveolar nerve

Terminals of lingual
nerve to tongue

Incisive nerves

Mental nerve at
mental foramen

Mylohyoid nerve

FIGURE 5.16
Nerves of the mandible.

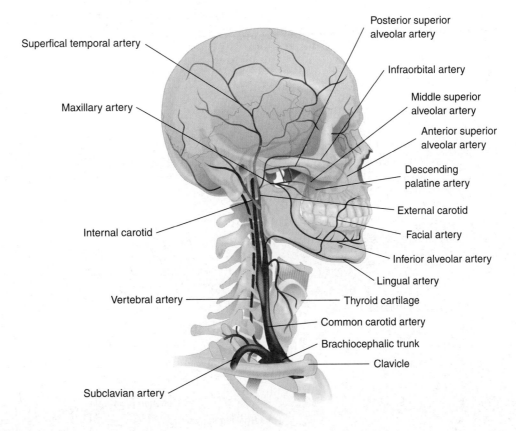

Superfical temporal artery

Maxillary artery

Internal carotid

Vertebral artery

Subclavian artery

Posterior superior
alveolar artery

Infraorbital artery

Middle superior
alveolar artery

Anterior superior
alveolar artery

Descending
palatine artery

External carotid

Facial artery

Inferior alveolar artery

Lingual artery

Thyroid cartilage

Common carotid artery

Brachiocephalic trunk

Clavicle

FIGURE 5.17
Arteries of the face and neck.

mandible to provide circulation to deep structures of the face. It subdivides into the mandibular, pterygoid, and pterygopalatine arteries. The mandibular branch supplies the lower teeth and chin. The pterygoid artery supplies the temporalis, pterygoid, masseter, and buccinator muscles. The pterygopalatine artery serves the posterior superior alveolar artery and the posterior maxillary teeth, the hard and soft palate, the pterygoid and pharynx, as well as the infraorbital artery, which goes to the face. It also supplies the anterior superior alveolar, which branches into the maxillary teeth. Arteries often travel along with nerves.

Veins of the Face

The veins of the face receive deoxygenated blood from capillaries and return blood to the heart. Their names are similar to those of the arteries with which they are closely related. For instance, the two primary veins in the neck are the external and internal jugular veins. These are further divided into superficial or deep veins.

Blood from the face and oral cavity drains into either the external or internal jugular vein. The external jugular vein drains facial structures including the eye, nose, lips, tongue, maxilla, and mandible. Deep veins include the internal jugular vein and the pterygoid plexus. The internal jugular vein is responsible for draining the brain, face, and neck, whereas the pterygoid plexus drains into the maxillary vein, which then drains into the internal jugular vein. Major veins of the face and neck include the internal jugular and external jugular veins (Figure 5.18).

The pterygopalatine fossa is extremely vascular. Occasionally during an intraoral anesthetic injection, a blood vessel becomes pierced causing a localized mass of blood to accumulate called a hematoma. The vessels most commonly associated with a hematoma are the pterygoid plexus veins, the posterior superior alveolar vessels, and the inferior alveolar vessels. The patient will notice swelling and discoloration, or bruising, which will last 7 to 14 days. If the hematoma is noticed immediately, the dentist will apply direct pressure to the area. The patient can be instructed to apply ice following the dental appointment and to take analgesics as necessary for comfort.

How can an infection in the oral cavity spread to other structures of the body?

Professionalism

As a dental assistant it is always important to present a professional image in both words and actions. When speaking with patients, coworkers, and supervisors, remember to speak slowly and clearly. Ask questions when you are unsure and never assume. Positive and professional communication occurs by speaking clearly and by listening to what others are saying. One's body language can send positive or negative nonverbal messages. Smile and be pleasant.

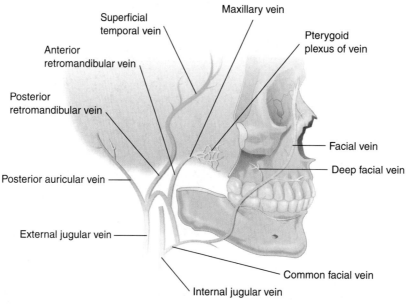

FIGURE 5.18
Veins of the face and neck.

SUMMARY

This chapter defined the anatomy and functions of the major parts of the head and neck. The anatomic landmarks of the maxilla and mandible are mandatory for the dental assistant to know in order to properly perform his or her duties.

The brain is protected by bones of the cranium and face, which have muscles attached to them that allow for movement, including mastication and facial expression. The junction of the mandible and maxilla is at the temporomandibular joint, which is an encapsulated joint that functions through several important muscles. Other muscles of importance in dentistry include those in the neck, and under and around the tongue.

Dental assistants need to understand the many parts of the oral cavity and how they collectively function. Dental assistants need to be aware of delicate tissues as the oral cavity is evacuated, when radiographic exposures are performed, and when impressions are taken.

Salivary glands produce the saliva necessary for digestion and also cleanse the mouth. The paranasal sinuses are air-filled spaces within bones. The lymphatic system removes excess fluid, transports fats, and fights infection. Recognizing nerve and blood vessels of the circulatory system will provide the dental assistant with the knowledge required to aid the dentist and therefore help patients.

KEY TERMS

- **Alveolar process:** The part of the mandible and maxilla that contains the tooth sockets. p. 75
- **Articulate:** To join together. p. 74
- **Bruxism:** Grinding of the teeth. p. 78
- **Cancellous bone:** Bone that is more spongy or porous than dense bone. p. 75
- **Crepitus:** A crackling or grinding sound. p. 79
- **Foramina:** Openings in bone allowing for passage of nerve and blood vessels. p. 73
- **Glenoid fossa:** A shallow depression within the temporal bone. p. 74
- **Insertion:** The movable end of a muscle. p. 79
- **Mandible:** The bone of the lower jaw. p. 77
- **Masseter:** The principal muscle of mastication that closes the mouth. p. 79
- **Mastication:** The act of chewing. p. 79

- **Maxilla:** Two bones that form the upper jaw. p. 75
- **Maxillary tuberosity:** A rounded prominence of bone located posterior to the maxillary molars. p. 75
- **Mentalis:** Muscle of the chin that protrudes the lower lip and wrinkles the skin. p. 81
- **Origin:** The fixed attachment of a muscle. p. 79
- **Sialolith:** A stone in a salivary duct. p. 86
- **Suture:** An immovable line of union between two bones. p. 74
- **Temporomandibular joint:** The encapsulated synovial joint between the temporal bone of the skull and the condyle of the mandible. p. 78
- **Xerostomia:** Dryness of the mouth caused by an abnormal reduction in salivary secretion. p. 84
- **Zygomatic:** Pertaining to the cheekbone. p. 73

CHECK YOUR UNDERSTANDING

1. The bone of the cranium that articulates with the other cranial bones, binding them together, and is shaped like a butterfly with extended wings is the
   a. parietal.
   b. sphenoid.
   c. temporal.
   d. occipital.

2. The part of the maxilla and mandible bones that contains tooth sockets is called the
   a. alveolar process.
   b. tuberosity.
   c. zygomatic process.
   d. palatine process.

3. The bone forming the cheek is the
   a. vomer.
   b. inferior turbinate.
   c. lacrimal.
   d. zygomatic.

4. The longest and strongest bone of the face is the
   a. hyoid.
   b. maxilla.
   c. occipital.
   d. mandible.

CHECK YOUR UNDERSTANDING (continued)

5. The TMJ is formed by the union of which two bones?
   a. temporal and maxilla
   b. temporal and mandible
   c. turbinate and mandible
   d. turbinate and mylohyoid

6. The point at which the end of a muscle attaches to a fixed structure is the
   a. origin.
   b. insertion.
   c. cartilage.
   d. ligaments.

7. Match the muscle with its definition:

   _____ surrounds the mouth and puckers the lips

   _____ compresses cheeks to keep food in contact with teeth

   _____ wrinkles the chin and pushes the lower lip up

   _____ closes the jaw and pulls it forward
   a. temporalis
   b. orbicularis oris
   c. buccinator
   d. mentalis

8. The largest salivary gland is the
   a. parotid.
   b. sublingual.
   c. submandibular.
   d. Stensen's.

9. The disorder xerostomia is also known as dry mouth and is caused by
   a. chemotherapy.
   b. radiation therapy.
   c. antidepressants.
   d. antihistamines.
   e. all of the above.

10. The word parts *gloss, glossa,* and *glossal* mean "relating to the
    a. tongue."
    b. cheek."
    c. lips."
    d. gingiva."

INTERNET ACTIVITIES

- Go to http://uwmsk.org/tmj/anatomy.html and watch a Quicktime video of the hinge and glide motion of the temporomandibular joint.

- Go to www.oralcancerfoundation.org to understand treatments your patients who have cancer may go through, treatment side effects in the oral cavity, and aids to help your patients cope.

WEB REFERENCES

- Human Anatomy Online   www.innerbody.com/index.html
- Loyola University Medical Network   www.meddean.luc.edu/Lumen/MedEd/GrossAnatomy
- Data Face   http://face-and-emotion.com/dataface/anatomy/head_lateralview.jsp
- Get Body Smart.com   www.getbodysmart.com/ap/skeletalsystem/skeleton/axial/skull/quizzes/markings/sutures/animation.html
- The University of Michigan Medical School   http://anatomy.med.umich.edu/nervous_system/infratem_tables.html
- Cranial Nerves   http://mywebpages.comcast.net/wnor/cranialnerves.htm

The Face and Oral Cavity

Learning Objectives

After reading this chapter, the student should be able to:

- Define intraoral and extraoral.
- Describe major anatomic landmarks of the face and oral cavity.
- Discuss functions of the oral cavity.
- Identify major structures of the oral vestibule and the buccal and alveolar mucosa.
- Identify and describe parts of the hard and soft palates.
- Explain structures of the tongue and floor of the mouth.
- Describe oral leukoplakia.

Preparing for Certification Exams

- Identify intraoral and extraoral anatomy.
- Recognize and note any abnormal findings on the face and within the oral cavity.

Key Terms

Ala	Palate
Buccal	Pharynx
Commissures	Philtrum
Extraoral	Tragus
Intraoral	Uvula
Labial	Vermilion border
Linea alba	

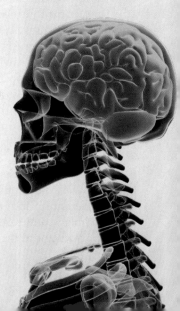

Understanding dentistry

requires an awareness of the structure and function of facial features and oral tissues, both **extraoral** (outside the mouth) and **intraoral** (inside the mouth). The dentist is often the first health care provider with the opportunity to take a thorough health history and perform an examination of the mouth and associated tissues.

The oral cavity is divided into an area outside the teeth and the oral cavity proper. Within the oral cavity proper are the hard palate, soft palate, tongue, and floor of the mouth. Examination of the dental patient is not limited to the oral cavity. Much information is obtained from inspection of the face and general appearance of an individual. Observation and palpation of soft tissues of the face and neck, as well as inspection of the interior structures of the mouth, are used to identify disease. It is important for the dental assistant to understand facial and oral anatomy in order to recognize when an abnormal condition exists so the dentist may be alerted. Identifying landmarks on the face also aids the dental assistant during radiographic procedures.

Landmarks of the Face

Landmarks of the face include the front of the head from the eyebrow to the chin including the skin, muscles, and structures of the forehead, eyes, nose, mouth, cheeks, and jaw. The forehead is also called the frontal eminence. At either end of the corners of the eye are the inner canthus and the outer canthus, which are folds of tissue formed by the meeting of the upper and lower eyelids (Figure 6.1). The bridge of the nose is often called the nasal bridge. Between the nose and the upper lip is a vertical groove with two slight ridges in the skin. This area is called the **philtrum.** The winged flare of the nostril is known as the **ala,** and the prominence of cartilage tissue anterior to the ear opening is called the **tragus.** The cheek bone is also known as the zygomatic arch. The chin is called the mental protuberance. Facial features incorporate the body of the mandible and the area where the mandible meets the ramus or the angle of the mandible. The size and shape of

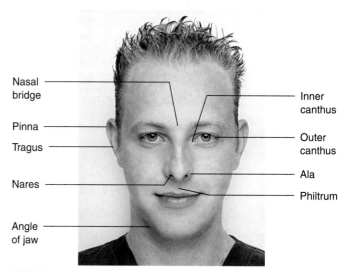

FIGURE 6.1
Landmarks of the face.

facial features are determined genetically through the genes of both parents.

During a dental examination, the dentist is looking for changes from the normal appearance of healthy tissue. Diseases and disorders that can directly or indirectly affect oral tissues include metabolic diseases, such as diabetes, cancers of the head and neck, immune disorders such as AIDS or ulcerative colitis, and developmental defects such as cleft lip or cleft palate. Techniques used by dental health care providers that are designed to aid in the diagnosis of disease processes include x-rays, observation and palpation of soft tissues, and laboratory studies.

Why does the dental exam include looking at facial features as well as the mouth?

The Oral Cavity

The oral cavity extends from the border of the lips to the junction of the hard and soft palate above, to the circumvallate papillae on the tongue below, and is divided into specific areas. It includes the lips, upper and lower vestibules, alveolar ridges, alveolar mucosa, buccal mucosa, and gingiva (Figure 6.2). The oral cavity is important in the complex functions of speech, taste, mas-

Dental Assistant **PROFESSIONAL TIP**

To ensure that proper procedures are followed, knowledge of oral soft tissues, the tongue, and structures on the floor of the mouth is important for the dental assistant to obtain. Familiarity with tissues near the soft palate will help the dental assistant protect delicate structures, prevent stimulating the patient's gag reflex during intraoral procedures, and ensure the best possible patient comfort.

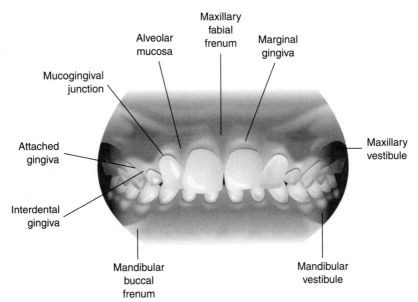

Mucogingival junction

Alveolar mucosa

Maxillary fabial frenum

Marginal gingiva

Attached gingiva

Maxillary vestibule

Interdental gingiva

Mandibular buccal frenum

Mandibular vestibule

FIGURE 6.2
View of gingivae and associated anatomic landmarks.

tication, digestion, and swallowing. Each structure in the mouth contributes to its overall function. The oral cavity also functions as an alternate airway.

What structures of the oral cavity provide humans with the capability of speech? What structures of the oral cavity provide chemoreception?

Functions of the oral cavity include:

- *Mastication:* chewing by the teeth and tongue
- *Digestion:* through the salivary amylase enzyme, which breaks down carbohydrates into smaller molecules
- *Chemoreception:* through the taste buds on the tongue, which react to certain chemical stimuli providing the sense of taste
- *Speech:* by the use of the lips, tongue, cheeks, and larynx
- *Swallowing:* by means of the hard and soft palates and tongue

The Lips

The lips are two highly sensitive mobile folds of tissue composed of skin, muscle, minor salivary glands, and mucous membrane. They surround the oral orifice to form the anterior boundary of the oral cavity. The upper and lower lips are joined at the corners of the mouth or **commissures.** The transitional area between the skin of the face and mucous membrane of the lip (pink portion) is called the **vermilion border.** The mucous membrane of the lip is referred to as the vermilion zone. The more

Life Span Considerations

The texture of the lips is normally smooth, soft, and resilient with minimal fissuring in young individuals. As people age and experience environmental factors, the lips may have more wrinkles and the tissue covering will become more thin and transparent. The dental assistant should stress to patients how medicated lip moisturizer with sun block can help prevent serious problems in the future.

pigment people have in their skin, the darker the color of the lips will be. Lips are very vascular, meaning that they contain many blood vessels, which are near the surface. The lips also contain sensory receptors, which are useful in judging the temperature and texture of food.

Oral Vestibules

When the lips are pulled away from the teeth and gingiva the oral vestibule can be seen. The oral vestibule is the entrance to the mouth that lies between the lips and teeth in front, and between the cheeks and teeth on both sides. It includes the labial mucosa, labial frenula, buccal mucosa, and buccal frenula. The vault-like space in the oral vestibule is called the vestibular fornix. Between the lips and teeth is labial mucosa. **Labial** is a term meaning "toward the lips." This area is rich with blood vessels and contains minor salivary glands. In the middle of both upper and lower vestibules are folds of tissue extending from the midline of the labial mucosa to the alveolar mucosa.

Buccal Mucosa

Mucosal tissues are smooth, shiny, wet, and thin. Buccal mucosa lines the entire inside of the cheeks and is important for mastication. **Buccal** means "toward the cheek." At the middle of the buccal mucosa in most individuals is a long, horizontal, raised white line or fold of tissue next to where the teeth come together. This is called the **linea alba** or occlusal line (Figure 6.3).

The buccal mucosa frequently has prominent yellow spots. These are sebaceous glands, or oil-secreting glands, called Fordyce's granules. Present in the buccal maxillary and buccal mandibular vestibules are lateral frenula, also called buccal frenula, opposite the canine and premolar (Figure 6.4 and Figure 6.5).

What might occur if a patient's denture did not fit the frenula correctly? **?**

Alveolar Mucosa and Gingiva

The mucous membrane continues from the vestibule over the tooth-supporting bone to the neck areas of the teeth. This area includes the alveolar mucosa, covering the alveolar ridge, and the gingiva, formed tightly around the teeth. The gingiva is subdivided into attached gingiva and free gingival tissues. The lighter pink or salmon-colored gum tissue is called attached gingiva because it is firmly attached to the underlying bone. The darker pink tissue is called free gingiva, and it is not firmly attached to the underlying bone. The junction between them is called the free gingival groove. The area where the attached gingiva meets the alveolar mucosa is called the mucogingival junction. Free gingiva extends into the interdental spaces as gingival papilla and is adapted around each tooth. Healthy gingiva has an orange-peel texture called stippling (Figure 6.6).

The Oral Cavity Proper

Many important anatomic structures exist within the oral cavity proper. The oral cavity proper is the space

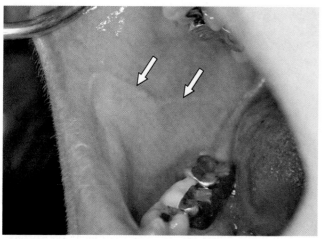

FIGURE 6.3
Linea alba.
Image courtesy Instructional Materials for Dental Team, Lex., KY

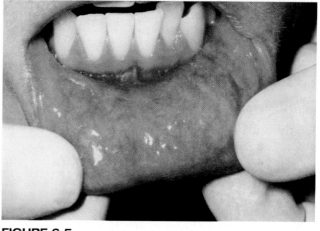

FIGURE 6.5
Mandibular frenum.

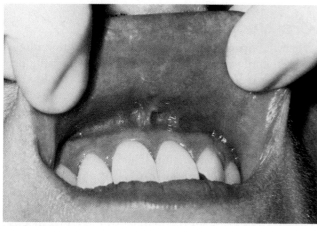

FIGURE 6.4
Maxillary frenum.

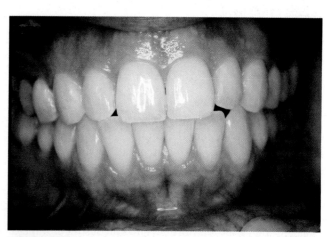

FIGURE 6.6
Healthy gingiva.

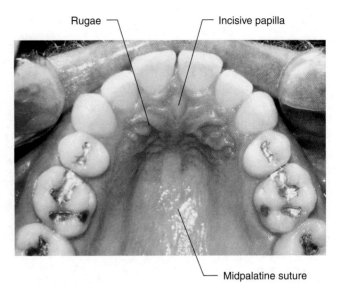

FIGURE 6.7
Landmarks of the hard palate.

within the maxillary and mandibular dental arches leading to the pharynx. The **pharynx** is a passageway for both food and air. Within the oral cavity proper are the hard palate, soft palate, tongue, and floor of the mouth. Both the hard and soft palate are lined with mucous membranes containing numerous salivary glands that lubricate the mouth and throat. Each of these structures is important in the complex functional capability of the oral cavity.

Palate

The **palate**, also known as the roof of the mouth, separates the nasal and oral cavities. It consists of a tough, rigid part at the anterior two-thirds of the palate, the hard palate, and a soft fleshy part posteriorly, the soft palate. A narrow elevated ridge extends along the entire midline of the palate from the incisive papilla in front to the tip of the uvula in the back of the mouth. This is called the palatine raphe (or median palatine suture).

Hard Palate

The hard palate is covered by thick firm mucosa adhering to the underlying bone. Located just behind the central incisors on the hard palate, over the incisive foramen, is a rounded projection of tissue called the incisive papilla (Figure 6.7). Behind the incisive papilla are palatine rugae, which are small irregular ridges or folds of mucous membrane extending outward on both sides of the palatine raphe. The hard palate curves to form a vault. The mucous membrane covering the hard palate is keratinized, or hardened tissue, and is firmly attached to the underlying bone and therefore not movable. This tissue becomes more flexible toward the gingival areas. Posterior to the last maxillary molar is a prominent ridge called the alveolar maxillary tuberosity. The maxillary tuberosities are tough, hard lumps of bone behind the upper teeth on both sides of the dental arches.

Soft Palate

Soft palate mucosa is thin and nonkeratinized. The gag reflex is strong in this area and may become stimulated if the dental assistant places the high-volume evacuator too near the back of the mouth, causing irritation of the soft palate. A thick cone-shaped fold of mucous membrane attached to the back of the soft palate that extends downward at the back of the mouth is the uvula (Figure 6.8). Muscles draw the soft palate and uvula upward during swallowing. This action closes the opening between the nasal cavity and the pharynx, preventing food from entering the airway. The uvula provides an important boundary between the oral cavity, the nasal cavity, and the oropharynx (Figure 6.9). On each side of the soft palate extending downward are the pillars of fauces, also called the tonsillar pillars. The pillars of fauces are two vertically directed projections that descend from the soft palate.

What could happen if the dental assistant placed the high-volume evacuator near tissues of the soft palate?

Structures of the Tongue

The tongue consists of a body and a root, or base, connected by muscles to the hyoid bone below, the mandible in front, and the styloid process behind. It is a voluntary muscular structure attached to the floor of the mouth by a fold of tissue called the lingual frenulum. The tongue is also joined to the floor of the mouth by mucous membranes. The tongue functions as a digestive organ by providing movement of food during mastication and assisting in swallowing. Sensory functions include speech and taste. This extremely muscular organ provides for an amazing degree of flexibility and is vital to communication.

The base and body of the tongue are separated by a shallow V-shaped groove, the terminal sulcus, which varies among individuals. Along the midline of the tongue's top surface is a slight groove called the median sulcus. The dorsum or top surface of the tongue (Figure 6.10) is covered

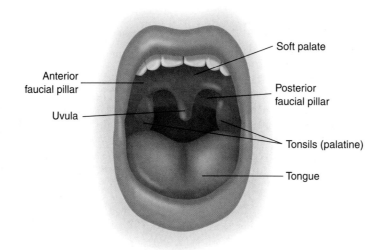

FIGURE 6.8
The soft palate.

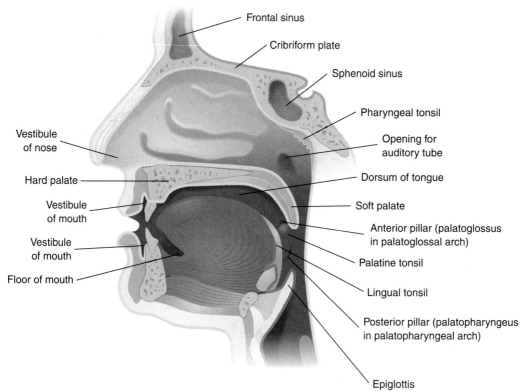

FIGURE 6.9
Lateral view of nasal and oral cavities.

with mucous membranes and numerous rough projections called papillae, which provide friction to help handle food. These papillae also contain taste buds. There are four types of papillae located on the tongue surface (Figure 6.11) (Table 6-1):

- Filiform
- Vallate or circumvallate
- Fungiform
- Foliate

Filiform papillae are slender structures that project up, forming a velvety covering on the tongue. Their function is mechanical as they have no sensory purpose. Performing the sensory function of taste are the vallate, fungiform, and foliate papillae. Vallate papillae are the largest and most prominent. They are paired and located on the back of the tongue, set into a deep pocket and surrounded by a trench into which some minor salivary glands secrete. Vallate papillae possess well-defined V-shaped sensory taste bud cells. Fungiform papillae are

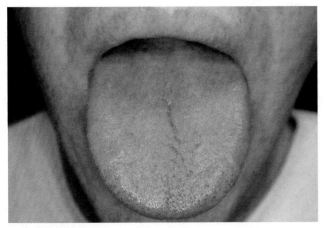

FIGURE 6.10
Dorsal surface of tongue.
Image courtesy Instructional Materials for the Dental Team, Lex., KY

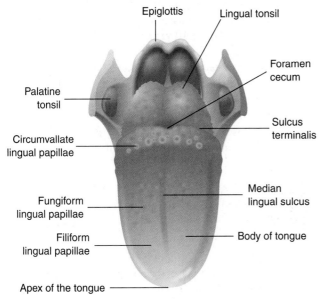

FIGURE 6.11
Papillae of the tongue.
Image courtesy Instructional Materials for the Dental Team, Lex., KY

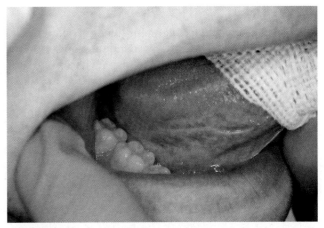

FIGURE 6.12
Right border of the tongue.
Image courtesy Instructional Materials for the Dental Team, Lex., KY

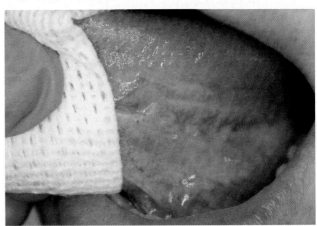

FIGURE 6.13
Left border of the tongue.
Image courtesy Instructional Materials for the Dental Team, Lex., KY

mushroom-shaped taste buds located at the tongue's center. Foliate papillae carry taste buds set into sides of the tongue and their shape is leaf-like. Note that the word *papilla* is singular, whereas *papillae* is plural.

The floor of the mouth allows unrestricted mobility of the tongue. The ventral surface, or underneath the tongue, is smooth with a thin membrane through which the lingual veins are visible. In the middle of the underside of the tongue is a distinct elevated mucosal fold called the lingual frenum, which attaches the tongue to the floor of the mouth. (Figure 6.12 & Figure 6.13)

Problems of the tongue that may occur in patients include:

• Pain upon movement and protrusion
• Temporary discoloration
• Inflammation
• Suspicious lesions
• Cancer

TABLE 6-1 Papillae of the Tongue

Papillae	Shape	Location	Sense
Filiform	Slender projections	Tip of tongue	No taste buds
Vallate (circumvallate)	V-shaped	Base of tongue	Contain taste buds
Fungiform	Mushroom shaped	Center of tongue	Contain taste buds
Foliate	Leaf-like	Sides of tongue	Contain taste buds

The Floor of the Mouth

In front of the lingual frenulum (or frenum), on each side, are two slight protuberances containing openings for saliva ducts from the submandibular (Wharton's ducts) and sublingual glands (ducts of Rivinus). These are called sublingual caruncles. Spreading out from each side of the lingual frenulum are fringed projections called the fimbriated folds (or plica fimbriata). The condition of having a short lingual frenulum is called ankyloglossia or being tongue-tied. It causes interference in sucking and use of the tongue during speech. It may be treated surgically if necessary. Figure 6.14 shows the floor of the mouth.

What are the names of the papillae on the tongue that contain taste buds? What would happen if a person was born with a short lingual frenulum?

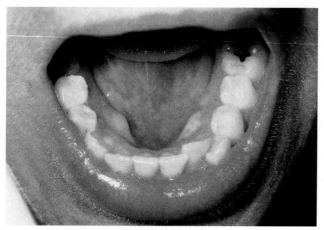

FIGURE 6.14
Floor of the mouth.

Oral Cancer and Other Conditions

Problems within the oral cavity include cancer. Many types of tumors can develop in the oral cavity. Some of these tumors are benign or noncancerous. Unlike cancerous tumors, benign or noncancerous tumors do not typically invade other tissues and spread to other parts of the body. Some growths in the oral cavity start off harmless but can later develop into cancer. These are known as precancerous conditions.

A complete exam, performed by the dentist, includes an inspection of the patient's oral soft tissues and tongue to screen for oral cancer as well as other conditions. Oral leukoplakia is a thickened white patch that cannot be rubbed off and cannot be associated with any physical or chemical causative agent except tobacco. Leukoplakia is a lesion that sometimes becomes a cancerous tumor that invades and destroys other tissue. Factors most frequently blamed for the development of leukoplakia include tobacco use, alcohol consumption, chronic irrita-

tion, candidiasis, vitamin deficiency, endocrine disturbances, and possibly a virus. Oral leukoplakia is considered potentially malignant and is more common in men than in women. Approximately 80% of oral leukoplakia patients are older than 40 years.

Oral piercing has become a popular form of self-expression but does come with risks. Risks related to oral piercing procedures include pain, infection, prolonged bleeding, blood clots, swelling, possible nerve damage, and bloodborne disease transmission. For many, the swelling of the tongue is a common side effect. In extreme cases a severely swollen tongue can close off the airway and prevent breathing. Jewelry-related complications that may be seen by dental health care providers are damage to the oral cavity such as fractured teeth, injuries to gingival tissues, bone loss, interference with normal oral function, excessive saliva, allergic reactions to metal, and blood poi-

soning. The possibility also exists that the jewelry may come loose and become a choking hazard. The dental assistant must ensure that all oral piercing jewelry is removed by the patient prior to exposure to x-rays because such jewelry will block oral anatomy on radiographs.

SUMMARY

The process of digestion begins when the mouth receives food and mechanically reduces the size of solid particles and mixes them with saliva. The lips, cheeks, tongue, and palate surround the mouth, which includes a chamber between the palate and tongue called the oral cavity, as well as a narrow space between the teeth, cheek, and lips called the vestibule.

The lips are highly mobile structures that surround the mouth opening. Their normal reddish color is due to the many blood vessels near their surface. The palate forms the roof of the oral cavity and consists of a hard anterior part, the hard palate, and a soft posterior part, the soft palate. Different types of mucous membranes line

the oral cavity. The buccal mucosa, labial mucosa, and alveolar mucosal tissues each have specialized functions.

The tongue is primarily composed of muscle and is attached to the floor of the mouth via the lingual frenulum and other mucosal tissues. The tongue aids in mixing food particles with saliva during chewing and moves food toward the pharynx during swallowing. Rough projections called papillae on the tongue surface contain taste buds. An important number of anatomic landmarks are also located beneath the tongue.

All oral tissues are examined as part of an oral cancer screening.

KEY TERMS

- **Ala:** Winged flare of the nostril. p. 94
- **Buccal:** Toward the cheek. p. 96
- **Commissures:** The corners of the mouth. p. 95
- **Extraoral:** Outside the mouth. p. 94
- **Intraoral:** Inside the mouth. p. 94
- **Labial:** Toward the lips. p. 95
- **Linea alba:** A long fold of tissue along the buccal mucosa next to where the teeth come together. p. 96
- **Palate:** The roof of the mouth. p. 97
- **Pharynx:** Passageway for air and food. p. 97
- **Philtrum:** A vertical groove between the nose and upper lip. p. 94
- **Tragus:** The prominence of fleshy tissue anterior to the ear opening. p. 94
- **Uvula:** A fold of mucous membrane attached to the back of the soft palate. p. 97
- **Vermilion border:** Transitional area between the skin of the face and mucous membrane of the lip. p. 95

CHECK YOUR UNDERSTANDING

1. An important facial landmark the dental assistant will use during radiographic procedures is the
   a. philtrum.
   b. nasal bridge.
   c. ala.
   d. tragus.
   e. both c and d.

2. The corners of the mouth are called the
   a. vermilion zone.
   b. commissures.
   c. fornix.
   d. alveolar mucosa.

3. Match the function with the correct parts of the oral cavity:

   _____ hard and soft palate

   _____ lips, tongue, cheeks, larynx

   _____ salivary enzymes

   _____ taste buds

   _____ teeth and tongue
   a. mastication
   b. digestion
   c. chemoreception
   d. speech
   e. swallowing

CHECK YOUR UNDERSTANDING (continued)

4. The term meaning "toward the lips" is
   a. buccal.
   b. frenula.
   c. fornix.
   d. labial.

5. The term meaning "toward the cheek" is
   a. buccal.
   b. frenula.
   c. fornix.
   d. labial.

6. Healthy gingiva has what texture?
   a. shiny
   b. dark pink
   c. like an orange peel
   d. translucent

7. The fold of mucous membrane extending downward at the back of the mouth is the
   a. pillar of fauces.
   b. incisive papilla.
   c. rugae.
   d. uvula.

8. Match the following papilla structure of the tongue with its definition:

   _____ largest papilla and V-shaped

   _____ slender projections at the tip of the tongue

   _____ shaped like a mushroom

   _____ located on the sides of the tongue and are leaf-like
   a. foliate
   b. vallate
   c. fungiform
   d. filiform

9. The tongue is attached to the floor of the mouth by the
   a. lingual frenulum.
   b. buccal fold.
   c. fimbriated fold.
   d. caruncles.

10. Factors most frequently blamed for the development of oral leukoplakia are
    a. tobacco use.
    b. alcohol consumption.
    c. chronic irritation.
    d. all of the above.

◉ INTERNET ACTIVITIES

- Go to www.oralcancerfoundation.org/dental/slide_show.htm to see slides of an oral exam.
- Go to www.oralcancerfoundation.org to understand treatments available for cancer and what the dental patient will experience from the treatment.
- Go to www.ghorayeb.com/PicturesOralCavityThyroidandParathyroid.html to see pictures of oral and throat cancer.

◉ WEB REFERENCES

- A.D.A.M. Healthcare Center http://adam.about.com
- American Cancer Society www.cancer.org
- emedicine from WebMD http://emedicine.com/ent/topic731.htm
- Louisiana State University Health Sciences Center www.medschool.lsuhsc.edu
- Net Wellness: Consumer Health Information www.netwellness.org/healthtopics/dentalseniors/tobaccocancerODA.cfm
- Procter and Gamble's Premier Portal for Dental Professionals www.dentalcare.com
- University of Arkansas for Medical Sciences: Department of Neurobiology and Departmental Sciences www.uams.edu/neuroscience_cellbiology
- University of Michigan Medical School: Medical Gross Anatomy www.med.umich.edu/lrc/coursepages/M1/anatomy/html/surface/head_neck/oral_cavity.html
- Virginia Commonwealth University: School of Dentistry www.dentistry.vcu.edu

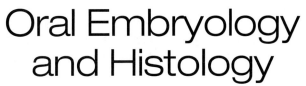

Oral Embryology and Histology

Learning Objectives

After reading this chapter, the student should be able to:

- Define the terminology associated with oral embryology and histology.
- Name the three stages of embryonic development.
- Describe the process of facial and palatal development.
- Understand the stages of tooth development.
- Explain eruption and exfoliation of the primary dentition.
- Determine the eruption dates for both primary and permanent dentitions.
- Describe the tissues that compose the teeth.
- List and define the components of the attachment unit.
- Explain the gingival unit and describe the composing tissues.

Preparing for Certification Exams

- Recall the approximate time that the teeth begin developing in utero.
- Calculate the approximate eruption and exfoliation dates for primary dentition.
- Predict the eruption dates of the permanent dentition.

Chapter Outline

Key Terms

Alveolar crest	Enamel organ
Alveolar socket	Histology
Ameloblasts	Lamina dura
Anatomical crown	Lining mucosa
Apex	Masticatory mucosa
Apical foramen	Odontoblasts
Cementoblasts	Periodontium
Clinical crown	Primary dentin
Dental lamina	Pulp
Dental papilla	Secondary dentin
Dental sac	Stomodeum
Dentin	Succedaneous teeth
Dentinal tubules	Tertiary dentin
Embryology	Zygote

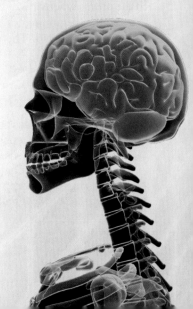

By understanding the concepts of embryology and histology, the dental assisting student will learn how teeth and their supporting structures are formed and understand their functions. The information covered in this chapter provides the working dental assistant with the abilities to recognize the current situation of the patient's oral cavity and to rationalize clinical treatment given to the teeth and their supporting structures.

Oral Embryology

Embryology is the study of how a human being develops through three stages before birth. Embryonic development begins with the fertilization of an egg cell by a sperm cell, known as conception. Fertilization normally occurs in the fallopian tube of the female reproductive organs. This begins gestation, which is the period of time between conception and birth. The average human gestation period lasts between 38 and 40 weeks after the last menstrual period. Once a sperm penetrates the ovum, it forms a protective coating that inhibits other sperm from penetrating the egg as well.

The first stage in embryonic development is the **zygote** stage, which begins with the union of the sperm and ovum. The sperm and ovum have each brought to the union 23 chromosomes that will join together for a total of 46. This merging of chromosomes is known as meiosis (Figure 7.1).

After fertilization, the zygote divides into 2 halves. Those 2 halves divide again to create 4, the 4 become 8, the 8 become 16, and this division continues until the mass consists of about 100 sections. It is during this division period that the zygote travels from the fallopian tube to the uterus where it will become imbedded in the lining.

By the beginning of the second week the zygote becomes an embryo. The embryo is the second stage in

Professionalism

As a dental assistant, it is important not to judge patients regarding the condition of their oral cavity. Judging a patient is not conducive to building rapport. Instead of judging them, educate patients on methods to assist them in improving the conditions of their oral cavity. Most patients want to learn to improve the condition of their oral cavity, but are often too afraid to ask questions.

Dental Assistant   PROFESSIONAL TIP

Part of your job as a dental assistant will be to educate your patients on how to clean and maintain their oral structures. It is valuable for the assistant to understand the oral structures on a professional level; however, the patient will not understand professional jargon. It is important that the dental assistant be able to communicate instructions and procedures to the patient using simple terms that can be easily understood.

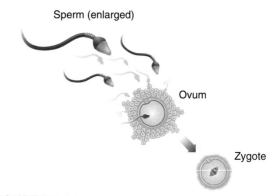

FIGURE 7.1
The union of the sperm and egg creates the zygote, after meiosis has occurred.

development, a stage that continues through the eighth week. By the third week of the embryonic stage, the embryo consists of cells that form three primary embryonic layers. The cell is the basic building block of the human body: cells form tissues, groups of tissues form organs, and groups of organs form integrated systems that ultimately make complex life possible.

The third and final stage in development is the fetal phase, which begins at the ninth week and continues until birth. During the fetal phase all of the major body systems are in place. The fetus will continue to grow and the systems will mature, making it possible for the baby to survive outside of the mother's body after birth (Figure 7.2) (Figure 7.3).

When does embryonic development begin?

Primary Embryonic Layers

During the second stage of development, the primary embryonic layers form. These layers are the:

• Innermost layer, called the endoderm
• Middle layer, called the mesoderm
• Outer layer, called the ectoderm

These primary embryonic layers are composed of specialized cells that will eventually become the tissues,

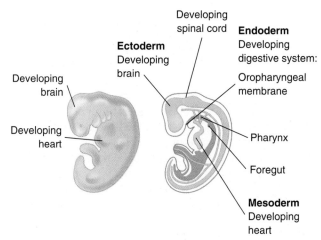

FIGURE 7.2
The embryo during the fifth week of development.

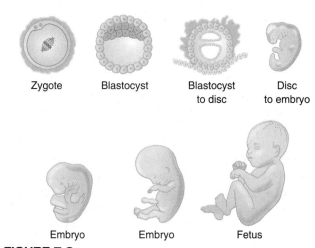

FIGURE 7.3
Phases of prenatal development.

organs, and systems of the human body. The lining of the lungs, structures of the urogenital system, and the lining of the gastrointestinal systems arise from the endoderm. The dentin, pulp, and cementum of the teeth arise from the mesoderm layer. Also initiated by this layer are the bones, cartilage, muscle, kidneys, and cardiovascular and reproductive systems. The oral epithelium, the enamel of the teeth, the lining of the oral cavity, the skin, and the nervous system arise from the ectoderm layer.

The embryonic period is a crucial time in development because it is when the foundations for all future organs and systems are being laid. This phase occurs early in gestation when the mother may not realize she is pregnant. During gestation, the mother's body is the environment in which the baby develops; therefore, everything the mother does—or does not do—can affect the development of the embryo. This includes nutrition, stress, drug and alcohol use, and the mother's medical and dental health.

Development of Facial Structures

By the third week of the embryonic phase, the embryo has evolved from a mass of cells into a tadpole-like structure consisting of the three embryonic layers. The primitive brain and spinal cord already are evident. The primitive spinal cord appears as a tail at the opposite end of the brain structure. When viewing the embryo from a frontal position, a large prominence is apparent. This prominence is the forehead area known as the frontal prominence. At this stage of development the embryo is approximately three to four millimeters in length. An embryo at four weeks is shown in Figure 7.4.

Even at this primitive stage, the precursors of what will become facial structures are evident, as is the **stomodeum** (primitive mouth). There are folds of tissue situated below the frontal prominence and the stomodeum of the embryo. These folds of tissue are known as the pharyngeal arches. As the development of the embryo continues, the first three folds of tissue will become orofacial structures. The first pharyngeal arch, also known as the mandibular arch, will become the bone of the mandible or lower jaw, as well as the lower lip and muscles of mastication. As growth continues in the posterior region of the mandibular arch, the maxillary process will develop from this arch as well. The maxillary process will form the maxilla, which includes the upper jaw area, hard palate, and palatine and zygomatic bones.

Development of the Hard and Soft Palates

During the fourth week of prenatal development, two small concave areas, called nasal pits, appear on the lower frontal prominence. As the nasal pits are forming, folds of tissue surrounding these pits are also developing.

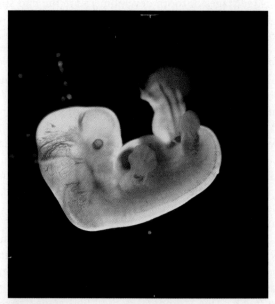

FIGURE 7.4
Embryo at four weeks. Note eyes and stomodeum.
Photo Lennart Nilsson/Albert Bonniers Forlag

The folds of tissue are known as the medial and lateral nasal processes. These medial and lateral nasal processes grow toward the midline, forming the area of tissue where the maxillary central and lateral incisors will eventually be situated. This area is considered to be the primary palate or premaxilla. The maxillary processes will develop into the remainder of the hard and soft palates.

Development of the hard and soft palates begins during the fifth week of prenatal development. During the sixth or seventh week of embryonic development, the maxillary processes grow toward the center of what will become the oral cavity, eventually fusing with the primary palate to complete the hard palate. A lack of fusion in any area of the hard palate is known as a cleft palate (Figure 7.5).

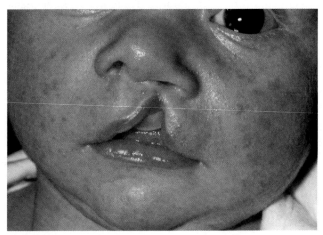

FIGURE 7.5
Newborn with a cleft palate.

Formation and Growth of the Teeth

The three stages of tooth development are the bud stage, cap stage, and bell stage.

The Bud Stage

The first indications of tooth formation are evidenced during the sixth week of embryonic development, with an increase in the growth of cells covering the primitive oral cavity. These cells are known as the epithelium. The growth of the oral epithelium is known as the **dental lamina**. This is a gradual expansion of the oral epithelium, beginning first with the anterior region and gradually expanding into the posterior area. This thickening band of oral epithelium follows the curves of the primitive oral cavity that will become the future dental arches.

During the eighth week of embryonic development the dental lamina continues to thicken in 10 specific areas on both upper and lower dental arches. These thickened areas are tooth buds that will ultimately form the primary teeth. This is known as the "bud stage." As the buds continue to grow they begin protruding away from the dental lamina. As it continues to grow, the outer portion of the bud becomes concave, giving the bud a "cap-shaped" appearance.

The Cap Stage

The concavity of the buds projecting from the enamel organ becomes more pronounced as growth continues. This leaves the middle portion void. At the same time the connection between the cap area and the enamel organ becomes thinner. The **enamel organ** develops during the cap stage and forms the enamel of the teeth. The oral epithelium and the dental organ tissues are developed from the ectoderm of the primary embryonic layers. This differentiation begins prior to the bud, cap, and bell stages.

The **dental papilla** arises during the cap stage from a connective tissue called mesenchyme, which is formed from the mesoderm of primary embryonic layers. During the cap stage, the dental papilla becomes the dentin and pulp of the tooth. As the enamel organ and dental papilla continue to develop, the mesenchyme compresses and encases the voided area, creating a capsule called the **dental sac**. The dental sac becomes the cementum of the tooth and the periodontal ligament.

Other than dental papilla what other structures develop from the mesoderm layer?

The Bell Stage

During the bell stage, the enamel organ is now bell shaped in appearance, and the voided area that occurred during the cap stage now takes on the shape of the tooth it will become. The bell stage begins with a process called histodifferentiation. During histodifferentiation cells differentiate into specialized cells that will form specific tooth structures. These cells include:

• **Ameloblasts:** Epithelial cells become cells that specifically form the enamel
• **Odontoblasts:** Part of the dental papilla that become cells that specifically form the dentin
• **Cementoblasts:** Cells from the inner portion of the dental sac that become cells which specifically form the cementum

Ameloblasts and odontoblasts will lay down the enamel and dentin within the concavity of the bell, forming the shape and size of the tooth it is to become.

The stages of tooth development are shown in Figure 7.6.

Eruption and Exfoliation

After the teeth have passed through the aforementioned stages, they must be able to achieve their working positions within the oral cavity. For that to occur, the teeth have to make their way through bone, connective tissue, and gingival tissue. This process is called eruption. Once eruption has taken place, the tooth continues to erupt until reaching the opposing tooth on the opposite arch. This is known as active eruption. The schedule in which the teeth erupt into the oral cavity varies; however, the dental assistant should be aware of the general timelines, as shown in Figure 7.7 for primary dentition and Figure 7.8 for permanent dentition.

Exfoliation is the normal process by which the primary teeth are shed to make room for the succedaneous teeth. The **succedaneous teeth** are the permanent teeth that succeed or replace the primary teeth in the oral cavity. The succedaneous teeth develop in the same manner in which the primary teeth developed. They go through the bud stage, cap stage, bell stage, and the eruption process.

While the dental lamina is evolving into a primary tooth, another projection of the dental lamina is present. This projection is the successional lamina. The successional lamina produces permanent teeth to replace primary teeth. During exfoliation the roots of the deciduous or primary teeth are resorbed until there is nothing to hold the tooth in the socket. As the succedaneous tooth is forming in the dental sac beneath the primary tooth,

(A) Initiation
Bud stage

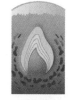

(E) Apposition
Maturation stage

(B) Proliferation
Cap stage (begins proliferation, histodifferentiation, and morphodifferentiation)

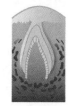

(F) Calcification

(C) Histodifferentiation
Bell stage

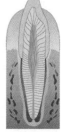

(G) Eruption

(D) Morphodifferentiation

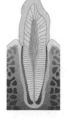

(H) Attrition

FIGURE 7.6
Life cycle of the tooth.

the roots of the deciduous tooth are being resorbed by osteoclasts (Figure 7.9). Osteoclasts are found on the dental sac and are the cells responsible for destroying cementum, bone, and dentin; therefore, they play a vital role in exfoliation of the primary teeth.

The first of the permanent teeth to erupt into the oral cavity are the mandibular first molars, thus beginning the mixed dentition stage where both primary and permanent teeth are present in the oral cavity. All of the permanent molars are nonsuccedaneous teeth, meaning they have no predecessors. They are able to erupt when the jaw has grown enough to make eruption possible. The first permanent molars erupt distal to the last primary molar in each quadrant, the second permanent molar will erupt distal to the first, and the third distal to the second. It is important to note that the succedaneous teeth replacing the primary molars are premolars, not molars.

Upper deciduous teeth

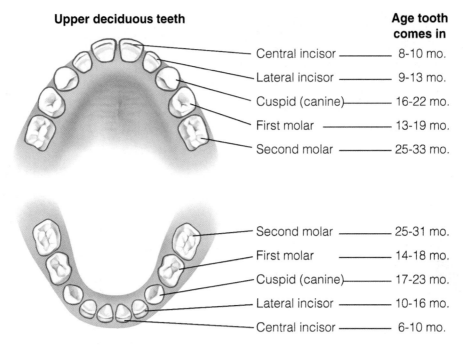

	Age tooth comes in
Central incisor	8-10 mo.
Lateral incisor	9-13 mo.
Cuspid (canine)	16-22 mo.
First molar	13-19 mo.
Second molar	25-33 mo.
Second molar	25-31 mo.
First molar	14-18 mo.
Cuspid (canine)	17-23 mo.
Lateral incisor	10-16 mo.
Central incisor	6-10 mo.

Lower deciduous teeth

FIGURE 7.7
Eruption schedule for the primary dentition.

Are the permanent molars considered to be succedaneous teeth?

?

Oral Histology

Histology is the study of the composition and function of tissues. The basic anatomic structure of each tooth consists of a crown and root(s). The crowns of the teeth are covered externally with enamel, whereas the roots are covered externally with cementum. The enamel and cementum of the tooth come together at the cervical line of the tooth, called the cementoenamel junction (CEJ). The **anatomical crown** is the entire portion of the tooth that is covered by enamel. The anatomical root is the portion of the tooth covered by cementum. The **clinical crown** is the portion of the tooth that can be seen above the gingiva in the oral cavity, even on a newly erupted tooth where just a sliver of the crown is visible.

In healthy, adult dentition, the cervical third of each tooth remains covered by the gingiva. Anything below the gingiva is considered to be the clinical root. A tooth may have more than one root. The tooth with a division that divides the root in two is called a bifurcation, and a tooth with a division into three roots is called a trifurcation. Each root tapers toward the end to form a peak called the **apex**. There is an opening in the apex of each root that allows blood, lymph, and nerve supply access to the tooth (Figure 7.10). This opening is known as the **apical foramen**.

Tissues of the Tooth

Four types of tissues make up a tooth:

- Enamel
- Dentin
- Cementum
- Pulp

The first of these three are hard tissues, whereas the pulp is a soft tissue.

Enamel

Enamel is the hardest tissue of the body and completely covers the anatomical crown. It serves to protect the softer underlying tissues during mastication (chewing)

Preparing for Externship

In a dental assistant course, a lot of material is learned and some of the material such as oral embryology and histology can be challenging to remember. Prior to going on their externships, some individuals may benefit from a review of certain portions of their studies. Reviewing the information will ensure that the knowledge necessary to perform well as a dental assistant is obtained.

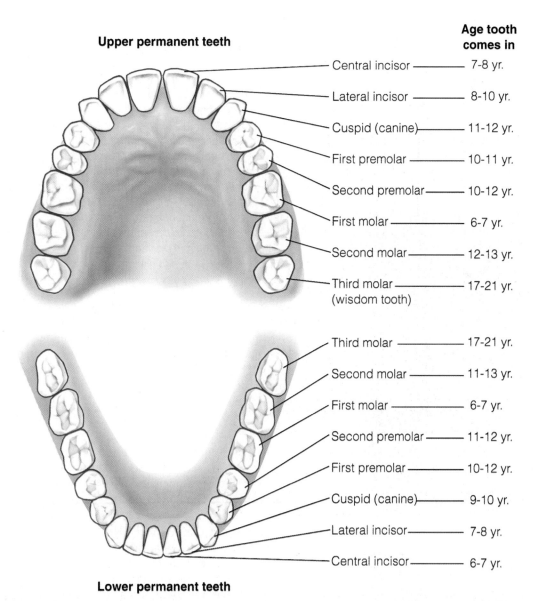

Upper permanent teeth

Tooth	Age tooth comes in
Central incisor	7-8 yr.
Lateral incisor	8-10 yr.
Cuspid (canine)	11-12 yr.
First premolar	10-11 yr.
Second premolar	10-12 yr.
First molar	6-7 yr.
Second molar	12-13 yr.
Third molar (wisdom tooth)	17-21 yr.
Third molar	17-21 yr.
Second molar	11-13 yr.
First molar	6-7 yr.
Second premolar	11-12 yr.
First premolar	10-12 yr.
Cuspid (canine)	9-10 yr.
Lateral incisor	7-8 yr.
Central incisor	6-7 yr.

Lower permanent teeth

FIGURE 7.8
Eruption schedule for the permanent dentition.

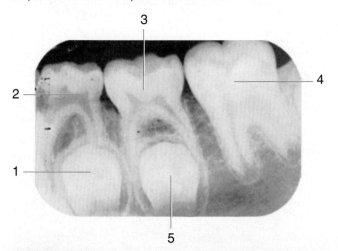

FIGURE 7.9
Radiograph of mixed dentition with resorption of primary roots:
(1) unerupted first premolar, (2) primary first molar, (3) primary second molar, (4) permanent first molar, and (5) unerupted second premolar.

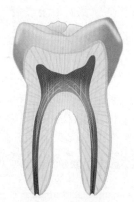

FIGURE 7.10
Tooth structures for an anterior and posterior tooth.

and also from invading bacteria (Figure 7.11). As the most densely mineralized tissue of the human body, enamel is able to withstand crushing forces up to 100,000 pounds per square inch (ppi). It is composed of 96% inorganic matter and 4% organic matter. The main component of enamel is hydroxyapatite, which consists mainly of calcium.

The color of enamel varies depending on the thickness and mineralization. The thicker the enamel, the lighter the color will appear. Enamel also has a translu-

cent quality, allowing some light to pass through it. Enamel is smooth, making it difficult for bacteria and food to stick to the teeth, hence giving the teeth a self-cleaning quality. During the decay process, enamel weakens and breaks down. Once enamel has been broken down or decayed, it is unable to repair itself, unlike many tissues of the body.

Dentin

Dentin makes up the bulk of the tooth and is found in both the crown and root areas of teeth. The coronal portion is covered by enamel, and the root portion is covered by cementum. Primary dentin is formed prior to tooth eruption. Dentin is a hard-mineralized tissue, harder than bone, but softer than enamel. Dentin is generally yellow in color and is a somewhat flexible material, which helps cushion the enamel. It is composed of 70% inorganic material and 30% organic material.

Dentin has microscopic canals running through it called dentinal tubules (Figure 7.12). These canals extend from the dentinoenamel junction into the pulp tissue.

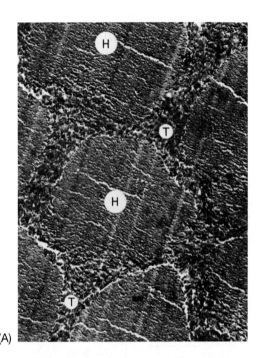
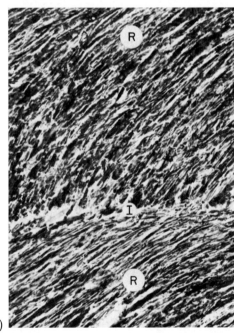

FIGURE 7.11
Microscopic views of enamel. (a) Micrograph showing head (H) and tail (T) relationship. (b) Micrograph showing two rods (R) and inter-rod area (I).

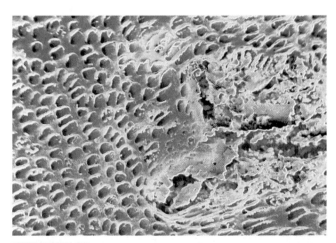

FIGURE 7.12
Microscopic view of tooth decay. The tiny holes in the dentine are dentinal tubules.

Each dentinal tubule contains a fiber known as Tome's dentinal fibril that serves to transmit stimuli to the pulp of the tooth. Dentin is also capable of some growth and repair, unlike enamel. Dentin will continue to grow and add to itself as the tooth matures. This added dentin is called **secondary dentin.** The secondary dentin can be seen in the pulp chamber area. The pulp chamber on a newly erupted tooth is larger than that of an older tooth. As the tooth grows, the pulp chamber becomes smaller. Reparative or **tertiary dentin** is sometimes formed due to trauma or decay.

Why is the presence of enamel important on a human tooth?

Cementum

Cementum is a bone-like connective tissue that covers the dentin area on the roots of the teeth and joins with the enamel at the CEJ. The composition of cementum is approximately 50% inorganic and 50% organic. The cementum serves as an attachment to anchor the tooth to the alveolar bone via the periodontal ligament. Cementum is yellow in color and lacks the shine and translucency of enamel.

There are two types of cementum: cellular and acellular. Acellular cementum covers the upper two-thirds of the root, whereas cellular cementum covers the apical third of the root. Cellular cementum can reproduce itself and over time will become layered by compensating for the natural attrition or by the wearing away that occurs to enamel. The cementum is also part of the attachment unit and serves to connect the teeth to the periodontal ligament. The periodontal ligament contains fibers called Sharpey's fibers, which are imbedded into the cementum.

Pulp

The dental **pulp** is the lifeline of the tooth and is composed of blood and lymph vessels, nerve and connective tissue, and also odontoblasts, the dentin-forming cells. Pulp is a soft tissue and red in color. Pulp tissue is located in the center of the tooth, is completely surrounded by dentin, and usually follows the shape of the tooth in form (Figure 7.13).

Pulp is divided into two structures: the pulp chamber, which is located in the coronal area, and the pulp canals, which run the length of the root. Blood brings nutrients and oxygen to the tooth, lymph tissue filters the fluids within the tooth, and nerve tissue transmits pain stimuli to the brain, all via the apical foramen.

Supporting Structures

The supporting structures or **periodontium** are those tissues that support and surround the teeth in the oral cavity. The periodontal tissues serve to nourish and protect

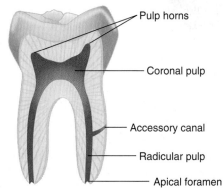

FIGURE 7.13
Structure of the pulp.

the teeth. The tissues of the periodontium are subdivided into two categories: the attachment unit and the gingival unit.

Attachment Unit

The attachment unit consists of four components (Figure 7.14):

* Alveolar processes of the maxilla
* Alveolar processes of the mandible
* Cementum
* Periodontal ligament

The alveolar process, also known as the alveolus, is the area of the maxilla and mandible bones in which the teeth are held. The **alveolar socket** is the opening within the alveolar bone that houses the roots of the teeth. The teeth do not sit directly on the bone itself, but are connected to the bone by the periodontal ligament. The socket is lined with a dense bone called the **lamina dura.** The lamina dura is a compact bone that is also known as the cribriform plate. The process of bone separating from one socket to another is called the interdental septum. The process of bone separating the root area of a multi-rooted tooth is called the interradicular septum.

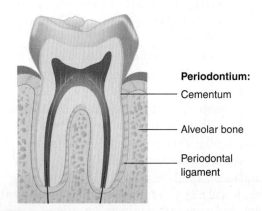

Periodontium:
Cementum

Alveolar bone

Periodontal ligament

FIGURE 7.14
Supporting structures of the teeth.

The highest areas of the alveolar bone are peaked areas called **alveolar crests.** These crests stay fairly consistent with the CEJ in a healthy oral cavity. However, if there is bone loss due to periodontal disease, it will become evident when the alveolar crests begin to flatten out.

The periodontal ligament (PDL) is the fibrous connective tissue that attaches the roots of the teeth to the alveolar bone. Fibers from this ligament are imbedded in both the cementum and the lamina dura. These fibers are known as "Sharpey's fibers." The periodontal ligament serves to support and stabilize the teeth within the sockets, enabling them to maintain their proper space, and acts as a shock absorber that cushions the teeth from the extreme forces that occur during mastication. The periodontal ligament also provides nourishment to the teeth.

Gingival Unit

The gingival unit consists of those specialized epithelial structures that line the oral cavity and surround the teeth. It is made up of free and attached gingivae. The free gingivae are gum tissues that form the gingival sulcus. The attached gingiva is the firmly attached gum tissue extending from the base of the free gingivae to the alveolar mucosa. The **lining mucosa** is thin, delicate tissue that covers the areas inside of the cheeks, vestibule, and soft palate and the area under the tongue. The lining mucosa is a supple tissue not attached to bone. Below the lining mucosa is a submucosa that contains many blood vessels, which gives the tissue a bright red appearance.

Masticatory mucosa is composed of a dense thick mucosa, designed to withstand the trauma of mastication. It covers the gingiva, the hard palate, and the dorsum or upper surface of the tongue.

SUMMARY

Embryology is the study of how a human being develops through the three stages before birth. It involves the development of the orofacial structures. It is important for the dental assistant to understand the oral embryology stage and how the structures of the oral cavity develop, including the eruption and exfoliation processes.

Histology is the study of the composition and function of tissues. By understanding the composition and function of tissues, dental assistants can comprehend the

procedures performed to restore the teeth and tissues. The tissues found in the oral cavity serve a variety of functions, including the breaking down of food to begin the digestive process. Speech is also an important function of the oral cavity. The teeth and tongue are vital in the role of speech. The more the dental assistant understands the concepts presented in the study of oral embryology and oral histology, the more competent the dental assistant will be in providing care to the dental patient.

KEY TERMS

- **Alveolar crest:** The highest peak in the alveolar process. p. 112
- **Alveolar socket:** The opening within the alveolar bone that houses the roots of the teeth. p. 111
- **Ameloblasts:** Enamel-forming cells. p. 106
- **Anatomical crown:** The portion of the tooth that is covered with enamel. p. 108
- **Apex:** Peaked tip at the end of each root. p. 108
- **Apical foramen:** Opening in the apex of each root. p. 108
- **Cementoblasts:** Cementum-forming cells. p. 106
- **Clinical crown:** The portion of the crown that is visible in the oral cavity. p. 108
- **Dental lamina:** Growth of the oral epithelium that will eventually form the teeth. p. 106
- **Dental papilla:** Tissue from the mesoderm layer that will form dentin and pulp. p. 106
- **Dental sac:** Capsule that contains the developing tooth; it will also form the cementum, periodontal ligament, and some alveolar bone. p. 106

- **Dentin:** Tissue that makes up the bulk of the tooth; it is covered by cementum on the root and enamel on the crown. p. 110
- **Dentinal tubules:** Microscopic canals running through dentin. p. 110
- **Embryology:** The study of how a human being develops through three stages before birth. p. 104
- **Enamel organ:** Tissue arising from the ectoderm layer that will form the enamel. p. 106
- **Histology:** The study of the composition and function of tissues. p. 108
- **Lamina dura:** Compact bone that lines the socket of the alveolar process. p. 111
- **Lining mucosa:** A thin delicate tissue that covers the inside of the cheeks, vestibule, soft palate, undersurface of the tongue, and floor of the mouth. p. 112
- **Masticatory mucosa:** A dense thick mucosa that is designed to withstand the trauma of chewing; it covers the hard palate, tongue, and gum tissue. p. 112
- **Odontoblasts:** Dentin-forming cells. p. 106

KEY TERMS (continued)

- **Periodontium:** Tissues that surround and support the teeth. p. 111
- **Primary dentin:** Dentin formed prior to tooth eruption. p. 110
- **Pulp:** Tissue composed of blood and lymph vessels, nerve and connective tissues, and odontoblasts. p. 111
- **Secondary dentin:** Dentin formed after tooth eruption that remains for the life of the tooth. p. 111
- **Stomodeum:** A primitive mouth. p. 105
- **Succedaneous teeth:** The permanent teeth that replace the primary teeth. p. 107
- **Tertiary dentin:** A reparative dentin that forms in response to injury or irritation. p. 111
- **Zygote:** The first stage in embryonic development. p. 104

CHECK YOUR UNDERSTANDING

1. What dental tooth tissue arises from the ectodermic layer?
   a. enamel
   b. dentin
   c. pulp
   d. periodontal ligament

2. Which of the following is the first stage in embryonic development?
   a. zygote
   b. embryonic
   c. fetal
   d. gestation

3. During which week of embryonic development does the first sign of tooth development occur?
   a. 1st
   b. 6th
   c. 10th
   d. 15th

4. In what stage of development does the oral epithelium thicken in 10 areas of each dental arch?
   a. bud stage
   b. cap stage
   c. bell stage
   d. fetal stage

5. The process by which the primary teeth are shed to make room for the permanent teeth is known as
   a. mastication.
   b. active eruption.
   c. exfoliation.
   d. gestation.

6. What is the name of the tooth tissue that makes up the bulk of the tooth?
   a. enamel
   b. dentin
   c. pulp
   d. cementum

7. At approximately what age does the first primary tooth erupt into the oral cavity?
   a. 9 months
   b. 7 months
   c. 1 year
   d. 18 months

8. What are dentin-forming cells called?
   a. odontoblasts
   b. ameloblasts
   c. osteoblasts
   d. cementoblasts

9. At what age does the first permanent molar erupt into the oral cavity?
   a. 4 years
   b. 6 years
   c. 10 years
   d. 12 years

10. What is the portion of the alveolar bone called that separates one tooth socket from another?
    a. interdental septum
    b. lamina dura
    c. interradicular septum
    d. cribriform plate

INTERNET ACTIVITIES

- For further information on tooth eruption, visit http://www.ada.org/public/topics/tooth_eruption.asp
- Conduct further research to learn more about cleft palates at www.pedisurg.com and www.operationsmile.org

WEB REFERENCES

- Doctor NDTV www.doctorndtv.com
- Family Doctor Books www.familydoctor.co.uk
- The Visible Embryo www.visembryo.com/baby

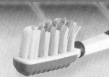

8

Tooth Morphology

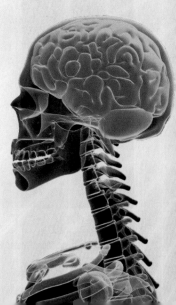

As a dental assistant, not only is it important to learn procedures necessary to assist the dentist, it is just as important to be familiar with the development and structure of the oral cavity. Oral histology is the study of the tissues of the teeth, the surrounding structure, and the functions of teeth in the mouth. In this chapter, the dental assistant will become familiar with the development of these tissues and surrounding structures to aid in the understanding of their function for the lifetime of a person's dentition. (See Chapter 7 for information on the embryonic development of the human body.)

Histology of Tooth Development

There are two sets of teeth in the life span of every human body. Deciduous teeth are the first set of teeth. They are also called primary teeth, baby teeth, or milk teeth. **Dentition** describes the teeth of the mouth in the dental arch. The **primary dentition** begins to emerge in the mouth around the sixth month of age (Figure 8.1). By age 3, full

Dental Assistant   PROFESSIONAL TIP

Your patients' prenatal health will significantly impact the health of their children's teeth. Locate community organizations that can provide information regarding the importance of prenatal health. Keep a list handy that includes the organizations' names, addresses, and telephone numbers for your pregnant patients. Caring about the dental patient and taking the initiative to locate this information will be greatly appreciated by both your employer and your dental patients.

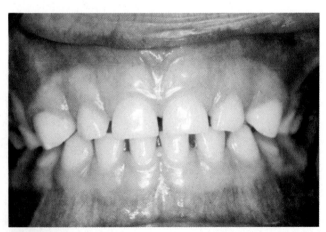

FIGURE 8.1
View of primary teeth.
Image courtesy Instructional Materials for the Dental Team, Lex., KY

Patient Education

Most parents are not aware of how important good dental care is to the health of the baby and the baby's teeth. What the mother eats affects her baby's developing teeth. Slight deficiencies in the mother's diet and dental health may cause changes in the baby's tooth formation that will leave a tooth at greater risk for decay later in life. At birth, the baby has all his unerupted primary teeth and many permanent teeth at different stages of development. During pregnancy good dental care and an adequate diet is necessary for optimal oral development of the baby and his teeth.

Patient and parent education are important during the prenatal growth process for healthy dental oral tissues and developing teeth. Educating the dental patient in making wise nutrition and food choices during pregnancy can help avoid malnutrition that may bring on hypoplasia, a condition characterized by inadequate development of an infant's tooth enamel. Remind pregnant mothers to consume dairy products, which are the best source for calcium, the main building block of bones and teeth. Also make nutritional suggestions that include foods in the patient's diet that are good sources of calcium and vitamin D, phosphorus, vitamins A and C, and protein. Some examples include milk, yogurt, cheese, dried peas and beans, dark leafy greens, fortified cereals, whole grains, peanut butter, and juices. Always have the patient consult with her physician.

eruption has occurred for all 20 primary teeth. Around the age of 6 years, the 32 permanent teeth, also referred to as secondary teeth or adult teeth, begin to erupt and start the **succedaneous** ("comes after") process of taking the place of the primary teeth through the natural pushing out, or exfoliation, of the teeth.

All primary teeth have a succedaneous permanent replacement. Primary molars are replaced by permanent premolars. Until all primary teeth are fully exfoliated and have been replaced by the succedaneous permanent teeth, the mixture of primary and permanent teeth in the mouth is described as **mixed dentition** (Figure 8.2). Once all of the permanent teeth have erupted, the dentition is referred to as **permanent dentition** (Figure 8.3).

How many teeth do adults have? When does a child begin to lose his or her baby teeth? What is the difference between deciduous and succedaneous?

Stages of Tooth Development

Tooth production or development, termed **odontogenesis**, is the process of the creation of each tooth. For a healthy dentition to develop, the enamel, dentin, cementum, and

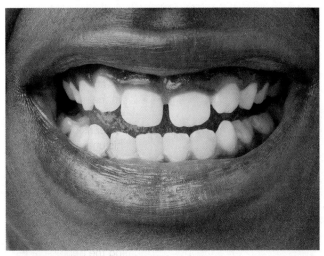

FIGURE 8.2
View of mixed dentition.

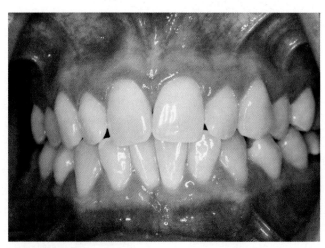

FIGURE 8.3
View of permanent dentition.
Image courtesy Instructional Materials for the Dental Team, Lex., KY

periodontium must all develop during appropriate stages of fetal development. Every tooth progresses through certain developmental stages as it grows. The first signs of tooth development occur around the fifth to sixth week of the embryonic phase. By the seventh week all primary dentition has developed as well as the beginning stages of the permanent dentition. At birth approximately 44 teeth will already be in various stages of development (Figure 8.4).

There are seven stages describing this progression. The stages, discussed in the following subsections, are named by the meaning of their terminology (Figure 8.5).

Stage 1: Initiation

The first stage in the process of odontogenesis, also known as the bud stage, is termed **initiation**. The dental

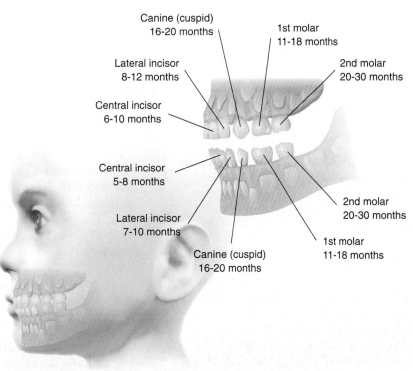

FIGURE 8.4
Development stages indicated for erupted primary dentition with permanent unerupted dentition.

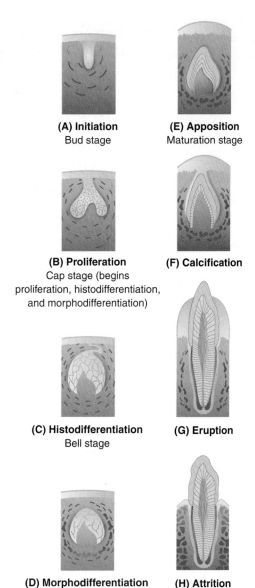

(A) Initiation
Bud stage

(B) Proliferation
Cap stage (begins
proliferation, histodifferentiation,
and morphodifferentiation)

(C) Histodifferentiation
Bell stage

(D) Morphodifferentiation

(E) Apposition
Maturation stage

(F) Calcification

(G) Eruption

(H) Attrition

FIGURE 8.5
Stages of tooth development.

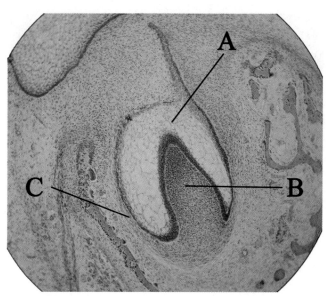

FIGURE 8.6
Histologic picture taken of tooth bud with (A) enamel organ, (B)
papilla, and (C) follicle.
Courtesy wikipedia.org

lamina, a membrane surrounding a small growth of epithelium (oral tissue), gives form to the tooth or tooth bud (sometimes called the tooth germ) to begin development. The bud stage is distinguished by the manifestation of cells that initiate a tooth bud.

Stage 2: Proliferation

The second stage in the process of odontogenesis, also known as the cap stage, is termed **proliferation**. Proliferation begins during the fourth and fifth month of pregnancy. Small tooth buds begin to develop at different times until all 20 deciduous teeth are evident. Deciduous teeth begin to form during the sixth to eighth week of an embryo's development.

Stage 3: Differentiation

The third stage in the process of odontogenesis, **differentiation**, is also known as the bell stage. During this stage changes begin to occur in two different ways. First, the tooth bud begins to take on a different shape. This is called morphodifferentiation. Second the tissue makeup begins to change, called histodifferentiation (see Chapter 7 for more information on histodifferentiation). In the differentiation stage various tissues of the tooth begin to progress and perform. The foundation and shape of the teeth change from the cap stage into the early bell stage.

The tooth bud is organized into three parts: the enamel organ, the papilla, and the follicle (Figure 8.6). The enamel, or dental, organ is made up of ameloblasts, which produce enamel-forming proteins that cover the tooth. Enamel is the hardest substance in the human body. The dental papilla is made of odontoblasts, which form the outer portion of the dental pulp. These cells form dentin, which creates the bulk of the tooth.

The dental follicle (dental sac) is the covering of the tooth bud. The tooth bud contains three important elements: cementoblasts (cells needed for the development of cementum that covers the root of the tooth), osteoblasts (cells required in building bone for the alveolar bone and alveolar plate), and fibroblasts (cells needed in forming connective tissue for the periodontal ligament).

One can also often differentiate the function of cells by examining their name's suffix. The suffix *-blast* means "building up" and the suffix *-clast* means "destroying" (as in *osteoclasts;* see discussion in Chapter 7).

Stage 4: Apposition

The fourth stage in the process of odontogenesis, **apposition**, is known as the mature stage or crown stage. In the apposition stage, tissue and tooth formation occurs. The hard tissues (enamel and dentin) start to develop during this stage. The crown of the tooth also takes shape during this stage. Throughout the mouth, all teeth go through this same process. In earlier developmental stages enamel cells divided and multiplied to increase the overall bud size. This process stops in the fourth stage, and mineralized hard tissue begins to form. By the end of this stage, enamel has completed the mineralization process in tooth formation.

Stages 5, 6, and 7: Calcification, Eruption, and Attrition

The fifth stage in the process of odontogenesis, **calcification**, is the hardening and setting of tooth tissues. This process occurs in the final formation of the enamel, dentin, cementum, and periodontium.

Enamel formation usually occurs in two stages: the secretory and maturation stages. During the secretory stage, enamel proteins are produced and secreted. Once this occurs, this organic matrix creates a partially mineralized enamel. It is in the maturation stage that enamel mineralization is completed. The enamel growth proceeds outward away from the center of the tooth.

Dentin development is also known as dentinogenesis. It is the first characteristic feature of the crown stage. Dentin formation occurs prior to the development of enamel. Four main types of dentin are associated with the different stages of dentin development: mantle, primary, secondary, and tertiary dentin.

Cementogenesis is the formation of cementum, which occurs near the latter part of a tooth's development. As mentioned in Chapter 7, the two types of cementum are acellular, which occurs first, and cellular, which forms after the majority of the tooth development is complete. As mineralization occurs the fibers of the periodontal ligament attach to the cementum. This process aids in growth, attachment, and support of the tooth to the alveolar bone.

The supporting structure of the tooth is known as the periodontium. The periodontium is composed of alveolar bone, periodontal ligaments, gingiva, and cementum. The cementum is the only component of the periodontium that is actually part of the tooth structure. The alveolar bone surrounds the roots of the teeth, providing support, while forming the socket. The periodontal ligaments provide the anchor from the bone to the cementum, while the gingiva, commonly known as "gums," surrounds the teeth.

The sixth stage is known as the **eruption** stage. Tooth eruption is the process of a tooth breaking through the gum tissue to grow into place in the mouth and become visible. Although tooth eruption occurs at different ages for different people, general eruption age guidelines are listed in Tables 8-1 and 8-2. There are three stages in tooth eruption. The first, the deciduous or primary dentition stage, occurs when only the primary teeth are visible. During this stage the first permanent tooth erupts into the mouth. At this point the teeth are in the mixed dentition stage. When the last primary tooth falls out of the mouth, and only permanent teeth remain, the teeth are in the permanent dentition stage. Children going through this stage may experience some discomfort due to the loss of primary teeth and the eruption of permanent dentition.

The seventh and last stage is the **attrition** stage. The natural wear that happens over the life span of a tooth is called attrition. It occurs when the occlusal surfaces of the teeth begin to wear down from normal functions such as chewing and speaking. There are many reasons why a tooth can wear away. When newly erupted anterior teeth in the permanent dentition begin the eruption stage, the chewing surfaces or incisal edges of the teeth appear with

TABLE 8-1 Developmental Timeline for the Primary Dentition

Primary Teeth	Maxillary (Upper) Teeth				
	Central Incisor	Lateral Incisor	Canine	First Molar	Second Molar
Initial calcification	14 wk	16 wk	17 wk	15.5 wk	19 wk
Crown completed	1.5 mo	2.5 mo	9 mo	6 mo	11 mo
Root completed	1.5 yr	2 yr	3.25 yr	2.5 yr	3 yr
	Mandibular (Lower) Teeth				
Initial calcification	14 wk	16 wk	17 wk	15.5 wk	18 wk
Crown completed	2.5 mo	3 mo	9 mo	5.5 mo	10 mo
Root completed	1.5 yr	1.5 yr	3.25 yr	2.5 yr	3 yr

TABLE 8-2 Developmental Timeline for the Permanent Dentition

Permanent Teeth	Central Incisor	Lateral Incisor	Canine	First Premolar	Second Premolar	First Molar	Second Molar	Third Molar
Maxillary (Upper) Teeth								
Initial calcification	3–4 mo	10–12 mo	4–5 mo	1.5–1.75 yr	2–2.25 yr	at birth	2.5–3 yr	7–9 yr
Crown completed	4–5 yr	4–5 yr	6–7 yr	5–6 yr	6–7 yr	2.5–3 yr	7–8 yr	12–16 yr
Root completed	10 yr	11 yr	13–15 yr	12–13 yr	12–14 yr	9–10 yr	14–16 yr	18–25 yr
Mandibular (Lower) Teeth								
Initial calcification	3–4 mo	3–4 mo	4–5 mo	1.5–2 yr	2.25–2.5 yr	at birth	2.5–3 yr	8–10 yr
Crown completed	4–5 yr	4–5 yr	6–7 yr	5–6 yr	6–7 yr	2.5–3 yr	7–8 yr	12–16 yr
Root completed	9 yr	10 yr	12–14 yr	12–13 yr	13–14 yr	9–10 yr	14–15 yr	18–25 yr

three rounded ridges known as mamelons (Figure 8.7). Mamelons are not present on the primary teeth. To date, no clear definitive answer has been reached as to why this is the case. Mamelons aid in tooth eruption and are worn down shortly after eruption by attrition.

Attrition is seen commonly in older patients whose teeth have been worn down by repetitive chewing that flattens the biting surface. Shortening the teeth height can remove contours necessary in mastication. Concerns beyond the natural wearing process can be corrected through the use of mouth guards to help to reduce the excessive occlusal wearing process associated with bruxism. Crowding or space issues in the mouth can cause interference with and occlusal trauma of the biting surfaces that can further damage teeth due to repetitive wearing down of an area on a tooth. Orthodontic treatment may be needed to help correct tooth placement in order to address the crowding or space issue that is causing the attrition.

How can prenatal care affect a child's teeth?

Abnormalities of Tooth Development

A number of tooth abnormalities can occur during the tooth development stages. These include the following:

- *Amelogenesis imperfecta,* known as dental enamel hypoplasia, is an incomplete formation of the dental enamel caused by vitamin deficiency, infectious disease, birth injury, trauma, or local infection. In mild cases of amelogenesis, small grooves, pits, and fissures are seen in the enamel. Deep horizontal rows of pits are visible in severe cases. Extreme cases can involve the absence of enamel.

- *Anodontia,* a complete lack of tooth development, is a rare genetic disorder that appears at birth.

- *Dens in dente* is an irregularity of the tooth, resembling a "fold" in the enamel that occurred during the early stages of tooth development. It is typically found on upper lateral incisors on the lingual or tongue side of the tooth.

- *Dentin dysplasia* is a hereditary disorder of dentin formation.

- *Dentinogenesis imperfecta* is a condition of tooth development in which the dentin shows discoloration of the teeth, ranging from grays to a brownish color. The dentin is poorly formed. The teeth are soft and can wear down quickly.

- *Fluorosis* occurs from exposure to excessive fluoride during tooth development, causing yellowing of teeth, white spots, and pitting or mottling of enamel (Figure 8.8).

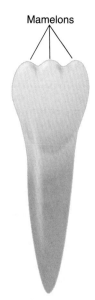

Mamelons

FIGURE 8.7
The three mamelons present on the mandibular central incisor.

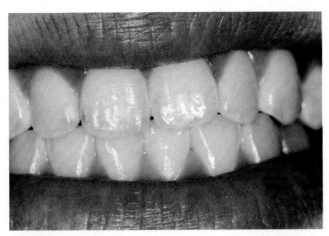

FIGURE 8.8
Fluorosis.

- *Fusion* happens when two teeth become one tooth and/or are joined together during development and during the bud stage of tooth development (Figure 8.9). The tooth may be connected at the enamel, at the roots, or by both.
- *Germination* is when a single tooth separates to form two crowns on a single root, occurring in the bud stage during development (Figure 8.10).
- *Hypodontia* is a lack of some tooth development. Hypodontia is a common developmental abnormality. For example, the congenital absence of third molars or wisdom teeth is very common.
- *Hyperdontia* involves a single extra tooth in the mouth, common where the incisors are located in the upper dentition. Hyperdontia is thought to be linked to an excess of dental lamina in the early development stages of the tooth. Linked causes of hereditary factors along with some evidence of environmental factors may lead to this condition.

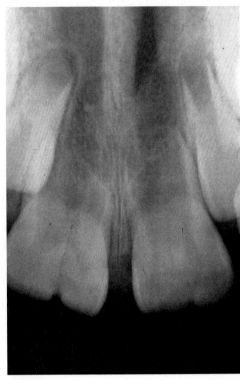

FIGURE 8.10
A radiograph of germination.
Courtesy Department of Pathology, University of Missouri–Kansas City School of Dentistry

- *Macrodontia* is the term used to describe abnormally large teeth; it can be associated with mental retardation growth abnormalities (Figure 8.11).
- *Microdontia* is the term for uncommonly small teeth. It is usually limited to just one or two teeth. A common heritable dental trait is the "peg-shaped" upper lateral incisors, also sometimes found in small third molars.
- *Supernumerary teeth* are extra teeth. **Supernumerary teeth** can be erupted or impacted. Heredity may play a role in the occurrence of this anomaly as well as hyperactivity of the dental lamina at the time of the initiation stage in tooth development.

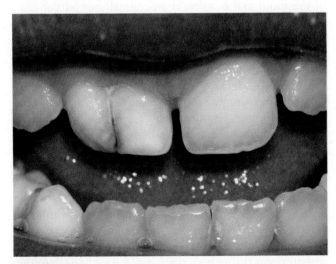

FIGURE 8.9
Teeth fused to form one large tooth.
Courtesy wikipedia.org

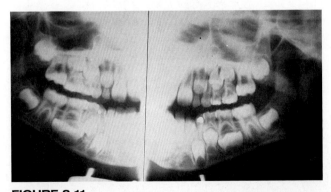

FIGURE 8.11
Radiograph of macrodontia.
Courtesy Department of Pathology, University of Missouri–Kansas City School of Dentistry

What are the seven stages of tooth development? Explain how you would describe these stages to a patient's parents.

Hard Tissues of the Teeth

The human dentition has four different types of teeth: incisors, canines, premolars, and molars. All teeth have the same tissue structure, as well as anatomic and structural landmarks (Figure 8.12).

Enamel

Enamel is a hard covering and is thicker on the biting surfaces of the teeth than on the nonbiting surfaces. The enamel is harder on the biting surfaces of teeth to give them the strength and durability to resist fracture due to the occlusal forces placed on the teeth from biting. Enamel consists of calcium and phosphate and is the strongest living tissue in the human body. Tooth enamel has a number of unique structural characteristics. The basic unit of enamel is called an enamel rod (Figure 8.13). An enamel rod, also known as an enamel prism, is a tightly packed mass of mineralized organic material in an organized pattern. It lies parallel to and extending from the dentinoenamel junction to the outer surface, creating a smooth hard shell surrounding the dentin of the tooth's crown. The enamel matrix is produced by ameloblasts and called the Tome's process, which guides the process of ameloblasts or enamel matrix to lay down layers of rods. As the second layer begins to form, the first layer becomes harder and the process continues until the last layer is formed.

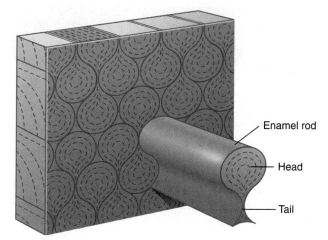

FIGURE 8.13
Structure of an enamel rod.

Enamel contains brownish stripes or lines of Retzius. These are developmental identification marks similar to those found in a tree trunk, indicating stages of tooth development. These incremental lines have areas of diminished calcification caused by short pauses in the development of the enamel. *Enamel spindles* indicate short dentinal tubules that have crossed over into the enamel and fused during the enamel mineralization process. The enamel rod endings or enamel tufts are irregular groupings of undercalcified enamel resembling small brown brushes. The thin structures of longer, narrower enamel tufts are called enamel lamellae and are developmental cracks or imperfections that extend toward or into the dentin.

Dentin

Dentin is the main tissue surrounding the pulp or nerve of the tooth and is softer than enamel, but harder than cementum and bone. Dentin can be described as forming the bulk of the tooth. It is slightly yellowish-brown and gives bulk to the tooth. The thickness of dentin is what determines the various shades of tooth enamel. The thicker, more dense the dentin is, the darker or more yellowish-brown gray the tooth shade will appear to the eye. The thinner, less dense the dentin is, the lighter or more translucent the tooth shade will appear to the eye. Dentin is found in both the root and crown of the tooth. Dentin is sensitive to tactile (touch), thermal (temperature), and chemical stimulation.

There are two identifying hollow structures in the dentin. Tubules, also known as Tome's dentinal tubules, extend from the dentinoenamel junction to the pulp chamber (Figure 8.14). The tubules conduct pain stimuli and nutrients throughout the tissue. Inside of each tubule lies a fiber known as Tome's dentinal fibril that assists with the regulation of nutrition and conveys sensation.

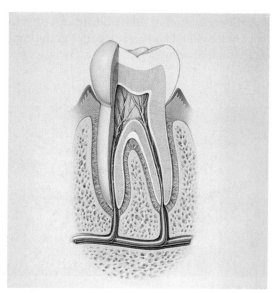

FIGURE 8.12
Parts of the tooth.

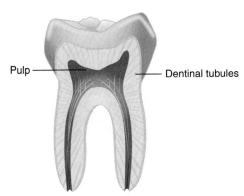

FIGURE 8.14
Dentinal tubules.

As previously stated in Chapter 7 and to serve as a review, there are three types of dentin: primary dentin, which is newly formed dentin; secondary dentin, which occurs when the tooth is maturing; and tertiary dentin or reparative dentin, which can occur whenever irritation to the tooth occurs due to attrition, trauma, or decay. Tertiary dentin may be irregular and begins to form under the disturbed site to provide protection to the pulp.

Pulp

The pulp is the nerve of the tooth, and includes soft and vascular tissue that is found in the center of the tooth surrounded by the dentin. The pulp is encased in the pulp chamber, which is located in the crown portion of the tooth. The pulp canals extend from the pulp chamber to the apex of the tooth. The pulp is a defense center for the tooth alerting the tooth to stimulus, temperature and chemical changes, vibration, and bacteria invasion that is relayed to the brain. The pulp produces cells called fibroblasts that develop connective tissue. The pulp is the life of the tooth. When the pulp dies or becomes necrotic (necrosis is the death of a cell) due to disease or injury, the tooth is no longer vital (alive).

Cementum

The cementum is a thin bone-like tissue that covers the root and meets the enamel tissue at the cementoenamel junction (CEJ), which is located at the neck of the tooth. The main function of the cementum is to anchor the tooth to the bony wall of the socket by connective tissue fiber called Sharpey's fibers, otherwise known as the periodontal ligament. Cementum will meet directly with the enamel in 30% of teeth, overlap the enamel in 60% to 65% of teeth, and may not meet the enamel, leaving a small portion of dentin exposed to oral fluids, in 5% to 10% of teeth. These areas can be sensitive to temperature changes and to metal instruments.

Formation of the Periodontium

The tissue surrounding the teeth is called the periodontium. The periodontium is composed of three separate tissues that aid in its goals of anchoring, supporting, and protecting the teeth. The three separate tissues include the periodontal membrane, the alveolar bone, and gingival tissues.

Periodontal Membrane

The periodontal membrane, more commonly known as the periodontal ligaments, is made up of bundles of dense and fibrous connective tissue that connect or attach the tooth between the alveolar bone and the cementum of the tooth. The connective tissues are referred to as the Sharpey's, gingival, interdental or transseptal, and alveolar fibers.

Alveolar Bone

The alveolar bone or sockets for tooth placement provide support to the teeth. Alveolar bone or alveolar process is composed of an alveolar socket and cortical plate (thick covering of compact bone). The alveolar socket is lined with a cribriform plate lining over the lamina dura.

Gingiva

The gingiva is surface tissue in the mouth that surrounds and protects the teeth as well as the underlying tissues. The gingiva is generally known as the gum tissue. It has various attached and free gingival epithelial layers that help protect the tooth and underlying tissues. The mucogingival junction is where the attached gum tissue and movable mucous membrane attaches and meets. It is indicated by a color change between pink gingiva to red mucosa. The free gingival groove is a depression on the gingiva that corresponds to the sulcus depth. This groove is not always present but serves as a demarcation between the free gingiva and the attached gingival. The sulcus is the open space between the tooth and the free gingival tissue, almost like the space between one's neck and shirt collar. The gingival crest or gingival margin is the coronal part of free gingiva. The interdental papilla is the triangular gum tissue that is positioned between the teeth and area beneath where the contacts of the teeth meet.

What type of tissue, including tissues of the tooth, exists in the mouth to help protect the teeth and the tooth socket?

Dentition Periods

The human body produces two sets of teeth in a lifetime. Dentition describes the natural teeth in a dental arch. In a lifetime the human body will go through three different dentition periods: primary, mixed, and permanent.

Primary Dentition

Primary teeth, deciduous teeth, milk teeth, and the commonly used *baby teeth* are terms used to describe the first set of human dentition. There are 20 teeth when all are fully erupted. As these teeth fall out, 32 permanent, adult, or secondary teeth replace them. Eruption dates for the primary teeth vary from 6 months up to about 3 years of age. Some infants get them earlier than others.

The deciduous teeth play a very important role in the proper alignment, spacing, and occlusion of the permanent teeth. Baby teeth hold space in the jaw for the adult teeth. If a baby tooth is lost too early, the teeth beside it may drift into the empty space. Then when it's time for the adult teeth to come in, there may not be enough room. This can make the teeth crooked or crowded. The eruption times begin with the primary mandibular (lower) central incisors and complete the eruption or "teething" process with the second primary molar.

Table 8-3 lists additional information about the ages when exfoliation occurs in the primary dentition.

Mixed Dentition

The transition from primary to permanent dentition is referred to as mixed dentition. Mixed dentition occurs when there are primary teeth and permanent teeth present in either dental arch at any time. The development toward full permanent dentition begins with the eruption of the four first permanent molars, and replacement of the lower deciduous central incisors by the permanent lower central incisors. The pressure of the developing permanent teeth causes the roots of the baby teeth to resorb or dissolve. Without a root there to anchor into the jaw, the baby teeth become loose and ultimately fall out. Complete resorption of the deciduous tooth roots

Cultural Considerations

Many cultures are not educated in the importance of oral hygiene for children's teeth. This can be tough on the primary dentition due to premature loss of deciduous teeth. Explaining the necessity for baby teeth retention and their role in proper jaw and speech development will help parents make decisions regarding the repair of decayed teeth versus extracting them. Prevention of tooth decay so that primary teeth exfoliate naturally is very important.

permits **exfoliation** of that tooth and future replacement by the succedaneous permanent teeth.

This dentition period can be a difficult adjustment time for children for various reasons. Individuals differ greatly in dental development and tooth size, which are determined predominantly by heredity. Children may notice color and size differences in their teeth. Baby teeth are whiter than adult teeth, and permanent teeth have larger crown sizes than the primary teeth they replaced, at times causing crowding of the teeth as they erupt and shift into their positions. Mixed dentition exists from approximately 6 to 12 years of age.

Permanent Dentition

The permanent teeth begin to develop within the jaw around the ages of 2.5 to 6 years and continue to grow

Life Span Considerations

During the mixed dentition stage, life for children can be tough. Teeth take on different shades and sizes as well as missing teeth and crowding. This is commonly known as the "ugly duckling" stage. Educating children and their parents on what to expect regarding the general stages of development and what the final outcome will produce can be helpful.

TABLE 8-3 Primary Tooth Eruption and Exfoliation Ages

Primary Dentition	Eruption Age		Exfoliation Age	
	Maxillary	Mandibular	Maxillary	Mandibular
Central incisors	6–10 mo	5–8 mo	7–8 yr	6–7 yr
Lateral incisors	8–12 mo	7–10 mo	8–9 yr	7–8 yr
Canines	16–20 mo	16–20 mo	11–12 yr	9–11 yr
First molars	11–18 mo	11–18 mo	9–11 yr	10–12 yr
Second molars	20–30 mo	20–30 mo	9–12 yr	11–13 yr

Preparing for Externship

Prepare for your externship by becoming familiar with the types of patients who frequent the dental practice where you will be externing. Educate yourself in the specialty area that you will be practicing. For example, if you work for a pediatric dentist, you will need to be able to educate parents and answer "frequently asked questions" such as these:

- *When do I start caring for my baby's teeth?* The incorporation of good oral hygiene into the daily routine should begin even before the first tooth erupts. A parent can use a warm, moist washcloth to go over the gingiva to wipe away any remnants of milk or debris. When the first sign of a tooth appears, it is especially important to care for that tooth. Milk allowed to pool around the tooth, or teeth, makes teeth susceptible to decay even at an early age. In addition to the washcloth, commercial products are available that can assist the parent in taking care of the teeth.
- *What is teething?* Teething is usually considered as the time when a child has a tooth that is trying to erupt from the gingiva. This is often referred to as the "cutting of teeth." Often, the infant or child may experience painful, swollen gums. Some pediatricians, although not all, often see a correlation between teething and diarrhea and fever associated with the erupting tooth.
- *Why are baby teeth important?* Baby or primary teeth serve several purposes. They assist in the mastication of food substances, speech development, and space maintenance for the future eruption of the permanent teeth.

Visit your externship location. Find out what the practice's focus of dentistry is. Ask what and how the dental assistant is utilized in patient education. Knowledge is a powerful communication device between the dental assistant and his or her patients.

until fully erupted (see Figure 8.3 earlier in this chapter). Between the ages of about 6 years old and again around 12 to 14 years old, the jaw grows. The permanent teeth erupt into their place, replacing the primary teeth. The permanent molars are considered nonsuccedaneous teeth because they do not replace any primary teeth, but erupt behind them in the posterior of the arches.

Table 8-4 lists additional information about the ages when exfoliation occurs in the permanent dentition.

How would you explain the differences in the three dentitions of tooth development if you were having to explain it to a parent of one of your younger patients?

TABLE 8-4 Permanent Tooth Eruption Ages

Permanent Dentition	Eruption Age	
	Maxillary	Mandibular
Central incisors	7–8 yr	6–7 yr
Lateral incisors	8–9 yr	7–8 yr
Canines	11–12 yr	9–10 yr
First premolars	10–11 yr	10–12 yr
Second premolars	10–12 yr	11–12 yr
First molars	6–7 yr	6–7 yr
Second molars	12–13 yr	11–13 yr
Third molars	17–25 yr	17–25 yr

SUMMARY

Prenatal growth is an important time in the development of the oral cavity. This is when the stages of teeth development begin as well as the formation of other organs in the body. It is very important for the entire dental team to be aware of the structures and functions that occur throughout a lifetime. Dental assistants must be conscious of the different stages of tooth development. By having knowledge of prenatal growth and the course of development of oral embryology, the dental assistant will be able to communicate effectively with dental patients and their families regarding questions or concerns about changes occurring in the oral cavity.

Professionalism

One of the fun things about being a dental assistant is having the time to talk with patients. Patient education and communication are what sets fantastic dental assistants apart from good dental assistants. When the dental assistant has confidence and knows how to comfort a patient, that is when the dental assistant has moved from being a career dental assistant to being a professional dental assistant.

KEY TERMS

- **Apposition:** The process in which tissue and tooth formation occur; fourth stage of tooth development. p. 119
- **Attrition:** The wearing away of the chewing surface of the teeth during their normal function; final stage of tooth development.   p. 119
- **Calcification:** The process in which tissue becomes hardened due to calcium deposits; fifth stage of tooth development.   p. 119
- **Dentition:** Tooth arrangement; in position.   p. 116
- **Differentiation:** Changes in the function of cells in the tooth bud and development of teeth occurs; third stage of tooth development.   p. 118
- **Eruption:** The process of a tooth breaking through the gum tissue to grow into place in the mouth; sixth stage of tooth development.   p. 119
- **Exfoliation:** The normal process of losing, shedding, or falling out of primary teeth.   p. 124

- **Initiation:** The bud stage or start of tooth development; first stage of tooth development.   p. 117
- **Mixed dentition:** Mixture of permanent and primary teeth present in the mouth at same time; exists until all primary teeth fall out.   p. 116
- **Odontogenesis:** Tooth production; the origin and formation of the tooth.   p. 116
- **Permanent dentition:** Second set or succedaneous teeth.   p. 116
- **Primary dentition:** First set of 20 teeth; also called deciduous or baby teeth.   p. 116
- **Proliferation:** Production of new parts, the bud and early cap stages of tooth development.   p. 118
- **Succedaneous:** Refers to permanent teeth that replace primary teeth.   p. 116
- **Supernumerary teeth:** Extra teeth.   p. 121

CHECK YOUR UNDERSTANDING

1. Which of the following terms describes the teeth of the mouth in the dental arch?
   a. primary teeth
   b. dentition
   c. resorption
   d. exfoliation

2. By age 3 full eruption has occurred for all primary teeth. How many primary teeth are there?
   a. 16
   b. 20
   c. 22
   d. 32

3. In which of the following stages does the dental lamina, a membrane surrounding a small growth of epithelium, give form to the tooth or the tooth bud to begin development?
   a. proliferation
   b. initiation
   c. apposition
   d. attrition

4. Congenital missing teeth are
   a. missing from birth.
   b. missing after primary exfoliation.
   c. missing from permanent eruption.
   d. replacements for supernumerary teeth.

5. Which of the following abnormalities refers to uncommonly small teeth that may have the characteristic "peg shape" and usually occur on the upper lateral incisors?
   a. fused teeth
   b. microdontia
   c. macrodontia
   d. hypodontia

6. What is the strongest living tissue in the human body?
   a. mucous membrane
   b. permanent teeth
   c. tooth enamel
   d. alveolar bone

7. Which of the following teeth are not present in the primary dentition?
   a. incisors
   b. canines
   c. premolars
   d. molars

8. Which of the following is not a type of dentin?
   a. primary dentin
   b. secondary dentin
   c. permanent dentin
   d. reparative dentin

CHECK YOUR UNDERSTANDING (continued)

9. The development toward full permanent dentition begins with the eruption of which four teeth?
   a. central incisors
   b. canines
   c. first premolars
   d. first molars

10. The function of cementum is to anchor the tooth to the bony wall of the socket by connective tissue fiber called
   a. Sharpey's fibers.
   b. gingiva.
   c. interdental papilla.
   d. pulp chamber.

INTERNET ACTIVITIES

- Educational handouts are excellent sources for patient education. Various information, topics, and tips are available that can be sent home with your patient for reference. These handouts are fun to do, and patients enjoy obtaining information to reference later. Create your own handouts if necessary to provide further information to your patients. For a handout example, visit the following website: http://dentalcare.com/soap/patient/index.htm

- Read the excellent review "Lab Exercises: Tooth Development" at http://cellbio.utmb.edu/microanatomy/digestive/tooth.htm
- Go to the search engine www.google.com, enter "cleft palate," and use the results to research the information on this deformity.
- Research embryology at www.babycenter.com

WEB REFERENCES

- Abnormalities of Teeth http://dentistry.umkc.edu/practition/assets/AbnormalitiesofTeeth.pdf
- American Academy of Pediatric Dentistry www.aapd.org
- Preventive Care for Child Development www.craigentinny.co.uk/Children/tooth_development.htm

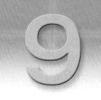

Dental Charting

Chapter Outline

- Dental Arches
- Dentition Periods
  —Primary Dentition
  —Permanent Dentition
- Types and Functions of Teeth
- Tooth Surfaces
- The Morphology of Teeth
- Angles and Divisions
- Stabilization of the Maxillary and Mandibular Arches
  —Occlusion
  —Malocclusion
- Tooth Numbering Systems
  —Universal Numbering System
  —Palmer Notation Method
  —FDI World Dental Federation Notation System
- Cavity Classification
- Dental Charting Procedures

Learning Objectives

After reading this chapter, the student should be able to:

- State the names and surfaces of primary and permanent teeth.
- Identify anatomic features and functions of various teeth.
- Describe the difference between ideal occlusion and malocclusion.
- Recognize common charting symbols and abbreviations.
- Distinguish between the different dental charting systems.
- Demonstrate the application of dental charting.

Preparing for Certification Exams

- Chart existing restorations and conditions.

Key Terms

Anterior	Lingual
Buccal	Mesial
Charting	Occlusal
Deciduous	Overbite
Distal	Overjet
Facial	Pit
Fissure	Posterior
Fossa	Proximal
Incisal	Quadrant
Interproximal	Succedaneous
Labial	

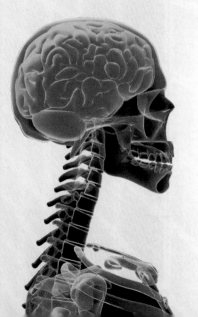

The term charting usually refers to any entry made in a patient's chart. In dentistry, however, the term generally refers to recording the dentist's findings when examining a patient's mouth. The dentist dictates these findings very quickly and with technical terminology. The dental assistant must be familiar with the terms, symbols, and abbreviations used in order to record the exam efficiently and accurately. This chapter focuses on the anatomic features of the teeth, including their various components and how they work together for oral health. The names and surfaces of the teeth will be discussed along with how they are used for dental charting procedures.

Dental Arches

The upper jaw is the maxillary arch or the maxilla. The lower jaw is the mandibular arch or the mandible. The mouth is further divided down the midline of the body, which then divides the mouth into four equal parts called quadrants. (**Quadrant** means one-fourth.) Teeth are described as being located in one of the four quadrants:

- Maxillary right quadrant (Quad 1): teeth 1–8
- Maxillary left quadrant (Quad 2): teeth 9–16
- Mandibular left quadrant (Quad 3): teeth 17–24
- Mandibular right quadrant (Quad 4): teeth 25–32

Dentition Periods

Normally, a human grows two sets of teeth during a lifetime. The first set of teeth, often called baby teeth, are properly named the primary or deciduous dentition. Primary teeth are shed as the jaw increases in size and are replaced by permanent dentition, which is designed to last the entire lifetime of an individual.

Dental Assistant PROFESSIONAL TIP

All states have regulations regarding direct/indirect supervision by a dentist. For indirect supervision, the dentist must first direct charting to be performed by the dental assistant. Upon direction of the dentist a competent dental assistant may begin charting existing restorations of a patient's mouth before the dentist arrives in the treatment room, if allowed by the state dental practice act. Using x-rays, the dental chart, colored pencils, and a mouth mirror, an efficient and motivated dental assistant can save time by beginning this procedure.

Primary Dentition

The first set of teeth to erupt through the gingival tissues into the mouth is the primary or deciduous dentition (Figure 9.1). The word **deciduous** means "to shed." Teeth begin forming before birth. The tooth buds are present in the maxilla and mandible. Usually the first teeth to appear in the mouth are the mandibular central incisors at around 6 months of age. By 1 year of age, the deciduous molars begin to erupt. All 20 primary teeth are usually present by age 3. There are five primary teeth in each quadrant: two incisors, one canine, and two molars.

The eruption pattern for the deciduous dentition is:

1. Central incisors
2. Lateral incisors
3. Deciduous first molars
4. Canines
5. Second molars

Eruption times can vary. There is a mixed dentition period that begins when the first permanent molars erupt at around age 6. Between 6 and 7 years of age, there are 20 deciduous teeth, 4 permanent first molars, and 28 permanent tooth buds in various stages of development. If deciduous teeth are retained too long, lost too soon, missing, or impacted by other teeth, the permanent dentition will be affected.

Permanent Dentition

The second set of teeth to erupt into the mouth is 32 permanent teeth, which replace the primary dentition. They are called the permanent dentition (Figure 9.2).

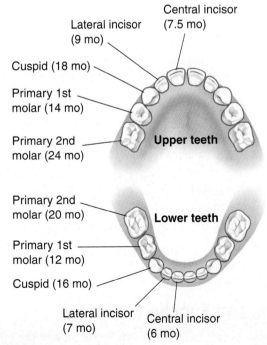

FIGURE 9.1
Primary dentition.

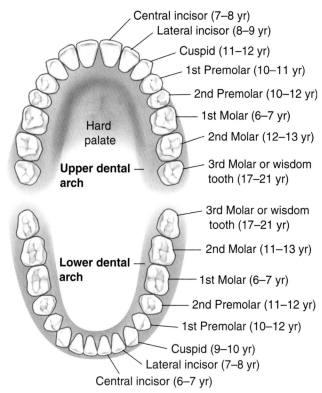

FIGURE 9.2
Permanent dentition.

The permanent teeth that replace deciduous teeth are called succedaneous teeth. **Succedaneous** means "to replace" or "succeed." There are eight permanent teeth in each quadrant: two incisors, one canine, two premolars, and three molars.

The permanent first molars usually erupt into the mouth at about age 6. From about age 6 until about age 12, all primary teeth loosen and are replaced by permanent teeth. The permanent first molars are the most important teeth for the development of adult dentition because they are the key to proper occlusion. The maxillary and mandibular occlusal relationships are established when the last of the deciduous teeth are lost. The mesiobuccal cusp of the maxillary molars should occlude with the central grooves of the mandibular molars. The permanent molars are nonsuccedaneous because they do not replace any primary teeth.

How many teeth are there in the permanent dentition? How many teeth are in the primary dentition? Which teeth are in the permanent dentition that are not in the primary dentition?

Types and Functions of Teeth

The tooth positioned immediately to the side of the midline is the central incisor, which occupies the central location in the arch. To the side of the central incisor is the lateral incisor. Next to the lateral incisor is the canine, due to its long cusp and location at the corners of the mouth. Next to that is the first premolar, then the second premolar. These are called premolars because they precede the molars. Following the second premolar is the first molar, followed by the second molar, then the third molar.

The **anterior** teeth are in the front of the mouth, whereas the **posterior** teeth are located in the back of the mouth. Anterior teeth include the central incisors, lateral incisors, and canines. The incisors have thin sharp edges and are used for biting and cutting. Canines are located at the corners of the mouth, have a single cusp, and are designed for cutting and tearing food. Canines have strong heavy roots and are useful as a guide in occlusal relationships, and for retaining prostheses.

The premolars and molars are posterior teeth. Premolars have two to three cusps, which are used to hold and crush food. The molars are wider and somewhat flat for chewing and grinding solid masses of food. Premolars have one to two roots with features similar to those of molars. Maxillary molars have three roots, two buccal roots, and one palatal root. Mandibular molars commonly have only two roots. Molars have four major cusps and somewhat flat occlusal surfaces.

Which teeth are considered anterior and which teeth are in the posterior of the mouth? Why are the molars shaped wide and flat?

Tooth Surfaces

Not only must the dental assistant be able to name and locate a tooth, he or she must also be able to identify various surfaces on a tooth, as shown in Figure 9.3. Each tooth has five surfaces. The **mesial** surface of a tooth is the surface facing toward the midline of the arch. The **distal** surface is the opposite of a mesial surface and is facing away from, or distant from, the midline. The **lingual** surface is the surface of a tooth next to the tongue. The **incisal** edge is only found on anterior teeth, and is the biting or cutting surface. The **occlusal** surface of a tooth is the chewing surface of posterior teeth only. The **facial** surface is the tooth surface toward the face. The **labial** surface is the tooth surface toward the lips of the anterior teeth only, and the **buccal** surface is next to or toward the cheek of posterior teeth only.

In dentistry common abbreviations are used to identify a single surface or a combination of two or more surfaces. A cavity may be referred to as being simple, compound, or complex. A simple cavity is one that involves only one surface. A compound cavity involves two surfaces, and a complex cavity involves three or more surfaces. When two or more surfaces are involved, the combined surfaces become one name and the letter *o* replaces the *-al* ending of the first surface. The common

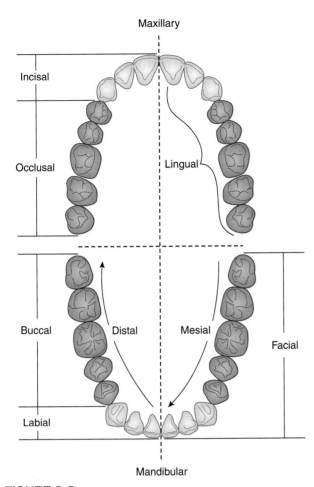

FIGURE 9.3
Tooth surfaces identified on the maxillary and mandibular arches. Posterior teeth are noted in brown.

TABLE 9-1 Abbreviations for One Tooth Surface

Tooth Surface	Abbreviation	Definition
Mesial	M	Surface of tooth toward the midline
Distal	D	Surface of tooth away from the midline
Lingual	L or Lg	Surface of tooth next to the tongue
Facial	F	Surface of tooth toward the face
Labial	La	Surface of tooth toward the lips
Buccal	B	Surface of tooth next to the cheek
Occlusal	O	Chewing surface of posterior teeth
Incisal	I	Biting or cutting edge of anterior teeth

TABLE 9-2 Abbreviations for More Than One Tooth Surface

Tooth Surfaces	Abbreviation
Mesio-occlusal	MO
Disto-occlusal	DO
Mesio-occlusodistal	MOD
Occlusobuccal	OB
Mesio-occlusodistobuccolingual	MODBL
Mesioincisal	MI
Distoincisal	DI
Occlusolingual	OL

abbreviations for one tooth surface are listed in Table 9-1 and for more than one tooth surface in Table 9-2.

Name the location of the following tooth surfaces: mesial, distal, occlusal, incisal, buccal, labial, and facial. What is the abbreviation for each of these surfaces?

The Morphology of Teeth

As discussed in Chapter 8, morphology is the study of the shape and form of teeth. The dental assistant must be familiar with several anatomic features of teeth and their terms. **Proximal** surfaces are tooth surfaces that are adjacent to each other in the same arch. Each tooth has two proximal surfaces: one is mesial and the other is distal. The proximal surface is the part of the tooth that touches the tooth next to it. This is also called a contact point. Between the proximal surfaces is the **interproximal** space. Dental professionals sometimes use the terms *proximal* and *interproximal* interchangeably. Some of the interproximal space is filled in by part of the gingival tis-sue called the interdental papilla. The V-shaped space extending in different directions from the contact point is referred to as the embrasure.

Embrasures extend to the facial, lingual, apical, and occlusal surfaces of a tooth, as shown in Figure 9.4. They are important because they allow food to be forced away from the contact areas, reduce the forces of occlusion, and permit a slight amount of stimulation to the gingiva. The cusp tips and incisal edges align so that there is a smooth curve of the maxillary and mandibular arches when the jaws are viewed from the side. This curvature of the occlusal plane is called the curve of Spee (Figure 9.5).

A tooth cusp is a point or peak on the occlusal surface of a premolar or molar and on the incisal edge of a canine. A ridge is any elevation on the surface of a tooth and is named according to its location and form such as

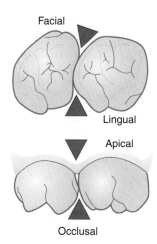

FIGURE 9.4
Tooth embrasures extend to the facial, lingual, apical, and occlusal surfaces.

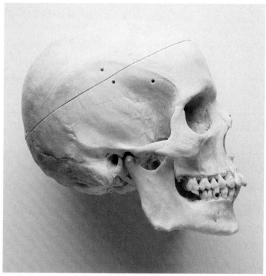

FIGURE 9.5
Curve of Spee.
Philip Dowell © Dorling Kindersley

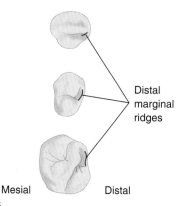

FIGURE 9.6
The marginal ridges of a central incisor, biscuspid, and molar.

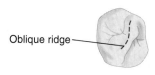

FIGURE 9.7
A maxillary first molar with the oblique ridge identified.

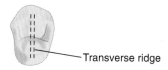

FIGURE 9.8
A maxillary right first bicuspid with the transverse ridge identified.

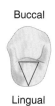

FIGURE 9.9
A triangular ridge identified on the occlusal surface of a maxillary second bicuspid.

a buccal ridge, an incisal ridge, and a marginal ridge. Marginal ridges are rounded borders of enamel that form the edges of the occlusal surface of premolars and molars on the mesial and distal sides of a tooth (Figure 9.6). An oblique ridge runs diagonally across the occlusal surface of maxillary molars (Figure 9.7). Two triangular ridges that join and cross the occlusal surface of a posterior tooth form a transverse ridge (Figure 9.8). Triangular ridges run from the tips of the cusps of the premolars and molars to the central pit of the occlusal surface (Figure 9.9).

A developmental groove is a shallow groove or line on the surface of a tooth. It represents the junction of primary parts during the developmental growth of the tooth. Buccal and lingual grooves are developmental grooves found on a tooth. A **fossa** is an irregularly shaped depression on the surface of a tooth. Pits and fissures are pinpoint or linear faults that are defects in the formation of a tooth. A **pit** is a small pinpoint depression on the sur-

face of a tooth caused by the failure of the union of developmental grooves (Figure 9.10). A **fissure** is a deep furrow running along a developmental groove.

Located at the gingival third on the lingual surface of an anterior tooth is a convex prominence of enamel called a cingulum. A mamelon is one of three prominences located on the incisal edge of a newly erupted incisor (Figure 9.11). Mamelons usually wear away and flatten over years of use.

Why are the contact areas the same as the proximal areas? What anatomic areas of a tooth would most easily collect plaque?

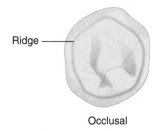

FIGURE 9.10
A permanent first bicuspid with occlusal pits identified.

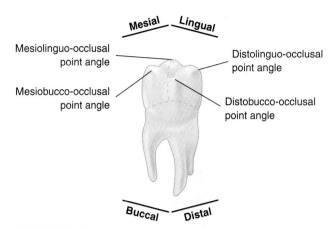

FIGURE 9.12
Line and point angles.

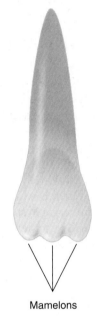

FIGURE 9.11
A newly erupted maxillary incisor showing mamelons on the incisal edge.

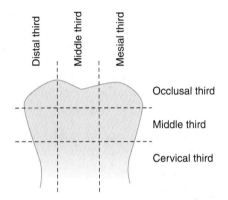

Angles and Divisions

It is helpful to understand teeth in terms of angles and divisions. The junction of any two surfaces of a tooth forms a line angle. A line angle is named by combining the names of the two surfaces. For example, *mesiolingual* and *mesiobuccal* are names of line angles. A point angle is formed by the junction of any three surfaces of a tooth and is named by combining the names of the three surfaces (Figure 9.12). The mesio-occlusobuccal point angle or the disto-occlusolingual point angle are examples.

Often for descriptive purposes, each surface of the tooth is divided into thirds, and each third is named according to the area in which it lies (Figure 9.13). The root is divided into the apical third, the middle third, and the gingival or cervical third. The crown may be divided into thirds in a parallel direction to the occlusal or incisal edge. Each tooth has an occlusal (or incisal) third, a middle third, and a gingival or cervical third. The crown is divided again vertically or longitudinally into a mesial third, middle third, and distal third.

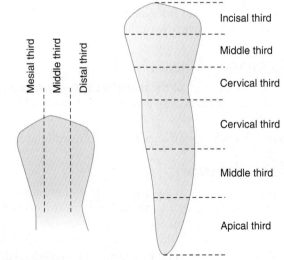

FIGURE 9.13
Tooth divisions.

What is the difference between a line angle and a point angle?

Stabilization of the Maxillary and Mandibular Arches

Properly aligned teeth stabilize each other. When teeth are lost or unable to erupt, the adjacent teeth shift and the teeth on the opposite arch supraerupt into the available space, causing malocclusion. Primary teeth are guides for permanent teeth. When children lose deciduous teeth prematurely, those more distal in the arch or the permanent first molars often drift forward, not leaving sufficient space for other permanent teeth to erupt into the mouth.

The teeth may drift, tip, or rotate if a primary tooth is lost prematurely. Occlusion changes with the shedding of primary teeth and the succession from primary to permanent dentition.

Occlusion

Occlusion is the relationship of the teeth on one dental arch to those teeth on the opposite arch. An ideal molar cusp and buccal relationship as described by Dr. Edward H. Angle, the "father of orthodontics," is for the mesiobuccal cusp of the maxillary first molar to fit into the buccal groove of the mandibular first molar.

Angle's classifications of occlusion are as follows:

Class I: Neutro-Occlusion

- Mesiobuccal cusp of the maxillary first molar fits into the mesiobuccal groove of the mandibular first molar.
- Also called *mesiognathic profile.*

Class II: Disto-Occlusion

- Mesiobuccal cusp of the maxillary first molar is mesial to the mesiobuccal groove of the mandibular first molar.
- Mandible appears to slightly retrude and maxilla appears protrusive; also called an overbite or retrognathic profile.

Class III: Mesio-Occlusion

- Mesiobuccal cusp of the maxillary first molar is distal to the mesiobuccal cusp groove of the mandibular first molar.
- Mandible is prognathic; also called an underbite.

Malocclusion

Malocclusion refers to an improper fit and misalignment of the teeth and jaws. A malocclusion is any degree of irregular contact of the teeth in the upper jaw with the teeth of the lower jaw; this includes overbites, underbites, and cross-bites. The maxillary teeth may overlap teeth in the mandibular arch. When the overlap is vertical, it is called an **overbite**. When the overlap is horizontal, it is called an **overjet**. Malocclusion can be caused by genetics or environmental factors. Some causes of malocclusion include the following:

- Small jaw size and large teeth
- Small teeth and large jaw
- Excessive thumb sucking beyond age 5
- Early or late loss of primary teeth
- Mouth breathing
- Tongue thrust when swallowing

How many types of occlusion did Dr. Angle identify and what are the differences between them? What is the difference between an overbite and an overjet? **?**

Tooth Numbering Systems

Numbering systems have been developed in order to create a standard way of referring to particular teeth. Two systems are commonly used in the United States. The Universal Numbering System has been adopted by the American Dental Association and is used by most general dentists and some orthodontists. Some U.S. orthodontists, pediatric dentists, and oral surgeons use the Palmer Notation Method. Internationally, the FDI World Dental Federation Notation System is widely used.

The Universal Numbering System and the FDI World Dental Federation Notation System are compatible with computer electronic charting, whereas the Palmer Notation Method is not used for computer charting.

Universal Numbering System

With the Universal Numbering System, the permanent teeth are numbered 1 through 32 (Figure 9.14), and the primary teeth are lettered from A through T (Figure 9.15). Each tooth has only one number or letter that refers only to that specific tooth. Tooth number 1 is the tooth farthest back on the right side of the patient's upper

Legal and Ethical Issues

A patient's chart is a valuable legal record and must be protected. Charts should never be left lying around. After use they must be returned to their proper place. They should also be stored where they are protected from fire, damage, and loss. If the patient's dental history and personal information are stored electronically, security should be put in place to ensure privacy. For example, security systems for dental records should limit access by unauthorized personnel, provide backup storage of records, and protect patients from disclosure without their consent. Human error accounts for the majority of data security problems. Employers are extremely cautious when hiring dental personnel in order to ensure confidentiality of patient information.

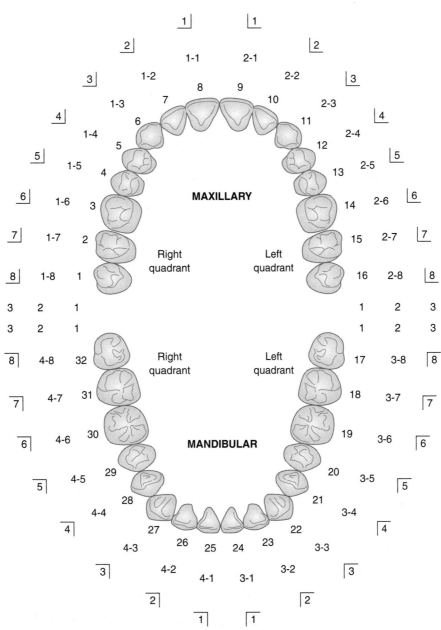

FIGURE 9.14
Tooth numbering system for permanent dentition.

jaw. Numbering continues along the upper teeth toward the front and across to the tooth farthest back on the top left, which is tooth number 16. The numbers continue by dropping down to the lower jaw. Tooth number 17 is the tooth farthest back on the patient's left side, on the bottom. Numbering continues again toward the front and across to the tooth farthest back on the bottom right, which is tooth number 32.

In this system, the teeth that should be there are numbered. If there are missing wisdom teeth, the third molars, then tooth numbers 1, 16, 17, and 32 would be missing and you would begin counting at tooth number 2.

In children, the system uses uppercase letters instead of numbers. A child's first tooth on the upper right would

be tooth A, and following the same order the last tooth on the lower right would be tooth T.

Palmer Notation Method

Using the Palmer Notation Method, the mouth is divided into four equal sections called quadrants. The numbers 1 through 8, and a unique symbol, are used to identify the teeth in each quadrant. The numbering runs from the center of the mouth to the back. For example, tooth number 1 is the incisor and the numbers continue to the right and back to the third molar, which is tooth number 8. The numbers sit inside an L-shaped symbol used to identify the quadrant (see Figure 9.14). The "L" is right side

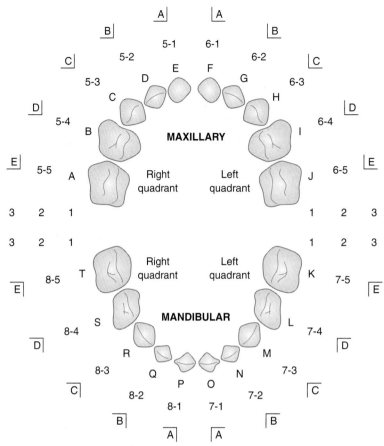

FIGURE 9.15
Tooth numbering system for primary dentition.

up and backwards for teeth in the upper right quadrant. The teeth in the upper left quadrant use a backward, but right side-up "L." For the lower quadrants, the "L" is upside down. Following the same order as for permanent teeth, primary teeth are lettered A through E in each quadrant with the same "L" symbols used to identify each quadrant (see Figure 9.15).

FDI World Dental Federation Notation System

The FDI (Federation Dentaire Internationale) World Dental Federation Notation System is a two-digit notation system that is commonly used internationally. For permanent teeth, the first digit designates the quadrant: 1 is for the upper right quadrant, 2 is upper left, 3 is lower left, and 4 is lower right. For the second digit, 1's are central incisors, 2's are lateral incisors, 3's are canines, 4's are first premolars, and so on, up through 8's, which designate third molars. The resulting tooth identification is a two-digit combination of the quadrant and tooth. For example, the upper right central incisor is 1-1 and the left is 2-1 (see Figure 9.14). The lower left permanent first molar is 3-6; however, it is not pronounced "thirty-six," but "three-six"; 1-1 is "one-one," not "eleven." The numbering for primary teeth using the FDI system is sim-

ilar. The difference is that the tooth two-digit combination starts with the number 5. For instance, the upper right quadrant first digit is 5, 6 is upper left, 7 is lower left, and 8 is lower right.

What are the most common types of dental charts used in the United States? How are the primary teeth lettered with this system? How are the permanent teeth numbered with this system?

Cavity Classification

Decay is the term commonly used to describe the disease process that results in destruction of tooth structure; *caries*, however, is the proper term to use when describing this process. Damage resulting from caries is technically known as a carious lesion. Caries can attack any surface of a tooth and often attacks more than one surface at a time. It can also attack root surfaces of a tooth if they are not properly protected by bone and gingiva.

Dr. G. V. Black, known as the "grand old man of dentistry," developed a system of cavity classification and preparation in the early 1900s that is still used today

G.V. Black's Classification of Dental Caries and Restorations		
Class	**Description**	**Pictorial View**
I	Pits and fissures of anterior and posterior teeth.	
II	Proximal surface of posterior teeth. Commonly involves occlusal surface.	
III	Proximal surface of anterior teeth not involving the incisal edge.	
IV	Proximal surface of anterior teeth involving the incisal edge.	
V	Cervical (gingival) 1/3 of the facial or lingual surface.	
VI	Incisal edge of anterior teeth or cusp tips of posterior teeth.	

FIGURE 9.16

G. V. Black's classification of dental caries and restorations.

(Figure 9.16). This system makes it possible to quickly and accurately describe the type and location of a cavity. To understand this system, the dental assistant must know what areas of the mouth and type of teeth will be involved. If necessary, refer to the abbreviations listed in Tables 9-1 and 9-2 as you read about the following classifications:

- *Class I:* all pits and fissures (B pit, L pit, O pit, OB, OL)
- *Class II:* caries of the occlusal and proximal surfaces of a posterior tooth (MO, DO, MOD, MODL, MODB, MODBL, MOB, MOL, DOB, DOL)
- *Class III:* caries of the proximal surface of an anterior tooth (M or D)
- *Class IV:* caries of the proximal and incisal edge of an anterior tooth (MI, DI)
- *Class V:* caries on the smooth surface at the gingival one-third of all teeth (F, L, B)
- *Class VI:* caries not due to the decay process, such as an abraded edge or cusp

---

What is the difference between Class III and Class IV cavities? Why are OB and OL cavities Class I and not Class II?

Professionalism

All dental health care providers should tend to their own oral health through periodic dental exams and radiographs so as to ensure that dentition and restorations are sound and remain caries free.

Dental Charting Procedures

It is always important to ensure that a medical history is completed first for every patient. Make sure the correct date and year are recorded. To record information manually in a patient's chart, be sure to use black ink to make entries under the services rendered area of the patient's chart. In the charting section make notations in colored pencil.

The dental assistant must know the terms the dentist will be using and be ready to use proper symbols to record the findings associated with the patient's mouth and dentition. The dental assistant must pay attention, listen carefully, and not be afraid to ask questions about anything he or she doesn't understand completely. Dental charting must be accurate. A mistake could cause the patient considerable pain and trouble.

Technology has created new opportunities for dentistry. Computer software programs are standardizing digital charting. Many software programs provide for oral charting methods, using a microphone, which frees the hands of dental health care providers, therefore offering more efficiency and less chance for cross-contamination of

Preparing for Externship

Review charting procedures before beginning your externship. Go through specific terms and definitions. Practice full mouth charting as often as you can so that you become more efficient and familiar with the symbols and abbreviations. Practice charting the mouths of fellow classmates in order to become as proficient as possible.

Life Span Considerations

As we age our dental restorations go through much wear and tear and often need to be replaced. Some patients may not realize this, so the dental assistant may need to explain that although dental restorative materials are excellent, they are not as good as the original tooth structure and do not last forever.

infectious organisms. A patient's chart can be easily accessed in a computer database and updated at each visit. Paperless dental records are becoming more popular because they save time and are an efficient means of storing patient records.

If done manually, dental charting is done with red and blue pencils. Solid blue or a blue outline is used to show existing restorations. Amalgam fillings that are in place and in good condition are solid blue. Composite fillings that are in place and in good condition are outlined in blue. Solid red is used to show caries or other conditions that require attention. Solid blue outlined in red is used to show that restorations are present but need

to be replaced. The need for replacement could be caused by faulty margins, fracture of a restoration or tooth, or recurrent decay. Examples of various dental charts are shown in Figures 9.17 through 9.20.

The dental assistant should be able to chart:

- Caries
- Single and multiple surface existing fillings (restorations)
- Missing teeth
- Teeth needing to be extracted
- Impacted teeth, both full and partial impactions
- All types of crowns, porcelain and gold
- Bridges, both present and required
- Partial and complete dentures
- Abscessed teeth
- Endodontically treated teeth, existing and required

What is used to record services rendered entries in a patient's record? What color is used to note treatment that is needed? What color denotes existing restorations?

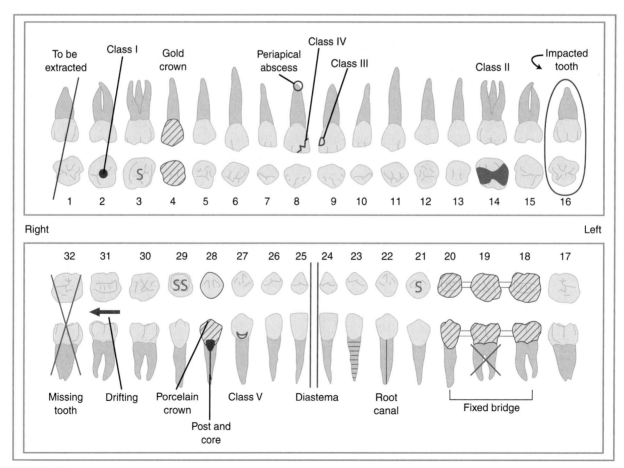

FIGURE 9.17
Example of an anatomic style dental chart with conditions of the mouth charted on a digital diagram.

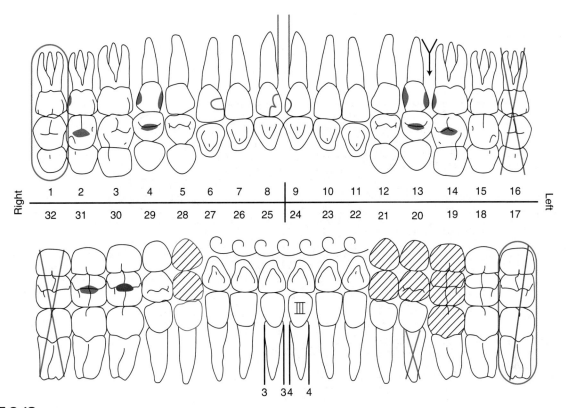

FIGURE 9.18
Example of an anatomic diagram with conditions of the mouth charted.

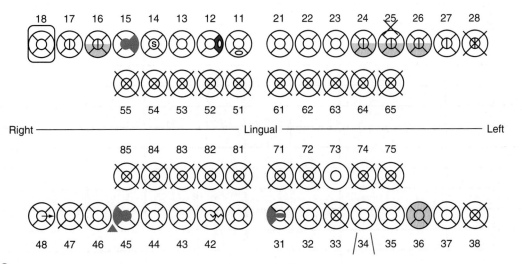

FIGURE 9.19
Charting using the geometric style chart and the international system.

DIAGNOSIS AND TREATMENT PLAN

PATIENT NAME	NITROUS LEVEL *(Verify level each time)*
	MEDICAL ALERT
PATIENT ACCOUNT NO.	PRE-MEDICATION

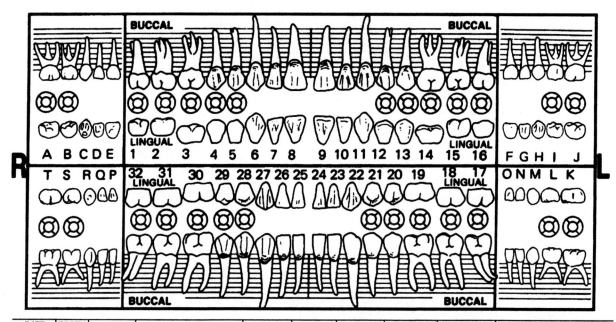

DATE DIAG.	TOOTH NO.	SURFACE	SERVICE NECESSARY	FEES	EST. INS. FEES	SEQUENCE OR PHASE	UNITS NEXT APPT.	DATE NEXT APPT.	COMMENTS

® Pride Institute   FORM 006   (03.97)   1.800.925.2600   www.prideinstitute.com

FIGURE 9.20

Example of a diagnosis and treatment plan form.

Courtesy Pride Institute—complete patient records for the dental office

SUMMARY

Both primary and permanent dentitions are important for an individual's oral and overall health. The primary teeth are replaced by permanent teeth, which are designed to last a person's lifetime. Each tooth has specific characteristics and functions. The dental assistant must understand the various anatomic parts and structures of each type of tooth and must be able to identify each tooth surface. Occlusion is how the teeth come together. Occlusion changes with development, maturity, and aging.

Dentistry uses abbreviations to quickly and easily recognize and name tooth surfaces and cavity classifications. The Universal Numbering System makes it possible to quickly identify specific teeth. In this system the permanent teeth are numbered 1 through 32 and the primary teeth are lettered A through T. The dental assistant must listen carefully in order to record the conditions of the patient's mouth as they are called out by the dentist.

Electronic charting via computer is being used as often as paper records. Charting software provides new opportunities for dentistry and standardizes data recording. It is an excellent visual for the dental team and is often used to provide a visual in educating patients about their dental conditions.

Cultural Considerations

Often, once the dentist discusses treatment options with a patient and leaves the area, patients will ask the dental assistant what he or she thinks they should do. Sometimes a language barrier prevents patients from understanding the treatment options. The dental assistant plays a significant role in making sure that patients understand what choices they have. Dental assistants need to ensure that their ideas regarding dental health coincide with the philosophy of the dentist who employs them so that the best decision can be made and communicated to the patient.

KEY TERMS

- **Anterior:** The front of the mouth or the front teeth.   p. 130
- **Buccal:** Surface next to or toward the cheek of posterior teeth.   p. 130
- **Charting:** The process of recording information about the patient's mouth and dentition.   p. 129
- **Deciduous:** The first set of teeth in a human; also known as primary.   p. 129
- **Distal:** Surface of tooth away from the midline.   p. 130
- **Facial:** Surface of tooth toward the face.   p. 130
- **Fissure:** A deep furrow running along a developmental groove.   p. 132
- **Fossa:** An irregularly shaped depression on the surface of a tooth.   p. 132
- **Incisal:** The biting or cutting edge of anterior teeth.   p. 130
- **Interproximal:** The space between adjacent contacts of teeth in the same arch.   p. 131

- **Labial:** Surface of tooth toward the lips.   p. 130
- **Lingual:** Surface of tooth next to the tongue.   p. 130
- **Mesial:** Surface of tooth toward the midline.   p. 130
- **Occlusal:** Chewing surface of posterior teeth.   p. 130
- **Overbite:** A vertical overlap of the maxillary teeth with the mandibular arch.   p. 134
- **Overjet:** A horizontal overlap of the maxillary teeth with the mandibular arch.   p. 134
- **Pit:** A small pinpoint depression on the surface of a tooth that is caused by the failure of the union of the developmental grooves.   p. 132
- **Posterior:** The back of the mouth.   p. 130
- **Proximal:** Place where a tooth contacts its neighbor in the same arch.   p. 131
- **Quadrant:** One-fourth of the mouth.   p. 129
- **Succedaneous:** Teeth that replace primary teeth.   p. 130

CHECK YOUR UNDERSTANDING

1. What is the term for the first set of teeth a human receives?
   a. primary
   b. maxillary
   c. permanent
   d. deciduous
   e. a and d

2. How many teeth are there in the permanent dentition?
   a. 20
   b. 32
   c. 28
   d. 30

CHECK YOUR UNDERSTANDING (continued)

3. The distal surface of a tooth is
   a. close to but not touching it.
   b. away from the midline.
   c. under the gingiva.
   d. touching the tongue.

4. What is the name of the tooth surface that cuts or tears?
   a. occlusal
   b. labial
   c. incisal
   d. buccal

5. The teeth that have occlusal surfaces are the
   a. incisors.
   b. canines.
   c. premolars.
   d. molars.
   e. both c and d.

6. What surface of the tooth is being touched by the tongue?
   a. mesial
   b. distal
   c. occlusal
   d. lingual

7. A composite restoration would be
   a. charted in solid blue.
   b. outlined in blue.
   c. charted in solid red.
   d. charted in solid blue and outlined in red.

8. Tooth number 14 is found in which quadrant?
   a. upper right
   b. upper left
   c. lower right
   d. lower left

9. A Class V cavity is located at the
   a. pits and fissures.
   b. occlusal surface.
   c. gingival one-third.
   d. proximal surface.

10. Caries can attack
    a. one surface.
    b. two or more surfaces.
    c. root surfaces.
    d. all of the above.

INTERNET ACTIVITY

- Go to http://patterson.eaglesoft.net/cnt_c_reschart.html to see a demonstration of dental software uses.

WEB REFERENCES

- Colgate® Professional.com   http://colgateprofessional.com
- The University of Texas Medical Branch   www.utmb.edu
- The Dental Place   www.brushfloss.com/faq.htm

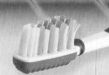

10

Oral Pathology

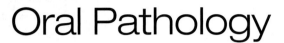

Learning Objectives

After reading this chapter, the student should be able to:

- Describe the classic signs of inflammation.
- Identify oral lesions according to their appearance and location.
- Identify oral diseases and lesions related to biological, physical, and chemical agents.
- Explain conditions associated with the tongue.
- Describe oral lesions associated with HIV/AIDS.
- Recognize the oral conditions that are related to developmental disturbances.
- Describe various disorders affecting the oral cavity.

Preparing for Certification Exams

- Define oral pathology.
- Describe the inflammation process.
- Identify placements of oral lesions in relation to the oral cavity.
- Describe oral lesions.
- Describe the oral conditions related to developmental disturbances.
- Identify lesions of oral neoplasms.
- Identify oral lesions associated with HIV and AIDS.
- Distinguish between systemic and localized infection.

Key Terms

Abscess

Aphthous ulcers

Basal cell carcinoma

Candida albicans

Carcinoma

Exudate

Herpetic whitlow

Hyperplasia

Kaposi's sarcoma

Leukoplakia

Obturator

Sarcoma

Squamous cell carcinoma

Tori

Chapter Outline

- Diseases and Conditions Affecting the Oral Cavity
  - The Effects of Infection on the Oral Cavity
  - Recognizing Abnormal Conditions in the Oral Cavity
- Oral Lesions
  - Lesions Below the Oral Mucosa Surface
  - Lesions Lying Above the Mucosal Surface
  - Lesions Lying Flat or Even with the Oral Mucosa Surface
  - Lesions Lying Flat or Above the Oral Mucosa Surface
  - Oral Manifestations from Biological Diseases
  - Oral Manifestations Due to Physical Causes
  - Oral Piercings
  - Oral Manifestations Caused by Chemicals
- Conditions of the Tongue
- Oral Cancer
  - Neoplasms
- Oral Conditions Due to HIV and AIDS
- Developmental Disorders
  - Tooth Development Disturbances
- Miscellaneous Disorders
- CDC Rankings of Evidence
- Environmental Infection Control

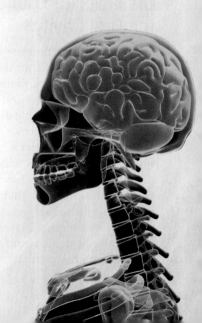

Oral pathology is defined as the

study of diseases that occur in the oral cavity. The practice of oral pathology includes research; diagnosis of diseases using clinical, radiographic, microscopic, biochemical, or other examinations; and management of patients. It is one of the nine specialties officially recognized by the American Dental Association and the federal government. Because of this recognition, it has its own national certifying board, the American Board of Oral and Maxillofacial Pathology.

A basic knowledge of oral pathology is important for a dental assistant to acquire. This knowledge provides the ability to distinguish between normal and abnormal findings in the mouth. The head and neck regions as well as the oral cavity are common places for abnormal findings. Oral pathology includes descriptions of abnormalities and diseases of the oral cavity. Abnormal conditions found in the mouth can be caused by many different disturbances, such as biological, chemical, hormonal, or nutritional effects. Even too much stress in a patient's life can precipitate a condition that may be exhibited within the oral cavity.

Diseases and Conditions Affecting the Oral Cavity

Signs and symptoms of systemic or infectious diseases may be exhibited within the oral cavity. Some systemic diseases such as measles, mumps, or tetanus can involve the oral cavity. Measles and mumps are considered to be childhood communicable diseases, but adults are susceptible to these diseases as well. In the early stage of the disease, measles affect the oral cavity by an outbreak of small erythematous macules with white necrotic centers that are called Koplik's spots. Mumps is a viral infection of the parotid glands that is characterized by painful swelling of the salivary glands and the bilateral swelling of the parotid glands (Figure 10.1).

Tetanus is an acute infectious disease caused by the toxin of the tetanus bacillus microorganism. Tetanus can

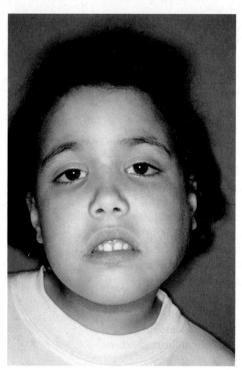

FIGURE 10.1
The effects of mumps on the parotid glands.

be localized at the wound site or can manifest in a person's muscles or joints. The first symptom tetanus causes in the head or neck is stiffness of the jaw, also known as "lockjaw." The person who has lockjaw could have difficulty swallowing due to the effect that tetanus has on muscles in the neck and throat.

The Effects of Infection on the Oral Cavity

The body has a number of mechanisms to protect itself from injury. Intact skin or mucosa is one such mechanism that provides a barrier against injury or invading organisms. Tears, urine, diarrhea, and saliva are considered to be other types of protection as evidenced by their flushing actions. When the body responds to disease and injury, it involves a process in which specialized cells in

---

Dental Assistant PROFESSIONAL TIP

Before being able to recognize abnormal conditions in the oral cavity, the dental assistant must have a good understanding of what normal conditions appear like in the oral cavity. As a dental assistant, the terms associated with pathological conditions of the head and neck should be understood and be part of everyday professional communications in the clinical setting. This understanding and daily usage will allow the dental assistant to converse professionally with others about these conditions. It is very important to remember that a dental assistant must never diagnose a disease and inform the patient; instead, the dental assistant must always discuss the concern with the dentist.

the area of the disease or injury release chemicals. These chemicals cause an inflammatory process that is part of the immune response. One of these chemicals is called histamine. Histamine helps to bring about the inflammatory process by increasing the blood flow to the area involved, which in turn causes redness (erythema) and heat. The increased blood flow floods the capillaries, causing the excess fluid to seep into the tissues and cause the condition of edema. Edema is a common swelling from fluid that can accompany an injury or a disease. Pain may accompany the swelling as the nerve endings become stimulated by the released chemicals.

Inflammation occurs regardless of the type of injury incurred. The extent and duration of an injury determines how much and how long the inflammatory process stays in the body. Inflammation may remain localized at the site of the injury or, if the injury is extensive, the inflammatory process may become systemic and spread throughout the body. If the injury is minimal, then the inflammatory process may be defined as acute inflammation, meaning of short duration. Chronic inflammation occurs when the injury is extensive or long lasting. This type of inflammation can lead to further tissue injury. When chronic inflammation becomes systemic, the classic signs of inflammation are present as well as the systemic signs of fever, increased white blood cells, and swelling of the lymph nodes (Figures 10.2 and 10.3). If the body is unable to protect itself, usually it is because the immune system is not functioning properly. When the immune system does not function properly, the body is then susceptible to the invasion of other microorganisms and diseases that are known as opportunistic.

Recognizing Abnormal Conditions in the Oral Cavity

Dental assistants have an important role in recognizing abnormal conditions in the oral cavity and observing changes in the patient's skin and oral mucosa. The dental assistant may be the first person in the dental office to see

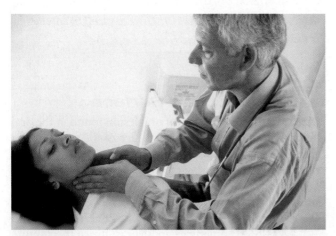

FIGURE 10.2
Checking a patient for swelling of the lymph nodes.

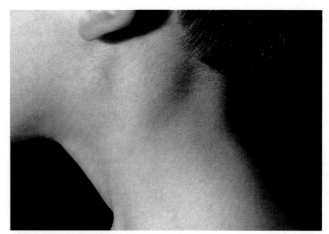

FIGURE 10.3
Swelling of the lymph glands is called lymphadenopathy.

the patient's mouth, for example, when taking x-rays for an initial exam. The dental assistant should be alert to recognize the signs of any abnormal pathology. When working in four-handed dentistry during a dental examination, the dental assistant is positioned on one side of the patient, while the dentist is positioned at the head of the patient. The dental assistant's position provides a different view of the oral cavity than that of the dentist; therefore, the dental assistant may view an abnormal condition that the dentist is not able to see from his or her view of the oral cavity. Though the dentist is responsible for making the diagnosis, the dental assistant can discreetly point out the area of concern to the dentist. The dental assistant should study the appearance of normal oral conditions in order to recognize what is abnormal.

Oral Lesions

An oral lesion is defined as any abnormal tissue appearing in the mouth. During a clinical examination, if a lesion is noted, the dentist will palpate the area with his or her fingers and perform a visual examination of the suspicious area. Lesions in the oral cavity can be found in these locations:

- Below the surface of the oral mucosa
- Above the surface of the oral mucosa
- Flat or even with the oral mucosa
- Raised or elevated above the oral mucosa

The classification of lesions helps to establish if the changes in the tissues are normal occurrences or if the changes in the tissues are abnormal and should be studied further. Tissue changes can result in various types of oral lesions. Lesions are categorized into four different classifications: size, appearance, texture, and location on the surface of the mucosa. When palpating the lesion, the dentist will describe the texture of the lesion as either soft, firm, semifirm, or fluid filled. The lesion is also determined to be either fixed (found in bone or on hard tissues) or movable (found within or on soft tissues). The lesion will also be described by its color: red, white, pink, brown, black, gray, salmon, or blue-black.

The next step in classifying a lesion is to obtain a measurement of its size. Lesions are measured by using the millimeter end of a periodontal probe or by using a centimeter ruler in order to describe the length, width, and height of the lesion. The dentist may further describe the lesion by its surface texture as being corrugated or wrinkled, by determining whether the surface is smooth or rough, or by checking whether it is elevated above the surface of the mucosa.

Radiographs are another examination method employed by dentists to help diagnose conditions that cannot be seen clinically. Radiographs can help determine the developmental stage of a lesion. Depending on the stage of the lesion, the radiograph may show light (radiopaque) or dark (radiolucent) areas of the lesion. Radiographs are used to determine if the lesion is in the bone and/or tissue.

A very useful diagnostic method for detection of lesions is the VELscope. The VELscope is a handheld device that emits a safe blue light into the oral cavity. The light provides a direct visualization of tissue fluorescence. Any suspicious tissue will appear dark due to loss of fluorescence.

To further aid the diagnosis of an oral lesion, the dentist may perform a biopsy. A biopsy is a surgical method that aids in the diagnosis of a lesion. The type of biopsy depends on the type of tissue that is involved and where the lesion is located. Some of the most common forms of biopsies performed include:

- A punch biopsy, in which a small disk-shaped amount of the lesion is removed
- An incisional biopsy, in which a sample of tissue or cells is removed
- An excisional biopsy, in which the entire lump of the lesion is removed, along with a border of normal tissue that surrounds the lesion that is defined by the depth, length, and width of the existing lesion
- A brush biopsy, in which cellular material is collected on a small brush, which is then transferred to a glass slide. This particular biopsy is noninvasive and is a simple chairside procedure. It is used to determine if an oral lesion has any cancerous cells

In addition to these types of biopsies, an important diagnostic tool is the ViziLite method of applying a toluidine dye to the affected mucosa. The dye shows where suspected lesions are on the oral surface. This specific test checks for certain kinds of cancer. The biopsy is then sent to a pathology laboratory where a pathologist examines the biopsy with a microscope. The pathologist further diagnoses the biopsy by identifying the etiology or the cause of the disease.

The dentist provides background about the lesion in a written report to the pathologist by describing what he or she observed clinically in the oral cavity. Other information that is important to document and report to the pathologist includes general information on the patient's health and current medications, how long the lesion has been present, if it is painful, and if the patient can indicate the cause of the lesion.

In order for the dentist to make an accurate diagnosis, he or she must gather clinical information that pertains to the patient and the patient's condition or lesion that is present. The dentist relies not only on the clinical findings, but on the patient's medical and dental history, radiographic surveys, and existing symptoms and conditions. Each piece of information is a necessary component of being able to provide a diagnosis for a patient. Sometimes, the dentist must use a differential diagnosis when there is more than one possible cause for a condition. A differential diagnosis is a systematic approach that includes the consideration of all likely causes of the patient's given symptoms. The dentist then proceeds to rule out the less likely causes. This process helps the dentist make a final diagnosis.

During the oral examination, the dental assistant assists the dentist by recording clinical information obtained from the patient's oral examination. The dental assistant also prepares the patient for necessary x-rays, develops the x-rays, and mounts the x-rays correctly. If the patient is scheduled for a biopsy during the appointment, the dental assistant sterilizes the necessary instruments and items for the procedure. Once the tissue specimen has been collected, the dental assistant fills out the necessary form that accompanies the specimen, then puts the form along with the specimen container into a specified and labeled container for mailing to the laboratory.

After the surgical procedure has been performed, the dental assistant will need to discuss with the patient post-operative instructions and home health care instructions before the patient is released. The dental assistant also cleans the operatory and performs disinfection of the operatory in preparation for the next scheduled patient.

Why is the accurate documentation of a patient's clinical examination so important to the patient's overall oral health?

Lesions Below the Oral Mucosa Surface

An ulcer is a common type of oral lesion found in the oral cavity that extends below the surface of the oral mucosa (Figure 10.4). Its appearance is similar to the shape of a crater. An ulcer may be very small or it can be as large as several centimeters. The presence of an ulcer means that the epithelium has lost its continuity. The center of an ulcer is often a grayish to yellow color that is surrounded by a red border. Sometimes an ulcer is due to the rupture of an elevated lesion, such as a pustule or vesicle.

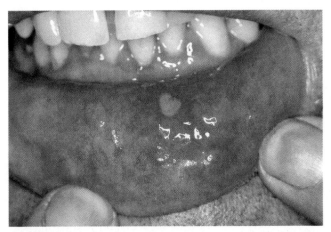

FIGURE 10.4
An ulcer found in the mouth.

An erosion (a sore or wound) of the soft tissue is usually due to a mechanical injury such as chewing. An erosion has ragged or uneven margins and may be painful, though it does not extend through the epithelium to the deeper tissues. If the erosion is irritated continually, it will not heal and it can then become an ulcer.

A cyst is an example of a lesion that extends below the mucosal surfaces. A cyst can be fluid filled or semi-solid. The material found in a cyst is not always infectious. A common cyst in the oral cavity is usually found around the crown of an unerupted tooth. The most common teeth that are affected by cysts are impacted third molars. This type of cyst is considered to be a developmental cyst that is related to the development of the tooth. The cyst forms when the crown of the tooth is completely formed and calcified, but has a thin enamel epithelium. Fluid tends to accumulate between the crown and the thin enamel epithelium. This cyst is known as an odontogenic or dentigerous cyst. Dentigerous cysts can form around the crowns of other unerupted or impacted teeth besides third molars, such as supernumerary teeth. Upon radiographic examination, this type of cyst appears as a radiolucency around the crown of the tooth. Treatment for a patient who has a dentigerous cyst often involves complete removal of the cyst as well as the tooth. If the cyst is not removed, it will continue to enlarge, causing damage to the surrounding bone and tissues.

Badly decayed teeth can result in an **abscess**. An abscess is an area that has a concentration of pus or **exudates** (dead cells and cellular debris) as a result of an infection by bacteria. An abscess can be either a periodontal abscess or a periapical abscess. When the infection from the bacteria affects the soft tissues of the periodontium, it is called a periodontal abscess. The patient who has a periodontal abscess may show signs of swelling and pain, have swollen gingival tissues, and the tooth may extrude (move upward from the gingiva) or feel loose. The treatment for this condition is to incise the periodontal pocket and drain the exudate (pus). Upon radiographic examination, the dentist will view the radi-

ographs for a radiolucent area next to the tooth, which may indicate a periodontal abscess or a cyst.

The periapical abscess forms at the apical or terminal end of a root of a tooth. The patient who has a periapical abscess may show signs of severe pain, sensation of pressure, redness, or have a fistula. A fistula is the body's way of creating a passageway for drainage of the abscess to the external surface of the gingiva. In this type of abscess, the inflammation has extended beyond the tooth apex into a localized area. All of the tissue in this area is destroyed because of the acidic environment. If an abscess is left untreated, the infection at the terminal end of the root(s) of the tooth can spread into the bloodstream and travel via the bloodstream, affecting numerous body systems and possibly causing life-threatening medical condition(s). Treatment for a periapical abscess may include antibiotic therapy, extraction of the tooth, or root canal therapy. Radiographically, a periapical abscess will appear as a radiolucency at the apex of the root of the tooth (Figure 10.5).

Lesions Lying Above the Mucosal Surface

A blister or a vesicle is a raised, fluid-filled area that results from some type of trauma or disease. The fluid in a blister is for the protection of the underlying damaged tissue. Blisters can vary in size, whereas vesicles remain small. Blisters are rarely seen in the oral cavity. A fluid-filled blister that is more than one-half inch in diameter is called a bulla.

A pustule is a small elevated yellow lesion on the skin or mucosa that contains pus, which is like a type of blister. During its noninfective stage, it can look similar to a stye (small bump) or look similar to pustules on the skin of a person with acne. A lesion that ranges in size from a pinhead to less than one-half inch in diameter is called a papule. This elevated lesion is also seen above the surface of the skin or above the surface of the mucosa. Papules

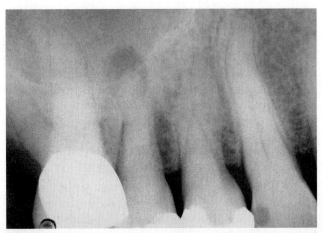

FIGURE 10.5
Radiograph showing a periapical cyst with a large abscess at its root.

are solid lesions that do not contain fluid. They are defined by by their shape and how they are attached. Papules may appear as pointed or rounded lesions or they can have flat tops. If the papule is attached by a slender stalk, it is called a pedunculated lesion. If the base is as wide as the lesion, then it is said to be a sessile lesion. Its surface can be pigmented, smooth, or bumpy in appearance.

A bruise or a hematoma is a lesion that resembles a blister, but is filled with blood caused by a ruptured blood vessel. A hematoma following a dental injection can happen if a blood vessel is infiltrated during the injection. When this condition occurs, the dentist will apply pressure to the site.

Lesions Lying Flat or Even with the Oral Mucosa Surface

An area of skin that appears different in texture or color is called a patch. A macule appears as a different color or texture on the skin. Purplish or reddish-brown areas or spots of discoloration are called purpura. Purpura can range in size from a small pinhead diameter up to one inch. Purpura are caused by bleeding into the tissues. Small purpura are called petechiae, whereas larger areas are called ecchymosis or bruises.

Lesions Lying Flat or Above the Oral Mucosa Surface

A small lump of tissue, either firm or soft, and more than one-quarter inch in diameter is called a nodule. A nodule can form beneath the tissues or in the upper layers of tissues and can be seen as a small lump at the skin surface.

A tumor is an abnormal growth that can be either benign (noncancerous) or malignant (cancerous). The medical term used for tumor is *neoplasm* (new growth). A neoplasm forms from an abnormal accelerated growth of cells. A lesion that is associated with chronic inflammation and the formation of a neoplasm or tumor is known as a granuloma, which may contain granulation tissue. A granuloma can be found on gingival tissue as a swollen area or it can be seen radiographically at the apex of a nonvital tooth. Repeated trauma to an area can result in a lesion called traumatic granuloma. As an example, this can occur when someone impinges on the tissues repeatedly while brushing her teeth.

Oral Manifestations from Biological Diseases

Many different microorganisms can cause lesions and oral diseases. Actinomycosis is a chronic infection caused by an anaerobic (without oxygen) bacterium (Figure 10.6). The bacterium, *Actinomyces israelii*, is a common, usually nonpathogenic organism found in the throat and nose. *Actinomyces* causes disease when it is introduced into tis-

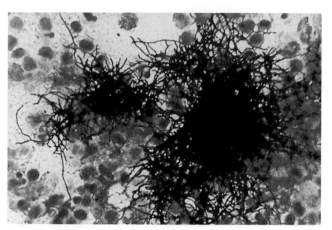

FIGURE 10.6

A Gram-stained specimen from a patient with actinomycosis. The lesion included yellow granules containing *Actinomyces israelii*. Reprinted by permission of INFECTIONS in MEDICINE, Vol. 9, No. 9, 1992. Copyright © 1992 SCP Communications, Inc.

sues by trauma, surgery, or infection though it is unclear why this organism occasionally causes disease. The most common form of the disease is the formation of abscesses that drain via a sinus tract. This lesion first presents as a painful swelling and then later produces pus with yellow granular discharge. Eventually, the abscess breaks through the skin surface to produce drainage. Treatment for actinomycosis is long-term use of high doses of antibiotics.

Tuberculosis (TB) is the infectious disease that causes primary lung infection. It is caused by the organism *Mycobacterium tuberculosis,* which is spread by droplet infection from an infected person's cough. If infected, after a few weeks, the symptoms emerge as fever, chills, fatigue, weight loss, malaise, and persistent cough. Under a microscope the biopsy sample of the affected area will show a TB granuloma. The tongue and palate are the common sites for the tuberculosis lesion in the oral cavity. The lesion can occur anywhere in the oral cavity; even in the bone, as osteomyelitis (inflammation of the bone marrow). The lesions are painful, nonhealing, and slowly grow into large ulcerations that can be either very deep or superficial.

A Mantoux test, also known as a tuberculin skin test, is given to determine if a person has been exposed to or is infected with tuberculosis (Figure 10.7). This test is performed by injecting pure protein derivative (PPD) with a sterile needle and syringe into the top layer of the skin on the inner surface of the forearm. Two to three days later, the skin reaction is measured. This test will show positive results (a large reddened and swollen skin reaction) if the person has been exposed to *Mycobacterium tuberculosis*; however, this does not mean that the person has the active disease. It just means that they have been infected with the TB germs and that they have a chance of becoming ill. Sometimes, people can be exposed to TB germs without getting the actual disease.

Effective treatment for tuberculosis has been available since the 1940s. Though the reemergence of the disease was prevalent in crowded urban areas in the 1980s,

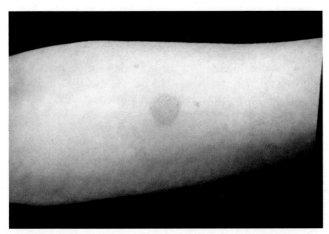

FIGURE 10.7
A patient who shows a positive Mantoux test for tuberculosis.

that reemergence was due to noncompliance of individuals for treatment therapy and for those who have human immunodeficiency virus (HIV) infection. Through public health efforts for tuberculosis treatment, the disease is reported to be on the decline for U.S.-born persons. The Centers for Disease Control and Prevention (CDC) has reported a 7.0% decline from 2005 and a 68% decline from 1993 for this category. However, the rates for foreign-born persons are reported to have increased. Other groups affected with high numbers of TB include migrant farmers and those individuals who are HIV positive.

For the dental health care worker, the practice of routine universal precautions is important to help prevent transmission of diseases from airborne droplet infections. Herpes labialis, commonly called fever blisters or cold sores, are found on and around the lips (Figure 10.8). These blisters are painful and can be solitary or appear in clusters. Herpes labialis is a form of the herpes simplex virus type 1 (HSV-1), which affects the body above the waist. In the work environment, this virus can last up to four hours on countertops or work surfaces. Dental assistants need to be aware that this virus is transmitted from the patient during the vesicular stage and during the crusted stage through direct contact and especially if barriers are not used.

If there is a break in the skin of the hands and this break in the skin is accessible to the virus, **herpetic whitlow** may occur. Herpetic whitlow, which is extremely painful, occurs as a crusting ulceration on the fingers or the hands (Figure 10.9). If infected with herpes whitlow, the dental professional will most likely be unable to work due to the high rate of contagion associated with it. It is advisable to delay routine treatment until the lesion subsides.

Herpetic gingivostomatitis is a term used to describe a disease that is normally seen in children from ages 6 months to about 6 years. This disease is caused by HSV-1. It is characterized by painful, erythematous, swollen gingiva with multiple tiny vesicles on the skin around the mouth, on the lips, and on the oral mucosa. The vesicles progress into ulcers. The infection is passed from person to person through contact with saliva that contains the virus, which can occur, for example, if two individuals drink out of the same glass or use the same eating utensil.

Herpes simplex virus type 2 (HSV-2) may appear in the oral cavity but usually affects the body below the waist with genital herpes. Anyone who has vesicular ulcerations for more than a month should be tested for immunodeficient diseases, such as HIV.

The varicella zoster virus causes chickenpox and shingles, both of which are contagious. Chickenpox is highly contagious. It causes vesicular and pustular lesions on the skin and on the mucous membranes (Figure 10.10). Headache, fever, and malaise are common systemic symptoms that accompany chickenpox. Recovery occurs in two to three weeks. The vaccine developed for chickenpox is called Varivax and may be given to children ages 6 months to 12 years.

Herpes zoster or shingles is a reactivation of the varicella zoster virus in adults. It manifests as painful clusters of unilateral lesions that can last up to five weeks. Although the lesions will resolve within five weeks, the

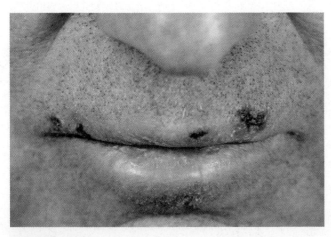

FIGURE 10.8
Cold sores caused by herpes simplex.

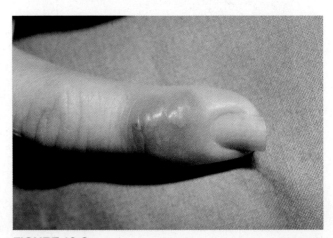

FIGURE 10.9
Herpetic whitlow.

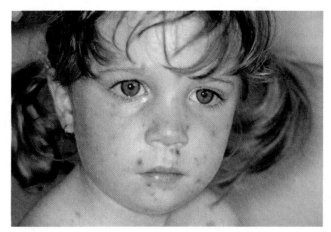

FIGURE 10.10
A child with chickenpox.

pain from inflammation to the nerve endings may last for several months. Adults who have a weakened immune system or who take immunosuppression drugs are prone to shingles. When someone has chickenpox, the virus stays or lies dormant in the nerve tracts along the spine and then reactivates as shingles at a time when the person's immune system is weak. Shingles on the face can have various effects, as seen in Figure 10.11. Treatment for shingles is aimed at relieving the symptoms. In 2006 a vaccine for shingles, called Zostavax, was approved by the U.S. Food and Drug Administration (FDA).

Aphthous ulcers known as canker sores are common ulcerations that can recur in the oral cavity (Figure 10.12). The tendency to develop these ulcers is inherited, though other factors may be causative. These ulcers are not contagious and patients may have from one to six sores at a time. Aphthous ulcers last from 10 to 14 days. Clinically, these ulcers appear circular with yellow necrotic centers that have red (erythematous) halos. The cause is unknown, but trauma from accidents as well as trauma resulting from dental appointments, stressful situations, food allergens, vitamin deficiencies, or hormonal changes are associated with the recurrence of aphthous ulcers.

There are three types of recurrent aphthous ulcer lesions: minor, major, and herpetic forms. Minor aphthous ulcers are less than one centimeter in diameter and occur more commonly in the anterior portion of the mouth. Usually, an individual will experience a burning sensation 1 to 2 days before the lesions appear. Healing from these lesions may take 7 to 14 days. Major ulcers (also called Sutton's disease) are more than one-half inch in diameter and take longer to heal than minor ulcers and

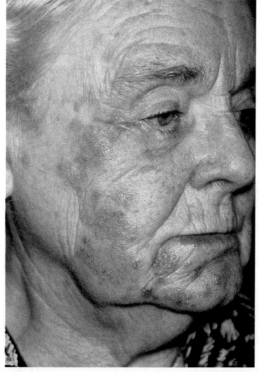

FIGURE 10.11
An older woman affected with shingles. Notice how the virus has affected the mandibular branch of the trigeminal cranial nerve, which supplies the jaw.

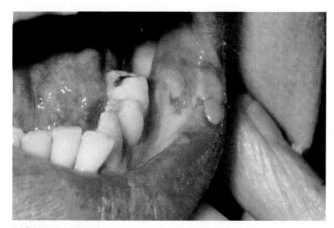

FIGURE 10.12
Aphthous ulcer on the inside of a patient's lower lip.

can leave scars. Herpetic ulcers are a rare form of ulcers that have clusters of dozens of smaller ulcers and can develop anywhere in the oral cavity.

Oral Manifestations Due to Physical Causes

Some conditions in the oral cavity result from physical causes. For instance, ulcerations due to self-induced trauma to the tissues include bites to the inside of the cheek, accidental falling involving striking the mouth, or even wearing an ill-fitting dental appliance. During dental care, the dental team should be careful to not induce trauma while using dental instruments, high-volume evacuators (HVEs), or cotton rolls. The dental assistant must watch constantly the transfer of materials and instruments to and from the mouth of a patient during dental care. For instance, gingival ulcers can be induced during dental procedures when removing overly dry cotton rolls. If removed quickly, the dry cotton can pull on and peel off the epithelial layer of the mucosa. Before removing cotton rolls, the assistant should wet the cotton rolls and remove slowly.

Hyperplasia (tissue overgrowth) due to denture irritation is usually caused by an ill-fitting denture that rubs an area in the oral cavity, causing it to become irritated and sore. If the irritation is not corrected, the irritated tissue will soon become folds of excess tissue, termed epulis fissuratum. If the irritation is in the palatal area, the rugae can swell and become nodular. This can be resolved if the patient leaves the dentures out for a few days. The treatment for an ill-fitting denture is to adjust the denture or in some cases remake the denture. Placement of soft liners is another option in some cases. Temporarily, an over-the-counter local anesthetic ointment can be prescribed by the dentist to ease the pain.

Amalgam tattoo occurs when amalgam particles are induced into the gingival tissue and become trapped during a restorative or surgical procedure. The gingival tissue in this area develops a blue or gray color. No treatment is necessary when this happens, because it is harmless to the patient. To prevent it, however, the dental assistant should thoroughly rinse the area after a restorative or surgical procedure is completed in order to remove the excess particles. The use of a dental dam during a dental procedure can also help.

Radiation treatment injury may result from radiation treatment received and administered for the treatment of cancer. Mucous membranes and the glands of the oral cavity and in the head and neck region are especially sensitive to radiation effects. Dental implications from radiation treatments are usually specific to the area that is exposed. Because radiation therapy kills cancer cells by shrinking blood vessels, the blood vessels in the radiated area will not support the blood flow that is needed for normal healing to take place.

Radiation mucositis occurs when radiation received for treatments of head and neck cancers affects the blood vessels, bones, and salivary glands. Mucositis is quite painful and the mucosa appears erythematous and ulcerates, making it difficult for the patient to eat and swallow. Xerostomia (the reduction of or the absence of saliva) usually develops after radiation treatments. Xerostomia can result in an increase of caries to all tooth surfaces, with the cervical or gingival surfaces being most susceptible. For this reason, patients should be encouraged to have all necessary dental treatments completed before starting any kind of radiation treatment. Patients with xerostomia should use daily fluoride treatments.

Demineralization of the teeth and the lack of saliva make the teeth more sensitive to hot and cold stimuli. Patients may also experience a loss of taste because of damage to the taste bud cells. The patient's ability to taste certain things returns slowly while other tastes do not. Complications from radiation treatments can affect the patient's ability to speak, swallow, eat foods due to xerostomia (dry mouth), or open the mouth (trismus). When a patient experiences loss of saliva, the dentist may recommend a saliva substitute. Saliva substitutes mimic saliva and provide relief for patients with xerostomia. Saliva substitutes are available in swabs, sprays, gels, and lozenges.

For children with cancer, defects in tooth development are a common effect of radiation treatment. Ulcerations in the soft tissue are another type of radiation injury. Osteoradionecrosis (death of bone) is probably one of the most severe effects of radiation treatments. This happens because the body ceases to have the ability to withstand trauma from the radiation treatment. If a patient needs extractions, the extraction procedure should be performed before the patient has radiation treatments, due to the danger of fractures or breaking the bone. One of the most successful treatments for osteoradionecrosis, hyperbaric oxygen therapy, was first proposed in the 1960s. It is very similar to the idea of using atmospheric chambers with deep-sea divers. Though the tests performed in the 1960s were inclusive, in the 1970s, head and neck surgeons who dealt with osteonecrosis and the damage of the maxilla and mandible came to recognize that hyperbaric oxygen therapy was quite effective (Figure 10.13). They found that treating patients with this therapy actually increased the oxygen saturation to the affected areas, cut down on infection levels, increased the blood supply flow, and helped in the healing process.

Oral Piercings

Piercings of the tongue and of the face and other body structures have become a popular form of body art among various segments of the population (Figure 10.14). The risk for infection of pierced tongues is high due to the various types of bacteria that are found in the oral cavity. Also, accumulation of plaque on the jewelry itself can be detrimental to the overall oral health of the individual. Jewelry in oral piercings should be removed every day and cleaned thoroughly.

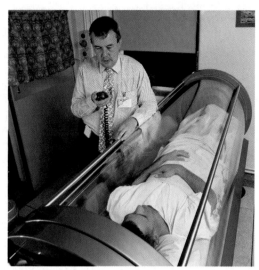

FIGURE 10.13
Hyperbaric oxygen therapy.

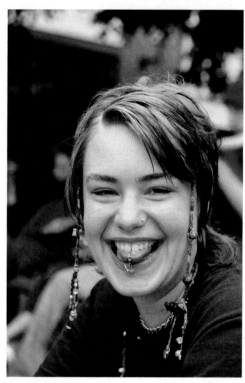

FIGURE 10.14
Tongue piercing.

Another popular site for piercings is the lips and the vermilion border of the lips. Dental complications arising from piercings of the tongue and lips can include chipped or broken teeth, local or systemic infections, and tissue damage or scarring. For tongue and lip piercings, the patient should be instructed to rinse for 60 seconds with an alcohol-free antimicrobial mouth rinse multiple times every day. After each meal the individual should also rinse with a saline solution for 10 to 15 seconds. A soft toothbrush should be used on the tongue, teeth, and tongue jewelry, and the toothbrush should be replaced every month.

Oral Manifestations Caused by Chemicals

Many chemicals are used in dental treatments. Some of these chemicals are caustic and can cause chemical burns in the oral cavity, though the dental team is very careful to utilize dental materials properly. Patients sometimes induce their own chemical injuries through self-use of chemicals such as tobacco. Tobacco contains a number of chemicals that are carcinogenic, and tobacco can cause oral lesions, especially if chewed.

Aspirin burns and nicotine stomatitis are also commonly seen in the dental office. Aspirin burns occur when an individual places aspirin directly on the gingival tissue. This may be done due to a toothache or may simply be the way the patient administers the aspirin to himself or another (child, elderly). The aspirin burns the gingival tissue and causes a lesion that is white and rough in texture. The tissues become quite sore and the necrotic tissue may slough off and result in a large ulcer. This ulcer generally heals in 7 to 21 days. Patients should be educated on the effects of localized aspirin use.

Nicotine stomatitis is a lesion caused by the effects of the heat and chemicals on the gingival tissues in a concentrated area; for example, it is seen more frequently in pipe smokers than cigarette smokers because the pipe is usually placed in the same area of the mouth. The lesion it causes begins as a red area in response to the irritation of the chemicals in the smoke and the heat. If the irritation continues then the gingival lesion progresses to a reddish-white, hyperkeratinized nodule. This condition will clear up within a couple of weeks if the patient stops smoking.

Snuff tobacco or smokeless tobacco is a mixture of 28 cancer-causing agents, plus powdered tobacco and other substances made for inhalation by nose or placed in a wad into the mouth between the lip and the gum. It contains nicotine and is addictive. The lesion produced as a result of the use of snuff tobacco is located in the vestibule, usually in the mandibular anterior area. It appears as a wrinkled, white, thickened tissue. This lesion is identified as leukoplakia or smokeless tobacco patch. The severity of the lesion depends on how often the smokeless tobacco is used. Some of the lesions associated with the continued use of smokeless tobacco are speckled leukoplakia, erythroplasia, tobacco-associated keratosis, carcinoma *in situ*, verrucous carcinoma, and invasive squamous cell carcinoma. These oral cancers are about four times more likely to occur in users of smokeless tobacco than nonusers. Prognosis for the patient with one of these lesions varies depending on the location and size of the lesion.

Smokeless tobacco is known to be a significant health risk. The CDC reports that currently 3% of adults are smokeless tobacco users, and that it is used at least 6% more by men as compared to the 0.4% in women. High school age students are an estimated 8% of the users, and middle school students rank at 3%.

Conditions of the Tongue

Hairy tongue is a condition in which the filiform papillae on the tongue become elongated and hair-like (Figure 10.15). When the papillae on the tongue appear white in color, the condition is called white hairy tongue. When the papillae become stained with food, tobacco, or other microorganisms, the papillae on the tongue will appear dark or black in color. This condition is called black hairy tongue. A hairy tongue is usually associated with the use of mouth rinses, antibiotics, or chemotherapeutic drugs.

Gingival hyperplasia is an overgrowth of the connective tissue over the teeth. It is a fibrous mass that can be caused by medication (such as Dilantin), orthodontic braces, plaque, or irritants. If the overgrowth becomes a problem, the tissue can be removed surgically. Normally,

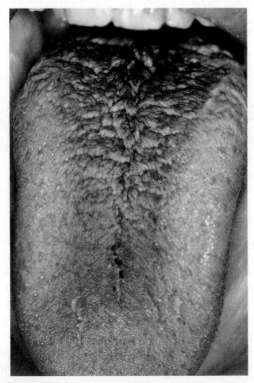

FIGURE 10.15
Hairy tongue.

if the irritant cause is removed, the condition will improve. Scurvy, a vitamin C deficiency, is also an example of gingival hyperplasia. In this condition, the person's gums swell, become spongy and red, and bleed very easily. Vitamin C is the treatment for scurvy.

Pregnancy gingivitis affects about 5% of pregnant women. During pregnancy the gingival tissues enlarge. When a woman's hormone levels go back into balance, the condition resolves itself. While the condition exists, good oral hygiene practices are of particular importance. This helps control the gingivitis and oral bleeding that can occur with the condition.

Another condition that can be related to pregnancy is that of pyogenic granuloma. The exact cause of this condition is unknown. Many variations of pyogenic granuloma occur in children and in adults. A pyogenic granuloma that often arises in pregnancy, usually on the gingiva or elsewhere in the oral mucosa, is termed the *pregnancy tumor*. Pyogenic granuloma can also be found in men as well as women who are not pregnant. It can range in size from a few millimeters to several centimeters.

Environmental effects from many common items found in our environment can have negative effects on prenatal development. Negative environmental effects are called *teratogens*. Diseases, use of drugs during pregnancy, and exposure to hair dyes, herbicides, and even cleaning fumes can also have negative effects. Noninfectious maternal conditions, such as alcoholism, diabetes, stress, anemia, and use of over-the-counter medications, all have negative effects on prenatal development. Additionally, the timing of the exposure to a teratogen is critical to the amount of impact on prenatal development. Teratogens do more damage if exposure occurs at the time when the baby's organ systems are developing. If a person suspects that she may be pregnant, she should avoid teratogens.

Puberty gingival enlargement occurs during adolescence due to the hormonal changes occurring in the body. This condition appears similar to pregnancy gingivitis in that the gingival tissue enlarges and bleeds easily; it also appears soft and swollen. It is more common in girls than in boys and will correct itself when the hormonal level is again in balance.

Glossitis is a term that means inflammation of the tongue. With glossitis, the filiform papillae are absent from the tongue, making it appear smooth or bald. The tongue may become sore and the patient may have difficulty in swallowing. Usually, the patient has a lack of the vitamin B complex. To correct this condition, the patient should eat a well-balanced diet and/or take B vitamins.

Geographic tongue is often a painless condition of the tongue that presents an ever-changing irregular pattern on the dorsal and lateral surfaces of the tongue (Figure 10.16). Sometimes this irregular pattern is found on the mucosal surfaces in addition to being on the tongue. When this happens this condition is known as ectopic geographic tongue. Geographic tongue is an inflammatory condition that presents with loss of filiform papillae in patches surrounded by an elevated white or yellow border. This condition can have periods of remission, and treatment is unnecessary. Geographic tongue can occur at any age, though it affects women more often than men. Occasionally, a patient will report a burning feeling when eating or drinking foods that are acidic.

A fissured tongue has a wrinkled appearance and is deeply grooved (Figure 10.17). The cause of a fissured tongue is not known. No treatments are necessary, although the patient who has a fissured tongue needs to be sure to clean the deep groove(s) thoroughly of debris.

Angular cheilitis is a lesion that appears at the corners (or *commissures*) of the mouth (Figure 10.18). It affects both the mucous membranes and the skin and is

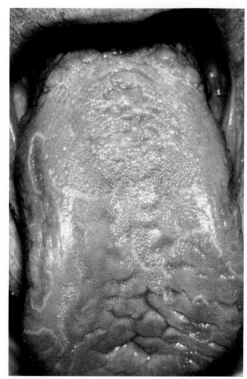

FIGURE 10.17
Fissured tongue.

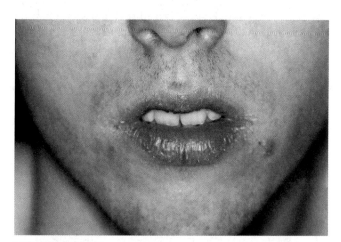

FIGURE 10.18
Angular cheilitis.

caused by a vitamin B complex deficiency. Angular cheilitis also happens if a denture patient loses vertical dimension and overcloses the mouth, which allows the saliva to pool in the corners of the lips. This pooling of saliva gives microorganisms an excellent place to grow. The **Candida albicans** fungus is often found in this area, which can cause opportunistic fungal infections.

Bifid tongue appears as an extra tag of muscle at the tip of the tongue when the two halves of the anterior two-thirds of the tongue fail to fuse. If the tag is large enough and annoying to the patient, surgery can be performed to remove it; otherwise it is left.

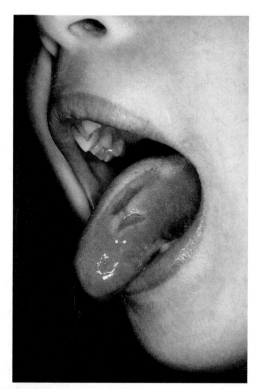

FIGURE 10.16
Geographic tongue.

Oral Cancer

Oral cancers are fatal if not found early enough or if left untreated. Oral cancers are frequently undetected in their earliest stages because the patient often has no pain or symptoms. One of the most common areas for cancer is the vermilion border on the lip. In the oral cavity, the growth of white lesions, red lesions, ulcers, masses, or unlikely areas for pigmentation are suspect for oral cancer.

Neoplasms

The medical terminology for a tumor is a *neoplasm*. A neoplasm may stay benign or become malignant or cancerous. Many lesions that manifest in the oral cavity have the potential to become malignant. Early diagnosis and treatment could save a patient's life. Early diagnosis and treatment of any white patch on the oral mucosa are very important, because white patches or **leukoplakia** (Figure 10.19) can lead to the development of a malignant lesion. Leukoplakia can be caused by chronic irritation or trauma, but usually the cause is unknown. It does vary in appearance from a fine white transparency to a thick leathery or warty-type plaque. It is firmly attached to underlying tissue and cannot be removed by rubbing or scraping of the tissue. Usually, there is no pain with leukoplakia unless there is a secondary infection or an ulceration. A biopsy is recommended for further diagnosis.

Erythroplakia is a term used to describe any red patch of tissue in the oral cavity not associated with inflammation. It is commonly seen on the soft palate, retromolar pad area, or the floor of the mouth. This lesion is usually seen in patients over the age of 60 who have chronically used tobacco and alcoholic beverages. This lesion is of great concern because when biopsied they are typically premalignant or malignant. In the very early stage, an erythroplakia can be surgically removed. In later stages, the patient must have the lesion treated with radiation and chemotherapy.

Lichen planus (Figure 10.20) is another lesion that can appear in the oral cavity. It is a common inflammatory disease of the skin and mouth that is usually asymptomatic and is a reaction to more than one factor (stress, genetics, autoimmune factors, infection, or the use of drugs). Normally, this lesion appears on the lower leg or ankle as a flat-topped lesion that is dark red or purplish in color. It is accompanied by mild to severe itching. In the oral cavity (reticular lichen planus), it begins as small white papules that group together and form interlacing white lines that are commonly found on the buccal mucosa and are known as Wickham's striae. It can also affect the tongue and it lasts longer than on the skin. Although lichen planus in the oral cavity is difficult to treat, it causes minimal problems. More severe forms of lichen planus in the mouth can cause burning, redness, blisters, and ulcers. Treatment for lichen planus is topical steroid therapy.

Carcinoma (Figure 10.21) is a cancerous lesion of the epithelium (tissue that lines the mouth) that spreads into bone and connective tissues. Carcinomas metastasize (travel) to other parts of the body as well as to the cervical lymph nodes. This lesion first appears as a white plaque or ulcerated area, although some carcinomas can be red in color and very smooth.

Adenocarcinoma is a malignant salivary gland tumor that is located beneath the oral mucosa in the oral cavity. Clinically, this tumor appears as a lump or a bulge and is given a specific name according to its location.

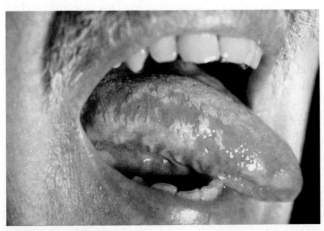

FIGURE 10.19
Oral hairy leukoplakia.
Courtesy PD Dr. P. Itin, Kantonsspital Basel

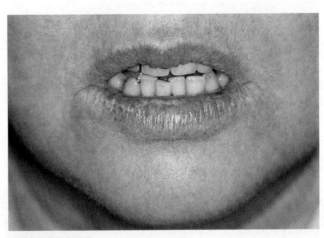

FIGURE 10.20
Lichen planus.

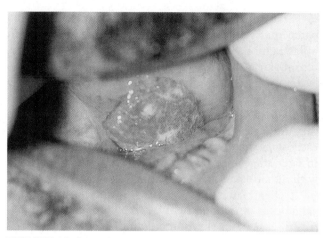

FIGURE 10.21
Carcinoma.

Sarcoma is a malignant neoplasm that begins in supportive and connective tissue such as bones. In the oral cavity this cancer may start in the jaw bones, but will often spread into the soft tissues. An osteosarcoma is a malignant tumor that involves bone.

Squamous cell carcinoma is a malignant neoplasm that spreads or metastasizes into surrounding tissues or into the lymph nodes of the body. It first appears as a thick white plaque that develops into an ulcerated area in the soft tissues of the mouth, primarily on the floor of the oral cavity under the tongue, on the sides or borders of the tongue, and in the soft palate and the tonsil area. As the ulcerous lesion grows, it has a distinct rolled border around the center tissue, and as it continues to grow, the mass rises above the surrounding tissue.

Basal cell carcinoma (Figure 10.22) is a type of skin cancer found commonly in areas on the head and neck that are exposed to the sun. People with fair complexions are more susceptible to basal cell carcinoma. Lips, neck, ears, face, and head are common areas where basal cell carcinomas begin. This lesion begins as a nodule then ulcerates. As it continues to grow, the center becomes a

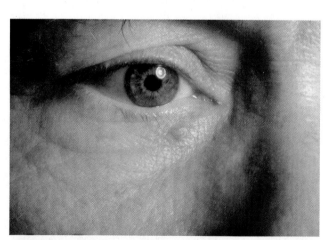

FIGURE 10.22
Basal cell carcinoma on the face.
© Mediscan

crater while the borders rise. This lesion does not metastasize and can be removed by surgery. Patients commonly develop more than one lesion, so careful clinical examinations are required at their recall appointments.

A **papilloma** is a benign neoplasm of the squamous epithelium. Papillomas can occur after an individual has been infected with a virus. This lesion has the appearance of a cauliflower and is white to red in color. Papillomas should be surgically removed along with a small amount of normal epithelium cells.

When a patient has continued trauma to an area in the oral cavity, it can lead to the growth of a benign tumor of connective tissue cells called a **fibroma**. Normally, a fibroma can be found on the buccal surface next to where the teeth occlude. In the oral cavity, fibromas are a smooth, dome-shaped lesion that is pink in color. Fibromas can be surgically removed if troublesome to the patient or they can be left alone with no treatment.

A lesion is detected under the tongue in the oral cavity of a 32-year-old male construction worker. What type of lesion do you suspect it may be? How would you find out for sure? What are the treatment options? **?**

Oral Conditions Due to HIV and AIDS

Patients who have HIV have a deficient immune system. Patients who have a deficient immune system have a much harder time with opportunistic microorganisms, such as *Candida albicans*. These patients ultimately have more disease conditions because their immune systems cannot fight off opportunistic infections. HIV is transmitted by sexual contact with an infected person or via infected blood and blood products. Infants born to mothers who have HIV may also have HIV. The end stage of the HIV disease is when the patient develops acquired immunodeficiency syndrome (AIDS). Oral lesions are common features of the HIV infection and of AIDS and are caused by opportunistic infections, tumors, and autoimmune-like diseases (Figure 10.23).

Atypical gingivitis or hypertrophic gingivitis is a characteristic of a patient who has HIV. This lesion presents as a bright red line along the border of the free gingival margin. The patient may have an accelerated attachment loss. This type of gingivitis is present without plaque being an issue. The HIV patient can also develop small, pinpoint bruising called petechiae that are located on the gingiva.

Periodontitis presents as inflammation in the gums and then spreads to the periodontal ligaments and bone. In the HIV patient periodontitis resembles ulcerative lesions that are found in acute necrotizing gingivitis. Other symptoms include swelling, intense erythema on the free and attached gingiva, intense pain, spontaneous bleeding, bad breath, cratering, and necrosis of the inter-proximal areas.

Kaposi's sarcoma is a malignant bluish-purple vascular tumor. This cancer is aggressive and progresses rapidly. The lesion is flat or nodular. As the tumor grows it becomes a hemorrhagic neoplasm. The patient has bleeding and pain in the advanced stage. This lesion can appear all over the body as well as in the intraoral cavity (Figure 10.24).

Kaposi's sarcoma is indicative of the patient having AIDS and may be the first sign/symptom for the dental professional and the patient toward diagnosis of the condition. Treatment for this cancer is low-dose radiation or chemotherapeutic drugs.

Developmental Disorders

A wide range of developmental disturbances can take place in the human body during the stages of embryo development. Developmental disturbances can result in

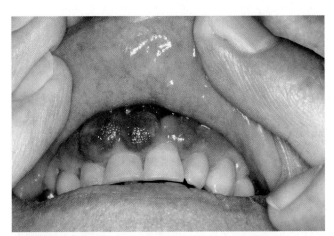

FIGURE 10.23
Gingival lymphoma in an AIDS patient.

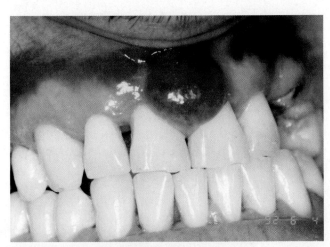

FIGURE 10.24
Kaposi's sarcoma on the gums of a mouth.
Courtesy of B.C. Muzyka and M. Glick

deformities of the body. Some conditions are inherited (determined by genetics); other conditions are congenital (present at birth). Teratogens such as alcohol, drugs, or disease (e.g., the mother having syphilis while pregnant) can have negative effects on fetal development and result in birth defects when the baby is born. As stated earlier, the timing of the exposure to a teratogen is critical to its impact on prenatal development, as are the dose amount and the genotype of the mother and of the fetus.

Cleft lip and cleft palate are two of the most common developmental disturbances. If the disturbance is severe enough, these conditions can cause the person difficulty with speaking, eating, swallowing, and so forth. A cleft palate occurs when the primary palate and the palatal shelves do not fuse or grow together. A cleft lip results when the medial nasal process and the maxillary process do not fuse or grow together. A cleft lip and cleft palate can occur separately or together (Figure 10.25). Treatment for cleft palate is the construction of an **obturator**, which is a prosthetic device that the patient wears to aid in swallowing. In some cases, surgery may be performed in an attempt to partially or fully close the cleft.

A short lingual frenum that extends to the tip of the tongue is called ankyloglossia (meaning tongue-tied). A patient who has ankyloglossia has limited movement of the tongue, which can affect the person's speech.

Why might the use of a prosthetic device be important to a patient with cleft palate?

Tooth Development Disturbances

Ameloblastoma is a slow-growing, aggressive tumor that develops with pieces of the dental lamina that failed to disintegrate after the tooth buds were formed. It invades

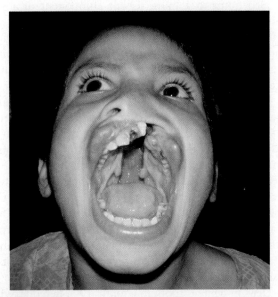

FIGURE 10.25
A child with bilateral complete cleft lip and palate.
Image courtesy Instructional Materials for the Dental Team, Lex., KY

the surrounding tissues and it can cause extensive damage. If this tumor occurs in the maxilla, it can cause death due to its infiltration into vital structures. Ameloblastomas are usually asymptomatic. In 75% of individuals, they are typically found during routine dental x-rays. Upon radiographic examination, this tumor appears as a multiocular soap bubble or it can have a honeycomb appearance. Ameloblastomas can occur anywhere in the jaw, although they are more commonly found in the mandible molar and ramus area. In the maxilla, they are most often found in the molar region. As ameloblastomas grow, they cause expansion of the bone and must be removed by surgery.

Amelogenesis imperfecta is an inherited condition of the teeth in which defects occur during the formation of enamel. The enamel is discolored, partially missing, or extremely thin. The teeth are much more susceptible to dental caries without the normal amount of enamel.

Anodontia is the developmental condition in which all teeth are congenitally missing. This condition is rare and affects primary teeth, permanent teeth, or both.

Hypodontia is a common developmental anomaly that affects primary and permanent teeth, although the permanent teeth are more commonly affected. In the maxillary arch, the third molars and the maxillary laterals are usually the teeth that are missing or never develop. In the mandibular arch, the second premolars are commonly missing or never develop. In the primary dentition, the mandibular incisor is the most common missing tooth.

Missing teeth may be hereditary. To diagnose congenitally missing teeth, a careful clinical examination and a radiographic examination along with a thorough patient medical history are necessary. Missing teeth may result in problems with a patient's occlusion, causing drifting or tilting in the remaining teeth. Missing teeth can also point to a more serious component of a syndrome. A syndrome is a collection of symptoms that occur together to become part of another more serious condition. Other factors such as jaw lesions during infancy or radiation therapy can affect the development of teeth and even cause lack of teeth.

When the enamel appears bluish in color or opalescent, this condition is called dentinogenesis imperfecta. This disorder of tooth development causes discoloration of the teeth. During the formation of the dentin, mutations alter the proteins that are involved. Teeth with this defective dentin are weak, discolored, and more likely to decay and break. This is a hereditary condition that appears in both primary and permanent dentition. Radiographically, when a patient has dentinogenesis imperfecta you will be able to see the obliterated pulp chambers and root canals (Figure 10.26). Clinically, these patients present with attrition due to the lack of enamel.

Dens in dente ("tooth in a tooth") is a hereditary factor that commonly affects the permanent maxillary lateral incisor. During the cap stage of tooth development, the

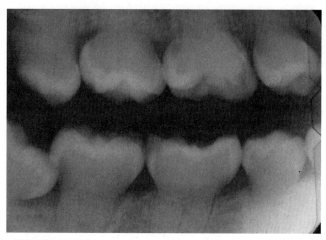

FIGURE 10.26
A radiograph of dentinogenesis imperfecta.
Courtesy Department of Pathology, University of Missouri–Kansas City School of Dentistry

enamel organ extrudes into the dental papilla. Radiographically, the infolding can extend to within the pulp cavity, the root, and sometimes the root apex (Figure 10.27). Clinically, it is characterized by an unusual barrel-shaped or peg-shaped crown. It is associated with other dental anomalies, such as taurodontia, microdontia, supernumerary teeth, gemination, and dentinogenesis imperfecta. Endodontic treatment is the recommended treatment.

Supernumerary teeth are extra teeth most often seen in the maxillary dentition. These teeth are smaller than normal teeth and may occur as a single tooth or in mul-

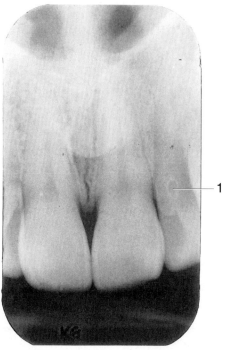

FIGURE 10.27
Dens in dente.

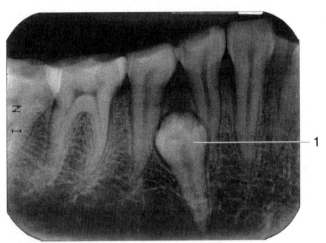

FIGURE 10.28
Radiograph of unerupted supernumerary teeth.

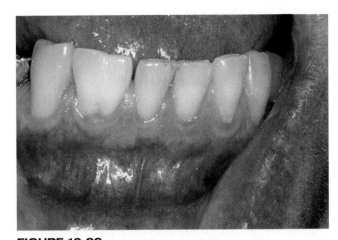

FIGURE 10.29
Gemination.
Courtesy Department of Pathology, University of Missouri–Kansas City School of Dentistry

tiples, either lingually, buccally, or facially. The most common teeth affected are the mesiodens, located between the maxillary central incisors near the midline. Most supernumerary teeth are embedded in the gingiva but some do erupt (Figure 10.28).

An enamel pearl is an uncommon occurrence. It is a round pearl-like structure of enamel located near the root bifurcation or trifurcation area on the root of the maxillary molars and close to or at the cement–enamel junction. Upon clinical examination, the enamel pearl may appear as calculus, but can be seen radiographically as a small spherical radiopacity. Radiopacity pertains to the passage of the x-ray beam through the enamel pearl. Because it is a dense structure, it resists the passage of x-rays, which in turn will show a light or white spherical shape on the radiograph near the root bifurcation or root trifurcation.

Fusion occurs when one or more teeth join together at the outside length of the tooth or teeth, or they join only at the roots or share a root canal. The teeth may have separate crown indentations and appear broader. This condition is most often observed in the anterior mandibular deciduous teeth.

Gemination appears similar to fusion, but in this condition the tooth bud attempts to divide and the indentation is clearly visible on the incisal or occlusal surface of the tooth (Figure 10.29). Gemination is seen in primary dentition more than permanent dentition and most often appears in the mandibular deciduous incisors and in the maxillary incisors in the permanent dentition. Upon clinical examination, gemination presents as two crowns joined together by a notched incisal area. Upon radiographic examination, this tooth shows a single root and one pulp canal (Figure 10.30). Treatment for this anomaly is challenging as well as an aesthetic problem of altering the tooth so that it appears to be a normal size and shape. Twinning is the condition in which the process of gemination is successful and two separate teeth are formed from one tooth bud. The second tooth is a clone of the original tooth.

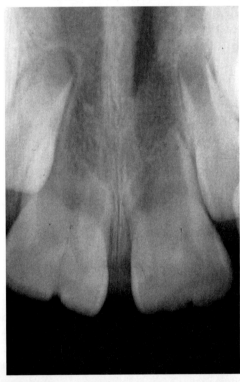

FIGURE 10.30
Radiograph showing gemination.
Courtesy Department of Pathology, University of Missouri–Kansas City School of Dentistry

Concrescence is another condition that is common with permanent maxillary molars. This disorder is the union of the root structure of two or more teeth by cementum. Concrescence may be caused by traumatic injury or crowding of teeth during the maturation stage of tooth development.

Microdontia teeth are abnormally small teeth usually seen in patients with Down syndrome, in patients who have congenital heart disease, or in patients affected by congenital syphilis. This condition is also associated with pituitary dwarfism. Usually, microdontia is limited to one or two teeth, but in certain cases the entire dentition may show effects of this condition. The teeth most commonly affected are the maxillary laterals.

The condition in which the teeth are abnormally large is called macrodontia and is seen either in the entire dentition in certain cases or in only one or two teeth.

Neonatal teeth are present at the time of birth or within the first month. Neonatal teeth are shed quickly because they have no root formation. Often these teeth will be removed because if left there is a chance the baby could choke on the teeth when they are shed.

Ankylosis is a condition in which the deciduous teeth are fused to the cementum and the dentin preventing exfoliation, thereby affecting the eruption of the permanent tooth. Primary molars are the most common teeth affected by this condition. Ankylosed teeth are confirmed by radiographs of the suspected tooth (Figure 10.31). The treatment for the ankylosed tooth is extraction, which allows for eruption of the permanent tooth.

Impacted teeth are any teeth that remain unerupted beyond the normal eruption time. The most common teeth that are impacted include the maxillary and mandibular third molars, the maxillary canines, supernumerary teeth, and the maxillary and mandibular premolars. Fully impacted teeth are usually "locked" in bone due to excessive curved roots or angled positions that do not allow these teeth to erupt. These bony impactions can be fully impacted (not visibly seen on the oral cavity). Partially impacted teeth can involve the soft tissues as well as the bony tissues (partial crown of the tooth is visible in the oral cavity).

Radiographic examination of impactions is necessary before any surgery or extractions in order to check positions and angles of these teeth (Figure 10.32). Fully impacted teeth should be surgically removed. Partially impacted teeth can sometimes be extracted without surgery. Removal of fully or partially impacted teeth helps to prevent formation of cyst or tumors, resorption of adjacent teeth, infections, and fractures of the bone.

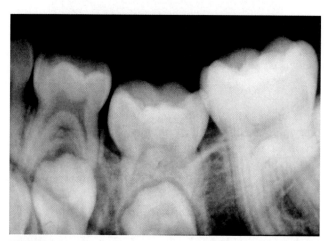

FIGURE 10.31
Radiograph of ankylosis of a deciduous molar.
Image courtesy Instructional Materials for the Dental Team, Lex., KY

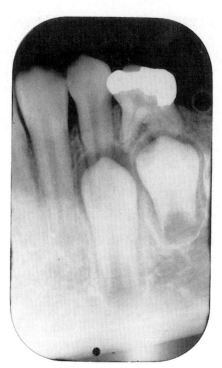

FIGURE 10.32
Radiograph of impactions in mixed dentition.

Miscellaneous Disorders

Other disorders that the dental assistant may see in the oral cavity can be grouped as miscellaneous disorders. The abnormal wearing away of tooth structure is called abrasion. Patients who exhibit abrasion have repetitive habits that wear away tooth structure. Toothbrush abrasion is a common type of abrasion. This is caused by the patient brushing the teeth too vigorously or with a hard bristle brush.

Attrition is the normal age-related wearing away of tooth structure. The motion of chewing contributes to attrition in dentition. The use of chewing tobacco makes attrition worse, as does bruxism, an oral habit that is characterized by clenching or grinding of teeth. Bruxism tends to worsen when patients are experiencing high levels of stress in their life. Many people are not aware that they have bruxism. The nightly grinding and clenching contributes to damage of the periodontal ligament and contributes to temporomandibular joint disorders.

Temporomandibular disorders can also occur due to accidents, diseases of the joints, and malocclusion. Symptoms of temporomandibular disorders include pain around or in the ear, headaches, and difficulty chewing and opening the mouth (Figure 10.33). Treatments for temporomandibular joint disorders depend on the severity of the condition.

Acute necrotizing ulcerative gingivitis (ANUG; also known as Vincent's infection and trench mouth) is a painful condition of the gingival tissues brought on by reduced local resistance of the gingival area and caused by microbial overgrowth of several organisms, of which *Borrelia vincentii* (a spirochete) is a recognized microor-

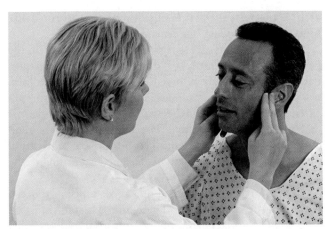

FIGURE 10.33
Palpating the temporomandibular joints.

ganism. The history of ANUG goes back to the days of Hippocrates. In 1999, the American Academy of Periodontics used a classification system for ANUG, which is now known as necrotizing periodontal disease (NUG). Poor hygiene, poor nutrition, lack of sleep, and stress are all factors that precipitate this infection. NUG is seen more readily in adolescents and college students, because this age group tends to have more incidence of poor oral hygiene habits and poor nutrition, as well as little sleep, which can contribute to a lower body defense against infection. A foul odor accompanies this condition because the gingival tissues are dying and sloughing or peeling.

The patient who has NUG must be treated with antibiotics, a deep thorough debridement, and cleaning. After the debridement and cleaning, the dental hygienist will explain instructions to this patient for home care and then provide the patient with written instructions. This includes a regimen of saline rinses, chlorhexidine rinsing, toothbrushing, and flossing. The patient must understand that the condition will not go away when the pain is eliminated. The dental assistant explains the underlying infection and how NUG recurs if the condition is not treated.

A patient has necrotizing ulcerative gingivitis. What causes this painful condition?

Professionalism

All of the duties that a dental assistant performs during dental procedures are viewed not only by the dental team but also the patients themselves. Therefore, professionalism is a must in both language skills and the way in which other members of the dental team are addressed. A dental assistant who has high ethical standards will also exhibit punctuality and dependability in working as a team member. Patients do appreciate a caring attitude from their dental assistant.

A mucocele occurs as the result of trauma to a minor salivary gland. The mandibular anterior lip is a common site where a mucocele begins, usually due to the patient accidentally biting the tissue. If this trauma occurs at the site of a minor salivary gland, the swelling may cause the duct to close off and trap the secretion causing the tissue to appear to "bubble." Sometimes only the gland may be affected. This can happen when a stone-like particle blocks the saliva duct, causing the gland to fill with fluid. The gland can be opened and the fluid expressed. Usually, the gland and the duct will be removed if the condition reoccurs.

Another condition called varix is similar to that of varicose veins except it is found in the oral cavity, usually on the ventral surface of the tongue on either side of the midline. These veins appear distended and sometimes nodular and are thought to be related to the weakening of the blood vessel wall and may be more prominent in elderly patients. The blood vessels become weakened and distended and appear as a deep, dark purple color. No treatment is necessary for varix.

Eating disorders can affect a patient's dentition. Dental assistants are often the first dental team member to screen the patient with an eating disorder. Issues related to the patient's dental problems may be indicative of an eating disorder. If certain oral cavity issues are present, the dentist may diagnose the patient as having an eating disorder. Patients with the anorexia nervosa disorder have an intense weight loss of 15% or more of their total body weight and they have an aversion to food (Figure 10.34). In essence, they starve because they are afraid of being fat.

In the bulimic stage of the disease, the patient indulges in food binging and then purging (vomiting). Because of the frequent vomiting, stomach acid can wash over the teeth and gingiva. Repeated vomiting can cause a significant and permanent loss of dental enamel. Teeth may become ragged and chipped, and dental cavities may increase. Dental management of the patient with an eating disorder includes encouraging the patient to seek professional treatment, promoting the daily use of fluoride toothpaste, and urging the patient to rinse immediately after vomiting to lessen the effects of the acid on the teeth.

Although its symptoms are somewhat similar to those of a stroke, Bell's palsy is not related to a stroke. It is named for Sir Charles Bell, a Scottish surgeon in the 19th century who first described this condition. Bell's palsy causes temporary paralysis or weakness of the facial muscles on one side of the face, causing a drooping eyelid, dryness or tearing of the eye, drooping of the corner of the mouth, and drooling. Many scientists believe this condition results from a viral infection. Sometimes the patient experiences pain in the ear on the affected side. The patient's sense of taste may be diminished and sounds may be perceived as unnaturally loud. Usually, this condition will clear up on its own, but corticosteroid

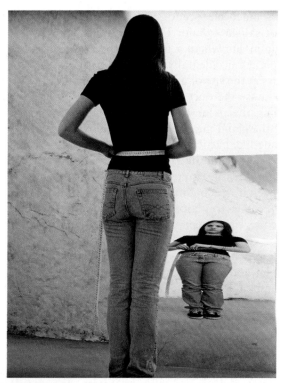

FIGURE 10.34
Anorexia nervosa: A distorted view of one's body.
Image courtesy Instructional Materials for the Dental Team, Lex., KY

drugs can be given to reduce inflammation of the trigeminal nerve and analgesics can be given for symptoms of discomfort. The trigeminal nerve helps to control the sensory perception of the face and of the head region. In rare cases, both sides of the face may be affected.

Torus palatinus and torus mandibularis define the areas for oral tori. **Tori** are hard bone growths that have a thin tissue covering (Figure 10.35). Tori palatinus are located in the maxillary arch close to the midline of the hard palate, but can be located on the lateral borders of the palate also. Tori mandibularis are located in the mandibular canine or premolar region in the mandibular

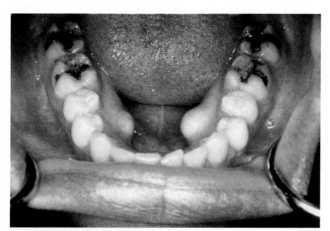

FIGURE 10.35
Bilateral mandibular tori.
Image courtesy Instructional Materials for the Dental Team, Lex., KY

arch. Sometimes the actual position of the tori can cause food debris to collect underneath them.

These growths are surgically removed only if the patient needs a denture or other prosthetic appliance. Patients are generally referred to an oral and maxillofacial surgeon for evaluation and impressions if the tori are extensive. The patient is then referred back to his dentist to have impressions taken. The dental office will send these impressions to the dental laboratory for fabrication of the prosthesis, which will be designed according to the patient's needs.

These growths can be a nuisance, especially if the patient needs radiographs. The dental assistant must be careful in the placement of the intraoral radiographic film. Wrong placement of the intraoral film can cause the patient discomfort because the film can abrade or cut the thin tissue covering the tori.

When placing radiographic films on a patient who has mandibular tori, what must the dental assistant consider?

CDC Rankings of Evidence

When treating dental patients with oral pathology conditions, it is important for the dentist and the dental team to work with the patient to achieve positive outcomes. Treatment choices for oral pathology conditions depend on many factors specific to the disease or lesion being treated. Outcomes are usually based on the type of treatment chosen and on the patient's commitment to personal care and preventive measures. Sometimes if the disease or condition is uncommon or rare, the condition must be researched. Two organizations that continually research diseases and continually update statistical data gathered on disease conditions are the Public Health Department and the Centers for Disease Control and Prevention (CDC). These two organizations work closely together.

The CDC works to promote health and to improve the quality of life by preventing and controlling disease, injury, and disability. State and local public health departments collect data from physicians and dental offices by means of surveys or reports on the occurrence of medical disease or dental diseases. These statistical data help to provide information on recognizing serious outbreaks, epidemics, or even pandemic diseases for various demographic areas.

The data also help to rank diseases and the seriousness of the disease, thereby giving the CDC the information needed on how to proceed. For example, if a county shows a higher incidence of dental caries than the surrounding counties, the public health department will launch an investigation as to why that one county has a higher incidence of dental caries. If the incidence of dental caries happens to be tied to an infection, then this infection may be ranked and the information passed on to the CDC. The CDC will work closely with public health departments to provide the best safeguards or treatment methods for infection or disease. For instance, the CDC has provided new research on infection control methods that affect the dental office and the medical office, allowing for better practice of infection control methods and disease containment.

Environmental Infection Control

The universal disinfection technique for cleaning and disinfecting surfaces, use of an ultrasonic machine, sterilization of dental instruments in an autoclave, and sterilization monitoring are all techniques and aids that help to reduce the exposure to microorganisms in the dental office. The use of personal protective equipment by the dental staff, the use of rubber dam materials during dental procedures, and the use of barriers on all contact surfaces are practices that help to ensure infection control within the dental office environment.

Staff training in infection control methods is a way to ensure that all procedural guidelines are followed. By learning and incorporating the routine steps for infection control, the dental staff helps to eliminate mistakes or omissions of steps in providing aseptic techniques and therefore reduces the chance of cross-contamination in the dental office. An environment free of pathogens reduces the danger of infection or disease for all concerned.

SUMMARY

Attentiveness by the dental assistant to a patient's oral health can help bring attention to potentially abnormal conditions. Early discovery of lesions can help to avert further dental or medical problems for the patient. A primary goal for a dental assistant is to attain a thorough knowledge of normal and abnormal conditions concerning the oral cavity and to provide the patient education for at-home care associated with the oral condition.

Cultural Considerations

Dental assistants are exposed to a broad range of patients from any number of different cultural backgrounds. Patients' language skills and social customs can have a major influence on how your patients perceive their dental treatments. Taking a language class, preferably a language that is used by at least some of the dentist's patients, would be a start toward removing the communication barrier between you and your patients.

KEY TERMS

- **Abscess:** A collection of pus in a localized area. p. 147
- **Aphthous ulcers:** Painful ulcers appearing in the oral cavity as a circular lesion with a yellow center and a red outline or halo; sometimes referred to as a canker sore. p. 150
- **Basal cell carcinoma:** Cancerous lesion that does not metastasize; most commonly found on areas of the skin that have been exposed to the sun. Occurs more often in individuals with fair skin tones. p. 156
- *Candida albicans:* An oral yeast infection presenting as a thick, white covering on oral mucosa; also called moniliasis. p. 154
- **Carcinoma:** Cancerous lesion of the epithelium (tissues that line the mouth) that spreads into bone and connective tissues. p. 155
- **Exudate:** Cellular debris from an infection; the drainage of pus. p. 147
- **Herpetic whitlow:** Painful crusting ulcerations on the fingers or hands resulting from exposure to the herpes virus. p. 149

- **Hyperplasia:** Excess folds of tissue that result from an ill-fitting denture. p. 151
- **Kaposi's sarcoma:** Malignant bluish-purple vascular tumor; an opportunistic neoplasm that may occur in people with HIV infection. p. 157
- **Leukoplakia:** Usually a precipitating factor for cancer; appears as a white leathery patch that cannot be identified as any other white lesion. p. 155
- **Obturator:** Constructed prosthetic device designed to close a congenital or acquired opening in the palate. p. 157
- **Sarcoma:** Malignant neoplasm beginning in supportive and connective tissue such as bones. p. 156
- **Squamous cell carcinoma:** Malignant lesion that metastasizes (travels) into surrounding tissues or into the lymph nodes of the body. p. 156
- **Tori:** Oral maxillary, mandibular, or palatal bone growths projecting outward from the surface. p. 162

CHECK YOUR UNDERSTANDING

1. Chemical agents cause all of the following except
   a. pustules.
   b. nicotine stomatitis.
   c. aspirin burn.
   d. hairy tongue.

2. In the first stage of syphilis, the lesion that appears is called a
   a. split papule.
   b. mucous patch.
   c. chancre.
   d. gumma.

3. The condition in which the facial muscles are temporarily paralyzed, with no known cause, is called
   a. anorexia nervosa.
   b. Bell's palsy.
   c. AIDS.
   d. ANUG.

4. When the tooth, cementum, or dentin fuses with the alveolar bone, the resulting condition is known as
   a. ankylosis.
   b. amelogenesis imperfecta.
   c. anodontia.
   d. fusion.

5. A vitamin B complex deficiency can result in a condition known as
   a. hairy tongue.
   b. Fordyce's granules.
   c. *Candida albicans.*
   d. angular cheilitis.

6. When the third molars do not fully erupt into the oral cavity, these teeth are said to be
   a. not present.
   b. impacted.
   c. malpositioned.
   d. misaligned.

7. When two separate teeth are grown from one tooth bud, the process is called
   a. a clone.
   b. fusion.
   c. dens in dente.
   d. twinning.

8. In this developmental condition the patient has limited movement of the tongue:
   a. syphilis
   b. herpes labialis
   c. ankyloglossia
   d. Hutchinson's incisors

9. Caused by a chemical agent, this lesion has a white color and rough feeling with soreness after the agent is removed from the root area of a tooth and before healing is complete.
   a. lichen planus
   b. snuff tobacco lesion
   c. aspirin burn
   d. gingival hyperplasia

10. The term for congenitally missing is
    a. neonatal teeth.
    b. developmental problems.
    c. amelogenesis imperfecta.
    d. anodontia.

INTERNET ACTIVITY

- Go to www.aad.org to find and view images of lichen planus of the mouth. Discover what foods can aggravate this condition.

WEB REFERENCES

- National Institute of Neurological Disorders and Stroke www.ninds.nih.gov
- National Institute of Allergy and Infectious Diseases www.niaid.nih.gov
- Colgate World of Care www.colgate.com
- Merck & Co., Inc. www.merck.com
- Centers for Disease Control and Prevention www.cdc.gov
- University of Iowa, Oral Pathology Image Database www.uiowa.edu/~oprm/AtlasHome.html

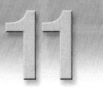

Microbiology

Learning Objectives

After reading this chapter, the student should be able to:

• State the accomplishments of the scientific pioneers in microbiology.

• Define common terminology used in microbiology.

• List the major groups of microorganisms.

• Describe common viral diseases.

• Name common bacterial diseases.

• Discuss the primary bacterial component in dental plaque.

• Demonstrate understanding of the microorganisms that cause disease.

Preparing for Certification Exams

• Provide patient preventive education.

Key Terms

Acquired immunodeficiency syndrome (AIDS)

Aerobic bacteria

Anaerobic bacteria

Bacteria

Candidiasis

Facultative bacteria

Hepatitis

Human immunodeficiency virus (HIV)

Microbiology

Pathogenic

Penicillin

Spore

Streptococcus mutans

Tetanus

Tuberculosis

Viruses

Chapter Outline

• Pioneers in Microbiology
  —Robert Hooke
  —Anton van Leeuwenhoek
  —Louis Pasteur
  —Robert Koch
  —Alexander Fleming

• Major Groups of Microorganisms
  —Algae
  —Bacteria
  —Fungi
  —Protozoa
  —Rickettsaie
  —Viruses

• Viral Diseases
  —Herpes
  —HIV and AIDS
  —Hepatitis

• Bacterial Diseases
  —Anthrax
  —Botulism
  —Tetanus
  —Tuberculosis
  —Pneumonia
  —Dental Plaque

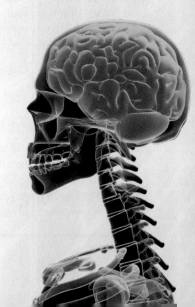

Microbiology is the branch of science concerned with the study of living organisms too small to be seen with the naked eye. Microorganisms perform many functions that are beneficial for other forms of life. Bacteria assist in food digestion and are important in the production of foods including bread, cheese, and yogurt. The term *biodegradable*, meaning "broken down by living things," refers largely to the work of bacteria. Other microorganisms pose a threat to human health and other living organisms. These are called **pathogenic**, or disease-producing, microorganisms. Early scientific discoveries in microbiology paved the way for understanding diseases and development of vaccines to help mankind fight life-threatening illnesses.

Pioneers in Microbiology

The major pioneers in microbiology had curiosity, persistence, and independence. They taught themselves and us about microbiology. Their determination created breakthroughs in microbiological science and formed foundations for development of medicines, food production, and a clearer understanding of our environment.

Robert Hooke

The science of microbiology started with the invention of the microscope. The English scientist and inventor Robert Hooke reported observations with a primitive microscope. He is credited with discovering cell theory in 1665. He observed cork under a microscope and described a matrix of cylindrical-like shapes. From this discovery Hooke proposed that all living things are composed of cells.

Dental Assistant   PROFESSIONAL TIP

A thorough health history must be taken for every patient. This ensures that other health needs are being met for the dental patient. Sometimes a person will see her dentist, who may then refer the individual to another health care provider for a medical consult or clearance before dental treatment may continue.

Anton van Leeuwenhoek

In the Netherlands in 1673, Anton van Leeuwenhoek described a world of microorganisms in a drop of rainwater. He noticed that the drop contained tiny creatures that he called "animalcules." These creatures were bacteria. Due to van Leeuwenhoek's observations, he became known as the first person to study microorganisms.

Louis Pasteur

Louis Pasteur (Figure 11.1) was probably the greatest biologist of the 19th century. In 1864 he successfully showed that life can only be generated from existing life of the same species. Pasteur also showed that fermentation, a process used in baking and brewing, was caused by microorganisms. As a result of his work he went on to develop the process for sterilizing milk, which was named after him: pasteurization.

Pasteur was able to prove the following:

- Airborne microbes cause disease.
- Microbes can produce spoilage in food.
- Microbes can be killed by heating the liquid in which the microbes exist.

He believed that microbes could spread disease among humans and is credited with the development of vaccines, including rabies and anthrax vaccines. Pasteur also identified and eliminated disease in silkworms, which saved the silkworm industry at that time.

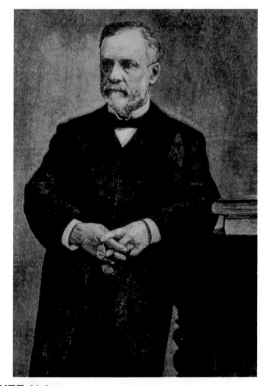

FIGURE 11.1
Louis Pasteur.

Robert Koch

Robert Koch is credited with developing germ theory. He identified the microbes that cause anthrax, tuberculosis, and cholera. Koch discovered that the anthrax microbe could produce spores that lived for a long time and then developed into the anthrax germ that could infect other animals. He devised a method of proving which germ caused an infection and perfected the technique of growing pure cultures of bacteria. In 1881 he began to work on one of the worst diseases of the 19th century: tuberculosis.

Eventually his research techniques began to be used by others throughout the world to discover how to treat many diseases. Koch's procedure for defining the agent of any disease consists of four steps:

- *Step 1:* Isolate the suspected agent from the diseased victim.
- *Step 2:* Grow the agent in a pure culture.
- *Step 3:* Infect a healthy host and show that the organism produces the clinical disease.
- *Step 4:* Isolate the same organism from the new victim.

Alexander Fleming

In 1928 Alexander Fleming, a Scottish bacteriologist, turned a ruined culture into one of the greatest medical advances in history. One of Fleming's bacterial cultures became contaminated with a patch of mold. Before throwing out the culture dish he noticed that no bacteria were growing near the mold. His keen observations led to the isolation of **penicillin**, the first antibiotic.

What are some beneficial functions that microorganisms perform? Who discovered penicillin? What did Louis Pasteur prove?

Major Groups of Microorganisms

Single-celled organisms are numerous and nearly everywhere, including in the bodies of larger creatures, such as human beings. Humans are in constant contact with microbes; in fact, our health and survival are closely tied to theirs. This relationship is often mutually beneficial, but some of humanity's most deadly diseases stem from microorganisms. The bubonic plague killed one-third of the population of Europe during the Middle Ages. The major groups of microorganisms consist of algae, bacteria, fungi, protozoa, rickettsia, and viruses.

Algae

Algae are one-celled marine plants that are the lowest form of plant life. Algae contain chlorophyll and are found in freshwater, saltwater, and in moist places on land. They are plants without roots, stem, or leaves and vary in size from microscopic forms to massive seaweeds.

Bacteria

Bacteria are small unicellular microorganisms. Nearly all bacteria are encased in a porous but rigid cell wall that protects them and gives the different types of bacteria their characteristic shapes. The most common bacterial shapes are rod-like bacilli, spheres called cocci, and corkscrew-shaped spirilla (Figure 11.2).

Bacteria are normally very small. About 250,000 average-sized bacteria could gather on the period at the end of this sentence. Bacteria reproduce through a simple form of cell division called binary fission in which the cell divides into approximately two equal parts. Under ideal conditions, a bacterium can divide every 20 minutes. A group of bacteria growing in one place is called a colony. Colonies of bacteria may descend from a single cell (Figure 11.3).

Spores

Certain species of bacteria, called **spores**, have the ability to develop layers of protective membranes. Sensing an uncomfortable environment, the bacterium replicates its genetic material to protect itself and becomes surrounded by a tough outer coating or capsule. This is called a daughter cell. The mother cell will disintegrate, releasing a spore with layers of protective protein membranes. Within these membranes the dormant bacterium is able to survive for weeks, even years, through drought, heat, chemicals, and even radiation. As soon as conditions become more favorable again—for example, when more water or more food is available—the bacterium "comes to life" once more, transforming from a spore back to a

FIGURE 11.2
Examples of spherical, rod-like, and curved bacteria shapes.
Daniel Pyne © Dorling Kindersley

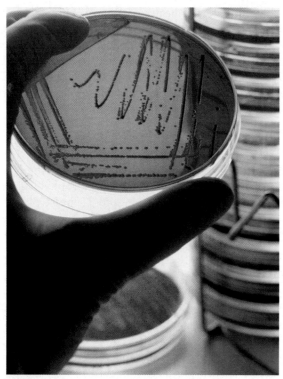

FIGURE 11.3
Bacteria colonies in a culture plate.

cell. The size, shape, and location of a spore in the cell are all identifying genetic characteristics. The spores of bacteria are difficult to destroy because they are very resistant to heat and require prolonged exposure to high temperatures to kill them. Examples of diseases caused by spore-forming bacteria are anthrax and tetanus.

Bacteria's Oxygen Requirements

Depending on the type of bacteria, the bacteria are either destroyed by oxygen or thrive on it:

- **Aerobic bacteria** depend on oxygen to survive.
- **Anaerobic bacteria** are destroyed by contact with oxygen.
- **Facultative bacteria** have the ability to adjust to particular circumstances and can live with or without oxygen.

These classifications of bacteria are based on the types of reactions they use to generate energy for growth

Cultural Considerations

Due to language barriers some patients may not understand how easy it is to prevent the spread of disease. Dental assistants need to stress to parents how important it is to ensure their children are immunized against common childhood diseases. These inoculations are available at no or low cost at all state and county health departments.

and other activities. Anaerobes multiply well in dead tissue. Multiplication of aerobic or facultative organisms in association with anaerobes in infected tissues lowers the concentration of oxygen and develops a habitat that supports growth of anaerobic bacteria.

For survival and reproductive success, different species of bacteria often rely on close relationships with each other. A collection of bacteria occupying the same physical habitat is called a community. One example of a community of microorganisms is a biofilm. Biofilms have been implicated in many infections including those present in the oral cavity. Microbial communities depend on and help each other to survive. As aerobic bacteria grow, they consume oxygen, and create a more favorable environment for anaerobic bacteria. The effects of the biofilm community are more toxic than those of the individual microorganisms.

Gram Stain

The Gram stain is a staining technique that distinguishes two types of cell wall construction in bacteria. This enables them to be classified as either gram positive or gram negative. The cell walls of gram-negative bacteria include an additional outer membrane. Gram-positive bacteria retain the stain, whereas gram-negative bacteria are almost colorless due to a more complex composition of the cell wall. This outer membrane is sometimes toxic to mammals, providing one mechanism by which some bacteria cause disease. The antibiotic penicillin works best on gram-positive bacteria.

What is the ability some bacteria have that allows them to survive in unfavorable conditions? What type of bacteria can live with or without oxygen?

Fungi

Fungi is a general term used to denote groups that include mushrooms, yeasts, and molds. They may invade living organisms, including humans, as well as nonliving organic substances. Of the 100,000 identified species of fungi, 100 are common in humans, and more than 10 are pathogenic. Most fungal infections are superficial and mild, though persistent and difficult to eliminate. Some may become life threatening, especially in older debilitated or immunosuppressed people.

Examples of fungal infections include oral candidiasis, tinea corporis, and tinea pedis. Oral **candidiasis** (Figure 11.4) is caused by the fungus *Candida albicans*. *Candida* is part of the normal flora of mucous membranes, but could spread in some people who are prescribed antibiotic therapy. It is usually a harmless condition in children called oral thrush. Candida is characterized by creamy, white-colored patches on the oral mucosa and is treated with antifungal drugs. Tinea is a

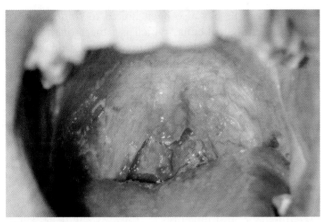
FIGURE 11.4
Oral candidiasis.

name applied to many different kinds of fungal infections of the skin. Tinea corporis is also called ringworm and is sometimes acquired from animals. Tinea pedis is known as athlete's foot.

Protozoa

Protozoa are single-celled microorganisms and the lowest form of animal life. Protozoa are more complex than bacteria and are self-contained. They attach themselves to other objects or organisms. Approximately 30 protozoa are disease-producing organisms, or pathogenic, to humans. Examples of these include amebic dysentery, malaria, and *Giardia*.

Why might a patient who is prescribed antibiotics for a bacterial infection also need to receive an antifungal medication? **?**

Patient Education

A simple fact that must be understood by the dental patient is that antibiotics kill bacteria, not viruses. Doctors often prescribe antibiotics partly due to patient demand. Antibiotic resistance occurs when evolutionary mutations in bacteria allow them to survive these powerful drugs, making the drugs much less effective in the future. This worsens the problem by producing bacteria with a greater ability to survive our strongest antibiotics. Also, when a patient does not finish taking a prescription for antibiotics, drug-resistant microbes not killed in the first days of treatment can multiply and cause the next treatment of drugs to be less effective. Ensure that your patients understand they must finish any antibiotic medications prescribed by the dentist for a bacterial infection even if they feel better before completing the prescription.

Rickettsiae

Rickettsia is a type of microorganism that causes various diseases such as typhus and Rocky Mountain spotted fever. Rickettsia is like a virus since it requires other living cells for growth but it is also like bacteria that requires oxygen. The rickettsia microorganism is susceptible to antibiotics.

Viruses

Viruses are the smallest microorganisms at approximately 1/1000 of a millimeter in diameter. They cannot move or grow and are dependent on their host cells. Their protein coat enables them to penetrate the cells of a specific host. Once inside the host cell, the viral genetic material produces components of new viruses, which attack neighboring cells. Viruses responsible for the common cold attack membranes of the respiratory tract, those causing measles infect the skin, and the rabies virus attacks nerve cells. Other diseases caused by viruses include chickenpox, influenza (the flu), measles, rubella, and mumps. Antiviral agents may destroy host cells as well as viruses.

Attributes of viruses include these:

* Viruses reproduce only inside of a host cell.
* They are more simplistic than cells.
* They require an electron microscope in order to see them.
* They are unable to grow or reproduce on their own.
* They have a protein coat that is specialized to enable the virus to penetrate the cells of hosts.
* Each type of virus is specialized to attack a specific host cell.

Viral Diseases

Viruses cannot reproduce outside of a living cell and have evolved to transmit their genetic information from one cell to another for the purpose of replication. Viruses often damage or kill the cells that they infect, causing disease in the infected organisms. Three common viral shapes are shown in Figure 11.5.

The antibiotics that are effective against bacterial infections are useless against viruses, although some promising antiviral drugs are being developed. Four antiviral drugs that have been approved by the Food

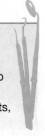

Preparing for Externship

Health care providers must protect themselves from contagious diseases. Dental assistants need to keep up to date on their immunizations for measles, mumps, and rubella (MMR) and HBV, annual flu shots, and TB tests.

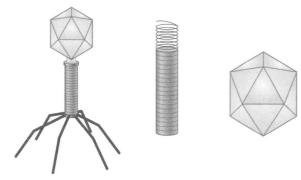

FIGURE 11.5
Various virus shapes.

and Drug Administration for treatment of influenza are amantadine, rimantadine, zanamivir, and oseltamivir. Each of these has specific indications and directions for use and is not always effective for all types of flu viruses.

Herpes

Herpes simplex virus type 1 (HSV-1) is one type of herpes virus that occurs in mucous membranes of the mouth and lips. With HSV-1, painful fever blisters, called vesicles, may develop inside the mouth on the buccal mucosa and gingiva, or on the lips and skin around the mouth. In unusual cases these vesicles may occur on the head and neck. This virus is spread by direct contact with the lesions. Another type of herpes virus transmitted through sexual contact, producing similar sores on or near the genitals, is herpes simplex virus type 2 (HSV-2).

The herpes virus secures permanent residence in the body, erupting periodically, usually during times of stress, as infectious sores. Clinically, HSV-1 and HSV-2 lesions cannot be distinguished from each other. One can acquire HSV-1 oral infections or HSV-2 genital infections through oral–genital contact. Location is the only difference between the two types of herpes. Symptoms of herpes are called outbreaks that can be treated with antiviral ointments.

HIV and AIDS

The devastating disease **acquired immunodeficiency syndrome (AIDS)**, which cripples the body's immune system, is caused by the **human immunodeficiency virus (HIV)**, which attacks a specific type of white blood cell that controls the body's immune response. HIV destroys the CD4 T-cells that are required for the proper functioning of the immune system. AIDS is the late stage of the HIV disease.

Many of the problems faced by people infected with HIV result from failure of the immune system to protect them from opportunistic infections. Opportunistic infections are caused by organisms that do not usually cause disease in a person with a healthy immune system. HIV attacks organs such as the kidneys, the heart, and the

brain. This virus has also been linked to some types of cancers such as leukemia, which is cancer of the white blood cells. HIV is only transmitted through direct contact of a mucous membrane with a body fluid containing the virus. It is spread through blood, semen, vaginal fluid, breast milk, and other body fluids. To ensure that dental team members are protected from contracting diseases such as HIV through their patients, it is important during dental procedures to wear personal protective equipment such as gloves, mask, and a face shield.

Hepatitis

Hepatitis is a viral infection that affects the liver. There are at least six different types of hepatitis viruses and they are lettered A through G. The most common types are hepatitis A, hepatitis B, and hepatitis C. Hepatitis A virus (HAV) is an acute infection and people usually improve without treatment. Acute infections have a rapid onset, severe symptoms, and last a short period of time. Hepatitis A is found in the feces of HAV-infected people and is spread from one person to another by putting something in the mouth that is contaminated. This can happen when people who prepare foods do not wash their hands after using the toilet.

Hepatitis B and C can cause a chronic persistent infection that leads to chronic liver disease. Chronic illnesses have a slow and long-lasting progression. Both hepatitis B (HBV) and hepatitis C (HCV) are found in the blood and certain body fluids. They are spread when a person comes in contact with the blood or body fluids from an infected person. Exposure to blood in any situation can be a risk for transmission of these two viruses. Vaccines are available to prevent hepatitis A and B, but not for HCV.

The liver processes everything an individual consumes and is therefore susceptible to injury by chemicals that enter the bloodstream such as cleaning chemicals when workers do not wear proper clothing to provide respiratory protection. Some of these chemicals are difficult to eliminate and can cause toxic hepatitis with symptoms similar to viral hepatitis. Liver inflammation usually subsides within days or weeks after exposure to the chemical is stopped.

Life Span Considerations

Older patients are especially vulnerable to respiratory infections such as influenza or pneumonia. It is important to note that older people may have fewer or different symptoms than younger people have. An elderly person who experiences even a minor cough and weakness for more than a day or so should seek medical help to ensure that the condition does not become life threatening.

Bacterial Diseases

Some bacteria pose a threat to human health. These pathogenic bacteria create toxic substances that cause disease symptoms. Some bacteria are especially virulent, meaning very potent and able to overcome defense mechanisms. Infectious diseases caused by bacteria include anthrax, botulism, gonorrhea and syphilis, Lyme disease, meningitis, pneumonia, *Streptococcus* bacterium, which comes in many forms that produce a variety of diseases, and tuberculosis.

Anthrax

Anthrax is an acute infectious disease caused by the spore-forming *Bacillus anthracis*. It most commonly develops in animals, but can also occur in humans if exposed to the infected animal or tissue from an infected animal or it can be acquired by inhaling anthrax spores. It is not contagious and cannot be spread from person to person.

Botulism

Botulism and tetanus produce toxins that attack the nervous system. These bacteria are anaerobes that survive as spores until introduced into a favorable environment. Botulism is a lethal form of food poisoning. A sealed container of canned food that has been improperly sterilized provides a haven for botulism bacteria. These anaerobes produce a toxin so potent that a single gram could kill 15 million people.

Tetanus

Tetanus, also known as lockjaw, is caused by bacteria often found in soil. The bacteria enter the body through wounds in the skin. A deep puncture wound, through which tetanus bacteria enter the body, also protects the bacteria from contact with oxygen. As the bacteria multiply, they release their paralyzing poison into the bloodstream. Tetanus is caused by *Clostridium tetani*, a gram-positive, spore-forming bacteria.

Tuberculosis

Tuberculosis (TB) is a bacterial disease affecting the lungs and is known as pulmonary TB. Tuberculosis is caused by *Mycobacterium tuberculosis* bacteria. It is spread through the air when a person with untreated TB coughs or sneezes. It is the leading cause of death in the world from a single infectious disease. Symptoms of TB include a low-grade fever, night sweats, fatigue, weight loss, and a persistent cough.

A positive tuberculin skin test can indicate an active case of TB or prior exposure to the disease. A chest x-ray is required to confirm the diagnosis of tuberculosis. Some people do not have obvious symptoms of the disease. A person may have a latent TB infection and cannot spread the infection to others. Treatment usually includes taking antituberculosis medication for several months. People with active TB must complete a course of treatment for six months or longer.

Pneumonia

Pneumonia is an inflammation of the lungs caused by bacteria, viruses, fungi, and other microorganisms. The severity of pneumonia depends on which organism is causing the infection. Symptoms often begin suddenly with chills, fever, a persistent cough, and chest pain. Pneumonia is usually triggered when a patient's defense system is weakened, most often by a simple viral upper respiratory tract infection or a case of influenza. Such infections do not cause pneumonia but alter the mucous membranes, allowing bacterial growth that makes the person even more ill. Yearly influenza vaccines are a preventive measure to help fight the possibility of contracting the flu and the possible complication of acquiring pneumonia. Viral pneumonias are usually not very serious, but they can be life threatening in very old and very young patients, and in people whose immune systems are weak.

Dental Plaque

Surrounding the cell walls of some bacteria are sticky capsules, or slime layers, composed of protein. These capsules help certain disease-causing bacteria to escape detection by their host's immune system. The slime layers, or capsules, allow the bacteria that cause tooth decay to adhere in masses to the smooth surface of a tooth. This slime forms the basis of dental plaque. Poor oral hygiene allows plaque to multiply into bacterial colonies that, if left on the teeth and gingiva long enough, release their by-products and acids on oral structures. Dental plaque is also called dental biofilm, which refers to a complex community of several varieties of bacteria that may reach a thickness of 300 to 500 cells on the surfaces of teeth, resulting in dental disease due to bacterial activities.

The primary bacteria that cause tooth decay are **Streptococcus mutans** bacteria. *Streptococcus mutans* bacteria initiate development of dental caries because their activities lead to colonization of the tooth surfaces, plaque formation, and demineralization of tooth enamel. After the initial weakening of the enamel, various oral bacteria gain access to interior regions of the tooth. *Lactobacilli*, *Actinomyces*, and various other bacteria are secondary invaders that continue the destruction process. *Streptococcus mutans*, *Streptococcus sanguis*, and *Actinomyces viscosus* species are early colonizers of the tooth surface that produce fermentable carbohydrates as waste by-products, which are then fermented by other neighboring species of bacteria. *Lactobacillus* bacteria in plaque produce lactic acid from the fermentation of sugars and other carbohydrates in the diet of the host. The

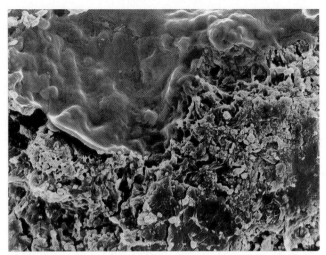

FIGURE 11.6
Bacterial colonies of dental plaque.

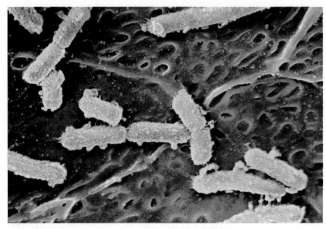

FIGURE 11.7
Close-up view of plaque bacteria.

metabolic and structural interactions between different plaque microorganisms are a complex ecological niche. Breaking up these bacterial communities on the teeth by brushing and flossing will prevent their formation (Figures 11.6 and 11.7).

Numerous studies indicate that *Streptococcus mutans* bacteria can be transmitted from a parent or another caregiver to an infant or child through sharing of saliva if the adult has a high concentration of *Streptococcus mutans* in his or her mouth. The mode of transmission may be through either direct or indirect contact. The transfer occurs by direct contact when a child is allowed to put fingers into the parent's mouth and then back into his or her own mouth. Cleaning a pacifier or bottle nipple that has fallen by cleaning it with the parent's own saliva before giving it back to the infant is another method of transfer, as is kissing. Indirect contact occurs through shared contaminated objects such as eating utensils, toothbrushes, cups, and even toys. Parents and caregivers should practice good oral hygiene and avoid habits that could transmit bacteria. Any caretakers can infect a child with this potentially destructive bacterium. The degree of transmission will vary based on the degree of infection of the parent, caregiver, or playmate, the frequency of contact, and the diet and immune system of the child.

Which microorganism is the smallest? What is the primary bacterial component in dental plaque?

SUMMARY

The only way some organisms can be seen is by using a microscope. The study of these organisms is called microbiology. Microorganisms are found almost everywhere. Some need oxygen to grow and stay alive, and some live well without oxygen. By studying microbes, pioneering scientists have achieved remarkable success in understanding life processes and disease control. They led the way to vaccines that have nearly eliminated several dreaded childhood diseases.

Although some microbes play an important part in our daily lives by keeping us healthy, other microorganisms cause infection and disease. The major groups of microorganisms are algae, bacteria, fungi, protozoa, rickettsia, and viruses. Several common, as well as life-threatening, diseases are caused by bacteria and viruses. Disease-causing microbes are very good at adjusting to new environments, which makes it difficult to find a way to eliminate them. Dental health care providers must be aware of these microorganisms in order to protect themselves from the possibility of infection and to ensure no infectious microorganisms are transmitted to patients through cross-contamination.

KEY TERMS

- **Acquired immunodeficiency syndrome (AIDS):** Disease that destroys the body's immune system.   p. 170
- **Aerobic bacteria:** Bacteria that depend on oxygen to survive.   p. 168
- **Anaerobic bacteria:** Bacteria that are destroyed by contact with oxygen.   p. 168
- **Bacteria:** Small one-celled microorganisms.   p. 167

KEY TERMS (continued)

- **Candidiasis:** Disease caused by the fungus *Candida albicans*; also called oral thrush. p. 168
- **Facultative bacteria:** Bacteria that can live with or without oxygen. p. 168
- **Hepatitis:** A viral infection that affects the liver. p. 170
- **Human immunodeficiency virus (HIV):** A virus that attacks a specific type of white blood cell that controls the body's immune response. p. 170
- **Microbiology:** The study of living organisms too small to be seen without a microscope. p. 166
- **Pathogenic:** Disease producing. p. 166

- **Penicillin:** The first antibiotic. p. 167
- **Spore:** Layers of protective membranes formed by some bacteria. p. 167
- *Streptococcus mutans:* The primary bacteria found in dental plaque. p. 171
- **Tetanus:** Disease caused by bacteria often found in soil; the bacteria often enter the body via a wound in the skin. p. 171
- **Tuberculosis:** A bacterial infection that affects the lungs. p. 171
- **Viruses:** The smallest microorganisms. p. 169

● CHECK YOUR UNDERSTANDING

1. What are some of the useful attributes of bacteria?
   a. food digestion
   b. production of bread
   c. production of cheese
   d. all of the above

2. Name bacteria associated with dental plaque.
   a. *Actinomyces sanguis*
   b. *Streptococcus sanguis*
   c. *Clostridium tetani*
   d. both a and b
   e. all of the above

3. Bacteria divide by a process called binary fission. How frequently can they divide in ideal conditions?
   a. every 20 minutes
   b. every 30 minutes
   c. every 2 hours
   d. every 24 hours

4. Bacteria are shaped like
   a. rods.
   b. spheres.
   c. corkscrews.
   d. all of the above.

5. A technique that distinguishes two types of cell wall construction in bacteria is called Gram-
   a. stain.
   b. positive.
   c. negative.
   d. spore.

6. What type of microorganism causes oral candidiasis?
   a. fungus
   b. protozoa
   c. rickettsia
   d. bacteria

7. Which microorganisms reproduce genetic material inside their host cells?
   a. bacteria
   b. protozoa
   c. viruses
   d. algae

8. What is the name of the virus that causes inflammation of the liver?
   a. HSV-1
   b. HSV-2
   c. HIV
   d. HBV

9. The primary microbe that initiates dental disease is
   a. plaque.
   b. *Candida.*
   c. *Streptococcus mutans.*
   d. tuberculosis.

10. Tuberculosis is spread by a person
    a. coughing.
    b. sneezing.
    c. sweating.
    d. a and b.

● INTERNET ACTIVITY

- Take a virtual tour of the bacteria museum at
  http://bacteriamuseum.org/niches/wabacteria/
  bacteria.shtml

WEB REFERENCES

- The Guardians.com   www.theguardians.com/ (once at the site click on microbiology on the right-hand bottom corner)
- Loyola University Health System: Microbiology & Immunology
  www.meddean.luc.edu/lumen/DeptWebs/microbio/med/gram/tech.htm
- Open Wide: Oral Health Training for Health Professionals
  www.mchoralhealth.org/OpenWide/mod1_3.htm and www.mchoralhealth.org/OpenWide/mod1_4.htm

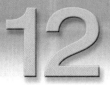

Dental Disease and Infection Control

Learning Objectives

After reading this chapter, the student should be able to:

- Define a pathogen.
- Identify the steps in the chain of infection.
- Identify the categories of occupational exposure.
- Explain the difference between chronic, acute, and latent infections.
- Describe disease transmission in the dental office.
- Explain universal and standard precautions.
- Discuss the purpose of an exposure control plan.
- Describe the importance of infection control in the dental laboratory.
- Demonstrate and describe hand hygiene techniques.
- Discuss waste management in the dental office.

Preparing for Certification Exams

- Perform proper hand hygiene.
- Wear suitable personal protective equipment for the appropriate situation.
- Maintain aseptic conditions.
- Understand and follow the bloodborne pathogen standard.
- Dispose of biohazard wastes and other types of waste in the dental office.

Chapter Outline

- The Chain of Infection
  - Virulence
  - Types of Infections
  - Stages of an Infection
  - Modes of Disease Transmission
- The Immune System
  - Recommended Immunizations for Health Care Personnel
- Disease Transmission in the Dental Office
- Roles and Responsibilities of the CDC and OSHA in Infection Control
  - CDC's *Guidelines for Infection Control in Dental Health-Care Settings*
  - OSHA Bloodborne Pathogens Standard
  - Universal Precautions
- Exposure Control Plan
  - Exposure Prevention and Management
  - Engineering and Work Control Practices
- Environmental Infection Control
  - Chemical Disinfectants
  - Surface Barriers
- Infection Control Practices
  - Personal Protective Equipment
- Additional Infection Control Practices
  - Controlling Cross-Contamination in the Dental Laboratory
  - Laser Plumes
  - Infection Control in Dental Radiology
- Waste Management in the Dental Office
  - Waste Classifications
- Special Considerations from the Centers for Disease Control and Prevention
  - *Mycobacterium Tuberculosis*
  - Creutzfeldt-Jakob Disease and Other Prion Diseases

Key Terms

Active immunity

Bloodborne pathogens

Droplet transmission

Engineering control

Exposure control plan

Innate immunity

Latent infection

Opportunistic infection

Other potentially infectious materials (OPIM)

Passive immunity

Personal protective equipment (PPE)

Standard precautions

Universal precautions

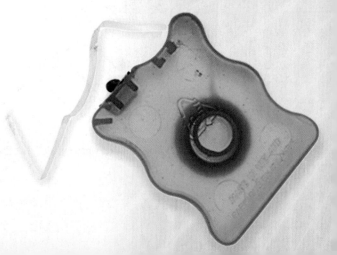

Dental health care workers are at risk of exposure to infectious blood and body fluids. For this reason, it is important for the dental assistant to understand the types of infection and how infection is transmitted. Protecting oneself and the dental patient can be achieved by following the guidelines of infection control established by the Centers for Disease Control and Prevention (CDC). In addition to the CDC's guidelines, the bloodborne pathogen standards established by the Occupational Safety and Health Administration (OSHA), including disposal techniques for disposing of infectious and hazardous waste, must be followed to protect the entire dental team and all patients.

The Chain of Infection

Pathogens are disease-causing microorganisms. In order for an infection to occur, certain steps or factors must be present. These factors make up the chain of infection (Figure 12.1). Understanding the chain of infection can assist the dental assistant in preventing the spread of infection.

To have an infection, six factors must exist:

1. A pathogenic organism such as a virus, bacterium, fungus, protozoa, or rickettsia.
2. A location of the infectious source or reservoir, such as equipment, a person, food, or animals.
3. A way for the infectious source to leave or exit the reservoir, such as an individual coughing or sneezing without covering the mouth.

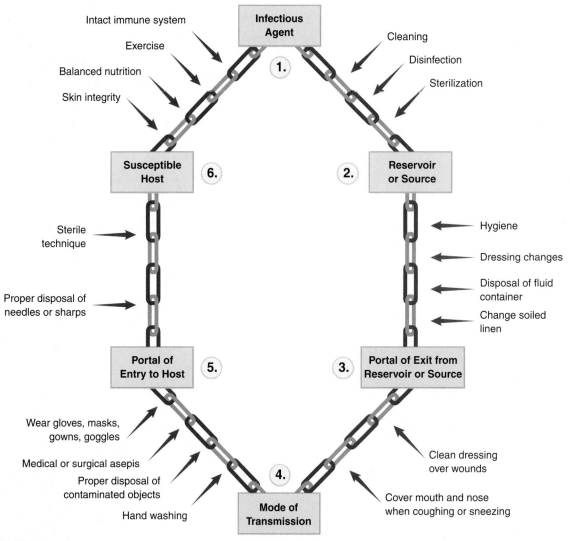

FIGURE 12.1
The chain of infection.

4. A mode of transmission that can occur through methods such as touching, breathing, or ingesting pathogens.

5. A portal of entry, in other words, a way for the pathogen to enter the body. The mouth and nose are portals of entry for airborne diseases. Needlesticks, cuts, or a break in the skin are portals of entry for **bloodborne pathogens.**

6. The presence of a susceptible host. A susceptible host is a person who is unable to resist the high number of microorganisms or pathogens. This person's immune system is usually compromised, which causes the pathogens to invade, resulting in illness. Once the microorganism is inside the host, it begins to break down the cell function. This can cause an infection depending on the virulence of the pathogen.

Virulence

Virulence is the reproducing power of a pathogen (Figure 12.2). The human body, including the oral cavity, contains normal flora or bacteria. Normal flora in the oral cavity can be pathogenic or nonpathogenic. Usually the body adapts to this flora; however, if the flora increases in number or is transferred to sites in the body where such microorganisms are not normally present, then illness may occur. The basic categories of microorganisms are:

- Bacteria
- Fungi
- Protozoa
- Rickettsiaie
- Viruses
- Prions

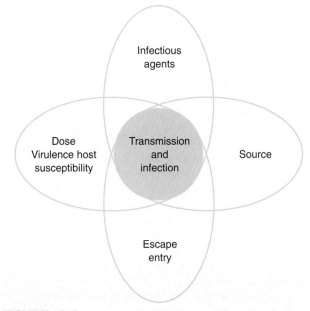

FIGURE 12.2
Virulence.

To reduce the amount of exposure to microorganisms during dental treatment, a dental dam and high-volume evacuation are used along with a preprocedural rinse with an antimicrobial. (See Chapter 26 for information on dental dams and oral evacuation systems.)

What are the links to the chain of infection? What is normal flora and does it cause infection?

Types of Infections

Four main types of infections can occur in the chain of infection: acute, chronic, latent, and opportunistic infections. Infections may be a combination of more than one of these types. Acute infections have a short duration. The symptoms, which can be severe, are usually of quick onset soon after the infection. The common cold is an example of an acute viral infection.

Unlike the short-lived acute infections, chronic infections can live in the human body for an indefinite period of time. The person with a chronic infection may not show any symptoms of the disease but may be a carrier. Examples of chronic infections are hepatitis C (HCV) and the human immunodeficiency virus (HIV).

A **latent infection** is one that "hangs on," but the symptoms come and go. The herpes virus that can appear in cold sores or genital herpes is an example of a latent infection. Once the virus enters the body, it lies dormant until certain conditions such as an illness or stress bring it to the surface. **Opportunistic infections** are usually caused by nonpathogenic organisms that attack individuals with weakened immune systems. These infections are common in patients with AIDS and those with diabetes.

Stages of an Infection

There are four basic stages of infection:

- *Incubation stage:* the initial entrance of the pathogen in the body
- *Prodromal stage:* the appearance of "early symptoms"
- *Acute stage:* when the symptoms are at their peak and the person is obviously ill

• *Convalescent stage:* the recovery phase. The microorganisms begin to decline and are being destroyed by the body's defenses

Modes of Disease Transmission

Disease can be spread in many ways. The primary modes of disease transmission in dentistry are direct contact, indirect contact, and droplet infection. Parenteral, bloodborne, airborne, food and water, and fecal–oral routes are also modes of disease transmission, but are not common in the field of dentistry.

Direct contact transmission occurs by touching an infected lesion or coming in contact with contaminated blood and other bodily fluids such as semen and saliva. An individual who has small cuts or breaks in the skin is at a higher risk of contracting the disease once direct contact has been made. This is why it is important for dental team members to wear proper personal **protective equipment (PPE)** during any activity where potentially infectious fluids are involved.

Indirect contact occurs when an individual comes in contact with inanimate materials such as contaminated instruments, items, and surfaces. An example of indirect contact is when a dental assistant touches a dirty instrument or dental chair that has been contaminated with saliva. Appropriate use of PPE, disinfection, and sterilization can prevent indirect contact transmission. Indirect contact can also result in the transmission of disease.

Droplet transmission, also known as inhalation transmission, occurs through contaminated spray and spatter from use of a high-speed handpiece. Spray and spatter can occur when using instruments in the dental office. PPE such as gloves, mask, eyewear, and protective clothing will help prevent droplet infection.

Parenteral transmission can occur through needlesticks, cuts, bites, and other breaks in the skin. *Parenteral* means "through the skin." Bloodborne pathogens can be transferred through this mode. Some pathogens are considered bloodborne because they are carried in the blood and bodily fluids. These pathogens can be transmitted through direct and indirect contact with the blood and bodily fluids of an infected person. Improper sterilization of instruments and improper needle handling can spread bloodborne pathogens. HIV, HCV, and hepatitis B (HBV) are common bloodborne pathogens that are of concern to dental health care workers.

Airborne disease is another method for disease to be transmitted and occurs when a host inhales a pathogen. Airborne pathogens are particles that have evaporated in the air and can be inhaled by the health care worker. For example, a cough from someone can transmit the flu airborne. Protective eyewear and masks are required to prevent airborne transmission.

Many diseases are transmitted by contaminated food or water. Tuberculosis, botulism, and staphylococcal and streptococcal infections are spread this way. Tuberculosis can be spread through coughing and sneezing on a person or surface. Properly washed and cooked foods and use of appropriate hand hygiene techniques help eliminate this type of transmission.

Fecal–oral transmission occurs most often with health care or daycare workers who change diapers frequently or those who assist in cleaning individuals. If an individual does not use effective hand hygiene techniques after coming in contact with feces, possible transmission can occur. This transmission is extremely rare in a dental setting; however, health care workers must always remember to wash their hands after using the restroom.

What is the appropriate PPE for airborne transmission? What is the difference between airborne and droplet transmission?

The Immune System

The immune system is the body's defense against invasion of infectious organisms. The immune system offers the body protection against disease. This protection is called immunity. Humans have three types of immunity: innate,

---

Life Span Considerations

Forty to 50 years ago, infection control practices were almost nonexistent. Due to this fact, many of your older patients may not be familiar with the importance of infection control. For example, the patient who arrives at your reception desk and proceeds to remove his broken denture and place it on your desk may not think twice about it. However, you can politely inform the patient of your infection control policy and request that he hold onto the dentures until the patient is taken back to the treatment area. Once the patient leaves the desk area, be sure to disinfect the desk.

Cultural Considerations

A patient's culture can significantly impact his or her beliefs on how disease is transmitted and on the importance of practicing infection control techniques. As a dental assistant it is important to be sensitive to a patient's culture. Sometimes based on the patient's culture, further education may be required. Education may include teaching the patient about how infection control methods such as hand washing make a difference in minimizing disease transmission. Encourage patients to utilize these methods in their own personal lives.

adaptive, and passive. Everyone is born with **innate** (or natural) **immunity.** Many of the microorganisms that affect animals do not harm the human body because of innate immunity. Innate immunity includes the external barriers of the body such as the skin and mucous membranes, which are the first line of defense in preventing diseases from entering the body.

Another type of protection for the human body is that of **active** (or adaptive) **immunity** or artificially acquired immunity. This type of immunity develops throughout one's life. Active immunity involves the lymphocytes and develops as children and adults are exposed to diseases or immunized against diseases through vaccination. Vaccinations are created from diseased organisms that are genetically altered to eliminate the harmful effects. The vaccine is then injected into the body where antibodies are formed from the vaccine.

Passive immunity is "borrowed" from an outside source and lasts for a short period of time. For example, antibodies in a mother's breast milk provide the infant with a temporary immunity from diseases to which the mother has been exposed. This can help protect the infant against infection during the early years of childhood while the infant's own immune system is maturing.

Figure 12.3 illustrates these three types of immunity, as well as a fourth, less common type: passive artificial immunity.

Recommended Immunizations for Health Care Personnel

According to the CDC, health care workers are at a high risk for acquiring and/or transmitting HBV, influenza, measles, mumps, rubella, and varicella. All of these diseases can be prevented with immunizations. OSHA requires that employers make HBV vaccinations available to all employees who have potential contact with blood or other infectious materials within 10 days of assignment. Those employees who decline the vaccination must document and sign a declination statement. The declination statement must contain the same information as required in the sample provided in OSHA guidelines. All health care workers must be educated on the risks of exposure and on infection control policies prior to signing the declination statement.

Here is a standard hepatitis informed refusal statement:

> I understand that due to my occupational exposure to blood and other potentially infectious materials I may be at risk of acquiring hepatitis B virus (HBV) infection. I have been given the opportunity to be vaccinated with the hepatitis B vaccine, at no charge to myself. However, I decline hepatitis B vaccination at this time. I understand that by declining this vaccine, I continue to be at risk of acquiring hepatitis B, a serious disease. If in the future I continue to have occupational exposure to blood or other potentially infectious materials and I want to be vaccinated with hepatitis B vaccine, I can receive the vaccination series at no charge to me.

The statement is signed and dated by the employee and a witness. Offices may use different forms for informed refusal; this is just one example.

Employees have the right to refuse the HBV vaccine and/or any postexposure evaluation and follow-up. It is important to note, however, that the employee needs to be properly informed of the benefits of the vaccination and postexposure evaluation through training. The employee also has the right to decide to take the vaccination at a later date if he or she so chooses.

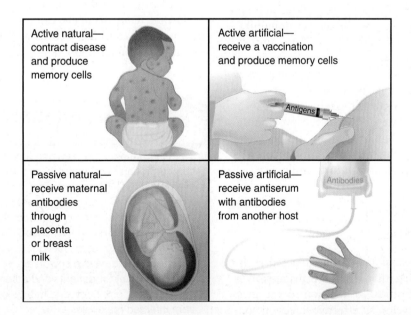

FIGURE 12.3
Types of immunity.

The CDC recommends the following vaccinations for dental health care workers:

- *Hepatitis B:* A series of three doses; two doses one month apart and the third dose five months after the second dose. A hepatitis B surface antibody titer (to make sure the body developed immunity to hepatitis B) is recommended after three doses of vaccine for persons in risk groups such as health care workers who could be exposed to blood and bodily fluids.
- *Rubella:* One dose, no booster required.
- *Measles:* One dose, no booster.
- *Influenza:* Annual vaccination.
- *Tetanus-diphtheria:* Booster every 10 years.
- *Polio vaccine.*
- *Varicella.*

Immunizations greatly reduce the number of diseases to which health care workers are susceptible. Immunizations are an essential part of prevention and infection control programs. OSHA requires the employer to offer and pay for hepatitis immunizations. For a large number of new dental assistants, the cost of certain immunizations is covered inclusively with their school tuition. However, some schools require immunizations upon acceptance into a dental assisting program. Some states require that immunizations be up to date prior to the dental assistant beginning his or her externship. The local health department or private physician can provide the immunizations needed. Dental health care workers should maintain copies of their immunization records to show as proof of immunization to future employers.

Disease Transmission in the Dental Office

Ensuring that dental professionals are vaccinated is the first step toward ensuring that disease transmission is minimized in the dental office. In addition to vaccines, the dental office must develop an effective infection control program that reduces the risk of exposure to and the spread of infectious microorganisms. The following are paths for contamination in the dental setting:

- Patient to dental team
- Dental team to patient
- Patient to patient
- Dental team to dental team
- Dental team to community
- Community to dental office to patient

Cross-contamination from patients to dental health care workers can occur through direct contact with blood and saliva. Breaks in the skin and small tears in protective gloves allow pathogens from patient's bodily fluids to invade the dental worker. Intact gloves and proper hand hygiene are control measures for this path of transmission.

Droplet infection and indirect contact are other paths of microorganism transmission from patients, so it is important for dental assistants to wear masks, gloves, safety glasses, and a face shield to protect themselves from inhalation of pathogens.

Practicing safe needle and instrument handling and using ultrasonic cleaners and antimicrobial cleaners are also ways to reduce the amount of pathogens to which the dental worker is exposed.

The pathway of contamination from dental team member to patient is rare, but very possible. Contamination can occur if the dental assistant does not follow proper infection control procedures.

Pathogens can also be transferred from patient to patient, by improper handling, cleaning, and sterilizing of instruments and treatment room surfaces and through use of inaccurate hand hygiene techniques. Patient-to-patient transmission occurs through indirect contact, for example, when an instrument used on one patient is not sterilized prior to using it on another patient.

Dental team members can also transmit disease to each other by touching records or the dental unit when wearing contaminated gloves. The dental assistant should not document, file, or handle dental records with contaminated gloves.

The dental team can also transmit disease to the community. This pathway can occur when pathogens from patients leave the office on laboratory appliances or equipment needing repairs. Pathogens can also leave the office on the clothing of dental office employees. The CDC recommends that dental health care workers change out of their work attire prior to leaving the office. It is further recommended that the clothing be laundered at the office so as to reduce the spread of infection to the community, including the dental team's family members.

Contamination from community to dental office to patient can occur through the community water system. Microorganisms can enter the dental office through the community water system that supplies water to dental waterlines. Organisms colonize in the waterlines and form a biofilm, which can spread disease through the use of handpieces and air/water units. Waterborne diseases such as Legionnaires' disease can be caused by various types of bacteria from the public water supply. These organisms stay stagnant in the water that is left in the waterlines and suction lines of the dental unit. It is important for the dental health care worker to understand how to minimize the transmission of disease from the community through waterlines and dental units because the bacteria can cause opportunistic infections especially in individuals with lowered immune systems. (See Chapter 19 for information on dental unit waterlines and waterborne diseases.)

How do patients transfer pathogens between patients? How can the dental team avoid transmitting diseases to the community?

Roles and Responsibilities of the CDC and OSHA in Infection Control

According to the CDC it is estimated that in the United States 9 million people work in health care professions. That number includes 168,000 dentists, 112,000 hygienists, and 218,000 dental assistants. The CDC provides guidelines specifically for dental health care workers regarding infection control. Publications such as *Morbidity and Mortality Weekly Report* (MMWR) and *Guidelines for Infection Control in Dental Health-Care Settings* provide recommendations designed to prevent or reduce the potential for disease transmission in the dental office. Table 12-1 provides some definitions used when discussing infection control that will be helpful as you read the following paragraph.

The CDC recommendations are categorized based on scientific data, rationale, and applicability; in other words, infection control procedures are categorized based on the potential to transmit disease. Researchers

TABLE 12-1 CDC Infection Control Definitions

Occupational exposure	Defined as "reasonably anticipated skin, eye, mucous membrane, or parenteral contact with blood or OPIM that may result from the performance of the employee's duties"
Blood	Defined as human blood, human blood components, and products made from human blood
Other potentially infectious material (OPIM)	Defined as the following human bodily fluids: saliva in dental procedures, semen, vaginal secretions, cerebrospinal, synovial, pleural, pericardial, peritoneal, and amniotic fluids; bodily fluids visibly contaminated with blood; along with all bodily fluids in situations where it is difficult or impossible to differentiate between bodily fluids; unfixed human tissues or organs (other than intact skin); HIV-containing cell or tissue cultures, organ cultures, and HIV- or HBV-containing culture media or other solutions; and blood, organs, or other tissues from experimental animals infected with HIV or HBV

from the CDC study various procedures and test them in controlled settings to determine the transmission possibility. They then rank each procedure to indicate the possibility of transmission and state the recommended infection control procedure that should be followed. The dental team can use this information to help guide itself when establishing proper infection control protocols that provide the team members and the dental patient the most protection.

CDC's Guidelines for Infection Control in Dental Health-Care Settings

To communicate clearly to dental health care professionals, the CDC has created categories that indicate what type of infection control should be established for each dental procedure. The following categories and recommendations are published in the CDC's *Guidelines for Infection Control in Dental Health-Care Settings*:

- *Category IA:* Strongly recommended for implementation and strongly supported by well-designed experimental, clinical, or epidemiologic studies. For example: Place used disposable syringes and needles, scalpel blades, and other sharps in appropriate puncture-resistant containers. This procedure is categorized as IA and IC, which is strongly recommended, and mandated by state and federal regulations.

- *Category IB:* Strongly recommended for implementation and supported by experimental, clinical, or epidemiologic studies and a strong theoretical rationale.

For example: Dental health care workers should receive infection control training upon hiring and then annually thereafter. Also prior to performing a new task or procedure, training should be conducted.

- *Category IC:* Required for implementation as mandated by a federal or state regulation or standard. For example: Each dental office must develop a comprehensive postexposure management and medical follow-up program. This mandatory program must be in place in the event a dental health care worker gets exposed to bloodborne pathogen infectious materials.

- *Category II:* Suggested for implementation and supported by suggestive clinical or epidemiologic studies or a theoretical rationale. For example: All health care workers should keep their fingernails short with smooth, filed edges. This is a *suggested,* not mandatory, task/procedure.

- *Unresolved issue:* No recommendations. Insufficient evidence or no consensus regarding efficacy exists. For example: When treating patients with Creutzfeldt-Jakob disease and other prion diseases, standard or universal precautions should be used. No additional recommendations are provided because the disease is still being studied.

In addition to the categories just discussed, the CDC's *Guidelines for Infection Control in Dental Health-Care Settings* also cover these topics as taken from the *MMWR:*

- Use of standard precautions
- Work restrictions for health care personnel with infectious diseases
- Postexposure management of occupational exposures to bloodborne pathogens
- Hand hygiene products/surgical hand asepsis
- Latex hypersensitivity and contact dermatitis
- Sterilization of unwrapped instruments
- Dental radiology infection control
- Preprocedural mouth rinses
- Oral surgery procedures
- Laser plumes
- Tuberculosis
- Infection control program evaluation

Note that the CDC and OSHA both provide research, guidance, and regulations for the safety and health of employees. OSHA, however, is a regulatory agency that provides lawful standards that employers must follow to protect employees. Failure to follow OSHA regulations can result in fines or closures. In contrast, the CDC is not a regulatory agency; its standards are recommendations, not mandates. The CDC's guidelines, however, have become the standard of care throughout the dental field, so it is very important that the dental team follow these guidelines. The regulations established by OSHA and the guidelines set forth by the CDC are published to protect the health and safety of employees and patients and apply to all dental health care personnel.

OSHA Bloodborne Pathogens Standard

As part of its overall Occupational Safety and Health Standards, on December 6, 1991, OSHA put into effect the Bloodborne Pathogen standard. This standard is designed to protect workers in health care occupations from the risk of exposure to bloodborne pathogens, such as HIV and HBV. This standard protects all employees who are at risk of occupational exposure to blood or **other potentially infectious materials (OPIM).** Per OSHA's requirements, employers must develop an exposure control plan that details how the standards will be implemented and how employees will be trained to protect their health.

Both the employer and employee have the responsibility of complying with the OSHA Bloodborne Pathogen standard. The employee must go through OSHA training in a cooperative manner, obey policies and standards, and use universal or standard precautions when handling blood and OPIM. Employees must wear appropriate PPE, use safe work practices and engineering controls, maintain clean work areas, and report any unsafe conditions to their employer.

Universal Precautions

The intent of **universal precautions** is to treat all human blood and some bodily fluids as infectious. The CDC has taken this concept further by applying it to all bodily fluids and secretions regardless of whether blood is present. This concept allows dental health care workers to treat every patient as if they are infectious and to take **standard precautions** for all patients. Standard precautions include the use of PPE and other protective equipment such as finger guards while suturing. By using the same precautions with everyone, the risk of exposure to pathogens is reduced. If an exposure to pathogens should occur, however, OSHA's Bloodborne Pathogen standard provides steps to manage the exposure.

OSHA studies show that saliva contains blood, which could contain pathogens (disease-causing bacteria). Because of this, the dental team must treat saliva as a potentially infectious material. This means that both universal and standard precautions must be followed. As with blood, the dental assistant should never touch saliva with ungloved hands. In fact, both universal precautions and standard precautions apply when contact is made with any of the following:

- Saliva
- Blood

- All bodily fluid secretions, regardless of whether or not they contain blood
- Nonintact skin (breaks in skin)
- Mucous membranes

Exposure Control Plan

The **exposure control plan** explains the specific exposure determination for employees to help minimize occupational exposure to bloodborne pathogens. Occupational exposure refers to anticipated cuts, needlesticks, or contact with blood or saliva based on the employee's job tasks. These tasks are listed in three categories:

- *Category 1* is for dental assistants, hygienists, dental laboratory technicians, and dentists. All tasks involving blood, saliva, and body tissues are included in this category.
- *Category 2* is for the receptionist and business assistant. These tasks do not usually include exposure to blood and bodily fluids, but occasionally these types of employees will perform some tasks from Category 1. For example, a receptionist might fill in for a chairside assistant or process instruments. Universal precautions and work practices controls are explained to Category 2 personnel in the event they handle a contaminated record or perform a chairside assist.
- *Category 3* is for individuals such as a dental office's insurance assistant and accountant. Performance of these tasks does not include exposure to blood or bodily fluids at any time.

In the exposure control plan, many ways to control exposure are explained, such as using universal precautions and PPE, establishing engineering and work control practices, addressing general housekeeping issues, providing information on hepatitis B vaccination, establishing a postexposure evaluation and follow-up procedure, and addressing education, training, and recordkeeping issues.

The employer must provide infection control and safety training to all personnel who may come in contact with blood, saliva, or other infectious materials. The employer must keep records of all training that include the date, the topic, the trainer, and the names of all employees who attended. The training records should be kept for three to five years.

Exposure Prevention and Management

The best way to prevent occupational exposure to blood is to minimize contact through the use of environmental controls. Environmental controls are those procedures that are used to prevent the spread of infection from surfaces and instruments. The use of disinfectants and sterilizing techniques prevent disease transmission. However,

exposures can occur when the skin is exposed to infectious blood, mucus, saliva, or other bodily fluids through a needlestick or cut in the skin. Exposure can also occur with nonintact skin such as chapped hands or hands with dermatitis. According to the CDC, skin injuries among dental personnel usually occur outside the patient's mouth, involve small amounts of blood, and are usually caused by needles, burs, or other sharp instruments.

The majority of exposure incidents in the dental field are preventable. This is where the use of engineering controls is helpful. An **engineering control** is the use of a device that minimizes the risk of exposure to infectious material. Examples include the use of single-handed, needle recapping techniques and disposal of sharps in OSHA-approved sharps containers.

If an incident does occur, certain procedures must be followed. First aid should be administered as soon as possible. The wound should be washed with soap and water; any mucous membranes should be flushed with water. Applying bleach or disinfectants to the wound is not recommended. Exposed personnel should immediately report the exposure incident to the infection control monitor, who will begin the referral and documentation steps. A dentist or other dental health care worker knowledgeable in infection control practices is usually assigned to be the infection control monitor. This person is responsible for the day-to-day management of creating and maintaining a safe work environment and providing new and recurrent training in infection control to the dental team.

When addressing an exposure incident, it is important to immediately conduct an evaluation of what occurred and what measures were or were not taken to avoid the situation. The evaluation should include the following steps:

- *Evaluate the practice of engineering controls and the work practices that are in place.* For example, if the dental assistant was exposed through a needlestick, an investigation should take place to establish how the dental assistant handled the needle and if appropriate recapping procedures were followed.
- *Investigate to determine the presence of protective equipment or clothing used at the time of the exposure incident.* For example, if a dental assistant was exposed during a procedure, an investigation should be conducted to determine if the dental assistant was wearing approved gloves, mask, eyewear, or a fluid-resistant gown during the procedure.

An evaluation of the control method policies should also be conducted when an incident occurs. When an incident occurs, it is important to take note of what current policies are in place and whether other policies or control methods should be implemented to more effectively ensure that the dental team and patients are protected.

Immunizations and proper infection control practices are the primary means of prevention for occupational exposure to pathogens. Written policies for reporting exposure incidents guide employees about how to report exposure incidents. Evaluation, counseling, treatment, and medical follow-up should be available to all employees. All written policies should be consistent with state and federal regulations regarding exposure management.

In the event of an exposure incident, specific management steps are required by the OSHA Bloodborne Pathogen standard, as listed in Table 12-2.

The employer must keep a confidential medical record on file that should include the employee's name, Social Security number, proof of HBV vaccine or signed refusal, and, in the event of an occupational exposure, documentation of the exposure incident and a copy of the postexposure follow-up report.

Engineering and Work Control Practices

OSHA mandates that specific work practices be in place to prevent exposure from occurring. These practices are called engineering and work control practices and they are designed to minimize and reduce the risk of exposure. The term *engineering controls* refers to controls that isolate bloodborne pathogen hazards from the workplace. These controls include the use of sharps disposal containers (Figure 12.4), self-sheathing needles (Figure 12.5), and safer medical devices, such as sharps with engineered sharps-injury protections and needleless systems. Work control practices that dental assistants must comply with include proper hand hygiene, no two-handed recapping of needles, no eating or drinking in patient areas, minimizing splatter of blood and OPIM,

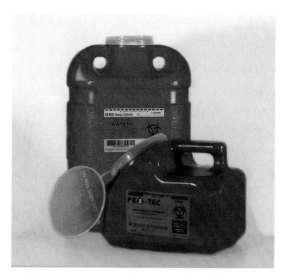

FIGURE 12.4
Sharps container.

TABLE 12-2 OSHA's Postexposure Evaluation and Follow-Up for Exposure to Bloodborne Pathogens

Step 1:	Employee reports exposure incident to supervisor. Supervisor documents the route of exposure and how it occurred.
Step 2:	Employer sends employee to health care provider. Employer provides a copy of the job description of the employee, an incident report, and source of patient's identity and HBV/HIV status if known.
Step 3:	Health care provider obtains consent from the employee and the patient and arranges for testing to be done. The employee and patient receive blood test for HIV and HBV.
Step 4:	Employer notifies employee of the results of the testing and discusses any further required treatment.
Step 5:	Employer provides postexposure prophylaxis such as blood test, vaccines, and medicines as required. Counseling must be offered and paid for by employer.
Step 6:	Employer evaluates reported illness and documents the evaluation and places the final evaluation in the employee's record. These are confidential medical records. The employee's record must be maintained by the employer for 30 years from the last date of employment.
Step 7:	Evaluating medical doctor sends written opinion to employer to include that the employee was informed of results and if any further evaluation is needed.

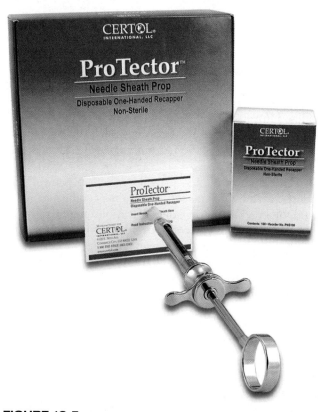

FIGURE 12.5
ProTector™ needle sheath prop.
Courtesy Certol International, LLC

using leakproof containers, and properly decontaminating and sterilizing equipment.

To avoid possible needlesticks, OSHA and the CDC advise against two-handed recapping and bending or breaking of needles prior to disposal. There are alternative methods to traditional two-handed needle recapping. For instance, the dental assistant can use one hand to slip the needle cover back on the needle; this is known as the "scoop" method. Another method is to use a holder to hold the needle cap, while recapping the needle with one hand. The use of a disposable cardboard needle shield helps to prevent inadvertent sticking. (See Chapter 28 for information on dental syringes and needles.)

Dental assistants can minimize injury from contaminated sharps by adhering to the following procedures:

- Always point the sharp end of the instrument away from the body.
- Pass scalpels and syringes with the sharp end away from the body and the dentist.
- Avoid using the two-handed technique to clean sharps at the dental chairside and never use the two-handed needle recapping.
- Dispose of used needles and other sharps immediately after the procedure in a biohazard, leakproof, puncture-resistant container.
- Never overfill or put hands in a sharps container.
- Wear puncture-resistant utility gloves during treatment room cleanup and when handling dirty instruments.
- Remove scalpel blades and needles with a mechanical device such as a hemostat.

Environmental Infection Control

OSHA requires dental treatment offices to protect employees and patients from bloodborne pathogens. While sterilization is the action of choice to kill pathogens (see Chapter 17 for sterilization procedures), it is not always practical or feasible. When sterilization is not feasible, surface disinfectants and barriers are used to inactivate or remove pathogens from certain surfaces. These environmental surfaces (Figure 12.6) are categorized as follows:

- *Touch surfaces:* surfaces that are touched and contaminated during a dental procedure; for example, light handles, chair/unit controls, and x-ray exposure buttons. If these surfaces are touched, they must be disinfected after the patient's treatment, or a barrier must be used during treatment. A barrier is a fluid-resistant disposable cover such as plastic wrap or plastic bags that cover surfaces. The barriers get disposed of after each patient treatment. If a surface has barriers, then ideally that surface doesn't need disinfecting. An assistant must be careful not to touch the underlying surface with the contaminated barrier when removing and disposing of the barrier.
- *Transfer surfaces:* surfaces that usually come in contact with contaminated instruments; for example, instru-

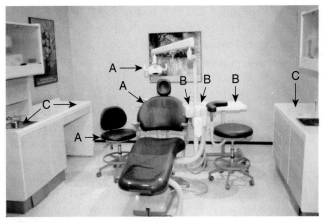

FIGURE 12.6
(a) Touch surfaces, (b) transfer surfaces, and (c) splash and spatter surfaces.
Image courtesy Instructional Materials for the Dental Team, Lex., KY

ment trays and handpiece brackets. (A handpiece bracket holds the dental handpiece in place when not in use.)

- *Splash, spatter, and aerosol surfaces:* all of the remaining surfaces in the dental treatment room that may have been contaminated with a spatter of blood or saliva.
- *Housekeeping surfaces:* floors, walls, and sinks that are cleaned with regular household cleanser. These surfaces have a lower risk for disease transmission.

Cleaning is the first step of any disinfection process. Cleaning removes organic matter and visible soils. Scrubbing with detergents and rinsing with water removes a large amount of microorganisms or bioburden. Bioburden is the microbial material on surfaces before decontamination. Removing all visible blood and inorganic and organic matter from surfaces is just as critical as disinfecting. If a surface cannot be cleaned adequately, then it should be protected with barriers.

Some things to consider when cleaning and disinfecting the treatment areas are the amount of direct patient contact, type and frequency of hand contact, potential aerosol spray contamination, and dust. Dust on surfaces allows microorganisms to stick, which could potentially cause disease transmission. The more direct patient contact and exposure to pathogens, the higher the risk to the dental health care worker. For this reason, it is important for dental health care workers to understand environmental infection control measures to protect themselves as well as their patients. The CDC publishes and ranks recommendations for environmental infection control. The general recommendations for environmental infection control include the following:

- The dental assistant should follow manufacturers' instructions for using Environmental Protection Agency (EPA)-registered disinfectant (EPA-registered disinfectants are discussed in the next section). According to the CDC this requirement is categorized as Categories IB and IC, meaning that this instruction is mandated by federal or state regulation and all dental health care workers are required to follow it.

- Chemical liquid sterilants should not be used for disinfecting environmental surfaces. This recommendation falls under CDC Categories IB and IC, meaning this instruction is mandated by federal or state regulation (see earlier discussion). It is important for the dental worker to understand that if a liquid sterilant is not used properly, then the risk of cross-contamination is increased.
- Dental health care workers must wear appropriate PPE when cleaning and disinfecting. CDC Category IC has been established for this environmental infection control, which means that it is mandatory. The use of proper PPE will protect the health care worker from any infectious material and the caustic disinfecting solution.

The recommendations by the CDC for cleaning clinical contact surfaces are as follows:

- Surface barriers should be used when possible, especially on hard-to-clean areas. Barriers should be changed between patients. This procedure is not mandatory, although it is suggested by the CDC. If barriers aren't used, then it is imperative that all surfaces be disinfected.
- An intermediate-level disinfectant should be used when surfaces are not barrier protected or when surfaces are visibly soiled with blood or OPIM. This procedure is strongly recommended by the CDC.

Housekeeping surfaces such as floor, walls, and sinks should be cleaned with water and an EPA-registered hospital disinfectant cleanser. Mops and cloths must be cleaned after use and then allowed to dry before the next use. Use of disposable mop heads or cloths is suggested. A fresh cleanser should be prepared according to the manufacturer for use throughout the day. Walls, blinds, windows, and other areas that collect dust should be regularly cleaned. It is the responsibility of every dental assistant to accomplish housekeeping duties, and the responsibility of the infection control monitor to provide a schedule and ensure that these tasks are completed.

Chemical Disinfectants

The EPA registers disinfectants. The products used in the dental office must have an EPA approval shown on the labels and must provide information as to whether the solution sterilizes or disinfects and what types of microorganisms are destroyed. The contact time for each product should also be stated on the label. The contact time is the amount of time the disinfectant must remain on the surface in order to deactivate microorganisms prior to it being wiped off. The disinfection levels should also be on the labels. The disinfection levels approved by the EPA and CDC are high, intermediate, and low.

- A high-level disinfectant is a tuberculocidal that kills most but not all bacterial spores. This is used for items that are heat sensitive and must be submerged in the disinfectant.
- An intermediate-level disinfectant is also tuberculocidal, but usually doesn't kill bacterial spores. It does kill most viruses.
- A low-level disinfectant kills some viruses and fungi.

Characteristics of disinfectants include antimicrobial chemicals that come in six types:

- Antibiotics (kills microorganisms on or in the body)
- Antiseptics (kills microorganisms on the skin)
- Disinfectants (kills microorganisms on environmental surfaces)
- Sterilants (kills all microorganisms)
- Bacteriostatic (slows or inhibits the growth of bacteria)
- Bacteriocidal (kills bacteria)

When reading labels on disinfectants, it is important to understand the terms used to distinguish the different types. For instance, if the label indicates the presence of a "viralcidal," this means that the product will kill at least some viruses. A disinfectant with a "bactericidal" will kill at least some bacteria. Fungicidal disinfectants kill some fungi, tuberculocidal disinfectants kill the tuberculosis bacteria, and sporicidal disinfectants kill bacterial spores (which means it is a sterilant).

Each product has advantages and disadvantages; no one product meets all needs. For instance, one disadvantage of some disinfectants is that they can stain and corrode instruments. Read the labels carefully and choose the one that best suits the needs of your office.

The universal technique for cleaning and disinfecting surface areas is the *spray, wipe, spray technique*. The surface is sprayed first, and then wiped to remove dust and bioburden. Then the surface area is sprayed and the disinfectant left on for the recommended amount of contact time, as indicated by the manufacturer. Disinfectants usually stay on for 3 to 10 minutes before removal. The dental assistant may also perform the *wipe, discard, wipe technique* using disinfecting towelettes. Many dental offices are moving away from aerosol sprays and switching to disinfecting towelettes.

The following is a list of disinfectants that may be used in the dental office:

- Quaternary amine/low concentration alcohol-based disinfectants come in spray or towelette wipes. One such disinfectant is Cavicide. This is an effective, ready-to-use, multipurpose, broad-spectrum solution for surface disinfection. It is noncaustic and designed to clean and disinfect.
- Chlorine dioxide is a high-level, EPA-registered disinfectant used on items that don't corrode easily. It is tuberculocidal but can damage metals and fabrics. Dis-

infection time is 5 to 10 minutes, but when used as a sterilant disinfection can take 6 to 10 hours. When using chlorine dioxide, protective eyewear, gloves, masks, and clothing are required, as well as good ventilation.

- Glutaraldehyde is a high-level, EPA-registered disinfectant and sterilant. Some glutaraldehydes are corrosive to metals. It is important to always follow manufacturers' directions regarding contact time for disinfecting and sterilizing. Glutaraldehyde works well as a sterilant on items that can be submerged but not heated. As a sterilant, it takes up to 6 to 10 hours to kill microorganisms. Protective masks, utility gloves, eyewear, and protective clothing that is impervious to fluid must be worn when handling it. Glutaraldehyde fumes can be toxic, so proper ventilation is also required.

- Iodophors are an intermediate-level, EPA-registered disinfectant (Figure 12.7). One of the key ingredients is iodine, which is red and can stain countertops and clothing. As a surface disinfectant, an iodophor can take from 5 to 25 minutes to activate. It is corrosive to some items and has a short shelf life. Solutions need to be changed every three days. PPE including utility gloves should be worn while using this disinfectant.

- Sodium hypochlorite is an intermediate-level, EPA-registered disinfectant. This can be regular household bleach (Figure 12.8). For use in the dental office, it should be mixed in a 1:10 dilution. This solution must be mixed daily. It is very effective against a broad spectrum of microorganisms. It works in about 10 minutes as a surface disinfectant, but can be very corrosive to metals. PPE including protective eyewear must be worn

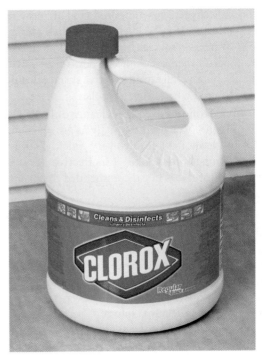

FIGURE 12.8
Sodium hypochlorite.

because sodium hypochlorite is very irritating to the eyes and it can create toxic fumes if mixed with other cleaning solutions. Good ventilation is essential.

- Phenolics are used as an intermediate-level, EPA-registered disinfectant (Figure 12.9). Phenols are carbolic acid, one of the first recognized disinfectants. Joseph Lister, a surgeon, used carbolic acid as an antiseptic more than 100 years ago to reduce infections from surgeries. Carbolic acid is destructive to tissues, so over the years these

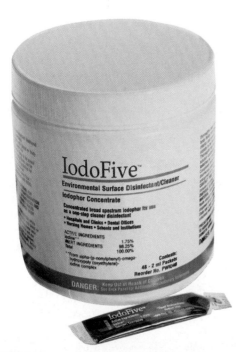

FIGURE 12.7
IodoFive™ disinfectant jar and unit dose packets.
Courtesy Certol International, LLC

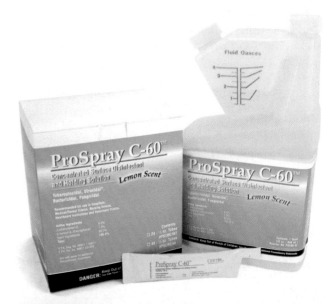

FIGURE 12.9
ProSpray C-60 ™ synthetic phenol disinfectant.
Courtesy Certol International, LLC

compounds have been synthesized, and are now referred to as synthetic phenols. Phenols are tuberculocidal and have a 10-minute contact time. Some come in premixed spray bottles; others are diluted. They can be corrosive to materials, but overall are an effective surface disinfectant. PPE is required when using phenols.

- Isopropyl alcohol is used as a cleaner only. Prior to the 1980s, alcohol was used routinely as a surface disinfectant, but alcohol evaporates very quickly, so its short surface contact time makes it ineffective as a disinfectant. Therefore, it is not recommended for disinfection in dental offices.

Many of these disinfectants come in wipes (Figure 12.10) and liquid spray. The various types of surface disinfectants are summarized in Table 12-3.

It is acceptable to use paper towels or gauze to wipe down surfaces. Note that paper towels are more cost effective. It is not acceptable, however, to keep gauze soaking in a disinfectant solution because the cotton fibers in the gauze may inactivate or absorb certain

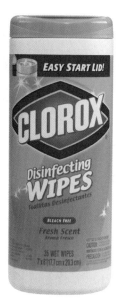

FIGURE 12.10
Disinfectant disposable wipes.
Courtesy The Bosworth Company

TABLE 12-3 Surface Disinfectant Reference (Organization for Safety and Asepsis Procedures)

Product Classification	Brand Name	Dilution (RTU = Ready to be Used. NTM = Need to Mix)	TB Claim (Contact Time on Surface to Inactivate TB)
Citric acid Hydroxyacetic acid, diproopylene glycol *n*-butyl ether	Lysol IC	RTU	10 min
Iodophors Alpha-omega-hydroxypoly iodine	IodoFive	NTM 1:213	10 min
Phenolics (alcohol based) Tertiary amylphenol plus ethyl alcohol	Coe Spray II DisCide Spray	RTU RTU	6 min 10 min
Phenolics (water based)	Birex DisCide Germicidal Foaming Cleaner ProSpray Spray Surface Disinfectant ProSpray Wipes	NTM 1:256 RTU RTU RTU	10 min 10 min 10 min 10 min
Quaternaries plus alcohol Diisobutylphenoxyethoxyethyl dimethylbenzyl ammonium chloride; isopropanol	Cavicide Spray CaviWipes Clorox Disinfecting Spray Lysol IC Maxispray Plus Sanitex Plus Spray Sani-Cloth Plus Wipes	RTU RTU RTU RTU RTU RTU RTU	5 min 3 min 10 min 10 min 5 min 6 min 5 min
Sodium Hypochlorite Chlorine Bleach	Clorox Germicidal Spray Clorox Germicidal Wipes	RTU RTU	30 sec 2 min
Other Sodium Bromide and Chlorine	Microstat 2 Tablets	2 tablets/1qt. water	5 min

Source: Adapted from OSAP Surface Disinfectant Chart 2008.

Procedure 12-1 Disinfecting a Treatment Room

Equipment and Supplies Needed

- PPE (utility gloves, eyewear, mask)
- Intermediate-level disinfectant
- Paper towels or 4 × 4 gauze

Procedure Steps

1. Put on PPE. *Rationale:* To prevent contact with chemicals.

2. Prepare disinfectant according to manufacturer's instructions.

3. Spray towels with disinfectant and wipe surfaces (precleaning).

4. Spray disinfectant on clean paper towel or gauze. Allow disinfectant to contact surface for the recommended amount of time.

5. If surface is still wet after contact time, wipe dry with clean towel.

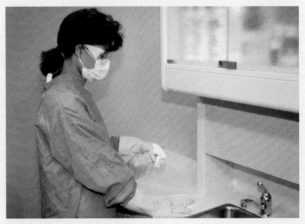

Disinfecting the operatory.
Image courtesy Instructional Materials for the Dental Team, Lex., KY

6. When using disinfectant wipes, follow manufacturer's instructions, don appropriate PPE and wipe surface, discard towelette, wipe surface with new towelette, allow to dry.

germicides. If gauze is used then ensure they are saturated at the time of use. For instructions on how to disinfect a treatment room see Procedure 12-1.

Surface Barriers

One way to manage surface contamination so that areas do not have to be precleaned and disinfected before reuse is through the use of surface barriers. Barrier protection of surfaces and equipment prevents contamination of clinical contact surfaces. Barriers should prevent the leakage of fluid and keep microorganisms such as saliva and blood from soaking through to the contact area. Clear plastic wrap, bags, tubes, or other materials impervious to moisture are appropriate surface barriers. Some of these plastics are made to fit on the dental chair or handpiece hoses, light handles, and x-ray tube head (Figure 12.11). These areas are commonly touched during treatment so the use of these plastics helps prevent pathogenic contamination.

Barrier coverings become contaminated so they should be removed and discarded between patients while the dental assistant is gloved. Once the contaminated barrier has been removed, the dental assistant should examine the surface to ensure it did not become soiled. The touched surfaces should be disinfected only if contaminated. After removing gloves and washing hands, the dental assistant should place clean barriers prior to the next patient's arrival. If barriers are not used, all surfaces should be cleaned and disinfected with an EPA-approved disinfectant between each patient. For instructions on placing and removing surface barriers see Procedure 12-2.

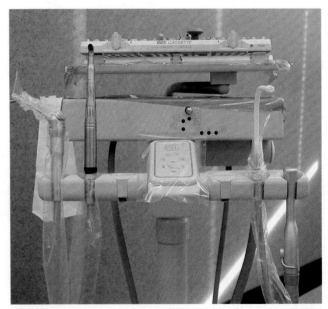

FIGURE 12.11
Equipment covered with barriers.

What is the difference between universal and standard precautions? What are the three engineering controls used to reduce the risk of bloodborne pathogen exposure? What is an advantage of a surface barrier?

Procedure 12-2 Placing and Removing Surface Barriers

Equipment and Supplies Needed

- Antimicrobial soap
- Utility gloves
- Plastic surface barriers

Procedure Steps

1. Wash and dry hands using proper hand hygiene techniques.

2. Select appropriate surface barriers for clean surface.

3. Place barrier securely on dental chair or other surface so it does not fall off. If barrier comes off, then the surface will require disinfecting.

4. Wear utility gloves to remove contaminated barriers; discard barrier in contaminated or general waste container. (Check state laws regarding disposal of contaminated barriers.)

5. Remove, wash, disinfect, and dry utility gloves. Then wash hands.

6. Apply fresh surface barriers for the next patient.

Preparing for Externship

As you participate in your externship be aware of the different ways dental offices manage their infection control programs. Keep an open mind and be willing to learn new techniques and enhance the techniques you learned in school.

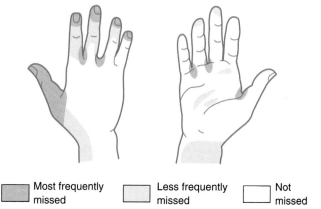

	Most frequently missed		Less frequently missed		Not missed

FIGURE 12.12
Hand hygiene: Areas missed during hand washing.

Infection Control Practices

The goal of a good dental infection control program is to provide a safe working environment that reduces the risk of infections among patients and dental personnel. A successful program depends on the standards developed, the monitoring of infection control practices, and documentation of occupational exposure to blood and OPIM. According to the CDC, periodic observational assessments, checklists to document procedures, and reviews of dental practice protocols provide the office an opportunity to improve their practices.

Hand hygiene is considered the single most critical measure in reducing the risk of transmitting organisms because it reduces pathogens on the hands. The skin contains transient microorganisms on the layers of skin that can easily be removed by the simple act of washing one's hands. Hand washing, however, must be properly performed; Figure 12.12 shows areas that are often missed during hand washing.

The method of hand hygiene depends on the procedure to be performed and the amount of contamination that may be possible. For example, for routine procedures (nonsurgical), an antimicrobial soap or an alcohol-based hand rub works well. Liquid soap with hands-free controls is preferred over bar soap because bar soap has been found to have many pathogenic organisms surrounding it. Hands should be vigorously rubbed together with enough soap to create lather. Hands and fingers should be lathered for no less than 15 seconds, followed by a rinse with cool or tepid water. Prior to putting on gloves, hands should be dried.

Antiseptic hand cleaner in conjunction with clean cloth/paper towels or antiseptic towelettes are examples of acceptable alternatives to running water. However, when these types of alternatives are used, employees must wash their hands (or other affected areas) with soap and running water when visibly soiled.

The CDC publishes information on the various methods of hand hygiene, the duration of time, and the indications for use of specific procedures, as summarized in Table 12-4 and outlined in Procedure 12-3.

Lotions are a good defense against transmission of pathogens. Frequent hand washing causes skin to become dry and crack, resulting in contact dermatitis. When the skin is damaged, it allows more colonization of bacteria. These skin irritations can be greatly reduced by using lotions. Petroleum-based lotions can cause the integrity of the latex gloves to weaken. Lotion manufacturers can be contacted to inquire about which lotions interact with gloves and dental materials.

TABLE 12-4 CDC Hand Hygiene Methods

Method	Cleaning Agent	Purpose	Duration of Wash	Indications
Routine hand wash	Water and plain soap	To remove dirt and microorganisms	15 sec	Prior to and after treating patients (before and after gloving)
Antiseptic hand wash	Water and antimicrobial soap	Destroy transient microorganisms; reduce resident flora (bacteria)	15 sec	Prior to and after treating patients; before and after gloving; after touching surfaces that can potentially get contaminated
Antiseptic hand rub	Alcohol-based hand rub	Remove and destroy transient microorganisms; reduce flora	Rub hands until dry	Same as above (hand washing is the most effective method that prevents contamination) Waterless hand cleanser can be used if hands are not visibly soiled
Surgical antisepsis	Water and antimicrobial soap	Remove or destroy transient microorganisms; reduce resident flora	2–6 min	Before putting on sterile gloves for surgical procedures

Source: Adapted from the CDC's *Guidelines for Infection Control in Dental Health-Care Settings.*

Fingernails can break the integrity of latex gloves. It is recommended that fingernails be kept short so health care workers can thoroughly scrub underneath the nails. A majority of the microorganisms that have been found on hands have been found underneath the nails. Long nails are also likely to rip the gloves, which increases the possibility of pathogen transmission.

Artificial nail wearers have a greater number of microorganisms beneath the nails than those who do not wear artificial nails. Also, like long nails, artificial nails have a tendency to rip latex gloves. Nails painted with fingernail polish do not increase the number of microorganisms on the hand, however, chips in the nail polish can harbor bacteria.

It is good practice to keep nails clean, short, and well groomed to reduce the risk of pathogen transmission. In addition to keeping one's hands and nails in good shape, removing jewelry will help to ensure the integrity of latex gloves. Studies have shown that heavy colonization of bacteria occurs under rings. Rings and other hand jewelry can make donning gloves difficult and cause them to rip and tear. Jewelry should not hinder the proper wearing of gloves and other PPE.

Personal Protective Equipment

Personal protective equipment (PPE) is designed to protect the skin, eyes, nose, and mouth from potential exposure to blood and infectious bodily fluids. The use of handpieces, air/water syringes, and ultrasonic scalers causes a spray that is composed of water, blood, saliva, tooth particles, and other debris. The spatter lands on the floor, chair, patient, dentist, and dental assistant, so it is important to protect both the patient and the dental team from possible exposure.

The primary protective equipment for health care workers include gloves, masks, protective eyewear, face shields, and protective gowns and jackets (Figure 12.13). All PPE should be removed prior to leaving the patient treatment area. Reusable PPE, such as protective eyewear, should be disinfected between patients and when visibly soiled. The financial responsibility for repairing, replacing, cleaning, and disposing of PPE rests with the employer. If laboratory jackets or uniforms are intended to protect the employee's body or clothing from contamination, they are to be provided by the employer.

OSHA requires that PPE be removed prior to leaving the work area. Although the "work area" must be determined on a case-by-case basis, a work area is generally considered to be an area where work involving occupational exposure occurs or where the contamination of surfaces may occur.

Protective Eyewear Masks and Face Shields

Infectious diseases can be transmitted through various methods including the mucous membranes of the eyes. Some viruses and bacteria can cause conjunctivitis. Those types of viruses and bacteria are adenovirus, herpes simplex, and *Staphylococcus aureus*. Also, systemic infections such as hepatitis and HIV can be transmitted through the mucous membranes. These infectious microorganisms are introduced directly through blood splashes or droplets from coughing or from touching one's eyes with contaminated hands or objects. Some common types of eye protection are as follows:

- *Goggles:* Vented side shield goggles should fit snugly across the brow; many styles fit over prescription glasses. Goggles do not protect other parts of the face.

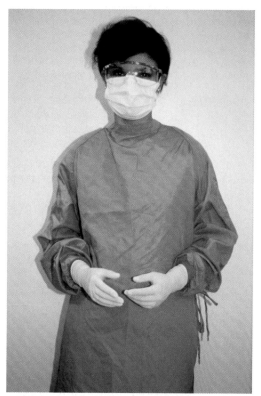

FIGURE 12.13
Dental assistant in PPE.
Image courtesy Instructional Materials for the Dental Team, Lex., KY

- *Face shields:* The face shield should have head and chin protection and wrap around the face to the ear. This reduces the likelihood of splashes into the eyes. A mask should be worn with a face shield.
- *Safety glasses:* Safety glasses that fit snugly on the face provide impact protection and side protection. If choosing between safety glasses and goggles, the goggle is the protection of choice.

Surgical masks that cover both the nose and the mouth are required when aerosol spray from handpieces and air/water syringes are used. The surgical mask protects the dental assistant from inhaling infectious organisms. Masks protect against organisms with a 95% efficiency rate according to the CDC. Masks can become contaminated with the spray of oral fluids or when touched with contaminated gloves. If the mask becomes wet, it should be changed as soon as possible. Wet masks lose their effectiveness. The mask should be changed with every patient. Masks should never be left dangling around one's neck or from the ear but rather should be removed and discarded after use.

When airborne isolation procedures are required for patients with tuberculosis, a National Institute for Occupational Safety and Health (NIOSH)-certified particulate-filter respirator should be used. Protective eyewear and face shields should have appropriate side shields to protect against droplet, spray, and spatter transmission. If a face shield is worn, a mask must also be worn for protection.

Procedure 12-3 CDC Recommendations for Hand Antisepsis and Hand Washing

Supplies Needed
- Alcohol-based hand rub
- Antimicrobial liquid soap
- Hand/nail scrub brush
- Paper towel

Procedure Steps for Alcohol-Based Hand Rubs
1. Apply hand rub in palm of hand.

2. Rub hands together.

3. Be sure all surfaces of hands and fingers are covered with the rub. Rub until dry on the hands and fingers.

Procedure Steps for Hand Hygiene
1. Wet hands first.

2. Apply soap to hands.

3. Use brush to scrub fingernails on each hand.

4. Rub hands together vigorously for 15 seconds.

5. Cover all surfaces of hands and fingers with soap, washing from top to bottom of each finger and thumb.

6. Rinse hands with cool water. This helps close the pores and keep skin intact.
   Avoid rinsing with hot water. It may increase the risk of dermatitis.

7. Dry with clean, disposable paper towel.

8. Use paper towel when touching the faucet to turn off the water. Dispose of paper towel in general waste.

continued on next page

Procedure 12-3 *continued from previous page*

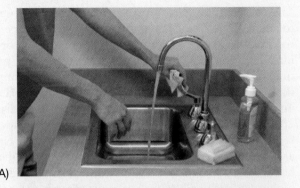
(A)

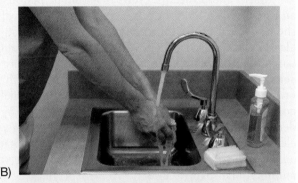
(B)

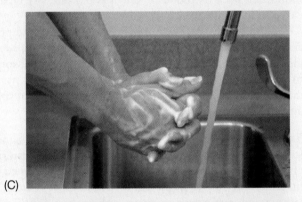
(C)

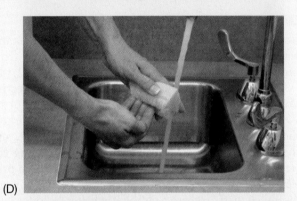
(D)

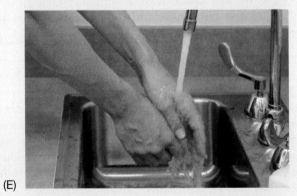
(E)

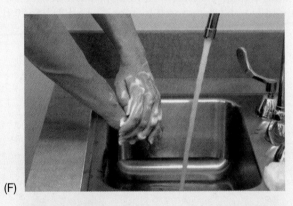
(F)

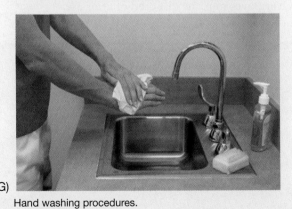
(G)

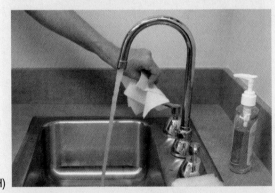
(H)

Hand washing procedures.

With the current use of lasers and high-intensity lights, the risk to eye injury is great. Special light filter glasses should be worn during operation of lasers and high-intensity lights.

Masks and protective eyewear should be put on and adjusted prior to putting on gloves. Each individual should have a proper fit to minimize the need to adjust glasses while gloved. The use of eye protection should be based on the reasonable anticipation of exposure to aerosols and spatter. Face masks in combination with eye protection devices such as glasses with solid side shields, goggles, or a chin-length face shield should be worn by all dental team members when contact with contaminated elements may be possible. Eyewear may be decontaminated with a chemical disinfectant after washing with antimicrobial soap.

Gowns or Lab Coats

Gowns or lab coats should be worn to prevent contamination of street clothes and to protect the skin from exposure to blood and bodily fluids (Figure 12.14). OSHA states that employers must provide protective clothing that is worn and laundered in the office or by a commercial laundering service. Dental workers change into uniforms when they arrive at the office, and change out of protective clothing prior to leaving the office. OSHA requires sleeves to be long enough to protect forearms from exposure. Health care workers should change protective clothing when it becomes visibly soiled and penetrated by blood or other bodily fluids. Disposable lab coats are available; however, they can be expensive.

Gloves

The wearing of gloves prevents contamination from touching blood, saliva, and mucous membranes and reduces the risk of transmission. Gloves are one of the most important factors in preventing the spread of infectious diseases. The wearing of gloves does not eliminate the need for hand hygiene. Hands should be washed immediately prior to donning gloves and immediately after removal of gloves because gloves can have microscopic defects or get torn during procedures. If the hands are free of visible bioburden, use of an alcohol-based hand sanitizer is permitted between glove changes. If bioburden such as blood or saliva is present, the health care worker must use soap and water.

Certain gloves are required for certain tasks and procedures. Examination gloves (latex and nonlatex), overgloves, sterile surgical gloves, and utility gloves are some of the different types of gloves with which dental assistants should be familiar. Gloves come in a variety of sizes and should be available to all health care workers.

Examination Gloves Examination gloves are designed for single procedures. Examination gloves are nonsterile and are ambidextrous, which means they are designed to fit either the left or right hand. These gloves come in latex, vinyl, and nitrile, with or without powder (Figure 12.15). These gloves also come in different flavors and are usually used in a pediatric office.

Overgloves Overgloves are made of clear, thin plastic and they resembles food handlers' gloves (Figure 12.16). These are to be worn over the treatment glove. An overglove would be used, for instance, when the dental assistant needs to retrieve materials out of the cabinet, make a chart notation, or answer the phone. In such cases, the overglove is worn to prevent contamination to other areas. This is a temporary use glove and is not designed to replace latex, vinyl, or nitrile gloves. Overgloves must be disposed of after use.

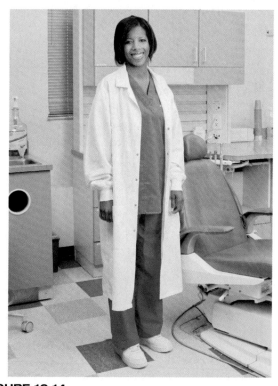

FIGURE 12.14
Dental assistant in scrubs.

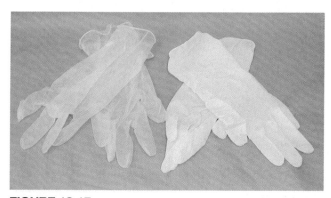

FIGURE 12.15
Vinyl gloves and latex gloves.

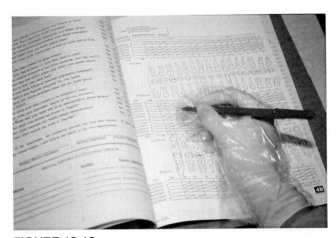

FIGURE 12.16
Overgloves.
Image courtesy Instructional Materials for the Dental Team, Lex., KY

Prepackaged Sterilized Gloves Prepackaged sterilized gloves are intended for one-time use in surgical procedures. The prepackaged sterilized gloves come in pairs, labeled right and left. These are disposable gloves that are stronger and more form fitting than examination gloves. They come in latex and latex-free versions.

Utility Gloves Utility gloves are similar to inexpensive household cleaning gloves; however, they are stronger and designed to protect the health care worker's hands from sharp instruments and disinfectants (Figure 12.17). These gloves are used when disinfecting the operatory and instrument processing area. Utility gloves should never be used in patient treatment. Utility gloves should be sprayed with disinfectant after use. Utility gloves that can be autoclaved are preferred to ensure that cross-contamination will not happen.

Gloving When donning a glove it is important to maintain asepsis and not contaminate other surfaces such as counters, drawers, and dental records. Gloves should be within reach or easy access of dental personnel.

The following procedure describes the method of gloving:

- Pick up the glove for the nondominant hand at the folded or cuffed area (this is actually the interior of the glove). Pull the glove onto the hand.
- Place the gloved nondominant hand under the fold of the dominant hand glove and pull it onto the dominant hand.
- The dominant gloved hand should then be placed under the folded portion of the nondominant gloved hand. The glove should then be pulled up on the arm (Figure 12.18).

Gloves should not be stored near heat or direct sun. Storage in heat or direct sun can result in a higher risk of tears in the gloves. A cool, dark place is sufficient for storage and the expiration date should be monitored.

Glove Integrity Studies by the CDC conclude that gloves develop defects within 30 minutes to 3 hours, depending on the type of procedure and glove used. A specific time for changing gloves during a procedure has yet to be determined, although dental personnel must change gloves immediately after a rip or tear occurs.

It is very common for dentists and dental assistants to come in contact with chemicals and materials that could compromise the integrity of the gloves. Latex gloves can interfere with the setting of certain vinyl polysiloxane impression materials. It is important to consult the glove manufacturer for the chemical compatibility of the gloves used. If the integrity of a glove is compromised, in other words, if it is punctured or torn, both gloves should be removed immediately (Figure 12.19), hands washed and dried, and new gloves donned. Other factors affecting latex glove integrity include the use of petroleum products on the patient's lips or in the hand lotions used by dental personnel. For this reason it is important to read labels to determine if mineral oil or other petroleum ingredients are used.

Examination and surgical gloves are disposable and should never be washed and reused. Soaps and disinfectants have a deteriorating effect on the gloves. This is

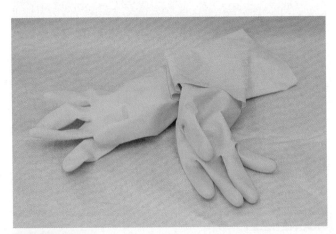

FIGURE 12.17
Utility gloves.

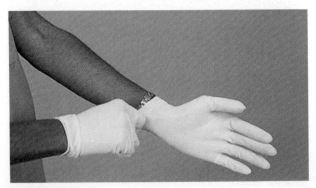

FIGURE 12.18
Donning gloves.

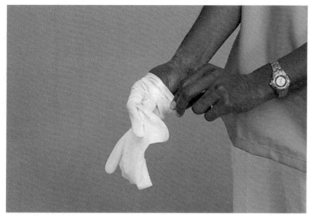

FIGURE 12.19
Removing gloves.

known as "wicking" and allows the chemical to penetrate through to the skin. Figure 12.20 shows a dental assistant in PPE donning gloves.

Which type of glove should be used when handling dirty instruments? What procedure is followed if a latex glove tears during dental treatment? If a face shield is worn, is a mask necessary? **?**

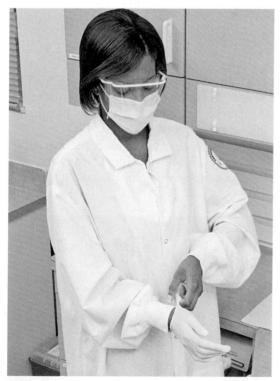

FIGURE 12.20
Assistant donning PPE.

Latex Allergies Many patients and workers have latex allergies. According to the CDC, Type 1 hypersensitivity latex allergy can be very serious. The symptoms can begin immediately on contact with latex and sometimes last for hours. Common symptoms include runny nose, sneezing, itchy eyes, hives, and itching or burning on the skin. Severe symptoms include difficulty breathing, coughing, cardiovascular ailments, and anaphylaxis. Natural rubber latex proteins are attached to glove powder. When the gloves are donned and removed, the powder can be inhaled and affect many allergic patients.

Irritant contact dermatitis or Type IV hypersensitivity can result from frequent use of hand hygiene products and continued glove use. This often begins as a rash and is usually confined to the area of contact (Figure 12.21). Nonlatex gloves and other materials should be on hand in the dental office for those workers and patients who have latex allergies. Nitrile and vinyl, low powdered or nonpowdered gloves, are good to use with latex sensitivities, as well as nonlatex dental dams and disposable prophy cups.

Additional Infection Control Practices

It is now recommended that, prior to any dental treatment, patients use an antimicrobial mouth rinse to reduce the number of microorganisms present. According to the CDC, preprocedural mouth rinses decrease the number of microorganisms in the bloodstream during invasive procedures. Because of the decreased number of microorganisms, there is a decrease in the amount of organisms present in aerosols and spatter from the dental handpiece and ultrasonic scalers, which reduces the risk to the dental health care provider. CDC studies state that no scientific evidence is available to indicate that preprocedural mouth rinses prevent clinical infections, but these rinses do reduce the number of microorganisms.

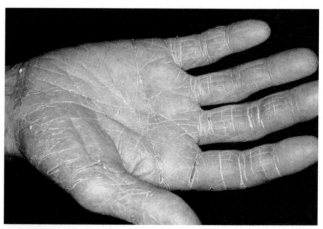

FIGURE 12.21
Irritant dermatitis.

Controlling Cross-Contamination in the Dental Laboratory

Controlling cross-contamination in the dental laboratory is just as important as controlling it in a dental treatment room. Even though most laboratory technicians do not have direct contact with patients, they do have indirect contact due to the impressions sent from dental offices. When the dental health care worker sends a laboratory item such as an impression off-site, according to the CDC, the individual must provide information in writing about the methods used to clean and disinfect the item. At a minimum the type of disinfectant and exposure time are required to be in writing. Laboratory technicians should also wear appropriate PPE and use standard precautions. Lab counters and work surfaces must be kept clean and disinfected using the same environmental techniques used in the dental treatment area.

The chairside assistant disinfects dental impressions (Figure 12.22). These impressions must be disinfected immediately after removal from the patient's mouth. The assistant sprays an approved disinfectant on the impression prior to placing it in a plastic bag. Many dental laboratory materials give off hazardous aerosols, so the laboratory technician needs to be aware of the prevention methods available to avoid contracting diseases. One such hazardous aerosol is beryllium. Laboratory technicians can develop chronic beryllium disease if they inhale the dust from beryllium. Items such as crowns, bridges, and denture frameworks are made from an alloy (mixture of metals) containing beryllium. It is important that all PPE be used when working in the dental laboratory.

The CDC has published specific guidelines for dental laboratories. The guidelines include the following:

- Use PPE when handling items received in the laboratory.
- Prior to handling specimens in the laboratory, one must clean, disinfect, and rinse all dental prostheses and materials including impressions, bite registrations, occlusal rims, and extracted teeth.
- Include information regarding disinfection techniques when laboratory cases are sent off-site.
- Clean and autoclave heat-tolerant items that are used in the mouth.

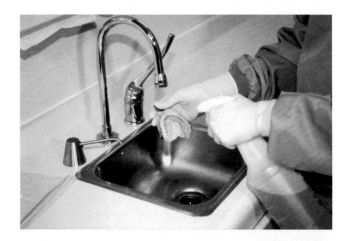
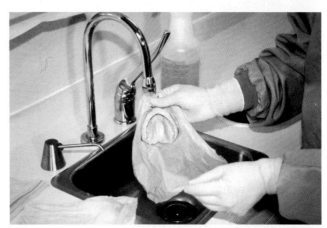
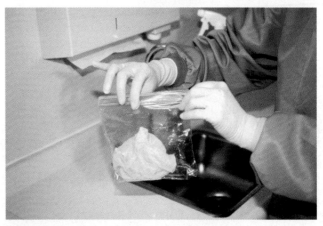

FIGURE 12.22
Steps used to disinfect dental impressions.
Image courtesy Instructional Materials for the Dental Team, Lex., KY

Laser Plumes

With the use of lasers becoming more prevalent in the dental office, the increased risk of disease transmission has also become more prevalent. When a laser is used, the thermal destruction of tissue creates a smoke by-product called a plume. The plume releases hydrogen cyanide, formaldehyde, tissue debris, viruses, and odors. The thought is that disease can be transmitted through aerosol and inhalation. HIV and the human papilloma virus have been detected in laser plumes.

Dentists should be aware of and advise their staff about the potential hazards of laser plumes. The use of standard precautions, high filtration surgical masks, and full face shields can protect dental workers. Special suction units that collect the plume particles and exhaust systems can also protect the dental health care provider from inhaling plume aerosols.

Procedure 12-4 Infection Control in the Darkroom

Supplies Needed

- Paper towel
- Gloves
- Plastic bag or paper cup
- Lead foil container

Procedure Steps

1. Place paper towel and cup next to processor in the darkroom. The paper towel is a barrier for the work surface.

2. Wash hands and put on new gloves.

3. Ensure safety light is turned on before touching the contaminated film.

4. Open the film packets and allow film to drop on paper towel.

5. Allow lead foil to drop in lead foil container. (Lead foil is considered an environmental hazard and should not be discarded in general waste.)

6. Place empty film packets in cup, remove gloves, and discard both.

7. Place films in the processor with bare hands, being careful to touch the edges only.

8. If the films had a plastic barrier, it would have already been removed outside of the darkroom with gloved hands. In the darkroom the film packets can be opened with bare hands.

Infection Control in Dental Radiology

Radiography rooms and darkrooms are sometimes overlooked when it comes to infection control. When dental assistants expose and process radiographs, the same infection control procedures used in treatment rooms must be used. The room is prepared by precleaning, disinfecting, and placing surface barriers where appropriate. When the procedure is complete the surface barriers must be removed and any contaminated surface areas must be disinfected. (For more information on infection control measures during processing, see Chapter 30.)

Protocol for darkroom procedures should be in place to eliminate the transmission of pathogens. The CDC publishes recommendations and guidelines for dental radiology infection control:

1. Wear gloves when exposing radiographs and handling contaminated film.
2. Use heat-tolerant or disposable intraoral film holding devices. Clean and sterilize between patients.
3. If film barrier pouches are used, the film packets should be removed from the contaminated pouch, and the film should be placed in a disposable container.
4. Transport contaminated film to the darkroom in a disposable container to prevent contamination.

Once the exposure room is disinfected and gloves removed, the dental assistant transports the cup with contaminated film to the darkroom. The dental assistant should not enter the darkroom with contaminated gloves; this increases the chance of disease transmission to the darkroom door, countertops, and processor. Pro-

tective barriers should be used on surfaces and equipment that may be contaminated. Digital radiography sensors should be either heat sterilized, disinfected with a high-level disinfectant, or barrier protected between patients. Infection control procedures should also be followed when using a daylight loader on the processor (Procedure 12-4 and Procedure 12-5).

Why do dental laboratory technicians need to worry about infection control if they do not see patients directly?

Waste Management in the Dental Office

OSHA's bloodborne pathogen standard requires that all waste be disposed of according to federal, state, and local guidelines. The CDC guidelines require dental offices to develop a medical waste management program. It is also required that dental health care workers be trained in the appropriate handling of waste disposal and be informed of the health risks involved with handling such waste.

Waste Classifications

The different types of waste determine how it is processed and handled. In most offices waste should be separated into regulated and unregulated waste (Figure 12.23). It is important to understand the types of waste so that employees can dispose of it properly.

Procedure 12-5 Infection Control with a Daylight Loader

Supplies Needed

- Paper towels
- Two pairs of gloves
- Disposable cup or plastic bag
- Lead foil container

Procedure Steps

1. After exposing film and placing contaminated film in cup, remove gloves and wash and dry hands.

2. Place a barrier (paper towel or plastic barrier) inside, on the bottom of the daylight loader.

3. Place the cup with contaminated film, a clean pair of gloves, an empty cup, and the lead foil container in the daylight loader.

4. Place clean hands into the sleeves of the loader, then put on clean gloves.

5. Open film packets and drop film into empty cup, drop lead foil in container, and then place contaminated film packets back into contaminated cup.

6. After the film packets are opened, remove gloves by turning them inside out.

7. Insert film into processor with bare hands.

8. When the film has been loaded, remove hands from loader.

9. Don clean gloves, open top of the loader, and remove and discard contaminated items.

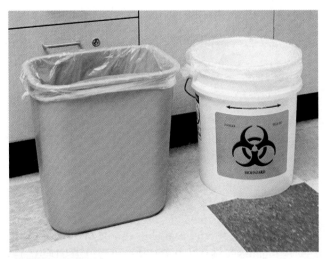

FIGURE 12.23
Unregulated (left) and regulated (right) waste containers.

- *General waste:* This type of waste is unregulated waste and should be disposed of in covered, durable plastic containers. These containers should be lined with plastic bags. General waste includes paper towels and mixing pads.

- *Contaminated waste:* This waste has been in contact with blood and bodily fluids and includes barriers and patient napkins. In some states this waste is disposed of in general waste. In other states it is disposed of as regulated or infectious waste. When disposing of this waste, appropriate PPE, such as gloves, mask, and eyewear, must be worn.

- *Infectious waste (regulated waste):* The CDC's Bloodborne Pathogens standard defines regulated waste as liquid or semiliquid blood or OPIM; items contaminated with blood or OPIM that could release liquid or semiliquid if squeezed; and items that are caked with dried blood or OPIM. Contaminated sharps and soft tissue and extracted teeth are also classified as regulated waste. If extracted teeth are not returned to the patient, then they should be disposed of as regulated waste. Regulated waste is incinerated, so it is crucial that teeth with amalgam restorations not be disposed of in this manner. If the extracted tooth contains an amalgam restoration, then it requires special disposal. Refer to local and state regulations regarding disposal. According to the CDC, regulated waste should be placed in containers that are:

  — Closable

  — Constructed to contain all contents and prevent leakage of fluids during handling, storage, transport, or shipping

  — Color-coded or have a warning label that includes the universal biohazard symbol with the term "Biohazard" on it (Figure 12.24) (Such symbols must be included on bags/contaminated laundry, refrigerators that store blood or OPIM, and contaminated equipment.)

  — Closed prior to removal to prevent spillage or protrusion of contents during handling, storage, transport, or shipping

- *Hazardous waste:* Hazardous waste can hurt the environment. Certain materials used in the dental office are classified as hazardous waste. Scrap amalgam, fixer solution, and lead foil from the x-ray film packs are examples of hazardous waste. Extracted teeth with amalgam restorations are classified as hazardous

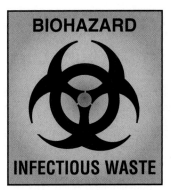

FIGURE 12.24
Biohazard symbol.

because of the mercury in the amalgam, and infectious because of the tooth.

What is the difference between hazardous and infectious waste? When can contaminated waste be disposed of in general waste containers?

Special Considerations from the Centers for Disease Control and Prevention

The risk of transmission of *Mycobacterium tuberculosis* and Creutzfeldt-Jakob disease is relatively low in the dental setting. However, because the dental health care worker and the infected patient share the same air and both conditions are infectious, the CDC determined that the subject be brought to the attention of health care workers for their protection and their patients' protection.

Mycobacterium Tuberculosis

Patients infected with *M. tuberculosis* may need dental treatment from an outpatient dental office. It is impor-

tant for the dental team to understand the disease and how to manage these patients. *M. tuberculosis* is a bacteria carried through airborne transmission such as coughing, sneezing, and speaking. These airborne particles can remain in the air for many hours. The infection occurs when a susceptible person inhales droplets containing *M. tuberculosis*. Individuals with latent tuberculosis (TB) usually have no symptoms and are not infectious. These individuals, however, can develop the disease later in life if they do not receive treatment for the latent infection.

For patients who know they have active TB, the CDC recommends that elective dental treatment be delayed until they are noninfectious. For those patients requiring urgent dental care, TB transmission can be controlled via administrative controls, environmental controls, and the use of personal respiratory protection. The CDC published the following guidelines for *M. tuberculosis*:

- Dental health care workers should be educated on the signs, symptoms, and transmission of TB.
- Dental health care workers should receive a TB skin test.
- Dental offices and personnel should follow the CDC recommendations for a TB infection control plan. *M. tuberculosis* can live for years on dental records and charts.

Creutzfeldt-Jakob Disease and Other Prion Diseases

Creutzfeldt-Jakob disease (CJD) is a group of progressive, fatal, neurologic disorders. These transmissible spongiform encephalopathies affect humans and animals, and CJD is commonly known as *mad cow disease*. It is caused by a pathogen called a prion. Prions are isoforms of a normal protein (see Chapter 11). Prion diseases have an incubation period of several years but can be fatal within one year of diagnosis. Potential infection of oral tissues in CJD patients is an unresolved issue; however, the use of standard precautions is recommended.

● SUMMARY

Infection control is always changing and improving for the safety of the dental team and patients. The OSHA Bloodborne Pathogen standard and the CDC guidelines for infection control are important to every dental office and health care facility. Various methods are available to protect both the patient and the dental team. These

efforts range from the wearing of proper PPE to disposing of waste properly. It is the responsibility of each dental practice to follow the regulations and standards established by the CDC and OSHA to maintain a safe environment for both the patient and the dental team.

KEY TERMS

- **Active immunity:** Immunity that is artificially acquired from immunizations; sometimes called adaptive immunity. p. 179

- **Bloodborne pathogens:** Organisms transferred through blood or bodily fluids that cause infectious disease. p. 177

- **Droplet transmission:** A disease that occurs from splash or splatter to the mucosa (mouth/eyes) or non-intact skin. p. 178

- **Engineering control:** The use of a device that minimizes the risk of exposure to infectious material. p. 183

- **Exposure control plan:** A plan that explains exposure determination for employees to help minimize occupational exposure to bloodborne pathogens. p. 183

- **Innate immunity:** The general protection that humans are born with; also known as natural immunity. p. 179

- **Latent infection:** An ongoing infection with recurrent symptoms. p. 177

- **Opportunistic infection:** An infection that is normally caused by a nonpathogenic organism in people with weakened immune systems. p. 177

- **Other potentially infectious materials (OPIM):** Items that have been in contact with fluids and tissues designated by the Centers for Disease Control and Prevention as possibly capable of spreading disease. p. 182

- **Passive immunity:** Immunity from an outside source that lasts for a short time. p. 179

- **Personal protective equipment (PPE):** Protective clothing, masks, gloves, and eyewear used to protect health care workers from exposure to bloodborne and airborne pathogens. p. 178

- **Standard precautions:** A standard of care that protects health care workers from pathogens that are spread by blood and other potentially infectious material. p. 182

- **Universal precautions:** Precautions used to protect patients and health care workers from coming into contact with contaminated bodily fluids. p. 182

CHECK YOUR UNDERSTANDING

1. The main reason a mask is used during dental treatment is to
   a. protect from odors.
   b. minimize the need for safety glasses.
   c. protect from aerosols and spatter.
   d. breathe better.

2. Once an alginate impression is sprayed with disinfectant, it should be
   a. autoclaved.
   b. air dried.
   c. soaked in water.
   d. sealed in a plastic bag.

3. When working with lasers or high-intensity lights, the dental assistant should
   a. spray with disinfectant.
   b. use special light-filtering safety glasses.
   c. wear sunglasses.
   d. look directly into the light to position it correctly.

4. Which category of employee job tasks do dental assistants fall under?
   a. I
   b. II
   c. III
   d. IV

5. Which type of gloves are worn during patient treatment?
   a. overgloves
   b. latex
   c. nitrile
   d. b and c

6. The type of immunity that everyone is born with is called
   a. passive immunity.
   b. innate immunity.
   c. adaptive immunity.
   d. active immunity.

7. A mask should be replaced
   a. when it gets wet.
   b. once a day.
   c. with every patient.
   d. a and c

8. Which of the following is not regulated waste?
   a. blood-soaked gauze
   b. extracted tooth
   c. used patient napkin
   d. anesthetic needle

CHECK YOUR UNDERSTANDING (continued)

9. The cost of an employee's HBV vaccination is the responsibility of
   a. the employee.
   b. OSHA.
   c. health insurance.
   d. the employer.

10. Which of the following is not a control measure for preventing disease transmission from the dental patient to dental team?
    a. hand washing
    b. masks
    c. gloves
    d. disinfecting waterlines

● INTERNET ACTIVITIES

- Search for more information on infection control in dentistry and infection control updates by accessing the *Morbidity and Mortality Weekly Report,* December 2003. This issue includes the CDC's *Guidelines for Infection Control in Dental Health-Care Settings.* Many resources are available to you including a PowerPoint slide show to enhance understanding. The slide show is located at www.cdc.gov/OralHealth/infectioncontrol/guidelines/slides/009.htm.

Search www.cdc.gov, and then enter *infection control in dentistry* in the search block to review the slide show.

- For further study on disease transmission in the dental office, go to www.OSAP.org and obtain the video "If Saliva Were Red." This video provides a clear picture of how diseases can be transmitted during routine dental care if proper infection control practices are not used.

● WEB REFERENCES

- Centers for Disease Control and Prevention (CDC)   www.cdc.gov
- Environmental Protection Agency   www.epa.gov
- Food and Drug Administration   www.fda.gov
- Occupational Safety and Health Administration (OSHA)   www.osha.gov
- Organization for Safety and Asepsis Procedures   www.osap.org

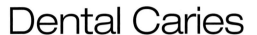

13

Dental Caries

Learning Objectives

After reading this chapter, the student should be able to:

• Discuss and explain the caries process.

• Identify the four areas of tooth structure where caries occur.

• Explain the causative bacteria of dental caries.

• Describe demineralization and remineralization.

• Compare and contrast the types of dental caries.

• Explain the importance of saliva.

• List the types of dental caries detection methods.

• Discuss the methods of caries intervention.

• Explain the caries risk assessment test.

Preparing for Certification Exams

• Provide patient preventive education and oral hygiene instruction.

Key Terms

Biofilm

Caries

Cariogenic agent

Cariology

Cavitation

Demineralization

Gross or frank caries

Incipient caries

Lactobacilli

Mutans streptococci

Pellicle

Plaque

Rampant caries

Remineralization

Root surface caries

Xerostomia

Chapter Outline

• The Caries Process
  —Tooth Anatomy
  —Bacterial Infection
  —Plaque, Pellicle, and Biofilm
  —Demineralization and Remineralization
  —Types of Carious Lesions and Locations

• The Importance of Saliva
  —Chemistry of Saliva
  —Protection Provided by Saliva

• Diagnosis of Caries
  —Dental Instruments
  —Radiographs
  —Visual Appearance
  —Indicator Dyes
  —Laser Caries Detector

• Methods of Caries Intervention

• Risk Assessment of Caries

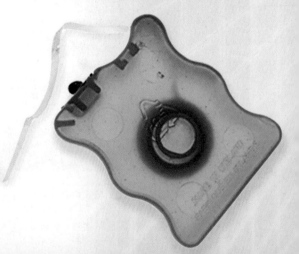

Dental caries (tooth decay) is a pandemic health problem. It affects all ages and socioeconomic groups (Figure 13.1). It has affected humans since prehistoric times. Dental caries is the most common chronic disease in children. In the general population, it is only second to the common cold, and it is more prevalent than asthma. When left untreated, it flourishes and becomes destructive to the teeth and oral environment. The prevalence of this disease was increasing on a worldwide basis until the late 1970s and early 1980s.

In the 1930s it was discovered that adding fluoride to drinking water significantly decreased the prevalence of caries. Therefore, fluoride was first added to the public drinking water in Grand Rapids, Michigan, in 1945. A long-awaited decline came with the understanding of the caries process and protocols for prevention and intervention of dental caries. With the addition of trace amounts of fluoride added to public drinking water and educational programs for the public and trained dental professionals, dental caries is on a slow decline. Although today the dental profession better understands this bacterial infection, it is still a worldwide problem.

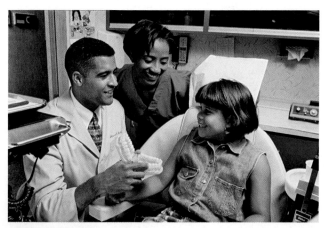

FIGURE 13.1
Caries affects all people.

The Caries Process

Cariology is the study of the caries process, also known as the formation of dental decay. The caries process is the primary reason general dentistry became necessary. Caries is an infectious disease that results in the localized destruction of the teeth. The dental profession can now fight to prevent this disease process instead of waiting to treat the results of its destruction. Although dentistry has improved greatly in the past decades, the dentist must still diagnose and the dental team must continue to treat tooth decay. Figure 13.2 shows a healthy occlusal surface. Compare that view with the photograph shown in Figure 13.3. Figure 13.3 shows what dental decay appears like on the occlusal surface.

Tooth Anatomy

It is important for the dental assistant to be able to recall tooth anatomy in order to understand how the caries process occurs and how the destructive bacteria that cause decay affect the different structures of the tooth. Enamel is the hardest tissue in the human body and is able to withstand the extreme forces needed to chew food. It is primarily made of hydroxyapatite crystallites

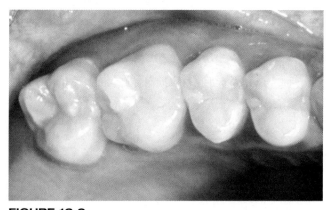

FIGURE 13.2
Occlusal view of healthy enamel.
Image courtesy Instructional Materials for the Dental Team, Lex., KY

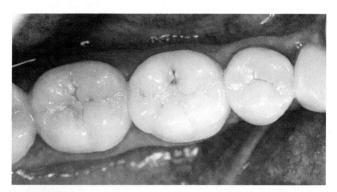

FIGURE 13.3
Occlusal view of carious enamel.
Image courtesy Instructional Materials for the Dental Team, Lex., KY

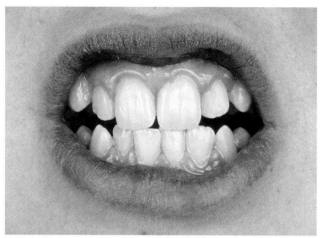

FIGURE 13.4
Dental plaque made evident with disclosant.

that are organized into long rods or prisms consisting mostly of calcium. Water flows between the prisms, carrying acids in and minerals out of the enamel. The hydroxyapatite is the material lost in the caries process. Unlike bone, the enamel does not contain reparative cells, but remineralization is possible.

Underneath the enamel is a softer material, dentin, that makes up the majority of the tooth structure. Dentin is harder than bone but not as hard as enamel. It contains less calcium and more water than enamel, which means it is more susceptible to decay than enamel. The root surfaces of the teeth are covered with cementum. The function of cementum is to allow for the connective tissue to anchor the tooth to the bone and soft tissues. Cementum is the softest of the three tooth components and most susceptible to decay. (See Chapter 8 for a more in-depth description of tooth anatomy.)

Bacterial Infection

Dental caries is a bacterial infection. The two primary bacterial groups are **mutans streptococci** (MS) and **lactobacilli** (LB). MS and LB are stimulated by fermentable carbohydrates (sucrose, fructose, and glucose) and produce large amounts of acids. The organisms that cause caries are known as **cariogenic agents**. MS is found in all humans regardless of race, culture, or geographical location. Newborns are not born with MS. The bacteria are transmitted by saliva, usually the parents' saliva. If the parents are found to have high levels of MS, the children usually have the same high levels of the bacteria. MS and LB contribute to dental caries via different means. MS is associated with the onset of caries, whereas LB is associated with the active destruction of tooth structure.

Plaque, Pellicle, and Biofilm

Plaque, also now known as **biofilm**, is a sticky, tooth-colored material composed almost completely of bacteria and their by-products (Figure 13.4). Plaque is not food debris as widely believed. It is a highly organized layering of microorganisms. The layering begins with a cell-free film of salivary proteins, called the **pellicle**, that protects the enamel, reduces the friction between the teeth, and possibly creates an environment for remineralization.

Next, the microorganisms begin to attach to the pellicle in an organized manner. MS is the first bacteria to adhere to the pellicle and begin plaque formation. Once MS has taken hold, LB begins to attach and then any number of other microorganisms to create plaque (Figure 13.5). There are hundreds of millions of microorganisms in just one milligram of plaque, whereas there are less than 1% of these microorganisms in one milligram of saliva. Obviously, plaque is the caries-causing culprit.

Demineralization and Remineralization

The caries process is an ever-changing system characterized by periods of **demineralization** and **remineralization**. Demineralization is the loss of calcium and phosphate from the hydroxyapatite crystallites in the enamel (Figure 13.6).

The enamel appears normal when wet but opaque when desiccated or dried. The surface also remains a normal smooth texture, but the hardness of the enamel is softened.

Remineralization occurs when calcium and phosphate are redeposited in the demineralized region (Figure 13.7). The majority of enamel rods remain after demineralization, providing a framework for the salivary ions to return to the enamel. The presence of fluoride encourages the precipitation of calcium and phosphate. This enamel is now more resistant to later caries attacks. Arrested lesions (remineralized areas) are often discolored brown, black, or even green. They should not be restored unless cosmetically unacceptable or the lesion penetrates into the dentin.

Types of Carious Lesions and Locations

The three types of carious lesions are:

1. Incipient caries
2. Gross or frank caries
3. Rampant caries

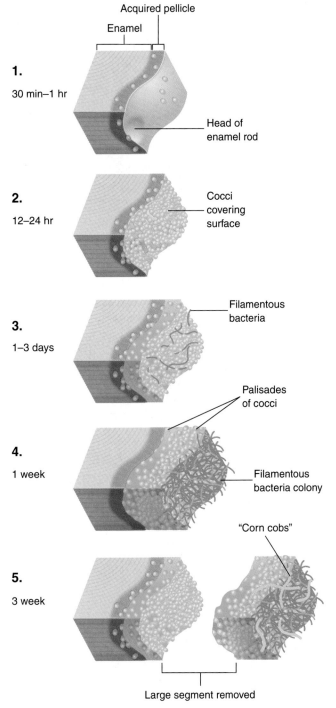

FIGURE 13.5
The formation of plaque beginning with the clean enamel followed by the pellicle. Mutans streptococci adhere to the pellicle followed by lactobacilli.

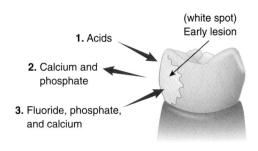

1. The tooth is attacked by acids in plaque and saliva.

2. Calcium and phosphate dissolve from the enamel in the process of demineralization.

3. Fluoride, phosphate, and calcium re-enter the enamel in a process called remineralization.

FIGURE 13.6
Demineralization followed by remineralization.

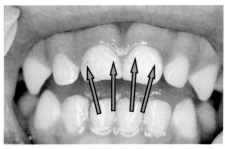

(A)   **Demineralization**

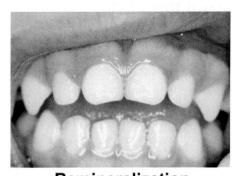

(B)   **Remineralization**

FIGURE 13.7
(a) Demineralized enamel and (b) remineralized enamel.
Images courtesy Instructional Materials for the Dental Team, Lex., KY

Incipient caries is the initial stage of decay where the enamel begins to demineralize (Figure 13.8a). The **gross or frank** caries is an obvious **cavitation** (a cavity or hole in a tooth or tissue), often resulting in severe loss of tooth structure (Figure 13.8b).

Rampant caries are multiple lesions throughout the mouth usually demonstrating cavitations (Figure 13.8c). This condition is often due to excessive and frequent eating or drinking of fermentable carbohydrates or xerostomia, chronic dry mouth. Baby bottle tooth decay is a good example of rampant caries. (See the discussion of pediatric dentistry in Chapter 47.) In the United States, abuse of a drug called methamphetamine, also known as meth, is on the rise. The oral effects of this drug are devastating. The teeth of a methamphetamine user have a distinctive caries pattern resembling the rampant caries of baby bottle tooth decay. This oral presentation is referred to as "meth-mouth."

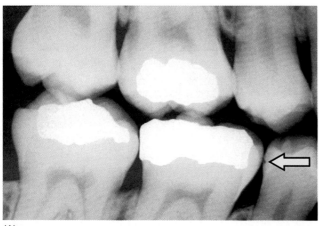

(A)

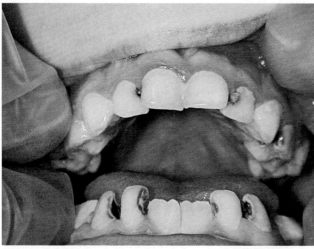

(B)

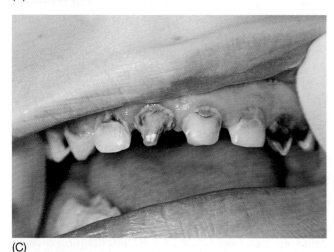

(C)

FIGURE 13.8
(a) Incipient caries, (b) gross or frank caries, and (c) rampant caries.
Images courtesy Instructional Materials for the Dental Team, Lex., KY

A formula has been developed for the development of caries:

Bacteria (SM) + fermentable carbohydrates + time = acid.

Acid (lowers pH) + tooth surface (decalcification) + time = decay.

Life Span Considerations

Patients of all ages have carious lesions. Babies with their first teeth commonly have caries, often known as baby bottle tooth decay. This is usually a rampant caries diagnosis. Many parents put their small children to bed with a bottle of milk or juice containing fermentable carbohydrates, allowing the caries process to occur on the primary teeth. It is important to educate expecting mothers and new parents to avoid giving their babies a juice or milk bottle in the bed.

Many young adults have increased incidence of decay due to dietary issues. The majority of patients over the age of 50 experience root surface caries. Geriatric patients often have poor dexterity and difficulty cleaning their teeth, not to mention medications that can cause caries to be prolific. Certain products and specialized toothbrushes may help these patients to control the caries process.

Therefore, decay cannot occur without bacteria or carbohydrates.

There are four clinical sites for caries onset:

1. Pits and fissures
2. Smooth surface
3. Root surface
4. Recurrent or secondary caries

Pits and fissures of teeth are the most susceptible areas for decay. The shape of pits and fissures vary greatly. Some even have an opening to the dentin. They are often hard to see and difficult to feel with the dental explorer. Smooth surface caries occurs anywhere else other than the pits and fissures, especially in the areas of contacting or proximal surfaces.

Root surface caries can occur on any surface of the root but usually on the buccal areas of gingival recession (Figure 13.9a). This caries condition is often seen in older populations because people are keeping their teeth longer and experiencing more recession as well as the loss of physical ability to perform oral hygiene properly.

Recurrent or secondary caries is found along the margins of failing restorations (Figure 13.9b). Bacteria can be harbored in the space between the tooth and the restoration, causing an area of decay and the need to replace the restoration. Contemporary restorations that are fluoride releasing seal the marginal area between the tooth and restoration, helping to decrease the incidence of recurrent caries.

Why do people get caries between their teeth? What information should you provide to help prevent this problem?

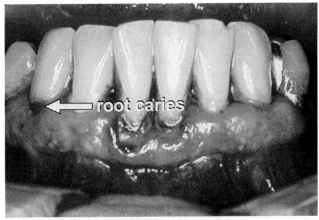

(A)

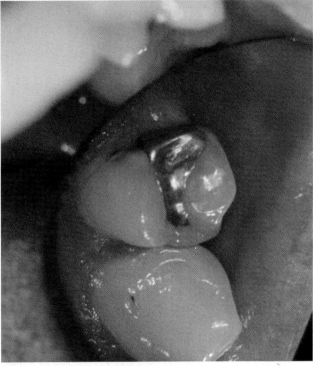

(B)

FIGURE 13.9
(a) Root surface caries and (b) photograph showing a recurrent carious lesion in a maxillary premolar at the gingivolingual aspect of a Class II amalgam restoration.

(a) Image courtesy Instructional Materials for the Dental Team, Lex., KY; (b) Mjor, IA, Clinical diagnosis of recurrent caries. *JADA* 2005; 136(10): 1426–33. Copyright © 2005 American Dental Association. All rights reserved. Reprinted by permission.

The Importance of Saliva

The human body produces approximately 1.5 liters of saliva daily that is vital to the health of the oral environment. Saliva has numerous functions including physical, chemical, and antibacterial protection. Saliva actually helps to remineralize tooth structure as well; therefore, diet is extremely important. The proper amount of calcium (CA) and phosphates (PH) required to remineralize tooth structure must come from good nutrition. Currently, teens especially, drink more soda than milk, which

changes the CA/PH ratio and, hence, decreases the chances of remineralization.

Chemistry of Saliva

Saliva is produced in and secreted from salivary glands. This fluid includes electrolytes such as sodium, potassium, phosphate, calcium, fluoride, and bicarbonate. Water, mucus, antibacterial compounds, and enzymes that aid in digestion are all important elements of saliva.

Protection Provided by Saliva

The water content of saliva provides much of the physical protection. The flow of saliva provided by the water coats the teeth, allowing for a cleansing effect that dilutes the acids and clears the plaque and carbohydrates. This flushing process is most effective during chewing, which produces large amounts of saliva. The thin layer of water and mucus provides a smooth surface, making it difficult for microorganisms to attach to the surface of the teeth.

Calcium, phosphate, and the other electrolytes found in saliva aid in chemical protection. These electrolytes are readily used in the remineralization process. Saliva has a buffering capacity that reduces the potential for acid formation. Other molecules in saliva raise the pH of plaque, reducing the ability of acids to form. Some patients experience **xerostomia** or abnormal dryness of the mouth due to insufficient amounts of saliva. This condition is often attributed to medications. Therapeutic radiation to the head and neck can cause the salivary glands to become fibrous or hardened, which also reduces saliva production. (See Chapter 5 for more information concerning xerostomia.) Numerous products are available to help patients increase salivation (Figure 13.10).

How does one's daily water intake affect one's saliva production?

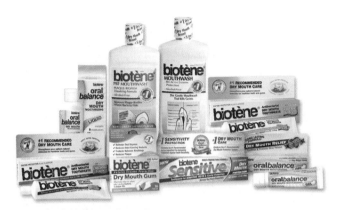

FIGURE 13.10
Products to increase salivary flow.
Courtesy of Laclede

Diagnosis of Caries

Proper diagnosis of dental caries is vital to the management of a patient's oral health. Many diagnostic tools are available to the dentist to accurately diagnose caries.

Dental Instruments

The dental instrument called the dental explorer has been the traditional means of detecting surface caries. The instrument is used by placing the sharp end into the suspected area of decay (Figure 13.11). If the instrument sticks into the enamel, caries is present. This method has faults because the use of fluoride increases the hardness

of enamel, and the instrument may just be wedged into a pit or fissure, causing it to stick.

The explorer may also cause a cavitation in enamel that had the possibility to remineralize. Although the use of the explorer is not perfect, it is still the most accepted means of caries detection. Occasionally, the dental hygienist will detect an area of caries with his or her instruments while cleaning at or below the gingiva (gums). The dentist must then confirm the presence of caries. (See Chapter 24 for a discussion of the various types of dental instruments.)

Radiographs

Radiographs (x-rays) are important in the diagnosis of interproximal caries. Although radiographs and the equipment to take radiographs have improved greatly with the invention of digital radiographs, small carious lesions are undetectable and identifiable lesions are usually larger than represented on the image (Figure 13.12). (See Chapters 29 through 32 for in-depth information on radiographs.)

Visual Appearance

Dentists are often able to diagnose caries simply by sight. The use of a dental mirror aids in viewing difficult areas of the mouth. Often, the dentist must distinguish between caries and a simple stain in the pits and fissures of the teeth. Remember, enamel is transparent, and caries may appear as a gray or other discoloration underneath the enamel. It is often helpful for the dentist, hygienist, or dental assistant to use an intraoral camera to digitally photograph the areas of suspected caries. By enlarging the image, recurrent or secondary caries are often seen adjacent to old restorations. Another positive aspect of this method is the ability to educate the patient by showing him or her the image of his or her own mouth on the computer screen.

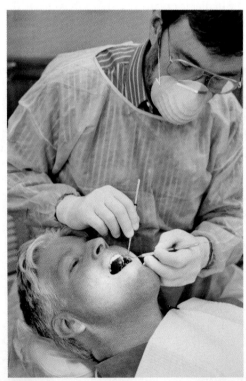

FIGURE 13.11
Dental explorer detecting decayed enamel.

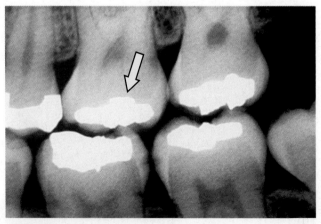

FIGURE 13.12
Radiograph indicating a carious lesion.
Image courtesy Instructional Materials for the Dental Team, Lex., KY

Indicator Dyes

A dye, used during removal of caries, helps the dentist to identify any remaining dentinal caries, especially in difficult-to-see or deep areas. If caries remain, the carious tooth surface will stain a different color, usually greenish-black or red. If the carious lesion is deep, the indicator dye may prevent the dentist from overexcavating the extensive lesion, preventing exposure of the pulp or nerve and blood vessels. Often, the dental assistant uses a syringe to place the dye onto the tooth surface and rinse it away for the dentist, who will observe the dye to determine if further excavation is necessary.

Laser Caries Detector

A rather new diagnostic tool is the laser caries detector, the DIAGNOdent (Figure 13.13). The DIAGNOdent consists of a handheld wand that is connected to a small unit. The wand is used to direct a laser beam of differing wavelengths into a suspected area of caries, usually in pits and fissures or easily accessible smooth surface caries as well as recurrent caries at the poor margin of a restoration. The laser beam measures changes in the density of the enamel and sends a numeric and audible alert.

Healthy tooth structure receives a very low number, whereas an area of large caries receives a higher number and a louder or longer audible alert. The laser is an alternative means to detecting caries while allowing the incipient lesions to possibly remineralize versus the use of the dental explorer, which, as mentioned, could create a cavitation in an incipient lesion. Depending on state dental laws, the dental assistant may use and record the numeric alert, which is then interpreted by the dentist. (Detection of caries is revisited in Chapter 21.)

Methods of Caries Intervention

All humans are at risk for dental caries, especially those who have experienced loss of tooth structure due to caries. In other words, people who have had caries earlier in their lives are at greater risk to have caries reoccur again somewhere in the mouth. It is only a matter of time before these individuals have new carious lesions. Therefore, the caries process should be disturbed and prevented. In modern dentistry, there are numerous means of preventing caries (Figure 13.14):

- A fluoride foam, gel, or varnish treatment is available in the dental office. Mouth rinse is found over the counter at the pharmacy to strengthen teeth and help to remineralize tooth structure.
- Antibacterial therapy is a means of destroying many of the bacterial colonies that cause caries. For example, chlorhexidine mouth rinses and doxycycline, a prescription antibiotic, help prevent oral infections.
- Change in diet for many patients will improve their ability to prevent caries. A decrease in fermentable carbohydrates such as soda pop, candy, dried fruit, honey, and starches can improve the oral environment. Occasionally, the dentist may refer a patient to a nutritionist or dietitian.
- Improved salivary flow with chewing gum containing the caries-fighting sweetener xylitol or over-the-counter products such as Biotene are good means of caries intervention.

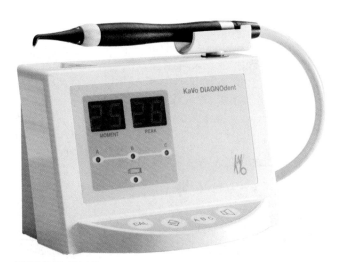

FIGURE 13.13
The DIAGNOdent.
Courtesy KaVo Dental Corporation

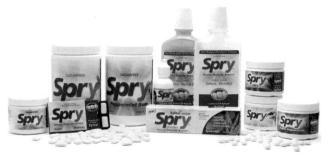

FIGURE 13.14
Products to intervene in caries process.
Courtesy of Xlear, Inc.

- Sealing of pits and fissures on the occlusal surfaces of primary and permanent dentition in patients who have exhibited the caries process will improve their chances of being caries free.
- Improved oral hygiene is imperative for all patients to avoid the caries process.

Can you think of other products you have used or seen to aid in caries intervention or prevention?

Risk Assessment of Caries

Some dentists use a caries risk test (CRT) to determine if a patient is a high-risk individual for dental caries. The test is usually performed in the office with a sample of the patient's saliva. The saliva is tested for pH and applied to an agar strip for bacterial growth. If the strip grows numerous colonies of bacteria, the patient is susceptible to the caries process and intervention techniques should be applied.

CRT kits may be purchased from a dental supply company and performed in the office or sent out to a lab. Unfortunately, CRT is not often found in private dental offices. CRT is most often found in public dental programs and educational settings. The dental assistant can perform this test. In the future, CRT may be used in pediatric dentistry to help identify children at high risk for dental caries so intervention and management of disease can begin early.

Cultural Considerations

Diet and dental hygiene vary greatly across different cultures. For patients from other countries or cultures, it may difficult to explain or have them accept the caries process. This is often due to different dental education and theories throughout the world. Not all cultures believe in Western dentistry. Try to be sensitive to these differences.

SUMMARY

Dental caries is a worldwide problem affecting all humans. Through advances in diagnostic technology and the understanding of the disease, dental professionals are able to provide better preventive care and educate patients and parents in hopes of someday eradicating this disease. Research is currently under way to find a vaccine for the caries-causing bacteria. Until a vaccine is found, diagnosis and treatment of carious lesions as well as preventive measures are the objectives of the dental team.

Professionalism

Listen carefully to the doctors and hygienists in the office and support their means of diagnosis and treatment plans for the patients. The patients are in your care as well. It is up to you and the doctors to help you stay educated in the latest techniques and patient care. Always maintain poise in the presence of patients and answer their questions with confidence.

KEY TERMS

- **Biofilm:** A thin layer of microorganisms (such as bacteria) that form on and coat various surfaces.   p. 205
- **Caries:** An infectious disease that results in the localized destruction of the teeth.   p. 204
- **Cariogenic agent:** Agent that causes caries.   p. 205
- **Cariology:** The study of the caries process.   p. 204
- **Cavitation:** The formation of cavities or holes in tissue or teeth.   p. 206
- **Demineralization:** The loss of minerals from the body or teeth.   p. 205
- **Gross or frank caries:** Obvious severe destruction of the tooth by decay.   p. 206
- **Incipient caries:** The initial formation of tooth decay.   p. 206
- **Lactobacilli:** Bacteria that produce lactic acid from fermentable carbohydrates.   p. 205

- **Mutans streptococci:** Bacteria with significant potential to cause dental caries.   p. 205
- **Pellicle:** A thin layer of salivary proteins coating the surface of the teeth.   p. 205
- **Plaque:** A sticky, usually tooth-colored film on teeth that is formed by and harbors bacteria and their byproducts, also known as a biofilm.   p. 205
- **Rampant caries:** Quickly developing decay apparent throughout the mouth.   p. 206
- **Remineralization:** The restoring of minerals to tooth structure.   p. 205
- **Root surface caries:** Decay found on the root surfaces of teeth.   p. 207
- **Xerostomia:** Abnormal dryness of the mouth due to insufficient amounts of saliva.   p. 208

CHECK YOUR UNDERSTANDING

1. Dental caries affects
   a. children.
   b. geriatric people.
   c. low socioeconomic groups.
   d. adolescents.
   e. all of the above.

2. Caries-causing bacteria include
   a. *Escherichia coli* and mutans streptococci.
   b. *Streptococcus pneumoniae* and lactobacilli.
   c. mutans streptococci and lactobacilli.
   d. *Candida albicans* and *Escherichia coli*.

3. What two elements are lost in the demineralization process?
   a. phosphate and fluoride
   b. bicarbonate ion and proteins
   c. hydroxyapatite crystals and calcium
   d. calcium and phosphate

4. Baby bottle tooth decay is an example of what type of caries?
   a. incipient caries
   b. secondary caries
   c. rampant caries
   d. primary caries

5. Which method is not a common method of caries intervention?
   a. use of fluoride
   b. use of antibacterial agents
   c. change in diet
   d. rinsing with acidic mouthwashes

6. Which of the following is related to an increase in caries?
   a. xerostomia
   b. increase in sucrose
   c. radiation to the head and neck
   d. lack of proper oral hygiene
   e. all of the above

7. Saliva contains all of the following except
   a. enzymes.
   b. electrolytes.
   c. water.
   d. antibacterial compounds.
   e. all of the above.

8. Babies are born without the bacteria that cause dental caries but acquire the bacteria from their parents.
   a. true
   b. false

9. How is plaque arranged on the tooth surface?
   a. tooth surface—pellicle—mutans streptococci—lactobacilli—other microorganisms
   b. tooth surface—lactobacilli—mutans streptococci—pellicle—other microorganisms
   c. tooth surface—other microorganisms—mutans streptococci—lactobacilli—pellicle
   d. tooth surface—mutans streptococci—pellicle—other microorganisms

10. Mrs. Smith is seated in the dental chair. Her chief complaint is a brown spot on her tooth at the gum line. She reports no sensitivity or pain. You notice she has some recession of the gingiva. On use of the dental explorer, the explorer sticks into the dark spot. What is the dark spot on Mrs. Smith's tooth?
    a. area of demineralization
    b. area of remineralization
    c. area of root caries
    d. area of stain

INTERNET ACTIVITY

- Visit www.ada.org and search for educational interactive areas. Find the animation and games area to be able to show children and parents fun dental learning materials. Some dental offices visit schools and children care centers, and these online games may give you some good ideas for presenting educational material on tooth decay and prevention of tooth decay to children in a school setting or in the dental office.

WEB REFERENCES

- American Academy of Pediatric Dentistry   www.aapd.org
- American Dental Association   www.ada.org
- Centers for Disease Control and Prevention   www.cdc.gov
- National Institute of Dental and Craniofacial Research   www.nidcr.nih.gov

14

Periodontal Disease

Learning Objectives

After reading this chapter, the student should be able to:

- Describe healthy periodontium.
- Discuss the prevalence of periodontal disease.
- Define gingivitis and periodontitis and describe their clinical presentation.
- Explain the different types of periodontitis.
- Discuss the roles of dental plaque and calculus in periodontal disease.
- Describe how poor oral hygiene contributes to periodontal disease.
- Identify systemic health conditions related to periodontal disease.
- Explain how smoking affects the periodontium.

Preparing for Certification Exams

- Identify intraoral anatomy.
- Provide patient preventive education and oral hygiene instruction.

Key Terms

Calculus	Periodontium
Edema	Plaque
Erythema	Subgingival
Gingivitis	Sulcus
Furcation	Suppuration
Periodontitis	Supragingival

Chapter Outline

- Structure of the Periodontium
- Prevalence of Periodontal Disease
- Types of Periodontal Disease
  —Gingivitis
  —Periodontitis
- Oral Conditions Linked to Periodontal Disease
- Signs and Symptoms of Periodontal Disease
- Systemic Conditions Linked to Periodontal Disease
  —Cardiovascular Disease
  —Respiratory Disease
  —Diabetes Mellitus
  —Low Birth Weight and Premature Infants
  —HIV/AIDS
- Risk for Periodontal Disease
  —Genetic Marker for Periodontal Disease
  —Other Risk Factors

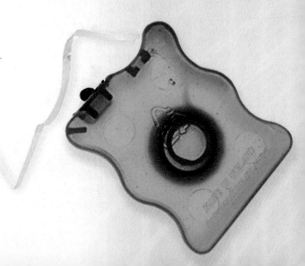

We live in a world inflicted with germs and diseases. Many are rare, but the common ones afflict most people sometime in their lives. One of these diseases is periodontal disease, a slow destructive bacterial infection of the gums and bone. Periodontal disease does not discriminate by sex, age, race, culture, or religion (Figure 14.1). We are all at risk of being affected by a form of periodontal disease whether it is gingivitis or chronic periodontitis. Most forms of periodontal disease can be avoided with the practice of good oral hygiene.

Structure of the Periodontium

It is important to understand the soft and bony structure, known as the **periodontium**, that surrounds and supports the teeth (Figure 14.2). The periodontium is composed of the following:

- Gingiva
- Epithelial attachment
- Periodontal ligament
- Cementum
- Alveolar bone

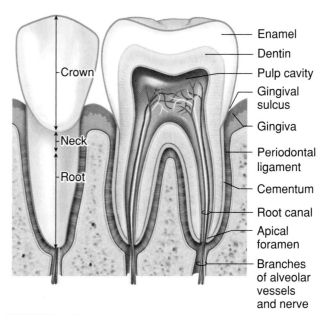

FIGURE 14.2
The anatomy of the tooth and supporting structures.

The gingiva is the soft tissue surrounding the teeth and covering the bone between the teeth. The **sulcus** is the small space between the tooth and the free gingiva. At the base of the sulcus is an area, known as the epithelial attachment, where the gingiva attaches to the tooth. Periodontal ligaments (fibrous attachments) connect the cementum of the roots to the supportive alveolar bone of the jaw. The purpose of the cementum is to anchor the tooth to the bone by providing the proper surface for the attachment of the periodontal ligament. Alveolar bone surrounds and supports the tooth in its position. All of the structures of the periodontium are vitally important to the health of the oral cavity.

Prevalence of Periodontal Disease

Periodontal diseases affect people of all ages. Nearly all adults and many adolescents and children have plaque and calculus on their teeth that contain the bacteria linked to periodontal diseases. Three out of every five teenagers have an early form of periodontal disease. Three of every four American adults have periodontal

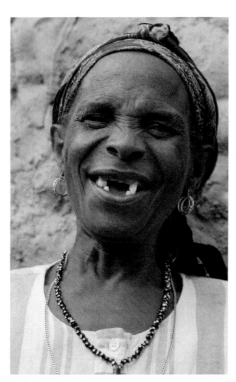

FIGURE 14.1
A woman with numerous teeth missing in the front.

Dental Assistant   PROFESSIONAL TIP

The dental assistant often records the clinical diagnostic findings. When recording notes for any of the members of the clinical team including the doctor, be very accurate. The clinical diagnostic information is extensive and is usually recorded at the initial exam. The clinical notes are part of the patient chart and are legal documents. If you do not clearly hear the team member, always ask him or her to repeat the information. Never guess what should be recorded.

disease. One of every two adults has moderate periodontal disease and one in eight adults has advanced periodontal disease resulting in tooth loss. Fortunately, tooth loss can be avoided with early detection and treatment of periodontal diseases. Most people have no idea they have this active disease process occurring in their mouth.

Types of Periodontal Disease

Periodontal disease encompasses both gingivitis and periodontitis and the various forms of both diseases. It is important for the dental assistant to recognize the characteristics of both diseases, to be able to instruct patients on improving daily home care, and to be able to answer their questions with confidence and assurance. There are seven basic forms of periodontal disease. These include gingivitis, chronic periodontitis,

Life Span Considerations

The prevalence and severity of periodontal disease increases with age. Thirty-three percent of people ages 55 to 64 have advanced periodontal disease. Periodontal disease is not directly related to the aging process. The increase in periodontal disease seen with aging is a result of lifelong cumulative effects. With modern dentistry and current treatments for periodontal disease, people may live their entire lives without periodontal disease and tooth loss.

aggressive periodontitis, periodontitis with systemic disease, necrotizing periodontal diseases, abscesses of the periodontium, and periodontitis associated with endodontic lesions (Table 14-1).

TABLE 14-1 Seven Basic Types of Periodontal Disease

Gingivitis	Seen at any age and defined by marginal gingival inflammation. Includes plaque-induced and non-plaque-induced gingival lesions.
Chronic periodontitis	Onset is seen at any age. Symptoms include inflammation of the periodontium, loss of epithelial attachment and periodontal ligament attachment, loss of bone, eventual tooth loss. • *Slight or early:* inflamed gingiva, early bone loss, site measurement of 3–4 mm (attachment loss of 1–2 mm) • *Moderate:* increased destruction of the periodontium, moderate bone loss, teeth become mobile, **furcation** (region of a multirooted tooth at which the roots divide) involvement, site measurement of 5–7 mm (attachment loss of up to 4 mm) • *Severe or advanced:* severe destruction of the periodontium, increased attachment loss, increased bone loss, increased tooth mobility, greater furcation involvement, site measurement of 7 mm or greater (attachment loss of more than 5 mm)
Aggressive periodontitis	Onset prior to age 35, but can affect older patients. Very rapid rate of periodontal destruction including bone loss, may have genetic relationship, usually bacteria specific. • *Prepubertal:* Onset is between eruption of primary teeth and puberty; localized forms not associated with a systemic disorder and generalized forms associated with blood disorders; symptoms seen as attachment loss around primary and permanent teeth • *Juvenile:* Generalized form is seen late in teenage years and associated with specific bacteria; localized form shows less inflammatory signs but is evident radiographically indicating bone loss around the first molars and anterior incisors
Periodontitis with systemic disease	Patient often has immune, genetic, or blood disorder affecting inflammatory response and tissue organization. Examples include leukemia, Down syndrome, and Papillon-Lefèvre syndrome.
Necrotizing periodontal diseases	Related to diminished systemic resistance to bacterial infection. Often seen with high stress and autoimmune diseases. • *Necrotizing ulcerative gingivitis (NUG):* sudden onset of pain, punched out necrotic papillae bleeding of gingiva, and bad breath • *Necrotizing ulcerative periodontitis (NUP):* clinical presentation of necrosis of gingiva, periodontal ligament, and supporting alveolar bone. Destruction is so extensive there is a lack of deep pocket formation. Associated more with immune disorders than NUG
Abscesses of the periodontium	Infection of the periodontal tissues with pus or **suppuration** formation. Often seen as a large blister filled with yellow to green pus and other fluids.
Periodontitis associated with endodontic lesions	A combination infection including the periodontium and the pulpal tissue of a tooth. Often seen on a radiograph as bone loss to the apex of a tooth.

The American Academy of Periodontology has created a classification system to describe and diagnose periodontal disease. The classification is based on the amount of destruction to the periodontium.

Gingivitis

Gingivitis is possibly more common than the common cold but is also one of the most easily treated inflammatory processes. **Gingivitis** is the first indication of periodontal problems and is noted by inflammation of the gingival tissues (Figures 14.3a, b). Only the free gingiva is affected, not the attached tissue or bone. Gingivitis is characterized by **erythema** (redness of the tissue) and **edema** (swelling as a result of excessive fluid in the tissue). The inflamed tissue tends to bleed easily, most notably during brushing. The gingiva may also appear loose around the contours of the teeth.

Plaque must usually be present for gingivitis to exist, but may be modified or exacerbated by systemic factors (Table 14-2). For example, female sex hormone changes may cause an increase in the symptoms of gingivitis. Dia-

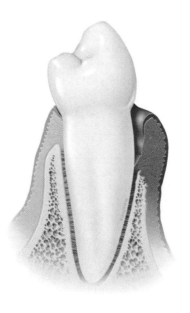

(A)

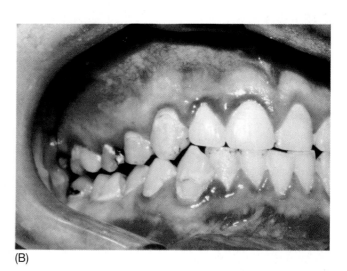

(B)

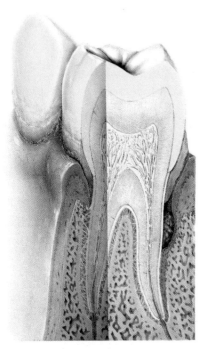

(C)

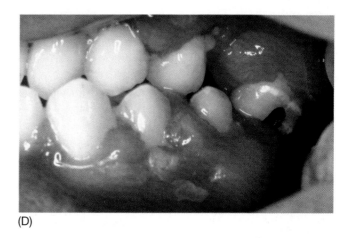

(D)

FIGURE 14.3
(a) Illustration of gingivitis. Notice the healthy tissue on the left and the inflamed gingival tissue on the right; (b) Gingivitis: plaque and inflammation of the marginal gingival tissues; (c) An illustration of periodontitis. This disease attacks the gum and bone around the tooth resulting in loss of the tooth; (d) Advanced periodontal disease.

TABLE 14-2 Dental-Plaque-Induced Gingivitis Modified by Systemic Conditions

Sex hormones	Changes in female sex hormones at puberty, pregnancy, and menopause exaggerate the response to plaque. Tissue may have an intense inflammatory response including edema, erythema, and pain but not attachment or bone loss. Many women report a localized gingival growth known as a pyogenic granuloma or pregnancy tumor.
Diabetes mellitus	Seen in patients with poorly controlled type 1 diabetes mellitus. Severity of gingivitis is related to blood glucose levels.
Blood disorders	Tissue is swollen, smooth, and spongy. It is bright red to purple in color. The papilla are the most obviously swollen red areas.
Medications	Numerous common medications create xerostomia, while others simply cause an exaggerated response to existing plaque. The symptoms usually first occur around the anterior teeth.
Nutrition	One of the first characteristics of vitamin C deficiency, also known as scurvy, is red, swollen, bleeding gingiva. Teeth may become loose. Symptoms are due to loss of the body's ability to make collagen.

betes mellitus, blood disorders, medications, and poor nutrition are other systemic factors affecting gingivitis. Non-plaque-induced gingival diseases do occur, but are rare. These include viral and fungal infections, allergic reactions, trauma, and genetic disorders.

Periodontitis

Periodontitis is defined as an inflammatory disease of the gingival tissues including loss of supporting bone (Figure 14.3c, d). This complex disease has numerous forms, all

Cultural Considerations

Many dental offices have a very diverse group of patients from many races, cultures, and religions. It is imperative to display accepting, nonjudgmental attitudes with each and every patient no matter what his or her beliefs and practices may be. These beliefs may affect the patient's health care practices and can sometimes be harmful. For example, some cultures believe they should never have blood in their mouth and, therefore, do not have their teeth cleaned below the gingival margin due to the bleeding of the gingiva. As much as possible, always encourage patients to practice good dental habits. At the same time, present this information without being disrespectful of your patients' cultures.

Legal and Ethical Issues

Periodontal disease has come to the forefront of dentistry in the last two decades as new information has surfaced. Unfortunately, numerous malpractice lawsuits have risen from failure of the dentist to diagnose and inform patients of their periodontal condition. It is extremely important to note all clinical findings at each appointment including instructions for oral home care. The clinical chart must be clear and complete so there is no mistake that the patient has been properly informed about periodontal disease or the potential for periodontal disease.

caused by groups of microorganisms in the mouth. The disease progresses from marginal inflammation to the loss of connective tissue attachments and eventually loss of the supporting alveolar bone. Periodontal disease is classified by the severity of the destruction of the supporting tissues and the location within the oral cavity where the destruction is occurring. Periodontitis may be chronic or aggressive. Chronic periodontitis indicates the destruction process of bone and other periodontal tissues surrounding a tooth, which can lead to more aggressive damage.

Gingival health is measured with a periodontal probe by placing the probe in the sulcus and recording the sulcus depth; this is known as a site. This deepened sulcus is now known as the periodontal pocket. Each tooth receives six site measurements. Chapter 45 discusses the periodontal examination and the role of the dental assistant in helping the dentist or hygienist develop the periodontal diagnosis and treatment plan. See Chapter 24 for more information on instruments used for periodontal procedures.

The extent of the disease is described as follows:

- *Localized:* Less than 30% of sites in the mouth are affected.
- *Generalized:* More than 30% of the sites in the mouth are affected.

The severity of the disease is described as:

- Slight or early
- Moderate
- Severe or advanced

Other Forms of Periodontal Disease

Systemic diseases are often associated with long-term periodontal disease. The gradual degeneration of periodontal tissues results in necrotic or dead matter creating ulcers and the formation of periodontal pockets. As the disease progresses, blisters form that contain pus and other by-products of the bacterial infection. Periodontal abscesses may appear along with periapical abscesses linked to infection within the pulp of the tooth as well as the surrounding periodontium.

Oral Conditions Linked to Periodontal Disease

Plaque is a sticky, tooth-colored film on teeth that is formed by and harbors bacteria and their by-products. When plaque builds up, it appears as a white mass following the gingival line along the teeth (Figure 14.4). The types of bacteria in plaque are different than the bacteria that cause dental caries, but they can be just as destructive to the soft and hard periodontal tissues.

Plaque is the leading cause of periodontal disease, often as the result of untreated gingivitis, although other factors are also involved.

Other factors include the amount of time the plaque is left undisturbed on the teeth and the patient's immune response to the bacteria. The bacteria produce enzymes and toxins that destroy the periodontium and cause an inflammatory response.

Calculus, also known as tartar, is a combination of calcium and phosphate salts from saliva that mix with plaque to form hard deposits on tooth surfaces. Calculus initially forms on the tooth surfaces nearest to salivary ducts. These areas are the lingual surfaces of the mandibular anterior teeth and the buccal surfaces of the maxillary molars. Even though these areas are the most common areas for calculus buildup, calculus can occur on all surfaces of the teeth. Calculus provides an excellent medium for more plaque to grow due to its rough surface. Calculus alone does not cause periodontal disease. It simply provides a place for plaque bacteria to thrive and destroy periodontium. A dental hygienist or a dentist must remove it with hand scaling instruments or an ultrasonic scaler. (See Chapters 24 and 45, respec-

tively, for details on dental instruments and periodontal procedures.)

Calculus is classified by its location on the tooth surface. Calculus above the free gingival margin is known as **supragingival** calculus, and calculus below the free gingival margin is known as **subgingival** calculus. Supragingival calculus is visible on examination and is often stained a dark yellow. It is found on the clinical crown of a tooth or on cementum of the roots if the periodontium has receded (Figure 14.5). Subgingival calculus is not obvious on visual examination. It is usually diagnosed upon periodontal examination or radiographic examination (Figure 14.6). This type of calculus is found on the cementum of the roots below the gingival margin and into the sulcus. It is often stained dark yellow, brown,

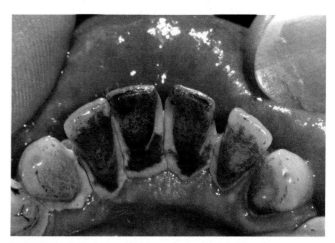

FIGURE 14.5
Calculus buildup on the surface of the teeth.

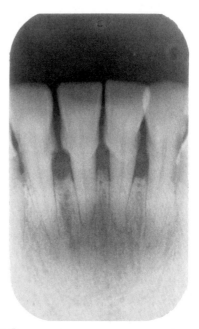

FIGURE 14.6
Radiograph showing large deposits of calculus around the necks of the teeth.

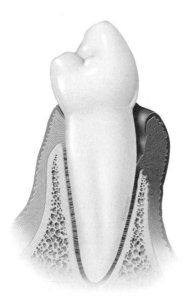

FIGURE 14.4
Bacterial plaque infecting the gingiva.

green, or black. These colors occur due to blood pigments from the periodontal inflammation created by the plaque trapped in the sulcus by the subgingival calculus.

Signs and Symptoms of Periodontal Disease

There are numerous signs and symptoms of periodontal disease. It is important for the dental assistant to know the adjectives describing the clinical appearance of diseased periodontium such as *red, swollen, spongy, bleeding*, and occasionally *painful tissue*. Diseased periodontal tissues exude a foul odor. Many patients will describe gingivitis or periodontitis not knowing they are describing a periodontal disease. One of the most important facts is that periodontal disease does not usually cause pain. Periodontal tissue may be described as either healthy or diseased. Table 14-3 compares healthy periodontium to diseased periodontium.

Systemic Conditions Linked to Periodontal Disease

Many systemic conditions (conditions that affect the entire body) are now known to be related to periodontal disease. Some of these conditions, such as HIV/AIDS, cause an increase in susceptibility to periodontal disease. On the other hand, periodontal disease may actually cause an increase in susceptibility to certain systemic diseases such as cardiovascular disease, respiratory disease, diabetes, as well as preterm delivery of low birth weight infants.

Cardiovascular Disease

In recent years, researchers have found that patients with periodontal disease have a greater chance of developing coronary heart disease than patients without periodontal disease. Periodontal disease causes a chronic inflamma-

Professionalism

In the dental field, procedures or clinical presentations can often be unpleasant, foul smelling, or surprising. It is important to maintain your poise and cease from making an unsightly face, rolling your eyes, or making some other unpleasing expression. Even though you are wearing a mask, the mask will not hide all of your expressions.

tory process in the mouth, allowing for high concentrations of pathogens to enter the bloodstream. This occurs whenever the gingiva is made to bleed. The pathogens attach to fatty deposits in the bloodstream and contribute to clot formation in the arteries, causing strokes and heart attacks. People with periodontal disease have 3.6 times greater risk for coronary heart disease and 3 times greater risk for a stroke. In fact, those with periodontal disease have a 1.5 to 2 times greater risk for a fatal cardiovascular event. If a patient has existing coronary disease, then periodontal disease may increase the severity of the cardiac condition.

Respiratory Disease

The bacteria in the oral cavity associated with plaque and calculus may be inhaled, creating a greater risk for respiratory infections. This bacterium changes the internal lining of the respiratory system, allowing for other pathogens to invade and cause a respiratory infection such as pneumonia. As with existing cardiovascular diseases, individuals with an existing respiratory condition may have their condition exacerbated due to periodontal disease. These respiratory conditions include chronic bronchitis, emphysema, asthma, and other chronic obstructive pulmonary diseases.

Diabetes Mellitus

Individuals living with diabetes have a higher than normal risk of periodontal disease linked to a lack of blood sugar control. In other words, persons with diabetes who have poor blood sugar control demonstrate periodontal disease more often and more severely than diabetics with good blood sugar control. Actually, well-controlled diabetics have the same risk for periodontal disease as persons without diabetes. Diabetic children are also at risk for gum problems. Therefore, the best protection against periodontal disease is good diabetic control.

Low Birth Weight and Premature Infants

All infections are cause for concern among pregnant women because they pose a risk to the health of the baby. Studies suggest that periodontal disease is a considerable

TABLE 14-3 Healthy Periodontium versus Diseased Periodontium

Healthy	Diseased
Pink	Red, magenta, purple, white, cyanotic
Firm	Spongy, loose, boggy, edematous, swollen
Stippled and smooth	Shiny, eroded, nodular, hyperkeratotic, fibrous
Knife-edge, flat, snug, pointed, pyramidal	Edema, fibrous, clefting, festooning, rounded, rolled, bulbous, cratered, blunted
Teeth firmly anchored	Teeth mobile and separating

risk factor for low birth weight and premature infants. Pregnant women who have periodontal disease may be seven times more likely to have a baby born too early and too small.

Research is ongoing to confirm how periodontal disease may affect pregnancy outcomes. Researchers believe that periodontal disease triggers increased levels of biological fluids that induce labor. Evidence indicates that women whose periodontal condition worsens during pregnancy have an even higher risk of having a premature baby. Researchers have established that treatment for periodontal disease significantly reduces the risk of having a preterm birth or a low birth weight infant.

HIV/AIDS

HIV and AIDS are viral infections that affect people around the world. Individuals with HIV/AIDS cannot effectively fight infections including periodontal disease. Due to the lack of a sufficient immune system, the gingiva becomes increasingly inflamed around the margins of all teeth. If the patient has poor oral hygiene, the progression of periodontal disease is swift and may result in severe bone and tooth loss in a very short period of time. Patients with HIV/AIDS also have a high risk for developing necrotizing ulcerative gingivitis or periodontitis. Oral hygiene visits should increase to help prevent these patients from progressing to a more severe form of periodontal disease.

Risk for Periodontal Disease

Dentists can assess patients' risk for periodontal disease, including its severity and onset, as discussed in the next two subsections.

Genetic Marker for Periodontal Disease

A recent development in risk factor assessment is the discovery of a genetic marker highly associated with periodontal disease. This discovery has resulted in a test for an individual's susceptibility for periodontal disease known as the Periodontal Susceptibility Test (PST). The PST is a saliva-based test that identifies a specific gene associated with periodontal disease. Approximately 30% of the population tests positive for this gene.

The dental assistant can perform the PST. A piece of DNA filter paper is used to collect saliva. The filter paper is sent to a DNA laboratory for analysis and the results are returned to the dentist. Once the PST has identified patients at high risk for periodontal disease, the dentist can determine the need for aggressive treatment and discuss improved home oral hygiene with the patients.

How does subgingival calculus get so deep into the sulcus? How can it be avoided?

Other Risk Factors

Other risk factors for periodontal disease affect the onset and severity of the disease. Bacterial plaque must be present, but other factors such as smoking, stress, medications, osteoporosis, poor oral hygiene, and local factors contribute to periodontal disease (Table 14-4).

Smoking has a tremendous impact on the periodontal tissues. It creates an environment for periodontal-causing bacteria to thrive. Smokers have deeper periodontal pockets, increased calculus formation, greater bone loss, and increased tooth loss. According to the Centers for Disease Control and Prevention, 41.3% of smokers over the age of 65 are toothless as

TABLE 14-4 Other Risk Factors for Periodontal Disease

Smoking	Smoking is an important risk factor. It causes greater loss of bone, deeper periodontal pockets, increased calculus formation, and increased tooth loss. The toxins in cigarettes provide an environment in which periodontal bacteria thrive. Smokers do not exhibit the inflammatory response of red bleeding gingiva due to the reduced blood flow to the gingiva caused by constriction of the blood vessels. Smokers also do not heal as well as nonsmokers.
Stress	Studies show a relationship among stress, poor coping skills, and periodontal disease. In particular, individuals with high financial stress and poor coping skills show a greater risk of severe periodontal disease.
Medications	Numerous medications cause xerostomia, which in turn creates increased plaque buildup, leading to periodontal disease. These patients need to visit the dental hygienist more frequently to be well monitored.
Osteoporosis	Osteoporosis is a disease in which the bones become porous and brittle. Studies have found a link between alveolar bone loss and osteoporosis. Loss of estrogen is also a factor in alveolar bone loss.
Poor oral hygiene	Lack of daily oral hygiene is a tremendous factor in the development of periodontal disease. Plaque left on the teeth daily compounds to form a haven for bacteria that leads to periodontal diseases. It is extremely important to maintain good oral home care, which leads to decreased risk of periodontal diseases.
Local factors	Local factors are items in the oral cavity placed by another individual. Overhanging margins of fillings and crowns, orthodontic appliances, removable partial dentures, and intraoral body piercings all provide areas for plaque to collect and lead to periodontal disease.

compared to only 20% of nonsmokers. Smokers also experience slow healing after periodontal therapy or oral surgery. The dental assistant should be aware of the effects of smoking on the periodontal tissues and have the ability to discuss smoking cessation with smoking patients.

Preparing for Externship

Before your first day of externship, ask the office manager or clinical manager to explain the doctor's philosophy and the office mission. The philosophy and mission are the underlying goals and beliefs of the office. Take this information to heart and treat each patient and coworker with the utmost respect.

SUMMARY

Periodontal diseases include both gingivitis and periodontitis. These bacterial infections affect all age groups. Important research has revealed periodontal disease to be related to many systemic conditions including cardiovascular disease, diabetes mellitus, and respiratory conditions. Recent developments have even shown a genetic marker for periodontal disease. Plaque and calculus are definitely contributing risk factors providing a medium for bacterial growth that can result in destruction of the periodontium.

The American Academy of Periodontology has created a classification system to help standardize the clinical diagnosis of periodontal disease. The types of periodontal disease range from the very curable gingivitis to the more destructive chronic periodontitis and aggressive periodontitis. The seven types are affected by numerous risk factors, but all are caused by groups of microorganisms. If left untreated, periodontitis leads to great loss of soft and bony tissues, eventually causing tooth loss. It is important for the dental assistant to know the signs and symptoms of the various periodontal diseases in order to provide the best care for all patients.

KEY TERMS

- **Calculus:** A hard deposit on tooth surfaces; in the presence of plaque, calculus is formed by calcium and phosphate salts from saliva; also called tartar. p. 218
- **Edema:** The presence of abnormally large amounts of fluid in the tissues (swelling). p. 216
- **Erythema:** Redness of the tissues, often due to inflammation. p. 216
- **Gingivitis:** Inflammation of the gingiva. p. 216
- **Furcation:** The region of a multirooted tooth at which the roots divide. p. 215
- **Periodontitis:** Inflammatory disease of the gingival tissues that involves loss of supporting bone. p. 217
- **Periodontium:** Soft and bony supporting structure of tissues that surrounds the teeth. p. 214
- **Plaque:** Sticky, tooth-colored film on teeth that is formed by and harbors bacteria and their by-products. p. 218
- **Subgingival:** Referring to the area below the gingival margin. p. 218
- **Sulcus:** Space between the tooth and the free gingiva. p. 214
- **Suppuration:** The formation of pus; often in the gingival sulcus related to inflammation. p. 215
- **Supragingival:** Referring to the area above the gingival margin. p. 218

CHECK YOUR UNDERSTANDING

1. Periodontal disease is defined as
   a. caries on the smooth surfaces of the teeth.
   b. inflammatory disease of the periodontium including gingivitis and periodontitis.
   c. inflammatory disease of bone only.
   d. viral disease of the soft tissue of the cheeks and lips.

2. Gingivitis generally presents as
   a. red, swollen, and bleeding gingiva.
   b. pink, firm, and rolled gingiva.
   c. punched-out papillae.
   d. red, firm, and spongy bone loss.

3. Cardiovascular disease (CVD) is a very serious condition. How does periodontal disease relate to CVD?
   a. The inflammatory disease in the mouth allows pathogens to enter the bloodstream and attach to fatty deposits to clog the arteries.
   b. The calculus breaks off the teeth and is swallowed, allowing pathogens to enter the blood through the stomach.
   c. Pathogens enter the body through contaminated foods and fluids entering the bloodstream through the stomach and eventually into the heart.
   d. CVD and periodontal disease are not related.

CHECK YOUR UNDERSTANDING (continued)

4. Which of the following structures does not belong to the periodontium?
   a. cementum
   b. epithelial attachment
   c. free gingiva
   d. enamel
   e. periodontal ligament

5. Individuals living with uncontrolled diabetes have a higher than normal risk of all the following except
   a. periodontal bone loss.
   b. tooth loss.
   c. swollen bleeding gingiva.
   d. all of the above.

6. Periodontitis is defined as
   a. inflammation of the pulpal tissues.
   b. a viral disease of the soft tissue of the cheeks and lips.
   c. an inflammatory disease of the gingival tissues that includes loss of supporting bone.
   d. recession to the level of the alveolar bone.

7. All of the following are categories of chronic periodontitis except
   a. slight or early.
   b. moderate.
   c. severe or advanced.
   d. necrotic.

8. Dental-plaque-induced gingivitis modified by systemic conditions includes all of the following except
   a. nutrition.
   b. stress.
   c. medications.
   d. medications.
   e. sleep depravation.

9. Juvenile periodontitis is characterized by lack of inflammatory response, but shows moderate to severe bone loss around the first molars and anterior incisors.
   a. true
   b. false

10. Periodontitis is characterized by all of the following except
   a. edema.
   b. erythema.
   c. pain.
   d. bone loss.

● INTERNET ACTIVITY

- Visit www.perio.org. Locate the page defining periodontal (gum) disease. Find *"Do you have periodontal disease? Take a quiz and find out"* highlighted in red. Click on this statement and follow the instructions for the self-evaluation quiz. If you answer yes to any of these questions, consult your dentist immediately and report your findings.

● WEB REFERENCES

- American Academy of Periodontology   www.perio.org
- American Dental Association   www.ada.org
- Diabetes and Periodontal Disease   www.seniorhealth.about.com
- HIV and Periodontal Disease   www.hivdent.org
- Mayo Clinic   www.mayoclinic.com
- National Institute of Dental and Craniofacial Research   www.nidcr.nih.gov

15

Oral Health

Learning Objectives

After reading this chapter, the student should be able to:

- State the primary role of a dental assistant regarding oral health education.
- List risk factors for dental disease.
- Discuss the use of fluoride and the controversy surrounding it.
- Demonstrate the topical application of fluoride for a patient.
- Explain how proper nutrition prevents oral diseases.
- Discuss the bacterial components in dental plaque and the formation of calculus.
- Demonstrate the use of disclosing agents.
- Describe how to calculate a plaque score.
- List the proper techniques of toothbrushing and flossing.
- Demonstrate oral hygiene instruction for a patient.

Preparing for Certification Exams

- Demonstrate oral hygiene instruction for a patient.
- Demonstrate topical fluoride treatment for a patient.

Key Terms

Bridge threader

Calculus

Fluoridation

Fluorosis

Gingivitis

Halitosis

Sulcus

Systemic fluorides

Topical fluoride

Chapter Outline

- Patient Education
  - Prevention

- Fluoride
  - History of Fluoridation
  - Optimum Fluoridation
  - How Fluoride Works
  - Encouraging Fluoride Use
  - The Fluoride Controversy

- Nutrition and Dental Caries
  - Eating for Health

- Plaque Control Program
  - Disclosing Dental Plaque
  - Toothbrushing
  - Flossing
  - Oral Hygiene Aids

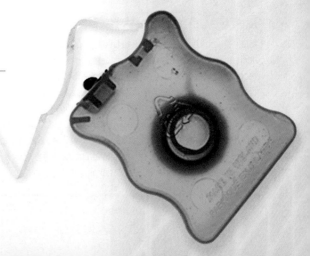

Oral health is essential to the general overall health of the body. The primary function of a dental assistant is to educate and motivate patients to understand the importance of oral health care and preventive dentistry. During dental visits the effectiveness of a patient's oral health care and nutrition is assessed to determine the patient's needs. The dental assistant discusses with the patient how often the patient should brush his or her teeth and use dental floss.

It is important for the dental assistant to know how to best educate each patient on how to maintain optimal long-term oral health. Proper oral health is achieved through the benefits of fluoride as it relates to preventing dental caries and eating a balanced diet. The vast majority of dental disease can be prevented by daily plaque removal techniques. The dental assistant is responsible for teaching each patient oral hygiene instructions to include proper toothbrushing and flossing techniques used to keep the teeth clean.

Although the single most important measure to prevent dental disease is home oral hygiene, regular dental checkups are necessary to identify and treat problems as soon as possible. Once dental caries is present, a restoration is necessary for the tooth in order to prevent further problems such as caries reaching the pulp chamber within

Dental Assistant PROFESSIONAL TIP

Many studies have been done to link periodontal disease and problems such as cardiovascular disease, diabetes, and low birth weight. One recent study provided evidence that preventing or curing periodontal disease can reduce the inflammation that leads to atherosclerosis within the blood vessels and suggests that brushing and flossing may also help prevent heart disease. The dental assistant can help patients with their overall physical health by providing them with an appreciation of how bacteria in the mouth can affect the entire body system and how easy it is to remove bacterial plaque daily.

Life Span Considerations

An increasing number of older patients are keeping their natural teeth longer due to the use of fluoride and better knowledge about prevention. Some patients in this age group require special consideration because reduced mobility and dexterity may make daily oral hygiene difficult. The dental assistant must be patient and work with each patient individually to help them maintain their home dental care effectiveness.

the tooth and creating serious discomfort and further dental infections. Checkup appointments with the dentist provide the opportunity to ensure optimum oral health is being maintained.

Patient Education

According to the U.S. Surgeon General, oral diseases are among the most common health problems affecting individuals in the United States. Factors such as personal self-care behavior, diet, tobacco and alcohol use, and the availability of fluoridated water influence oral health.

A better understanding of risk factors for oral diseases is necessary in our communities. By age 17 more than 80% of adolescents will have cavities. Periodontal diseases range from mild forms of gingivitis to severe forms of periodontitis that result in tooth loss. According to the National Institute of Dental and Craniofacial Research, an estimated 80% of Americans currently have some form of periodontal disease. The Centers for Disease Control and Prevention (CDC) reports that more than 50% of the U.S. population 30 years of age and older have **gingivitis,** a reversible inflammation of the gingiva, and more than 52% of those 20 years and older have this oral disease.

Tobacco use is proven to be a significant risk factor in the development of periodontal disease, and its use can lower the success of periodontal treatment. People with poorly controlled diabetes are at a higher risk for developing infections including periodontal disease. Some medications such as antidepressants and some heart medications can reduce the flow of saliva, which has a protective effect on the teeth. Illnesses such as AIDS and cancer along with their treatments can seriously affect oral health. Minorities, the elderly, and children of low-income families have fewer preventive visits with the dentist and therefore experience a lack of preventive care that is correlated with poorer oral health. Warning signs for periodontal disease are tender, red, or bleeding gingiva (Figure 15.1) and a constant bad taste or bad breath.

Dental caries and periodontal diseases are caused by microorganisms found in dental plaque. These microorganisms cause diseases that can destroy tissues surround-

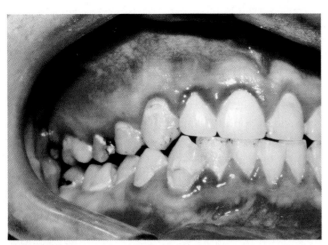

FIGURE 15.1
Signs of gingivitis: tender, red, bleeding gums.

Patient Education

The dental assistant has a unique opportunity to educate each patient at every visit. Recent studies by microbiologists suggest that brushing teeth and using dental floss may help prevent heart disease. Reducing inflammation caused by gingivitis and periodontal disease can also reduce the inflammation that leads to atherosclerosis, which is thickening of the walls of the arteries due to a buildup of cholesterol.

ing teeth and ultimately result in tooth loss. Patients need to understand that controlling the numbers of these bacteria can provide an environment that leads to a healthy mouth. The primary bacterium in dental plaque that causes decay is *Streptococcus mutans*. This bacterium converts sugars and simple carbohydrates in the mouth into acid, which dissolves and weakens tooth enamel, causing tooth decay.

Oral hygiene instruction is a vital part of patient education. It is an ongoing process. To promote good oral hygiene, the dental assistant must help the patient understand what plaque is, where it is found, and how to remove it. After explaining what plaque is, methods of plaque removal should be explained to the patient. The dental assistant should stress that the patient is responsible for his or her own daily oral health care. The dental assistant must educate and motivate patients toward optimal oral health and therefore the best possible overall health.

The American Dental Association (ADA) recommends the following for good oral hygiene:

- Brush teeth twice a day for two minutes with a toothpaste containing fluoride.
- Clean between teeth daily with floss and/or an interdental cleaner.

- Eat a balanced diet and limit between meal snacks.
- Visit the dentist regularly for professional cleanings and oral exams.

A patient needs to learn how to keep bacterial plaque under control to help reduce oral diseases. This is where the dental assistant can be incredibly valuable. The dental assistant is an educator and motivator for each patient. The dental assistant encourages patients in the prevention of oral disease. Individual risk factors for dental disease must be identified for each patient as early as possible.

Among young children, the dental hygiene and oral health education of the mother have a significant influence on the child's risk for developing dental caries. Health of the primary teeth affects the health of the permanent teeth as they erupt into the mouth. A child with dental caries in her deciduous teeth is at a much higher risk of developing decay in the permanent dentition. Factors specific to a person's susceptibility to tooth decay include levels of cariogenic bacteria, the level of saliva present, proper diet and sugar consumption, individual immune factors, exposure to fluoride, and home care.

Prevention

Prevention has received increased attention, effectively replacing restorative concepts as the major focus of dentistry. If dental caries is prevented, tooth restorations are unnecessary. Teaching preventive dentistry to avoid oral disease includes motivating patients toward nutrition and dietary control as well as home care and the use of fluoride. Communication will be unique to each individual but imperative to each person's general health and well-being and should begin as soon as possible.

Tooth decay is the most chronic disease among children. Dental caries begins at an early age. According to the CDC, 42% of children ages 6 to 19 have caries or a restoration in their permanent teeth. Another national survey found that nearly 20% of children between the ages of 2 and 4 had tooth decay, and by age 17 almost 80% had experienced dental caries. Low-income families have the lowest rate of dental care. Untreated decay may cause pain, absence from school, underweight, and poor appearance that can greatly reduce a child's self-esteem and later success in life. The radiographs in Figures 15.2, 15.3, and 15.4 shows various types of dental decay.

More than two-thirds of adults ages 35 to 44 have lost at least one permanent tooth due to dental caries or periodontal disease, and older adults suffer from the problem of root caries. Although public education and promotion of preventive health care are widespread, successful outcomes are most likely to occur with specific interventions targeted to those at the highest risk for developing caries. These interventions include:

- Educating mothers regarding oral health during prenatal visits
- Incorporating oral health into well-baby care

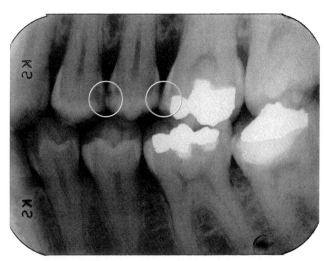

FIGURE 15.2
Radiograph of carious lesions.

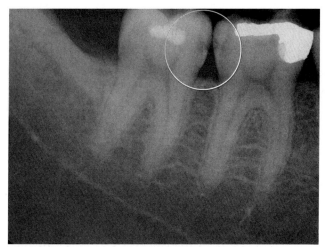

FIGURE 15.3
Radiograph of interproximal caries.

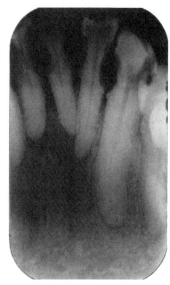

FIGURE 15.4
Radiograph of rampant caries.

- Screening 1-year-old children to identify those at high risk and ensure they are followed up with preventive regimens
- Educating patients on proper toothbrushing and flossing techniques and why they must be accomplished daily
- Providing fluoridated toothpaste for infants and children
- Providing topical fluoride for infants, young children, and older adults
- Applying sealants for children susceptible to caries
- Providing dental care including radiographs to low-income families

The CDC and the ADA stress that increasing access to preventive and restorative services for children and adults results in a decrease in the incidence of dental disease.

Child's First Visit to the Dentist

The ADA and the American Academy of Pediatric Dentistry recommend a first visit to a dentist when a child is about 1 year old. The majority of children who see a dentist for the first time are between the ages of 3 and 5 years. The recommendation for an earlier first visit is so that early childhood dental caries may be recognized sooner and preventive measures taught to children and parents in a timely manner before problems become extensive.

Baby Bottle Decay

Tooth decay in infants and young children most often occurs in the maxillary anterior teeth but may affect other teeth. A baby's teeth can decay soon after they first erupt into the mouth. The decay may even enter the underlying bone structure, which can hamper development of the permanent teeth. This problem is frequently referred to as baby bottle tooth decay. This kind of decay is caused by long-term exposure of a child's teeth to liquids containing sugars. When a child consumes a sugary liquid, acid attacks the teeth and gingiva. Even formula and breast milk can cause decay when in prolonged contact with the teeth.

Bottles containing juices are the most common cause of baby bottle tooth decay especially if allowed at bedtime. Parents must be educated not to put children to bed with anything but water in a bottle and should take their infant to the dentist just after the first tooth appears.

Ages 2 to 6 Years

Between 2 and 3 years of age, children should have all of their primary dentition. The importance of good nutrition should be emphasized to children and their parent or guardian. Oral hygiene instruction should be taught geared to this age group. Most children in this age group are not able to understand the use of words such as "on top of," "inside," and "behind." Therefore, methods such as showing audiovisuals or pictures should be utilized for teaching these younger patients. Each child must receive individual instruction, and the parent should also join in on the process.

Children can be helped to clean teeth properly by standing behind them while they are looking into a mirror and showing them exactly how to brush in a systematic manner. The dental assistant should show the child as well as the parent how to make sure each area in the mouth is cleaned. Young children should be given positive reinforcement and continual demonstration and supervision to learn and appreciate plaque removal.

Methods of educating this age group on care of the teeth include the use of cartoons to teach children and using the child as a model when demonstrating toothbrushing.

Children under 7 years old lack the motivation for toothbrushing and have poor manual dexterity for reducing oral plaque on their own. Therefore, parents must take an active role to ensure their child's teeth are cleaned (Figure 15.5). When this habit is taught early in life, it becomes naturally ingrained in the daily routine of the child. Children need a simple method to clean their teeth. The dental assistant may show younger patients and their parents how to brush in three steps: Clean the chewing surfaces first, then the outer surfaces next to the cheek and lips, and then the inner surfaces on the upper and lower arches.

Ages 7 to 12 Years

Effective plaque removal techniques can be reinforced when the child takes an active part in his or her oral hygiene education. School-aged children should be educated in oral self-care according to their physical and psychological development. By age 7 most children have the manual dexterity necessary to proficiently use a toothbrush. In this age group the permanent first and second molars erupt into the mouth.

The importance of healthy habits, nutrition, and self-care should be addressed to parents with increasing involvement of the child in the discussion and decision making. This is the age when dental floss should be intro-

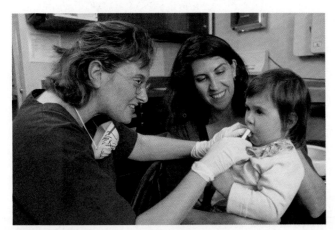

FIGURE 15.5
Dental assistant teaching a parent how to clean a child's teeth.

duced as part of oral health care. Preventive treatments such as placing sealants on the first permanent molars are ideal procedures for many young patients (see Chapter 49).

Adolescents

Teenagers should be guided toward a healthy lifestyle, which includes counseling on risky behaviors such as tobacco and alcohol use. Good-quality patient care occurs when the dental assistant advises a patient on factors affecting oral health so that the patient can make informed decisions.

A central focus of personal oral hygiene should be one-on-one interaction between the patient and the dental health care provider. This interaction should inform patients of their own responsibility for maintaining their oral health and be documented in the dental record to help the entire dental team become aware of each patient's needs.

Adults

The necessity of oral health must be communicated continually to patients when they visit the dental office. Educating patients on oral hygiene saves dollars for dental treatment that can be prevented by conscientious home care. Patients need help and encouragement toward improving their use of dental floss and their toothbrushing techniques. It is important to make each patient aware that they are ultimately responsible for improving and maintaining the health of their oral tissues.

A patient can be motivated by emphasizing that money and discomfort may be saved by preventing the need for dental treatment through conscientious daily home care to include daily brushing and flossing. Adults also need to schedule periodic cleanings by a dentist or dental hygienist to reduce the amount of bacterial plaque on the teeth and gingival tissue in order to help maintain optimum oral health.

What is the percentage of adults who have gingivitis? What is a major risk factor for development of periodontal disease? Who is responsible for daily oral health?

Fluoride

In 2005 the U.S. Surgeon General said, "Community water fluoridation is the single most effective public health measure to prevent dental decay and improve oral health over a lifetime for both children and adults." The ADA and CDC agree with him and are trying to reach populated areas that do not have access to this method of fighting dental disease. These organizations are encouraging all communities to adopt water **fluoridation**, the adding of fluoride to the public water supply. Fluoride is a mineral that occurs naturally in soil and all water sources such as lakes, rivers, and oceans. When ingested some of the fluoride is absorbed by the body tissues and deposited in the teeth and bones.

History of Fluoridation

In 1945, Grand Rapids, Michigan, became the first community to adjust the fluoride content in the public water system to the level effective for prevention of tooth decay. Since then more than 170 million Americans, including residents of 44 of the nation's 50 largest cities, have benefited from optimally fluoridated water. When rates of documented tooth decay in communities with and without fluoride in the water supply were compared, the evidence proved the ability and effectiveness of fluoride to decrease tooth decay in children. Other cities rapidly adopted this interceptive means of preventing caries.

Optimum Fluoridation

Water fluoridation is the addition of fluoride to raise the natural concentration of fluoride in a community's water supply up to the level recommended by the U.S. Public Health Service for the best possible dental health. The optimum level is approximately 1 part per million (1 ppm), or 1 part fluoride per 1 million parts of water. One part per million is the equivalent of about 1 cent in $10,000. Some water supplies already contain fluoride naturally. For others it is intentionally added to the water supply. Not all communities add fluoride to the water; therefore, parents should visit their child's pediatrician if a fluoride supplement is needed.

How Fluoride Works

Dental caries, commonly known as tooth decay, is an infectious disease in which acids from bacteria dissolve the enamel of a tooth. This often results in pain and loss of tooth structure. Fluoride works by keeping the tooth strong and preventing the loss of minerals from the enamel as well as facilitating the remineralization or uptake of minerals into the tooth.

Children from birth through 14 years of age benefit the most from **systemic fluorides.** Systemic fluorides are delivered to the tooth surface via the bloodstream of the body. Fluoride is then built into the enamel structure of the developing tooth, making it more resistant to acids. People susceptible to caries will also benefit from a **topical fluoride,** which is fluoride that is applied to the surface of tooth enamel. For those whose water does not contain fluoride, fluoride drops and vitamins are available. People at risk and in need of fluoride include:

- Adults with a high incidence of root caries
- People who experience an extremely dry mouth
- Patients who wear orthodontic braces
- All people who have a history of excessive tooth decay

Topical Fluoride

Fluoride is added to most toothpaste formulas. Fluoride may also be applied as a gel in the dental office following a routine coronal polishing of the teeth by placing trays over the teeth (Figure 15.6 and Procedure 15-1). Fluoride varnish is becoming a very popular type of fluoride that can be given to younger children because it has no harmful side effects with digestion of the product. Fluoridated mouth rinses are available for home use for those patients over 6 years of age and adults who are especially vulnerable to decay. Home care fluoride gels for those who are highly susceptible to caries are applied by means of trays or brushes.

Encouraging Fluoride Use

The CDC works with state and national agencies to improve the quality of water fluoridation and to implement fluoridation in new communities. During the past 60 years, damage caused by tooth decay has been drastically reduced primarily through the use of fluoride. The activities of the CDC to promote fluoride use include:

- Issuing *Recommendations for Using Fluoride to Prevent and Control Dental Caries in the United States*
- Providing fluoridation training to state drinking water system engineers, dental directors, and other public health staff members
- Managing an Internet-based system that helps states monitor the quality of fluoridated water systems
- Educating people throughout the country on the appropriate use of fluoride products

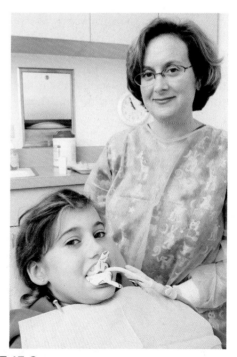

FIGURE 15.6
Dental assistant placing trays with topical fluoride into a patient's mouth.

Procedure 15-1 Applying a Topical Fluoride

Equipment and Supplies Needed

- Basic setup: mirror, explorer, cotton pliers
- Saliva ejector, high-volume evacuator (HVE) tip, air/water syringe tip
- 2 × 2 gauze squares
- Topical fluoride solution
- Proper size fluoride trays
- Watch with a second hand

Procedure Steps

1. Seat the patient upright in the dental chair and adjust the headrest. Place the patient napkin around the neck. Explain the procedure to the patient and instruct the patient to not swallow the fluoride.

2. Ensure the disposable fluoride trays will cover all teeth but not extend too far distal.

3. Fill both trays about one-third full with topical fluoride. Show the patient how to use the saliva ejector.

4. Dry the teeth with 2 × 2 gauze squares or by blowing air with the air/water syringe.

5. Insert the loaded fluoride trays carefully. Place one on the lower arch and the other on the upper arch. Move the trays around to disperse the fluoride.

6. Place the saliva ejector between the arches and have the patient gently close.

7. Look at the second hand on your watch to ensure the fluoride treatment is in place for the entire specified time. Most fluoride treatments require one full minute.

8. Remove the trays and quickly use the HVE to completely remove all fluoride from the teeth. Tell the patient not to swallow.

9. When dismissing the patient, tell her that she may spit into the sink, but instruct her not to rinse or drink anything for at least 30 minutes to allow the fluoride to work.

10. Be sure to enter the fluoride treatment procedure and patient instructions in the patient's dental record.

The CDC further recommends that all persons should know the fluoride concentration in their primary source of drinking water and whether it is below optimal, optimal, or above the optimal level. The CDC suggests parents and caregivers must have this information to protect their children and that in the areas where natural fluoride is below the optimal level, fluoride supplements should be considered.

When the natural fluoride concentration is greater than 2 ppm, the CDC suggests that alternative sources of drinking water should be used. The CDC recommends that all persons receive frequent exposure to small amounts of fluoride. They also recommend that preschool-aged children be supervised when using toothpaste to encourage children to spit out excess paste and minimize the amount swallowed (Figure 15.7).

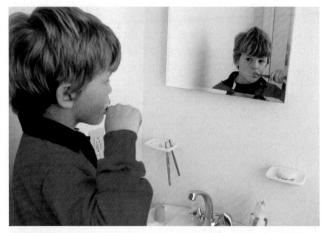

FIGURE 15.7
Children must be supervised to ensure they don't swallow too much fluoride.

The Fluoride Controversy

Adding fluoride to public water supplies has been controversial since it began. The intention of fluoridation is to improve oral health. Those opposed to public fluoridation say that the mineral is toxic and that its toxicity far outweighs its benefits. Therefore, people in many cities in the United States have voted to keep fluoride out of the water supply. Those opposed to fluoridation view it as an infringement of their personal rights and believe that it causes health problems.

Studies about the negative effects of fluoridation are inconclusive. In order for adverse effects of fluoride to result, an extremely large amount of fluoride would need to be consumed. If large amounts of fluoride are consumed, dental **fluorosis** (visible discoloration of tooth enamel with white or brown spots and enamel surface defects called mottling) may occur (Figure 15.8). Proponents of fluoridation consider it to be a safe, simple, and cost-effective public health measure to reduce incidents of dental caries. Debate on this topic will continue as will the research.

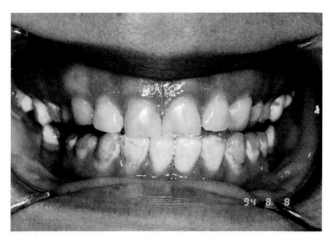

FIGURE 15.8
Dental fluorosis from too much fluoride.

What is the optimum level of fluoride according to the U.S. Public Health Service? How does fluoride strengthen the tooth? What is dental fluorosis? **?**

Nutrition and Dental Caries

A primary function of dental health care providers is to be educators. Dental assistants have an important responsibility to educate patients on the advantages of good nutrition. It is important to encourage a healthy lifestyle for each patient, at each visit. Part of a healthy lifestyle is consuming a diet that includes essential nutrients for proper functioning of the body. All food eaten goes through the mouth. Bacteria present in the mouth thrive on sugars and starches found in many foods. When the teeth are not cleaned after eating, plaque bacteria use the sugar and starch to produce acids that can destroy the enamel surface of the tooth, which in turn softens and erodes the enamel. Enamel breakdown leads to tooth decay. If erosion spreads through the enamel, pain and sensitivity may result. This can cause infection of the nerve or pulp inside the tooth.

Eating for Health

The more often a person eats and the longer foods are in the mouth, the more damage occurs. Due to this fact the amount of snacks one eats should be limited. Each time food containing sugar or starch is eaten, the teeth are attacked by acids for 20 minutes or longer. When snacks are consumed, the snacks should be nutritious and should be chosen from the five major food groups, such as:

- Breads, cereals, and other grain products
- Fruits
- Vegetables
- Meat, poultry, and fish
- Milk, cheese, and yogurt

Foods that are eaten as part of a meal cause less harm. More saliva is released during meals, which helps wash foods from the mouth and reduce the effects of acids. Foods to avoid include:

- Soft drinks
- Diet drinks (because they contain phosphoric acid)
- Excessive fruit drinks
- Coffee or tea with sugar
- Chocolates and candy (especially those that sit in the mouth to dissolve)
- Large amounts of dried fruit or citrus fruits

People who consume too much soda and not enough nutritional beverages are prone to tooth decay and may experience serious ailments later in life, such as diabetes and osteoporosis. Drinking carbonated soft drinks regularly can contribute to erosion of tooth enamel. Soft drinks contain sticky sugars that bacteria in the mouth can use as an energy source.

A diet low in important nutrients makes it more difficult for the body's immune system to fight off infection. Dairy products provide calcium and vitamin D for strengthening teeth and bones. Breads and cereals supply B vitamins for growth and iron for healthy blood, which contributes to healthy gum tissue. Fruits and vegetables containing vitamin C, among other important nutrients, are essential for maintaining healthy gingiva. Lean meat, fish, poultry, and beans provide iron and protein for overall good health, and magnesium and zinc for teeth and bones (Figure 15.9). Drinking lots of water and keeping the mouth moist washes away food and neutralizes plaque.

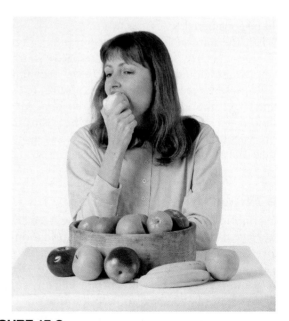

FIGURE 15.9
Choosing the right foods is important for health.
© Dorling Kindersley

Which foods are less harmful to teeth enamel? What are some foods that should be avoided?

Plaque Control Program

Dental plaque is a sticky, colorless, almost invisible mass of bacteria that contain by-products. It is constantly forming on teeth. Saliva, food, and fluids combine to produce these deposits that collect on teeth where the teeth and gingiva meet. This buildup of plaque is the primary factor in periodontal disease. Fighting plaque is a lifelong part of good oral health care.

Plaque begins forming on teeth 4 to 12 hours after brushing. Calcium and phosphate bind to form crystals on the teeth. These calcium phosphate crystals eventually harden within the plaque matrix, forming calculus. **Calculus**, also called tartar, is hardened plaque, a mineralized deposit on teeth formed by saliva, debris, and minerals that can trap stains and cause discoloration. It creates a strong bond that can only be removed from teeth through professional scaling procedures. Calculus formation makes removal of new plaque and bacteria more difficult.

Individuals vary greatly in their susceptibility to plaque and tartar. Calculus formation may be slight, moderate, or severe. The bacteria in plaque use carbohydrates to produce acids that can attack tooth enamel. The decaying action of plaque bacteria depends on its ability to adhere to tooth surfaces and to hold acids on the teeth. After many acid attacks, tooth enamel may break down, forming a cavity. A biofilm is a diverse community of microorganisms found on the tooth surfaces (Figure 15.10). Breaking up these bacterial communities on the teeth by brushing and flossing will prevent their formation.

Patients with dentures need to be made aware that their dentures should be removed and brushed with den-

ture toothpaste or even soap and water because dental plaque and calculus form on dentures as well as real teeth. Ordinary toothpaste is too abrasive and may scratch the denture material. Dentures should be soaked in cold water when not worn. Hot water should never be used since it can cause warping of the dentures. Patients with dentures should also brush their gingiva, tongue, and palate with a soft brush in the morning before inserting their dentures, and again at night when they take them out to sleep. Dentures should not be worn all night because the oral tissues need to be cleaned and allowed to rest without being covered. Fungal infections in the mouth can occur if dentures are never taken out.

Disclosing Dental Plaque

Disclosing solutions can help patients see dental plaque that is sticking to all surfaces of the teeth, including the spaces between the teeth and under the gums (Figure 15.11). Disclosing solutions are available in tablet form, as a liquid, or on swabs (Figure 15.12). Disclosing agents use a red dye to temporarily stain plaque. Some disclosing agents produce a bright red stain that can discolor clothing, and some people with allergies may be sensitive to the dye. The dental assistant should read the manufacturer's directions before using these products. Some disclosing solutions will dye more recent plaque red and older deposits that have calcified will become a purple color. The patient should be informed that the disclosing solution is temporary and that any discoloration of the lips and tongue will dissipate very quickly.

Oral hygiene instruction is part of the ongoing process of patient education. To promote plaque control by the patient, it is important to help the patient understand what plaque is, where it is found, and how to remove it. Once the patient understands this information, then a plaque

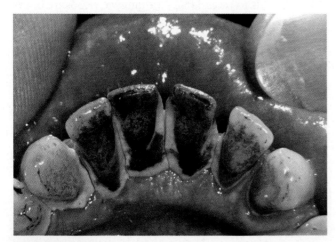

FIGURE 15.10
Bacterial plaque colonies collect on the gingival tissues.

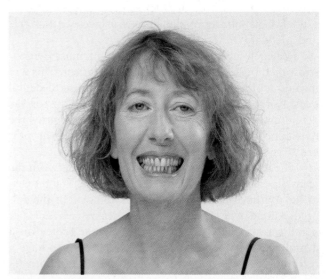

FIGURE 15.11
Dental plaque made visible with disclosing solution.
Jules Selmes © Dorling Kindersley

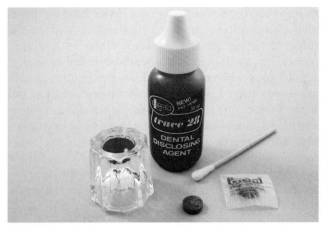

FIGURE 15.12
Examples of liquid and tablet disclosing agents.
Image courtesy Instructional Materials for the Dental Team, Lex., KY

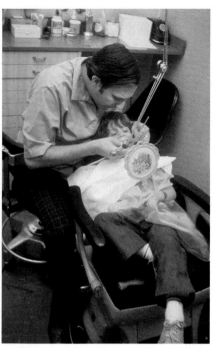

FIGURE 15.13
Patient watching while dental assistant teaches oral hygiene.

control program is developed for the patient with realistic goals set for plaque removal.

After educating the patient about plaque, the patient should receive a toothbrush. The patient should then show the dental assistant how the patient typically brushes his or her teeth. After the patient has demonstrated his or her brushing techniques, the dental assistant should use disclosing tablets or solutions to disclose the plaque in the patient's mouth. The patient should be given a hand mirror in order to see the presence and location of plaque that was missed during the patient's brushing. The patient should be able to see where the dye has stained plaque and debris, which is typically along the gingival margin and between the teeth.

A plaque score can be taken using a tooth chart to note the presence of plaque. The dental assistant indicates in red on the tooth chart where plaque is located on each tooth surface. The plaque score is estimated as the percentage of tooth surfaces present that are plaque free. A goal of 80% or more plaque-free surfaces is attainable and adequate for most people.

When necessary, the dental assistant must demonstrate methods of plaque removal to the patient. This will include toothbrushing techniques and the use of dental floss. As the patient watches with the use of a mirror, the dental assistant should use a toothbrush to remove the red-stained plaque while also showing proper toothbrushing techniques (Figure 15.13).

The effectiveness of dental floss to clean between the teeth may also be demonstrated at this time. The redness of the toothbrush and the successful removal of the colored plaque will help the patient realize why proper home care is important. Recording plaque scores on a dental chart enables the patient and the office to have a record of the patient's status and can be used to motivate the patient to achieve a lower level of plaque. A high plaque score is a predictor for the patient's likely caries risk and need for future restorations.

Toothbrushing

Plaque must be removed from the teeth through the mechanical action of proper toothbrushing. Teeth should be brushed for at least two minutes twice a day, and flossing should be accomplished at least daily. Most people brush for less than a minute and not always in the correct manner. The dental assistant should help the patient develop a systematic approach to brushing his or her teeth and recommend establishing a routine that works for the patient. Toothbrushing must become a habit in order to be successful.

Horizontal scrubbing with pressure applied to gingival tissues must be avoided. This type of brushing can cause trauma to the gingival tissues and the teeth. Horizontal movement with excessive pressure will cause damage that leads to recession of the gingiva, exposure of the root surface, and wearing away of enamel. This is called toothbrush abrasion or mechanical abrasion. The dental assistant should emphasize to patients the importance of maintaining a circular motion rather than back and forth movement and the use of soft bristles. Horizontal motions should be used only to clean the occlusal surfaces of the teeth.

Because every mouth is different, various techniques for toothbrushing have proven to be effective. Generally, most dentists recommend a circular technique for brushing. This includes brushing only a small group of teeth at a time and gradually cleaning the entire mouth. It is best to start by leaning the toothbrush against the gingiva and then moving to the facial or buccal surfaces of the tooth, massaging the gingival tissues, and stimulating blood circulation while cleaning the gingival sulcus. The dental assistant should tell the patient to use vertical movements away from the gingiva.

The primary recommended toothbrushing methods are the Bass, Stillman, Charters, rolling stroke, and Fones' techniques. The Bass technique for brushing teeth requires the bristles of the toothbrush to be pointed at a 45-degree angle where the teeth and gingiva meet. The bristles should gently slide into the gingival **sulcus**, the space between the gingiva and tooth, and be moved slightly with a circular motion and then lifted away from the tooth surface. This method is most often recommended for patients with periodontal disease. The Stillman technique includes a 45-degree angle toward the gingival sulcus using a rolling vibratory motion to pull the bristles downward in a vertical motion (Figure 15.14a). The toothbrush is also placed at a 45-degree angle for the Charters method and the brush swept toward the apex of the tooth in a circular vibrating motion with a rolling stroke then used to pull bristles

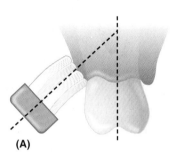

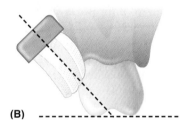

FIGURE 15.14
(a) Stillman method and (b) Charters method.

toward the occlusal surface (Figure 15.14b). The toothbrush is placed with the bristles parallel to the tooth and pointed at the gingiva and rolled gently toward the tooth during the rolling stroke method. The Fones' technique has the teeth closed with the toothbrush placed toward the teeth and moved in large circles at the tooth and gingiva of both arches then using circles at the palate and lingual areas. The Fones' technique is easier to perform by children who lack manual dexterity for more complicated movements.

The teeth should be brushed in a consistent pattern so that no areas of the mouth are missed. Proper toothbrushing is accomplished by:

- Placing the toothbrush tips at a slight angle toward the gingiva on two to three teeth at a time
- Using gentle touch to remove plaque from the teeth at the gum line
- Cleaning all surfaces of the teeth on the upper and lower jaws including:

    1. The inner surface next to the tongue (lingual)
    2. The chewing surfaces (occlusal)
    3. The surfaces next to the cheeks and lips (buccal and facial)
    4. The anterior lingual surfaces

- The surface of the tongue should be scrubbed to prevent bad breath (**halitosis**).

Recommended toothbrushing techniques are presented in Table 15-1.

Patients with Special Needs

People with special needs should also learn toothbrushing techniques. When teaching patients with special needs, it is important to be patient and provide enough time to explain the techniques. With repetitive practice these individuals should be able to master the techniques shown to them by the dental assistant.

TABLE 15-1 Toothbrushing Methods

Method	Bristle Position	Description
Bass technique	The toothbrush bristles are placed at a 45-degree angle to the tooth toward the gingival sulcus.	The bristles are moved in a circular motion allowing the bristles to get into the sulcus for at least 10 strokes.
Stillman technique	The toothbrush is placed at a 45-degree angle at the gingiva where it meets the tooth surface.	A rolling vibratory motion is used to pull the bristles downward and back and forth in a vertical motion.
Charters technique	The toothbrush is placed at a 45-degree angle to the tooth where it meets the gingiva.	The brush is swept toward the apex of the tooth in a circular vibrating motion, and a rolling stroke is then used to pull bristles toward the occlusal surface.
Rolling stroke	The toothbrush is placed with the bristles parallel to the tooth and pointed at the gingiva.	The toothbrush should be swept from the gingiva and rolled gently toward the tooth.
Fones' technique	With the teeth closed, the toothbrush is placed toward the teeth.	The toothbrush is moved in large circles at the tooth and gingiva of both arches, then large circles are used at the palate and lingual areas.

The patient's guardian should also learn how to help the special needs patient with oral home care. The patient, the patient's guardian, and the dental assistant should stand in front of a mirror. The dental assistant should stand behind the patient using one hand to support the chin or head, if necessary, and the other hand to help the patient brush. If the patient can hold the toothbrush, then he should brush alone. The dental assistant will need to supervise, observe, and correct brushing technique discrepancies. Use only a pea-sized drop of toothpaste or no toothpaste. If the patient cannot hold the toothbrush or refuses to do so, the dental assistant can perform the brushing for the patient. The dental assistant should pay special attention to problem areas such as along the gingival margin and next to the tongue.

After brushing is completed the patient should be shown how to rinse expectorate into the sink. If the patient has difficulty rinsing, suggest that the patient wear an apron to avoid getting his clothes wet. Teach the patient to first open his mouth over a sink, slowly pour water into the mouth, and let the water flow out naturally so the foam from the toothpaste is rinsed out. Working with patients with special needs and their guardians takes time and persistence but many such patients can learn simple tooth cleaning techniques.

Toothbrushes

Several toothbrush styles are available. The ADA recommends a toothbrush with soft round-ended, multitufted nylon bristles. A toothbrush should be relatively small so it fits easily into the mouth and large enough to avoid the need for prolonged brushing (Figure 15.15). The brush should be sturdy enough to clean the teeth and stimulate the gingival tissues but not so hard that the gingiva is damaged. The ADA recommends that a toothbrush be replaced every three to four months or sooner if the bristles become frayed.

The mechanical action of disturbing the bacterial colonies in plaque can be accomplished by any toothbrush, but many are specifically designed for cleaning the gingival sulcus, including powered toothbrushes. Powered toothbrush styles vary with their effectiveness. Manufacturer's directions must always be followed when using these products. Numerous studies have compared the effectiveness of manual and powered toothbrushes.

Both are equally as effective if used for at least two minutes twice a day. Strong evidence suggests that improvement in dental disease prevention is seen in patients after they begin using an electric toothbrush. Powered toothbrushes may increase motivation for children who think brushing is boring and for those with poor manual dexterity. Powered toothbrushes are available in a variety of styles (Figures 15.16, 15.17, and 15.18) and with an assortment of electrical components and actions designed to remove plaque:

- Brush head moving laterally from side to side
- Adjacent tufts rotating in opposite directions from each other
- Brush head rotating in one direction then in the other direction
- Brush head rotating in one direction
- Bristles vibrating at ultrasonic frequencies
- Brush imparting an ionic electrical charge to the tooth surface

One of the main reasons people don't brush effectively is because they don't brush long enough. To help alleviate that problem, manufacturers have incorporated timers into their products. Timers available on most powered toothbrushes also inform patients of the proper length of time that they should spend on tooth surfaces. Some electric toothbrushes signal at intervals indicating the length of time each quadrant should be cleaned.

Whichever toothbrush is preferred by the patient, instructions on its use should be explained by the dental assistant to ensure it is being used properly and effectively for plaque removal techniques. The dental assistant should become familiar with the many different powered toothbrushes available and recommended by the dentist.

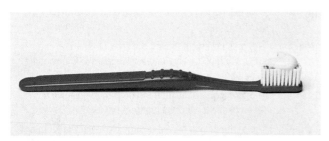

FIGURE 15.15
Manual toothbrush.
© Dorling Kindersley

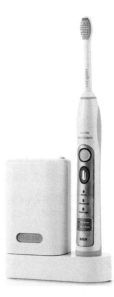

FIGURE 15.16
Sonicare toothbrush.
Courtesy Philips Sonicare

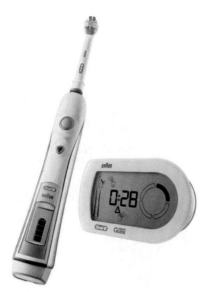

FIGURE 15.17
Oral-B Triumph with Smartguide powerbrush.
Image used with permission of Procter and Gamble, makers of Oral-B brushes

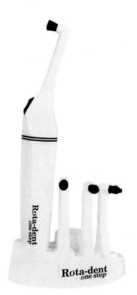

FIGURE 15.18
Rotadent brush system.
Courtesy of Pro-Dental, a Zila Company

Toothpaste

Another term for toothpaste is dentifrice. The ADA recommends use of a fluoride-containing dentifrice to help the tooth retain calcium and slow the production of acids that attach to the teeth. Most toothpastes not only contain fluoride, but some toothpaste manufacturers have formulations that aid in plaque control and prevent the buildup of calculus. Certain types of chemicals called pyrophosphates help to decrease calculus buildup by stopping the growth of crystals on the tooth surface and preventing new crystals from forming. Other toothpastes contain sodium hexametaphosphate, which is a pyrophosphate formulated to not only inhibit calculus, but also to loosen

extrinsic stains. Triclosan is an antibacterial product that is an ingredient in certain toothpastes that inhibits plaque growth and therefore gingivitis. While plaque can be brushed away, toothpaste manufacturers must prove to the ADA that their paste prevents gingivitis in order to make that claim. Tartar control toothpastes will not remove existing calculus but do help prevent further buildup. The only way to remove hardened plaque or calculus is by a professional cleaning in the dental office.

Toothpaste also contains abrasives designed to clean and polish teeth. Abrasives found in toothpaste include silica, alumina, calcium, or baking soda. If a toothpaste is too abrasive, it may damage teeth by scratching them and creating a place for bacteria to accumulate. Whitening agents may also be added to toothpaste. Whitening agents such as hydrogen peroxide may help the brightness of teeth, but should be used with caution so as not to damage the gingiva or cause sensitivity to cold over a long period of use. Whichever toothpaste is used, in order to be used effectively, it must remove destructive plaque every 24 hours, before it begins to develop and harden into calculus.

Flossing

Despite toothbrushing, decay-causing bacteria remain between teeth, in the interproximal spaces, where toothbrush bristles cannot reach. Therefore, flossing is required to remove plaque and food particles from between the teeth and under the gingival margin. When flossing, patients should be instructed to follow these steps:

- Pull off about 18 inches of dental floss and wind most of it around the middle finger on one hand and wind the remaining amount around the same finger of the other hand.
- Hold floss tightly with about 1 inch between the thumbs and forefinger.
- Gently slide the floss between the teeth, being careful not to snap it into the gingiva.

Cultural Considerations

Explaining oral hygiene procedures to non-English-speaking patients can be challenging. Many pamphlets and other visual aids are available in other languages that will help you explain what you want to say. Teaching proper toothbrushing and flossing techniques does not necessarily require words. You can show your patients how to brush and floss by having them watch you with the use of a mirror perform these tasks on their mouth. Disclosing solution is a great visual tool to explain how tooth surfaces can be missed when cleaning them.

- Curve the floss into a "C" shape against the tooth when it reaches the gingival tissues (Figure 15.19).
- Shape the floss gently against the tooth and move it up and down until a squeaking sound is heard.
- Wrap the floss onto one finger as you go, using a new clean piece of floss between each space.
- Clean behind back teeth with the floss.
- Use more floss when necessary to provide at least one inch of working space for patient control (Figure 15.20).
- Floss all teeth at least once a day.

If a person hasn't used dental floss before, explain that her gingiva may bleed or become sore for a few days. The soreness should subside if flossing is gently and regularly performed.

Dental floss is available as waxed or unwaxed and in plain, mint, cinnamon, or grape flavors. Patients with tight contacts between their teeth will benefit from the use of waxed floss. Some waxed floss brands also have fluoride incorporated into the wax. The importance of using floss to remove plaque deposits daily must be emphasized to patients. Children as well as adults may be motivated to floss more frequently by using the flavored floss that is available.

Oral Hygiene Aids

Many types of oral hygiene aids are available for patients to use depending on each individual's needs (Figure 15.21). It is the responsibility of the dental assistant to teach patients how to properly use interdental aids.

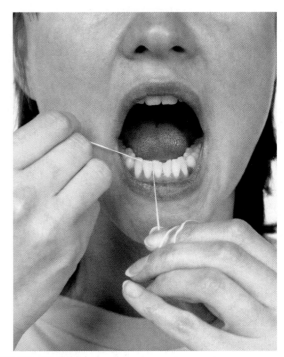

FIGURE 15.20
Keep the floss taut and guide it between the teeth.
Andy Crawford © Dorling Kindersley

Toothpicks, interproximal brushes, interdental stimulators, oral irrigators, and mouthwashes are all aids to oral hygiene.

Interproximal brushes are available in different sizes and shapes. They can be conical or cylindrical. The dental assistant should instruct the patient to place the bristles in the interproximal space to clean the area. They are indicated for patients with large spaces between their teeth and for patients with fixed prostheses, implants, or orthodontic appliances.

Interdental cleaning aids help remove food and debris that is caught between teeth. Toothpicks and wooden dental stimulators are effective when moistened and used carefully to massage the gingiva. Caution

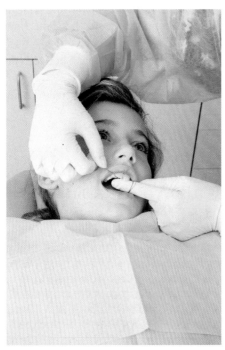

FIGURE 15.19
Floss wrapped around a tooth in a "C" shape.

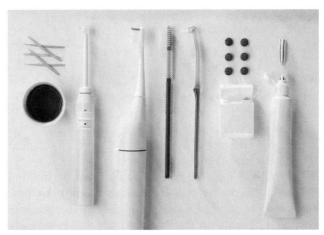

FIGURE 15.21
Interdental cleaning aids.

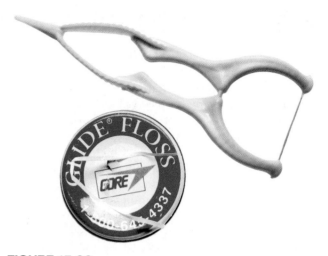

FIGURE 15.22
A bridge threader used to pull floss around orthodontic appliances.

should be taken to avoid causing any damage to the gingival tissues. Interdental stimulators are made of rubber or flexible plastic in a cone shape. They are placed in the interproximal space and used to massage and reduce inflammation and help blood circulation to the gingival tissues.

Using irrigating solutions or rinsing once or twice a day with an antiseptic mouth rinse has been demonstrated to reduce plaque and gingivitis. Antiseptic mouthwashes such as chlorhexidine gluconate must be prescribed by a dentist to control oral pathogens. These have proven to be very effective against the microorganisms that cause gingivitis. Antiseptic mouthwashes are unacceptable for use over a long period of time, however, because they will stain the teeth and may impair taste for the patient.

If a patient has a removable prosthetic appliance, it must be removed after meals and thoroughly brushed. If a patient has a fixed prosthesis, the patient will need to be taught how to use a **bridge threader** to thread dental floss through to clean underneath a bridge (Figure 15.22). The teeth on each side of a fixed bridge must be cleaned.

Teaching patients to correctly use oral hygiene aids is a primary responsibility of the dental assistant. The dental assistant must understand how each aid is utilized in order to educate patients on how to use them. The patient must understand how to maintain the investment she has in the restorations placed in her mouth and in what manner her oral health can best be preserved.

Xylitol

Xylitol, an extract from the bark of birch trees, is a naturally occurring substance that tastes like sugar and has no aftertaste. Research has shown that xylitol actually reduces the incidence of tooth decay. This substance works on the bacteria that cause decay, specifically on mutans streptococci. An acidic environment is an ideal atmosphere for the bacteria that cause decay to thrive. The acid dissolves the calcium and phosphorous matrix that makes up tooth enamel and breaks their molecular bonds. If fluoride is present, the calcium and phosphorus bind together with a molecule of fluoride and form a stronger unit. Xylitol changes the acidic environment of the mouth and therefore suppresses the activity of mutans streptococci, resulting in less harm to the dentition. The bacterium also does not receive the sugar needed to survive.

Consuming xylitol in large amounts may create unwanted side effects, such as an upset stomach or diarrhea, but the amount of xylitol found in many sugarless chewing gums and sugarless breath mints is extremely small. Scandinavian studies show that chewing one or two sticks of gum containing xylitol for five minutes three times a day after meals can reduce tooth decay up to 62%.

What is dental plaque? How soon after brushing does plaque begin forming on the teeth? What do the bacteria plaque colonies live on?

SUMMARY

Proper diet and meticulous plaque control help preserve teeth for a lifetime and will affect one's general overall health as well as one's dental health. Simple carbohydrates and sugar in any form contribute to the colonization of plaque. The most important plaque control method is toothbrushing and it should be established as a daily routine from early childhood. Children with healthy mouths chew more easily and gain more nutrients from foods. They learn to speak more quickly and clearly.

Community water fluoridation is cost effective and benefits everyone. It is the most efficient way to prevent one of the most common childhood diseases—tooth decay. Dental diseases are caused by microorganisms found in plaque. These microorganisms cause disease that can destroy healthy tissue and ultimately result in tooth loss.

Plaque control is the removal and prevention of all soft deposits on the teeth and gingival tissues. Motivating patients toward the awareness that they are ultimately responsible for improving and maintaining the health of their oral tissues is the primary duty of the dental assistant. Educating patients on the negative effects of poor nutrition, tobacco use, and neglect is part of overall general and oral health education. The dental assistant uses diagrams, charts, models, slides, videos, pamphlets, and other means to educate dental patients.

KEY TERMS

- **Bridge threader:** Used to thread dental floss to clean underneath a bridge or other dental appliance. p. 237
- **Calculus:** Hardened plaque, a mineralized deposit on teeth formed by saliva, debris, and minerals; also called tartar. p. 231
- **Fluoridation:** The process of adding fluoride to the public water supply. p. 227
- **Fluorosis:** White or brown discolorations of tooth enamel with surface defects called mottling. p. 229

- **Gingivitis:** Reversible inflammation of the gingiva. p. 224
- **Halitosis:** Bad breath. p. 233
- **Sulcus:** Space between the gingiva and tooth. p. 233
- **Systemic fluoride:** Fluoride that is delivered to the tooth via the body's bloodstream. p. 228
- **Topical fluoride:** Fluoride treatment that is applied to the surface of tooth enamel. p. 228

CHECK YOUR UNDERSTANDING

1. What is caused by the microorganisms found in dental plaque?
   a. caries
   b. periodontal disease
   c. gingivitis
   d. all of the above

2. To promote oral hygiene, the dental assistant must help the patient understand which of the following?
   a. what plaque is
   b. where plaque is found
   c. how to remove plaque
   d. all of the above

3. What might occur to a child with untreated decay?
   a. pain
   b. weight loss
   c. poor appearance
   d. low self-esteem
   e. all of the above

4. Between what ages should children have all of their primary dentition?
   a. by 2 years
   b. 2 to 3 years

   c. 8 to 9 years
   d. 7 to 12 years

5. At what age should a child first see a dentist?
   a. 1 year old
   b. 2 years old
   c. 3 years old
   d. 4 years old

6. What is the optimum level of fluoride according to the U.S. Public Health Service?
   a. 1 part per million
   b. 2 parts per million
   c. 3 parts per million
   d. none of the above

7. In which of the following ways can fluoride be absorbed into the body?
   a. systemic
   b. topical
   c. a and b
   d. none of the above

CHECK YOUR UNDERSTANDING (continued)

8. How long are the teeth attacked by acids each time we eat food that contains sugar or starch?
   a. 5 minutes
   b. 10 minutes
   c. 15 minutes
   d. 20 minutes

9. What do the bacteria in plaque use to produce acids that can erode tooth enamel?
   a. fluoride
   b. carbohydrates
   c. calculus
   d. disclosing agents

10. How should dental plaque buildup be removed from the teeth?
   a. brushing
   b. flossing
   c. interproximal aids
   d. all of the above

INTERNET ACTIVITIES

- Watch several animations regarding tooth eruption and proper brushing and flossing at www.ada.org/ada/index.asp. Search "tooth eruption" and then look for the animation link.
- Go to www.fluoridealert.org/carlson-interview.html to listen to audio clips against fluoridation by a renowned research scientist and Nobel Prize winner.
- Watch a video on proper toothbrushing techniques at www.expertvillage.com/videos/how-brush-techniques.html

WEB REFERENCES

- American Academy of Periodontology   www.perio.org/consumer
- American Dental Association: Oral Health Topics   www.ada.org/public/topics/cleaning.asp
- ANGLEFIRE   http://anglefire.com/az/sthurston/xylitol_natural_sweetener.html
- Crest Oral B Patient Education   http://dentalcare.com/soap/patient/english/menu.htm
- The Dental, Oral, and Craniofacial Data Resource Center: Periodontal Diseases   http://drc.hhs.gov/report/pdfs/section3-diseases.pdf
- Flesh and Bones: Prevention of Periodontal Disease   www.fleshandbones.com/readingroom/pdf/864.pdf
- Head Start Information and Publication Center   www.headstartinfo.org
- Medline Plus   www.nlm.nih.gov/medlineplus/gumdisease.html
- Odontocat: Prevention   http://odontocat.com/angles/prevplacaang.htm
- WebMD   www.webmd.com/hw/dental/hw12228.asp
- Xylitol.org   www.xylitol.org

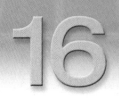

16

Oral Nutrition

Chapter Outline

- Functions of Six Major Nutrients
  —Water
  —Carbohydrates
  —Fats
  —Proteins
  —Vitamins
  —Minerals
- Diet Modification
  —Diet Modifications for Infants and Toddlers
- Diet Analysis
- Reading Food Labels
- Eating Disorders
- Healthy Eating Habits

Learning Objectives

After reading this chapter, the student should be able to:

- List the six key nutrients.
- Identify the function of each of the six key nutrients.
- Describe how to modify diets.
- Explain how to read basic labels found on food packaging.
- Identify signs and symptoms of eating disorders.

Preparing for Certification Exams

- Provide patient preventive education and oral hygiene instruction.

Key Terms

Anorexia

Bulimia

Carbohydrates

Fats

Minerals

Nutrients

Obesity

Proteins

Vitamins

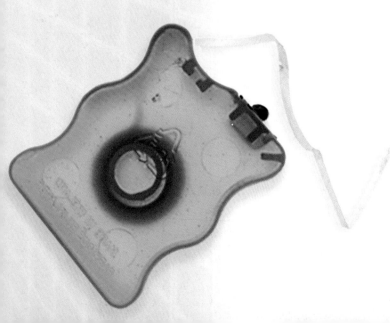

The human body needs six essential key **nutrients** on a daily basis. The U.S. Department of Agriculture (USDA) publishes a chart that provides information on the amount of nutrients that each individual should consume on a daily basis. As a health care professional, dental assistants will have patients who do not practice good nutritional habits. Some patients may even show signs and symptoms of eating disorders.

To provide nutritional advice to the dental patient, the dental assistant needs to be familiar with the effects of nutrition on oral health. As a dental assistant, knowledge regarding healthy eating habits can positively affect not only one's own health but can be passed on to patients in order to assist them in gaining healthier dietary habits. Good eating habits provide the body with more energy and the ability to prevent sickness and disease.

Functions of Six Major Nutrients

The six essential nutrients are water, carbohydrates, fats, proteins, vitamins, and minerals. The USDA recently created a new food pyramid with a list of recommended daily allowances (RDAs) for each food group (Figure 16.1). These food groups contain the essential nutrients required by the human body to function efficiently. From 1946 to 1992 the USDA's food pyramid contained four basic food groups. The new pyramid suggests that a healthy diet contains a variety of foods and that food portion sizes and

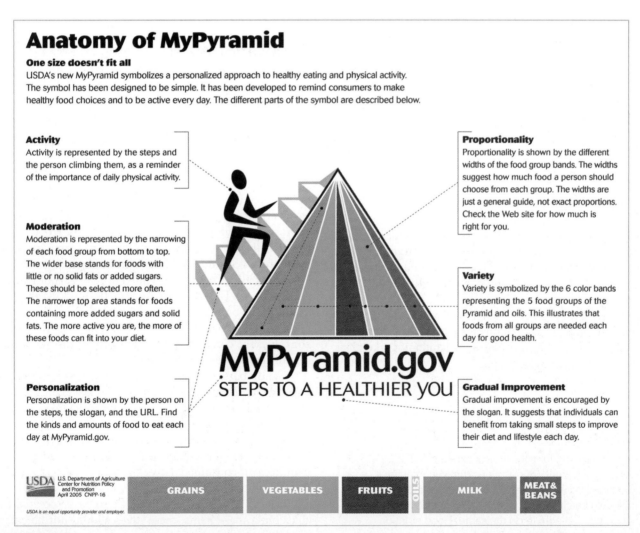

FIGURE 16.1
U.S. Department of Agriculture 2005 revised food pyramid.

Dental Assistant PROFESSIONAL TIP

It is important for the dental team to be able to identify potential diet deficiencies when seeing patients. Patients do not always notice the physical changes in their appearance unless they are brought to their attention. The oral cavity is one of the first places an abnormality caused by a nutritional deficiency will appear.

Cultural Considerations

Your patients' culture can significantly impact the importance they place on nutrition. Take the time to learn about the views of other cultures. This knowledge will help when trying to communicate dietary issues to your patients.

numbers of servings should be based on one's age, size, and activity level. These government RDAs are suggested to the public to track and maintain one's personal daily intake in order to stay healthy.

The RDAs have been created to help people further understand appropriate body weights and consumption of proteins, vitamins, and minerals. The Food and Nutrition Board of the National Academy of Sciences created the RDAs. Information about RDAs can be ordered through the National Academy Press, Washington, DC, at http://www.nap.edu/.

What are some ways for the body to obtain water?

Water

Water is the most essential nutrient our bodies need in order to survive. The body can typically survive 30 days or more on just water alone. The human body consists on average of 90% water. Water controls body temperature. When overheating is an issue, the body produces perspiration or sweat for a cooling effect. Perspiration not only cools the body, it also eliminates toxins from the body. Transportation of cells or nutrients would not take place without adequate water supply.

Preparing for Externship

When preparing for your clinical experience, be prepared to ask plenty of questions that you may have about nutrition. Dental assistants who have developed their own healthy eating habits are more likely to encourage patients to do the same. Good nutrition leads to a healthy oral cavity.

The recommended daily amount of water intake for an adult is eight 8-ounce glasses a day. Other sources can also provide this essential nutrient. For instance, fruits and vegetables contain the highest amounts of water in the food category. Great food sources for water include iceberg lettuce, watermelon, pineapple, tomatoes, and oranges.

Expelling or eliminating water from the body occurs through urination, exhalation, perspiration, and fecal elimination. Severe headaches, muscle cramps, dizziness, nausea, and fatigue might be symptoms of dehydration or lack of water intake.

Edema, also referred to as swelling, is the body responding to excessive amounts of water. This happens for a number of reasons including medications, heart conditions, a lack of protein, and pregnancy. When an individual develops edema, he should consult his physician to determine the best course of action.

What does it mean to be lactose intolerant? If an individual is lactose intolerant, what symptoms might she experience?

Carbohydrates

Carbohydrates are a source of energy for the body. Due to recent diets supporting the idea of low or no carbohydrates, carbohydrates have received a bad reputation. These nutrients, though, are beneficial to the body as long as the daily amounts are regulated. "Carbs," as they are typically referred to, are the body's primary source of energy.

Carbohydrates are divided into two categories: refined carbohydrates and complex carbohydrates. Carbohydrates are typically derived from plants. Refined carbs come from sources such as fruit (fructose), milk (lactose), berries (glucose), and beer (maltose). Glucose is the primary energy source for the brain. Complex carbs come from vegetables and from grains such as oats, barley, and wheat. The recommended dose of carbohydrates revised by the USDA in the April 2005 food pyramid, is as follows: 6 ounces of grains, 16 ounces (2 cups) of fruit, and 24 ounces (3 cups) of vegetables a day. An individual consumes the correct amount of healthy carbs by following this recommended daily dose.

Candy bars, energy drinks, sodas, and granola bars are often used by people as sources of quick energy. These are referred to as cariogenic foods, meaning they encourage the creation of decay. They also have little or no nutritional value. Large doses of these cariogenic foods are not beneficial to the dentition. They can lead to rampant decay if consumed daily. The acids created from the carbohydrates break down or decalcify the enamel. In addition to the dental problems that can be created by consuming these items, these items should not be eaten on a daily basis because studies show that they can contribute to fat storage.

Health Issues Resulting from Misuse of Carbohydrates

Misuse of carbohydrates can lead to a number of health issues such as lactose intolerance, hyperglycemia, hypoglycemia, alcoholism, and dental caries. For instance, low blood sugar can cause cravings for alcohol especially after a rush of simple carbohydrates.

Many disorders can be controlled by diet or with the help of a physician who can prescribe medications to control the symptoms. In some cases, if symptoms are not controlled, more serious health problems can occur.

Lactose Intolerance   Lactose intolerance has become a common condition. Some people believe lactose intolerance is a result of animal hormones in foods being ingested by humans, causing the inability to break down the sugar lactase. Lactose intolerance is a lack of enzymes to break down milk sugars. This condition can affect individuals later in adulthood. Studies show that more babies are being born with lactose intolerance.

There are various levels of this deficiency. Some individuals can eat yogurt, cow cheeses, or cow milk–based creams, whereas others cannot eat any cow milk–based products. Some signs and symptoms of the deficiency include painful bloating with flatus, diarrhea, nausea, and in some cases a skin rash.

Hyperglycemia and Hypoglycemia   Hyperglycemia and hypoglycemia are opposites. Hyperglycemia occurs when an excessive amount of glucose is deposited into the blood. Usually a blood glucose level over 120 mg/dL is considered to indicate the presence of hyperglycemia. Hypoglycemia occurs when there is an insufficient amount of glucose in the blood. A blood glucose level below 70 mg/dL is considered hypoglycemia. Both conditions are associated with diabetes.

Diabetes mellitus is an insufficient amount of insulin secretion. There are two types of diabetes. An individual with type 1 diabetes is insulin dependent. An individual with type 2 diabetes is noninsulin dependent and the diabetes is controlled by diet and/or medications other than insulin. More than 20 million new cases of diabetes are reported each year.

Diabetes cannot properly process starchy foods or sugars due to the lack of insulin. Medical researchers continue to make new discoveries on the causes and treatments available for diabetes. Causes of diabetes include weight, hormonal changes, and family history. Hormonal changes during pregnancy can also cause diabetes. This type of diabetes is called gestational diabetes.

There are many prediabetic signs and symptoms of diabetes including red swollen gingiva, a strong craving for water, excessive urination, numbness in hands or feet, blurred vision, strong cravings for sweets, fatigue, yeast or skin infections, and cuts or bruises that will not heal. If one suspects the possibility of diabetes, a glucose test, called a fasting plasma glucose (FPG) test, can be performed. All forms of diabetes must be treated. Untreated cases have been linked to loss of limbs and death.

Alcoholism   Alcoholism can affect carbohydrate intake. When processed by the body, alcohol is converted into a sugar or carbohydrate that can affect the blood sugar/insulin levels in the body. This, in turn, causes the alcoholic to crave more alcohol due to the low blood sugar after the body has used the alcohol for quick energy. Alcoholism depresses the nervous system due to overusage of alcohol-based products.

The abuse of alcohol can make the mucosa appear very red, shiny, and spongy. During a routine probing, an alcoholic's gingiva is very likely to bleed. Years of alcohol abuse can lead to liver disease (cirrhosis), stomach and intestinal cancers, heart disease, and circulatory disease. Signs of alcoholism include withdrawal from friends and family, spending large sums of money at a bar, forgetfulness, daily drinking, lack of basic hygiene, slurred speech, missed appointments, and the odor of alcohol seeping from the pores of the skin.

Although there is no medical cure for alcoholism, one option for combatting alcoholism is to become a member of the Alcoholics Anonymous organization. The use of an antiabuse medication may also help some individuals control their alcohol cravings.

Caries   Caries, also referred to as tooth decay or cavities, are caused by refined carbohydrates left in the mouth. The refined carbohydrates feed the lactobacilli and mutans streptococci bacteria that cause tooth decay. Cariogenic foods can be removed by brushing and flossing twice a day with the use of fluoride dentifrice (toothpaste). The use of a fluoride rinse is another way to fight decay.

How can high cholesterol be controlled?

Fats

Fats, also known as lipids, work like carbohydrates by helping to produce energy. Functions of fats include formation and repair of brain and nerve tissues. Fatty tissue is found in every membrane of every cell in the body. Without it, the human body would not function properly. Fat protects the joints and organs from injury and provides insulation to the body from extreme temperature changes. Fats take time to digest, leaving one with a feeling of bloating or fullness. Though the word *fat* has often been considered bad, fats are a necessity.

Fats are divided into two categories: unsaturated and saturated. *Fatty acids* is another term that can be used to describe saturated and unsaturated fats. Unsaturated fats are useful to the body and are divided into two types: polyunsaturated and monounsaturated. Polyunsaturated fats come from plant sources such as soybeans, corn, and safflowers. Monounsaturated fats are derived from seeds and nuts such as peanuts, olives, and walnuts. Saturated fats come from animal foods such as bacon, butter, chicken, whole milk, and eggs.

Saturated fats become lucid or clear when exposed to heat. It is during the cooling process of saturated fats or when set at room temperature, that they become opaque and solid. Animal fats can harden and block the blood vessels in arteries, causing high cholesterol, heart attacks, strokes, and high blood pressure. Excessive fat intake has been linked to breast cancer, obesity, heart disease, and colon cancer.

Cholesterol

Cholesterol is typically found in animal products. Cholesterol helps with the metabolism of vitamin D in the body and the production of certain hormones. Too much cholesterol in the body will store itself in the gallbladder and in the heart, contributing to gallstones and arteriosclerosis. Serum cholesterol is the level of cholesterol found in the blood. A normal level for an average adult is 200. Anything higher is considered high cholesterol.

Several medications have recently been released on the market to control high cholesterol. Some natural methods that have been suggested for lowering cholesterol include drinking more grapefruit juice, taking garlic, and consuming more grains and fruits. It has been proven that those who increase fruits and grains in their diets flush out more cholesterol than those who do not eat enough of them.

Proteins

Proteins are used for energy and for muscle and tissue construction and repair. Proteins also help to control water balance in the body. Great sources of protein include soy, meats, and cheeses. Animal protein is recommended because the structure in animals is much like that of human beings. Protein can also be found in foods such as almonds, peanuts, beans, and milk.

The two types of proteins are incomplete and complete proteins. Complete proteins are valuable to the body. They supply all of the necessary amino acids for energy and growth. There are two different types of amino acids: essential amino acids and nonessential amino acids. Essential amino acids come from sources of food such as nuts, whole grains, vegetables, dairy products, and meats. Nonessential amino acids are derivatives of essential amino acids and are manufactured by the body. Incomplete proteins have minimal value, because they lack certain amino acids. Incomplete and complete proteins can be used in combination with each other to make the proper complete protein dosage.

Through laboratory tests, physicians can observe the levels of protein excreted in the urine or feces. This can help the physician observe how the body is breaking down protein. Nitrogen is released in the human body and presents in urine and fecal matter. The amount of nitrogen found in a person's food intake should be equal or close to equal in the individual's urine and fecal output. Equal amounts simply mean old tissues are being replaced daily. When the right amount of nitrogen is not found in the urine, an imbalance is present and tissues are not being repaired adequately. This might also be a sign of an illness or of a major bodily repair, as can happen with an injury or surgery.

Deficiencies caused by lack of protein do not occur very often in the United States. However, protein deficiencies are common in economically challenged countries where proper nutrition is not always available. Kwashiorkor is a condition caused by a protein deficiency found throughout African villages. Kwashiorkor can cause stunted growth, lack of pigmentation in the skin or hair, muscle atrophy, and swelling in the liver. Severe edema (water retention) in the face, hands, and legs is usually a sign of a protein deficiency.

Proteins help to manufacture other substances found in the body, such as hormones (which regulate growth), enzymes (which help to break down other nutrients and foods), and antibodies (which help us to fight toxins). Proteins also aid in respiratory function. Newborn babies at birth are susceptible to viruses and disease because their protein counts are low. Breastfeeding of infants is recommended since this helps to build antibodies that help fight infections. During the lactation process, the mother loses fat at a higher level than normal, so ingestion of extra protein is recommended to replace what is lost. It would not be unusual to have a new mother eat six small meals a day (one meal every four hours) to keep her protein levels up.

What is the difference between vitamin A_1 and Vitamin A_2? What are some sources for obtaining vitamin A?

Vitamins

Vitamins and their positive benefit to the body have been around for hundreds of years or more. Some vitamins were accidentally discovered; others were drawn from various sources and then studied on diseased patients to see what type of response would occur. A Polish scientist, C. Funk, coined the term we use today, *vitamin.*

Vitamins come from natural (organic) sources, and assist the body with the growth and repair of tissues. Vitamins also regulate certain functions. The two types of vitamins are fat-soluble and water-soluble vitamins. Excess amounts of fat-soluble vitamins can be stored in tissues; excess water-soluble vitamins are excreted.

Four special fat-soluble vitamins are taken into the body in a manner similar to that in which fat enters the body. These four vitamins—vitamins A, D, E, and K (ADEK for short)—enter the body through the small intestine. An illness may cause the body difficulty absorb-

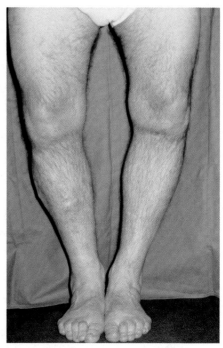

FIGURE 16.2
Middle-aged man with rickets.

ing vitamins, thus making it important for the patient to take vitamin supplements.

Vitamin A is the number one vitamin for healthy skin, hair, and eyes. Great sources of vitamin A are plant products that are green or yellow in color. These pigmented shades are referred to as carotenoids. Vitamin A has also been found in animal products. Another term used to describe vitamin A is retinal.

There are two different forms of this vitamin: vitamin A_1 and vitamin A_2. Vitamin A_1 is found in organic earthy sources, and vitamin A_2 comes from the skin of freshwater fish only. Either source will provide the same use in the body. Food sources containing vitamin A_1 and/or vitamin A_2 include spinach, squash, fish, carrots, liver, and egg yolk. Deficiencies for vitamin A are vision problems (night blindness) and severely dry skin. If vitamin A is taken in excess, hair loss, dizziness, and headaches or liver problems could occur.

Vitamin D is the most essential vitamin for healthy teeth and bone formation. Cow milk and soy milk products contain high amounts of this vitamin and should be taken daily. The USDA recommends three servings of dairy a day. Sources for vitamin D include whole milk, eggs, natural sunlight, and fish liver oils. Signs and symptoms of excessive amounts of vitamin D include weight loss and calcium deposits in the gallbladder and kidneys. The deficiency linked to vitamin D is rickets (Figure 16.2). Rickets is a severe bone deformity caused by lack of vitamin D during bone formation. If it is caught early, the severity of this deformity can be kept from progressing. Rickets is rarely found in the United States, but is found in areas such as India, Asia, and Africa.

The loss of vitamin D can also lead to other conditions such as osteoporosis or osteomalacia. Osteomalacia is the decalcification of bone, causing the bone to become soft. It causes bowing in the legs and/or arms and a decrease in height. This condition has been linked to genetics, poor diet, and lack of sun exposure. Osteoporosis occurs when the bones lose their inner strength or density. Causes of osteoporosis include poor diet, thyroid diseases, chemotherapy treatments, anorexia, and genet-

ics. Signs of osteoporosis include spinal pain, bone fractures (from falls), and a decrease in height.

Vitamin E assists fatty acids from oxidizing and is great for skin cell regeneration. Vitamin E can be purchased in liquid form. It can be placed on the skin for cuts, burns, discoloration, and dryness. Some sources for vitamin E include milk, eggs, wheat germ, vitamin E gel caps, and green leafy vegetables. Vitamin E deficiency occurs in a small percentage of individuals and occurs mostly in infants. It can appear as neurologic disorders and anemia.

Vitamin K is the fourth fat-soluble vitamin. Vitamin K is essential for natural blood clotting and kidney function. Liver is a great source of vitamin K because it contains large amounts of this vitamin. Other sources include soy products, cauliflower, and oats. Individuals with a deficiency in vitamin K can be more prone to hemorrhaging.

Water-soluble vitamins are the second type of vitamins. Water-soluble vitamins are absorbed by the blood. The blood cleanses itself constantly, which in turn diminishes the amount of water-soluble vitamins absorbed by the body. Water-soluble vitamins are not easily absorbed, and many of these vitamins are lost when high heat is applied to food due to the cooking process. In conjunction with minerals they help with growth, repair, and normal body functions. Table 16-1 provides descriptions of vitamins that are considered water soluble.

Minerals

Minerals are derived from elements found in the earth's crust. Minerals come in two different forms: macrominerals and microminerals. Macrominerals are minerals

TABLE 16-1 Water-Soluble Vitamins

Vitamin	Source	Purpose	Results of Deficiencies
Thiamin (B$_1$)	Meat, grains, and nuts	Assists in maintaining great muscle tone and helps to regulate a healthy appetite and metabolism.	Heart conditions, digestive issues, and beriberi (fatigue, paralysis, diarrhea, and nerve disturbances); excessive amounts can be very toxic.
Riboflavin (B$_2$)	Meat, green vegetables, and grains	Metabolizes other nutrients and helps to give energy.	Delayed growth, skin inflammation, lesions that appear around the mouth (*cheilosis*) or nose, stinging sensations that can be felt in the eyes or genital area.
Pyridoxine (B$_6$)	Grains, organ meats, nuts, oats, and soy	Helps to form red blood cells, maintain sodium and potassium levels.	Anemia; excessive amounts can cause loss of feeling in the extremities.
Cobalamin (B$_{12}$)	Eggs, seafood, organ meats, broccoli, and grains	Used by the body for protein synthesis, builds red blood cells and healthy nervous system function.	Anemia, lack of coordination, and digestive disorders.
Biotin	Grains, soy products, organ meats, and milk	Assists with the breakdown of protein and fatty acids.	*Glossitis* (swelling of the tongue), insomnia, muscle cramps, and hair loss.
Ascorbic acid (vitamin C)	Oranges, lemons, tomatoes, berries, and green vegetables	Used for healthy blood vessels, prevention of bacterial infections, and as a healing agent.	*Scurvy* (edema, severe dry skin, hemorrhage, and bruising).
Folic acid (folate)	Oats, green vegetables, legumes, organ meats, and eggs	Important for brain and nervous tissue formation and metabolism.	Mild developmental issues, digestive disorders, or brain dysfunction; excessive amounts can cause convulsions.
Niacin	Liver, grains, fish, eggs, and milk	Essential for healthy intestinal tract and nervous system function and metabolism.	*Pellagra* (confusion, hallucinations, diarrhea, digestive dysfunction, and scaly skin); excessive amounts of niacin are released into the urine.
Pantothenic acid	Grains and liver	Assists in the formation of hormones and metabolism of fats and proteins.	Insomnia, headaches, and nausea.

that are used by the body in large quantities. Microminerals are the total opposite of macrominerals: they are used by the body in small quantities. Table 16-2 provides descriptions of 13 important macrominerals and microminerals.

Diet Modification

Certain medical conditions may require modification of a patient's diet. Diet modifications might include consumption of less sodium, no sugar or no meat, consideration of food allergies, or a low-cholesterol diet. For instance, a patient with a heart condition should consume less sodium, and the diet of a person with diabetes limits sugar consumption.

Adults who cannot eat refined sugar may be at an increased risk for developing hypoglycemia or could become severely obese due to complications with diabetes. If an individual is unable to eat refined sugar, her diet can be modified by using an artificial sweetener. The amount of artificial sweeteners consumed, however, must also be monitored because they should not be consumed in large dosages. Some artificial sweeteners have been known to

cause headaches, diarrhea, skin rash, muscle cramps, dizziness, metabolic disorders, and liver problems.

Cancer patients are encouraged to increase the antioxidants in their diets. Antioxidants come from minerals and vitamins that naturally occur in certain foods such as blueberries, oranges, and green leafy vegetables. These antioxidants decrease the oxidation of cells affected during chemotherapy treatment. Diet modifications fall under the responsibility of a physician, a registered dietician (RD), a dietetic technician (DT), a licensed practical nurse (LPN), or a registered nurse (RN).

Diet Modifications for Infants and Toddlers

From birth, newborns are given a specific diet. This diet takes into account both the infant's lack of digestion capability and the desire to avoid activating the onset of any allergies. Certain allergies that children can develop are allergies to seafood, sugars, nuts, and honey/syrup.

Seafood contains trace amounts of mercury, which can be very toxic to a small child, causing a debilitating illness or even death. Seafood, however, is very high in

TABLE 16-2   Macrominerals and Microminerals

Macrominerals

Magnesium	Used for the breakdown of other minerals. Works in conjunction with vitamin D for bone and tooth formation.
Phosphorus	Controls energy levels that come from carbohydrate and proteins. Also regulates healthy muscle function and DNA (deoxyribonucleic acid).
Sulfur	Essential in the use of protein. Without it, the breakdown in protein would not occur.
Sodium	Works much like chlorine and potassium for fluid balance.
Calcium	Important for healthy teeth/bones and muscle function.
Potassium	Needed for normal muscular function and maintaining the body's electrolyte levels.
Chloride	Works in conjunction with potassium to maintain fluid balance. Supplies the mouth with enzymes for food breakdown and increases waste elimination.

Microminerals

Selenium	Similar to the function of vitamin E; helps to repair tissue. It has most recently been found to contribute to weight control.
Iron	Found through the systems of the body. More than half of all iron in the body is found in the blood, and the remainder is found in other organs such as the spleen and liver. Iron forms hemoglobin in the blood.
Copper	Found in the hair to give color and assists with regeneration of red blood cells.
Zinc	A major component in producing several enzymes found in the body.
Fluoride	Provides the dentition with protection from tooth decay. When ingested during pregnancy, it binds itself to the enamel structure, making it more resistant to decay
Iodine	Important for thyroid function. The thyroid controls levels of growth in the body.

vitamin A, which is essential for healthy eyes, skin, and gingival tissue. Therefore, a vitamin supplement can be taken as a substitute or the amount of fruits and vegetables could be increased. Red and orange vegetables are recommended because they are usually high in vitamin A.

Certain sugars have to be avoided by small children due to the fact that the digestive tract cannot yet process them. If a child consumes too much refined sugar, he can develop a loose stool or diarrhea.

Eating nuts at an early age can increase the chances of developing a nut allergy. Older children and adults should avoid nuts if it is known that they have a nut allergy. The older the individual is, the higher the possibility of a severe response from a peanut allergen. The allergy response may come in the form of a skin rash, inflammation of the skin, swelling in the throat (making it hard to swallow or breathe), fever, and diarrhea or vomiting.

Syrups and honey contain spores that can cause forms of botulism, which is a form of food poisoning. When food poisoning occurs in an adult, the individual usually recovers. In small children, however, food poisoning can be fatal. Small children have a weak or nonexistent immune system, which does not allow them to fight bacteria. Symptoms of nausea, vomiting, dizziness, and fatigue may be treated with antitoxins.

Diet Analysis

A written medical document called a diet analysis can be created to help patients monitor what they eat and provide ways to improve their daily diet or overall health. Newer testing to determine a diet analysis can be done through DNA testing.

When utilizing a diet analysis, the patient is typically asked to keep a five- to seven-day journal of everything that he eats and drinks. The doctor may also provide a record to the patient on which he records how much exercise he is performing daily. The diet analysis is a visual educational aid that can be utilized to educate the patient on his nutritional intake of the RDAs from each food group. For liquid consumption, patients should record fluid intake and what type. The journal may include a section to record how much sleep the patient has been averaging.

Reading Food Labels

Because sustaining good nutritional habits is important for one's overall physical health, it is important for the dental patient to understand the importance of reading food labels (Figure 16.3). Food labels are located on the side of food boxes or the back of plastic bag packaging.

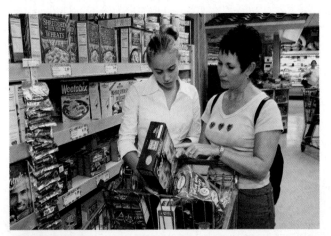

FIGURE 16.3
Reading nutrition label on a box of cereal.

Professionalism

If you find that you are not clear on why a doctor has changed a patient's diet or modified the patient's medication, be sure to ask the doctor to clarify. Be a professional by writing it down and asking the doctor when there is time available after the day has finished. It is considered inappropriate to ask questions during a procedure because this can cause patients concern regarding the treatment being performed. Asking questions during a patient's treatment may make you appear unprepared to practice your skills or ill-mannered.

Legal and Ethical Issues

It is not the job of the dental assistant to diagnose a patient's condition. Diagnosing patient conditions must be left to the dentist or registered dental hygienist. If a condition, such as an eating disorder, is suspected the dental assistant can privately share this information with the dentist, who can then address the issue with the patient as needed.

What are some signs of anorexia? Is a cure available for this condition?

Eating Disorders

Eating disorders that severely affect one's oral hygiene include anorexia nervosa and bulimia nervosa. Psychologists have found that most individuals who develop these eating disorders have tried many other ways of dieting before there is total loss of control in how to properly modify their diets to lose weight.

Recent surveys indicate that anorexia nervosa is becoming an increasingly common problem among our youth and adults. Teenagers especially feel the pressures of trying to fit in and look like famous individuals presented on magazine covers and television (Figure 16.4).

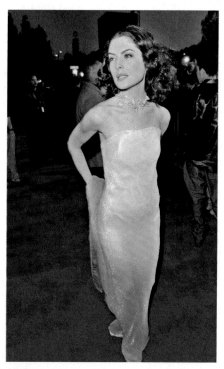

FIGURE 16.4
Actress Lara Flynn Boyle: An image of a famous person who teenagers may try to emulate.

Food labels are in a black outlined box usually in black print near the package bar code. This type of labeling should list all of the nutritional value of the food contained in the package and the ingredients. Fresh foods such as vegetables and fruits rarely have food labels attached to them. Food labeling is normally reserved for prepackaged foods.

Starting from the top of the food label, the first entry is the serving size. Serving sizes are determined based on USDA recommendations for daily serving sizes. Underneath the serving size, the container serving size is listed, showing how many total servings are in the package. The third line contains the number of calories per serving for that particular product.

Food labels rarely give exact measurements when it comes to calories. It is the buyer's responsibility to know how to figure out the actual totals. Figuring the amount of calorie intake is important. An example of how this is done is provided in the following example:

If one serving is 8 ounces and each serving is 100 calories, the calorie consumption for three servings would equal a total of 300 calories.

The middle section of a food label lists the daily value percentages of cholesterol, fat, sodium, carbohydrates, proteins, and sugar provided by one serving. This section is measured in terms of grams, which is almost always abbreviated as "g." Some labels use milligrams (abbreviated "mg"); 1,000 milligrams = 1 gram. This percentage system is also based on the USDA's RDAs. The percentages tell how much of the RDA of that particular item is being obtained from that particular food product.

Fat and calories are listed in two different sections that need attention when screening labels. Calories and fats are not the same thing, and calorie intake can come from more than one source such as protein, carbohydrates, and fat. For individuals with conditions such as high blood pressure, diabetes, and kidney complications, a diet that is low in sodium content and cholesterol content may be required. The amount of sodium and cholesterol in foods can be determined by reading food labels.

These images present the idea that everyone should be thin. Although anorexia is predominantly a female eating disorder, men can also suffer from this disease. **Anorexia** is characterized as the condition in which someone thinks and sees oneself as obese. Due to the distorted body image that a person with anorexia has, the individual consumes as little food as possible in order to lose whatever fat she may have.

Anorexia rarely starts as a sudden starvation. It starts out slowly with the individual noticing that she needs to lose just a few pounds. The individual may begin with eliminating one meal a day to see what weight loss might occur. When an achieved amount of weight loss has occurred, the individual will decrease the amounts of the other two remaining meals or totally eliminate another meal until she is down to just drinking fluids or eating scraps of food to fill her stomach.

The number one most obvious sign of anorexia is rapid weight loss. The results of anorexia and the severe nutritional deprivation that occurs with this condition include hair loss, tooth decay, and Raynaud's phenomenon (pain in the extremities with poor blood circulation due to constriction of the blood vessels causing numbness, tingling, and skin discoloration). Signs of anorexia include constant exercise, meals found thrown away in the garbage, trouble concentrating, cancellations to appear for group activities, and eating alone.

Another eating disorder is **bulimia**. The condition of bulimia is exhibited by an individual who self-induces vomiting after eating. Vomiting, however, is not always used to expel food. Sometimes the individual uses laxatives, diet pills, and diuretics (water pills) to excess. Signs of bulimia include overuse of diet pills or laxatives, lesions on the mucosa, bad breath, chemical erosion on the teeth, and swollen glands. Erosion, particularly on the lingual surfaces, is a good indicator that a person is binging and purging.

The cause of bulimia has been linked to individuals who have experienced some type of abuse. Bulimia is very common among females in their teens. Due to the loss of proper nutrition, bulimia, like anorexia, can lead to hair loss and body aches and pains.

Both eating disorders can lead to heart damage, hospitalization, and even death if left untreated. The dental assistant is often the first to see the oral condition of a patient. If the assistant suspects an eating disorder, he or she should consult the dentist before any oral treatment is performed. If the dentist suspects bulimia or anorexia because of the patient's poor oral health, he or she may refer the patient to a therapist or disorders clinic for evaluation. It is not mandatory for the patient to attend treatment; however, the dentist can decline to perform dental care on the patient until the patient seeks help. It is mandatory for a dentist to inform the parents if the patient is a minor.

A person is classified as overweight if she possesses more fatty tissue than recommended by the federal government. To be overweight means that a person still has control over achieving weight loss by increasing exercise, proper diet, and decreasing stress. **Obesity** can be defined as a condition of a person who is 20% over the desired weight for height and build. Individuals who are obese are at high risk for diseases such as diabetes, vascular disease, heart disease, and some cancers. Due to the issues related to obesity, some individuals include obesity in the category of eating disorders. This disorder affects the dentition by increasing the levels of decay due to excessive sugar and acid (juices and soda) in the diet. For extremely obese patients, counseling and hospitalization may be important treatment options. Utilizing professionals who can monitor the patient's diet and keep the individual on track for maintaining a proper weight may be helpful. Obese individuals need to be reconditioned to learn how to make safe and healthy food choices.

Healthy Eating Habits

Eating healthy does not mean that food cannot taste good. It means that attention should be paid to making wise food choices. Teaching children at a young age that eating healthy is important is crucial for both the child's current and future health (Figure 16.5). Each meal should contain healthy choices of fruits, grains, and vegetables. Snacks should include items such as fruit rather than the less healthy choice of potato chips or chocolate.

Cooking healthy requires food to be baked rather than fried. Rather than using unhealthy options for seasonings such as butter, creams, or salt, some great alternatives are available that can add good flavors to food. For instance, lemons tend to give food a similar flavor to that of salt. Lemons not only contain essential vitamins, but can also help with maintaining water weight gain. Low-sodium salts found in most stores offer an alternative to regular salt.

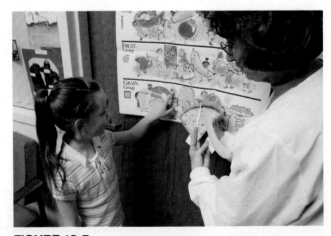

FIGURE 16.5
Teaching a child good nutritional habits.

SUMMARY

Unfortunately, America is considered the most obese country in the world. The type of food a person consumes as a child and later as an adult can significantly impact one's oral health. On a daily and weekly basis, individuals often consume too much sugar or sodium. To help dental patients monitor their eating, drinking, and exercise habits, a food journal may be a helpful suggestion. Keeping a weekly journal can assist individuals in monitoring the consumption of water, fruits, vegetables, grains, and dairy products. A food journal also helps people realize where they could decrease their intake of cariogenic foods, which in turn helps to decrease the development of decay in the mouth. The USDA provides a complete and current list of recommendations for children and adults at www.usda.gov.

KEY TERMS

- **Anorexia:** Common eating disorder for the male and female teen population. Involves daily starvation and excessive exercise to prevent weight gain. p. 249
- **Bulimia:** Eating disorder in which overeating is followed by vomiting. p. 249
- **Carbohydrates:** Sugars and starches used for energy. p. 242
- **Fats:** Nutrients used for body insulation and energy; also known as lipids. p. 243
- **Minerals:** Found in the earth's crust and also used like vitamins for body functions. p. 245
- **Nutrients:** Obtained from food and used by the body for various daily functions. p. 241
- **Obesity:** Condition of a person who is 20% over the desired weight for height and build. p. 249
- **Proteins:** Nutrients used for muscle tissue construction and repair; come from sources such as meat, eggs, and nuts. p. 244
- **Vitamins:** Nutrients derived from natural sources such as plants; they are needed for healthy body functioning and prevention of diseases. p. 244

CHECK YOUR UNDERSTANDING

1. The recommended daily allowance for servings of fruit is
   a. 2.
   b. 4.
   c. 3.
   d. 1.

2. Which age group does bulimia affect the most?
   a. elderly
   b. toddlers
   c. middle age
   d. teens

3. Which fruit not only contains essential vitamins but can also help maintain water weight gain?
   a. lemons
   b. pears
   c. bananas
   d. apples

4. Which of the following is not a vitamin?
   a. iron
   b. ascorbic acid
   c. riboflavin
   d. cobalamin

5. Which of the following is a nutrient we need in our diet?
   a. water
   b. fats
   c. proteins
   d. all of the above

6. This condition is a result of vitamin C deficiency.
   a. goiters
   b. rickets
   c. scurvy
   d. kwashiorkor

7. How many fat-soluble vitamins are there?
   a. 10
   b. 4
   c. 6
   d. 13

8. Which food is very high in vitamin K?
   a. liver
   b. carrots
   c. apples
   d. corn

CHECK YOUR UNDERSTANDING (continued)

9. Which is not a common sign of anorexia?
   a. fast weight loss
   b. empty food packages
   c. hair loss
   d. numbness in the extremities

10. Which one helps to produce energy?
    a. fats
    b. proteins
    c. carbohydrates
    d. water

INTERNET ACTIVITY

- Go to the website for the U.S. Food and Drug Administration at http://www.cfsan.fda.gov/~dms/foodlab.html and discover more on how to learn about nutritional facts found on food labels.

WEB REFERENCES

- Diseases Info   http://phoenity.com/diseases/pellagra.html
- Medical Images: ADAM   http://medicalimages.allrefer.com/large/scurvy-corkscrew-hairs.jpg
- Otolaryngology Houston: Geographic Tongue   www.ghorayeb.com/TongueGeographic.html
- United States Department of Agriculture: MyPyramid.gov   www.mypyramid.gov
- Web4Health   http://web4health.info/en/answers/ed-pictures.htm
- www.thyroidimaging.com   http://web.tiscali.it/thyroidimaging/pic_gozzonod3.htm

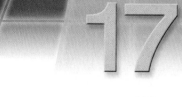

Instrument Processing and Sterilization

Chapter Outline

- Introduction to Instrument Processing
  —Sterilization versus Disinfection

- Classification of Patient Care Items
  —Patient Protection

- Transporting and Processing Contaminated Patient Care Items

- Instrument Processing Area
  —Workflow Pattern

- Precleaning Instruments
  —Hand Scrubbing
  —Ultrasonic Cleaner
  —Washer/Disinfector
  —Lubrication and Corrosion Control
  —CDC Guidelines for Cleaning Contaminated Instruments

- Packaging and Storing of Materials
  —Packaging Materials
  —Storing of Sterilized Instruments

- Sterilization Monitoring
  —Biological Indicators
  —Sterilization Documentation
  —CDC Guidelines for Sterilization Monitoring

- Methods of Sterilization
  —Steam Sterilization
  —Flash Sterilization
  —Dry Heat Sterilization
  —Chemical Vapor Sterilization

- Sterilization Failures

- Handpiece Sterilization

Learning Objectives

After reading this chapter, the student should be able to:

- Explain the difference between critical, semicritical, and noncritical items.
- Discuss how critical, semicritical, and noncritical items are processed.
- List the process of transporting contaminated patient care items.
- Describe instrument cleaning techniques.
- Describe the safety procedures for using the ultrasonic cleaner.
- Determine the appropriate packaging materials for sterilizing dental items.
- Demonstrate the use of biological monitors and internal indicators.
- Describe the different methods of sterilization.
- Demonstrate the use of an autoclave.
- Explain the use of chemical liquid sterilants.
- Describe how to sterilize dental handpieces.

Preparing for Certification Exams

- Prevent cross-contamination and disease transmission in all areas of the dental office.
- Prepare dental instruments and equipment for sterilization.
- Use appropriate method for sterilization of dental instruments and equipment.
- Properly store all instruments.
- Transport instruments in a manner that prevents disease transmission.
- Use appropriate system for sterilization monitoring.
- Demonstrate proper steps in packaging instruments.
- Clean and disinfect instruments wearing appropriate personal protective equipment.

Key Terms

Autoclave	Holding solution
Biological indicators	Noncritical items
Critical items	Semicritical items
Disinfection	Sterilization
Dry heat sterilizer	Time-related sterilization
Event-related sterilization	Ultrasonic cleaner
Flash sterilization	Washer/disinfector

Since the 1980s, infection control has been a serious issue among dental and health care workers. Instrument processing is one of the most important key areas of infection control for the dental team. Instrument processing involves the transporting of contaminated instruments and the processing, packaging, and sterilizing of instruments, while maintaining asepsis and infection control guidelines. This chapter will describe the rationale behind the Centers for Disease Control and Prevention (CDC) guidelines and steps to keep patients, the dental team, and the office safe from contamination.

Introduction to Instrument Processing

The processing of instruments consists of multiple steps designed to prepare contaminated instruments for reuse. Instrument processing itself is not a difficult task, but the steps must be performed correctly in order to minimize disease transmission from patient to patient as well as from patient to staff. These procedures or steps must be performed with attention to detail to prevent disease transmission. The basic instrument processing procedures include eight steps: transporting, cleaning, drying/lubricating, packaging, sterilizing, storing, and delivering of processed instruments, as well as sterilization monitoring.

Sterilization versus Disinfection

It is important to have a general understanding of the methods used to kill microorganisms when processing contaminated patient care items. **Sterilization** is a process that kills all living microorganisms, and it can be accomplished through heat sterilization and chemical liquid sterilization.

Professionalism

Working in the instrument processing section of a dental office is a very important job. The dental assistant may be asked to work in this area for an extended amount of time to ensure that the dental assistant understands and comprehends the importance of processing instruments correctly. Take the time to learn the procedures of proper infection control.

Sterilization can be monitored for the ability to kill bacterial endospores, the most difficult living organisms to destroy, by using live spore tests. These tests use harmless spores; however, they are just as resistant to sterilization as the more dangerous spores. **Disinfection** kills disease-producing microorganisms, but not endospores. Disinfection is used for items that are not invasive and do not have contact with blood or other body fluids. (See Chapter 12 for more information on disinfection.)

Monitored heat sterilization is the ideal method for processing instruments. However, some items are heat sensitive and are sterilized using a chemical liquid. Chemical liquid takes longer to sterilize instruments and cannot be monitored for quality assurance as can the heat method.

According to the CDC, certain items must be sterilized and certain items disinfected. The CDC's general recommendations state that only Food and Drug Administration (FDA) approved medical devices should be used for sterilization and that the manufacturer's instructions should be followed. These instructions include:

1. Clean and heat sterilize critical and semicritical dental instruments prior to each use. (See next section for a discussion of critical and semicritical instruments.)
2. Allow packages to dry in the sterilizer before handling, to avoid contamination.
3. Avoid use of liquid chemical sterilants and high-level disinfectants for holding solutions.

Classification of Patient Care Items

To determine the least amount of processing required for patient care items, and the potential risk of infection, a classification system is used. This system is mandated by the CDC; the categories of patient care items are critical, semicritical, and noncritical (Table 17-1).

Life Span Considerations

Regardless of your patient's age, race, or nationality your patient's safety is of utmost concern. The sterilization of dental instruments is critical to their health and safety. Studies are being conducted using lasers to sterilize specific dental instruments. One study looked at how contaminated endodontic reamers can be cleaned with the use of a laser at various levels of energy. The instruments were read for microorganism growth; the results indicated that there was no growth at a low laser level. This is a huge breakthrough in the sterilization field. Not only are lasers becoming more prevalent in the medical and dental field, but the use of lasers may minimize the use of pollution producing sterilizers. It is an exciting time to be a dental assistant!

TABLE 17-1 Classification of Instruments

Category	Definition	Examples
Critical	Penetrates soft tissue; contacts bone; enters into or contacts bloodstream or other normally sterile tissue.	Surgical instruments, scalers, scalpel blades, surgical dental burs
Semicritical	Contacts mucous membranes, but will not penetrate soft tissue; contacts bone; enters into or contacts the bloodstream, or other normally sterile tissue of the mouth.	Dental mouth mirror, amalgam, condenser, reusable dental impression trays, dental handpieces
Noncritical	Contacts intact skin.	Blood pressure cuff, radiology PID, stethoscope, pulse oximeter

Source: Adapted from *Centers for Disease Control and Prevention's Guidelines for Infection Control in Dental Health-Care Settings,* 2003.

Critical items are those that penetrate soft tissue and come in direct contact with bone, blood, and other body fluids. Critical items include surgical instruments (scalpels, forceps, bone chisels), periodontal scalers, surgical and dental burs, and manual cutting instruments. These items pose the biggest risk of disease transmission and, therefore, must be heat sterilized.

Semicritical items come in contact with mucous membranes or nonintact skin, and they do not penetrate soft tissue or bone or enter into the bloodstream. Dental mouth mirrors, amalgam condensers, dental impression trays, plastic instruments, handpieces, and items that are not intended to penetrate the skin are all examples of semicritical items. Most semicritical items in dentistry are heat tolerant and, therefore, should be heat sterilized. If the item is heat sensitive, however, it should be processed with an Environmental Protection Agency (EPA) approved high-level disinfectant.

Even though handpieces are classified as semicritical, the handpiece must be heat sterilized between each patient. Handpieces do not penetrate the mucous membrane, but the rotating burs on their ends do and can cause splatter of potentially infectious materials.

Noncritical items are those instruments that do not come in direct contact with body fluids. These items pose the least risk of disease transmission because they only come in contact with intact skin, which works as a barrier to microorganisms. Cleaning followed by disinfection with an EPA-approved disinfectant is an adequate procedure for noncritical instruments. Noncritical items include radiograph position-indicating devices (PIDs), blood pressure cuffs, face bows, dental dam frames, and pulse oximeters.

Patient Protection

To provide the highest level of patient protection, all reusable instruments and handpieces must be sterilized with heat between patients. If an item is not heat tolerant and cannot be sterilized at all, then it should be discarded after patient use. Many disposable dental items are on the market today to help prevent disease transmission. It is important to use standard precaution methods when handling any contaminated items. Universal or standard precautions are techniques used to prevent cross-contamination of microorganisms. This means treating every patient as if he or she is infected; in other words, the dental assistant uses the appropriate personal protective equipment (PPE) for each and every patient.

How would a noncritical item be cleaned or sterilized?

Transporting and Processing Contaminated Patient Care Items

Health care workers can be exposed to microorganisms through percutaneous injury, contact with cuts or abrasions on the skin, and contact with the mucous membranes of the eyes, nose, or mouth. The CDC guidelines for receiving, cleaning, and decontaminating patient care items follow:

1. Use work practice controls to minimize exposure potential by carrying instruments in a covered container instead of handling loose contaminated instruments.
2. Use ultrasonic cleaners or washer/disinfectors to remove debris, improve effectiveness of cleaning, and decrease worker exposure to blood.
3. Use work practice controls that minimize contact with sharp instruments if manual cleaning is necessary. (For instance, use long-handled scrub brushes.)
4. Wear puncture- and chemical-resistant utility gloves when cleaning and decontaminating all items or areas that are contaminated.
5. Wear appropriate PPE (mask, eyewear, gown, and gloves) to minimize splash and spatter contamination during cleaning or decontamination of all items or areas that are contaminated.

Instrument Processing Area

According to CDC guidelines, the instrument processing area should be a designated area with easy access from all dental operatories. The instrument processing area is divided into four separate sections: (1) receiving/cleaning/decontamination, (2) preparation and packaging, (3) sterilization, and (4) storage.

The processing area should be kept out of patient view. It should not be part of a common hallway or near the reception area. The flooring should be an uncarpeted, hard surface. The area should not have doors to the outside or windows that open since this can increase the presence of dust. Good ventilation is key to control the heat generated by the sterilizers. The design of the processing area should include many outlets, proper lighting, water, and air/vacuum lines for flushing handpieces. Hands-free soap dispensers and foot-operated controls help minimize cross disease transmission when handling contaminated items. The processing area may vary in shape and size; however, it should have separate contaminated and clean areas. Consider the following basic guideline from the CDC on instrument processing:

1. Designate a central processing area. Divide the area physically or spatially into distinct areas:

   a. *Receiving, cleaning, and decontamination:* high contamination area; utility glove and full PPE needed.

   b. *Preparation and packaging:* medium contamination area; utility glove and full PPE needed.

   c. *Sterilization:* low contamination; utility gloves and full PPE needed to load sterilizer. Start the sterilizer and empty after cycle completion with clean hands.

   d. *Storage:* low contamination; clean hands.

Train all dental health care workers to employ work practices that prevent contamination of clean areas.

Workflow Pattern

To maintain the four separate areas of the instrument processing area, a linear or U-shaped design is encouraged (Figure 17.1). This type of design enhances how

Dental Assistant PROFESSIONAL TIP

As a new dental assistant, obtain a copy of the CDC's *Guidelines for Infection Control in Dental Health-Care Settings.* Become extremely familiar with this document so you have a better understanding of how to maintain a safe environment for both the dental patient and the dental team.

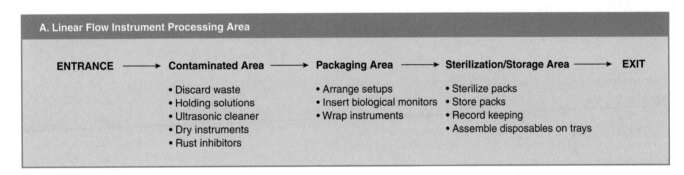

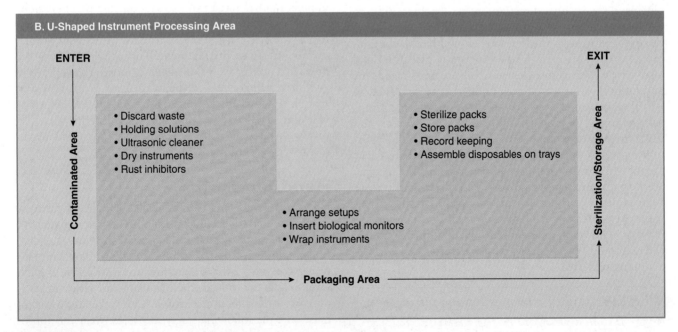

FIGURE 17.1
Instrument processing workflow areas: (a) linear and (b) U-shaped.

Procedure 17-1 Processing Contaminated Instruments

Equipment and Supplies Needed

- PPE (utility gloves, mask, protective eyewear and clothing)
- Contaminated instruments
- Holding solution
- Ultrasonic cleaner
- Instrument sterilization wrap
- Sterilizer

Procedure Steps

1. After patient dismissal, discard all contaminated disposables in dental operatory.

2. Wearing PPE, including utility gloves, transport instruments to processing area. Use container to transport loose instruments.

3. Submerge instruments in a holding/precleaning solution. (Dishwasher soap works well because it is low foaming.) This step can be skipped if the assistant has time to place the instruments in the ultrasonic cleaner immediately.

4. After disinfecting dental treatment room, return to processing area and rinse holding solution off of instruments.

5. Place instruments in ultrasonic cleaner. Do not hand scrub instruments. (Instrument cassettes can also be placed in a washer/disinfector.)

6. Determine which instruments will be heat processed and which will be processed in the chemical liquid sterilant.

7. Dry and lubricate handpieces and hinged instruments to prevent corrosion.

8. Wrap and prepare instruments according to the type of sterilization process used.

9. Load into sterilizer.

10. Store sterile instrument packages in a storage place away from contaminated instruments.

---

instrument processing procedures are handled and also helps prevent contamination to the operator and other items in the area. Each of these areas should be clearly labeled with a sign for identification; all dental health care workers must be trained on the work practices to prevent contamination of the clean areas.

Regardless of the pattern, the processing should always flow in one direction, never backtracking to another area. For example, as the dental assistant enters the processing area, the first stop should be the contaminated area. This area is where waste is discarded and also where ultrasonic cleaners, lubrication, cleansers, and holding solutions are maintained. The area next to it is the packaging area. In this area, instrument setups are arranged, biological indicators are placed, and instruments are wrapped. From there the dental assistant moves to the sterilization/storage area where packs are loaded into the sterilizer for the recommended time. Sterile packs are removed from the sterilizer, sterile/clean disposables are assembled on trays, and sterile instrument packs are stored. This area is typically right next to the exit. The whole procedure flows in a linear pattern. There should be no reason to have sterile items in the contaminated area.

What is the significance of having a linear or U-shaped workflow in the instrument processing area?

Precleaning Instruments

Dental instruments are typically cleaned in three different ways: manually by hand scrubbing, with an ultrasonic cleaner, or with a washer/disinfector. Precleaning is an important step in processing instruments. Precleaning removes blood and saliva (bioburden) and reduces the number of microorganisms so that the instruments can be sterilized properly. In many dental offices it is not feasible for the dental assistant to clean the instruments immediately after patient treatment. That is why soaking the items in a **holding solution** can help loosen the debris and prevent it from drying on the instrument. Note, however, that even if instruments are soaked, the precleaning stage will still need to be completed before sterilization. To review the procedure for processing contaminated instruments see Procedure 17-1.

Hand Scrubbing

Hand scrubbing is not recommended by the CDC because of the potential for accidental exposure to microorganisms. With hand scrubbing, the chances of an injury are high because the dental assistant can easily slip and puncture his or her skin with a sharp contaminated instrument. If hand scrubbing is the only method available for cleaning, as is the case, for instance, for handpiece burs, then the assistant must take the following safety measures: wear the appropriate PPE (goggles, utility gloves, mask, and gown) (Figure 17.2); clean one instrument at a time, preferably

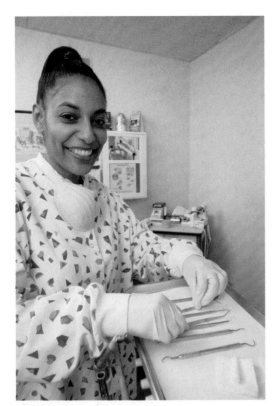

FIGURE 17.2
PPE, including utility gloves, must be worn while handling contaminated instruments.

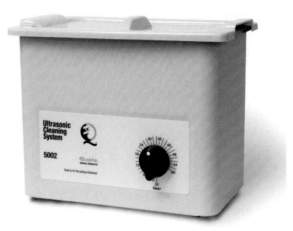

FIGURE 17.3
Quala 5002 ultrasonic cleaning system.
Courtesy Quala, a registered Trademark of American Dental Cooperative (ADC)

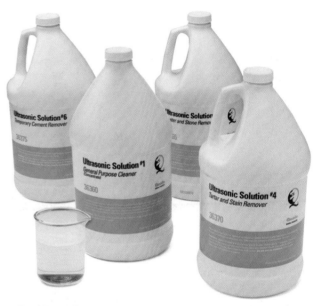

FIGURE 17.4
Liquid ultrasonic cleaner solutions.
Courtesy Quala, a registered Trademark of American Dental Cooperative (ADC)

using a long-handled brush that has been sterilized after each use; keep items below water level; and allow instruments to air dry. If the instrument is kept above water while being cleaned, it may generate more spatter. The federal Occupational Safety and Health Administration (OSHA) may have specific state requirements with regard to hand scrubbing of instruments. State guidelines should also be reviewed before using this procedure.

Ultrasonic Cleaner

The ultrasonic method is the preferred and safest method of cleaning instruments. It reduces the chance of cuts or puncture wounds that might result from hand scrubbing. **Ultrasonic cleaners** come in a variety of sizes to fit the needs of any dental office (Figure 17.3). The ultrasonic sound waves create bubbles and vibrations that dislodge debris from the instruments. A specially made antimicrobial solution added to the water helps clean the instruments more effectively (Figure 17.4). The solution also helps reduce the buildup of microorganisms in the solution. The solution is designed to provide enzyme activity to help remove debris.

The solution must be changed daily or more frequently if it becomes cloudy or visibly dirty, to prevent disease transmission. When emptying the dirty solution, a mask, gown, safety goggles, and utility gloves must be worn. Once the pan is emptied, it should be rinsed with clean water, disinfected with disinfectant, rinsed, and then dried.

Instruments and instrument cassettes are placed in the basket of the ultrasonic cleaner, the basket is then placed into the solution, and the lid is placed on to reduce spray and spatter of the contaminated liquid. The processing time ranges from 4 to 16 minutes depending on the brand of machine, amount of debris on the instrument, and whether the debris has dried. Instruments housed in a plastic cassette are processed longer than individual instruments because the cassette absorbs some of the energy of the cleaner. See Procedure 17-2.

After the cleaning cycle is complete, the instrument basket is removed and the basket and instruments are rinsed with water. Keep in mind that the ultrasonic cleaner and the instruments are still contaminated with microorganisms; the instruments are considered clean of debris and are ready to be dried, lubricated, packaged, and sterilized.

Procedure 17-2 Operating the Ultrasonic Cleaner

Equipment and Supplies Needed

- PPE (utility gloves, mask, protective eyewear and clothing)
- Ultrasonic cleaner
- Ultrasonic solution

Procedure Steps

1. Don PPE, including utility gloves, mask, and protective eyewear and clothing.

2. Remove instruments from holding solution. Remove lid from ultrasonic cleaner.

3. Ensure cleaner is filled with water and the appropriate ultrasonic solution. (Check manufacturer's instructions.)

4. Place loose instruments or instrument cassettes in ultrasonic basket; gently submerge into cleaner, carefully avoiding excess splash.

5. Replace lid and turn on cycle to desired time (typically between 6 and 12 minutes).

6. When the cleaning cycle is complete, remove basket and rinse with tap water.

7. Tip basket onto a clean towel, remove instruments, and replace basket and lid on ultrasonic cleaner.

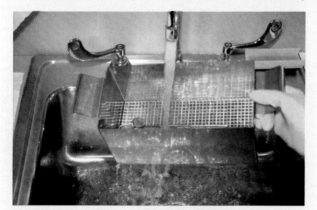

Instruments being rinsed prior to placement in ultrasonic cleaner. Image courtesy Instructional Materials for the Dental Team, Lex., KY

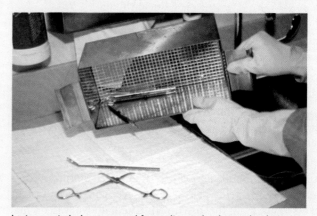

Instruments being removed from ultrasonic cleaner basket. Image courtesy Instructional Materials for the Dental Team, Lex., KY

PPE and utility gloves must be worn when handling contaminated instruments. Most instruments can be cleaned via the ultrasonic method; however, handpieces should never be submerged in liquid of any kind. Handpieces should be wiped free of debris, lubricated, and steam sterilized between each patient. (If necessary, the handpiece should be lubricated following the manufacturer's instructions.)

There is a way to test and monitor the ultrasonic cleaner to ensure that instruments are getting as clean as they should. To test the cleaner, hold a lightweight piece of foil half submerged into fresh, unused solution and run the unit for 20 to 30 seconds. If the part of the foil that was submerged has small dots or indentations, then the ultrasonic action is working properly. If it doesn't have the marks, then the unit may not be working properly and may require service. See Procedure 17-3.

Washer/Disinfector

Washer/disinfector machines resemble regular dishwashers; however, these particular washers are approved by the FDA for use in hospitals and dental offices to clean,

rinse, and disinfect patient care items (Figure 17.5). These machines reduce the handling of contaminated instruments. Loose instruments are placed in baskets or instrument cassettes. Washer/disinfector machines work

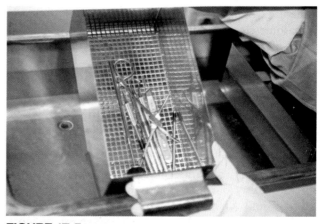

FIGURE 17.5
Assistant using a washer/disinfector.
Image courtesy Instructional Materials for the Dental Team, Lex., KY

Procedure 17-3 Testing the Ultrasonic Cleaner

Equipment and Supplies Needed

- Ultrasonic cleaner
- Fresh ultrasonic solution
- Foil

Procedure Steps

1. Use regular household aluminum foil; cut a piece to fit the width of the cleaner.

2. Prepare fresh cleaner solution and fill the ultrasonic tank according to manufacturer's directions.

3. Insert the foil vertically into the ultrasonic tank.

4. Hold the foil steady. Turn the machine on for 20 to 30 seconds.

5. If the machine is functioning properly, the entire foil surface will be covered with a tiny, uniform pebbling effect. If areas of more than 0.5 inch square show no pebbling, then the machine may need servicing.

---

similar to ultrasonic cleaners; however, they do more and can hold large amounts of instruments. When the washer cycle is complete, the dental assistant dons the appropriate PPE, including utility gloves; removes the dry instruments; and then packages, sterilizes, and stores them.

Table 17-2 provides a comparison of the three types of cleaning methods just discussed.

Lubrication and Corrosion Control

Instruments should be dried and lubricated to prevent rust and corrosion. If instruments are packaged in paper, the excess water should be shaken off to avoid weakening and tearing of the sterilizing packaging. Hinged instruments may require a lubricant prior to sterilizing to maintain proper opening of the instrument. Many instruments are made of carbon steel and will rust in a steam sterilizer. A rust inhibitor may be required to prevent corrosion. The rust inhibitor comes as a spray and also as a liquid into which the instruments can be dipped. Once this step is accomplished, the instruments must be packaged or wrapped.

CDC Guidelines for Cleaning Contaminated Instruments

The CDC provides the following guidelines for cleaning contaminated instruments:

1. Minimize handling of loose, contaminated instruments during transport to the instrument processing area.
2. Clean all visible blood and other contamination from dental instruments and devices prior to sterilization and disinfection.
3. Use automated cleaning equipment to remove debris, to improve cleaning effectiveness, and to decrease exposure to blood.
4. Wear puncture- and chemical-resistant utility gloves for instrument cleaning and decontamination.
5. Wear appropriate PPE.

Cultural Considerations

The Organization for Safety and Asepsis Procedures publishes infection control and instrument processing documents in Spanish. The CDC's *Guidelines for Infection Control in Dental Health-Care Settings* is published in Spanish. If Spanish is your native language, consider visiting these organizations on the Internet and reading the information offered.

TABLE 17-2 Comparison of Cleaning Methods

Method	Advantages	Disadvantages
Hand scrubbing	Effective only if performed properly.	Increased chance of injury. Spread of contamination through spatter. Time consuming.
Ultrasonic cleaning	Safer than hand scrubbing. Effectively cleans instruments. Reduces spread of contamination. More efficient than hand scrubbing.	Microorganisms build up in solution. Will not remove cement.
Washer/Disinfector	Reduces spread of contamination. Efficient. Effectively cleans instruments.	Not all instruments compatible with washer/disinfector.

TABLE 17-3 Types of Packaging Material

Sterilization Method	Packaging Material Requirements	Acceptable Materials
Steam autoclave	Should allow steam to penetrate.	Paper. Plastic. Cloth. Paper peel packages. Wrapped perforated cassettes.
Dry heat	Should not insulate items from heat. Should not be destroyed by temperature used.	Aluminum foil. Polyfilm plastic tubing. Wrapped perforated cassettes.
Unsaturated chemical vapor	Vapors should be allowed to precipitate on contents. Vapors should not react with packaging material. Plastics should not contact sides of sterilizer.	Wrapped perforated cassettes. Paper. Paper peel pouches.

Packaging and Storing of Materials

The purpose of packaging instruments for sterilization is to prevent them from becoming contaminated after sterilization and during storage. Unpackaged instruments are exposed to dust and contaminated aerosols, surfaces, moisture, and improper handling. The CDC suggests these guidelines for packaging instruments:

Preparation and Packaging

• Use internal chemical indicators in each package; use external indicators if internal ones cannot be seen from the outside.

• Use a container or wrapping compatible with the type of sterilization performed.

• Semicritical and critical instruments should be placed in packaging designed to maintain sterility during storage.

Sterilization of Unwrapped Instruments

• Clean and dry instruments before the sterilization cycle.

• Allow instruments to dry and cool in the sterilizer before handling.

• Semicritical instruments that will be used immediately can be sterilized unwrapped in a container system.

• Critical instruments intended for immediate use can be sterilized unwrapped if instruments are maintained sterile during removal from the sterilizer.

• Do not sterilize implantable devices unwrapped.

• Do not store critical instruments unwrapped.

Why should instruments be wrapped prior to sterilization?

Packaging Materials

Packaging material must be FDA approved. It is very important that only designated sterilization packaging material be used. Substitute materials and products may cause damage to the instruments and sterilizer and will not allow sterilization to occur. Products that should not be used are plastic wrap, foil, or paper that is not designed for heat sterilization. Only the specific materials that meet the need of the sterilizing process should be used. Table 17-3 lists the acceptable types of packaging materials for the various sterilization techniques. Many types of material are available such as self-sealed bags, heat-sealed bags, paper packaging, and paper/cloth wrap (Figures 17.6 and 17.7).

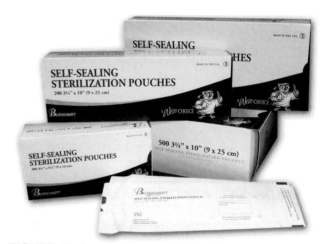

FIGURE 17.6
Self-sealing sterilizing packages.
Courtesy Burkhart Dental Supply

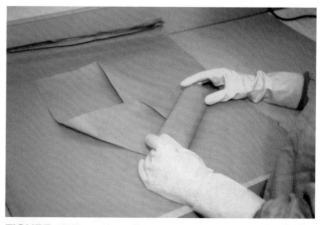

FIGURE 17.7
Blue sterilizing wrap.
Image courtesy Instructional Materials for the Dental Team, Lex., KY

Storing of Sterilized Instruments

Sterile instruments and materials should be stored in a closed area such as a cabinet or drawer (Figure 17.8). Dental items should not be stored under sinks where they may become wet. This can damage the integrity of the item. Sterilized items should remain wrapped until needed. Always store these items in a way that maintains the integrity of the packaging material. Do not overfill drawers or containers with instrument packs. This may cause ripping or tearing of the package.

Sterile instrument packs can be stored using either a time-related or event-related shelf life. The date of sterilization should be placed on the package when sterilizing. With **time-related sterilization,** the shelf life of instruments is identified with an exact expiration date. After this date, the item is considered outdated and should be repackaged and resterilized. With **event-related sterilization,** the shelf life of the sterile instrument is maintained indefinitely if packages are handled and stored properly. With the event-related method, packages are sterile unless ripped or damaged. If this occurs, then the instrument must be repackaged and resterilized. Damaged packages can collect dust and contaminated aerosols, so it is crucial that the dental assistant continually check for damaged instrument packs.

The CDC guidelines for storage of sterilized items are as follows:

1. Implement practices on the basis of time- or event-related shelf life for storage of wrapped, sterilized instruments and devices.
2. Place the date of sterilization and, if multiple sterilizers are used, write the sterilizer used on the outside package.
3. Examine wrapped packages of sterilized instruments before opening them to ensure the barrier wrap has not been compromised during storage.
4. Reclean, repack, and resterilize any instrument pack that has been compromised.

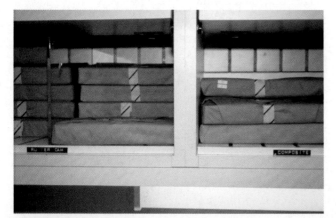

FIGURE 17.8
Instrument storage.
Image courtesy Instructional Materials for the Dental Team, Lex., KY

5. Store sterile items and dental supplies in covered or closed cabinets.

Why is a ripped, sterile instrument package considered nonsterile if it hasn't been used in someone's mouth?

Sterilization Monitoring

To ensure quality and effectiveness with sterilizers, sterilization monitoring is required. According to the CDC, this monitoring should include mechanical, chemical, and biological processes. Mechanical techniques include assessing the time, temperature, and pressure by observing the gauges on the sterilizer to ensure the correct temperature is met for proper sterilization. Check the manufacturer's instructions regarding temperatures and times. Correct temperatures and times are not a guarantee that sterilization has taken place, but incorrect readings could be an indication of a malfunctioning machine. Chemical indicators assess physical conditions such as time and temperature during the sterilization process. There are two different types of chemical indicators: external and internal.

- *External indicators:* These indicators, such as indicator tapes or special markings, are applied to the outside of the instrument package and change color when exposed to the heat of the sterilization process. However, this does not mean sterilization has taken place.
- *Internal indicators:* These indicators are placed inside each package and ensure that the sterilizing agent has penetrated the package and reached the instrument (Figure 17.9).
  — Single-parameter internal indicators only provide information on time or temperature.
  — Multiparameter indicators provide information on the presence of steam as well as time and temperature. Multiparameter indicators are only available for autoclaves (steam sterilizers), which are discussed in a later section.

Chemical indicators do not guarantee that the load of instruments has been sterilized. They can only indicate if the temperature did not get to the level it should have. If both mechanical and chemical indicators indicate there is a problem (time, temperature, no change in color, etc.), then the instrument load should not be processed in that particular machine.

Biological Indicators

Biological indicators are the most widely used method for sterilization monitoring (Figure 17.10). This method is also referred to as a *spore test* because it assesses the

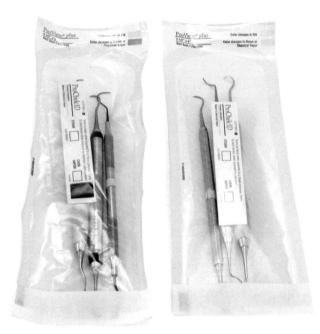

FIGURE 17.9
ProView® Plus sterilization pouches with ProChek® ID internal indicator strip before and after.
Courtesy Certol International, LLC

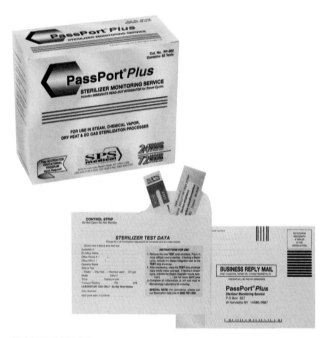

FIGURE 17.10
Biological indicators.
Courtesy SPS Medical Supply

sterilization process by killing known, highly resistant microorganisms. *Geobacillus stearothermophilus* spores are used for testing steam or chemical vapor. *Bacillus atrophaeus* are preferred for testing dry heat or ethylene oxide gas. Spore tests consist of strips of paper or vials that contain highly resistant bacterial spores. The CDC, American Dental Association (ADA), and Organization for Safety and Asepsis Procedures (OSAP) all highly rec-

ommend weekly spore tests for monitoring equipment. Individual state requirements should be checked. They may require weekly, monthly, or cycle-specific intervals, for instance, testing after every 30 or 40 hours of use.

Biological indicators are used in two ways: for in-office monitoring or for mail-in monitoring. In-office monitoring is more expensive and time consuming than mail-in monitoring because it involves purchasing supplies and equipment, analyzing the tests, and preparing the records. A more convenient approach is the mail-in sterilization monitoring service (Figure 17.11). The mail-in indicators come in an envelope with a control strip and a test strip. After the test strip is processed, the control and the test strip are mailed to the company, which analyzes it and sends the results immediately either through e-mail, fax, or telephone. See Procedure 17-4.

Biological indicators are placed in the sterilizer with a load of instruments and processed. The indicator is then analyzed against a control indicator. The control indicator should have growth of spores to confirm if live spores are present. The test indicator should be sterile after processing.

If a test reads positive:

- Remove sterilizer from use and review sterilization procedures (work practice and use of mechanical and chemical indicators) to determine if operator error is responsible.
- Retest sterilizer with a new biological indicator.
- If the indicator still reads positive, send sterilizer out for service maintenance.

Sterilization Documentation

It is important to keep accurate records of biological testing on the sterilizer. Check state guidelines for the length of time records must be maintained. At a minimum, documentation should include the following:

- Date and time of biological test
- Sterilizer and its identification number
- Sterilizing conditions: temperature and exposure time
- The individual conducting the test
- Results of the biological test
- Any malfunctions or repairs on the sterilizer

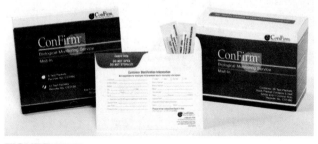

FIGURE 17.11
Mail-in biological monitoring system.
Courtesy Confirm Monitoring Systems, Inc.

Procedure 17-4 Performing Biological Monitoring

Equipment and Supplies Needed

- PPE (exam gloves, mask, protective eyewear and clothing)
- Biological indicator (spore test)
- Sterilizer bag/wrap
- Autoclave
- Sterilization monitoring log

Procedure Steps

1. Don appropriate PPE.

2. Put the biological indicator in a sterilizing bag.

3. Place in the center of the instrument load; place instrument packs in the sterilizer.

4. Process through a normal cycle.

5. Remove PPE; wash and dry hands.

6. Record date of test, type of sterilizer, temperature, time, and the name of the person doing the test.

7. When cycle is complete, remove processed biological indicator.

8. Mail processed indicator and control to the monitoring service.

9. Document results on log when received.

Legal and Ethical Issues

Read the following scenario and consider what you would do as a dental assistant.

The CDC recommends performing biological monitoring of sterilizers. OSHA recommends that this procedure be accomplished and recorded. The large dental practice where you are employed becomes short handed, so all of the instrument processing procedures are placed on one dental assistant. During a busy time, you offer to help record the recently faxed biological monitor results for the sterilizers. As you are reading the results, you notice that the results are more than one week old and one of the sterilizers has a positive report. You notice that the particular sterilizer is still being used. After informing the assistant, she tells you how busy she's been and that the positive report is probably nothing. She asks you to forget about it and to not tell anyone. She says she doesn't have time to run a new indicator. What should you do?

Answer: The lack of ethics may cause a patient to contract a disease because the sterilizer failed. Inform the assistant about the importance of biological indicators and offer to rerun the test since she is so busy. Inform the supervisor as well. Suggest that maybe a staff in-service training on the importance of the biological monitoring system might be helpful.

Always use the type of biological indicator that is compatible with the method of sterilization used. The microbes used for testing should also be stated/documented. *Geobacillus stearothermophilus* is used for the autoclave and chemical vapor sterilizers and *Bacillus subtilis* is used for the dry heat sterilizer. Check the manufacturer's instructions on the sterilizer being used.

Because instrument sterilization is the process that kills microorganisms, it is very important to ensure that the sterilizer is functioning properly. The safety of patients and dental health workers could be at risk if the testing and quality assurance of the sterilizer is not accomplished or is not accomplished properly.

CDC Guidelines for Sterilization Monitoring

Sterilization monitoring should include the use of mechanical, chemical, and biological monitors to ensure the effectiveness of the sterilization process. Mechanical techniques include monitoring the cycle time, temperature, and pressure by observing the gauges on the sterilizer and annotating these areas for each sterilizer load. Chemical indicators are used to assess the physical condition during sterilization, such as time and temperature. Biological indicators are the most widely accepted method for sterilization monitoring because they assess whether the sterilizer is killing highly resistant microorganisms. The following are basic steps from the CDC for sterilization monitoring:

1. Monitor each load with mechanical (time, temperature, and pressure) and chemical indicators.
2. Place a chemical indicator on the inside of each package and an exterior indicator if the internal one cannot be seen.
3. Place items correctly and loosely in sterilizer.
4. Do not use instrument packs if mechanical or chemical indicators indicate inadequate processing.
5. Monitor sterilizers at least weekly.

6. Use a biological indicator for every load that contains an implantable device.

7. If spore test is positive:

   a. Remove sterilizer from service and review procedures to determine error.

   b. Retest sterilizer.

   c. If results are negative, put sterilizer back into service.

8. If spore test remains positive:

   a. Do not use sterilizer until it has been inspected and test comes back negative.

Methods of Sterilization

Any item that is reusable for patient treatment must be sterilized between usage. The majority of items are heat sterilized; note, however, that some plastic items may not be heat tolerant, in which case a liquid chemical sterilant is used instead. Table 17-4 lists some of the most common heat sterilizers, which use steam, dry heat, and chemical vapors.

Steam Sterilization

A steam sterilizer or **autoclave** is used to sterilize instruments and dental items. Distilled water is used to create steam, producing a moist heat that kills microorganisms. The distilled water does not contain minerals or impurities. This helps to minimize rust and corrosion. The pressure of the machine pushes cool air out of the chamber and allows the steam to sterilize the instruments. The majority of autoclaves are set to reach maximum temperatures of 273+°F (121°C) with 15 to 30 pounds of pressure per square inch (psi). The autoclave is the most widely used sterilizer because it can sterilize a variety of dental instruments, including some plastics, handpieces, cotton rolls, and gauze. Packaging materials that work with steam include cloth, paper, nylon tubing, or wrapped metal/plastic cassettes. The main disadvantage of steam sterilization is that moisture may cause some high-carbon steel to corrode; however, the use of distilled water will minimize this and is required for most sterilizers. If rust or corrosion occurs, a rust inhibitor should be used. Foil, solid metal trays, and glass vials cannot be used in the autoclave because steam cannot penetrate through the pack to sterilize the instrument.

Loading and Unloading the Autoclave

Packages and cassettes should be loaded with space between them so the steam can penetrate to all instruments. If possible, items should be placed on their sides, not stacked on top of each other; stacking blocks the circulation of steam and can prevent air removal from the chamber (Figure 17.12).

It is important to allow instruments to dry in the steam sterilizer to maintain the sterility of the instruments. Wet packages can tear easily, causing the instruments to become contaminated. Bacteria from the air can penetrate the wet packages and be pulled into the package. This is called *wicking*.

TABLE 17-4 Heat Sterilization

Sterilizer	Temperature and Pressure	Time	Advantages	Disadvantages	Spore Test
Steam autoclave	250°F (121°C) at 15–30 psi	15–30 minutes	- Nontoxic - Time efficient - Penetrates packages	- Non–stainless steel items corrode - May damage plastics	Bacteria: *Bacillus stearothermophilus*
Statim sterilizer (autoclave)	Same as steam autoclave	3 minutes	- Quick sterilization of needed instrument	-Unwrapped or wrapped depending on the item - Must be used promptly after sterilization	Bacteria: *Bacillus stearothermophilus*
Dry heat (oven)	320°F (160°C) for 120 minutes 340°F (171°C) for 60 minutes	60–120 minutes	- No corrosion - Nontoxic - Items are dry after cycle	- Long cycle time - Door can be opened during cycle - Too hot for handpieces	Bacteria: *Bacillus subtilis*
Dry heat (rapid heat transfer)	375°F (190°C)	12 minutes wrapped; 6 minutes unwrapped	- No corrosion - Nontoxic - Time efficient	- Unwrapped items quickly contaminated after cycle	Bacteria: *Bacillus subtilis*
Chemical vapor	216°F (102°C); 270°F (132°C) is common; at 20 psi	20 minutes	- No corrosion - Time efficient	- May damage plastics - Hazardous chemical	Bacteria: *Bacillus stearothermophilus*

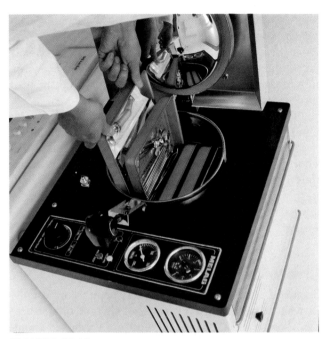

FIGURE 17.12
Assistant loading sterilizer.

Operation and Maintenance of the Autoclave

Steam sterilizers in dental offices usually have four main cycles: the heat-up cycle, the sterilizing cycle, the depressurization cycle, and finally the dry cycle. The steam is generated after the water is added, the sterilizer chamber is loaded with instrument packs, the door is closed, and the heat-up cycle starts. See Procedure 17-5.

The CDC calls for weekly monitoring of the steam sterilizer using a spore test. The inside of the steam sterilizer should be cleaned each day prior to being heated. A mild soap should be used to wash the surfaces, followed by a rinse of plain water. If this procedure is not done, minerals will collect on the chamber. Do not use any kind of abrasive cleaners on the sterilizer. Always follow the manufacturer's instructions.

Flash Sterilization

The **flash sterilization** procedure involves the use of a quick flash of heat to sterilize the instruments. It can be accomplished by steam, chemical vapor, and rapid heat transfer. Instruments may need to be unwrapped in order to be flash sterilized. Some of the newer machines, however, allow instruments to be bagged, so it is important to

Procedure 17-5 Operating the Autoclave

Equipment and Supplies Needed

- PPE (gloves, utility gloves, mask, protective eyewear and clothing)
- Autoclave
- Contaminated instruments
- Instrument lubricant
- Instrument packaging
- Distilled water
- Internal indicators

Procedure Steps

These are the general steps to operating the autoclave. Be sure, however, to check the manufacturer's instructions before proceeding because some models may not require all of these steps.

1. Don appropriate PPE (mask, eye protection, and utility gloves).

2. Lubricate instruments as needed.

3. Insert internal indicator in each package; seal package and label.

4. Remove contaminated utility gloves. Don clean exam gloves to touch the sterilizer controls.

5. Use distilled water to fill the chamber or tank up to "fill line." (Check manufacturer's instructions.)

6. Check pressure gauge to ensure it is at zero. Never open door if pressure gauge is not at zero.

7. Load autoclave with larger packages on the bottom. Don't overfill; ensure there is space between the packages so the steam can circulate.

8. Turn control valve to "fill." The chamber will fill with water.

9. Close and secure door.

10. Turn control valve to "Steam/Sterilize."

11. Pressure and temperature must be reached prior to setting the timer. (Remove PPE.)

12. After the cycle, vent the steam.

13. Allow instruments to dry and cool before removing from chamber.

14. Store cooled sterilized instruments.

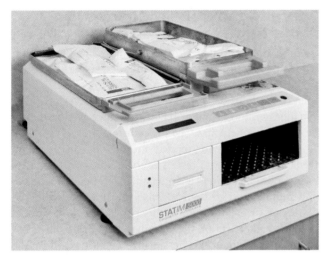

FIGURE 17.13
Sterilizer used for flash sterilization.

Preparing for Externship

Take the time to visit different dental offices and discuss and observe the instrument control practices being performed. It would also be a benefit to the dental assistant to know the information published in the CDC's *Guidelines for Infection Control in Dental Health-Care Settings.* The more information you are armed with when you go to your first dental office, the better able you will be to perform your job and ultimately help maintain the health of your patients.

follow the manufacturer's instructions. The Statim steam flash sterilizer does allow instruments to be wrapped. (Figure 17.13).

One disadvantage of flash sterilization is that as soon as unbagged instruments are removed from the sterilizer, sterility is compromised because of the bacteria and dust in the air. It is important to promptly use the instruments when removed from the sterilizer.

Dry Heat Sterilization

Dry heat sterilizers work at high temperatures (320° to 375°F) (190°C) to destroy microorganisms. Dry heat is considered safe for metal instruments because it does not dull instrument edges or corrode the instruments. Two types of dry heat sterilizers are available: static air and forced air (rapid transfer).

The static air sterilizer resembles a toaster oven. The heating coils in the bottom of the sterilizer cause the hot air to rise in the chamber. Because it is static air, it takes about one to two hours for the instruments to get hot enough to kill microorganisms; this includes the time required to warm up the sterilizer. The main disadvan-

tages of static air sterilizing are that it is very time consuming and the heat varies because the doors are not under pressure and can be opened during a cycle. Usually metal containers are used instead of paper/plastic wrapping because the sterilizer can get so hot it can melt or burn paper/plastic wrappings.

The forced air (rapid heat transfer) sterilizer uses high heat and forces it onto the instruments at a high rate of speed. This allows for quick transfer of heat, which reduces sterilizing times. Sterilization time after warm-up is 6 minutes for unpackaged instruments and 12 minutes for packaged instruments. For both methods of dry heat sterilization, the CDC recommends weekly spore testing.

Chemical Vapor Sterilization

Chemical vapor heat sterilizers (Chemiclave) usually have short sterilizing cycle times. This type of sterilization uses a special chemical solution in a closed chamber, under pressure. The hot chemical vapors kill microorganisms. The chemical contains formaldehyde (the active ingredient), ethanol acetone, ketone, water, and other alcohols. To avoid any burns or inhalation damage, the skin and eyes must be protected with the appropriate PPE. The sterilizer, if used, should be placed in a well-ventilated area away from patients. An advantage to using a chemical vapor sterilizer is that it reduces corrosion of carbon steel instruments because there is not enough water in the chemical to cause corrosion.

Chemical heat sterilizers require specific wrapping materials. Wrapped cassettes, paper/plastic peel pouches, and paper wrap are acceptable for reducing chemical absorption on the instruments. Items that are not acceptable for wrapping are closed containers, cloth, and also plastics, which might melt. Check your state guidelines for required ventilation and wrapping materials.

Operation of Chemical Heat Sterilizers

Instruments should be loaded and unloaded in the same manner as a steam sterilizer. The dental assistant should check with the manufacturer on the use of the chemical heat sterilizer. The Chemiclave goes through four different cycles: the heat-up/vaporization cycle, the sterilization cycle, the depressurization cycle, and the purge cycle. After the chemical solution is added, the instruments are loaded, the door is closed, and the heat cycle begins. The heat causes the chemical to vaporize, causing pressure in the chamber. The sterilization cycle then begins. The sterilizing temperature is maintained for at least 20 minutes. The chamber is then depressurized. Once the chamber is completely depressurized, the door is opened and the sterilizer is left to ventilate. When cooled, the instruments can be removed. See Procedure 17-6.

Procedure 17-6 Operating the Chemical Vapor Sterilizer

Equipment and Supplies Needed

- PPE (gloves, utility gloves, mask, protective eyewear and clothing)
- Contaminated instruments
- Internal indicators
- Sterilization bag/wrap
- Chemical sterilizer and chemical

Procedure Steps

1. Don appropriate PPE (mask, eye protection, and utility gloves).

2. Ensure instruments are free of debris and dry prior to packaging them.

3. Insert process indicator in package.

4. Remove contaminated utility gloves. Don clean exam gloves to touch sterilizer controls.

5. Ensure chemical is placed in the sterilizer. (Check manufacturer's instructions.)

6. Load chamber with instrument packs.

7. Set appropriate time, temperature, and pressure. (Remove PPE.)

8. Vent sterilizer.

9. Remove instruments when cool.

10. Store cooled sterilized instruments.

Chemical Solutions for Sterilization

Glutaraldehydes (liquid disinfectants) and chlorine dioxide liquids are used in dental offices and other health care facilities (Figure 17.14). The liquid chemical cannot be used for all medical materials. Certain cycle times will only disinfect, but not kill microorganisms. The liquid chemical solution is very toxic and corrosive, so it is important for the dental assistant to wear the appropriate PPE, including utility gloves. Plastic instruments that cannot be heat sterilized are usually immersed in a glutaraldehyde solution for at least 6.75 to 10 hours to kill any microorganisms. The lid must remain on the solution to prevent vapors from escaping. Instruments immersed in this solution must be rinsed with sterile water and dried with a sterile towel. Aseptic techniques must be followed.

Instrument sterility is compromised the moment it is removed from the solution. Due to this fact, it is important to handle each instrument aseptically. Immersion in liquid sterilants is not a recommended, common practice because this type of sterilization cannot be monitored. The dental assistant should maintain the solution by testing it with a chemical test kit, which is available from the manufacturer. The solution should be replaced per manufacturer's instructions, when the solution level is low, or when visibly dirty and cloudy. Once the dirty solution is discarded, rinse with a detergent and warm water, dry, and then fill with fresh solution. The wearing of the appropriate PPE during this process is important. Some of the newer models of chemical sterilizers have filtration devices that help reduce the amount of chemicals in the air. Formaldehyde monitoring badges are also available for dental health care workers who experience daily exposure to chemical sterilizers. This monitoring badge measures the exposure a dental assistant has to the

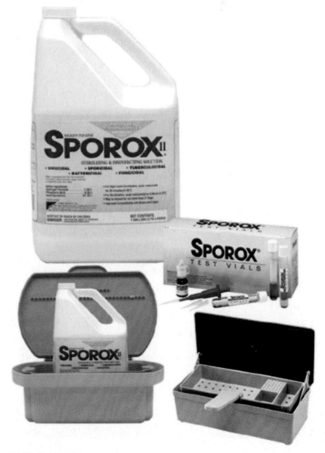

FIGURE 17.14
Sporox II high-level disinfectant/sterilant.
Courtesy Sultan Healthcare

Procedure 17-7 Sterilizing Handpieces

Equipment and Supplies Needed

- PPE (gloves, utility gloves, mask, protective eyewear and clothing)
- Moist gauze
- Handpiece lubricant
- Handpiece
- Dental unit
- Sterilization bag
- Internal indicator
- Autoclave

Procedure Steps

1. Keep the handpiece attached with bur after treatment. Don appropriate PPE (mask, eye protection, and utility gloves) and run the handpiece for 20 to 30 seconds to flush air/water lines.

2. Wipe off debris with moist gauze.

3. Clean/lubricate internal parts of handpiece. Use manufacturer's instructions for lubrication.

4. Reattach handpiece to unit; run lubricant through.

5. Insert handpiece and internal indicator in sterilizing bag. Remove contaminated utility gloves and don clean exam gloves before touching the sterilizer controls.

6. Place in autoclave or Chemiclave for the required time, temperature, and pressure.

7. Prior to using, ensure the handpiece is cool. Open the end of the bag and lubricate if recommended by manufacturer. The handpiece is now ready to use on the next patient.

---

formaldehyde. The badge is mailed to a monitoring service for determination of whether exposure is too high.

Sterilization Failures

There may be times when the sterilization process fails, and its failure is reported by the biological monitoring service. Many things can cause sterilization failure:

- Improper instrument cleaning
- Improper packaging (too much wrap)
- Improper sterilizer loading (instruments packed too tight)
- Improper timing (operator error; timing began prior to the sterilizer reaching the correct temperature)

To avoid sterilization failures, it is important for the dental assistant to follow procedures exactly.

Handpiece Sterilization

Dental handpieces need to be flushed, lubricated, and sterilized between patients. Because handpieces operate at high rates of speed, blood and saliva can get stuck in the smaller parts of the handpiece and not get cleaned properly, thus it won't get sterilized properly.

The outer shell of the handpiece should be wiped free of debris using moist, soapy gauze or alcohol gauze. A pressurized handpiece cleaner is used to flush the head of the handpiece. It is important to ensure that the handpiece has a bur in place prior to running it. However, some handpieces may not require this, so check the manufacturer's instructions first. Lubricate with the appropriate manufacturer's lubricant, dry and package the handpiece, and then sterilize it. Keeping the handpiece clean and free of debris will prolong its life.

Handpieces should only be sterilized in steam and chemical vapor sterilizers. The sterilizing temperature of the handpiece should not go above 275°F (121°C). Handpieces should be packaged in bags or wraps to protect against contamination while not in use. Avoid using the handpiece while it is still hot and avoid rapid cooldown. Rapid cooldown may stress the metal and break down the parts of the handpiece. See Procedure 17-7.

● SUMMARY

To maintain the health and safety of the dental team and patients, it is important for dental health care workers to know and understand the Centers for Disease Control and Prevention's dental infection control safety guidelines. Safety and health issues addressed by proper instrument processing include the packaging of instruments, the different types of sterilizers used in dental offices, and the methods of sterilization. The future holds many improvements in the areas of instrument processing and sterilization. Dental assistants should not only remain knowledgeable about how to properly handle and process instruments but should also stay abreast of the latest techniques and equipment used to maintain the health and safety of patients and the dental team.

● KEY TERMS

- **Autoclave:** Sterilizer that uses moist heat, under pressure. p. 264
- **Biological indicators:** Spore tests (vials or strips) that contain bacterial spores; used to determine if sterilization has occurred. p. 261
- **Critical items:** Items that penetrate soft tissue and directly contact bone, blood, and other body fluids. p. 254
- **Disinfection:** Process that prevents growth of disease-carrying microorganisms. p. 253
- **Dry heat sterilizer:** Sterilizer that uses heated, dry air to sterilize instruments. p. 266
- **Event-related sterilization:** Instrument packages that remain sterile unless an event causes contamination (i.e., wet or torn packages). p. 261
- **Flash sterilization:** Procedure that uses a quick flash of heat to sterilize instruments. p. 265
- **Holding solution:** Solution in which instruments are placed prior to placing them in an ultrasonic cleaner. p. 256

- **Noncritical items:** Items that come in contact with intact skin only. p. 254
- **Semicritical items:** Items that come in contact with tissues, but do not penetrate soft tissue or bone. p. 254
- **Sterilization:** A process that kills all living microorganisms; the ability to destroy all living organisms and endospores. p. 253
- **Time-related sterilization:** Type of sterilization in which the shelf life of instruments is identified with an exact expiration date. p. 261
- **Ultrasonic cleaner:** Cleaning system that loosens and removes debris by the use of sound waves in a liquid. p. 257
- **Washer/disinfector:** Automatic cleaning system designed to clean and disinfect instruments using a high-temperature cycle. p. 258

● CHECK YOUR UNDERSTANDING

1. Critical patient care items require
   a. cleaning.
   b. low-level disinfectant.
   c. sterilization.
   d. both a and c.

2. Which of the following is the proper way to load the autoclave?
   a. Pack instrument packages tight.
   b. Place packages on edges.
   c. Stack packages on top of one another.
   d. Sterilize one package at a time.

3. How often does the CDC recommend biological monitoring be performed?
   a. twice weekly
   b. monthly
   c. daily
   d. weekly

4. How often should the ultrasonic cleaning solution be changed?
   a. weekly
   b. twice weekly
   c. daily
   d. monthly

5. How should the dental assistant clean handpieces?
   a. Use an ultrasonic cleaner, bag, sterilize.
   b. Wipe off debris, lubricate according to manufacturer's direction, bag, sterilize.
   c. Rinse off debris in running water.
   d. Spray with disinfectant.

6. What is the procedure for handling ripped or torn sterilized instrument packages?
   a. Reclean, rebag, resterilize.
   b. Resterilize.
   c. Rebag and resterilize.
   d. None of the above.

7. Which type of sterilization is appropriate for handpieces?
   a. steam
   b. dry heat
   c. chemical liquid
   d. both a and b

8. Which of the following indicators ensure that sterilization has occurred?
   a. biological indicator
   b. internal process indicator
   c. mechanical indicator
   d. all of the above

9. The most effective way to clean instruments is with
   a. an ultrasonic cleaner.
   b. a washer/disinfector.
   c. hand scrubbing.
   d. both a and b.

10. Which type of gloves should be used when handling contaminated instruments?
    a. utility gloves
    b. exam gloves
    c. sterile gloves
    d. none of the above

⊙ INTERNET ACTIVITY

- Search the Organization for Safety and Asepsis website (www.osap.org) to research and learn more about current issues related to infection control.

⊙ WEB REFERENCES

- American Dental Association www.ada.org
- Centers for Disease Control and Prevention www.cdc.gov
- Infection Control Today www.infectioncontroltoday.com
- Occupational Safety and Health Administration www.osha.gov
- The Organization for Safety and Asepsis www.osap.org

18
Occupational Health and Safety

Learning Objectives

After reading this chapter, the student should be able to:

- Differentiate standards, regulations, and recommendations.

- Discuss the complementary roles of OSHA, the FDA, and the EPA.

- Explain how chemical exposure occurs and can cause harm.

- Describe the purpose and provisions of the Hazard Communication standard.

- List specific potential hazards found in dental practices.

- Explain information typically found on a hazardous material label.

- Identify the types of waste generated in a dental practice.

- Describe proper disposal procedures for waste found in dental practices.

Chapter Outline

- Types of Safety Standards
  —Regulatory Agencies
  —Advisory Agencies

- Hazardous Chemicals
  —Chemical Exposure
  —Hazard Communication Program
  —Achieving Safety Through Personal Action

- Waste Handling and Disposal

Preparing for Certification Exams

- Follow the standards and guidelines of occupational safety for dental office personnel, including those in the Hazard Communication standard by OSHA.

- Properly store, prepare, and use hazardous materials in accordance with the manufacturer's directions and in compliance with the OSHA Hazard Communication standard.

- Protect the patient and operator through the use of barrier techniques and safety equipment.

- Properly dispose of regulated waste generated in the dental office.

Key Terms

Compliance

Contaminated waste

Hazard Communication standard

Hazardous waste

Infectious waste

Material Safety Data Sheet (MSDS)

Recommendation

Regulated waste

Regulation

Standard

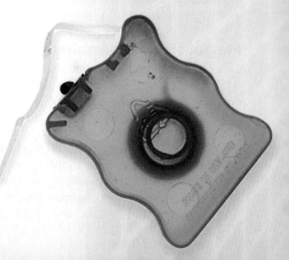

The most important safety

component in the dental office is each staff member's personal commitment to accept and practice safety standards and procedures. The dental assistant's commitment is particularly important because it is usually the assistant who prepares dental operatories, processes contaminated instruments, and maintains equipment.

Dentists often recognize the vital role assistants play in maintaining safety by designating a dental assistant to oversee the office safety program. Safety is maintained in two ways: development of **standards** that promote safety and practice of safe procedures. Standards and procedures are interdependent. Standards are designed to promote the use of safe procedures, just as safe procedures must be followed to ensure safety.

Types of Safety Standards

There are two types of standards: regulations and recommendations. **Regulations** are official standards of government agencies such as licensing boards. By law, regulations must be followed. Dental practices that are not in compliance with safety regulations are subject to enforcement through such means as fines, license suspension or revocation, or imprisonment.

Recommendations are official statements of government, professional, or voluntary agencies that provide guidelines for best practices. They offer advice based on evidence from the best available research. Compliance is voluntary. Although these types of safety standards are only advisory, most dental practices do comply with recommendations made by respected agencies such as the Centers for Disease Control and Prevention (CDC) and the American Dental Association (ADA) in order to provide the greatest safety for employees and patients.

Regulatory Agencies

The Occupational Safety and Health Administration (OSHA) promotes and enforces workplace standards designed to protect the health and safety of workers in the United States. Although OSHA regulations impact a wide range of physical, chemical, and infectious hazards, two standards related to the daily practice of dentistry are of particular importance to the dental assistant. The Bloodborne Pathogen standard (Standard 29 CFR 1910.1030) sets forth regulations designed to prevent

---

Dental Assistant   PROFESSIONAL TIP
Organize the tasks you perform to maintain office health and safety into a written one-page calendar format and then laminate it. In a busy professional office this will provide a quick reference you can use to ensure that you have remembered everything, to teach new dental assistants what needs to be done, and to educate patients who have read articles or seen television or Internet programs that raise dental office safety questions. Because the sheet is laminated it can be disinfected and used repeatedly.

disease transmission (see Chapter 12). The Hazard Communication standard (Standard 29 CFR 1910.1200) sets forth regulations to protect workers from such workplace hazards as chemical exposure and physical injury.

OSHA federally regulates all states; however, a state may develop and administer its own OSHA program. To operate its own program, the state must meet or exceed federal standards and receive OSHA approval. As of 2008, 25 states and territories administered and operated their own programs. It is important for the dental assistant to know whether there is a state or territorial OSHA program operating where the dental practice is located. Practices in such states must meet both federal and state OSHA requirements. Table 18-1 lists the states and territories with approved programs.

OSHA enforces its standards through an investigative and sanctions process. OSHA investigators have authority to enter a workplace and assess whether it is in **compliance** with the standards. If a dental practice is not in compliance, a citation may be issued for each violation. OSHA also has the authority to close the workplace if unsafe conditions are not corrected as specified. Most dental office inspections occur because an employee or patient files a complaint, randomly for a dental office with 11 or more employees, or by request of a dentist for a consultation visit.

When possible, OSHA inspectors prefer to assist dental practices to achieve compliance rather than issue citations for violations. Practices are cited when they do not achieve compliance by stated deadlines. To assist

TABLE 18-1 States and Territories with Federally Approved OSHA Programs

Alaska	Kentucky	New York*	Utah
Arizona	Maryland	North Carolina	Vermont
California	Michigan	Oregon	Virgin Islands
Connecticut*	Minnesota	Puerto Rico	Virginia
Hawaii	Nevada	South Carolina	Washington
Indiana	New Mexico	Tennessee	Wyoming
Iowa			

*For state and local government employees only.

practices in achieving compliance, OSHA provides free information about workplace hazards and safety procedures, general assistance, record-keeping guidelines, and posters and copies of the expected minimum standards.

The Environmental Protection Agency (EPA) issues regulations to protect human and environmental health. The EPA has a wide-ranging mission but its principal association with dentistry is twofold. It ensures the safety and effectiveness of disinfectants as part of its pesticide program, and it regulates waste materials, such as amalgam scrap, chemicals, and medical waste. The EPA regulates waste from the point of generation to the point of final disposal. Every handler, including the dental office, is responsible for ensuring proper final disposal.

To dispose of hazardous waste properly, dental offices hire hazardous waste disposal companies. It is extremely important for a dental office to hire a reputable hazardous waste disposal contractor. When waste is improperly discarded, the EPA has the authority to enforce site cleanup, disposal under acceptable conditions, and, when indicated, impose fines or file criminal complaints. Cleanup can cost many times the amount that would have been paid originally to dispose of the waste properly. Additionally, should a criminal complaint result, the negative effect on a dentist's reputation is a huge liability to the practice.

The Food and Drug Administration (FDA) regulates areas such as food, drugs, and medical/dental devices. In dentistry, items such as sterilizers, biological and chemical indicators, ultrasonic cleaners, dental units, personal protective equipment, and radiography equipment must be approved by the FDA. The FDA is responsible for reviewing the safety and effectiveness of the products it oversees, regulating their labeling, and ensuring that claims on the product labels are true.

Overall, OSHA, the FDA, and the EPA have complementary missions. OSHA seeks to protect the health and safety of employees, the FDA works to protect the health and safety of patients and the general public, and the EPA acts to protect the environment.

What responsibility does the dental assistant have in reporting any unsafe working conditions?

Advisory Agencies

Various advisory agencies provide recommendations for the best practices to protect both dental professionals and patients. These recommended practices are based on research that indicates how the best practices make a difference in patient and employee safety.

Government Advisory Agencies

The Centers for Disease Control and Prevention issues recommendations regarding best practices to protect human health and prevent disease. The CDC's 2003 *Guidelines for Infection Control in Dental Health-Care Settings* established the infection control procedures currently used in dental offices. The guidelines also discuss best practices for handling chemicals used in infection control procedures and other hazards such as injection needles. Even though the CDC does not have the authority to make laws or issue regulations, its recommendations are very influential.

The National Institute for Occupational Safety and Health (NIOSH) is a component of the CDC. NIOSH is responsible for conducting research; providing guidance, information, and services; and making recommendations for the prevention of work-related injury and illness. NIOSH and OSHA often work together toward the common goal of protecting worker safety and health. As a component of the CDC, when requested, NIOSH also cooperates with other injury and illness prevention organizations nationally and internationally to advance worker safety.

Professional Organizations and Association Advisory Agencies

The American Dental Association is a professional association of dentists and other dental personnel that advocates in the interest of public oral health and the dental profession. In service of this mission, it reviews and supports oral health research, accredits dental and allied dental education programs, and develops policies and recommendations related to oral health issues. The ADA publishes its findings, standards, and policies and serves as a resource for the dental profession and the public.

The ADA cooperates with the American National Standards Institute (ANSI) and the International Standards Organization (ISO) to develop and disseminate standards for dental materials. It also operates the ADA Acceptance Program. Manufacturers voluntarily submit information concerning a product's safety and effectiveness. The ADA Council on Scientific Affairs studies the safety, efficacy, and promotional claims for the product. A product deemed to be safe and effective earns the ADA Seal of Acceptance®. Manufacturers of accepted products can inform potential buyers of the product's acceptance through use of the acceptance seal on packaging and in advertisements. Both the public and dental personnel rely on the seal as an indicator of quality for products sold over the counter without a prescription.

The Organization for Safety and Asepsis Procedures (OSAP) is a global nonprofit association of dental professionals. It is dedicated to promoting oral health infection control and safety news, policies, and resources that are supported by evidence-based research. OSAP provides helpful publications, educational tools and programs, and answers to infection control and safety questions. OSAP also helps educators, researchers, companies, and patients with their dental infection control and safety needs.

The CRA Foundation (Clinical Research Associates) is a nonprofit national dental organization that evaluates dental materials, devices, and concepts for effectiveness and clinical usefulness. It conducts clinical and in-house research, publishes its findings in a monthly newsletter, and provides training courses for dentists and staff members. General practice dental personnel rely heavily on the information in the CRA newsletter and courses as a guide to what other clinicians are experiencing as they use particular materials and devices and to keep abreast of recent trends in material and device usage.

The American Dental Assistants Association (ADAA) represents professional dental assistants. It cooperates with other dental-related organizations to promote health and safety for dental assistants and the public.

State and local dental associations, including dental assisting societies, are often helpful in complying with regulatory issues that are specific to a particular area or state. These organizations can answer questions, work with a dental practice, and in some instances offer liaison to regulatory agencies. Table 18-2 summarizes agency and organization roles in promoting dental practice safety.

How can a professional dental assistant keep abreast of changes in regulations and recommendations regarding the safety of patients and the dental team?

Hazardous Chemicals

Dental practices use a variety of chemicals that can be hazardous. Chemicals can be hazardous because they are highly reactive, toxic, carcinogenic, corrosive, contaminated, combustible, or degraded. Highly reactive chemicals are unstable. An unstable chemical may combine with another chemical to create an unplanned hazard. Toxic chemicals are poisonous. Carcinogenic chemicals contribute to the development of cancer. Corrosive chemicals eat away other substances, such as tooth surfaces, restorative materials, soft tissue, equipment, countertops, and gloves. Contaminated chemicals contain infectious microorganisms and may spread disease. Combustible chemicals may burst into flame or explode.

Degraded chemicals have deteriorated in quality. A degraded chemical may be less effective or form hazardous by-products. Chemical degradation may be caused by exposure to:

TABLE 18-2 Summary of Agency Roles in Safety Assurance

Agency Acronym	Safety Role
ADA	Advocacy, standards, policies, recommendations, and programs to safeguard public oral health; administer Acceptance Program for over-the-counter products
ADAA	Advice, assistance, and advocacy for dental assistants
CDC	Recommendations for best practices to protect human health and prevent disease
CRA	Clinical evaluation of dental materials and devices; education of dental personnel
EPA	Regulations to safeguard the environment
FDA	Regulations to protect patients and the public
NIOSH	Recommendations to prevent work-related injury and illness
OSAP	Promote use of evidence-based dental infection control and safety procedures; educate dental personnel
OSHA	Regulations to promote worker safety

- Heat,
- Cold,
- Light,
- Moisture, and
- Storage of the chemical beyond its expected shelf life.

Chemical Exposure

There are two types of chemical exposure: acute and chronic. Acute exposure is exposure to a large amount of a chemical in a short time period. Chronic exposure is repeated exposure to a small amount of a chemical over a long time. What constitutes a large or small amount is dependent on the chemical under consideration. Whether a material actually causes harm depends on how readily it can cause damage, the exposed individual's susceptibility to it, the route of exposure, and the type and amount of exposure received. Chemicals can enter the body through inhalation, ingestion, or contact with the skin or mucous membrane.

Caustic agents (e.g., phenol) are strong acids or bases that can cause corrosion, irritation, and severe burns. They can enter the body by direct contact, inhalation, or ingestion. The initial sign of skin injury from phenol is whitening. This is later followed by deep damage. Caustics may be strong enough to eat through clothing and shoe leather; extreme care should be exercised when they are used. If phenol is accidentally spilled on the skin or splashed in the eye, the area should be immediately flushed with water for 20 to 30 minutes and any contaminated clothing should be discarded. Caustics should be stored in closed containers in a segregated area.

Hazard Communication Program

OSHA Standard 29 CFR 1910.1200, the **Hazard Communication standard,** sets forth regulations for safe handling of chemicals. This standard is often called the "Right to Know" law. It operates on the assumption that employees should know the hazards posed by any chemicals being used and how to minimize the hazards by handling all chemicals safely.

The standard requires the chemical manufacturer or importer to evaluate the hazards of any chemicals it sells and inform employers of the hazards. Responsibility for ensuring employee knowledge is placed on the employer. The employer must have or provide:

- Written policies and procedures that are accessible to all employees who have actual or potential exposure to chemicals.
- A comprehensive, current inventory of all chemicals used in the workplace.
- A complete file of current **Material Safety Data Sheets (MSDSs)**. Some manufacturers have MSDSs for all of their products. An MSDS is a written document that provides comprehensive information about a single chemical. Manufacturers are required to provide current English-language MSDSs to material purchasers. Figure 18.1 shows a sample MSDS.

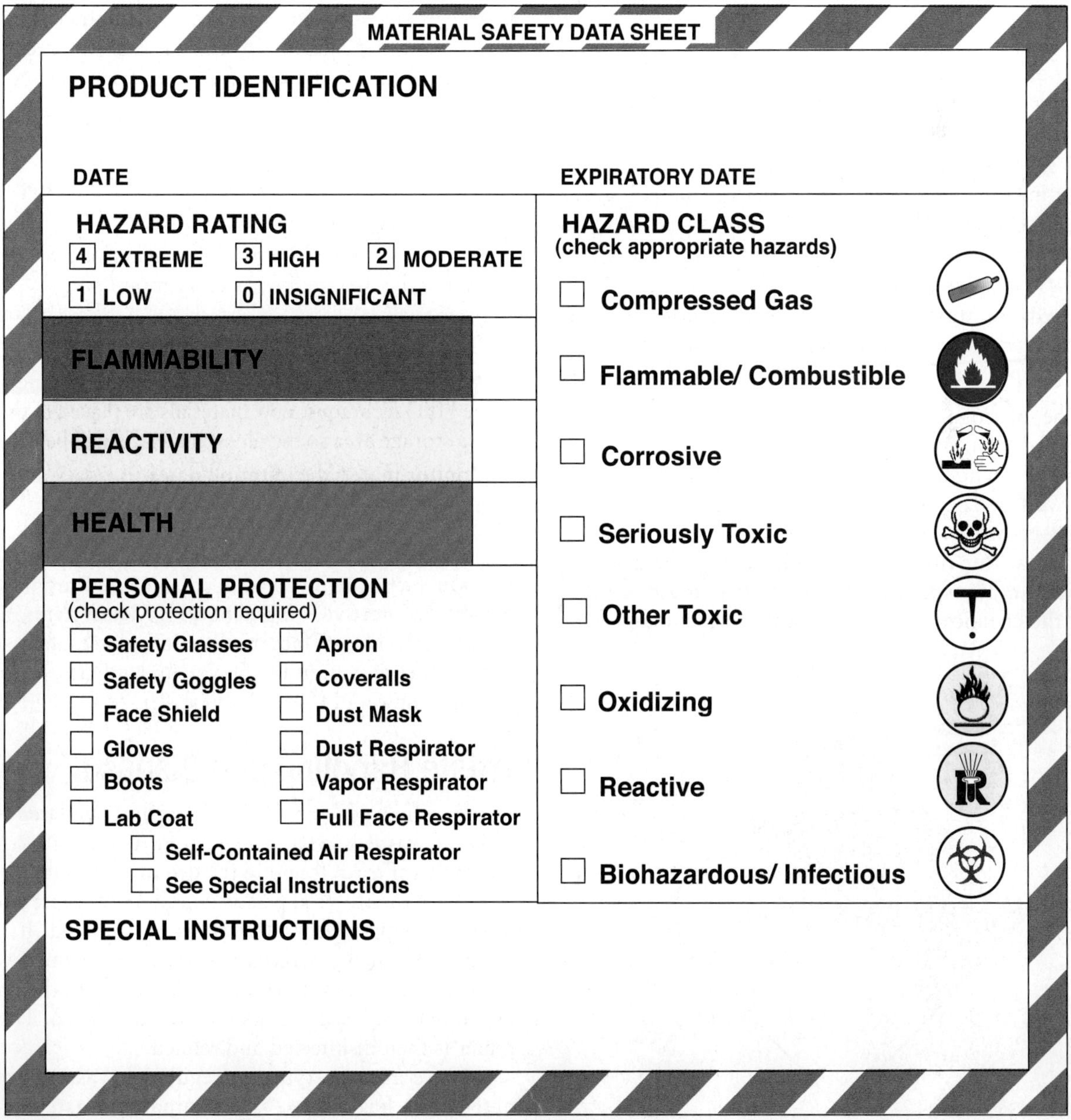

MATERIAL SAFETY DATA SHEET

PRODUCT IDENTIFICATION

DATE

EXPIRATORY DATE

HAZARD RATING

4 EXTREME 3 HIGH 2 MODERATE

1 LOW 0 INSIGNIFICANT

FLAMMABILITY

REACTIVITY

HEALTH

HAZARD CLASS
(check appropriate hazards)

- ☐ Compressed Gas
- ☐ Flammable/ Combustible
- ☐ Corrosive
- ☐ Seriously Toxic
- ☐ Other Toxic
- ☐ Oxidizing
- ☐ Reactive
- ☐ Biohazardous/ Infectious

PERSONAL PROTECTION
(check protection required)

- ☐ Safety Glasses
- ☐ Safety Goggles
- ☐ Face Shield
- ☐ Gloves
- ☐ Boots
- ☐ Lab Coat
- ☐ Apron
- ☐ Coveralls
- ☐ Dust Mask
- ☐ Dust Respirator
- ☐ Vapor Respirator
- ☐ Full Face Respirator
- ☐ Self-Contained Air Respirator
- ☐ See Special Instructions

SPECIAL INSTRUCTIONS

FIGURE 18.1
An example of a Material Safety Data Sheet (MSDS).

- Legible, English-language labeling of chemicals that informs employees of specified hazards and how to contact the manufacturer.
- Training of employees in proper storage, handling, and disposal of chemicals used in the workplace on initial assignment to the work area and when materials or procedures are changed.
- Records of training session agendas, attendees and their workplace titles, topics covered (including site-specific practices), and the qualifications of the trainer.

The National Fire Protection Association (NFPA) developed a hazardous chemical labeling system to provide a quick readout of the important hazard information in an MSDS. The system uses colored, diamond-shaped symbols to denote specific types of hazards (Figure 18.2). Numbers within the diamonds indicate the extent of each hazard and any special precautions that must be taken when the chemical is handled. Table 18-3 explains what

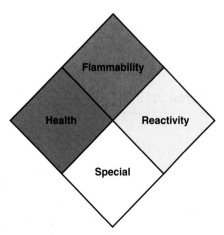

FIGURE 18.2
National Fire Protection Association hazard communication label.

the different colors and numbers on a hazardous materials label mean.

What responsibility does the dental assistant have when it comes to safety in the dental office?

Achieving Safety Through Personal Action

Nearly every procedure in dentistry requires the use of a material; some require several materials. Materials can be single chemicals or chemical combinations. The dental assistant must learn to practice safe material storage, handling, and disposal as a routine part of everyday dental assisting practice. Dental assistants are usually in charge of inventory control in the dental office. They prevent material problems by taking specific precautions. Dental assistants routinely perform these tasks:

- Read MSDSs to learn how to store, handle, and dispose of each material properly.
- Exercise care when using any material in the mouth.
- Practice rigorous infection control.
- Purchase only the amount of a material that can reasonably be used before its expiration date.
- Store materials in a cool, dry, dark area unless the MSDS for a specific material directs otherwise.
- Use "first in, first out" (FIFO) storage techniques. With the FIFO technique, new materials are placed in the back of a storage area so the oldest materials will be used first.
- Monitor material expiration dates.
- Discard expired materials.

To shield themselves from chemical exposure, dental assistants who are involved in patient care routinely wear personal protective equipment (PPE). These items include a uniform, lab coat, face mask, safety glasses, face shield, patient care gloves, utility gloves, and goggles. (For more information on PPE see Chapter 12.)

Waste Handling and Disposal

Dental offices generate both general and regulated waste. General waste is what a layperson would call "trash." Examples of trash found in the dental office include such items as paper towels, plastic cups, patient bibs, and disinfectant wipes. General waste is unregulated. It is collected in a sturdy, covered waste container lined with a bag that is impervious to fluids. At the end of the day the bag is removed, securely closed, and discarded. The container is then disinfected and relined.

There are two types of **regulated waste**: contaminated and hazardous. **Contaminated waste** includes infectious waste and sharps. **Infectious waste** consists of blood and body fluids and other potentially infec-

TABLE 18-3 Decoding a Hazardous Materials Label

Diamond Color	Hazard	Number	Information Indicated
Red	Fire	0	Does not burn
		1	Burns at temperatures above 200°F
		2	Burns at temperatures below 200°F
		3	Burns at temperatures below 100°F
		4	Burns at temperatures below 73°F
Blue	Health	0	Normal material
		1	Slightly hazardous
		2	Hazardous
		3	Extreme danger
		4	Deadly
Yellow	Reactivity	0	Stable
		1	Unstable if heated
		2	Violent chemical change
		3	Shock and heat may detonate
		4	May detonate spontaneously
White	Special precautions	OXY	Oxidizer
		ALK	Alkaline
		W/	Use no water
		ACID	Acid
		COR	Corrosive
			Radioactive

Life Span Considerations

Children may be fearful of the PPE a dental assistant wears; elderly patients may believe it is unnecessary. Adult patients may be fearful that the chemicals in dental amalgam will cause cancer or that fluoride is dangerous or that anything dental personnel will not directly touch should not be used on the tissues. Regardless of age, any patient who has safety concerns should receive a calm reply. The basic principles of patient management—validation of the patient's concerns, provision of correct information, response to what is really being said rather than simply the words spoken, and distraction of children when indicated—can be used with patients of all ages. The office safety procedures must remain unchanged, but the dental assistant's responses should leave the patient feeling fortunate the dentist and dental assistant provide only services research has shown to be safe and effective, and keep up with new procedures that increase patient and personnel safety.

tious material (OPIM). OPIM are defined by the CDC as follows:

- The following human bodily fluids: semen, vaginal secretions, cerebrospinal fluid, synovial fluid, pleural fluid, pericardial fluid, peritoneal fluid, amniotic fluid, saliva in dental procedures, any bodily fluid that is visibly contaminated with blood, and all bodily fluids in situations where it is difficult or impossible to differentiate between body fluids.

- Any unfixed tissue or organ (other than intact skin) from a human (living or dead). HIV-containing cell or tissue cultures, organ cultures, and human immunodeficiency virus (HIV)-containing or hepatitis B virus (HBV)-containing culture medium or other solutions; and blood, organs, or other tissues from experimental animals infected with HIV or HBV. (Dental offices do not handle all of these items, so dental OPIMs are often defined as blood and blood-stained materials, and pathological waste such as extracted teeth or excised tissue. Sharps include needles, orthodontic wires, and broken glass.)

Professionalism

Think about the many safety skills and attitudes you developed in the initial weeks of your education program that will help you fit seamlessly into a professional environment. From day 1 of your externship your sparkling cleanliness, neatness, professional attire, orderly manner of working, correct use of PPE, and conscientious performance of expected safety procedures will demonstrate that you accept your professional responsibility for helping to maintain patient and personnel health and safety.

A cheerful willingness to clearly answer patients' questions about safety standards and procedures will help you earn and keep their trust. Enthusiasm for communication of the values that underlie safety procedures helps create bridges that tell your patients you care.

Proper storage, handling, and disposal of hazardous materials, rigorous infection control, ensuring the water used in treatment is of acceptable quality, and knowing which document or organization to consult for safety advice enables your dental office to have confidence in and depend on you. Safety knowledge and skills quietly promote the professionalism of both you and the dental office in which you work.

- Infectious waste may be autoclaved and then treated as noninfectious.
- Sharps are disposed of whole and unbent in dedicated, puncture-proof, closable red containers marked with a biohazard symbol and located as close as possible to the area of use (Figure 18.3). They should be closed between uses. When a container is three-quarters full, it is sealed and sent to a sharps waste contractor for proper disposal.

Hazardous waste consists of hazardous and toxic chemicals and materials. Disposal procedures vary depending on which chemical is involved:

- The appropriate MSDS must be consulted for information regarding safe disposal of a particular chemical.
- Regardless of the disposal procedures required, all hazardous chemicals must be packaged in secure, leakproof containers, and labeled with the standard hazardous symbol and the name of the chemical (Figure 18.4).

Some waste items, amalgam scrap or an extracted tooth with an amalgam restoration, for example, may be both potentially infectious and hazardous. They are considered hazardous because they contain mercury. Amalgam scrap should be stored in a closed, unbreakable container labeled "Hazardous: Contains Mercury" and recycled. The scrap is potentially infectious if it has been in the mouth or recovered from a chairside wastewater line. Both the contaminated amalgam scrap and the extracted tooth would be classified as OPIM and hazardous. Neither the scrap nor the tooth can be autoclaved because that would generate hazardous mercury fumes. To address this hazard a two-step process is used: disinfection followed by shipment to a hazardous waste contractor for processing.

Disposing of hazardous waste can be costly. It is advisable to minimize the amount of hazardous waste the office generates. To accomplish this, the first rule is not to mix different waste materials. Dental practices typically hire waste contractors to properly dispose of hazardous mate-

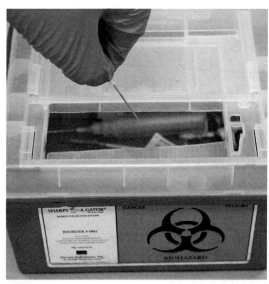

FIGURE 18.3
Biohazard container used for sharps.

HAZARDOUS WASTE

FEDERAL LAW PROHIBITS IMPROPER DISPOSAL

IF FOUND, CONTACT THE NEAREST POLICE OR PUBLIC SAFETY AUTHORITY OR THE U.S. ENVIRONMENTAL PROTECTION AGENCY OR THE CALIFORNIA DEPARTMENT OF TOXIC SUBSTANCE CONTROL.

GENERATOR INFORMATION:
NAME ____
ADDRESS ____ PHONE ____
CITY ____ STATE ____ ZIP ____
EPA ID NO. / MANIFEST DOCUMENT NO. ____
EPA WASTE NO. ____ CA. WASTE NO. ____ ACCUMULATION START DATE ____
CONTENTS COMPOSITION ____

PHYSICAL STATE ☐ SOLID ☐ LIQUID | HAZARDOUS PROPERTIES ☐ FLAMMABLE ☐ TOXIC ☐ CORROSIVE ☐ REACTIVITY ☐ OTHER ____

D.O.T. PROPER SHIPPING NAME AND UN OR NA NO. WITH PREFIX

HANDLE WITH CARE!

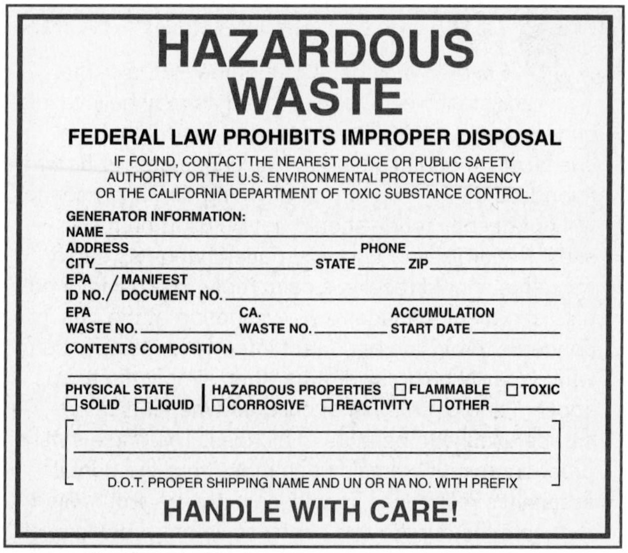

FIGURE 18.4
A hazardous material label must be attached to all hazardous waste containers.

TABLE 18-4 Dental Practice Waste Streams

X-Ray/ Photography	Office	Medicaments	Sterilants	Restorative Materials
Developer	Paper	Anesthetics	Cleaners	Amalgam
Fixer	Cardboard	Antibiotics	Disinfectants	Composites
Machine cleaners	Toner	Analgesics	Detergents	Bonding agents
Lead foil	Electronic devices	Administration equipment	Sterilants	Cements
Spent film	Ink cartridges		Water treatment chemicals	

rials. Prior to disposing of the waste, the hazardous waste contractor must separate mixed materials before processing them. The separation step is an additional, unnecessary expense that should be avoided if possible.

It is also helpful to separate the different waste streams. Waste streams are groups of hazardous materials normally generated from different types of tasks. For example, radiography procedures repeatedly generate developer, fixer, and film waste if chemical developing is used in the office. Table 18-4 gives a summary of the waste streams potentially generated in a dental office.

Each state may regulate disposal of particular types of waste even though the federal government does not. Different states may have very different policies and procedures. It is important to follow both state and federal waste disposal regulations.

How could you learn whether computers and printers used in the dental office for which you work are considered hazardous waste in your state?

Cultural Considerations

Safe interactions with dental patients from cultural backgrounds that are different from those of the office staff must encompass all areas, particularly communication. Visiting the dentist can actually be dangerous for patients who do not speak the same language as the office personnel. Consider the patient who speaks only Spanish who is receiving postoperative directions from a dental assistant who speaks only English. The directions are for the patient to take a particular medication once per day. In Spanish *once* means 11. A potentially serious, even deadly, situation could result from the patient's ingestion of massive doses of the prescribed chemical.

Patients must receive information they can understand. If your office does not have bilingual personnel on hand, using information from the Internet such as the information found at (www.freetranslation.com/) or (www.languageline.com/page/industry_healthcare/) can be helpful. Better yet, once you are settled in an office, identify the non-English language most commonly spoken in your area and enroll in classes to become bilingual.

SUMMARY

The dental assistant handles many potentially hazardous chemicals while providing dental assisting services. When stored, transported, used, and disposed of correctly, the materials used in dentistry are safe. The key is knowledge. Federal and state OSHA, FDA, and EPA programs provide a template of regulations. Other federal agencies and professional and voluntary organizations, such as the CDC, NIOSH, ADA, and OSAP, provide additional insight into the practices that help to ensure dental patient and personnel safety. Organizations, websites, publications, and personal consultants are available to provide help on such diverse topics as infection control, safe use of chemicals, proper storage and disposal of waste, and general issues of occupational health and safety. Regulatory agencies set forth rules and regulations that must be followed.

The dental assistant needs to learn as much as possible about the standards and best practices, then regularly complete safety procedures to implement them. It is the actual practice of specific procedures recommended for safe use of specific materials and devices that results in safety for dental patients and personnel.

◉ KEY TERMS

- **Compliance:** Adherence to official standards. p. 272
- **Contaminated waste:** Regulated waste that is potentially infectious and/or sharp. p. 276
- **Hazard Communication standard:** Statement of OSHA regulations regarding how the employer must protect employee health if hazardous chemicals are used in the workplace. p. 275
- **Hazardous waste:** Chemical waste that is potentially harmful to humans or the environment because it is highly reactive, toxic, corrosive, contaminated, combustible, carcinogenic, or degraded. p. 278
- **Infectious waste:** Regulated waste that has been in contact with blood or other body fluids. p. 276

- **Material Safety Data Sheet (MSDS):** Written document that provides comprehensive information about a chemical and information about how to contact its manufacturer. p. 275
- **Recommendation:** Official public or private agency statement of the best way to comply with a regulation. p. 272
- **Regulated waste:** Infectious, sharp, or hazardous waste. p. 276
- **Regulation:** Official government agency rule that must be followed. p. 272
- **Standard:** Official government agency statement of the regulations governing a specified issue. p. 272

◉ CHECK YOUR UNDERSTANDING

1. In what waste classification would you place blood-soaked, 2 × 2 gauze squares and what would that mean regarding how you should dispose of them?
   a. general waste—discard in closed, fluid-impervious bag
   b. hazardous waste—consult appropriate MSDS and follow its waste disposal directions
   c. OPIM—package, seal, autoclave, then treat as general waste
   d. both hazardous waste and OPIM—disinfect, then process as hazardous waste

2. As you are reviewing your patient's medical history you note that she is allergic to latex and many plastics. You are scheduled to take an impression for her. How can you determine whether it is safe for you to take the impression?
   a. Ask the office manager if you will incur any liability.
   b. Check ADA policies regarding use of the material.
   c. Ensure the material has FDA approval.
   d. Consult the MSDS for the material.

3. Your dentist employer has asked you to find out if a new material being considered for purchase is "accepted." Which of the following organizations' websites would you consult?
   a. CDC
   b. ADA
   c. NIOSH
   d. OSAP

4. You are checking your materials inventory to determine which ones can no longer be safely used. The items on hand include those listed below. If all dates refer to this year, which items should be discarded?

Material	Expiration Date
Alginate impression material	June 16
Impregum polyether impression material	May 12
Express vinyl impression material	August 4
Permlastic rubber base impression material	January 9
Alginot impression material	November 25

   a. Permlastic only
   b. Permlastic and Impregum
   c. Permlastic, Impregum, and alginate
   d. Permlastic, Impregum, alginate, and Express
   e. All materials with expiration dates through today.

5. The hazard label for the material you will be using in an upcoming procedure has a "1" in the yellow diamond. What precaution should be taken?
   a. Wear a sturdy respirator.
   b. Do not shake the material.
   c. Keep the material away from heat.
   d. Avoid using water near the material.

6. The safety of dental materials used in patient treatment is the legal responsibility of this agency.
   a. FDA
   b. ADA
   c. ISO
   d. OSHA

7. The purpose of using a safety labeling system for dental materials is to provide
   a. comprehensive information about a material.
   b. rapid, understandable information about a material.

CHECK YOUR UNDERSTANDING (continued)

c. a reliable means of locating information about the manufacturer.

d. warning information to prevent allergic reactions to the material.

8. The MSDS you have just consulted states the material in question should be stored away from light and heat. What chemical problem is this designed to prevent?
   a. dilution
   b. contamination
   c. corrosion
   d. degradation

9. Assume your state has a voluntary recycling program for paper and cardboard. What is this program?
   a. regulatory
   b. recommended

c. advised

d. cannot answer without more information

10. Which TWO requirements below must a state OSHA program meet?
    a. The state program must meet or exceed federal OSHA standards.
    b. The state program must be linked to a state EPA program.
    c. The state must agree to staff federal OSHA positions in the area.
    d. The state program must be approved by the federal OSHA agency.

INTERNET ACTIVITY

- As a professional dental assistant you will be responsible for educating patients about the correct use of commercial denture cleansers. Denture cleansers are hazardous materials. They are not expected to be used internally, but sometimes are, with disastrous results. Go online and locate the document entitled *Using Dental Cleansers Safely*. This information sheet will provide tips regarding what you need to teach your patients who use denture cleansers on how to use them safely. Start at www.fda.gov. To reach the document, remember you are searching for information about a device and dental practices.

WEB REFERENCES

- Centers for Disease Control and Prevention www.cdc.gov
- Food and Drug Administration www.fda.gov
- Environmental Protection Agency www.epa.gov
- Occupational Safety and Health Administration www.osha.gov
- National Institute of Dental and Craniofacial Research www.nidcr.nih.gov
- National Institutes of Health www.nih.gov

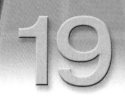

19

Dental Unit Waterlines

Learning Objectives

After reading this chapter, the student should be able to:

- Discuss how water is used during dental treatment.
- State the amount of bacteria allowed in drinking water compared to the recommended amount allowed in dental unit waterlines.
- Define biofilm and explain who may be at risk of infection from pathogenic microbes.
- List the unique properties of dental waterlines that encourage bacterial growth.
- Explain various methods for reducing bacterial contamination in dental waterlines.

Preparing for Certification Exams

- Perform sterilization and disinfection procedures.

Key Terms

Adhere

Biofilm

Colony-forming units (CFUs)

Immunocompromised

Laminar flow

Pathogens

Slime layer

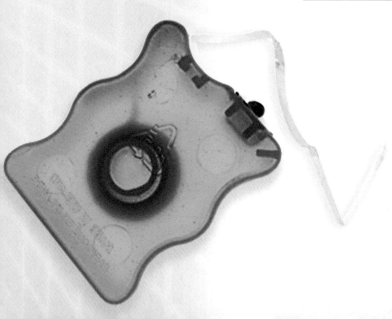

The oral health professions have traditionally assumed responsibility for assessing and improving the quality of health care provided to patients. Dental staff members should be familiar with the issue of dental unit waterline contamination and be prepared to discuss the issue with patients. Bacteria are a very persistent life-form. In their evolution bacteria have developed successful strategies for survival, including the ability to attach to surfaces and develop environments that allow them to grow and thrive. Dental unit waterlines present an ideal atmosphere in which bacterial colonies can grow.

There is currently no definable public health problem resulting from the presence of disease-producing microorganisms, called **pathogens,** in dental waterlines. However, the proven existence of disease-producing microorganisms and their by-products supports the dental industry's objective of improving water quality. Techniques already exist and more are being developed to help reduce bacterial growth in plumbing systems and dental unit waterlines. Dental assistants are responsible for following the standard procedures for maintenance and monitoring of water delivery systems set by the dental facility that employs them.

Introduction to Dental Unit Waterlines

Dental unit waterlines supply the water used during dental treatment (Figure 19.1). The water is used most often in high-speed handpieces, the air/water syringe, and the ultrasonic scaling unit. Water both cools and helps clear away debris when a tooth is being prepared for a restoration.

Standards for safe drinking water quality are established by different agencies, including the Environmental Protection Agency (EPA). Normal drinking water is usually allowed to have up to 500 **colony-forming units**

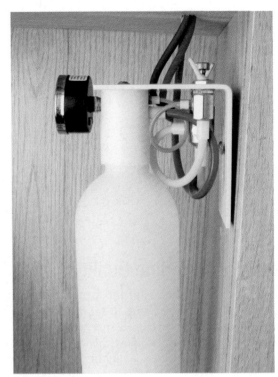

FIGURE 19.1
Dental waterline tubing.

(CFUs) of bacteria per milliliter; often, though, water pipes in homes are found to have many times that amount due to colonization of microorganisms. Water coming into buildings from city water supplies or wells is not sterile and contains a number of waterborne bacteria and trace amounts of organic nutrients that may support growth of the bacteria. Water found in drinking fountains, water coolers, and supposedly "pure" bottled water has been found to have thousands of CFUs per milliliter.

Many researchers have studied the bacterial content of tap water. A glass of water from a kitchen faucet sitting stagnant at room temperature is often teeming with bacteria due to increasing numbers of bacteria populations (Figure 19.2). People are exposed to potentially high concentrations of bacteria-laden water all the time from many different sources. Being constantly exposed to naturally occurring bacteria causes people to develop a resistance to these bacteria.

Dental Assistant PROFESSIONAL TIP

To ensure compliance with dental unit waterline standards and to minimize any risk to patients and to self, the dental assistant should become educated on effective treatment measures to ensure compliance with dental unit waterline standards. Visit the CDC and ADA websites to learn the guidelines suggested by these two organizations.

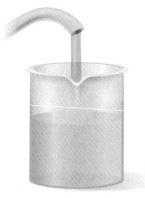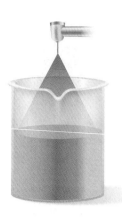

FIGURE 19.2
Tap water versus handpiece water.

History of Waterline Quality

Bacteria are a very successful life-form. Bacterial cells float freely in moist areas and, in the process of evolution, these cells have developed survival strategies and protective mechanisms that allow them to attach to surfaces. A discussion of water quality in dental unit waterlines was first initiated in 1965 but resurfaced in 1995 due to increased awareness of potential occupational hazards and concern about the increasing numbers of **immunocompromised** patients seeking dental treatment.

Immunocompromised patients are those with weakened immune systems due to age, smoking, heavy drinking, illness, or disease. It is more difficult to fight off invading microorganisms when a person's immune system is compromised. Patients with weakened immune systems should inform their dentist at the beginning of any treatment so the patient and dentist together can make the best treatment decisions. The American Dental Association (ADA) published a statement in 1995 on dental unit waterlines that challenged the dental industry to produce systems that can reduce the level of bacteria used in dental treatment water to 200 CFU/mL or fewer. This is the standard used in kidney dialysis machines.

What equipment in a dental office sprays water? What is water usually used for during dental treatments? Why do people not always become infected by microorganisms with which they come in contact? What types of individuals are particularly susceptible to infectious microorganisms?

Biofilm

Biofilm is a community of bacterial cells and other microbes that **adhere** to (hold onto) surfaces and form a protective matrix from their cell walls called a **slime layer.** Found in almost all places where moisture meets a suitable solid surface, biofilm can contain many types of

bacteria as well as fungi, algae, and protozoa. The continually replicating bacterial colonies form a protective slime layer produced by many microbial inhabitants while water within the biofilm carries nutrients to the cells within the film. The bacteria in dental plaque forms the most well-known oral biofilm. The formation of biofilm is a universal bacterial strategy for survival and optimum positioning with regard to available nutrients. In comparison with free-floating bacteria, the microbes in biofilm have superior resistance to disinfection.

Biofilms attach themselves to either inert or living surfaces and exist wherever surfaces contact water. Well-known examples are the slippery slime on stones found in rivers and ponds or the film on the inside of a vase that held flowers and water in it for a week. Some microorganisms floating freely in water will permanently stick to surfaces through the chemicals they secrete through their cell walls. These microorganisms cement themselves in colonies and shield themselves in slime.

Bacteria benefit by capturing nutrients from the water. Secondary bacteria will colonize with the primary microorganisms and use the waste products from their neighbors. Several species of bacteria can work together in complex cooperative communities to break down food supplies that no single species can digest alone.

Aerobic bacteria, that is, those that live only in the presence of oxygen, exist best on the surface, whereas an anaerobic bacterial layer may develop underneath the aerobic film. Anaerobic bacteria are able to live without oxy-

Cultural Considerations

We develop resistance to microorganisms to which we are constantly exposed. When providing dental treatment to patients from other countries, remember that they may not be as resistant to the microbes in our water as we are. In addition, some patients may have been routinely exposed to microorganisms in drinking water. Meticulous compliance with all methods for increasing water quality can prevent cross-contamination.

Life Span Considerations

As the population ages because of advancements in medical sciences and health care delivery systems, chronic and debilitating diseases have emerged that can weaken the immune system and make individuals more susceptible to infectious disease. Opportunistic diseases have become more commonplace. For these reasons, it is important for dental team members to focus on following procedures and guidelines that promote a healthy and safe environment for dental patients.

gen. A mature biofilm may take several hours to several weeks to develop. In the past microbiologists assumed that biofilms contained disorderly clumps of bacteria with no particular structure or pattern. New techniques to magnify biofilms without destroying the gel-like structures have enabled researchers to discover the complex organization of these communities (Figure 19.3).

Biofilm in Dental Waterlines

The amount of bacteria found in dental unit waterlines varies. The primary source of microorganisms in dental waterlines is the public water supply. Water from dental unit waterlines usually contains higher levels of bacteria than city water supplies, yet no widespread health problems have been associated with this water. Most organisms found in dental unit waterlines (DUWLs) are nonpathogenic for healthy patients and dental health care providers. A few studies have suggested that dental personnel who are continuously exposed to bacterial aerosols through high-speed handpieces and ultrasonic units have higher levels of certain bacterial antibodies than the general population. There are no documented serious health effects among patients or dental providers that can be directly related to contact with dental unit water.

The Uniqueness of Dental Unit Waterlines

Unlike household waterlines, dental unit waterlines provide living conditions that are particularly suited to biofilm formation. Ideal conditions for biofilm are highly dependent on particular water flow characteristics:

- Laminar flow
- Low flow rate

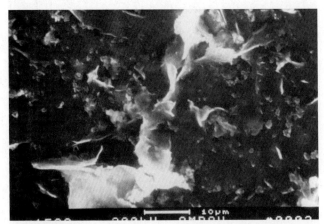

FIGURE 19.3
Scanning electron micrograph of microbial biofilm in a section of a high-speed handpiece waterline. Evidence of multiple coccal and bacillus forms is noted, with accumulation of extracellular material also present (¥1,500).
Murdoch-Kinch, C. A., et al., Comparison of dental water quality management procedures, *JADA* 1997; 128(9): 1235–1243. Copyright © 1997 American Dental Association. All rights reserved. Reprinted by permission.

- Low volume of use
- Small-diameter tubes
- High surface-to-volume ratio
- Long lengths of tubing
- Room temperature or warmer water
- Plastic tubing
- Dental water aerosols

Municipal water supplies have a turbulent flow, a high flow rate with high volume, and a larger diameter of pipes which create a low surface-to-volume ratio and are often made of copper. **Laminar flow** means the water flows fastest in the middle of the tube and slows toward the edge. Even when water is used during dental treatment, the flow rate is very low with little movement, which helps stagnation and encourages bacterial replication. The fact that dental units are unused overnight and during weekends further promotes microbial proliferation. The long lengths of narrow tubing used in DUWLs also lead to low volumes of slow-moving water. These flow characteristics are ideal for microorganisms because they ensure minimal disruption, which encourages further colonization.

Plastic waterlines, as opposed to copper pipes in homes, provide the ideal environment for enhancing bacterial growth and replication. The inside measurement of DUWLs is only 1/16 of an inch in diameter, which virtually guarantees that bacteria in the water have an opportunity to be in contact with the surface and attach themselves to the surface and grow. Some dental units even have heaters to keep the water warm for patient comfort. This condition also helps bacteria multiply. Dental personnel and patients are exposed to aerosols through the high-speed handpiece and ultrasonic units that spray water from the tubing into the air, forming airborne droplets that may be inhaled.

Why is biofilm so strong and difficult to destroy? What makes dental unit waterlines such an ideal environment in which biofilm can grow? How are dental personnel exposed to waterline biofilm?

Methods of Reducing Bacterial Contamination

Like all living creatures, bacteria require certain nutrients for growth and reproduction. Limiting these nutrients will limit bacteria growth, but even minute amounts of organic matter support many bacteria. Current technology cannot completely eliminate nutrient levels, but dental offices can routinely take many measures to reduce the bacteria in dental water used during treatment. Current standard precautions for dental treatment from the

Patient Education

Some patients may ask about bacterial contamination in dental waterlines. If patients ask, they should be given the facts. Patients should be told that biofilm is a thin layer of microorganisms that accumulate in common devices used to transport water, such as faucets and drinking fountains. Explain how the dental office maintains dental waterlines to utilize the best quality water available for dental equipment.

ADA, the Centers for Disease Control and Prevention (CDC), and the Organization for Safety and Asepsis Procedures (OSAP) include the following:

- Use a high-volume evacuator to remove water during treatment.
- Use a rubber dam for some procedures to prevent water from getting into the mouth.
- Flush out water from the dental lines for several minutes at the beginning of each day.
- Run the dental handpiece for 30 seconds between patients.
- Install sterilized handpieces and sterile or disposable syringe tips after flushing.
- Avoid heating dental unit water.
- Install and maintain antiretraction valves to prevent oral fluids from being drawn into dental waterlines.
- Properly maintain all waterlines.
- Always follow the manufacturer's recommendations for treating dental unit waterlines to avoid damage.
- Use a self-contained water supply.

The ADA has encouraged manufacturers of dental units to help solve the waterline problem. Some companies have created products that improve water quality in the waterlines (Figure 19.4). Not all existing products are approved by the Food and Drug Administration. Some options currently available to help solve the waterline problem include these:

- Use filters for the water (Figure 19.5).
- Use a separate water bottle/reservoir system.
- Use chemicals to disinfect the dental lines.
- Use a combination of ozone and silver ion catalyst to disinfect dental lines.

What are some methods that can be used in a dental office to reduce waterline contamination? Which methods must be accomplished by the dental assistant? **?**

Infection Control and Dental Unit Water

Although scientific reports have not linked illness to water passing through dental waterlines, it is important that waterline procedures be followed and documented on a regular basis. Dental offices have set procedures for cleaning and maintaining waterlines, and the procedures must be performed according to an established schedule. Failure to treat the waterlines when indicated will result in rapid regrowth of the biofilm.

Routine testing of the output dental water can be easily accomplished to ensure the effectiveness of each particular office protocol. Monitoring of dental waterlines may be accomplished by sending water samples to an

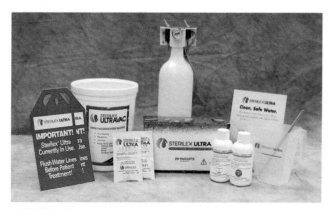

FIGURE 19.4
Water decontamination products.
Courtesy Sterilex Corporation

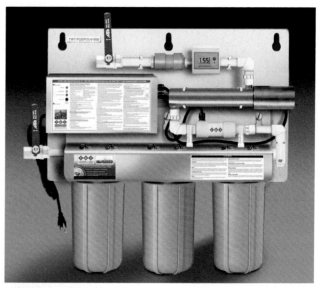

FIGURE 19.5
Water filtration systems.
Courtesy Triangular Wave Technologies, Inc.

outside microbiology lab or by using in-office kits. When an in-office kit is used, the water sample should be tested immediately.

To help reduce the number of microorganisms in dental treatment water, the ADA recommends that dentists follow the infection control guidelines of the CDC in addition to other precautions that may be in place. A combination of approaches will provide the best assurance of high-quality water. OSAP suggests that if a unit is going to be out of service for an extended period of time, it should be treated, air lines flushed out completely, and stored dry. Replacing waterlines is another alternative. For short periods of disuse, weekly treatments should be continued.

Maintenance Procedures for Dental Unit Waterlines

The dental assistant is responsible for performing proper maintenance procedures on dental unit waterlines. The protocol used depends on the water delivery system available and the preference of the dentist. Disinfecting independent water systems and waterlines can be accomplished by flushing with products such as 10% sodium hypochlorite, chlorhexidine gluconate, 95% ethanol, glutaraldehyde, hydrogen peroxide, or other recommended solutions. Note, however, that compatibility with equipment components is a concern. Sodium hypochlorite (common household bleach) may damage metal components in some dental units. Waterline antimicrobials must be registered with the EPA and the chemicals used must be compatible with various dental materials and oral tissues. In-line filter systems should be changed and monitored through a daily and weekly routine.

The dental assistant should develop a schedule for performing waterline maintenance and monitoring water to ensure harmful microorganisms are not present during patient treatment. The following steps should be followed to reduce any potential risk of dental unit waterline contamination:

- At the beginning of each day, purge all lines by removing handpieces, air/water syringe tips, and ultrasonic tips and run until no water remains.

- Add manufacturer-recommended disinfectant to the reservoir of the independent water system.

- After the recommended contact time, flush the disinfectant through the lines of handpieces, air/water syringe tips, and ultrasonic units until no longer visible (colored disinfectants), until monitoring devices such as pH strips no longer indicate the presence of disinfectant (colorless disinfectants), or for the recommended time, usually about 30 seconds to one minute.

- Run each high-speed handpiece, air/water syringe, and ultrasonic unit for 20 to 30 seconds after each patient to purge all air and water.

- Use sterile water or sterile saline solution when flushing open sites during invasive surgical procedures.

Filters may be installed between the waterline and the dental instrument to block the passage of microorganisms. The dental assistant should replace filters periodically depending on the amount of biofilm in the waterline. Compliance with waterline protocols must be monitored just as office sterilizers are monitored on a regular schedule.

Routine testing of the output dental water is easily accomplished using water testing products or services that ensure the effectiveness of waterline procedures. Dental equipment should be removed before water samples are taken. The dental assistant should wear gloves to avoid contamination of the water during testing procedures and carefully follow the product or service directions. (See Chapter 12 for a review of infection control procedures.)

How does the dental office know if methods of reducing waterline contamination are effective? What procedures should be followed if a dental unit is not going to be used for an extended period of time? What should be done if it will not be used for a short period of time? Is one method of water treatment enough to provide the best results?

SUMMARY

As awareness of infection control issues has increased, concern over dental unit waterline contamination has risen. Dental assistants must be knowledgeable regarding microbial contamination and biofilm formation in dental unit waterlines. Continuing education for all dental personnel should stress the need for improvement in the quality of water delivered to patients during treatment.

DUWL manufacturers play an important role by providing training and education on the proper use and maintenance of their systems. Several commercial options are available for improving dental unit water quality including independent water reservoirs, chemical treatment regimens, daily draining and cleaning, and the use of filters (Table 19-1). Research suggests that some combination of these strategies is necessary to control biofilm formation and achieve the desired level of water quality.

All dental unit water should be monitored weekly with an in-office monitoring kit or commercial water testing service. When used with a chemical treatment protocol, self-contained water systems or independent water reservoirs have demonstrated safety and efficacy.

TABLE 19-1 Some Commercially Available Chemicals and Devices for Waterlines

Self-Contained Water Systems	Chemicals and Chemical Delivery Systems	Sterile Water Delivery Systems	Water Purifiers	Water Monitoring Systems
A-Dec, Inc.	A-Dec, Inc.	Amadent	Crosstat/Waterclave	Millipore Corp.
AMPCO Dental	Anodia Systems	Lares Research	DCI International	Pall Medical
Anodia Systems	Dental Pure	Odonto-Wave	Germiphene Corp.	Waterclave
DCI International	Germiphene Corp.		Patterson Dental	
Frio Technologies	Micrylium Laboratories		Sterisil, Inc.	
Patterson Dental	Rowpar Pharmaceuticals			
Sterisil, Inc.	Sterilex			
	Sterisil, Inc.			

KEY TERMS

- **Adhere:** To hold onto a surface. p. 284
- **Biofilm:** A community of microorganisms that accumulates on surfaces in moist areas. p. 284
- **Colony-forming units (CFUs):** Unit of measure for numbers of viable bacteria per milliliter. p. 283
- **Immunocompromised:** Condition in which a person is at risk for a disease due to a weakened immune system. p. 284

- **Laminar flow:** Occurs when water flows fastest in the middle and slower on the edges of tubing. p. 285
- **Pathogens:** Microorganisms that are capable of causing disease. p. 283
- **Slime layer:** A matrix produced by some bacteria from their cell walls. p. 284

CHECK YOUR UNDERSTANDING

1. Normal drinking water is usually allowed to have how many colony-forming units (CFUs) of bacteria per milliliter?
   a. 200 CFUs
   b. 300 CFUs
   c. 400 CFUs
   d. 500 CFUs

2. The American Dental Association challenged the dental industry to produce systems that can reduce the level of bacteria used in dental treatment water to what level?
   a. 200 CFUs
   b. 300 CFUs
   c. 400 CFUs
   d. 500 CFUs

CHECK YOUR UNDERSTANDING (continued)

3. Why did dental unit waterlines become a concern?
   a. because of increased awareness of occupational hazards
   b. because of concerns about increasing numbers of immunocompromised patients
   c. because of so many personnel and patients becoming infected
   d. a and b only
   e. all of the above

4. What types of dental patients will have compromised immune systems?
   a. older patients
   b. those who smoke and drink alcohol
   c. transplant and cancer patients
   d. AIDS patients
   e. all of the above

5. Why is biofilm so strong and difficult to destroy?
   a. It is a community of bacterial cells and other microbes.
   b. It adheres to certain surfaces.
   c. It forms a protective layer.
   d. All of the above.

6. What is a slime layer?
   a. a protective matrix produced from bacterial cell walls
   b. a strategy for survival
   c. an antimicrobial
   d. a and b

7. State methods the dental assistant will use to reduce waterline contamination.
   a. Use a high-volume evacuator to remove water during treatment.

   b. Run the dental handpiece for 30 seconds between patients.
   c. Place sterile or disposable syringe tips after flushing the lines.
   d. Follow the manufacturer's recommendations for treating dental unit waterlines.
   e. All of the above.

8. What are some methods the dental office will use to reduce waterline contamination?
   a. filters or a separate water reservoir
   b. chemicals to disinfect the dental lines
   c. ozone and silver ion catalyst to disinfect dental lines
   d. a and b only
   e. a combination of a, b, and c

9. When should an in-office kit be used to test the dental unit water sample?
   a. immediately prior to chemically treating the water
   b. prior to replacing the filter
   c. it does not matter
   d. a and b

10. Bacteria that are able to live without the presence of oxygen are called
    a. aerobic bacteria.
    b. anaerobic bacteria.
    c. fungi.
    d. algae.

INTERNET ACTIVITY

- Go to www.sterilex.com for information on how to remove and prevent the formation of biofilm in dental unit waterlines.

WEB REFERENCES

- American Dental Association: Dental Unit Water Quality
  www.ada.org/prof/resources/topics/waterlines/art_cleaning_waterlines.pdf
- American Dental Association: Oral Health Topics A-Z   http://ada.org/public/topics/waterlines_faq.asp
- Foundations in Continuing Dental Education   www.nurseslearning.com/courses/fice/fde0033/c11/index.htm
- Organization for Safety and Asepsis Procedures   www.osap.org/displaycommon.cfm

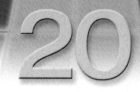

20

The Dental Office

Chapter Outline

- Dental Office Setting
- Administrative and Reception Area
- Dentist's Private Office
- Dental Staff Lounge
- Daily Routine Office Care
- Clinical Treatment Rooms
- Clinical Equipment
  —Oral Evacuation System and
   Central Air Compressor
  —Patient Dental Chair
  —Operator's Chair and Assistant's
   Stool
  —Dental Unit
  —Dental Cabinets
  —Dental Radiology Units
  —Small Equipment
- Central Sterilization Area
- Dental Laboratory Area

Learning Objectives

After reading this chapter, the student should be able to:

- Define key terms associated with the dental office.
- Explain the effect of the Americans with Disabilities Act on dental office design.
- Describe the different types of rooms typically found in a dental office setting.
- Discuss the importance of the reception area.
- Describe the purpose and design of dental treatment rooms.
- List and describe the use of common office equipment.
- Discuss the operations of the dental unit and its components.

Preparing for Certification Exams

- Perform preventive maintenance on the equipment and instruments in the dental operatory per manufacturer instructions.
- Maintain patients' right to privacy.
- Receive and dismiss patients and visitors inside the dental practice.

Key Terms

Consultation room

Dental chair

Dental operatory/treatment room

Dental unit

Handpieces

Rheostat

Subsupine position

Supine position

Triturate

Upright position

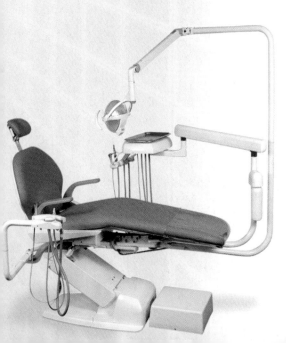

The design and size of a dental office are determined by the type of practice the dentist plans to build. One of the most important elements in designing a successful dental practice is for the dentist to consider the type of dentistry he or she will provide. For instance, if the dentist has decided to practice family dentistry there are elements such as child-proofing waiting rooms or providing a child-friendly waiting area separate from the reception area. If the dentist is to perform adult cosmetic services, the office design may reflect a more subtle, quiet atmosphere that is more appealing for adults.

The office design must reflect goals and incorporate all of the qualities needed to attract patients into a welcoming atmosphere. The appearance of the practice creates a statement about the dentist, the staff, and the quality of dental work being provided. Patients may judge the quality of the dental care provided by the practice based on the appearance of the office (Figure 20.1). First impressions are established through the appearance of the office as well as the first greeting from the dental team.

The dental office should be designed to provide a safe and stress-free work area to the office

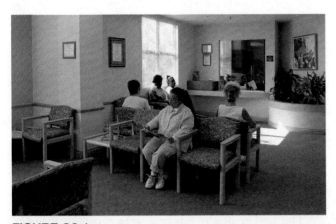

FIGURE 20.1
Dental office reception area.
Image courtesy Instructional Materials for the Dental Team, Lex., KY

staff as well as comfort to the patient before, during, and after dental treatment. The proper placement of office and dental equipment will help in ensuring that efficiency is achieved along with comfort for the dental team, patients, and visitors.

Dental Office Setting

The type of dental practice and the dentist preferences and needs determine the design goals when setting up an office. Practices range from small to large offices. Smaller offices typically have fewer treatment rooms than larger practices. Regardless of the number of operatories, several basic components go into designing a dental practice.

Most offices have a reception area, business office area, treatment rooms, sterilization area, laboratory, x-ray processing or darkroom, restrooms, and the dentist's private office. Additional rooms found in larger practices may include a consultation room, staff lounge, patient education area, storage area, manager's office, panoramic and x-ray room, shower and changing area, and computer room. According to Occupational Safety and Health Administration (OSHA) regulations, employers with incorporated businesses may not take home personal protective equipment. The employer is responsible to clean, launder, repair, and replace PPE. The choice by the employer to launder the PPE in the office rather than to send it out to a service or to use a commercial laundromat means that the office layout must accommodate the installation of a washer and a dryer.

Another change that has improved practice designs is the Americans with Disabilities Act, passed in 1990. This act emphasizes office designs that ensure anyone can move freely around an office without any obstructions. Table 20-1 lists some of the Act's office design modifications that help create a barrier-free office. For instance, doorways must now have openings large enough for wheelchairs to pass through freely. Specifications for office design under the Americans with Disabilities Act must comply with state and federal guidelines. Table 20-2 provides contact information for those who want to learn more about the Americans with Disabilities Act.

An atmosphere that is inviting and pleasant for the dental patient can be achieved in many different ways.

TABLE 20-1 Design Elements for a Barrier-Free Office in Compliance with the Americans with Disabilities Act

Designate a handicapped parking area.
Install sidewalks and curb access to accommodate wheelchairs and other devices.
Install access ramps to building and practice areas.
Widen doors and doorways to accommodate wheelchairs and other devices.
Install raised letters and braille over elevator controls.
Provide visual and sound alarms.
Install grab bars.
Install raised toilet seats and wider stalls.
Make paper towel dispensers accessible.
Install paper cup dispensers at water fountains.
Eliminate plush, low-density carpet.

TABLE 20-2 Contact Information for the Americans with Disabilities Act

Office of Americans with Disabilities Act
U.S. Department of Justice
P.O. Box 66118
Washington, DC 20035-6738
1-800-514-0301 voice
Internet website: www.usdoj.gov/crt/ada/adahom1.htm (ADA home page)
Internet website: www.access-board.gov

Some offices may choose a theme-type setting, whereas other offices may choose a more trendy type of setting. A detailed, organized dental practice is necessary in maintaining a professional atmosphere that draws new patients in and provides a reason for established patients to stay with the practice. Attention given to the office environment setting will help to establish that professional atmosphere.

Ideally, the office temperature should be set anywhere between 68° and 72°F. Well-established airflow and ventilation will help prevent and/or diminish odors associated with dentistry. Lighting is different in the various areas of the dental office. For instance, the clinical areas will require special lighting, such as the operating light used to illuminate the oral cavity. The reception area might have more subdued lighting.

Wall coverings and flooring should use soothing color tones and relaxing designs and be coordinated with the rest of the office decor. Infection control in the treat-

Cultural Considerations

Some patients who use wheelchairs can transfer themselves into the dental chair, but others need assistance. The extent of the dental assistant's involvement will depend on the patient's or caregiver's ability to assist in this transfer. Most people can be transferred safely from wheelchair to dental chair and back by using the two-person method. Learn about the two-person transfer at the "How to" Internet site at www.nidcr.nih.gov/HealthInformation/DiseasesAnd Conditions/DevelopmentalDisabilitiesAndOralHealth/ WheelchairTransfer.htm.

ment areas may require suitable materials that can be wiped down and easily cleaned, such as vinyl flooring or smooth surface walls. Therefore, the type of flooring should be carefully selected depending on where in the office it will be installed. For example, carpet should never be used in a treatment area because it is difficult to sanitize.

Controlling sounds within the dental practice from one room to another is important. Sound control ensures that noises associated with dental procedures are minimal and that patient privacy is maintained. Specified areas may be designated for discussing patient financial and personal information as set forth by the Health Insurance Portability and Accountability Act of 1996 (HIPAA). HIPAA regulates the privacy of patients.

Patient flow within the practice needs to be established to not only assist the office in preserving patient confidentiality but also to appropriately greet, treat, and dismiss the patients. Easy entry in and out of the dental office and clinical areas creates a perception of order. Regardless of the dental surroundings and atmosphere, the staff's smiles and caring attitudes will always set the most inviting tone for the dental patient within the dental practice.

What is a barrier-free office as set forth by the Americans with Disabilities Act?

Administrative and Reception Area

The administrative area in the dental office is a work space that is centrally located to enable effective communication with patients and the dental team. This area is the core section in the dental practice where business is conducted (Figure 20.2). The business office is convenient for the patient and allows the business manager and office assistants to be aware of all activities occurring in the dental office.

The design of the business area typically includes items such as desks, computers, photocopier, phone system, fax machine, calculators, business materials, and

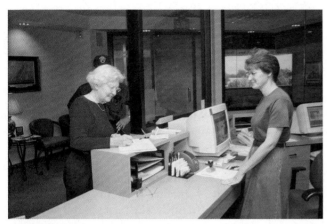

FIGURE 20.2
Business office and receptionist area.

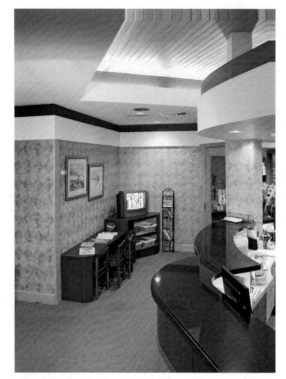

FIGURE 20.3
Dental reception room with child's area.

storage for patient records. No matter who works in the front office, all personnel should know how to operate front desk equipment. This area should be designed to accommodate all patient privacy rules and provide a secured location to conduct financial payment transactions with patients. Some offices provide a small private room, or **consultation room,** that is specifically designed to discuss financial arrangements and treatment planning. Other considerations of the business area include the following:

- Business assistants should face the reception area so they can make eye contact with patients as they arrive and leave the office.
- Items such as appointment cards and patient information should be easily accessible to the dental staff but confined to areas that are secure.
- Intercom systems should be placed in appropriate areas to provide effective communication between the administrative and clinical areas.
- Master controls for heating and air settings, music volume, and light settings should be within easy reach for quick access.
- Storage space for paper, pens, pencils, and telephone message pads should be provided to ensure that these items are available as needed.

The reception area or dental lobby is the gateway to the dental practice and is the area that patients first encounter. This area should be warm, inviting, and kept clean at all times. All patients entering the reception area should be immediately greeted by an office staff member. The décor of the dental office should be welcoming and be geared toward the type of patients the office is seeing. For example, if the dental practice serves children, small chairs, toys, and children's reading material should be available (Figure 20.3). Proper seating should be provided with small chairs for younger patients. The number of seating options made available in the dental lobby will be based on the size of the practice and how many

patients typically are waiting to be seen. It is important to consider spacing of seats. Most offices prefer to use chairs rather than couches in order to address personal space issues as well as privacy for completing required paperwork.

Dentist's Private Office

Many dentists have private office space. The dentist's office is an area where the dentist may consult privately with patients concerning dental diagnosis and treatment plans or have telephone conferences with other doctors or dentists concerning patients. The dentist may meet with the office manager or a staff member regarding patient care. The dentist's office is an area that must be respected and treated as a private area usually with a private entrance. Each dentist will set entrance guidelines that must be respected and followed by the rest of the dental team.

Dental Staff Lounge

This area of the practice will vary greatly from office to office. The dental lounge is a designated area for use by all clinical and administrative members of the dental team. This area is used for daily breaks, lunchtime, and sometimes for staff meetings. The dental lounge typically contains a table with chairs, refrigerator, sink, coffee pot, and personal storage areas. Some are equipped with changing facilities and a washer and dryer for laundering uniforms. The dental staff lounge may also include amenities such as computers and telephones for staff members to use during their breaks, a water cooler, and food/soda vending machines. This area is usually maintained by the dental team. A rotating schedule may be created in order to ensure that each member of the dental team participates in cleaning and maintaining the lounge.

Daily Routine Office Care

Routine office care and equipment maintenance is an important responsibility of the dental assistant. The following should be completed on a daily, weekly, or monthly basis or as required by the manufacturing instructions of the particular piece of equipment:

- Change and clean x-ray processing solutions and tanks (monthly or every 28 days).
- Ensure that x-ray solutions and water levels are maintained (daily).
- Change O-rings for air/water syringes when leaks occur (as needed).
- Ensure nitrous oxide and oxygen tanks stay full and replaced as needed (Figure 20.4) (daily).
- Clean the inside and outside surfaces of the sterilizer (weekly or more often if needed).
- Monitor and keep accurate records on the sterilizer's effectiveness (typically weekly).
- Change ultrasonic solutions (daily or more often if under heavy use and solution is cloudy or bloody).
- Change traps and filters throughout the dental office (as needed).
- Conduct small repairs (as needed).

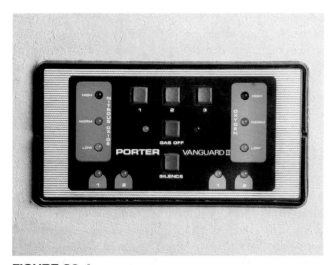

FIGURE 20.4
Nitrous oxide control panel that indicates level of both nitrous oxide and oxygen.

What is the responsibility of the dental assistant regarding opening and closing the office?

The dental assistant is usually responsible for the daily opening and closing of the clinical portions of the practice. Conscientious detail to tasks in the morning prior to opening can help to ensure a more organized and efficient day ahead. Due to the tasks that must be completed prior to patients arriving, the dental assistant typically arrives in the morning about 30 minutes prior to seating the first patient for treatment. To further understand the process of opening dental offices, see Procedure 20-1.

The end-of-day routine includes closing the office and preparing for the next day. The dental assistant usually helps with these tasks. Attention given to correctly closing down the clinical areas and equipment will prevent any undue wear and tear on the machines. The goal by completing the end-of-day tasks is to be ready for the patients the next time the office opens. To further understand how to close the office for the day and prepare it for the next day, see Procedure 20-2.

The ultimate goal in completing the tasks for opening and closing the dental practice is to minimize the loss of production time while patient care is being completed and to reduce the stress of the dental team through organization and efficiency.

Clinical Treatment Rooms

Clinical treatment rooms are considered the control center of the clinical portion of the dental practice and are where dental procedures are provided to the patient. These **treatment rooms** are also known as **dental operatories** (Figure 20.5). The size and type of dental practice usually indicates the number of operatories needed. In a general dental practice, there are usually two types of operatories: one for providing operative dentistry and the other for dental hygiene.

The dentist moves from operatory to operatory to deliver dental care. Easy access to, and similar setups

Preparing for Externship

It is important for the dental assistant to become familiar and confident with the use of dental equipment in the dental office. By becoming comfortable with the equipment not only does the dental assistant feel more confident, but this confidence is then translated to the patient. For instance, knowing how the dental chair operates prior to seating a patient, instead of learning while the patient is in the chair, will help in relieving any stress that the patient may be experiencing.

Procedure 20-1 Opening the Dental Office

Routine Steps

1. Arrive early enough to complete tasks needed to create an on-time and smooth flow for the daily patient schedule.

2. Turn on all master switches to lights, radiology and dental units, clinical computers, central air compressors, vacuum system, and regulator for nitrous oxide sedation system.

3. Flush water through waterlines for a minimum of two to four minutes.

4. Open valves on the nitrous oxide and oxygen tanks.

5. Turn on the x-ray film processor. Change water and replenish tanks to appropriate levels with processing solutions, as necessary.

6. Check the reception room for neatness, organize magazines and books, straighten chairs, turn on lights, and unlock and open patient doors.

7. Print and post copies of schedules in designated areas throughout office.

8. Check answering machine for messages.

9. Review patient schedule and ensure that all patient records and x-ray/laboratory results are available for patients on the day's schedule.

10. Dress in appropriate OSHA-required attire for the clinical treatment rooms. Perform a 60-second thorough hand washing.

11. Turn on and complete sterilization from prior day. Check sterilizer's fluid levels, complete any overnight and/or cold sterile procedures, and change disinfectant solutions as needed.

12. Prepare rooms for daily patients:
    - Check and restock supplies.
    - Place barriers.
    - Fill water reservoir/bottles.
    - Prepare tray and instruments for first patients.

13. Prepare operatory completely before seating patient.

14. Greet and seat patient on time for first appointment.

---

between, the operatories allows the dentist and dental staff to flow efficiently from one room to the next without disrupting the patient's comfort and promotes a smooth process for dental procedures to be performed. When designing a proficient clinical treatment area, special consideration should be given to both providing a private and comfortable atmosphere for the patient and mobility and comfort for the dental team.

Clinical Equipment

The equipment in the dental treatment room includes the dental chair, the dental unit, dental operating light, operator's stool, dental assistant's stool, cabinets (some may be mobile), x-ray machine, and various materials depending on the operator's preferences. Depending on the size, type of use, and provider preferences, other small equipment may be located within the operatory (e.g., cameras, computer equipment, and ultrasonic cleaner). Dental equipment is expensive to purchase and it is crucial to the practice that the equipment is always functioning properly. With attention to manufacturer care instructions and maintenance, dental equipment can last many years. A routine maintenance schedule for equipment is usually performed by the dental assistant. When equipment needs to be repaired, a dental equipment technician is called to repair large equipment;

Life Span Considerations

Allowing children to touch and feel dental equipment that is going to be used during their visit will help reduce their fear of the equipment. Let children hold the saliva ejector while it is on and play with it. Let them go up and down in the dental chair and show them how it is done. Create a fun routine for children's visits. Educating children about procedures and equipment in a fun manner will make their dental visits into positive experiences.

smaller equipment can be either mailed to the manufacturer or picked up by service representatives.

Oral Evacuation System and Central Air Compressor

The oral evacuation system (Figure 20.6), also known as the central vacuum compressor, provides suction to the oral evacuators or high-volume evacuators (HVEs) and saliva ejectors at the dental unit. Water is used often in dental procedures and needs to be removed from the oral cavity. This is done by using saliva ejectors or HVEs.

Saliva ejectors are less powerful, have less suction strength than the oral HVE, and are more comfortable

Procedure 20-2 Closing the Dental Office

Routine Steps

1. Wear appropriate personal protective equipment (PPE) for exposure control.

2. Complete operatory room cleanup and preparation. This may include:
   - Performing an extensive cleaning of the dental chair and dental unit
   - Flushing air/water syringes and handpieces
   - Running evacuation cleaner through vacuum lines
   - Cleaning traps and filters
   - Maintaining water reservoirs/bottle
   - Wiping down with disinfectants all surfaces in the operatory room

3. Sterilize all instruments and setup trays for the next day. Empty ultrasonic solutions and be sure all overnight or cold sterilization instruments are fully submerged into solutions.

4. Empty waste cans and replace fresh plastic liners.

5. Make sure all laboratory cases have been sent to the lab and next day cases have been checked in and received from the lab.

6. Complete processing, mount and file patient x-rays, turn off water supply to processor, and turn off/shut down according to manufacturer's instructions.

7. Wipe down with disinfectant solutions all surfaces and turn off darkroom lights, including safe light.

8. Turn off all master switches to equipment in the operatories, each radiology and dental unit, central sterilization, lights, computers, any small equipment that may have been used during the day, and regulator for nitrous oxide sedation system.

9. Close valves on the nitrous oxide and oxygen tanks.

10. Remove and dispose of PPE in appropriate container prior to leaving treatment area according to OSHA requirements.

11. Straighten reception area, lock patient doors, turn off any machinery and clean staff lounge, back up computers, turn off business equipment and computers, turn on answering machine, and ensure all charts have been pulled for the next day.

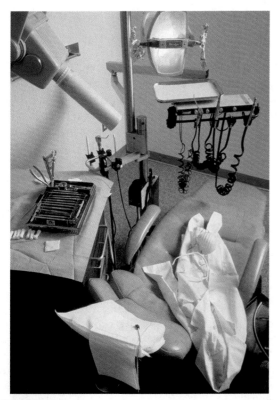

FIGURE 20.5
Dental operatory.

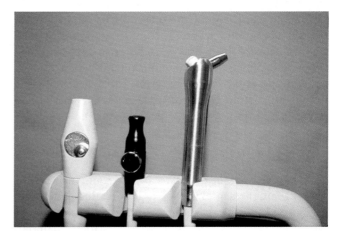

FIGURE 20.6
Oral evacuation system.
Image courtesy Instuctional Materials for the Dental Team, Lex., KY

for the patient in less invasive procedures such as applying sealants, cleanings, fluoride treatments, and use under dental dams. The saliva ejector is disposable and is made of a thin flexible tube with a wire in the tubing so that the tube can be bent into any shape to aid in positioning the suction in the patient's mouth.

High-volume evacuators are stronger and wider than the smaller saliva ejectors and are intended to remove debris such as old restorative materials or pieces of tooth as well as fluids. Evacuation tips are usually beveled at each end and come in metal styles that can be sterilized or in disposable plastics. (Note, however, that most offices now use disposable HVE tips for infection control reasons.) Both the metal styles and the disposables plastics are sturdy and do not bend. High-volume suction tips are used by the dental assistant to help keep saliva and water from obscuring the dentist's field of vision. The HVE tips are inserted into a handle at the end of a hose. There is an on/off valve at the handle that is used to open the suction tip for suction. The HVE tips are replaced between each patient. Infection control barriers are used to cover the handle and hoses. The filters and traps of the HVE and small saliva ejectors must be cleaned and maintained to keep the vacuums of these devices at full vacuum potential. The dental assistant should review service and manufacturers' instructions on all dental equipment used in the office to ensure that routine maintenance and repairs are taken care of correctly.

The central air compressor provides compressed air to the dental unit for air-driven handpieces and air/water syringes. Condensation in the air lines can be the cause of contaminants such as moisture, debris, and algae. Without proper maintenance, buildup can occur in the air lines and lead to possible damage of dental handpieces as well as possibly expel harmful microorganisms into patients' mouths. Special attention is required regarding routine maintenance. Repairs should be conducted by a licensed service technician.

The size of the air and vacuum compressors depends greatly on how many dental units in an office simultaneously require the use of the compressor. Due to size and the desire to minimize noise levels and enhance safety, compressor units are typically stored away from the main portions of the dental practice and usually in a soundproof room. Turning the power on to the central vacuum compressor and the central air compressor is usually one of the steps done when opening the office in the morning. At night when the office is closed the compressors are turned off. Some offices may even have timers that automatically power on and off the compressor according to the dental practice's office hours.

Patient Dental Chair

The **dental chair** is the center for all clinical and treatment activity. Its purpose is to provide comfort to the patient and to assist the operator and/or assistant in providing the most efficient treatment to the patient. Dental chairs are usually contoured in shape and are designed for the concept of four-handed dentistry that is performed in the sitting-down delivery style. Several parts to the dental chair aid in the patient's comfort and allow dental treatment to be delivered in an efficient manner (Figure 20.7):

- The body of the chair supports the patient's knees, buttocks, and both lower and upper back when the patient is properly seated.

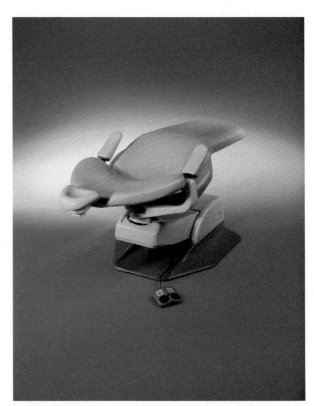

FIGURE 20.7
Patient chair with headrest, backrest, armrest, and leg support.

- The armrest can be raised and/or moved to the side, out of the patient's way, to allow for easy access into and out of the dental chair. The armrest comfortably supports the patient's arms and elbows.
- The headrest supports the patient's head and neck. The headrest also holds the patient's head securely in the appropriate position while treatment is being provided. It can be adjusted to position the patient's head lower or higher as well as to accommodate the patient's height by adjusting the headrest up or down.

What does it mean when the patient is placed into a supine position? What would it mean to be in a subsupine position?

- The dental chair has controls or a control panel that allows the entire chair to be moved up or down, recline the backrest, raise the knees, or do a combination of movements that adjusts the patient into a desired position for treatment. Three positions are used when treating a patient. The **upright position** is where the patient is seated with the dental chair back at a 90-degree angle. This position is used for patient entry and release from the dental chair. The **supine position** is where the patient is reclined in the dental chair with the patient's nose and knees at the same level. This position is used when the maxillary arch is being treated. The **subsupine position** is where the patient is reclined in the dental chair with the patient's head positioned lower than the feet. This position is used for emergencies rather than for dental treatment. The controls to the dental chair can be located on each side of the dental chair. In addition, a floor foot control can be used to operate the chair in the same manner as the side controls. The floor foot control can help in eliminating infection control barrier issues.

• A swivel lever allows the base of the chair to be rotated from side to side and left and right. This is important to adjust the patient's position for operator comfort.

The dental chair is made of materials that are comfortable to the patient, match office décor, and are easy to clean and disinfect between patients. The base of the dental chair is secured to the floor and should be cleaned and disinfected between patients. At the closing of the day, the dental chair should be left in the upright position and lifted up to the highest level possible allowing easy access for cleaning the area under the chair.

What is the difference between the operator's chair and the dental assistant's stool?

Operator's Chair and Assistant's Stool

Performing sit-down, four-handed dentistry at the sides of a patient's dental chair requires specialized chairs designed to support the bodies of both the operator and the dental assistant for sustained periods of time. The design of these chairs and stools may vary depending on the user's preferences; however, the features of the equipment need to meet the following guidelines:

Operator's Chair (Figure 20.8a)
• The seat on the chair is padded and needs to be either flat or contoured.
• The base should provide easy mobility and have four to five casters to prevent tipping.

• Beneath the chair, an adjustable lever should be available in order to allow the operator to modify the chair to a comfortable height from the floor.
• The chair needs to have an adjustable back for support to the operator.

Assistant's Stool (Figure 20.8b)
• The seat on the stool is padded, flat, and needs to be comfortable to the user.
• The base should provide easy mobility, should be broad, and have four to five casters to prevent tipping.
• The stool should be able to twist and turn, allowing easy access to counters, shelves, drawers, and the patient's side.
• The stool should have a foot ring for supporting the feet.
• Beneath the chair, an adjustable lever should be placed making it easy for the assistant to comfortably adjust the height and leg length.
• The stool may have an adjustable support arm to brace the assistant's torso or upper body in a fatigue-reducing posture. Assisting stools can have a back rest that is adjusted to support the lumbar region.

Both the operator's chair and the assistant's stool are made of materials that are comfortable to the users, match office décor, and are easy to clean and disinfect between patients.

Dental Unit

The **dental unit** consists of handpieces, air/water syringes, saliva ejector, high-volume evacuator, and ultrasonic scalers, along with numerous other options depending on the operator's preferences (Figure 20.9). Its basic function is to provide electrical and air-operated power to the hoses, attachments, and working parts of the unit.

There is a wide range of dental units. Some items to take into consideration when selecting a dental unit include space availability, preference of delivery system,

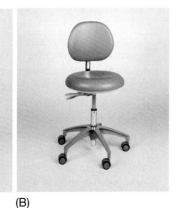

(A)   (B)

FIGURE 20.8
(a) Operator's chair and (b) assistant's stool.

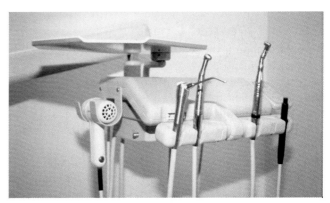

FIGURE 20.9
Dental unit.
Image courtesy Instuctional Materials for the Dental Team, Lex., KY

whether the operator is left or right handed, and whether a dental assistant is utilized at the patient's dental chair. The master switch controls the power to the entire unit. Each attachment has its own individual control for water and air pressure.

Types of Delivery Systems

The dental unit can be positioned in various places in the operatory. This is known as the delivery system. Some delivery systems mount to the floor or the wall, others mount to the dental chair, and some are on movable, mobile units.

* *Front delivery system:* Designed to allow equipment to be used over the patient's chest and in front of the operator and the assistant (Figure 20.10a).
* *Rear delivery system:* Designed to allow equipment to be used from behind the patient's head (Figure 20.10b).
* *Side delivery system:* Designed to allow equipment to be used from the operator's side (Figure 20.10c). The dental unit is either attached to a fixed or mobile unit that has an extendable arm to aid the operator in gaining access from the dental unit to the patient. With this system, the operator and assistant needs to have separate suction and air/water syringes.

Dental Handpieces

There are two types of dental **handpieces** on the dental unit: high-speed handpieces and slow or low-speed handpieces (Figure 20.11). They are attached to the hoses that are a part of the dental unit. It is important to ensure that the hoses do not become tangled or kinked. Each handpiece connection on the unit has two on/off switches; one that will prevent more than one handpiece from operating at the same time and one that controls the rheostat. The handpieces are operated by the foot control called a rheostat that controls the speed while performing dental treatment in the oral cavity.

The longevity of equipment can be sustained if proper care is provided. All handpieces are removed and

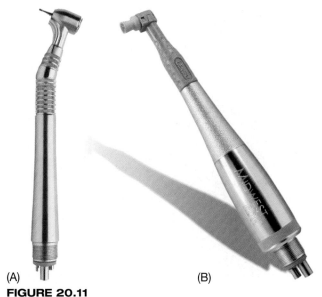

FIGURE 20.11
(a) High-speed and (b) low-speed dental handpiece.
Courtesy DENTSPLY Professional

sterilized after each patient. Prior to removing handpieces they should be flushed for one minute before and after each use. It is important to follow the manufacturer's instructions concerning the care and cleaning of the handpieces.

Rheostat

The **rheostat** is a foot-controlled or pedal device that is used to operate and control the dental handpieces from the dental unit. The disk-shaped rheostat is connected to the dental unit by a flexible power hose (Figure 20.12). To easily power dental unit attachments and handpieces, the rheostat is positioned on the floor at the base of the chair close to the operator. The operator uses his/her foot to press the rheostat to operate and control the speed of the high- and low-speed handpieces.

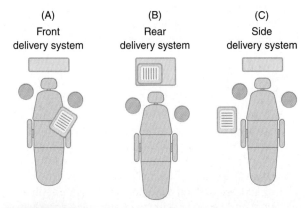

FIGURE 20.10
View of (a) front delivery system, (b) rear delivery system, and (c) side delivery system.

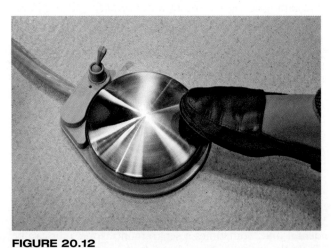

FIGURE 20.12
Rheostat.
Image courtesy Instuctional Materials for the Dental Team, Lex., KY

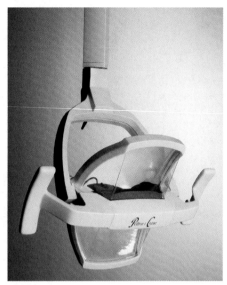

FIGURE 20.13
Operating light.

Operating Light

The operating light, also known as the dental light, provides the bright light necessary to see into the oral cavity during procedures (Figure 20.13). The operating light may be attached to the dental chair or mounted directly above the patient on the ceiling. The dental light is designed to have two handles, one on each side of the halogen bulb. Care should be taken not to shine the light into the patient's eyes. The operator and the assistant need to have easy access to adjust the light as needed during procedures. Cleaning, disinfecting, and maintaining the operating light should be done by carefully following the manufacturer's instructions.

Air/Water Syringe

The air/water syringe is attached to the dental unit and is necessary in most dental procedures. Air from the syringe is used to dry the surfaces in the oral cavity. Water is used to rinse surfaces in the oral cavity. A spray will result from the combined use of air and water to flush surfaces in the oral cavity. Infection control barriers are used to cover the tubing and handles of the air/water syringe while the tips are either sterilized or disposable. Sometimes the O-rings within the air/water syringe heads need replacement. This is particularly true if they begin to leak. It is also important to flush the air/water syringe before and after each patient, and at the beginning and end of the day.

Ultrasonic Scalers

Ultrasonic scalers are used during dental cleanings and produce a vibrating action that removes hard deposits such as calculus and other debris from the teeth. These tips are sleeved into a handle on a hose attached to the dental unit. Sometimes a separate ultrasonic unit can be specially connected to the dental unit as an add-on device. All handles and hoses should be covered with

infection control barriers and the ultrasonic tips sterilized between each patient.

What are the three different types of delivery systems?

Dental Cabinets

Operatories have cabinets to store supplies and materials needed when providing dental treatment. These cabinets vary in design depending on the preference or reason for their use. Some cabinets may open from both sides to easily retrieve patient trays, x-ray machines, or materials shared between two operatories. Mobile units are a type of cabinet that can be easily moved by the dental team. These units are typically stored against a wall and then pulled into position after the patient has been seated. All cabinets should be kept stocked and cleaned between patients.

All operatories should have cabinets with sinks for the operator and assistants to use. There are usually two sinks in an operatory, one for the dentist and one for the dental assistant. The dental assistant's sink will usually be foot controlled for the purpose of infection control. The sink area needs to have soap and a towel dispenser close by and should be easy to clean and disinfect between patients.

Dental Radiology Units

Radiology units are used to expose intraoral radiographs and digital radiographs. X-ray machines are part of operatories. The x-ray machine can be mounted to the wall or be housed in a cabinet. If the tube head is going to be shared between two treatment rooms, it can be placed in a cabinet that is situated between the two rooms. The cabinet doors can then be designed to swing open allowing easy access from both rooms. In all cases, the controls for the x-ray machine are found outside the treatment room. This ensures that the person taking the x-rays is not exposed to the radiation used when taking x-rays. The x-ray tube head and controls should be covered with infection control barriers. (See Chapter 12 for information on infection control barriers.) If problems arise with the equipment, use should be discontinued immediately and service should be provided by a certified dental service technician. (For further information related to radiology, see Chapter 29.)

Professionalism

Understanding and following routine equipment maintenance of dental equipment as recommended by the manufacturers' instructions will keep the equipment at peak performance without a lot of downtime and delays in the daily office schedule. Following and establishing a routine maintenance schedule is not only productive to the dental office schedule, but to the lifetime of the equipment.

Small Equipment

Various types of small equipment are found in the dental operatory. The dentist's preferences and types of treatments performed will dictate the type of small equipment necessary for the dental treatment rooms. Small equipment includes:

- An amalgamator (Figure 20.14) is a small machine used to **triturate** or mechanically mix dental amalgam for silver fillings and some dental cement. The amalgamator should be placed in an area that is easily accessible to the dental assistant. (For further information on the amalgamator, see Chapter 38 on general dentistry.)

- A curing light (Figure 20.15) is used to cure, harden, or set light-cured dental materials. Many different types of curing lights are available, depending on the operator's preference. Characteristics of a dental curing light are evaluated by the intensity, which is the speed of the light, and the spectrum, which is the heat generated by the light. Other amenities to consider when choosing a curing light include portability, digital timers, audio timers,

filters, protective eye shields, and different size interchangeable tips. The curing light can be mounted to a wall, set on a cabinet, or be cordless. The curing light could be integrated onto the dental unit. Because of light intensity and ultraviolet rays, special protective eyewear is necessary for the patient and a protective shield is necessary to prevent eye damage for the operator and dental assistant during the curing process. If the curing light is not working at full strength, the material will not set properly, which results in an inadequate outcome for the restorative material. Barriers are available to provide infection control and should be placed to reduce disinfection between patients. Manufacturer care and maintenance instructions should be referenced when changing the curing light bulb. (For further information on the curing light, see Chapter 38 on general dentistry.)

- An x-ray view box (Figure 20.16) is used by the dentist to read and diagnose dental radiographs. View boxes are placed on a shelf in a cabinet or can be mounted on the wall or in a cabinet. Radiographs are placed on a frosted glass cover that is encased with a light source that allows the radiograph to be easily viewed. The x-ray view box should be disinfected between patients as described in the manufacturer's instructions. The x-ray box should be kept away from direct sunlight to keep frosted glass from yellowing.

- The intraoral camera is a powerful and valuable diagnostic tool in the operatory for computer viewing of the patient's oral cavity. The intraoral handpiece or wand has a camera on the end that is placed in the patient's mouth and images are then transmitted to a computer screen for visual display. The computer can freeze images that can then be printed or stored in a patient's file for later referencing. This method of examining the oral cavity allows for visual education of the patient concerning conditions present in the patient's mouth while the dentist discusses treatment.

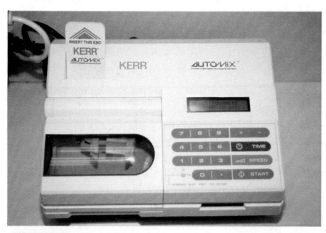

FIGURE 20.14
Amalgamator.
Image courtesy Instuctional Materials for the Dental Team, Lex., KY

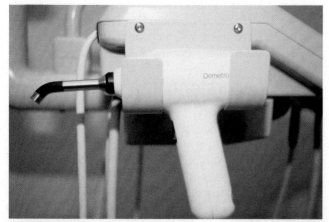

FIGURE 20.15
Curing light.
Image courtesy Instuctional Materials for the Dental Team, Lex., KY

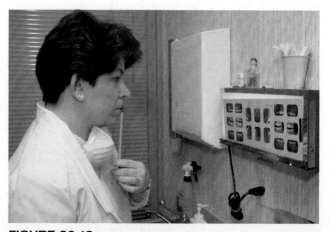

FIGURE 20.16
An x-ray view box is used by the dentist to read and diagnose dental radiographs.

Legal and Ethical Issues

Intraoral cameras are one of the best marketing tools for the dental office. In the best of situations, using the intraoral camera for informed consent is a standard of quality individual practices may want to invest in. By viewing the pictures taken with the intraoral camera, patients are given the opportunity to see the condition and discuss treatment and financial matters with the dentist. By being able to actually see the condition of the oral cavity, the patient may be more likely to provide consent for treatment. Once informed consent is provided, copies of the signed informed consent and a picture taken with the intraoral camera can be placed in the patient's chart. This information can later be provided to the insurance company to process payment or used to receive payment from the patient.

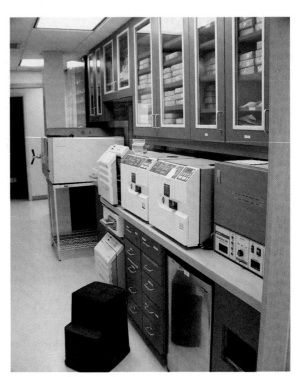

FIGURE 20.17
Central sterilization area.
Image courtesy Instructional Materials for the Dental Team, Lex., KY

- Air abrasion is the mechanical etching of the surface of a tooth. The benefits of air abrasion include removal of enamel, dentin, and restorative material gently without interfering with surrounding tissue. Air abrasion rarely requires anesthetics and provides more comfort to the patient than a dental handpiece because no vibration or heat is generated. Precautions are needed when using air abrasion. Some concerns the operator must be aware of include these: The production of high aerosol powder requires HVE suction to remove air debris. The production of air debris, in turn, raises the level of possible infectious disease in the surrounding environment, therefore infection control procedures must be followed. The improper use of a dental handpiece can cause damage to surrounding surfaces of the adjacent teeth. Patients need to wear protective eyewear and a drape over the entire face to reveal only the oral cavity. The lips need to be kept lubricated to prevent the drying effect of sodium bicarbonate.

- In many larger practices small computers may be located in the dental treatment areas. These computers are mainly used for storing digital x-rays, to update patient treatment notes, and to check patients' appointment times. Computers in the operatories are a valuable asset for enhancing the efficiency of an office.

What is the difference between an operating light and a curing light?

Central Sterilization Area

The sterilization area is centrally located near the operatory rooms but out of the view of patients (Figure 20.17). Infection control is closely monitored for the entire practice from this area. Work in this area includes the steril-

ization and maintenance of supplies as well as cleaning and storage of materials in preparation for reuse. The sterilization area is typically equipped with a sink, ultrasonic cleaning units, precleaning holding tanks, cold sterile holding baths, and some type of sterilizing unit. Infection control procedures are practiced in this area.

All contaminated items such as instruments, trays, and materials are sterilized and prepared for the next use in the central sterilization area. Some offices may store sterile patient trays, setups, and instruments in this area. The sterilization area should be well defined into three workspaces: a contaminated area (dirty), a clean area where the instruments are free of debris and ready to be separated for methods of sterilizing, and a sterile area (sterile) as defined in Chapter 17. This area should be kept clean, organized, and well ventilated due to chemical fumes and sterilizer exhaust.

Dental Laboratory Area

The dental laboratory (Figure 20.18) is organized and designed to accommodate laboratory procedures such as pouring impressions, trimming diagnostic models, creating custom trays, and preparing dental cases. The dental laboratory must be kept neat and organized at all times. This area of the dental practice is usually located in an isolated room that provides good ventilation. When handling specimens and laboratory equipment, it is important to follow infection control procedures and safety precautions. The dental staff should pay particular atten-

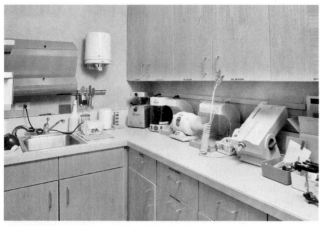

FIGURE 20.18
Dental laboratory.

tion to wearing safety glasses and a mask to help prevent dust and debris from causing injury while working with and around laboratory equipment. Some of the dental laboratory equipment includes the dental lathe and model trimmers, exhaust fan, dental stone vibrator, dental plaster and stone storage bins, and many more items that are discussed in depth in Chapter 37.

Why is it so important to follow the manufacturer's care and maintenance instructions for dental equipment?

SUMMARY

For a dental practice to operate efficiently, consideration must be given to the type of office design and materials. The design type and equipment chosen depends on the type of dentistry being practiced and the personal prefer-ences of the dentist. The dental assistant must be familiar with all types of equipment, which can vary among dental offices.

KEY TERMS

- **Consultation room:** Specified room or meeting area where diagnosis, financial information, treatment and/or treatment planning, as well as extensive personal or health-related issues are discussed concerning the patient.   p. 293
- **Dental chair:** The center for all clinical and treatment activity. The chair is designed for the patient's comfort and allows the operator and/or assistant to provide treatment to the patient in an efficient manner. p. 297
- **Dental operatory/treatment room:** Clinical or control area where dental treatment is performed.   p. 294
- **Dental unit:** Consists of handpieces, air/water syringes, saliva ejector, possibly an oral evacuator or ultrasonic scaler, along with numerous other options depending on operator's preferences.   p. 298
- **Handpieces:** Instruments that aid the dentist in tooth preparation and the removal of dental decay.   p. 299

- **Rheostat:** Foot-controlled or pedal device that is used to operate and control the dental handpieces.   p. 299
- **Subsupine position:** Position in which patient is reclined in the dental chair with the patient's head positioned lower than the feet. This position is also called the Trendelenburg position.   p. 297
- **Supine position:** Position in which patient is reclined in the dental chair with the patient's nose and knees at the same level.   p. 297
- **Triturate:** The mechanical combination of dental materials.   p. 301
- **Upright position:** Position in which patient is seated with the dental chair back at a 90-degree angle. This position is used for patient entry and release from the dental chair.   p. 297

CHECK YOUR UNDERSTANDING

1. Which of the following would best describe the features of the dental assistant's stool?
   a. adjustable height and backrest
   b. broad base, well balanced, and moves freely
   c. has a foot rest
   d. all of the above

2. In which area of the office would a patient's personal history, treatment plans, and financial information typically be discussed?
   a. treatment room
   b. dentist's private office
   c. consultation room
   d. front desk

CHECK YOUR UNDERSTANDING (continued)

3. When opening the office at the start of the work-day, which of the following tasks should the dental assistant perform?
   a. Turn on master switches to the central air compressor, vacuum units, sterilization equipment, dental units, and the radiograph and developing units.
   b. Turn on lights and computers.
   c. Check the daily schedule and ensure all dental instruments are sterile and ready for patient treatment.
   d. All of the above.

4. Why should the dental assistant arrive at the office 30 minutes prior to the first patient?
   a. to flush dental handpieces
   b. to set up the operatory
   c. to turn on equipment
   d. all of the above

5. What is the dental curing light used for?
   a. viewing the patient's oral cavity
   b. setting and hardening dental materials
   c. reading x-rays
   d. curing dental plaster

6. What is the foot pedal that controls the handpieces on the dental unit called?
   a. HVE
   b. amalgamator
   c. rheostat
   d. handpiece foot pedal

7. Who or what regulates the strict specifications that ensure dental office designs comply with state and federal guidelines?
   a. Justice Department
   b. Americans with Disabilities Act
   c. HIPAA
   d. local building permits office

8. Which dental team member is in charge of keeping the dental lounge clean?
   a. dentist
   b. dental assistant
   c. front desk receptionist
   d. all of the above

9. Who is responsible for the maintenance of the x-ray unit?
   a. certified dental service technician
   b. dental assistant
   c. dental repair person
   d. dental rover

10. The air compressor is used to provide service to which of the following?
   a. operation to the dental chair
   b. oral evacuation system
   c. power for dental light and amalgamator
   d. source for the air/water syringes and dental handpieces

INTERNET ACTIVITY

- Go to www.dentalcompare.com to review questions for designing an ideal dental practice.

WEB REFERENCES

- Henry Schein virtual tour of different dental office designs http://info.henryschein.com/Dental/OfficeDesign/DesignGallery

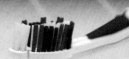

21

Examination and Care Planning

Learning Objectives

After reading this chapter, the student should be able to:

- Define patient record confidentiality.

- Explain how to correct an error on a patient's record.

- Demonstrate obtaining a medical history and how to document patient allergies.

- Discuss the order of precedence for an ideal care plan.

- Describe a thorough clinical dental examination to include intraoral and extraoral procedures.

- Demonstrate assisting a dentist during a dental examination.

- State what the SOAP format of a dental examination includes.

Preparing for Certification Exams

- Prepare patient records and receive and set up patients for examination, including seating, chair positioning, and placing the patient napkin.
- Demonstrate knowledge of patient record confidentiality.

Key Terms

Abrasion

Asymmetry

Attrition

Bruxism

Chief complaint

Comprehensive oral exam

Crepitus

Erosion

Etiologic

HIPAA

Objective evaluation

Palpation

Subjective evaluation

Chapter Outline

- Patient Record and Confidentiality
  - —Health Insurance Portability and Accountability Act
  - —Personal Data
  - —Dental and Medical History
  - —Clinical Examination and Progress Notes
  - —Retention of Records
  - —Transfer of Records
  - —Faxing Dental Records

- Creating and Maintaining the Patient Record
  - —Electronic Dental Record
  - —Recording Information in the Patient Record

- Patient Record Forms
  - —Personal Data
  - —Health History and Drug Allergies
  - —Visual Dental Chart of Existing Conditions
  - —Care Plan
  - —Progress Notes
  - —Miscellaneous Reference Data

- Obtaining the Health History

- Exam and Diagnostic Techniques
  - —Seating the Patient
  - —Comprehensive Examination
  - —Diagnostic Techniques

- Clinical Examination of the Patient
  - —Extraoral Examination
  - —Intraoral Examination

- Documentation of the Dental Examination
  - —Subjective Evaluation
  - —Objective Evaluation
  - —Assessment
  - —Plan

- Charting

- Care Plan Formulation
  - —Care Plan Presentation

- Documentation of Dental Treatment

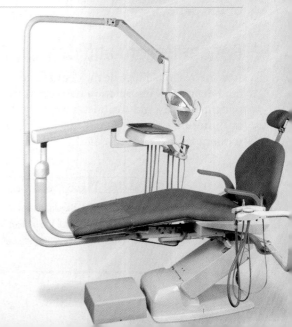

The planning of treatment for each patient is essential to the successful outcome of dental care and requires meticulous attention to detail. The primary purpose of care planning is to determine an appropriate sequence of dental treatment with anticipated short-term and long-term outcomes or prognoses. The outcome must be acceptable to the patient and the dentist. Patients should be encouraged to participate in care planning decisions, which will enhance their oral health as well as the overall health of their body.

To accomplish these goals, an effective relationship should be developed between the patient and the dental office. The patient must be assured of the confidentiality of all matters discussed. The need for thorough and precise record keeping cannot be overemphasized. This chapter discusses the confidentiality of patient information, the documents necessary to create a patient record, the importance of obtaining a thorough patient health history, and the essentials of a comprehensive patient dental examination. Following a complete exam and assessment by the dental clinician, a plan for how to proceed with dental care is formulated based on the needs of the patient.

Patient Record and Confidentiality

It is the responsibility of the dentist and staff to keep in confidence any information derived from a patient. All patient records and treatments are considered confidential information and should not be divulged to anyone without the patient's consent.

Dental Assistant PROFESSIONAL TIP

Always "inform before perform." Tell the patient what you are going to do before doing it. An example is to tell the patient that you are going to place the dental chair in a supine position before actually adjusting it.

Preparing for Externship

In preparation for externship, the dental assisting student should practice explaining to another student why certain dental procedures must be performed prior to other procedures. This exercise may also be used to practice communication and interaction between people. Dental assistants should be encouraged to discuss various treatment options, and explain to others the importance of ideal oral health.

The patient record is a legal document and must be maintained accurately and completely. The quality of dental records can be an important factor in cases of disagreement or lawsuits. Appropriate arrangements should be made for adequate physical security of patient records.

Several things must be taken into consideration regarding patient charts and records:

- Dental records must be maintained in a manner consistent with the welfare of the patient.
- Dental records should never be left where easy access by unauthorized individuals is possible. If visible to others, dental records should be placed facedown.
- Dental records must be returned to their proper location promptly following use and kept safe from fire, damage, and loss.

Dental records are permanent health records and need to be accurate, legible, and easy to understand.

Health Insurance Portability and Accountability Act

The primary purpose of the Health Insurance Portability and Accountability Act (**HIPAA**) is to protect patient confidentiality and to assure that patients know what is done with their health information. HIPAA rules require each person who maintains or transmits health information to adopt reasonable and appropriate administrative safeguards that address the following goals:

- To ensure the integrity and confidentiality of patient information
- To protect against any reasonably anticipated threat or hazards to the security or integrity of the information
- To protect against unauthorized uses or disclosures of the information
- To otherwise ensure compliance among staff

Dentists who transmit patient information via computer networks should exercise caution to guard against any breach of patient privacy.

The HIPAA regulations require every patient to sign an acknowledgment that they have received a notice of privacy practices. This acknowledgment form should be filed in the dental record. In addition, most practices will record this form in their computer system to track it electronically. In dental practices with multiple sites, a computer tracking system is beneficial because the dental record may not always be in the practice location when the patient comes for a visit. The patient has the right to receive an accounting of the names of the individuals and organizations that have received personal health information; this is referred to in HIPAA as the Accounting of Disclosures policy. For further information on HIPAA regulations, see Chapter 3.

Personal Data

Dental records must be meticulously kept for each patient and contain at minimum the following information:

- Name, date of birth, address, and, if a minor, name of parent or guardian
- Name and telephone number of person to contact in case of an emergency
- Place of employment
- Attitude toward dental treatment, including patient expectations about the care they receive

Figure 21.1 shows a sample of a patient health history form that can be used to record the information listed above.

Dental and Medical History

Dental records include information from the patient or the patient's parent or guardian regarding the dental and medical history. When a patient presents with a chief complaint, dental records should include the patient's reason for visiting the dentist. The **chief complaint** is the symptom or group of symptoms that represents the patient's reason for seeking care. The chief complaint is what brought the patient to the dental office such as a toothache, a sensitive area, a broken tooth or filling, or a routine examination.

Clinical Examination and Progress Notes

Dental records (Figure 21.2) will include chronological dates and descriptions of the following:

- Clinical examination findings, tests conducted, and a summary of all pertinent diagnoses
- Plan of intended treatment and sequence of care
- Services rendered and any complications from treatment
- All radiographs, study models, and periodontal charting, if applicable
- The name, quantity, and strength of all drugs dispensed, administered, or prescribed
- Name of dentist, dental hygienist, or other auxiliary who performs any treatment or service or who may have

contact with the patient regarding his or her dental health
- Documentation of informed consent, discussion of procedures and treatment options, and potential complications and known risks
- The patient's written consent to proceed with treatment
- Indications of patient allergies and other medical alerts; these must be clearly marked on either the electronic or paper record

Retention of Records

Dentists must maintain patient records in a manner consistent with the protection of the welfare of the patient. Most dentists keep records indefinitely. State laws dictate how long records must be kept, but typically dentists maintain patient dental records for a minimum of seven years after the date of the last examination, prescription, or treatment. Proper safeguards should be in place to ensure that manual and/or electronic records are protected from any destructive forces. When electronic records are kept, the dentist may keep either a duplicate hardcopy record or use an unalterable electronic record system.

Dental records are the legal property of the dentist. They may be duplicated if necessary for use by another dentist or subpoenaed for court cases. Upon request of a patient or another dental practitioner, a dentist should provide any information that will be beneficial for the future treatment of the patient.

Transfer of Records

The dental assistant must preserve the confidentiality of patient records in a manner consistent with protecting the patient's welfare. If another dentist or health care professional requires the patient's dental records, the dentist must obtain written permission from either the patient or patient's legal guardian to release the records. The permission must indicate if the record in its entirety is approved for release or if only part of the record is approved.

Once permission has been received, the dental office can make copies. The original record is never released. Dentists are allowed to charge a nominal fee for duplication of records, but may not refuse to transfer records. Copying of dental records may be the responsibility of the dental assistant.

Patients need access to the information in dental records for a variety of reasons. People move and may ask if they can take their dental records with them. They may also wish to consult with another dentist regarding proposed treatment. When a patient moves and is no longer seeking care through the dental office, the patient's record is stored with the archived patient records. Sometimes patients move back and seek out the dentist where they previously received treatment.

Patient Health History & Information

Patient Information

Date _8-21-2007_

Patient _John Doe_

Address _12121 Beautiful Smile St_
Lone Tree Colorado 80124

Sex ☑M ☐F Age _39_ Birthdate _1-1-68_

☑Single ☐Married ☐Widowed ☐Separated ☐Divorced

Patient SS# _332-33-3333_

Occupation _Stellar Marketing -VP_

Employer _Stellar Marketing_

Employer Address _3232 Happy Street_

Employer Phone _303-777-7777_

Spouse's Name _____

Birthdate _____ SS# _____

Occupation _____

Spouse's Employer _____

Whom may we thank for referring you? _____

Dental Insurance

Who is responsible for this account? _John Doe_

Relationship to Patient _Self_

Insurance Company _Delta Dental of Co_

Group # _2222_

Is patient covered by additional insurance? ☐ Yes ☑ No

Subscriber's Name _____

Birthdate _____ SS# _____

Relationship to patient _____

Insurance Company _____

Group # _____

ASSIGNMENT AND RELEASE

I, the undersigned certify that I (or my dependent) have insurance coverage with _John Doe_ and assign directly to Dr. Angela Osborn all insurance benefits, if any, otherwise payable to me for services rendered. I understand that I am financially responsible for all charges whether or not paid by insurance. I hereby authorize the doctor to release all information necessary to secure the payment of benefits. I authorize the use of this signature on all insurance submissions.

John Doe
Responsible Party Signature

Self   _8-21-2007_
Relationship   Date

Phone Numbers

Home _303-333-3333_ Work _720-444-4444_ Ext. _____ Spouse's Work _____

Mobile _303-222-2222_ Email _JohnDoe@Comcast.net_ Best time and place to reach you _anytime_

IN CASE OF EMERGENCY, CONTACT (Specify someone who does not live in your household.)

Name _Mary Doe_   Relationship _Mother_

Home Phone _303-555-5555_   Work Phone _____

Dental History

Reason for today's visit _Exam_
prophylaxis, X-rays

Former Dentist _Dr John Hurt_

City/State _Denver Colorado_

Date of last dental visit _2 years_

Date of last dental X-rays _2 years_

Place a mark on "Yes" or "No" to indicate if you have had any of the following:

	Yes	No
Bad breath	☑	☐
Bleeding gums	☑	☐
Blisters on lips or mouth	☐	☑
Burning sensation on tongue	☐	☑
Chew on one side of mouth	☐	☑
Cigarette, pipe, or cigar smoking	☐	☑
Clicking or popping jaw	☐	☑
Dry mouth	☐	☑
Fingernail biting	☐	☑
Food collection between the teeth	☑	☐
Foreign objects	☐	☑
Grinding teeth	☐	☑
Gums swollen or tender	☑	☐
Jaw pain or tiredness	☐	☑
Lip or cheek biting	☐	☑

	Yes	No
Loose teeth or broken fillings	☐	☑
Mouth breathing	☑	☐
Mouth pain, brushing	☑	☐
Orthodontic treatment	☑	☐
Pain around ear	☐	☑
Sensitivity to cold	☐	☑
Sensitivity to heat	☐	☑
Sensitivity to sweets	☐	☑
Sensitivity when biting	☐	☑
Sores or growths in mouth	☐	☑

How often do you floss? _never_

How often do you brush? _2 x day_

Angela Osborn DDS 9218 Kimmer Drive Suite #106 Lone Tree, CO 80124 303.799.9993 phone 303.799.9998 fax

FIGURE 21.1
Sample dental health history form.
Courtesy of Dr. Angela Osborn

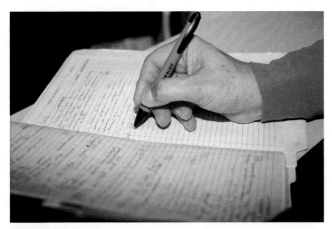

FIGURE 21.2
A patient record.
Image courtesy of Instructional Materials for the Dental Team, Lex., KY

When a patient is referred to another dentist or health care provider, the referring dentist may send records through the postal service or through e-mail. A patient may pick up her own records for consultation with another practitioner. If records are released for any reason to a patient, the patient should sign an acknowledgment that the patient is taking the records. The entry should be complete and accurate, stating specifically what records are being released, to whom, for what purpose, and the date should be indicated.

Radiographs are the property of the dentist. They can be duplicated for the patient to take to another dental facility. Diagnostic cast models, which are a record of a patient's condition prior to treatment, may be given to the patient or stored at the dental facility. Each dental practice has established procedures for handling requests from patients to see their dental records. Dental records may be requested via subpoena in cases of litigation.

If a patient's record has to be faxed, what precautions should be taken to ensure confidentiality?

Faxing Dental Records

Before sending medical or dental information via a facsimile (fax) machine, certain steps must be followed in order to protect patient privacy:

• Prior to faxing, be sure to obtain an authorization to release records. Make sure the release has been dated and signed by the patient or legal guardian.
• Only fax to a fax machine in a doctor's office or other secure area, not to machines in mail rooms or office lobbies. If necessary, call the receiving office prior to faxing the document to ensure the receiver is by the fax.
• Use a cover sheet that contains the warning: "The following material is strictly confidential; all persons are advised that they may be prosecuted under federal and

state law for sharing this information with unauthorized individuals."
• As soon as the fax has been sent, call the receiver and confirm that it was received.

What should be obtained from the patient before transferring records or giving out information regarding a patient?

Creating and Maintaining the Patient Record

A dental record must be created at the time of the patient's first appointment. Some dental facilities may mail the patient registration form and medical history for the patient to complete prior to the patient's first appointment. During the first call with a new patient, the patient should be instructed to complete the form and bring it with him to the appointment. This saves time for both the patient and the office. Each form must clearly state the patient's name.

A record of each patient visit is an essential part of dentistry. Accurate dental records help to ensure efficiency and completeness in the delivery of care. Good dental records facilitate high-quality care by making detailed and relevant patient information readily available to other health care providers. Dental records can play an important role in the identification of deceased persons if necessary. They also form the basis for retrieval of treatment details in the case of a dispute or the requirement to provide evidence in a court case. Dental records can also provide valuable information for teaching, education, and research. Typically forms in the patient's record are maintained in a chronological order, with the most recent information on top of previously recorded information.

Electronic Dental Record

Computers have been available in the dental office since the late 1960s. By the 1980s they had become a common practice management tool. As with the traditional patient record, the electronic dental record (EDR) is created during the first examination of the patient. The dental assistant enters information directly into the computer with a keyboard and mouse. Some digital systems support direct data entry based on voice recognition. During an examination the dental clinician can speak commands and information directly into the system. This software capability allows the clinician's hands to be free and assists in preventing cross-contamination.

Paperless dental records have many advantages. For instance, the cost of paper is eliminated, and storage, retrieval, presentation, and communication of computerized patient information becomes a more efficient method for keeping patient information. The principles that apply to handwritten records also apply to computer records. Digital dental treatment records must show who made each entry and when it was made. Security procedures, such as access to records only via a password, should be in place.

The ability to educate patients during a case presentation is excellent with a digital record. The dentist can develop care plans with the click of a mouse and determine the cost. Anatomically correct picture charts and digital radiographs assist the patient in understanding his or her dental condition as it is visually displayed on the computer screen. The patient can also take home a complete copy of his or her radiographs, chart, care plan, and fees. Electronic records help patients keep well informed about their dental needs.

In addition to digital patient records, computers are being used to produce radiographs and record dental charting. Advantages of digital radiographs include reduced radiation and chair time for the dentist and patient. Less money overall is spent on x-ray film, processing, and mounting. Digital radiographs have the ability to be enhanced by adjusting the contrast and color or by enlarging the images. Dental charting done on a computer can minimize human errors and can be done more quickly than with the manual method.

As charting software continues to develop, standards and formats will improve and enhance the electronic dental patient chart. There will be no need to look for a misfiled paper record. The electronic patient record is easily updated to reflect current changes in the medical or oral health status. If the patient is referred to a specialist, no copying and mailing, or faxing is necessary. The electronic transfer will save front-desk time as well as the patient's time and discomfort in an emergency situation.

A disadvantage to the electronic patient chart is that current standards have not yet established a norm for what must be included in the record.

Recording Information in the Patient Record

Accuracy of information recorded in the patient record is important regardless of whether the information is recorded manually or electronically. Dates for each patient visit must be recorded. Records must be accurate and concise and be promptly retrievable when required. They must be readily understandable by any third party such as another dental care provider.

For paper records, notations should be legible, written in ink, and contain no erasures or covered-up entries. Record entries should be legible and use consistent standard abbreviations. For manual entries, corrections made to records must not involve the removal of the original information. If the dental assistant needs to make a correction, he or she draws one line through the incorrect information and then writes the correct information next to the original entry. If an entry needs to be made after the fact, a new

dated entry must be made. The date used for this entry is the date the new information is entered. In this new entry the date of service that the new entry is discussing should be noted. The addition cannot be added to an old entry.

Notes should include details about materials used, any variations from the dentist's usual technique, and comments about the procedure. All comments should be noted in objective unemotional language. The detail should include the complexity or serious potential for complications. Complete record entries should reflect:

* Treatment advice that the patient was unwilling to accept
* Drugs prescribed (quantity, dose, instructions)
* Drugs administered (dose)
* Consents obtained for treatment
* Unusual results following treatment reported by the patient
* Estimates or quotations of fees
* Relevant comments by patients about concerns over offered treatments
* Comments or complaints by patients about treatment provided
* Annotations necessary following telephone conversations with patients

---

In what order should each form be placed in a patient's record? How might dental records be used to identify deceased persons?

Patient Record Forms

Patient record forms vary depending on the preference of the dentist, dental group, or hospital. Most entries on a dental patient's record are written in blue or black ink. Some entries requiring special emphasis may be placed in red ink. These include medical alerts and allergies. Most patient dental records are organized as follows:

* Personal data
* Health history and drug allergies
* Visual dental chart of existing conditions
* Care plan
* Progress notes
* Miscellaneous reference data

These types of patient record information are discussed in the following subsections.

Personal Data

The patient registration form contains personal data about the patient (Figure 21.3). It includes the name of the patient, date of birth, present address, and, if the patient is a minor, the parent or guardian's name. The

PATIENT REGISTRATION FORM
(Please Print)

Date: _____

Patient's
Name: _____   DOB: ____ / ____ / ____
         First   Middle   Last   Month Day Year

Address: _____   Phone: ____ / ____ - ____
          Street   City   State   Zip   (Area code)

Patient's SS#: ____-____-____   Driver's License #: _____   Occupation: _____

Method of payment (circle):   cash   check   credit card   insurance co-payment

Primary Insurance Co.: _____   Policy/Group #: _____

Medicare #: _____   Medicaid #: _____

Person
Responsible
For Payment: _____
              First   Middle   Last   Relationship

Address: _____   Phone: ____ / ____ - ____
          Street   City   State   Zip   (Area code)

Employer Name: _____   Dept: _____
                First   Middle   Last

Address: _____   Phone: ____ / ____ - ____
          Street   City   State   Zip   (Area code)

Spouse or
Nearest Relative: _____
                  First   Middle   Last   Relationship

Address: _____   Phone: ____ / ____ - ____
          Street   City   State   Zip   (Area code)

How were you referred to this office? _____

_____

Statement of Financial Responsibility: I, _____,
do hereby agree to pay all medical charges incurred by the above listed patient. I further understand
that these charges are my responsibility, regardless of insurance coverage.

Responsible Person's Signature: _____

FIGURE 21.3
Sample patient registration form.

patient registration form also usually includes the following information:

- Patient's telephone number
- Name and phone number of a person to contact in case of an emergency
- Patient's place of employment and work phone number
- Insurance information, including the policy number

Other information that is typically requested on the patient registration form includes the patient's attitude toward dental treatment, the patient's expectations regarding treatment, and any major concerns regarding the patient's teeth. The dental assistant must ensure that each new patient completes and signs the registration form. If the patient is a minor, the parent or guardian must sign this form for the minor.

Health History and Drug Allergies

The health history provides the dental clinician with detailed information about the patient's general health and date of last physical exam and must be updated at each and every visit. This form also asks the patient to provide the name, address, and phone number of the patient's primary physician. Other questions asked on the health questionnaire include:

- Is the patient currently under the care of a physician? If the answer is yes, the patient is asked to elaborate on what type of treatment and care are being received.
- What type of past and present health conditions has the patient experienced?
- What history, if any, does the patient have with smoking, drugs, or alcohol use?
- Is there any relevant family history relating to the patient's physical condition and history?

A sample health history, including information about drug allergies, is shown in Figure 21.4.

Allergies

Allergies can range from minor irritations to life-threatening emergencies. Patients may be allergic to certain medications.

Patient Health History & Information

Health History

Physician's Name: DR. Brenda Warren   Date of last visit: 6-12-2007

Place a mark on "Yes" or "No" to indicate if you have had any of the following:

Condition	Yes	No
AIDS	☐	☑
Anemia	☐	☑
Arthritis, Rheumatism	☐	☑
Artificial Heart Valves	☐	☑
Artificial Joints	☐	☑
Asthma	☐	☑
Back Problems	☐	☑
Bleeding abnormally, with extractions or surgery	☐	☑
Blood Disease	☐	☑
Cancer	☐	☑
Chemical Dependency	☐	☑
Chemotherapy	☐	☑
Circulatory Problems	☐	☑
Congenital Heart Lesions	☐	☑
Cortisone Treatments	☐	☑
Cough, persistent or bloody	☐	☑
Diabetes	☐	☑
Emphysema	☐	☑
Do you wear contact lenses?	☐	☑
Epilepsy	☐	☑
Fainting or dizziness	☐	☑
Fibromyalgia	☐	☑
Glaucoma	☐	☑
Headaches	☐	☑
Heart Murmur	☐	☑
Heart Problems	☐	☑
Hepatitis Type ______	☐	☑
Herpes	☐	☑
High Blood Pressure	☐	☑
HIV Positive	☐	☑
Jaundice	☐	☑
Jaw Pain	☐	☑
Kidney Disease	☐	☑
Liver Disease	☐	☑
Low Blood Pressure	☐	☑
Mitral Valve Prolapse	☐	☑
Multiple Sclerosis	☐	☑
Nervous Problems	☐	☑
Organ Transplant	☐	☑
Pacemaker	☐	☑
Women: Are you pregnant?	☐	☑
Due date ______ Are you nursing?	☐	☑
Psychiatric Care	☐	☑
Radiation Treatment	☐	☑
Respiratory Disease	☐	☑
Rheumatic Fever	☐	☑
Scarlet Fever	☐	☑
Shortness of Breath	☐	☑
Sinus Trouble	☐	☑
Skin Rash	☐	☑
Special Diet	☐	☑
Stroke	☐	☑
Swelling of Feet or Ankles	☐	☑
Swollen Neck Glands	☐	☑
Thyroid Problems	☐	☑
Tonsillitis	☐	☑
Tuberculosis	☐	☑
Tumor or growth on head or neck	☐	☑
Ulcer	☐	☑
Venereal Disease	☐	☑
Weight Loss, unexplained	☐	☑

Medications

List medications you are currently taking: none

Pharmacy Name: Walgreens

Phone: 303-888-8888

Allergies

- ☐ Aspirin
- ☐ Barbiturates (Sleeping Pills)
- ☐ Codeine
- ☐ Iodine
- ☑ Latex
- ☐ Local Anesthetic
- ☐ Penicillin
- ☐ Sulfa
- ☐ Other

Angela Osborn DDS 9218 Kimmer Drive Suite #106 Lone Tree, CO 80124 303.799.9993 phone 303.799.9998 fax

FIGURE 21.4
Sample patient medical health history.
Courtesy of Dr. Angela Osborn

Allergies to dental anesthetics, metals, latex, and any other allergies must be carefully documented in the patient's record. Most dental facilities will note allergies in red on the health history form. Patients should be asked what kind of allergic reaction they have experienced and the circumstances under which it occurred. For offices that have transitioned to electronic patient records, the medical health conditions and allergies will appear on the monitor of an EDR as an "Alert" to remind the dental team of the situation for a particular patient.

Visual Dental Chart of Existing Conditions

After the dentist has thoroughly reviewed and discussed the health history with the patient, the condition of the mouth is charted on a visual record, and current restorations and disease conditions are noted. The dental assistant uses red and blue pencils to note the condition of the patient's teeth. Electronic charting in the dental operatory is frequently done by voice recognition software. Digital dental charting may also be done manually by the dental assistant using a computer keyboard and mouse for entering information into the patient's record. (For more information on dental charting see Chapter 9.)

Dentists can choose from among many different styles of visual dental charts. The dental assistant must be able to chart on any type of tooth diagram available. The most common types of tooth diagrams use anatomic representations of teeth; others use geometric representations, and yet others use a combination of anatomic and geometric. The anatomic representation shows the tooth crown with a light indication of root structure. The drawings look like teeth and vary in the amount of tooth surface shown (Figure 21.5). Some drawings show only the crown of the teeth and some others show the crown and part of the root. The geometric representations do not really look like teeth. Instead the geometric representations consist of a series of circles, divided to represent the surfaces of the tooth. They include a simulation of the root structure of the permanent dentition.

Care Plan

The dentist will assess and diagnose dental disease within the patient's mouth and formulate a list of dental needs. The diagnosis uses scientific and skilled methods to determine the cause of a disease condition. Once a diagnosis has been made, the dentist forms a prognosis to predict the course of the disease or the outcome of treatment for the condition. The dentist designs a well-sequenced care plan that addresses the patient's dental circumstances.

Legal and Ethical Issues

To prevent misunderstandings, it is important to provide the dental patient with both a verbal and written explanation of the patient's care plan including information regarding fees. A copy of the plan should be kept with the patient's record. The care plan should also give an estimate of the likely short-, immediate-, and long-term costs; when payment is expected; and how it is to be made. The care plan may be divided into phases for financial reasons. These phases must be planned in an appropriate order, aiming to first eliminate any pain and discomfort and to control active disease.

The dentist's findings and recommendations are documented in the patient's record. The dental assistant, office manager, or care plan coordinator provides the patient with a written care plan (Figure 21.6). The patient is then informed of the expected cost of treatment. If the patient has health insurance, the patient is informed of any deductibles or copays that the patient will be required to pay out of pocket.

Progress Notes

At a minimum, progress notes include the date of the patient's treatment, the tooth being treated, and any treatment performed. The American Dental Association (ADA) procedure code and cost of treatment will often be noted on most progress notes. All entries placed in the record must be signed by the health care provider. Each entry must be legible, accurate, and detailed. There should not be any lines left open between entries.

Topics appropriate for entry into the progress notes include the following:

- Phone calls related to discussions with the patient
- Cancellations, broken appointments, late arrivals
- Conversations regarding treatment
- Symptoms, problems, diagnoses, and prognoses
- Compliance or noncompliance with treatments
- Assessments, treatments, and materials used during treatments
- Medications
- Response to treatments and care plans

Miscellaneous Reference Data

Various miscellaneous materials are placed in the patient's chart. An example would include the HIPAA privacy policy acknowledgment receipt that is signed by the patient (Figure 21.7). This part of the record may

DIAGNOSIS: MISSING TEETH and EXISTING PROBLEMS

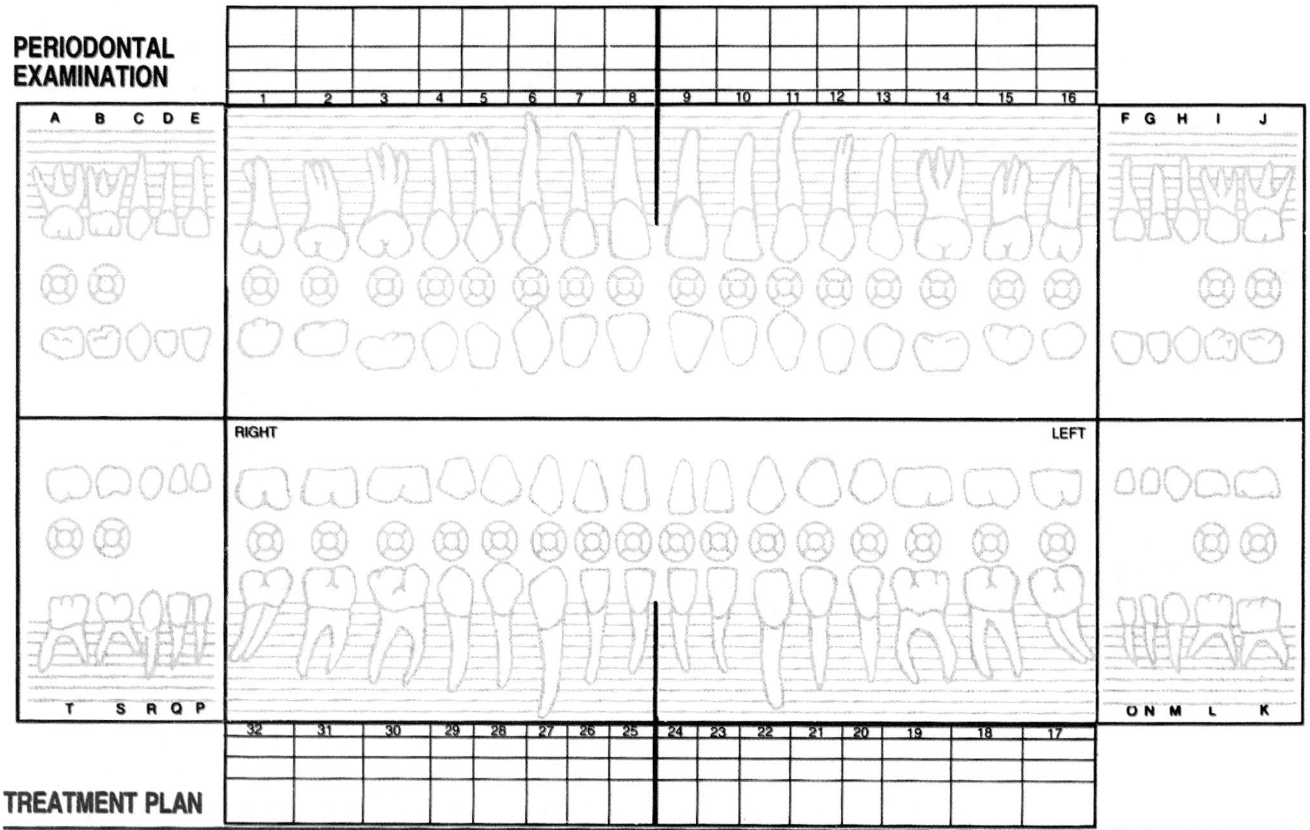

PERIODONTAL EXAMINATION

A B C D E

1 2 3 4 5 6 7 8 9 10 11 12 13 14 15 16

F G H I J

RIGHT

LEFT

T S R Q P

32 31 30 29 28 27 26 25 24 23 22 21 20 19 18 17

O N M L K

TREATMENT PLAN

DATE DIAGNOSED	TOOTH #	SUR-FACE	DESCRIPTION OF SERVICE	ADA CODE	FEE	CO-PAY	DATE DIAGNOSED	TOOTH #	SUR-FACE	DESCRIPTION OF SERVICE	ADA CODE	FEE	CO-PAY
			EXAMINATION										
			X-RAY: PANORAMIC: FMX: BWX:										
			DIAGNOSTIC MODELS										
			PROPHYLAXIS (CLEANING)										
			QUADRANTS SCALING & CURETTAGE										
			NITROUS-OXIDE GAS										

FIGURE 21.5

Sample clinical dental examination form.

Courtesy of Dr. Angela Osborn

COMPLETED TREATMENT

| | 1 | 2 | 3 | 4 | 5 | 6 | 7 | 8 | 9 | 10 | 11 | 12 | 13 | 14 | 15 | 16 | |

A B C D E   F G H I J

RIGHT   LEFT

T S R Q P   O N M L K

| | 32 | 31 | 30 | 29 | 28 | 27 | 26 | 25 | 24 | 23 | 22 | 21 | 20 | 19 | 18 | 17 | |

INITIAL PERIODONTAL EXAM:

GINGIVAL INFLAMMATION:	☐ Slight	☐ Moderate	☐ Severe
SOFT PLAQUE BUILDUP:	☐ Slight	☐ Moderate	☐ Heavy
HARD CALC. BUILDUP:	☐ Light	☐ Moderate	☐ Heavy
STAINS:	☐ Light	☐ Moderate	☐ Heavy
HOME CARE EFFECTIVENESS:	☐ Good	☐ Fair	☐ Poor
PERIODONTAL CONDITION	☐ Good	☐ Fair	☐ Poor
PERIODONTAL DIAGNOSIS:	☐ Normal	☐ Gingivitis	
PERIODONTITIS:	☐ Early	☐ Moderate	☐ Advanced

MUCOGINGIVAL DEFECTS #s: _____

CLINICAL DATA:

OCCLUSION: ☐ Class I ☐ Class II ☐ Class III ☐ Crossbite: _____

T.M.J. EXAM: ☐ Normal ☐ Popping ☐ Deviation ☐ Tooth Wear ☐ Pain

INITIAL SOFT TISSUE EXAM:

☐ Lips   ☐ Floor of Mouth   ☐ Palate   ☐ Tongue   ☐ Neck & Nodes

PATIENT'S TREATMENT DECISIONS:

☐ DOCUMENTATION OF DENTAL RECORD COMPLETED

☐ PATIENT INFORMED OF TX. RECOMMENDATIONS AND CONSENTS TO TX. (ALTERNATIVES DISCUSSED.)

☐ PATIENT WANTS NO TX. OR PARTIAL TX. INFORMED OF CONSEQUENCES AND RISKS INVOLVED.

INITIAL X-RAY FINDINGS:

X-RAYS TAKEN: ☐ FM-PAS ☐ BWX ☐ PANO. ☐ OTHER _____

	UR	UL	LR	LL
☐ NO BONE LOSS				
☐ SLIGHT BONE LOSS (04600)				
☐ MODERATE BONE LOSS (04700)				
☐ MAJOR BONE LOSS (04800)				
☐ BEGINNING FURCATION (04700)				
☐ ADVANCED FURCATION (04800)				
☐ OTHER: _____				

(QUADRANTS)

SHADE

Teeth	Upper	Lower
Cents		
Lats		
Cusp		
Posts		

PERIODONTAL SCREENING & RECORDING

SEXTANT SCORE   MONTH DAY YEAR

EXISTING PROSTHESIS:

MAX. _____ DATE PLACED: _____ CONDITION: _____

MAND. _____ DATE PLACED: _____ CONDITION: _____

REFERRALS:

PERIO: _____ ORTHO: _____ ENDO: _____

ORAL SURG: _____ M.D. _____ OTHER _____

NOTES

_____
_____
_____
_____
_____
_____

CONSENT

The undersigned hereby authorizes the Doctor to take X-rays, study models, photographs, or any other diagnostic aids deemed appropriate by Doctor to make a thorough diagnosis of the patient's dental needs. I also authorize Doctor to perform any and all forms of treatment, medication, and therapy that may be indicated. I also understand the use of anesthetic agents embodies a certain risk. I understand that my dental insurance is a contract between me and the insurance carrier, and not between the insurance carrier and the Doctor and that I am still fully responsible for all dental fees. These fees are due and payable at the time services are rendered unless prior financial arrangements have been made. I also assign all insurance benefits to the Doctor. Any payments received by the Doctor from my insurance coverage will be credited to my account, or refunded to me if I have paid the dental fees incurred. I further understand that a late charge will be added to any overdue balance. I understand that where appropriate, credit reports may be obtained.

PATIENT Signature (Parent of Child) _____ Date: _____ DENTIST Signature _____

315

Date: 08/21/2007

Angela Osborn
9218 Kimmer Dr. Suite 106
Lone Tree, CO 80124
(303) 799-9993

Page: 01

All Treatment Plans for John J Doe
12121 S.Beautiful Smile St
Lone Tree, CO 80124
(303) 333-3333

Plan#	Code	Description	Tooth	Surface	Date Prop.	Date Comp.	Fee	PatAmt	InsEst
T1	D2950	Core Buildup, Including Any Pins	30		08/21/2007		298.00	149.00	149.00
T1	D2740	Crown-Porcelain/Ceramic Substrate	30		08/21/2007		1081.00	540.50	540.50
T1	D2950	Core Buildup, Including Any Pins	31		08/21/2007		298.00	149.00	149.00
T1	D2740	Crown-Porcelain/Ceramic Substrate	31		08/21/2007		1081.00	540.50	540.50
T1	D2393	Resin-based composite - three surfaces, posteri	2	MOL	08/21/2007		289.00	57.80	231.20
							3047.00	1436.80	1610.20

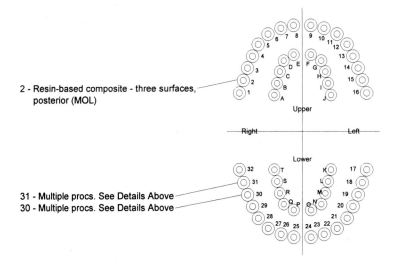

2 - Resin-based composite - three surfaces,
   posterior (MOL)

31 - Multiple procs. See Details Above
30 - Multiple procs. See Details Above

Primary Plan:				
Stellar Marketing/Delta Dental Co	Maximum Benefits:	**1500.00**	Benefits YTD:	**0.00**
Subscriber: **John J Doe**	Deductible:	**50.00**	Current Plan:	**1610.20**
	Ded. Met?	**No**	Remaining:	**0.00**

I recognize that this is an estimate only and is only valid for 3 months from date of proposal. The insurance coverage may vary from this estimated treatment calculation. I understand this is an estimate only and fully understand that I am ultimately responsible for payment in full for all treatment rendered.

Signature: _John Doe_   Date: _8-21 2007_

FIGURE 21.6
Sample completed patient treatment plan.
Courtesy of Dr. Angela Osborn

also contain referral letters from other dentists or physicians who have seen the patient. Other items may also be included in this section:

- Reports from consultations that occurred with other clinicians
- Clinical photographs of the patient, such as before/after treatment photos
- Copies of drug prescriptions given to the patient

- Documentation of informed consent for dental treatment signed by the patient

Information regarding a proposed procedure or care plan must be provided to the patient, and the patient must understand what she is consenting to. Disclosure of information and oral consent for minor procedures should be entered in the clinical notes. For major treatment, written consent forms acknowledge that the nature, implications,

Angela M Osborn DDS

ACKNOWLEDGEMENT OF RECEIPT OF NOTICE OF PRIVACY PRACTICES

I, ______________________________, have received a copy of this office's Notice of Privacy Practices.

____
{Please Print Name}

____
{Signature}

____
{Date}

For Office Use Only

We attempted to obtain written acknowledgement of receipt of our Notice of Privacy Practices, but acknowledgement could not be obtained because:

- ☐ Individual refused to sign
- ☐ Communications barriers prohibited obtaining the acknowledgement
- ☐ An emergency situation prevented us from obtaining acknowledgement
- ☐ Other (Please Specify)

____

____

____

This Form is educational only, does not constitute legal advice, and covers only federal, not state, law (August 14, 2002).

FIGURE 21.7
Sample acknowledgment of HIPAA privacy practices form.
Courtesy of Dr. Angela Osborn

and risks of the proposed procedure have been explained (Figure 21.8). This provides evidence that the information was given and consent granted.

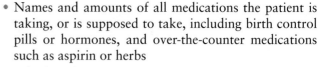

What color of ink should be used in the record to note the patient's allergies? What color ink should be used to write entries in the patient record? Who must sign the registration and consent forms if the patient is a minor?

Obtaining the Health History

A complete medical history must be obtained from each patient before beginning any dental treatment. Certain medical conditions may influence treatment and necessitate referral of the patient to a physician for further evaluation. Potential risks from dental treatment will be assessed before any treatment begins. To complement the medical history obtained at the first visit, the patient should be made aware of the need to advise the dentist of any change in his medical status during the course of his treatment. The dental assistant should always ask the patient at each appointment if there has been any change in his medical history. Most offices require the dental assistant to initial the health history to document that it was completed for the patient and verified by the assistant. If the patient is a minor, the parent or guardian must sign it.

A general medical history should contain information pertaining to:

- General health and appearance
- Systemic diseases and conditions such as cancer, cardiac conditions, history of rheumatic fever, diabetes, hepatitis, herpes, AIDS, and other contagious conditions
- Allergies and sensitivities to drugs
- Reactions to anesthetics
- Present medications and/or treatment
- Bleeding problems
- Nervous disorders
- Any other information pertinent to the formation of a care plan for the patient's health and safety; and also protect the staff and the public

Many patients unintentionally omit or distort answers. Patients should be told of the importance of a thorough medical history and its benefit to their dental health. Consideration and discretion are essential. The patient should be assured of the confidentiality of all matters discussed. The dental assistant may aid in completion of the health questionnaire by asking the patient for the following information:

- General health and date of last physical exam
- Name, address, and phone number of physician

- Names and amounts of all medications the patient is taking, or is supposed to take, including birth control pills or hormones, and over-the-counter medications such as aspirin or herbs
- Whether the patient is currently under the care of a physician and, if so, the patient's current health status

Why is a thorough medical history so vital for the patient? How often should the patient's medical history be updated?

Exam and Diagnostic Techniques

The ADA recommends a comprehensive exam for all patients who are new to a dental practice and an exam every year for established patients, that is, those who are already in the practice. The ADA defines a **comprehensive oral exam** as an extensive evaluation and recording of all extraoral, intraoral, and soft tissue findings. The ADA further defines a periodic oral exam as an exam that is done on established patients to determine any changes in dental and physical health status that have occurred after the patient's last comprehensive or periodic evaluation. A comprehensive exam lays the foundation for the routine (periodic) oral exam.

One role of the dental assistant is to listen to each patient and to document correctly patient concerns. The dentist then integrates this information into a comprehensive report that combines the patient's health history and oral findings. If health concerns are present the patient may be referred to his or her primary care physician.

Seating the Patient

Dental patients may be nervous, so the dental assistant plays a vital role in helping patients feel comfortable in the dental environment. Methods to achieve this include the following:

- Be friendly and use professional, positive communication skills.
- Familiarize the patient with the dental team by introducing each member by name.
- Ask the patient if there is anything that can be done to assist him in feeling more comfortable and relaxed.

Some dental offices ask the patient to use a prerinse before being seated. The dental assistant should ensure the patient uses the prescribed rinse for 30 seconds and has a tissue available to wipe his mouth following the procedure.

When the patient is seated, try to make the patient as comfortable as possible. Men can loosen or remove their ties. Sometimes just visiting with the patient about any topic helps put a person more at ease in the dental environment.

ANGELA OSBORN DDS
9218 KIMMER DRIVE
SUITE 106
LONE TREE, CO 80124
PHONE 303.799.9993
FAX 303.799.9998

GENERAL CONSENT

Thank you, for choosing our office for your dental care. We will work with you to help you achieve excellent oral health. While recognizing the benefits of a pleasing smile and teeth that function well, you should be aware that dental treatment, like treatment of any other part of the body, has some inherent risks. These are seldom great enough to offset the benefits of treatment, but should be considered when making treatment decisions.

Benefits of dental treatment can include: relief of pain, the ability to chew properly, and the confidence and social interaction that a pleasing smile can bring. Nonetheless, there are some common risks associated with virtually any dental procedure, including:

1. **Drug or chemical reaction.** Dental materials and medications may trigger allergic or sensitivity reactions.
2. **Long-term numbness (paresthesia).** Local anesthetic, or its administration, while almost always adequate to allow comfortable care, can result in transient or, in rare instances, permanent muscle numbness.
3. **Muscle or joint tenderness.** Holding one's mouth open can result in muscle or jaw joint tenderness, or in a predisposed patient, precipitate a TMJ disorder.
4. **Sensitivity in teeth or gums, infection, or bleeding.**
5. **Swallowing or inhaling small objects.**

While we follow procedural guidelines which most often lead to a clinical success, just like in any other pursuit in health care, not everything turns out the way it is planned. We will do our best to assure that it does. Please feel free to ask questions in regard to all dental procedures that are recommended to you.

I have read and understand the statement on this page:

John Doe _____   8-21-07 _____
Patient's NAME please print   Date

John Doe _____   8-21-07 _____
Patient's signature   Date

_____   _____
Parent's signature (if minor patient)   Date

FIGURE 21.8
Sample general consent form.
Courtesy of Dr. Angela Osborn

Procedure 21-1 Preparing the Patient for the Extraoral and Intraoral Dental Examinations

Equipment and Supplies Needed

- Basic setup: mirror, explorer, cotton pliers
- Periodontal probe
- Articulating paper and holder
- 2 × 2 gauze squares
- Patient record and black ink pen
- Dental chart and red/blue pencil or a computer that is ready to receive input

Procedure Steps

1. While escorting the patient to the treatment room, observe his general appearance, gait, speech, and eyes for anything unusual.

2. Seat the patient comfortably in the dental chair; adjust the headrest and light. Place the patient napkin around the patient's neck. Ensure the patient has eye protection.

3. Explain to the patient that the dentist is going to perform a complete dental exam, which includes gently feeling the face and neck with the hands and fingers and then performing an examination of the mouth.

4. Organize the dental record and chart on a flat surface, or set up the computer and prepare to document the examination as the dentist dictates his or her findings.

5. Tell the dentist that the patient is ready and prepare to record findings of the exam.

Professionalism

The most important concern in dentistry is the patient. Going to the dentist is distressing for some people. The dental assistant's positive attitude can help patients feel more at ease. Developing effective communication skills is a must for the dental assistant. You should be able to express yourself clearly and to listen effectively. Putting the patient at ease begins when you introduce yourself. Avoid words that might upset or frighten the patient, for example, *discomfort* is a better word than *pain*, *prepare the tooth* is better than saying *drill the tooth*. Courtesy, efficient attention to detail, and conscientious service are attributes of an outstanding dental assistant.

The dental assistant drapes the patient napkin around the patient's neck with the napkin holder, adjusts the headrest, and places the chair in the working position favored by the dentist. After the dental assistant has seated the patient and positioned the chair, the operating light should be turned on and the light beam focused beneath the patient's chin to avoid shining light into the patient's eyes. The light should then be turned off until the dentist is ready to begin the examination. When the dentist is ready, turn on the light and rotate the light up to the mouth.

Patients wearing lipstick should be given a tissue to remove it or any petroleum or mineral oil product that may cause degradation of latex and compromise the integrity of gloves worn by dental providers. Cocoa butter may be used as a lubricant for lips during dental procedures. Patients who are wearing corrective glasses should be asked to leave them in place during the exam; patients who are not wearing glasses should be given eye protection. See Procedure 21-1.

Comprehensive Examination

The mouth is a window into the body. Medical conditions may be discovered by a comprehensive dental exam before symptoms show up elsewhere in the body. Some medical conditions that the dentist may discover include these:

- Diabetes, especially poorly controlled or undiagnosed diabetes
- Hypertension or high blood pressure problems
- Cardiovascular problems
- Oral cancer
- Sinus problems
- Other diseases or disorders of the body such as leukemia

After completing a comprehensive examination on a patient, a long-term strategy for health and prevention of dental and systemic diseases can be established.

Diagnostic Techniques

When performing a visual examination, the dentist visually inspects the patient's lymph nodes in front of the ears, behind the ears, in the jaw area, beneath the chin, and around the neck. The dentist is looking for any pain, tenderness, or flexibility of the lymph nodes. The dentist usually palpates those areas to see if symptoms of pain and tenderness are present. **Palpation** is a process of examining by applying the hands or fingers to the external surface of the body to detect evidence of disease or abnormalities.

Once the lymph nodes have been checked, an exam of the inside of the mouth occurs. This involves evaluating the hard and soft palate, behind the molars, the floor of the mouth, frenum, the cheek surfaces, and the size, color, shape, and position of the tongue.

The dentist also completes a periodontal exam or screening by taking six measurements of each tooth sulcus or periodontal pocket depth. These pocket depths are recorded by the dental assistant on a specific form or electronically recorded into the computer. The periodontal examination includes documenting mobility of teeth, measuring bone loss, noting the presence of calculus, and documenting any bleeding, swelling, and gingival recession.

The dentist also examines the patient's bite, performing an occlusal screening to determine tooth occlusion, wear, chewing problems, pain in the joints and jaw areas, mouth opening abilities, and to check for temporomandibular joint problems.

What are some systemic conditions the dentist might discover during a comprehensive exam? What might the dentist do with this information?

Clinical Examination of the Patient

To provide a comprehensive oral exam, dentists use a systematic approach. A clinical examination of the patient includes a survey of the patient's general overall health. Vital signs are taken and documented in the patient's record. A physical examination of the head and neck region is performed by the dentist, the dental hygienist, or by the dental assistant if directed by the dentist. Hard and soft tissues in the oral cavity are examined for signs of disease. Determination of necessary radiographs and diagnostic cast models is assessed. The dentist also takes note of any harmful habits the patient may have and the patient's attitude toward care to the extent that it would affect dental treatment.

Extraoral Examination

The extraoral examination includes palpation of the temporomandibular joints and related structures as well as the lymph nodes (Figure 21.9). During the extraoral examination the patient will be asked to swallow. The dentist observes the patient for any distinguishing features or asymmetry of the face, and movement of the mandible during excursive movements (Figure 21.10). **Asymmetry** indicates a lopsided unevenness or irregularity in facial features that may be a disease condition.

Temporomandibular Joint Exam

A thorough temporomandibular joint (TMJ) examination includes palpation of several groups of muscles that

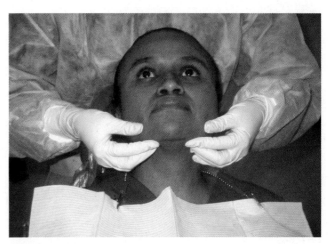

FIGURE 21.9
Palpating the submandibular nodes.
Image courtesy of Instructional Materials for the Dental Team, Lex., KY

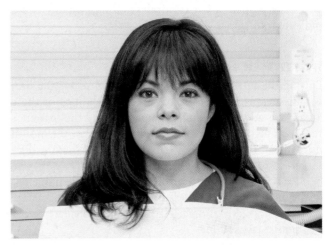

FIGURE 21.10
Visual exam of the patient's face for symmetry.

make up the TMJ (Figure 21.11). (For further information regarding the TMJ, see Chapter 5.) During the TMJ exam, these muscles are examined for soreness and sensitivity. The patient is asked to open and close her mouth and to move her mandible in various positions while the dentist palpates the TMJ muscles inside and outside of the mouth. The dentist observes how the patient's mandible opens and closes and moves from side to side, in order to look for any signs of deviation from the normal. The dentist listens for sounds such as crepitus or popping noises from the temporomandibular joint. **Crepitus** is a cracking or grating sound heard upon movement.

Examination of the Head and Neck

During the examination of the head and neck (Figure 21.12), the dentist examines the head to include the skin, hair, eyes, ears, and form of the face for signs of anything abnormal. Palpation is performed to identify conditions of the salivary glands, head and neck muscles, the carotid artery, and the lymph glands and nodes. These areas are

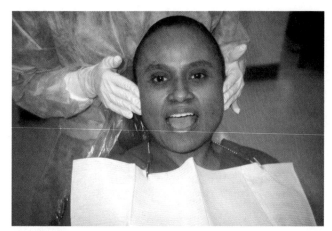

FIGURE 21.11
Palpating the TMJ.
Image courtesy of Instructional Materials for the Dental Team, Lex., KY

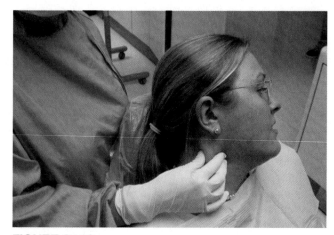

FIGURE 21.12
Palpating the sternocleidomastoid muscle.
Image courtesy of Instructional Materials for the Dental Team, Lex., KY

examined for any lumps or hardened areas. The dentist will also palpate for extraoral swelling, which would indicate infection.

Intraoral Examination

During the intraoral exam, the dentist observes the oral soft tissues as well as the teeth. Abnormalities of these areas are identified and documented in the patient's record. The dentist uses 2 × 2 gauze squares, the mouth mirror, an explorer, and a periodontal probe that the dental assistant has set out for the exam.

Prior to the intraoral examination, the dental assistant must ensure that all radiographs of the patient are mounted correctly and placed on the lighted view box for the dentist to examine.

Oral Soft Tissue Exam

An examination of the oral soft tissues includes the lips, tongue, and floor of the mouth (Figures 21.13, 21.14, and 21.15). The smile line and shape are observed during the oral soft tissue exam. The dentist uses the 2 × 2 gauze

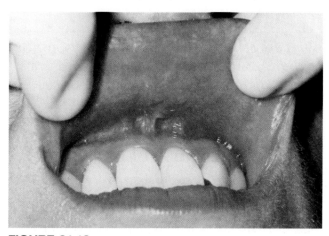

FIGURE 21.13
Examination of the oral mucosa and frenum.

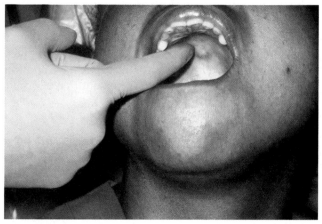

FIGURE 21.14
Palpating the hard palate.
Image courtesy of Instructional Materials for the Dental Team, Lex., KY

Life Span Considerations

Physical, functional, and cognitive deficits associated with chronic disease and aging can present many challenges to the dental health care team. By the year 2020, it is estimated that nearly 18% of the U.S. population will be 65 years of age or older. To provide the best possible care for these patients, the dental team must be aware of not only the physical and oral health needs and how to meet them, but how the patient's general and mental health may impact this care. Nutrition and self-care evaluations should be addressed as well. Integration of the elements of these geriatric assessments into the dental care plan should be evaluated in order to assess their impact on treatment outcomes.

to gently grasp the patient's tongue and lift it to observe conditions on the floor of the mouth and on the right and left sides of the tongue. The hard and soft palates are examined along with the uvula. Unusual conditions including lumps, inflammation, lesions, and discolorations on the mucosa are noted.

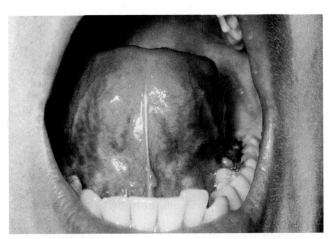

FIGURE 21.15
Examination of the tongue and floor of the mouth.

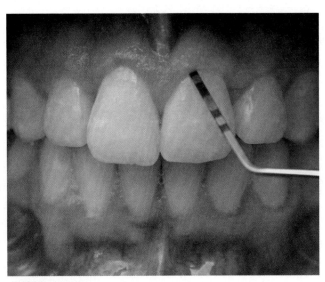

FIGURE 21.16
Examination of the periodentium.
Image courtesy of Instructional Materials for the Dental Team, Lex., KY

Hard Tissue Exam

A systematic assessment of all tooth surfaces is obtained using the dental explorer. During the hard tissue exam, the dentist looks for sound tooth structure, fractured teeth or those with loose or broken restorations, the presence or absence of caries, and the presence or absence of tooth surface loss.

Evidence of tooth abrasion, attrition, and erosion is recorded. **Abrasion** is the mechanical wearing away of tooth structure. Toothbrush abrasion is common and caused by using a toothbrush with hard bristles instead of soft bristles and by brushing the teeth improperly. **Attrition** is often a more normal wearing away of tooth structure over time. Examples of attrition include excessive grinding of the teeth, also called **bruxism**, or use of a pipe on the anterior teeth, which may wear them down. **Erosion** is chemical wearing away of tooth structure. Enamel may be worn down by stomach acid in patients with bulimia or those who suck on lemons. The clinical exam and important diagnostic findings of a patient's oral hard tissues will also note malaligned and displaced teeth.

Occlusal Exam

To examine the occlusion, the dentist asks the patient to close her teeth together. The dentist may use articulating paper, small pieces of carbon paper, to check the patient's bite in order to assess the pattern of occlusion. The patient is asked to close her teeth in centric occlusion.

During this portion of the exam, the dental assistant notes in the record whether the patient has a Class I, Class II, or Class III occlusion. (For further information regarding these classes, see Chapter 50.)

Periodontal Exam

A periodontal assessment includes pocket depth measurement all around the teeth. This exam includes noting the presence or absence of calculus, any gingival recession, and gingival bleeding (Figure 21.16). Areas where

Cultural Considerations

It may be necessary to meet with a patient on more than one occasion in order to provide further explanation and answer questions clearly regarding treatment options. Patients who have difficulty understanding English should be encouraged to bring someone with them who can help explain details of the dentist's diagnosis and prognosis so that the patient can make an informed decision regarding his or her dental health care choices. As often as possible, the dental assistant should use simple terms that the patient is familiar with and can understand.

the patient experiences food impaction, tooth mobility, and tooth migration are noted. (For further information on periodontal assessment, see Chapter 45.)

What instruments must the dental assistant lay out that the dentist will require during the clinical examination? What areas will be examined during the clinical examination?

Documentation of the Dental Examination

Clear documentation of the dental exam will describe the following:

- Present complaint
- Relevant history of the patient's condition
- Clinical findings

- Diagnosis of dental conditions
- Formulation of care plans
- Patient consent to treatment

A complete and up-to-date medical history must be confirmed at each appointment. All findings, observations made, and procedures performed for the patient must be noted in the patient's record. Any relevant communication with or about the patient should be documented. Drugs prescribed or administered must be entered on the record. Radiographs taken by the assistant or any communication between the dental assistant and the patient must also be entered. Each entry the dental assistant places in the patient's record should be followed by his or her initials.

The patient exam is most often performed in a methodical manner using the SOAP format:

- Subjective
- Objective
- Assessment
- Plan

Subjective Evaluation

As mentioned earlier, the reason for the patient coming to the dental facility is called the chief complaint. The chief complaint is part of the **subjective evaluation**, which is the part of the dental examination that consists of the patient's observations about why the patient decided to visit the dentist, not the observations of any of the dental team members.

The dental assistant should write as much of the patient-provided information down in the patient record as possible. Questions should be asked to gather enough information to assist the dentist in understanding the purpose of the patient's visit.

Objective Evaluation

An **objective evaluation** includes any observations regarding the patient made by members of the dental team. This can include observations such as swelling of the face, redness on the gingival tissues, and any exudates or fluid oozing around a tooth. Objective information also includes any radiographs taken of the patient's oral cavity.

Obtaining information for the objective evaluation often requires the dental assistant to ask questions of the patient so the dental assistant can make the necessary observations. For instance, if a patient comes into the office expressing concern regarding a tooth, the dental assistant should ask questions such as these:

- Where is the discomfort?
- What is the location of the painful tooth or area?

- Is the pain continuous or intermittent?
- Is the discomfort in the tooth spontaneous or provoked by hot or cold temperatures, or a combination of these stimuli?
- Does it hurt when you eat sweets?
- Does the discomfort linger after the stimulus that provoked it was removed?
- What is the character of the ache? Is it a dull throb, or more of a sharper ache?
- How, when, and where did the traumatic injury occur?

The answers to these questions help the dental assistant concentrate on certain areas that may lead to important observations about the patient's oral health. The dental assistant must thoroughly document any information obtained from a patient. This information is vital in assisting the dentist in determining the course of care.

Be aware that the patient might not be able to identify which tooth is bothering him. The discomfort may even be referred from one area to another.

Assessment

In the assessment part of the SOAP method, the dentist assesses findings during the examination and provides a diagnosis of the patient's condition. The doctor's assessment justifies the treatment that is needed for the patient's oral health. The dentist may perform tests on a tooth or teeth. The tests required may include palpation, heat or cold tests, an electric pulp test, or periodontal probing.

Plan

The care plan includes how to begin treatment, how future appointments should best be scheduled, the treatment that will be performed for the patient, and any prescriptions that may be needed. When determining and discussing a patient's care plan, the patient's financial situation is considered.

Care planning typically is done in the following general order from the most serious to the least serious dental conditions:

- Anything causing pain, such as extractions needed or abscesses present
- Catching caries before they become a problem; possibly temporary fillings
- Surgeries
- Periodontics
- Permanent restorations
- Fixed prosthodontics
- Removable prosthodontics
- Elective procedures
- Orthodontics

Charting

The dental assistant charts missing teeth and existing restorations in blue pencil. Caries, problem areas, and proposed restorations are charted with red pencil on paper or entered into the computerized patient record as the software directs. (For further information regarding charting, see Chapter 9.) During the charting part of the clinical exam, the dentist uses radiographs to determine:

- Oral conditions such as caries
- Restorations that are defective or those that are acceptable
- Missing teeth
- Cysts
- Periapical and periodontal abscesses present
- Other hard and soft lesions present in the patient's oral cavity

The periodontal status of the patient's mouth is often documented on a specialized form that emphasizes gingival conditions and bone level. (For further information regarding periodontics, see Chapter 45.) Existing conditions, including location and measurement of periodontal pockets, **etiologic** factors causing disease conditions, mobile teeth, and occlusal trauma, are noted on the periodontal form.

What color is used to chart the existing conditions in a patient's mouth? What color is used to chart problem areas in a patient's mouth?

Care Plan Formulation

Once the dentist's findings from the patient's history and diagnoses have been appropriately considered, a care plan is formulated to address the needs of the patient. The care plan is the projected series and sequence of dental procedures necessary to restore the oral health of the patient. The sequencing is based on the oral diagnosis and a complete evaluation of the patient. Potentially harmful or dangerous conditions will be taken care of first. An example of sequencing might be:

- Relief of pain and discomfort
- Elimination of infection, irritation, and traumatic conditions
- Treatment of extensive carious lesions and pulpal inflammation
- Prophylaxis and instruction in preventive care
- Periodontal treatment
- Elimination of remaining caries
- Necessary extractions
- Restorations and replacement of teeth
- Placement of the patient on a recall schedule to assess any further needs

Who presents the care plan to the patient? What type of patient disease condition will be treated first?

Care Plan Presentation

The dentist, office manager, dental assistant, dental hygienist, or care plan coordinator presents the care plan to the patient. An indication of the presentation must be included in the record. When the plan is complex, a comprehensive discussion with the patient (or guardian, if appropriate) should take place. This discussion will include:

- Dentist's diagnosis
- Prognosis of treatment
- Alternative plans for treatment
- Possible risks of treatment
- Expectant success of treatment
- Possible results if suggested treatment is not performed

Often, for risk management purposes, patients are asked to sign a form or the patient's record signifying that the care plan is understood and accepted.

Documentation of Dental Treatment

Information documented in a patient's record must be written legibly with the date and treatment rendered. Every date of a patient's visit must be noted. The following information, when relevant, should be written in ink:

- Type and amount of anesthetic administered or drugs prescribed
- Dental procedure described in detail
- Tooth number(s) and tooth surfaces
- Type, brand name, and amount of dental material used
- Detailed instructions given to the patient
- Notation of patient comments, positive or negative
- Information about any adverse event and how it was handled
- Initials of the health care provider

Making accurate and complete record entries is a crucial area of professional responsibility. A record entry must be made for every patient interaction that occurs. The importance of accurate record keeping cannot be overemphasized. The dental record document is primary evidence if legal action is taken against the practitioner and demonstrates that measures were taken to ensure patient confidentiality, safety, and the success of all treatment rendered. Adverse events are rare but must be documented because they may influence future dental treatment. These include allergic reactions to anesthesia or latex and other emergencies such as a heart attack or stroke.

SUMMARY

The best dental record is not one that is kept on paper or on a computer, but one that is complete and properly documented, including all necessary signatures. Before beginning dental treatment for a patient, a quality dental record must be created. The patient record contains various forms that provide detailed information about the patient. The dental assistant's role is significant during this process. Valid consent for treatment and an accurate and thorough medical history must be obtained from the patient. Patients must also be informed about the office privacy policy toward disclosing their personal information.

A care plan is formulated and documented by the dentist following a comprehensive clinical examination. The dentist makes the diagnoses of the patient's oral health according to conditions needing attention and prioritizes appropriate treatment to suit the best interests of the patient.

KEY TERMS

- **Abrasion:** The mechanical wearing away of tooth structure. p. 323
- **Asymmetry:** A lopsided unevenness or irregularity in facial features. p. 321
- **Attrition:** Wearing away of tooth structure over time. p. 323
- **Bruxism:** Excessive grinding of the teeth. p. 323
- **Chief complaint:** The symptom or group of symptoms that represents the patient's reason for seeking care. p. 307
- **Comprehensive oral exam:** An extensive evaluation and recording of all extraoral, intraoral, and soft tissue findings. p. 318
- **Crepitus:** A cracking or grating sound heard upon movement. p. 321
- **Erosion:** Chemical wearing away of tooth structure. p. 323

- **Etiologic:** Factors causing disease.   p. 325
- **HIPAA:** Health Insurance Portability and Accountability Act; requires that each person who maintains or transmits health information use appropriate administrative safeguards to protect against unauthorized uses or disclosure of patient information. p. 306
- **Objective evaluation:** Portion of dental examination that consists of any observations regarding the patient made by members of the dental team. p. 324
- **Palpation:** A process of examining by applying the hands or fingers to the external surface of the body to detect evidence of disease or abnormalities. p. 320
- **Subjective evaluation:** Portion of the dental examination that consists of the patient's observations about why the patient decided to visit the dentist. p. 324

CHECK YOUR UNDERSTANDING

1. HIPAA stands for
   a. Health Insurance Portability and Accountability Act.
   b. Health Information Personal Privacy Act.
   c. Hospital Identification Personality Privacy Act.
   d. Health Insurance Personal Accountability Act.

2. How should corrections to the patient record be made?
   a. Erase the entry in the record and write the correct word.
   b. Scratch out the mistake and place the correct entry next to it.
   c. Draw one line through the incorrect word and write the correct word.
   d. Use a white correction fluid to neatly cover the incorrect entry.

3. Dental records
   a. should never be left out in the open.
   b. must be protected and safe from fire and damage.
   c. are a permanent record.
   d. all of the above.

4. What information must be included on each form of the patient's record?
   a. name of the patient and date of entry
   b. name of the patient and patient's phone number
   c. patient's place of employment
   d. patient's date of birth

5. Dental records should be kept
   a. for one year.
   b. for three years.
   c. for seven years.
   d. according to state law.

CHECK YOUR UNDERSTANDING (continued)

6. In what order should dental forms be placed in the patient's record?
   a. most recent information on the bottom
   b. most recent information on the top
   c. in chronological order
   d. both b and c

7. The clinical dental examination includes palpation of
   a. each tooth.
   b. lymph nodes.
   c. TMJ muscles.
   d. salivary glands.
   e. b, c, and d only.
   f. all of the above.

8. The periodontal exam includes observation and testing of the
   a. gingiva.
   b. bone.
   c. periodontal pocket.
   d. all of the above.

9. Who presents the care plan to the patient?
   a. dentist
   b. office manager
   c. care plan coordinator
   d. any of the above

10. Entries in the patient record must be
    a. clear.
    b. accurate.
    c. legible.
    d. initialed.
    e. all of the above.

● INTERNET ACTIVITY

- To conduct further research on the American Dental Association standards for dental record keeping and forms, visit the following website: www.ada.org

● WEB REFERENCES

- Boston University School of Dentistry http://dentalschool.bu.edu
- Family Gentle Dental Care www.dentalgentlecare.com
- Medical College of Georgia: Syllabus of Clinical Procedures for Oral Diagnosis and Treatment Planning www.mcg.edu/SOD/oraldiag/SYLLBUS99.pdf

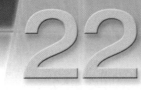

Caring for the Dental Patient

Chapter Outline

Learning Objectives

After reading this chapter, the student should be able to:

- Describe the elements of the patient record and the need for reviewing.
- Describe ways of developing patient rapport.
- Explain the process for greeting and seating the dental patient.
- Discuss the dental assistant's role in patient care.
- Describe the patient with possible dental anxiety and fear.
- Discuss how to care for the patient with dental anxiety.
- Identify various special needs of the dental patient.
- Identify specific ways to assist patients who have special needs.

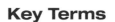

Preparing for Certification Exams

- Receive and prepare patients for treatment, including seating, chair positioning, and patient napkin placement.
- Demonstrate knowledge of ethics/jurisprudence/ patient confidentiality.

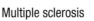

Key Terms

Angina pectoris	Muscular dystrophy
Emphysema	Phobia
Hypertension	Pulmonary disorders
Hyperthyroidism	Resorption
Hypothyroidism	Stroke (cerebrovascular accident)
Mechanical bruxism	
Multiple sclerosis	

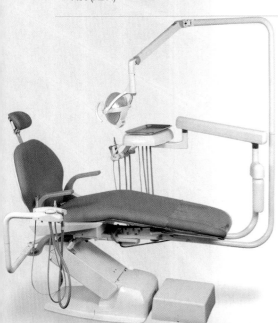

Care of the dental patient requires a team approach with each player on the team responsible for positive intervention with each patient. Many people today experience fear and anxiety when visiting the dentist. The fear and anxiety can come from past experiences that are often deeply rooted and difficult for the patient to overcome. As a result, many people resist seeing a dentist until they are experiencing a true dental emergency. The fearful patient who is seeking dental care is acting out of desperation and is likely to be resistant to any treatment beyond relief of the immediate problem. If the fearful patient is treated properly, however, the patient can gain trust in the dental team and may end up taking the necessary steps to regain oral health. The trust of the patient can be achieved through the support of a caring dental team.

Treatments for addressing patient fears are varied and include medication, hypnosis, and sleep specialty techniques. The patient with special needs could be a patient with dental anxiety, a person who uses a wheelchair, or a person who has a developmental disability. Each patient is an individual and must be treated with respect and kindness.

Establishing Patient Rapport

Rapport is a positive working relationship between people. The word *rapport* comes from the French word for "relationship." It is considered one of the most important aspects of human social interaction. It is the connection between people. Dental professionals must have the ability to assess the patient and be on the same level with the patient. This does not mean the dental professional should be condescending or look down on a person. Rather, it is the ability to build a relationship of mutual understanding and harmony. For example, a dental assistant who does not care about rapport will tell the patient what to do in factual terms. The dental assistant who cares about rapport will ensure that the message has been conveyed and that the patient has had an opportunity to ask questions or share small talk.

Ways to Build Rapport

General techniques for building rapport include using complementary body language, such as sincere eye contact, an open body stance, and welcoming gestures. In the dental practice, more specific techniques may be used such as a reassuring pat on the hand, clearly communicating what the patient should expect from the procedure, and ensuring that all of the patient's questions have been answered.

Natural kindness and empathy in allied health care are the foundation of effective patient rapport. For example, rapport has been shown to be a significant tool for educators. Learning is enhanced whenever a student has a good relationship with the teacher, as opposed to the student who does not get along with the teacher. Patient education is one of the most important features of successful dentistry because patients are the ones who must participate in the daily care of their teeth.

Another way to improve rapport with patients is to get to know them. Patients like to be called by their name in a friendly and respectful manner. Many dental assistants make notes about personal things patients have told them so that they can build a relationship with the patient by referring to these more personal issues on the patient's next visit. For instance, if an elderly patient comes in talking about her grandchildren, the dental assistant should make a note in the chart. The next visit the conversation can be resumed about the grandchildren. By doing so, the patient may feel more connected to the assistant because the assistant has shown a personal interest in the patient. It is important to patients for office staff to remember them and be happy to see them again.

Dental Assistant PROFESSIONAL TIP

The dental assistant will have many opportunities to participate in taking continuing education courses (CEU) throughout his or her career and is encouraged to do so by most dentists. Some CEU courses of benefit to the dental assistant are customer service, psychology of the dental patient, and caring for the person with a dental phobia.

Life Span Considerations

Many fears and anxieties of patients are not easily overcome. It can take years to recover from past fears related to a bad dental experience. The skilled dental team can be very helpful in assisting the patient with a dental phobia by being attentive to the patient's special needs. If the team is not skilled in caring for the patient with special needs it could cause the patient to not follow through with needed dental care.

There are other ways to build rapport with patients. Routine correspondence is generally well received by patients. Children often remember dentist visits due to the new toothbrush or piece of chewing gum they received. Some offices post pictures of their patients and postcards from vacationing patients. The general office ambiance can lend itself to a positive rapport.

What do you remember about going to the dentist as a child? As a dental assistant, how can you help patients feel more comfortable about seeing the dentist?

Reviewing the Patient Record

The most useful source of information about the patient is found in the clinical chart. In preparing for the day, clinical charts for the expected patients are pulled and prepared. It is important that the dental team look through each chart to prepare for each patient visit. Special attention should be paid to any previous incident, conversation, treatment, or problem such as a previous cancelled appointment, missed appointment, and any ongoing problem or other special condition. The chart also indicates what procedures will be performed during the expected visit.

As discussed in Chapter 21, the chart is a legal document and must be treated as such. It contains forms that must be filled out to provide complete and legal care of the patient. Consent forms, authorization forms, insurance forms, and personal information can be found in the patient chart. Law mandates that these records be kept up to date and be complete and accurate. This is critical because the dental record can be used in legal cases such as malpractice cases and cases involving forensics. In addition to fulfilling the requirements of the law, effective records management with routine review will make patients feel more secure. Good customer service ultimately results in better rapport between the patient and the dental team.

The patient chart also serves as a record for research since it is a complete and chronological account of services provided. Research leads to very important advances in dental care such as advances in the use of fluoride. In addition, research provides statistics that show the advantages of patients receiving regular dental care.

Quality Assurance

The chart must be evaluated periodically to ensure that it is complete and accurate. This process is called quality assurance. Because the patient is a consumer, it is wise to build in routine checks of random charts to detect any problems that could be causing customer dissatisfaction.

Utilizing a checklist as a reminder of the areas to assess in patient charts can be helpful. Important areas to review for proper entry include information on current medications the patient is taking, allergy information, and documentation of treatment plans. Quality assurance personnel look for each item on the checklist and report if any items are missing from any entry. Other quality assurance functions include maintaining emergency standards and maintaining checklists for office policies.

Health Insurance Portability and Accountability Act

The Health Insurance Portability and Accountability Act (HIPAA) is an act that was passed by Congress in 1996 to address security and privacy of health data. It established national standards for electronic health care transactions made by health/dental providers and health care plans. Protected health information (PHI) includes any information that can be used in some manner to identify the patient such as a Social Security number, zip code, or birth date. In April 2005, HIPAA security regulations were implemented for specifically protecting electronic health information (e-PHI). Dental practices are legally required to comply with the standards set by HIPAA. (For more information on HIPAA see Chapters 3 and 21.)

What implications may result if a patient's treatment is not documented?

Preparing the Treatment Area

Preparing the chart is the first step in ensuring that the treatment area is ready for the patient. The chart should always be placed in a secure location that is easily accessible to staff members. The patient chart should always be kept out of sight, away from the treatment area unless properly prepared with a barrier. The chart should only be handled with clean hands. Keeping a patient's chart "bibbed" means keeping the chart covered in order to protect patient confidentiality.

Patient charts are usually kept in the front office area away from the rest of the patients. Once a patient comes in to the office, the chart is then taken to the back office and kept in the operatory or near the dentist's desk. When preparing the chart, a fresh or blank progress note should be placed in the chart along with any necessary

Legal and Ethical Issues

The Health Insurance Portability and Accountability Act states that all patient personal information is to be kept private, which means it is not to be discussed outside the dental office with anyone.

financial forms. Progress notes contain information related to patient care. A new progress note is created each time a patient visits the office.

The Operatory

The treatment area, also known as the operatory, is the area of primary care. It consists of the dental chair, the operator and dental assistant chairs, the dental unit, the assistant cart, and a sink with counters and cabinets. The operatory, including all surfaces, must be clean prior to seeing patients. These areas should be disinfected and all required instruments and equipment should be sterilized and ready for use. New barriers should be placed on items such as the dental unit and hoses, chairs, counters, and dental light switches. A sphygmomanometer, stethoscope, and thermometer should be available in the operatory for taking patient vital signs.

Prior to escorting patients to the treatment room, ensure that a clear pathway exists from the reception area to the patient dental chair in the operatory. Tasks to be done in preparation for patients entering the operatory are as follows:

- Place the rheostat behind the patient's chair and push the operator and dental assistant chairs to the side.
- Raise the dental lamp out of the way and move any mobile carts.
- Position the chair to about knee-high (15 to 18 inches) from the floor. Position the back of the chair so it is tilted slightly back.
- Raise the arm of the dental chair.
- Place any x-rays on the view box, set any models on the counter, and set up the tray according to the procedure scheduled. A basic setup includes the mouth mirror, explorer, cotton pliers, cotton rolls, cotton-tip applicators, gauze sponges, lip lubricant, patient napkin and napkin clips, tissue, safety glasses, saliva ejector, evacuator, and air/water syringe tips.

Greeting and Seating the Patient

Once the treatment area has been prepared, it is time to retrieve the patient from the reception room. The patient should be identified by name as provided on the patient's chart. The dental assistant should be courteous and respectful to the patient while maintaining eye contact and smiling. Younger patients should be called by their first name or a nickname; whereas, elderly patients may prefer to be called by their title and surname. Prior to calling elderly patients by their first name, the dental assistant (DA) should ask permission to do so. Once the patient identifies himself to the DA, the dental assistant should introduce him- or herself to the patient. If the DA knows the patient, some type of reference can be made to indicate familiarity with the patient.

Escorting the Patient to the Treatment Area

Having identified the patient, the dental assistant should ask the patient to follow him or her to the treatment area and then watch how the patient stands up to determine if any physical difficulties are present. Try and read the patient's body language for any indications of fear or anxiety. While escorting the patient, lead the patient slowly, paying attention to the patient's gait and stance to determine if any other issues exist.

Once in the treatment area, ask if any of the patient's personal items need to be stored. This should be done as soon as the patient enters the treatment room. Place the items such as a purse, keys, wallet, or briefcase on a counter within view of the patient unless the office is equipped to lock the patient's personal effects in a locker or closet.

After the patient items have been stored, the patient should be prompted to freshen his mouth to serve as a pretreatment rinse. Offering mouthwash can help to make the patient feel more secure. It is also a preventive measure in infection control. Explain that this step is an infection control measure and that it lowers the amount of bacteria in the patient's mouth.

When escorting a patient back to the treatment area, what can the dental assistant do to help create a positive experience for the patient?

Seating and Preparing the Patient for Treatment

The time spent greeting the patient and taking him to be seated presents the best opportunity to boost rapport with the patient. It is a good time for small talk to convey to the patient that his overall well-being is important to the dental practice. It is ideal for making the patient feel more comfortable because it allows him time to talk. Some patients will talk about their fears and about the procedure that is about to be performed. Others will talk about more mundane things like the weather or any other topic that makes them comfortable. Regardless of the topic of conversation, it is important to use the seating time to get to know the patient and to try to make the experience as pleasant as possible.

The patient should be asked to sit in the chair and put his feet on the footrest. The patient needs to sit so that his back is against the back of the chair and his legs are fully supported by the chair. Lower the arm of the chair after the patient is seated. Ask the patient if the headrest is comfortable and make any adjustments necessary. If the patient is a female, offer tissue for the removal of lipstick; offer a drink of water and lip lubricant.

Prepare the patient napkin to go around the patient's neck. Place the napkin on the chest with the plastic side down toward the patient's clothing and secure the napkin with the napkin clips, using caution to avoid clipping the patient's skin or clothing. Position the napkin so that the majority of the bib is on the operator's side of the body. Offer the patient safety eyewear to don during the procedure (Figure 22.1). If the patient reports feeling cold or asks for a blanket, a drape or sheet can be offered to the patient.

While the patient is seated upright, vital signs should be taken, the patient's medical history should be reviewed, and the patient should be asked if he has any questions. Some dentists prefer to lower the chair themselves so they will have the patient remain seated upright until after the initial interview. Others dentists will ask the dental assistant to lower the chair. When lowering the chair, inform the patient when the chair is going to be reclined to place the patient in the supine position. The patient's knees should be raised to about the same level as the patient's nose. The chair's height may also be adjusted to meet the height of the operator's elbow, roughly eight inches above the seat of the operator's chair. Adjust the headrest so the neck is supported and ask the patient if he is comfortable.

The dental light should be placed so that it is centered over the area where the procedure will be performed. The lamp should be pointed away from the patient's face and pointed toward the bib. At this point the lamp can be turned on and then positioned to focus over the patient's mouth. It is important to not shine the light into the patient's eyes unnecessarily. The lamp should be three to five feet above the patient.

If the procedure is on the mandibular teeth, the light is raised straight above the patient and the beam is focused downward (Figure 22.2). If the maxillary teeth are the focus of the procedure, the light is lowered down and back and the beam is focused at an upward angle (Figure 22.3). It may be necessary to adjust the lamp dur-

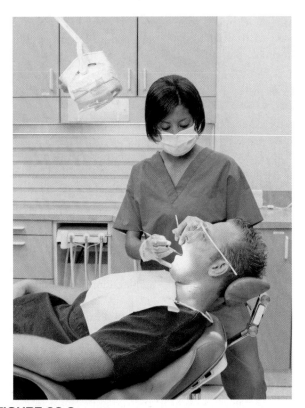

FIGURE 22.2
Dental light adjusted for the mandibular arch.

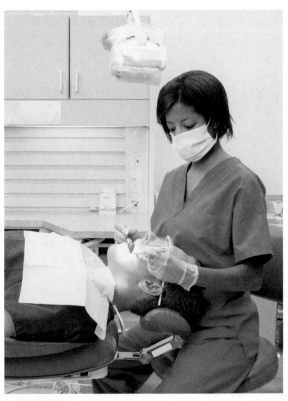

FIGURE 22.3
Dental lamp adjusted for the maxillary arch.

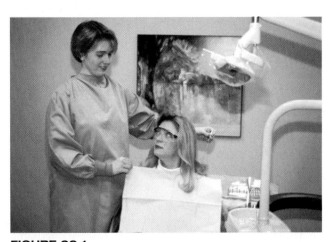

FIGURE 22.1
Patient prepared for treatment who is properly bibbed and wearing safety glasses.
Image courtesy Instructional Materials for the Dental Team, Lex., KY

ing the procedure periodically to keep the area of operation illuminated. Be cautious of the patient's positioning in order to avoid patient injury such as the patient hitting his head on the lamp.

Assessing Patient Needs

Assessing patient needs is an art perfected by experience. To begin assessing the needs of the patient, the dental assistant must look at certain physical clues. Many of these clues are often obvious such as a patient who has a distinct limp when walking. Some other clues are not so obvious, such as a patient who is deaf.

Children have special needs. If the patient is a child, certain changes must be made in order to provide the best dental experience. The patient's chart must contain consent forms signed by the patient's guardian or parent. Physical changes to the operatory area must be achieved to accommodate a child patient. Using booster seats and smaller equipment is an example of these adjustments. Make sure that items that would trigger anxiety (i.e., syringes for administering anesthetic) are completely out the view of the child patient. (For further information related to pediatric dentistry, see Chapter 47.)

A member of an efficient and patient-centered dental practice will begin to assess a patient's needs on sight. Once all accommodations have been made to get the patient to the operatory and positioned correctly, the dental assistant should inspect the oral cavity. Attention should be given to the shape of the bones and teeth. Any bone loss or obvious decay should be noted as well as the mechanics of the motion of the patient's mouth and any obvious abnormalities in the teeth and surrounding tissues. Such reports are based on observation, not on an attempt to diagnose. The general amount of saliva flow should be estimated. Once the assessments have been made, the dental assistant can be more prepared to anticipate the needs of the dentist and the patient.

Considerations for Pregnant Patients

When a patient is pregnant, considerations for her care and the treatment provided may need to be altered. For instance, sitting in a reclined position for a long period of time may be intolerable because it can lead to shortness of breath and fainting, especially during the third trimester. Scheduling short breaks and having the mother lie on her left side will relieve pressure on the aorta and may reduce the likelihood of maternal distress. Some pregnant women have digestive trouble such as morning sickness that is aggravated by the reclining position. Increased frequency in urination is also common in pregnant women, which means more frequent bathroom breaks for the patient.

Due to the harm that may be inflicted on the fetus, radiographs and medications are prescribed with cau-

tion, especially during the first trimester when the baby's vital organ systems are forming. The ideal time for dental treatment is the second trimester, because that is when the fetus is in the least danger and it is usually the most comfortable trimester for the mother.

Oral care is critical during pregnancy. Evidence is mounting that pregnant patients with periodontal disease are at a much higher risk for preterm and low birth weight babies. For this reason, pregnant women need to be educated about the necessity of impeccable home care and professional periodontal therapy. Gingival bleeding is not normal. It is a sign of infection that can endanger the health of both the mother and the baby. Increased hormonal levels exaggerate the effects of plaque, so normal home care measures may not be sufficient to prevent "pregnancy gingivitis." Routine cleanings are recommended for the pregnant patient with approval from the patient's primary care physician. When visited by a pregnant patient, the dental assistant is in an ideal position to review methods that the patient can implement to ensure good oral hygiene throughout the pregnancy.

Due to an increase in stomach acids, patients may have vomiting issues during pregnancy. Patients experiencing these issues can be told to rinse with a baking soda mixture to neutralize the acid, followed by brushing to avoid enamel damage. If the patient is experiencing nausea and vomiting in the morning, then the patient should be encouraged to brush and floss once the symptoms have diminished, such as in the afternoon or evening. It may also be a good idea for the patient to eliminate toothpaste, particularly if it leads to gagging. Pregnancy is an excellent time to talk with expectant mothers about the importance of good oral care for their new baby.

Considerations for Patients Who Have Sensory Impairments

It is important to assess whether or not a patient has sensory disabilities such as deafness or blindness. When a patient is deaf, a sign language interpreter may accompany the patient. If no interpreter is available, many deaf people can read lips very effectively. The key for the individual speaking is to stay positioned in such a way that the deaf patient can see the speaker's mouth.

Particularly for a deaf patient, it is important that the dental assistant provide all explanations prior to placing a mask over his or her mouth. Once the mask is on—and the lips are hidden—communication with a patient who is deaf is severely limited. To instruct the deaf patient during a procedure, the dental assistant will have to demonstrate what is desired of the patient or the DA can gently use his or her hand to show the patient what needs to be done. In other words, to open the patient's mouth wider the dental assistant may need to gently use his or her hands to guide the patient's mouth further open. On occasion, a pen or pencil and a pad of paper could be a helpful communication tool.

In contrast, patients who are blind can hear, so they can respond to voice commands. They may, however, require additional assistance with ambulation and with following pharmacological directions and written instructions for patient self-care.

Considerations for Patients with Language Barriers

A language barrier is another situation that can be assessed immediately. Many patients do not speak and/or understand English. In this situation, it is ideal for the patient to bring an interpreter, at least a relative or friend to translate. Even though there is a language barrier, courtesy and common respect are still required. Many professionals seek to learn some of the key words and phrases from the languages common to their regions. Many patient education brochures and flyers are also written in other languages and can be obtained to provide to non–English-speaking patients.

The Rights of All Patients

Most dental offices follow the Patient's Bill of Rights as designated by the federal government. Many institutions that offer patient care alter the statement as appropriate to address the specific needs of an individual practice. Most bills of rights have common features. The following examples represent some common features of rights that all patients have:

- The right to respectful treatment given by competent personnel, with respect and consideration of the patient's personal values and beliefs, which optimizes

Cultural Considerations

In the United States it is commonplace for people to visit a dentist for their dental care. Many people from other countries come to America for dental work as well. Because of increasing costs, however, more Americans are choosing to go to another country for their dental work. This is known as "dental tourism." Although some of the dental work performed in other countries is good, there are some significant risks. The standards are not the same for procedures and the use of infection control measures are typically minimal. These risks can lead to more serious dental issues in the future and often the work done in other countries must eventually be redone.

Other aspects of getting dental work done in foreign countries must be considered. For instance, most non-U.S. laws do not hold a dentist legally accountable for any dental treatment, which means that a dentist cannot be sued for malpractice regardless of the gross negligence incurred.

the patient's comfort and dignity, and is free from abuse or harassment.
- The right to be informed of one's rights as a patient at the earliest possible moment in the course of one's treatment.
- The right to privacy concerning one's dental care program. Case discussion, consultation, examination, and treatment are considered confidential and will be conducted discreetly.
- The right to confidentiality regarding all records pertaining to one's care except as otherwise provided by law or third-party contractual arrangements.
- The right to access all information contained in one's dental records, by the patient or designated/legal representative upon request.
- The right to receive all relevant information concerning one's diagnosis, treatment, and prognosis, including information about alternative treatments and possible complications.
- The right to be advised when one's case is being considered for an experiment or for research.
- The right to refuse any drugs, treatment, or procedure offered by the dentist.

What is the difference between a right and an obligation? What is the difference between a right and a responsibility?

Rights as Specified by the Americans with Disabilities Act (ADA)

The Americans with Disabilities Act of 1990 addresses the protection and rights of patients and employees who are physically and/or mentally challenged. These rights are addressed through titles. Titles I through IV are defined as follows:

- *Title I* addresses employment discrimination policies and procedures as they relate to the hiring of an employee with a physical disability.
- *Title II* supports the practice of making all facilities accessible for those with physical handicaps.
- *Title III* deals with making public accommodations for those with handicaps including access to equal services and goods.
- *Title IV* addresses telecommunications and other individual adaptive equipment made available for people with hearing, visual, and speech impairments.

The American Dental Association provides guidelines for patient rights. These guidelines can be found on the Internet (www.ada.org). This agency is involved in lobbyist activities to keep the rights of both the patient and the dental team protected.

The Role of the Dental Assistant

The role of the dental assistant is a versatile one. The dental assistant is required to assist in technical capacities and provide the human touch to patients—all in the same visit. The main focus of the dental assistant is to provide all of the necessary tools and instruments for the technical aspect of any dental visit. Providing emotional and sometimes physical support to accomplish the dental procedure is another role of the dental assistant. The dental assistant must perform all tasks within the boundaries of what is good and safe for the patient and the dental team. All tasks performed are bound to legal requirements and enhanced by good common sense.

The roles of the dental assistant are generally divided into three categories:

- Providing technical assistance to the dentist during treatment
- Providing education for patients and their families
- Recognizing and helping to alleviate patient anxiety and improving the patient's overall comfort

Functioning as a Member of the Dental Team

As a member of the dental team, it is important for the dental assistant to have good communication skills. Many dental teams engage in a practice known as the "daily huddle." The idea is that every day, the team meets to discuss the plan for the day's activities including each patient and the patient's individual needs. The information shared during the huddle ranges from treatment and procedures to patient financial considerations. These meetings can also provide an opportunity for performing team-building exercises and brainstorming about latest business trends.

Team membership and cooperation are skills that are imperative to master as a dental assistant. It is the competence of the dental assistant that is the backbone of the office. The role of the dental assistant is to assist in any way possible. The best way to assist is to do all that one can do and to continue to learn about unfamiliar areas. Once one knows how a procedure works, then one can offer the right assistance at the right time for the right patient with the right equipment. It is the role of the dental assistant to ensure quality customer service for the patient.

Caring for Patients with Special Needs

Some patients will present with obvious special needs. However, many of the special considerations needed are determined by asking the patient specific questions related to the patient's health needs and issues. For example, it is not possible to tell if a person has high blood pressure or diabetes by looking at the person. On occa-sion, certain diseases and conditions of the patient will require the dental team to make special accommodations. For this reason it is imperative to ensure that the patient's health history is updated at each visit and that vital signs are taken.

Senior Patients

Upon sight, the dental assistant can determine if a patient will need accommodation regarding anything related to age. Some senior patients, also known as geriatric patients, cannot tolerate sitting for the amount of time a procedure takes and may need to have the procedure done in increments rather than all at once. Some senior patients will need assistance with being seated or possibly helped with transporting medical equipment, such as an oxygen tank, into the operatory. Patients with pacemakers will need to be kept away from microwave activity including any microwave technology used to perform procedures. Extra care must be taken to individualize the accommodations made for each senior patient.

Statistics show that the life span of humans has increased over recent history. For example, before the 1800s a person's life span was about 40 to 50 years old. In addition to the increased longevity of today's elderly population, the total population today reflects an increase in the numbers of people that fall into the category of aging adults. Marked characteristics of the aging process can be divided into three categories:

- *Ages 65 to 74:* These are the youngest of aging adults. This group is beginning to include the older baby boomers. They are typically in fairly good health, still have their own teeth, and are more educated and more demanding of health services in general.
- *Ages 75 to 84:* This group is known for declining health where a series of medical problems are encountered. Some of them have retained their natural teeth, but a significant number of people in this age group have removable and/or fixed prostheses.
- *Ages 85 and beyond:* This group is considered to be very elderly. Many of these people have lost their natural teeth, and many believe that tooth loss is simply a matter of old age. Members in this category may have medical conditions that require premedication. Excessive oral health issues can be exhibited due to the amount of medications patients in this age group may be taking.

The dental team faces specific challenges in dealing with geriatric patients. Many oral health goals are the same for both young and old, but the aging process exhibited by elderly patients can provide challenges to the dental team. Increased prevalence of oral disease, multiple chronic diseases, and an increased use of prescription medications are some of the challenges faced by the elderly patient. The overall health of the mouth can affect many areas of life, such as personal self-esteem and appearance,

Professionalism

Professionalism is a learned behavior and is an ongoing process. The dental assistant is an integral part of the professional dental team. The entire dental team must work together as professionals focused on a team approach to better serve the needs of the patient. It is important to fulfill your role within the team by doing your job well and by helping others get the job done. Sometimes professionalism gets lost when employees forget to look out for and support each other.

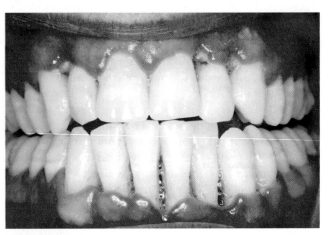

FIGURE 22.4
Root caries commonly seen in the elderly patient.
Image courtesy Instructional Materials for the Dental Team, Lex., KY

social and personal comfort, and nutrition. If the patient is having trouble chewing food or experiencing pain in the gums, the person may have multiple chronic medical conditions.

An indication that a patient has extensive medical problems can be reflected in the amount of medication the patient is currently taking. This information is discovered when the patient is asked about her past and present medical history. It is critical that a thorough interview be conducted for each patient, but especially for the elderly patient. Consider filling out a medication profile for each patient. Some medications can interact with a medication used by the dentist. The dentist must be made aware of the medications each patient is taking.

Some senior patients exhibit problems related to aging hands. Aging hands can make holding and maneuvering a toothbrush difficult. To ensure that the geriatric patient can continue to perform daily oral care, some form of adaptive equipment may be required. Toothbrushes with larger handles as well as electric toothbrushes are available and useful for senior patients, individuals with disabilities, or anyone who has problems with dexterity. (See Chapter 15 for more information on patient education and oral care.)

Many elderly people have certain characteristics they share when it comes to oral health. The common conditions seen are bone resorption, dark and brittle teeth, tooth decay, periodontal disease, and xerostomia. **Resorption** refers to the process in which portions of the alveolar ridge have shrunk and are no longer standing strong. This condition happens in patients who are fully or partially edentulous (without teeth).

Deposits of secondary dentin that have reduced the size of the pulp chamber over time cause dark and brittle teeth. When the pulp chamber is small and narrowed by the production of secondary dentin, the teeth are more susceptible to fractures due to the decreased size of the vital pulp in the tooth. Dental decay can happen at any stage of life, but the elderly are more susceptible as the gums begin to recede. When recession occurs the roots are exposed, and cavities can very easily develop in that area because the cementum covering the roots is much weaker than enamel (Figure 22.4).

Periodontal disease affects the surrounding gums and supportive structures of the teeth; it is on the rise among the elderly population (Figure 22.5). As more people are keeping their natural teeth longer, more periodontal disease is being diagnosed. Better hygiene and oral care can prevent this problem.

Xerostomia is a condition of having a dry mouth. It is caused by a decreased flow of saliva in the mouth. It is usually attributed to the effects of medications, but it can be a physiological problem or can be due to radiation or chemotherapy treatment as well. Prevention is critical with these types of conditions. Fluoride varnish, prescription fluoride pastes, or custom trays are useful in addressing these conditions.

Patients Who Use Wheelchairs or Walkers

Patients who use wheelchairs or walkers need additional assistance, a need easily assessed upon meeting the patient. The two basic types of wheelchairs are electric and manual. The electric wheelchair is battery operated, is very heavy,

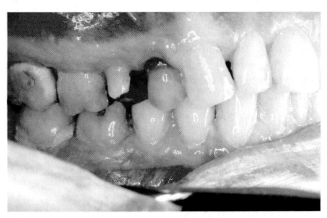

FIGURE 22.5
An elderly patient with commonly seen periodontal conditions.
Image courtesy Instructional Materials for the Dental Team, Lex. KY

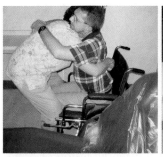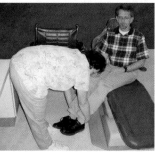

FIGURE 22.6
Assisting the patient from a wheelchair to the dental chair.
Images courtesy Instructional Materials for the Dental Team, Lex., KY

and requires additional space for maneuvering. Make sure the pathway to the operatory is clear of any clutter and allow plenty of time for the patient's visit. The manual wheelchair must be pushed for motion and steering.

When escorting a patient in a wheelchair to the operatory, ask the patient if he would like to wheel to the operatory of if he would like you to help him. Make sure the handbrake is in the locked position before the patient is transferred to the dental chair. If a patient transfer from the wheelchair to the dental chair is required, be careful of ergonomic considerations when helping a person in and out of the chair (Figure 22.6). If the transfer requires lifting, use a two-person lift or a gait belt. Many dentists are more amenable to treating the patient seated in the wheelchair.

Patients with Cardiovascular Disorders

Heart disease is the leading cause of death in men over 40 years old and women over 65 years old in America. It is also a problem that continues to rise in other countries. Heart disease is often treated with a number of prescribed medications. Information about a patient's heart condition is important for the dental team to discover. A weakened heart can lead to a variety of complications including the effects certain medications will have on the patient, how a patient may respond to a particular dental treatment plan, and the patient's stamina during a procedure. Recent research has shown that periodontal disease can lead to heart disease, especially in severe cases where the infection is left untreated.

Congestive heart failure is a condition in which fluids fill the heart and lungs, and the heart cannot pump blood to the other parts of the body. The patient with this condition becomes winded and tired very quickly. Sometimes these patients have a very wet cough and may feel like they are "drowning" in the reclining position, so they may not be able to lie flat on their backs for an extended period of time. Many of the medications prescribed for this disease have a diuretic effect, which causes increased urination.

Hypertension is the proper term for high blood pressure. High blood pressure means that the force of the blood is great against the walls of the artery. Factors associated with high blood pressure are heredity, stress, age, smoking, and obesity. Medications are usually given as treatment. Knowledge of the use of these medications is important to the dentist, who will need to ensure that any medications he or she may use during the dental treatment will be compatible with the existing medications. (For information related to the role of the dental assistant in monitoring patient blood pressure, see Chapter 23.)

Angina pectoris is a sophisticated title for sudden and sharp chest pain caused by reduced amounts of oxygen to the heart muscle. If the angina is unstable, the pain can begin at any time without much notice. Stable angina means that the patient is probably on medications and that the patient has the potential to have a serious heart condition such as a myocardial infarction or a heart attack. Patients with angina pectoris should have their medications with them at all times, and they should be readily available if chest pain occurs.

Endocarditis is inflammation of the inner lining of the heart. It affects the internal structures of the heart such as the valves. It is painful and requires antibiotics. If a patient has an infection or has been exposed to another individual with an infection, the bacteria can make its way into the bloodstream and then infect the lining of the heart where no white blood cells are located. In many cases the patient can get endocarditis more easily if a faulty structure is present within the heart such as a mitral valve prolapse.

For many years, dentists have prescribed antibiotics to patients with various heart conditions. These antibiotics must be taken prior to treatment to prevent the possibility of bacterial infections. The American Heart Association (AHA), however, has recently revised the guidelines to recommend that an antibiotic not necessarily be administered before dental treatment. It was historically given for any heart condition, but now the AHA claims that only certain heart conditions actually benefit from the administration of antibiotics. The AHA reports that the best line of defense is healthy gums and teeth.

Other problems with the circulatory system include blood disorders such as leukemia, anemia, and hemophilia. Leukemia is a malignancy of white blood cells. If a patient's body cannot fight infection, the dentist needs to know that. Anemia is either a shortage of red blood cells or a lack of oxygen in the red blood cells. It causes serious fatigue. Hemophilia is a disease characterized by a lack of clotting factors, resulting in possible excessive bleeding and the inability to stop bleeding once it starts. When a person with hemophilia bleeds, the individual must be given a blood clotting medication in order to stop the bleeding. Without medication, this condition could be fatal. Any patient with hemophilia must have a doctor's consultation before any invasive procedure is performed.

Patients with Neurologic Disorders

Neurologic disorders are problems with the nervous system including the brain, spinal cord, and any peripheral nerves. Common neurologic disorders are Alzheimer's disease, epilepsy, multiple sclerosis, cerebral palsy, and stroke. Alzheimer's disease is characterized by deterioration of mental abilities such as memory, judgment, intellect, and comprehension. Behavior problems can result from these impairments. The disease is progressive, meaning the condition continues to worsen. The best way to treat patients with Alzheimer's disease is to schedule the appointment at the best time of day for the patient's mental status and to try to have a familiar person accompany the patient during treatment. Because Alzheimer's disease is related to impaired mental function and memory loss, many patients suffer increased anxiety and fear during dental appointments.

Seizures are uncontrolled convulsions. The cause is not really known but certain factors are common to those people who have seizures. Drug use, head injury, brain tumors, and lead poisoning can cause seizures. Epilepsy is a disorder that is characterized by recurrent seizures.

There are typically two types of seizures: petit mal and grand mal. Grand mal seizures are also called generalized seizures. Some are preceded by a sudden smell of an unusual odor or a magnified sound or strange sensation in the extremities. Usually the aura is brief and most epileptics learn to recognize the aura as a sign of an impending seizure. The seizure itself usually causes the entire body to spasm, a loss of consciousness, and possibly incontinence. Petit mal seizures are not as noticeable. They are small absences from consciousness with only slight physical indications, such as eye rolling, a blank stare, or some minor twitching in the limbs.

Patients with a history of seizures must have a current history kept in the chart regarding seizure activity, medications used, and if there are any triggers that cause the seizures such as bright or flashing lights. If a patient has a seizure while in the office, it is important to ensure his safety by moving harmful objects out of the way. It is unnecessary and not advisable to place anything in the patient's mouth or to even touch the patient while he is seizing. If the patient has a seizure before an appointment, he may cancel the appointment, because having a seizure is physically exhausting. If the patient comes in within 24 hours or so after having a seizure, consider sending the patient home and rescheduling the appointment for a later date.

What would you do if a coworker had a seizure?

Multiple sclerosis is a neurologic disease that warrants extra attention in the dental office. It is a progressive weakening of the muscles due to nerve damage. The muscles will spasm without provocation, and a muscle relaxant or steroid treatment before a dental appointment could be in order. These patients are also heat sensitive and may have trouble getting to their appointments on hot summer days. Many of these patients use a walker or a wheelchair.

Patients who have had a stroke can be a challenge for the dental team. A **stroke**, also called a **cerebrovascular accident**, is a bleeding lesion or a tear in the brain. It causes paralysis, usually on one side of the body, slurred speech, double vision, headache, nausea, and vertigo or dizziness. If a person is having a stroke or a heart attack, an 81-mg aspirin should be administered immediately as long as there are no contraindications. Due to the possible paralysis after sustaining a stroke, the patient may not be able to tell if there is an ulcer present in the mouth. The patient might repeatedly bite her cheeks and tongue without knowing it. Because a stroke victim may be unable to move or detect sensation, food impaction can occur causing decay and/or gum disease. Some stroke victims also use modifications for ambulation such as a walker or a wheelchair.

Cerebral palsy (CP) is a neurologic disorder that encompasses a variety of neurologic physical disabilities. Its cause is attributed to disturbances in the brain during the fetal and infant stages of development. There are motor disturbances of sensation, cognition, communication, perception, and/or behavior. Many people with cerebral palsy also have epilepsy. The primary difficulty with a patient who has CP is the uncontrollable shaking and spasmodic jerking by the patient. Sometimes, the extent of the shaking requires the dental team to act very quickly and to reposition the structures within the operatory. Patients who have CP are also often unable to retain saliva in the mouth and have problems with drooling.

Patients with Pulmonary Disorders

Pulmonary disorders involve the lungs and the breathing process. Any patient who has trouble breathing could be problematic for the dental team, particularly during a treatment. Asthma, emphysema, and chronic obstructive pulmonary disease (COPD) are the most common pulmonary disorders encountered in the dental office. It is critical for the breathing-compromised patient to remain calm and minimize stress. Certain sedation medications can help keep the person calm, but it is important to ensure that these medications do not conflict with any other medications the patient may be taking.

An allergy is an immune response from the body. With allergies, the body encounters something that it considers foreign. The body is well equipped to fight diseases such as the common cold. The body is fighting in much the same way when it encounters an allergen such as dust, mites, pollen, animal dander, or certain foods or drugs. Most allergies are not serious and can be treated with an over-the-counter medication. Allergic rhinitis or a runny nose can be inconvenient for the dental team, but not a detriment. A serious allergic reaction, also known as anaphylaxis, can cause death and must be treated immediately. A common allergy seen in the dental office is latex allergy. Make sure the dental office can accommodate the patient who is sensitive to latex products by providing nonlatex products.

Asthma is a breathing condition characterized by the swelling of the body's air passages. Many patients who have asthma use an inhaler that is portable and can reduce the inflammation in the lungs. It is good practice for the dental assistant to ask the asthmatic patient to bring his inhaler to the appointment. Asthma can happen to any patient of any age. An asthma attack can be serious enough to stop the patient's breathing. If this happens during a visit to the dental office, you may need to activate the emergency response team or call 911.

Emphysema is almost the opposite of asthma in that it is the stretching out of the alveoli or the air sacs in the lungs. This person can get air in, unlike the patient who has asthma, but has difficulty getting the air out during the expiration phase of the respiratory cycle. Emphysema is most commonly seen in senior patients.

Chronic obstructive pulmonary disease is a term used to describe any ongoing disease that blocks the airways of the lungs. Chronic emphysema and chronic bronchitis are categorized as COPD, even though they are different problems. It is important for the patient with COPD to be calm during the dental visit. It might benefit the patient to use oxygen to ease her breathing, although oxygen flow should never exceed 3 mL/min to prevent shutdown of the breathing response or hypoxic drive. Nitrous oxide for pain management is not recommended for these patients, because of interference with the hypoxic drive.

Patients with Musculoskeletal Disorders

Arthritis and muscular dystrophy are the most commonly seen musculoskeletal disorders. Arthritis is inflammation of the joints. Any joint can become inflamed, and it is a condition seen mostly in the older patient. Once a joint becomes inflamed, the muscles and other connective structures can also become swollen and sore. Treatment for this condition is aspirin, anti-inflammatory medications, and steroids. The challenges the dental team face with these patients are possible mobility problems and the patients' inability to sit for long periods of time.

Muscular dystrophy is a group of diseases marked by progressive atrophy or a wasting away of the muscle tis-

sue. The atrophy leaves the person badly deformed and disabled. In the later stages of the disease, breathing can be compromised as muscles start to atrophy as well. At this stage, the gag and coughing reflexes can be ineffective so the dental team must be very careful to ensure the patient does not choke during treatment. Avoid the use of nitrous oxide, general anesthesia, and sedation therapy for patients with muscular dystrophy.

Patients with Endocrine Disorders

Endocrine disorders are problems with the glands that secrete hormones. Common endocrine glands are the thyroid, the pancreas, and the reproductive glands. Diabetes mellitus and thyroid problems are the endocrine disorders commonly dealt with in the dental office. The thyroid gland regulates metabolism and stimulates the passage of calcium into the bloodstream. Calcium is critical for the functioning heart and other organs. The thyroid can malfunction either by being overactive or underactive. If it is overactive, it is referred to as **hyperthyroidism**. This disease is more prominent in women than in men. A hypersensitivity to epinephrine and other anesthetics has been noted in hyperthyroidism. **Hypothyroidism** is a decreased function of the thyroid and can potentially aggravate a person's depression.

Diabetes mellitus is a very common disease in the United States. It is a condition in which blood sugar levels and insulin levels are unbalanced. This unbalance can be very dangerous. Typically patients can control this disease by either adjusting their diet or by taking prescribed medications. Extreme cases require the use of injected insulin for treatment. Diabetes is classified as follows:

- *Type 1 diabetes mellitus:* insulin-dependent diabetes
- *Type 2 diabetes mellitus:* non–insulin-dependent diabetes
- *Gestational diabetes:* occurs in pregnancy

Hypoglycemia occurs when the blood sugar is low, causing the person to stagger and talk oddly, appearing as if drunk and disoriented. If a patient is hypoglycemic, it is important to make sure the patient has eaten within an appropriate amount of time prior to the dental treatment. It is helpful to keep handy something with simple sugars such as orange juice, candy, or a can of soda. Should a patient show signs of hypoglycemia, give him a sweet as soon as possible and monitor.

The oral health of the diabetic is of concern to the dental team. Medications can cause xerostomia and related gingival and decay problems. The person with uncontrolled diabetes is much more susceptible to periodontal disease, and periodontal disease is an infection that makes control of blood sugar more difficult. Educating the patient with diabetes about the importance of good oral health as well as good glucose control is often the task of the dental assistant.

Patients with Developmental, Behavioral, and Psychiatric Disorders

Developmental disabilities are learning impairments (IQ under 70) that result from an event between birth and the age of 21. Certain developmental disabilities, such as Down syndrome, are a result of genetic deviations. Other disabilities are a result of problems during birth such as a fetus with the umbilical cord wrapped around his or her neck. Yet other disabilities result from injuries, for example, consider a normal 8-year-old boy who falls from a tree and lands on his head. If the injury impairs his ability to learn, he has experienced a developmental disability.

Common traits of a developmental disability that can create challenges to the dental team include limited communication skills and limited physical ability. Most of the people with developmental disabilities have difficulty talking or being understood, and because the learning process is affected, the dental team must not rely on verbal instruction alone.

Many patients with developmental disabilities are enrolled in local and state programs that manage the individual's needs. Because the funding comes from the government, many of these patients are on Medicaid and rely on assistance from others for their daily personal care. Many of these patients have rampant decay due to medications that decrease the moisture in the mouth, causing biofilm to build up into calculus. Calculus buildup also results from accumulated plaque biofilm if the person has poor oral care habits, which is also common in these patients. A decrease in the flow of saliva does not cause calculus, but it does increase caries due to the decrease in acid buffering.

Behavioral disorders is a term that represents a variety of problems. Behavioral disorders include hyperactivity, schizophrenia, psychopathic disorders, and eating disorders. Most of the time, behavior problems can be dealt with effectively through open and clear communication. A calm, truthful approach will suffice. A relationship of trust will be empowering as time goes on. In severe cases, the patient may need to be fully sedated before treatment can be provided. Some of the people who have behavior disorders will present orally with the same conditions seen in those with developmental disabilities, depending on how the disease affects their ability to maintain daily personal care.

Psychiatric disorders usually include anxiety, depressive, and bipolar problems. The manic-depressive person is either manic (i.e., the individual has too much energy) or depressed, which leads to the inability to be motivated. As a result, appointments are often missed and personal care is less than desirable. Anxiety disorders happen as a result of perpetual adrenaline release, causing the heart to race and breathing to be increased. It is an uncomfortable situation for the patient. A physician often administers medications to treat psychiatric disorders. The dental team must use caution when using general anesthesia and sedatives on individuals who have psychiatric disorders.

Patients with Dental Anxiety

Phobias are exaggerated internal fears held by people. The number one phobia in American culture is speaking in public. Many people who have this phobia will start sweating, get an upset stomach, and shake uncontrollably if they have to give a speech. The second most common phobia in the American culture is a fear of insects, particularly spiders. Seeing a dentist is also on the list of common phobias.

Dental phobias can be attributed to childhood dental trauma, parental fears passed down to a child, and feelings of suffocation. Many people will avoid going for dental treatment of any kind. Dental anxiety can be of a phobic nature or it can be a simple anxiety that can be managed by scheduling a patient as quickly as possible. Do not postpone or rearrange the appointments of these patients because increased waiting time may ultimately negate the courage it took on behalf of the patient to call in the first place. It can also decrease the level of trust between the patient and the dental team.

Some patients do not have a phobia but have nervousness to the point of requiring a sedative or nitrous oxide to help them relax. Alternative methods of reducing anxiety are being offered more routinely. These methods include acupressure, laser treatment, relaxing music from headphones placed on the patient, and televisions in the ceiling over the dental chair. Some dental practices are capitalizing on the widespread dental anxiety and marketing their practice as specializing in the treatment of anxiety.

Patients with Substance Abuse Problems

A considerable portion of American society engages in the use of drugs and alcohol. Even though alcohol and certain drugs are legal, abuse of legal and illegal drugs

Preparing for Externship

When preparing for your externship, it would be wise to review topics related to caring for the dental patient. Try to develop an awareness of how people look and act when they are comfortable as opposed to when they are uncomfortable. When with a patient, learn to watch the patient's eyes. The eyes can indicate a state of fear or can show that the patient is calm and comfortable.

poses certain challenges for the dental team. Alcohol abuse leads to improper nutrition and inconsistent daily personal care, which are detrimental for proper oral care. Patients who abuse drugs have the same issues as the alcoholic patient. Other problems exist for the drug abuser, depending on the type of drug that is abused. Epinephrine can be counteracted by drugs, which can lead to life-threatening reactions.

Extreme **mechanical bruxism** or grinding of the teeth (Figure 22.7), seen in amphetamine use, can lead to wearing away of cusps and the possibility of abfractions, in which a portion of the tooth is sheared off any surface except for the occlusal surface. This phenomenon is also seen in patients with bulimia.

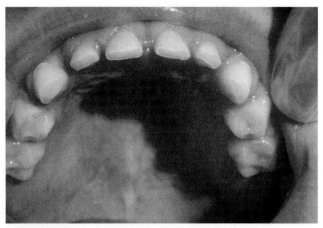

FIGURE 22.7
Attrition of the maxillary teeth due to bruxism.
Image courtesy Instructional Materials for the Dental Team, Lex., KY

SUMMARY

In conclusion, one of the key elements of effective dental treatment is patient care. All patients will be served better with honesty and careful consideration of any and all special conditions. Sincerely expressing kindness, working on individual rapport, and providing excellent services are the key features of a highly successful dental practice.

As a health care provider it is important that the dental assistant have self-awareness. Through self-awareness comes the ability to be sensitive to the needs of others. Some personality types exhibit an innate ability for this expression of care. Most people in an office setting will belong to a team of people that must work together to provide the greatest service. It is essential for the individuals on a team to help each team member become the best support for the patient. The best dental practices will be those that create trust in the patient.

KEY TERMS

- **Angina pectoris:** Sudden and sharp chest pain. p. 337
- **Emphysema:** A breathing condition characterized by the stretching out of the alveoli or the air sacs in the lungs. p. 339
- **Hypertension:** High blood pressure. p. 337
- **Hyperthyroidism:** Overactive thyroid function. p. 339
- **Hypothyroidism:** Underactive thyroid function. p. 339
- **Mechanical bruxism:** Excessive grinding of the teeth. p. 341
- **Multiple sclerosis:** Progressive weakening of the muscles due to nerve damage. p. 338

- **Muscular dystrophy:** A group of diseases marked by progressive atrophy or a wasting away of the muscle tissue. p. 339
- **Phobia:** Exaggerated internal fears held by people. p. 340
- **Pulmonary disorders:** Problems that involve the lungs and the breathing process. p. 338
- **Resorption:** Process that causes portions of the alveolar ridge to shrink. p. 336
- **Stroke (cerebrovascular accident):** A bleeding lesion or a tear in the brain. p. 338

CHECK YOUR UNDERSTANDING

1. What are some of the causes of dental phobias?
   a. childhood dental trauma
   b. parent fears passed down to child
   c. feelings of suffocation
   d. all of the above

2. What can the dental team offer fearful patients to reduce their fears?
   a. nitrous oxide sedation
   b. psychology classes
   c. headphones or a TV
   d. both a and c

CHECK YOUR UNDERSTANDING (continued)

3. When is the ideal time to discover a patient's special needs?
   a. just before an injection is given
   b. during the second appointment
   c. on initial contact with the office
   d. just after an injection is given

4. When and where is the best time for the members of the dental team to share information about patients who are having treatments/issues?
   a. in the morning huddle
   b. quickly and to the others at the front desk area
   c. on a notepad left in the staff room
   d. on a note placed on the chart just before the patient is brought back to the operatory

5. What is considered to be one of the most important aspects of human social interactions?
   a. a handshake
   b. a touch on the shoulder
   c. rapport
   d. patient education

6. Where is the patient's most important information found?
   a. driver's license
   b. birth certificate
   c. dental insurance card
   d. health history

7. In the morning huddle what is discussed and gone over so the entire team is informed?
   a. lunch schedule
   b. patient charts
   c. supplies that need to be ordered
   d. all of the above

8. The patient's chart is considered a _____ document.
   a. personal
   b. legal
   c. nonlegal
   d. public

9. What is the process of periodically reviewing and updating important items in a dental record called?
   a. quality assurance
   b. regular office maintenance
   c. catch-up
   d. random review

10. Which regulation requires that a patient's chart must be kept confidential?
    a. OSHA
    b. HIPAA
    c. JCAHO
    d. ADA

INTERNET ACTIVITIES

- Go to www.google.com, type in "dental phobic," and learn about dental phobia, dental fear, and dental anxiety.

WEB REFERENCES

- 1st Sedation Dentist .com www.1stsedationdentist.com/sedation-dentist-article26.shtml
- American Dental Association www.ada.org/prof/resources/pubs/jada/patient.asp
- Chet Day's Health & Beyond http://chetday.com/eftdentalanxiety.htm
- Michael C. Goldman DDS: Anxiety About Dental Care www.mgoldmandds.com/anxiety.htm

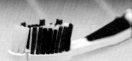

23

Vital Signs

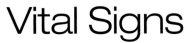

Learning Objectives

After reading this chapter, the student should be able to:

- List the vital signs commonly taken.
- Describe the factors that affect vital signs.
- Know the normal ranges for body temperature.
- Know the normal ranges for blood pressure.
- List common pulse sites.
- Discuss the characteristics of the pulse.
- Know the normal ranges for the pulse.
- Describe the characteristics of respiration.
- Know the normal ranges for respiration.
- Review the importance of proper documentation of vital sign findings.

Preparing for Certification Exams

- Take and record vital signs.
- Monitor vital signs.

Key Terms

Brachial	Inspiration
Bradycardia	Radial
Carotid	Sphygmomanometer
Diastolic	Systolic
Expiration	Tachycardia

Chapter Outline

- Factors That Affect Vital Signs
- Body Temperature
  —Methods of Taking Temperature
  —Normal Values
  —Types of Thermometers
  —Reading a Thermometer
  —Documentation
- Blood Pressure
  —Blood Pressure Equipment
  —Blood Pressure Readings
  —Normal Values
  —Documentation
- Pulse
  —Arterial Pulse Sites
  —Characteristics of the Pulse
  —Measurement and
    Documentation
- Respiration
  —Characteristics of Respirations
  —Taking Respirations
  —Documentation

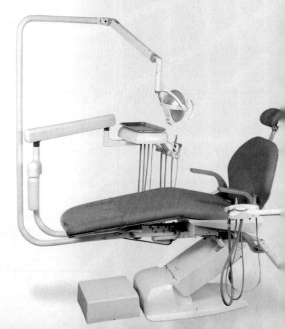

Vital signs consist of measurements of

a person's blood pressure, temperature, heart rate, and respirations. In addition to these common four vital signs, pain is now often considered the fifth vital sign. People are most familiar with vital signs as a result of going to a doctor's office. Taking one's vital signs is not an uncommon practice. Adults who exercise take their pulse rate to determine a maximum heart benefit. To check one's blood pressure, many individuals head to the grocery store pharmacy, which often have electronic blood pressure machines that provide a pressure check. Regardless of the common perceptions about vital signs, they are often taken routinely for medical evaluation before a dental procedure.

What external factors can you think of that might affect someone's vital signs?

Factors That Affect Vital Signs

Vital signs are measurements that reveal the status of a patient's general health. Vital signs are indicators necessary for life. They are:

- *Temperature:* the measurement of heat produced
- *Blood pressure:* the amount of pressure against the walls of the artery caused by the blood flow
- *Pulse:* the throbbing felt in the arteries as a result of the heartbeat
- *Respirations:* the act of inhaling and exhaling

These indicators are measured to detect changes in normal body functions. If any of these indicators register too high or too low, the person may have a serious disease or might just have been outdoors in hot weather.

Vital signs are affected by other factors such as anxiety, fear, pain, illness, anger, exercise, sleep, eating, and other physiological processes.

Some patients experience "white lab coat syndrome," so named because the very sight of a doctor's white lab coat can cause an increase in blood pressure related to anxiety about seeking professional help. If this happens to a patient, the dental assistant may have to wait a few minutes and retake the blood pressure, especially if successful attempts to relax and calm the patient have been made.

Normal ranges have been established for vital sign readings. Note, however, that if a patient consistently engages in cardiovascular activity such as jogging or cycling, the heart rate or pulse will be lower than normal because the heart muscle is stronger in those individuals.

Sleep alters vital signs because the body is at rest, so the heart pumps more slowly and, hence, the person's breathing is slower and deeper. The earlier in the day it is, generally the lower the body temperature.

Eating can affect vital signs because this physiological process requires energy. Some foods increase the blood pressure such as salt, which increases the body temperature, and hot chili peppers, which causes diaphoresis or perspiring.

Another physiological process that affects vital signs in women is that of reproduction. Both ovulation and pregnancy will cause the body temperature to rise. Aging is a physiological process that influences vital signs as well. Children have increased pulses, and the senior patient can have increased blood pressure.

External factors such as weather can increase a person's vital signs. When the weather is warmer, the body temperature is slightly warmer. The inverse is true as well: when the weather is colder, the body temperature is slightly cooler. Medications can also affect a person's vital signs. Some medications are designed to increase certain body functions and others are designed to decrease certain body performances. If an individual is taking medication, it is important for this person to routinely monitor her vital signs to ensure that no adverse affects are occurring.

Patient vital signs should be taken in the dental office routinely or according to office policy. It is critical to pay careful attention to patient history forms. Make sure they are filled out completely and accurately, ask patients about medications they may take, determine any known

---

Dental Assistant   PROFESSIONAL TIP

If the diaphragm on a stethoscope breaks, take a piece of exposed x-ray film and cut it to the size you need. Unscrew the ring around the diaphragm and remove the broken diaphragm. Replace it with the x-ray film. Screw the ring back into place and you have a temporary fix until the proper part can be ordered. Practice taking the pulse and respirations for 30 seconds each and multiply it by two to ensure correct readings.

Cultural Considerations

Some patients are very apprehensive about having medical procedures performed, even vital sign measurements, at the dental office. Simply explain to all patients calmly and concisely what you will be doing and why. All people appreciate being informed about what you are doing.

allergies, and pay attention to what patients say in order to correctly interpret the measurement of each vital sign.

Body Temperature

Body temperature is the degree of hotness or coldness of the body. The body temperature is regulated by the hypothalamus in the brain. In a healthy individual, one's body temperature varies throughout the day. However, during illness the body temperature increases in an effort to create a heated environment where microorganisms such as bacteria and viruses cannot survive. A dental patient who presents with a fever could have an infection in the teeth or the gums. Elevated temperature could indicate other illnesses as well. If a patient presents with an elevated temperature it is important to assess all other clinical indications that may be present.

What considerations might you need to consider when taking a child's temperature?

Methods of Taking Temperature

Four locations are commonly used for taking a temperature:

- *Orally* (by mouth)
- *Rectally* (in the anal canal)
- *Axillary* (in the armpit)
- *Tympanic* (in the ear canal)

The oral temperature is the most common route for taking a temperature in adults. The thermometer is placed under the tongue. The patient closes his lips around the thermometer and remains silent for the required amount of time according to the thermometer type. A rectal temperature is considered to provide the most accurate measurement; however, it is not as convenient as the other available locations. The axillary temperature is taken by placing the thermometer under the armpit. It is most commonly used for children and is considered the least accurate method.

The tympanic temperature is obtained by use of a specially designed electronic thermometer that is covered with a plastic sheath and fits into the ear canal (Figure 23.1). This method has gained in popularity. It is a great method for infants, children, and adults because it is quick and the location is more convenient and less embarrassing than the historically prevalent method of rectal temperature taking.

Normal Values

Normal value is the term given to temperature readings that are considered within a normal or healthy state. Because there are individual differences in people, these values are generally listed not as a single recording but as

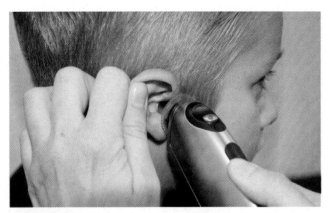

FIGURE 23.1
Tympanic thermometer.

a range. Normal temperature readings are listed below in the respective ranges:

- Oral: 97° to 99°F
- Rectal: 98° to 100°F
- Axillary: 96° to 98°F
- Tympanic: 97° to 99°F

Types of Thermometers

Thermometers have evolved over the years. The original thermometer was a person's hand. Moms would feel a child's head to determine if a fever was present. Today, although this practice is still common, for the sake of precision, utensils for measurement have been developed. Several types of thermometers are available:

- Glass
- Electronic
- Disposable
- Temperature-sensitive tape and band

Glass Thermometer

The glass thermometer (Figure 23.2) is a hollow glass tube filled with a heat-sensitive substance, such as mercury, that expands and rises up the tube when heat is applied. The substance contracts and moves down the tube once the tube is cooled. Shaking the thermometer can accelerate the process of moving the substance down. Note, however, that mercury is now considered a biohazardous material and in some states can no longer be used or purchased. Products are available that resemble mercury but are not dangerous. One benefit to a glass thermometer is—with proper cleaning—the ability to reuse it.

The shape of glass thermometers varies. Some have a long slender bulb and/or blue tip at the end, and others have a shorter stubby bulb and/or red tip. The long ones are for oral and axillary temperatures only, whereas the stubby one can be used orally, rectally, and in the axillary. The stubby one is usually reserved for rectal temperatures.

Procedure 23-1 Taking Temperature Orally

Equipment and Supplies Needed

- Digital thermometer
- Probe covers
- Waste container
- Pen and chart

Procedure Steps

1. Wash your hands.

2. Seat the patient and explain what you are about to do.

3. Place the thermometer in the probe cover and throw out the extra paper.

4. Turn the thermometer on.

5. With the patient seated, have the patient open his mouth and lift his tongue.

6. Place the thermometer under the tongue and have the patient close his mouth gently without biting down.

7. Leave the probe in place until it beeps, signaling the registration of the temperature.

8. Remove the probe from the patient's mouth.

9. Read the results from the thermometer.

10. Remove the probe cover and throw it in the trash.

11. Record the results in the patient's chart.

12. Put the thermometer in its proper storage place.

13. Wash your hands.

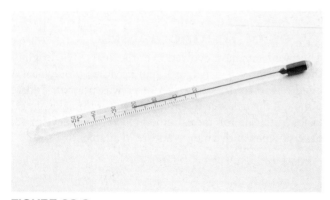

FIGURE 23.2
Glass thermometer.
Dave King © Dorling Kindersley

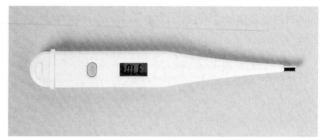

FIGURE 23.3
Electronic thermometer.
Trish Gant © Dorling Kindersley

One disadvantage to using a glass thermometer is the time it takes to obtain a reading: it takes anywhere from 3 to 10 minutes to obtain a reading on a glass thermometer depending on the site. For instance, oral temperatures take 2 to 3 minutes. Rectal temperatures take at least 2 minutes. Axillary temperatures can take as long as 10 minutes to register. Another disadvantage is that glass breaks easily. If a thermometer breaks, it can cause serious damage to the mouth or rectum. In addition, if a thermometer contains mercury, a patient could be poisoned and/or sustain lacerations to sensitive mucosal tissue.

Electronic Thermometer

The electronic thermometer (Figure 23.3) is battery operated and measures temperature in just a few seconds. The temperature appears in an LCD window on the front of the device. Many of these devices have rechargeable bat-

teries. A disposable probe cover is used to prevent the spread of disease, because these types of thermometers are reusable. For instructions on taking an oral temperature see Procedure 23-1.

The tympanic membrane thermometer falls into this category because the battery is recharged, a probe cover is used, and it takes 1 to 3 seconds to obtain a reading. Another example of an electronic thermometer is the digital thermometer. It is usually encased in plastic with a push-button operating button. It is battery charged and some devices store the last reading. A weak battery may give an inaccurate reading. The temperature takes about a minute to obtain and the thermometer automatically shuts itself off within about 10 seconds. Plastic probe covers are available to fit the electronic thermometer's shape.

Disposable Thermometer

Disposable thermometers (Figure 23.4) are white plastic strips that have chemical dots on them. Each dot turns blue at different levels of heat. The dotted end of the strip is

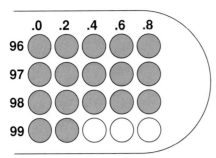

FIGURE 23.4
Disposable thermometer.

placed in the patient's mouth under the tongue. After 45 to 60 seconds, the dots that have heated sufficiently will turn blue. The dots are read much like reading a graph.

Temperature-Sensitive Tape and Band Thermometers

Temperature-sensitive tape or band thermometers (Figure 23.5) look like a piece of film. The tape or band is placed across the patient's forehead or abdomen. Within the number range marked on the tape, a rainbow-colored line appears and the number corresponding to the line is the reading. Note that these disposable bands only record temperature in whole numbers so they are less accurate than other types of thermometers.

Reading a Thermometer

Temperature is measured using the centigrade or Celsius scale or the Fahrenheit scale (Figure 23.6). Fahrenheit thermometers have long and short lines. Every other long line is marked in an even degree from 94° to 108°F. The short lines represent 0.2°. The long lines on a Celsius thermometer represent 1° and the short lines represent 0.1°. The Celsius range is from 34° to 42°. To read a glass thermometer:

- Hold the thermometer by the stem.
- Roll the thermometer so you can see the lines and the tops of the numbers.

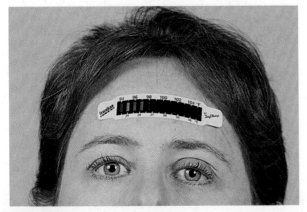

FIGURE 23.5
Temperature-sensitive tape thermometer.

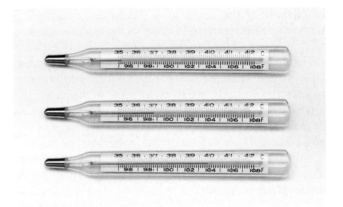

FIGURE 23.6
Fahrenheit and Celsius thermometers. Notice the difference in marked scores.

- Look inside the thermometer and slightly roll the thermometer until you see the silver or red line.
- Read the nearest degree mark to the end of the line.
- Read the nearest short line (even in Fahrenheit).
- Record your findings.
- Shake the thermometer down and cleanse according to office policy.

Documentation

The temperature reading is documented by writing down the number read from the thermometer followed by a degree symbol and indicating whether the scale was Fahrenheit (F) or Celsius (C). It is important to be very accurate by not transposing numbers or writing too hastily and making a mistake. Attention should be focused on the file in which you are writing to prevent accidents that could lead to mistaken diagnoses and improper treatment. Writing legibly is a must.

What can cause a person's blood pressure to be high?

Blood Pressure

Blood pressure represents the force of blood on the artery walls during the contraction and relaxation phases of the heart. The heart serves as the pump in the circulatory system. Freshly oxygenated blood is pushed out of the heart and sent out to the body via arteries to deliver the oxygen to the various cells throughout the body. Veins carry deoxygenated blood back to the heart for oxygenation and the cycle continues to form a complete circuit.

Blood pressure is an important vital sign because it indicates how hard the heart is working. Two sounds are produced for measurement: systole (the contraction phase of the heart) and diastole (the relaxation phase of the heart). Blood pressure is taken by crimping off the blood flow at the upper arm and listening through a stethoscope to the arterial sounds as the blood is allowed to flow again. The first heart sound is described as a sharp tapping. It is the first and highest number recorded, known as the **systolic** reading. Blood is allowed to resume regular flow slowly while continuing to listen to the artery. The last sound heard, the **diastolic** number, is described as a soft tapping sound in children, and the point where the sound disappears is the diastolic number in adults. This number represents the heart at rest, where tension is maintained as the heart's chambers are opened to receive more blood.

Blood Pressure Equipment

Two common instruments used in measuring blood pressure are the stethoscope and the **sphygmomanometer**, also called the blood pressure cuff. The stethoscope is a listening device designed to fit into the ear canals (Figure 23.7). Because the human ear canal points downward, it is wise for the dental assistant to point the earpieces away from one's body prior to putting the stethoscope into one's ear canal. This method points the sound directly into the eardrum for more clarity in hearing. The bottom portion of the stethoscope is known as the bell. Some stethoscopes are double sided with one side being smaller for use with pediatric patients. The sides of the bell are covered with a thin film called the diaphragm. The diaphragm is placed against the patient's arm at the location of the brachial artery. The brachial artery is located in the antecubital space (fold in the arm) halfway from the middle to the inner aspect of the elbow.

Life Span Considerations

Be sure to use a pediatric sphygmomanometer with children. Blood pressure readings are rarely taken on children but, if necessary, use the appropriate equipment. More commonly taken on children is a temperature. Tympanic thermometers are used most often with children.

The sphygmomanometer is a cuff that has an inflatable bladder sewn into the middle (Figure 23.8). It has a bulb that is used to inflate the bladder, controlled by a thumbscrew valve. The cuff is marked with a right and left arm indicator arrow to be placed over the respective brachial artery. Attached to the cuff is a measuring device of various types, aneroid, mercury, electronic, or digital. Mercury sphygmomanometers are the old-fashioned kind that can usually be seen mounted on the wall or on a rolling stand. As the sphygmomanometer bladder is pumped and the pressure of the arm cuff is increased, the mercury rises. As the pressure is released the mercury falls. Aneroid sphygmomanometers have a dial with a needle that moves clockwise around a circle as the pressure increases and decreases. An electronic sphygmomanometer electronically inflates the bladder, reads the pressure as it rises and falls, and displays the results on an LCD screen (Figure 23.9).

What happens if the sphygmomanometer doesn't fit properly?

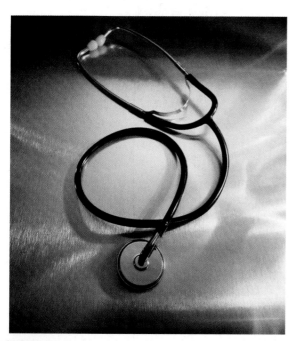

FIGURE 23.7
Stethoscope.

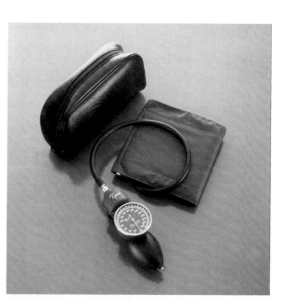

FIGURE 23.8
Sphygmomanometer with aneroid dial system.

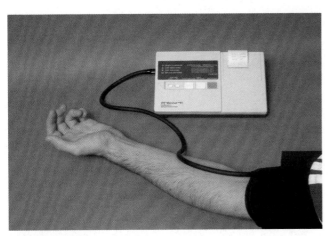

FIGURE 23.9
Automated electronic blood pressure device.

Blood Pressure Readings

The sphygmomanometer dial is marked with long and short lines to measure the level of mercury in millimeters (mm Hg). Every long line represents a multiple of 10 but only every other long line is marked with a multiple of 20 starting with 20 mm Hg and ending at 300 mm Hg. The short lines represent 2 mm. Make sure to remove any articles of clothing that would restrict the cuff.

Take the patient's brachial pulse for 30 seconds and double that number to get the one-minute reading. To this number add 40 and inflate the cuff to that number. For example, if the patient has a brachial pulse of 80, adding 40 would give an inflation number of 120. Inflate the cuff to this number. This method will give the health care provider an accurate inflation level. If the health care provider instead guesses at where to inflate the cuff, he or she may miss someone with high blood pressure.

If there is no heart sound, the pressure in the bladder is released slowly by unscrewing the valve. While the pressure is falling, the dial is watched to note the number the falling marker indicates when the first heartbeat is heard. The pressure in the bladder continues to be released and the heartbeats are heard clearly for an average of about 20 mm Hg until the last sound is heard. Take note of the corresponding number at the point of the first

Procedure 23-2 Measuring Blood Pressure

Equipment and Supplies

- Stethoscope
- Sphygmomanometer
- Disinfectant and gauze
- Pen and chart

Procedure Steps

1. Wash your hands.

2. Disinfect the earpieces of the stethoscope. Place both the stethoscope and working sphygmomanometer on the counter in the treatment room.

3. Seat the patient upright.

4. Explain in general terms what you will be doing.

5. Have the patient remove any long-sleeved shirt, sweater, or coat so the bend of the elbow is exposed. Locate the brachial artery (inside the elbow crease closest to the body).

6. Center the cuff according to the artery arrow found on the cuff. Position the cuff about one to two inches above the bend of the elbow. Close the inflator valve with the thumbscrew. Do not tighten too hard.

7. Find the brachial pulse with your first finger.

8. Pump the cuff until you cannot feel the pulse any more, and then pump the cuff another 20 to 30 mm Hg. This number will usually be between 160 and 180 mm Hg for a normal reading.

9. Put the stethoscope in your ears, pointing the earpieces forward.

10. Place the diaphragm of the stethoscope over the brachial artery and hold it in place with a thumb. Make sure the arm stays positioned at a straight angle.

11. Deflate the cuff slowly, at a rate of about 2 to 4 mm Hg per second by opening the thumbscrew slightly.

12. Listen. The first sound and its corresponding number represent the measurement of the systolic number.

13. Continue deflation of the cuff, listening to the pulse. The last sound marks the number of the diastolic reading. Continue deflating for another 10 millimeters to ensure that the last sound has been heard.

14. Open the thumbscrew all the way and let the air out of the bladder rapidly.

15. Removed the cuff from the patient's arm.

16. Disinfect the earpieces of the stethoscope.

17. Wash hands and record the procedure and the measurement on the patient's chart.

and last sounds because these are the numbers that are recorded for the blood pressure reading. Once the last sound is heard, the thumbscrew valve can be completely opened and the remaining air in the bladder released. The cuff is then removed from the patient. See Procedure 23-2.

Normal Values

According to the Joint National Committee on Prevention, Detection, Evaluation, and Treatment of High Blood Pressure, a normal reading for the systolic number is below 120 mm Hg, and for the diastolic number less than 80 mm Hg. High normal readings would be 120 to 139 mm Hg for systolic and 80 to 89 for the diastolic.

Stages of hypertension are as follows.

Hypertension	Systolic	Diastolic
Stage I (mild)	140–159	90–99
Stage II (moderate)	160–179	100–109
Stage III (severe to very severe)	above 180	above 110

A patient who has one reading outside of these ranges is not considered to be hypertensive (a condition of increased blood pressure) or hypotensive (a condition of decreased blood pressure) until an established pattern of irregular readings occurs.

Documentation

The blood pressure reading is recorded as the systolic number over the diastolic number. It is often written in fraction format (i.e., with a backslash between numbers) and the abbreviation "mm Hg" is used: 120/80 mm Hg. Note that the "mm Hg" abbreviation is rarely used anymore, but it is a good habit to get into using it. It is very important to record the proper reading in a legible way because the condition of the heart is indicated by this

Legal and Ethical Issues

A patient has come in for a surgical procedure requiring anesthesia. The dental assistant did not take a blood pressure. During the procedure, the patient starts to sweat and cannot catch his breath. These are typical signs of a heart attack. The procedure may have been delayed if the assistant had taken the proper vital signs. The vital signs are important in determining a patient's general health and must be taken before anesthesia is administered. Vital signs are to be taken at every visit, and the accuracy is of utmost importance. Accurate results are necessary so that the dentist can prescribe the proper treatment.

measurement. Also document the extremity and the side on which the blood pressure was taken, for example, "R" for "right" or "L" for "left" and "arm" or "leg."

So a complete blood pressure reading would be documented as follows: 120/80 mm Hg R arm.

Pulse

The pulse is the beat of the heart as felt through the walls of an artery. It is counted and reported as beats per minute. The pulse is indicative of the heartbeat even though the pulse is felt just slightly later than the heartbeats to allow for travel time of the blood.

Arterial Pulse Sites

Arteries pulsate throughout the body but certain sites are better for feeling the pulse by palpation or manually (Figure 23.10). The most common pulse sites include the **radial**, **brachial**, temporal, **carotid**, femoral, popliteal, dorsalis pedis, and apical sites. The location of each of these is further explained in Table 23-1.

Characteristics of the Pulse

The pulse has three characteristics commonly identified as the rate, rhythm, and volume. The rate is how fast the pulse is pounding. It is measured as the number of beats in a given minute. The rhythm refers to the time interval

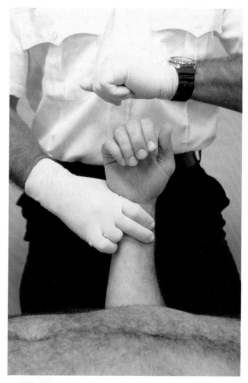

FIGURE 23.10
Taking a radial pulse.

TABLE 23-1 Common Pulse Sites

Pulse Site	Location	Comments
Radial	Located over the inner aspect of the wrist on the thumb side	Most commonly used site. With your index and middle fingers, not your thumb, follow the thumb line down the wrist to a bony protrusion. Pull your fingers toward the middle of the wrist slowly and allow them to fall into the divot. Feel for a pulse.
Brachial	Located over the inner aspect at the bend of the elbow known as the antecubital space	Look at the center of the antecubital space and at the innermost aspect of the elbow. Measure the pulse about halfway between the landmarks.
Temporal	Located on the side of the forehead	Commonly used in infants.
Carotid	Located on the right and left sides of the anterior neck	Commonly used in CPR. Locate the Adam's apple and feel for the curvature of the trachea. The tissue next to the trachea contains the pulse.
Femoral	Located at the inside of the upper thigh	Not commonly used.
Popliteal	Located at the back of the knee	Not commonly used.
Dorsalis pedis	Located at the upper surface of the foot between the ankle and toes	Not commonly used.
Apical	Located between the 5th and 6th ribs and approximately two to three inches to the left of the breastbone	Used in children under the age of 2 or for patients with an irregular heartbeat. Requires the use of a stethoscope.

between beats. It is described as regular or irregular or a skipping beat. Volume is the variance in the amount of pressure on the artery walls described as full, strong, bounding, weak, or thready.

Measurement and Documentation

Pulse is recorded as the number of beats counted in a minute's time. The count can be pure, meaning that the beats are counted for the full minute. Most professionals, however, count the pulse for only 30 seconds and multiply that number by two. The correct recording label is beats per minute, abbreviated as *bpm*. The average pulse range for adults is 60 to 100 bpm. If a person has a pulse of less than 60 bpm, the condition is called **bradycardia.** If the pulse is greater than 100 bpm, the condition is called **tachycardia.** The normal range for pulse in children ages 1 to 7 is 80 to 120 bpm.

What would you do if you could not find a pulse?

Respiration

Respiration is the act of breathing consisting of the **inspiration** (inhaling) of oxygen and the **expiration** (exhaling) of carbon dioxide. Respiration occurs both internally and externally. External respiration is the exchange between the body and the outside air. Internal respiration is the exchange of oxygen and carbon dioxide throughout the cells of the body.

Preparing for Externship

Dental assistant externs must be prepared to take vital signs. Students are required to practice taking vital signs on a regular basis so they will be well versed when they start their externships. Vital signs are taken on every patient, and the dental assistant must take accurate readings every time. Being prepared and showing initiative in fulfilling the nondental duties speaks volumes to the dentist and the office manager about the kind of employee you would make. When taking vital signs, you are physically very close to the patient. Make sure your hands are not too cold and your breath is fresh. Explain what you are doing in a pleasant and positive tone of voice to help make the patient feel comfortable.

Characteristics of Respirations

The characteristics of respirations are rate, rhythm, and depth. The rate is the number of breaths, both expiration and inspiration per count, during any given minute. The rhythm has either regular intervals of time between breaths or irregular periods of time between breaths. Depth depends on the amount of air taken in, described as deep or shallow.

Taking Respirations

Whenever a person knows his or her breathing is being watched, the individual subconsciously changes the patterns. The best way to obtain an accurate respiration rate is to count the breaths while the patient is unaware that

Procedure 23-3 Taking Pulse and Respirations

Supplies Needed

- Stopwatch
- Pen and chart

Procedure Steps

1. Wash your hands.

2. Seat the patient and explain what you are about to do, but do not mention that you will be counting the respirations. (A patient who knows she is being watched may change her breathing subconsciously.)

3. Ask the patient for her wrist.

4. Try to lay the wrist on the arm of the chair or a table nearby.

5. Locate the radial pulse by running your finger down the thumb to the first bony protrusion on the inner aspect of the wrist. Pull your fingers to the inside until they fall into the first divot. The pulse should be felt there.

6. Use the stopwatch to start counting the pulse.

7. Count for 30 seconds and remember the number.

8. Count the respirations for the next 30 seconds and remember the number.

9. Multiply the numbers by two and record the readings in the chart.

10. Pulse is recorded as the number after multiplying times two per minute.

11. Respirations are also recorded as the number after multiplying by two per minute.

12. Record any irregularity in pulse and/or breathing.

13. Wash your hands.

---

you are doing so. Many professionals will take the pulse for 30 seconds and then hold the patient's wrist to keep the attention away from the patient's breathing. For the next 30 seconds, breaths are counted. The respiration to pulse ratio is usually one to four or 12 to 20 respirations per minute in adults. See Procedure 23-3.

Documentation

The respiration rate is recorded as the number per minute. It is usually written as the number followed by a backslash and the word *minute* or the abbreviation *min;* for example, 18/min. It is also a common practice to note any irregularities in breathing such as labored breathing, wheezing, or shallow breathing.

If respiration is to be measured over the course of a minute, you can count for the full minute or you can count for 30 seconds and multiply that by two. What other increments of seconds would work and what would be the multiplier?

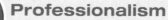

Professionalism

You must follow the dress code of the office or clinic where you work. A lab coat or scrubs is the usual attire. If a lab coat is worn, legs and feet must be covered. A personal policy of showing no skin is a good rule of thumb. The only exposed skin that patients are usually comfortable with are the arms from the middle of the upper arm to the hands, the neck to the middle of the breastbone, and your face. Your uniform and shoes should be clean and wrinkle free. Dental assistants should come to work clean, well groomed, and wearing little makeup or jewelry.

Fingernails should be clean and of a moderate length. The Centers for Disease Control and Prevention recommends that no nail polish should be used at all, because it can chip and harbor bacteria. Hair should be pulled back/restrained so it cannot fall into your mouth or eyes. If this is not done, it would be highly contaminated and would be an area that would cause cross-contamination to the patient or to you if you handled your hair with your hands in between patients. No facial or tongue piercing or visible tattoos are acceptable. They would not be considered professional in the field of dentistry.

SUMMARY

Vital signs consist of measurements of a person's temperature, blood pressure, heart rate, respirations, and pain. Temperature is defined as the balance maintained between heat produced by the body and heat lost. An increase in body temperature may be an indication of infection in the body. A tool known as a thermometer is used to measure the temperature precisely. Blood pressure is the measurement of the force of blood as it is pushed through the arteries by the contraction of the heart. It is expressed as the systolic reading over the diastolic reading. The pulse is the number of pulsations or beats felt through the arteries per minute. It can be strong or weak, regular or irregular. The respiration is the number of times a complete breath is taken in and released per minute. Respirations can be regular or irregular, shallow or deep.

KEY TERMS

- **Brachial:** Pertaining to the arm.   p. 350
- **Bradycardia:** A slow heart rate.   p. 351
- **Carotid:** The pulse felt at the neck on either side of the trachea.   p. 350
- **Diastolic:** The bottom number of a blood pressure reading; represents the amount of pressure during the relaxation phase of the heartbeat.   p. 348
- **Expiration:** The exhaled portion of a respiration.   p. 351
- **Inspiration:** The inhaled portion of a respiration.   p. 351
- **Radial:** Pertaining to the bone of the forearm.   p. 350
- **Sphygmomanometer:** Instrument used to take blood pressure readings; also known as the blood pressure cuff.   p. 348
- **Systolic:** The top number of a blood pressure reading; represents the force of the heart as it contracts.   p. 348
- **Tachycardia:** A fast heart rate.   p. 351

CHECK YOUR UNDERSTANDING

1. Bradycardia is a pulse rate lower than how many beats per minute?
   a. 40
   b. 50
   c. 60
   d. 65

2. What is the most commonly measured pulse rate?
   a. apical pulse
   b. brachial pulse
   c. radial pulse
   d. popliteal pulse

3. Which thermometers usually have digital readouts and are handheld?
   a. disposable
   b. electronic
   c. mercury-free glass
   d. glass

4. When taking a patient's pulse, it is best if you take it for how long?
   a. 10 seconds and then multiply by 10
   b. 15 seconds and then multiply by 4
   c. 30 seconds and then multiply by 2
   d. 60 seconds

5. An adult respiratory rate is how many breaths per minute?
   a. 10 to 15
   b. 16 to 20
   c. 20 to 40
   d. 25 to 40

6. When taking a blood pressure reading, what is the normal value for adult systolic pressure?
   a. less than 120 mm Hg
   b. less than 130 mm Hg
   c. less than 140 mm Hg
   d. less than 150 mm Hg

7. What does the term *bradycardia* refer to?
   a. slow breathing
   b. slow heart rate
   c. fast breathing
   d. fast heart rate

8. A stethoscope must be used to take which of the following pulses?
   a. apical pulse
   b. femoral pulse
   c. radial pulse
   d. temporal pulse

CHECK YOUR UNDERSTANDING (continued)

9. What type of thermometer measures body temperature inside the ear canal or the membrane of the ear?
   a. digital
   b. temperature-sensitive tape
   c. tympanic
   d. none of the above

10. _____ can raise or lower a pulse rate.
    a. Alcohol
    b. Nicotine
    c. Medications
    d. All of the above

● INTERNET ACTIVITIES

- Go to www.fi.edu/biosci/monitor/heartbeat.html. Listen to the heartbeats and take the quiz.

- Go to www.Joannabriggs.edu.au/best_practice/bp8.php. Summarize the Korotkoff sounds and rewrite the technique protocol in your own words.

● WEB REFERENCES

- University of Aberdeen: Video Tutorial www.abdn.ac.uk/medical/bhs/tutorial/tutorial.htm

24

Dental Instruments

Learning Objectives

After reading this chapter, the student should be able to:

- State the names, features, and functions of various dental hand and rotary instruments.
- List instruments used in the basic setup and their uses.
- Distinguish between the high-speed and slow-speed handpieces.
- Demonstrate connecting the straight attachment and contra-angle to a slow-speed motor.
- Identify categories of burs, their names, and numbers.
- Demonstrate placing burs into and removing burs from a high-speed handpiece and a slow-speed contra-angle.
- Discuss reasons for proper handpiece cleaning and lubrication.
- Describe the various types of instrument systems.

Preparing for Certification Exams

- Identify features of dental hand and rotary instruments.
- Prepare high-speed and slow-speed handpieces and burs.

Key Terms

Basic setup

Bevel

Carvers

Contra-angle

Dental handpiece

Fiber-optic system

Fulcrum

Straight attachment

Chapter Outline

- Identifying Hand Instruments
  —Hand Instrument Design

- Instrument Classifications
  —G. V. Black's Instrument Formula
  —Categories of Dental Instruments
  —Dental Examination Instruments
  —Restorative Instruments
  —Adjunctive Dental Instruments

- Rotary Equipment
  —Dental Handpieces
  —Dental Burs
  —Diamond Rotary Instruments
  —Finishing Rotary Instruments
  —Abrasive Rotary Instruments
  —Laboratory Rotary Instruments

- Instrument Systems
  —Cassette Systems
  —Tub and Tray Systems

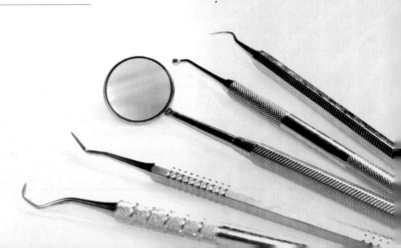

Dental instruments include

those used in the oral cavity by manual hand implementation and those used with mechanical devices. The dental assistant must know all instrument names and how they are utilized to effectively prepare for dental procedures. This chapter discusses individual dental hand instruments as well as the numerous dental rotary instruments used with power-driven handpieces. The name, special characteristic of each instrument, and its function is explained in order for the dental assistant to understand what is necessary to properly set up the instruments for general dental procedures.

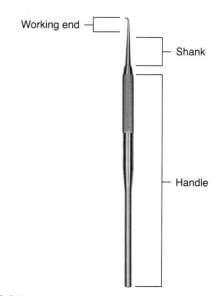

FIGURE 24.1
Parts of a single-ended dental hand instrument.
Courtesy Hu-Friedy

Identifying Hand Instruments

Dental hand instruments have a variety of functions including exploring, cutting, carving, placing, and condensing. Each working end is adapted to the function of the particular instrument. Hand cutting instruments are those instruments that are used manually by the operator as opposed to rotary cutting instruments, which are used with a mechanical device. Hand cutting instruments are used in conjunction with rotary instruments in order to refine cavity preparations. They may be applied to remove soft carious dentin. Hand cutting instruments have sharp cutting edges and are also used in cavity preparations during restorative procedures on teeth.

Hand Instrument Design

There are three basic components of a dental hand instrument. The longest part is the handle where the dental clinician holds the instrument during application. The shank joins the handle, and the working end, which consists of either a blade or a nib, is the tip of the instrument (Figures 24.1 and 24.2). A cutting instrument has a blade and a cutting edge, whereas a noncutting instrument has a nib and a face or point. The overall length of hand

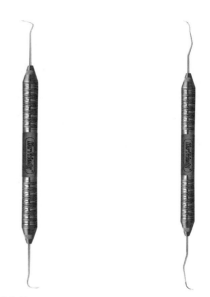

FIGURE 24.2
Point and blade working ends of a double-ended hand instrument.
Courtesy Hu-Friedy

instruments is approximately six inches. Identifying numbers are placed on the handles of each instrument along with the manufacturer's name.

Handle

Dental instrument handles are available in various shapes and sizes. They may be round, hexagonal, serrated, smooth, or padded. The handle is the part of the instrument that the operator grasps and is designed to give stabilization for grip and leverage. The operator grasps the handle of the instrument at approximately the lower one-fourth of the handle, near the shank, for balance and leverage. The ring finger of the operator's hand acts as a fulcrum to stabilize and direct the instrument into the

---

Dental Assistant   PROFESSIONAL TIP

For any dental assistant the task of learning all of the dental instruments and how they are used may seem overwhelming at first. However, reviewing this chapter combined with looking through manufacturers' catalogs and actually visualizing how and why a dental instrument is used will make learning easier.

hard and soft tissues without causing injury to the patient. The **fulcrum** is the pivotal point or finger rest support used to control a dental instrument. (See Chapter 25 for more details.)

When handing instruments to the dentist, the dental assistant must anticipate the dentist's needs. The dentist will signal the dental assistant when an instrument is to be passed. Instruments should be passed and received in careful and smooth flowing motions. During the transfer the dentist should not move the fulcrum or eyes from the treatment site. The dental assistant should grasp the new instrument at the nonworking end between the thumb and forefinger in a pen grasp close to the treatment area and parallel to the current instrument being used. The dental assistant's third and fourth fingers should be extended to receive the instrument from the dentist.

The assistant's hand serves two functions and is divided accordingly: the thumb, index finger, and middle finger together are the passing portion of the hand; the ring finger and pinky become the retrieving portion of the hand. The instrument must be passed correctly to allow the dentist to feel the handle of the new instrument between his or her fingers when ready to grasp it. When the exchange is complete, the dentist pivots the working end back into the working position. See Chapter 25 for more information on ergonomics, instrument transfer, and proper chairside positioning for the dental team.

Shank

The shank is straight or bent at an angle and connects the handle to the working end of the instrument (Figure 24.3). The angle is designed so that a specific area in the mouth can be reached with that particular instrument. The shank is tapered and may be straight, mono-angled (one angle), binangled (two angles), or triple-angled (three angles). The angulations must provide access to the

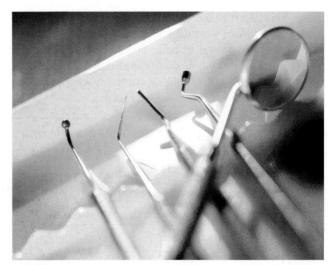

FIGURE 24.3
Instrument shank designs.

tooth to be operated on, whether in the anterior or posterior area of the mouth, and also afford balance and avoid breakage of the instrument.

Working End

The point, blade, or nib refers to the working end of an instrument (Figure 24.4). The working end of each dental instrument is designed to perform a specific function. The point or tip is used for diagnosis of dental conditions and to retract tissue. The blade of a hand instrument is a flat or rounded cutting edge and is most often at an angle. A slanted cutting edge is called a **bevel** and is used to place a distinct beveled angle at the enamel margins of cavity preparations. This portion of the instrument is designed to reach various areas of a tooth.

The nib is the noncutting portion of an instrument and may be smooth or serrated. Dental hand instruments

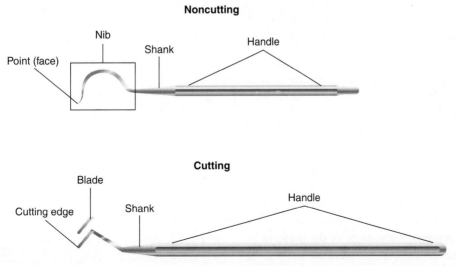

FIGURE 24.4
Beveled cutting edges of dental chisels.

are either single ended or double ended. Double-ended instruments have a working end on each side of the handle and are often designed in pairs that function as opposite angles of each other. Some double-ended hand instruments have varied styles of straight or curved working ends on each side and are various sizes (see Figure 24.2).

Where does the operator grasp the handle of a hand instrument? When the dental assistant passes an instrument, where should he or she be holding it so that the dentist may grasp the instrument in the proper location?

Instrument Classifications

Dr. G. V. Black, also known as the "grand old man of dentistry," made several major contributions to operative dentistry in the early 1900s. One of his developments was his classification of dental instruments. He classified instruments into six categories according to their function or use:

- Cutting instruments (hand and rotary)
- Condensing instruments
- Plastic instruments
- Finishing and polishing instruments (hand and rotary)
- Isolation instruments
- Miscellaneous instruments

Although some modifications have been made to these classifications, these basic categories should still enable the dental assistant to recognize instruments according to their function and identify them accordingly based on their distinguishing features.

G. V. Black's Instrument Formula

Using the metric system, Black developed a formula for dental instruments. In this formula Black identified the instruments according to a specific numbering arrangement. This was done to provide complete identification and duplication by manufacturers. These numbers provide manufacturers with exact measurements for producing dental instruments. Dr. Black's instrument system is expressed in a three- or four-number formula that is placed on the handle of each instrument. In the three-number formula:

1. The first number of the formula designates the width of the blade in tenths of a millimeter.
2. The second number describes the length of the blade in millimeters.
3. The third number represents the angle of the blade in relationship to the handle and is indicated in hundredths of a circle. (Hundredths of a circle are expressed as centigrade.)

For example, if the numbers on an instrument handle are 13-8-14, this would indicate the blade is 1.3 mm wide, the blade is 8 mm long, and the angle formed by the blade and the long axis of the handle is 14/100 of a circle (Figure 24.5).

When the cutting edge of an instrument is at an angle other than a right angle to the length of the blade, a fourth number is added to the basic three-number formula. The four-number formula is used for instruments such as gingival margin trimmers and angle formers, which have beveled cutting edges. This added number is expressed in centigrade, and represents the angle formed between the cutting edge and the central axis of the instrument handle. This fourth number is placed in the second position of the formula. The numbers on the handle would then read 13-80-8-14. The number 80 represents the cutting edge as being angled 80 degrees from the axis of the instrument handle.

Categories of Dental Instruments

Specific instruments are required for each type of dental procedure. Learning to identify instruments by their category of function allows the dental assistant to recognize each according to their use as well as physical characteristics. The major categories of dental instruments are:

- Examination
- Operative/restorative
- Adjunctive

Sterile dental instruments are always organized on the tray in their sequence of use from left to right, or from closest to the patient to farthest from the patient. The first instrument closest to the patient is always the mouth mirror, which is the primary instrument in every dental setup.

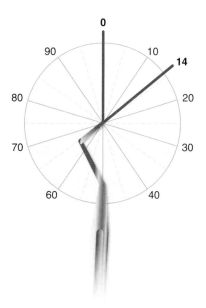

FIGURE 24.5
G. V. Black's instrument formula.

Dental Examination Instruments

Examination instruments are designed to be used specifically for examining the teeth and oral tissues. They may be used to examine the teeth or other structures during initial oral diagnosis or after placing a restoration. The basic dental examination setup, also known as the **basic setup,** consists of a mouth mirror, an explorer, and cotton pliers (Figure 24.6). These instruments are used in almost every dental treatment procedure. In addition to the basic setup, a periodontal probe, articulating paper, and 2 × 2 gauze squares may be used. A good light source from the overhead light is necessary for adequate vision when performing oral diagnostic procedures. The air/water syringe is frequently used to remove fluid and debris from tooth surfaces so they may be examined more accurately. As with all setups, the preference of the operator as well as treatment to be performed will dictate which instruments should be prepared.

Mouth Mirror

The mouth mirror enables the dental clinician to see, through reflection, surfaces of the teeth that cannot be seen with direct vision (Figure 24.7). Mouth mirrors may be plane glass mirrors or magnifying mirrors. They are

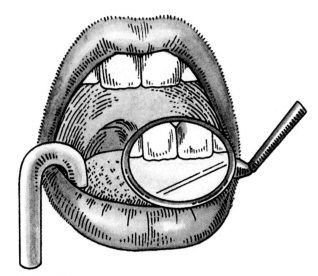

FIGURE 24.7
Mouth mirror.
Coral Mula © Dorling Kindersley

available in metal, fiberglass, or disposable plastic and have either a plane surface, front surface, or concave surface. The plane surface mirror has a silver coating on the back of the glass. This allows the light to be reflected from the glass and the silver layer which then provides a type of "ghost image." Mirrors with a front surface have a reflective coating on the top of the glass. The coating eliminates the ghost image, providing a clear view of the area being examined. The concave surface mirror magnifies the image. Metal mouth mirrors are designed as a cone and socket so that the mirror head can be replaced when necessary. The most common mouth mirror sizes are numbers 4 and 5. The mouth mirror has a wide range of uses (Figure 24.8):

- Allows for indirect vision
- Reflects light into dark areas of the mouth
- Retracts soft tissues of the tongue, cheek, and lips

Indirect vision is needed in certain locations of the patient's mouth where visibility is difficult or impossible such as maxillary posterior and lingual surfaces.

Without the mouth mirror, dental team members would experience poor body positioning that could lead to chronic muscular skeletal problems, especially of the back and neck muscles. Dental team members should sit with their backs straight and head fairly erect to prevent spinal problems.

It takes practice for the dental assistant to learn to use a mouth mirror for indirect vision, but it is mandatory when the dental assistant inspects the oral cavity. It also takes experience to realize how the mouth mirror can be utilized to reflect light into the oral cavity. There will be occasions when the dental assistant may want to use a mouth mirror to retract the cheek, tongue, or lips during a procedure in order to see the treatment area or

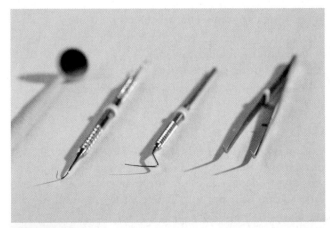

FIGURE 24.6
Basic setup.

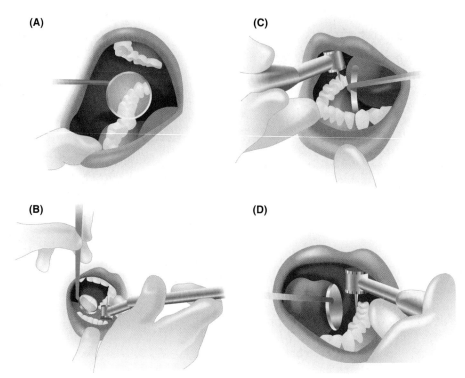

FIGURE 24.8
The mouth mirror being used for (a) indirect vision, (b) to reflect light into the oral cavity, and (c & d) retraction of the tongue, cheek, and lips.

to protect patient tissues from injury. A two-sided mirror allows one to retract and illuminate at the same time. For further information on how to use the mouth mirror correctly during procedures such as coronal polishing and dental sealants refer to Chapters 48–49.

Explorers

Dental explorers are sharp, pointed metallic instruments designed so that the various surfaces of the teeth may be

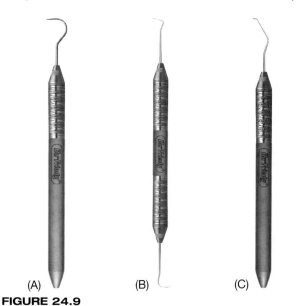

FIGURE 24.9
(a) Shepherd's hook explorer, (b) pigtail explorer, and (c) right-angle explorer.
Courtesy Hu-Friedy

conveniently reached with the tip. Explorers may be single or double ended. Double-ended explorers may be a combination of shapes with a different style at each end. There are a variety of explorer designs. The three most common designs are the shepherd's hook, the pigtail, and the right-angle explorer (Figure 24.9). The shepherd's hook explorer is a #23 explorer that ends in a semicircle tapering to a point at its end. The #2 pigtail explorer is also called a cow-horn. The #17 right-angle explorer is longer and straighter and has a right angle tip.

Explorers are used for diagnostic purposes, including the ability to penetrate defects in tooth surfaces and to remove debris from interproximal surfaces between the teeth. An explorer is also used for these other diagnostic purposes:

• Locating caries and enamel defects on tooth surfaces
• Locating supragingival and subgingival calculus (locating calculus subgingivally may only be accomplished by a dentist or dental hygienist)
• Locating faulty margins on dental restorations

Cotton Pliers

Cotton pliers (Figure 24.10) are tweezer-like metallic instruments that are either locking or nonlocking. The working end of a pair of cotton pliers consist of two tapered opposing portions. These pliers are supplied with serrated or smooth beaks. They are used for handling small cotton pellets, cotton rolls, small instruments, or other small items placed into or withdrawn from the

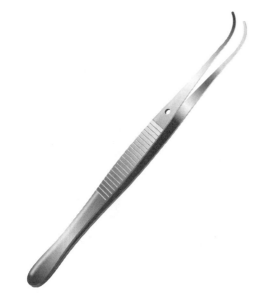

FIGURE 24.10
Cotton pliers.
Courtesy Hu-Friedy

mouth. The working end of cotton pliers is also used to carry medications, usually on cotton pellets, between the closed beaks for deposit in areas of the oral cavity. They may also be used to transport items from drawers and containers in the treatment room in order to avoid cross-contamination.

Periodontal Probes

Periodontal probes are used to determine the depth and outline of soft tissue pockets, in the gingival sulcus, between the gingiva and the tooth (Figure 24.11). This instrument is also used with light pressure to probe root contours when exploring for calculus and root roughness.

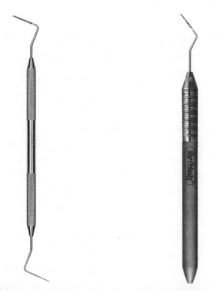

FIGURE 24.11
A double-ended periodontal probe and a single-ended periodontal probe. Both have indentations marked in millimeters.
Courtesy Hu-Friedy

They are single- or double-ended, slender, tapered flat or cylindrical instruments with indentations or color markers spaced in millimeters. Some instruments have a periodontal probe on one end and a #17 right-angle explorer on the other end that is used to locate calculus deposits. This instrument is commonly referred to as an *expro*.

Restorative Instruments

Many instruments are used to restore teeth, and these restorative instruments come in a wide variety of shapes and sizes. To be an effective dental assistant, it is important to be able to understand why, where, and when the dentist uses these types of instruments. Hand cutting instruments are used in the preparation of cavity walls and floors of the preparation. Amalgam restorative instruments consist of condensers, carvers, and burnishers. Composite resin placement instruments are designed to be used specifically with composite restorative materials. Additional, or adjunctive, instruments are also necessary during dental procedures in order to restore teeth to their proper function.

How should dental instruments always be organized on the tray? Which instrument is placed closest to the patient? What might happen if a clinician does not use the mouth mirror properly for indirect vision? **?**

Hand Cutting Instruments

Most restorative procedures require the use of hand cutting instruments. These instruments are designed with sharp cutting edges and are used for cavity preparation of various teeth in different parts of the mouth (Figure 24.12). Cutting or refining instruments include spoon excavators, chisels, hatchets, hoes, and gingival margin trimmers.

Spoon Excavators The spoon excavator is a double-ended instrument with a spoon or disk-shaped blade (Figure 24.13). The spoon is used primarily to remove debris, decay, and dentin from tooth preparations. The tips and sides of the spoon excavator are paired and designed to make a cutting or scooping action. Spoon excavators may also be used to remove temporary crowns or excess temporary and permanent cement.

Chisels Chisels, also called enamel chisels, are used to cleave or split enamel not supported by dentin along the lines of the enamel rods, and to smooth and sharpen cavity walls (Figure 24.14). Straight chisels have single bevels and straight shanks. Wedelstaedt chisels have single bevels and curved shanks. Binangle chisels have two distinct angles—one at the shank and one at the working end. This design allows access to tooth structure that would not be possible with straight chisels. Chisels are used with a pushing motion.

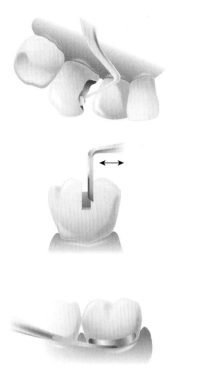

FIGURE 24.12
Dental hand instruments being used to remove carious dentin and to shape cavity preparations.

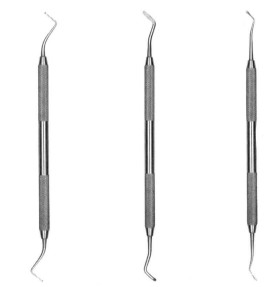

FIGURE 24.13
Double-ended excavators.
Courtesy Hu-Friedy

Enamel Hatchets   Like dental chisels, hatchets have single cutting ends or cutting edges on both ends (Figure 24.15). Enamel hatchet blades are set at a 45- to 90-degree angle from the shank. These instruments are designed to cleave or cut enamel along the lines of enamel rods and to prepare the walls and accessible margins of a cavity preparation.

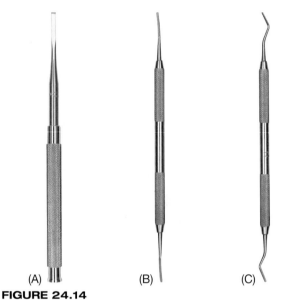

(A)   (B)   (C)

FIGURE 24.14
(a) Straight chisel, (b) Wedelstaedt chisel, and (c) binangle chisel.
Courtesy Hu-Friedy

Hoes   Dental hoes look like a miniature garden hoe (Figure 24.16). They are used with a pulling motion to smooth and shape the floor and sides of cavity preparations. Hoe blades are set at a 45- to 90-degree angle, almost perpendicular, from their handle.

Gingival Margin Trimmers   Gingival margin trimmers are modified hatchets that have working ends with opposite curvatures and bevels (Figure 24.17). As the name implies, they are used to trim, smooth, and shape the gingival floor of a cavity preparation in order to aid in retention of the restoration. Gingival margin trimmers are available in double-ended styles and are used in pairs. One working side is even numbered and the opposite side is odd numbered. The working end of an even-numbered instrument is beveled for use on the distal surface of a restorative preparation, whereas the odd-numbered end is angled for use on the mesial surface.

Sharpening of Hand Cutting Instruments   The efficiency of a dental hand cutting instrument is determined by the sharpness of its blade and the ability of the instrument to cut tooth structure. Instrument sharpening is a crucial task that must be carried out very carefully. The edge of the blade must be kept at the proper angle as it is sharpened because incorrect sharpening will alter the angle of a hand instrument and ruin its edge.

Instrument sharpening may be done manually with a flat Arkansas sharpening stone or an aluminum oxide stone. Sharpening may also be accomplished with cylindrical stones mounted on a slow-speed handpiece or lathe. The sharpening stone must be well lubricated with honing oil before being used to sharpen instruments. Safety glasses must be worn during this procedure and the dental assistant should never attempt to sharpen an instrument without first asking the dentist.

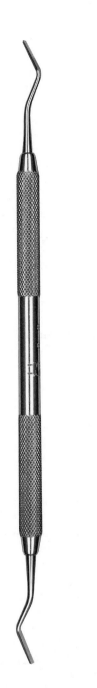

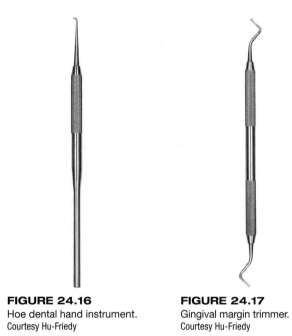

FIGURE 24.16
Hoe dental hand instrument.
Courtesy Hu-Friedy

FIGURE 24.17
Gingival margin trimmer.
Courtesy Hu-Friedy

packed before transferring to the dentist. After amalgam placement is completed, any remaining amalgam alloy should be ejected into the amalgam well so that no material is allowed to harden in the carrier barrel, which will make it unusable.

Condensers

Amalgam condensers, often called pluggers, are used to condense, or pack, amalgam filling material into the cavity preparation. The hammer-like working end is large enough to compress the soft amalgam without sinking into it. Condensers come in single- and double-ended designs (Figure 24.19). They have variously shaped and sized working ends, which may be smooth or serrated.

Carvers

After the amalgam is condensed, it must then be carved to approximately the same original tooth structure. **Carvers** have sharp cutting edges that are used to shape, form, or cut tooth anatomy into amalgam restorations. These instruments come in assorted shapes and sizes. Many carvers are designed for carving specific tooth surfaces. The discoid/cleoid (Figure 24.20) and Tanner #5 carvers are used on occlusal surfaces, whereas the interproximal and #1/2 Hollenback carvers (Figure 24.21) are designed for carving in between interproximal tooth surfaces. The Frahm amalgam carver (Figure 24.22) is sometimes called the acorn carver due to its shape and is used to quickly carve basic anatomy on occlusal surfaces. The dental assistant must learn the dentist's preference for carving instruments in order to have the desired instrument ready when needed.

FIGURE 24.15
Bi-bevel hatchet.
Courtesy Hu-Friedy

Amalgam Carriers

Amalgam carriers transport freshly prepared amalgam restorative material to the cavity preparation. They have hollow working ends, called barrels, into which the amalgam is packed for transportation. Both single- and double-ended carriers are available, with a variety of barrel sizes (Figure 24.18). When the lever at the top of the carrier is depressed, the amalgam is ejected into the cavity preparation.

When handed to the dentist, a poorly packed amalgam carrier may cause the material to fall out before it is ejected into the tooth preparation. It is the dental assistant's responsibility to ensure that the barrel is properly

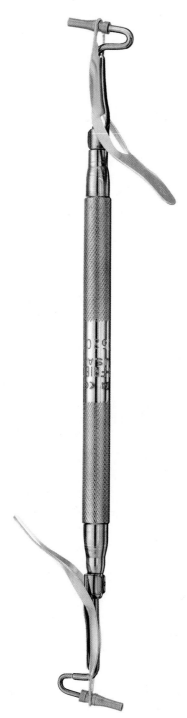

FIGURE 24.18
Double-ended amalgam carrier.
Courtesy Hu-Friedy

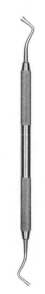

FIGURE 24.19
Double-ended amalgam condenser.
Courtesy Hu-Friedy

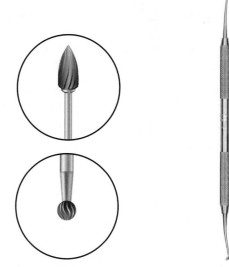

FIGURE 24.20
Discoid/cleoid amalgam carver with insert showing both ends of the instrument.
Courtesy Hu-Friedy

Burnishers

When the carving is complete the clinician may use burnishers to smooth and polish the amalgam restoration and to remove scratches left on the amalgam surface from the carving instruments. Burnishers have smooth rounded working ends and come in a variety of shapes including round, egg, football, and flat (Figures 24.23 and 24.24).

Plastic Filling Instruments

A variety of double-ended instruments make up this instrument group. They are used to transport and place dental cements, temporary filling materials, and insulating and pulp-capping materials. The working ends range from varying small cylinders to assorted angle and paddle-like shapes. These instruments are designed to place materials into the tooth while they are still in their plastic and pliable stage, before they harden. The most common is the Woodson #2, also called the Woodson metal plastic instrument.

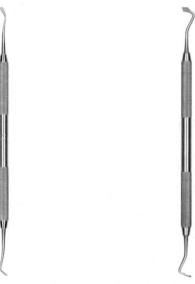
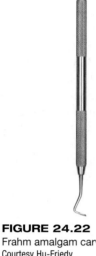

FIGURE 24.21
Hollenback amalgam carver.
Courtesy Hu-Friedy

FIGURE 24.22
Frahm amalgam carver.
Courtesy Hu-Friedy

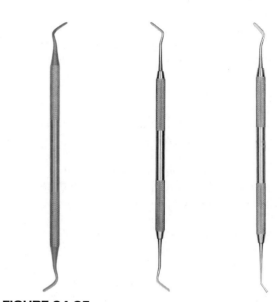

FIGURE 24.25
Composite resin instruments.
Courtesy Hu-Friedy

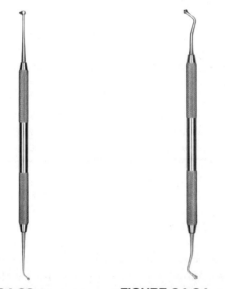

FIGURE 24.23
Egg and ball amalgam burnisher.
Courtesy Hu-Friedy

FIGURE 24.24
Acorn amalgam burnisher.
Courtesy Hu-Friedy

Composite Resin Instruments

Composite placement instruments used for condensing and contouring dental composite resin restorative materials are manufactured in anodized aluminum, aluminum titanium–coated stainless steel, or Teflon (Figure 24.25). Some composite resins contain hard particles and require strong condensing pressure, which causes abrasion and discoloration of the restorative material when metal instruments are used. Composite resin instruments are available in an assortment of designs and are often similar in design to the metal Woodson #2. These instruments allow for placement of composite materials without the composite resin sticking to the

instrument. A disposable brush is another instrument used for composite restorative procedures. This instrument is frequently used to apply liquids when etching and bonding are required.

Adjunctive Dental Instruments

Numerous accessory instruments are available and utilized by dental clinicians. Cement spatulas are single-ended stainless steel instruments used to mix cements, insulating bases, and temporary filling materials (Figure 24.26). Insulating base and pulp capping instruments have a small metal ball at the working end. They are used to mix, carry, and place insulating bases and are available

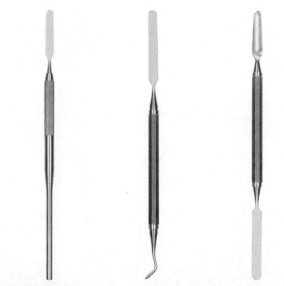

FIGURE 24.26
Cement spatulas.
Courtesy Hu-Friedy

as single- or double-ended instruments. A retraction cord is placed in the sulcus with a specialized gingival retraction cord packing instrument before impressions of an area are taken. The edges of the retraction instrument may be smooth or serrated.

Articulating paper forceps may be used to hold articulating paper when checking the patient's occlusion after filling material has been placed (Figure 24.27). Crown and bridge, or crown and collar, scissors are frequently used for many restorative procedures (Figure 24.28). These scissors may be curved or straight. The amalgam well is used to hold amalgam before it is picked up by the amalgam carrier. A glass dappen dish may be used to hold liquid and medications before transfer to the mouth. (See Chapters 43 and 46 for more information on oral surgery instruments.)

What will happen if a dental hand cutting instrument is improperly sharpened? What will happen if amalgam material is allowed to harden inside the barrel of the amalgam carrier?

Rotary Equipment

In early dentistry, preparing large cavities in hard tooth structure with hand cutting instruments was very slow and difficult. As rotary cutting instruments were developed, this procedure became easier. A rotary device is a power-driven revolving device that is used to cut enamel, dentin, or tooth restorative materials. With high-speed and slow-speed air turbine–driven rotary cutting instruments and newer electric motor handpieces, it is relatively easy to prepare large cavities in order to restore teeth to their proper function.

The rotary instrument group includes several small separate items. The high-speed and slow-speed motors, called dental handpieces, are used in conjunction with tungsten carbide, stainless steel, or industrial diamond burs. Rotary instruments are used to prepare carious lesions, finish restorations, trim dentures, polish teeth, and remove bone during oral surgery. These instruments are a vital part of most dental treatment procedures.

Rotary instruments are operated by a foot pedal that controls the power source and the amount of compressed air going to the handpiece, which activates and regulates the speed when rotary instruments are used. This foot pedal includes a rheostat for regulating the electric current. Many foot-control designs contain a toggle switch feature that is used to turn water to the handpiece on and off. Eye protection must be used when working with rotary instruments.

Dental Handpieces

The **dental handpiece** is a precision-built mechanical device designed for use with rotary instruments. Dental handpieces include burs, stones, wheels, and disks that are utilized during dental treatment. Handpieces may be air driven, electric, or compressed gas. Handpieces driven by compressed gas are used for surgical procedures.

The two types of dental handpieces are classified according to the revolutions per minute (rpm), or speed, at which they operate: high speed and slow speed (also called low speed). Both are operated by a compressed air system. The main function of the air is to rotate the air turbine drive. These devices convert highly pressurized air into mechanical energy, enabling burs, stones, wheels, and disks to rotate. High-speed handpieces are typically used to cut or prepare tooth structure, whereas slower speeds are necessary for polishing and finishing dental restorations.

The handpiece itself is a slender tube-shaped device that connects the bur with the driving motor (Figure 24.29). It is often lightweight and ergonomically designed.

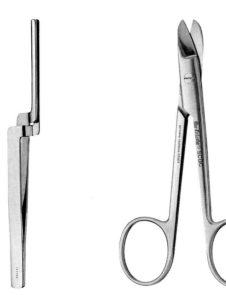

FIGURE 24.27
Articulating paper holder.
Courtesy Hu-Friedy

FIGURE 24.28
Crown and bridge scissors.
Courtesy Hu-Friedy

Legal and Ethical Issues

Proper cleaning, disinfection, and sterilization of rotary instruments is extremely important and a critical duty performed by the dental assistant. Improper cleaning could cause the transference of infectious microorganisms from one patient to another. If a patient becomes ill, and can prove the bacteria came from a contaminated dental instrument, it could potentially become a lawsuit against the dentist and the dental assistant. The dental assistant must consult the manufacturer's instructions for each type of handpiece and handpiece component for proper cleaning and maintenance procedures.

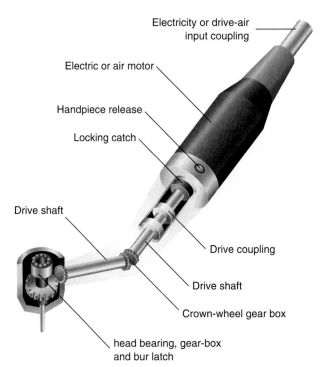

FIGURE 24.29
Parts and gears of a dental handpiece.

Manufacturers have been forced to develop handpieces that can withstand high-pressure steam sterilization. Couplings are used to connect the handpiece unit to the electric or air power source and cooling water through tubing and plumbing systems. Compressed air equipment combined with water delivery systems are subject to maintenance guidelines that must be followed. Handpiece tubing systems are available with two or four holes. Recently, fiber-optic illumination has been added to handpiece design in order to provide the dentist with a light source.

What is the dental assistant's job while the dentist is using the high-speed handpiece?

Cultural Considerations

Patients are concerned about dental treatments and about high-speed handpieces being placed in their mouth and vibrating their teeth. Patients want to be reassured that the dentist and dental assistant will perform necessary procedures efficiently and without causing harm. Patients who speak languages other than English must be informed about procedures and what to expect just as any patient would be. Part of a dental assistant's job is to reassure each patient before treatment begins. If the dentist approves, the patient may bring an interpreter along to help in understanding and communicating dental treatment needs.

High-Speed Handpieces

High-speed handpieces range from 380,000 to 400,000 rpm depending on the model and are used in cavity preparations to remove the bulk of enamel, dentin, or old restorations (Figure 24.30). High-speed handpieces are also used to prepare retention grooves and bevels within a cavity preparation and to create the cavity outline.

High-speed handpieces are designed to use smooth shank burs. All models work on the same basic principle:

> Burs are inserted into a metal friction grip chuck and held firmly by either manual tightening of the handpiece with a bur wrench or by a lever lock. The bur is rotated when air is forced into the head of the handpiece.

The high-speed handpiece uses a water system to cool the handpiece as well as to prevent heat damage to the tooth pulp. This water system also produces a fine spray mist, which aids in flushing debris from the treatment site. The dental assistant evacuates the water and also aids in retracting tissues of the mouth while the high-speed handpiece is being used by the dentist. (See Chapter 26 for more on oral evacuation and retraction.)

Constant preventive maintenance is essential in caring for handpieces. If they are not properly and frequently cleaned and lubricated, abrasives, such as finely ground tooth, metal, and other particles, will cause excessive wear and vibration. Proper lubrication of dental handpieces cannot be overstressed. Manufacturer's instructions must be read to understand the lubrication, cleaning, and sterilization or disinfection requirements of each dental handpiece. It only takes a few seconds for damage to be done to a handpiece due to improper or insufficient maintenance. High-speed handpiece heads may be standard or small and may contain a fiber-optic light system for better viewing of the treatment area.

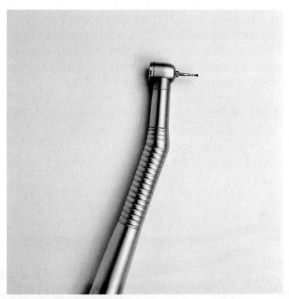

FIGURE 24.30
High-speed handpiece.

Fiber-Optic Handpieces

Fiber optics is often used with the high-speed handpiece in order to facilitate illumination of the oral cavity (Figure 24.31). **Fiber-optic systems** work by light traveling through long thin fibers of glass or transparent material to the head of the dental handpiece. The light travels through the fibers reflecting from wall to wall without generating heat. Fiber-optic lighting is useful to help identify and diagnose decay, stains, calculus, faulty restoration margins, and hairline cracks in a tooth. Maintenance of fiber-optic systems should be completed after each patient. A wet cotton swab with isopropyl alcohol should be used to clean both ends of the handpiece before sterilization. This prevents debris and handpiece lubricant from baking onto the fiber-optic surfaces.

Slow- or Low-Speed Handpieces

Slow-speed, also called low-speed, handpieces are the most versatile due to their wide variety of applications in dentistry. Slow-speed dental handpieces are used for removing caries, refining cavity preparations, performing coronal polish, and adjusting restorations and acrylics (Figure 24.32).

The slow-speed handpiece consists of a motor or power-driven unit and includes a large variety of attachments. Depending on the model of the handpiece, the speed will range from 5,000 to 80,000 rpm. The slow-speed handpiece includes the slow-speed motor and a straight attachment into which an assortment of rotary instruments or dental burs are fitted. Many slow-speed handpieces have a control ring on the handpiece motor base that, when turned, can control the direction of the bur or attachment rotation and may be noted as "F" for forward and "R" for reverse. When cleaning and lubricating the slow-speed motor and attachments, the solutions should be run alternately in forward and reverse to ensure complete cleaning and lubrication of all internal surfaces.

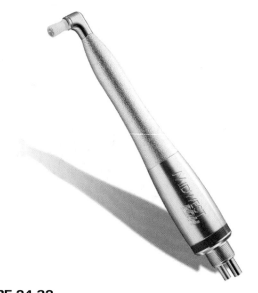

FIGURE 24.32
A slow-speed handpiece used for polishing.
Courtesy DENTSPLY Professional

Many slow-speed models have a method of quickly connecting and disconnecting the motor and slow-speed attachments to allow easy separation (Figure 24.33). Some units have a ring disconnect, while others have a button or indicator to depress. As with all handpieces and attachments, the manufacturer's directions must be followed for operation, cleaning, lubrication, and sterilization requirements.

Straight Attachments The slow-speed **straight attachment** for a handpiece (Figure 24.34) refers to a nose cone that is

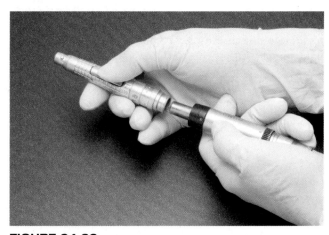

FIGURE 24.33
A straight attachment being removed from the slow-speed motor.

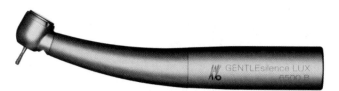

FIGURE 24.31
High-speed handpiece with fiber optics.
Courtesy KaVo Dental Corporation

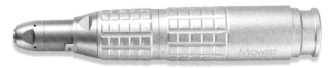

FIGURE 24.34
Straight attachment for the slow-speed handpiece.
Courtesy DENTSPLY Professional

connected to the motor and may be used independently with long shank burs or linked to other attachments. A contra-angle attachment, prophylaxis angle, or numerous accessory long-shank straight burs are fitted into this unit. The straight attachment is also used outside of the oral cavity for cutting and polishing fixed and removable prostheses.

The slow-speed straight attachment is assembled with the slow-speed motor and unit tubing at one end and to an adjunctive instrument on the other side. Frequent lubrication of the straight attachment keeps the internal rotating parts from overheating and prevents buildup of debris.

Contra-Angle Attachments   The term **contra-angle** describes the angle at the head of the handpiece attachment. This attachment changes the desired angle for better access to difficult areas within the oral cavity. The contra-angle attachment is used simultaneously with the straight attachment and slow-speed motor (Figure 24.35). The slow-speed contra-angle has a latch-type head into which the dental bur or other rotary instrument is placed. It functions to:

- Remove carious tooth structure
- Refine cavity preparations
- Adjust or polish restorations
- Adjust temporary or permanent prostheses

Prophylaxis Attachments   The prophylaxis attachment, also known as the prophy-angle, is also called the right-angle attachment. It is in a 90-degree angled shape and connects to the straight attachment of the slow-speed handpiece (Figure 24.36). It is used to polish the crown surfaces of the teeth. Prophy-angles can be metal, onto which a screw-type rubber cup or brush is attached, or they can be disposable, which has become a popular choice. Disposable prophylaxis angles reduce handpiece weight and save time because they eliminate the need for metallic angles, which must be cleaned, lubricated, and sterilized.

Handpiece Maintenance

Frequent and proper handpiece maintenance extends the life of a dental handpiece. Before each use, upon removal from its sterilized bag or when the manufacturer specifies, the slow-speed handpiece motor, straight attachment, contra-angle, and metal prophy-angle should be lubricated. The handpiece and attachments should be connected to the hose and run to blow out excess lubricant from the rotating parts. Most handpiece manufacturers recommend running the handpiece with a bur or blank chuck. Handpieces and attachments should be sterilized by steam autoclave. They should not be sterilized by dry heat unless specified by the manufacturer. No dental handpiece should ever be placed in an ultrasonic unit. Slow-speed contra-angle and metal prophy-angle heads should be disassembled, cleaned, and lubricated with appropriate solutions and then reassembled during pre- or poststerilization, depending on the manufacturer's directions.

General steps for high-speed handpiece maintenance are as follows:

1. Remove the high-speed handpiece from tubing.
2. Clean the outside with alcohol or a nonabrasive cleaning agent.
3. With the bur inserted place two to three drops of spray lubricant into the air drive port.
4. Reconnect the unit tubing to the handpiece and run it to eliminate excess oil from the turbine.
5. Remove the unit from the tubing and place in an autoclave bag and sterilize.
6. Allow to cool following sterilization.
7. Place bur in handpiece and place lubricant drops or spray into the air drive port.
8. Connect to tubing and run for 30 seconds to expel excess lubricant.
9. Wipe the excess lubricant from the handpiece with a clean 2 × 2 gauze.

Newer systems are available to dentistry for handpiece maintenance that automatically send cleaning solutions through the air and water lines, deliver the proper amount of oil to rotating components, and then purge excess fluid from the lines.

Air-Abrasion Technology

Through the use of air-abrasion technology, the dental clinician can gently strip away parts of the tooth surface with a handpiece that uses small particles of aluminum

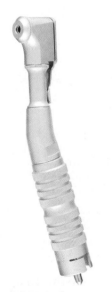

FIGURE 24.35
Contra-angle attaches to the slow-speed straight attachment and motor.
Courtesy Miltex, Inc.

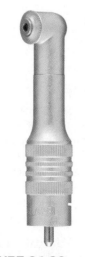

FIGURE 24.36
Prophy angles attach to the slow-speed straight attachment and motor.
Courtesy Miltex, Inc.

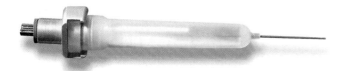

FIGURE 24.37
An air-abrasion dental handpiece.
Courtesy of North Bay/Bioscience LLC

oxide powder blown through very fine tips (Figure 24.37). The powder is forced out by a stream of compressed air and is used to remove small caries, stain, or plaque. This option does not require anesthetic. It is used to remove areas of early decay and to provide a better bond to tooth structure for pit and fissure sealants. This technique is called microdentistry because it allows much smaller cavities to be restored without "drilling" the tooth structure. Air abrasion is used in combination with the conventional dental handpiece as a complementary instrument.

Laser Technology

A more recent technological advance that has been developed is the laser (Figure 24.38). The U.S. Food and Drug Administration has approved use of the dental laser handpiece for treatment of soft tissues to remove lesions or tumors, to trim down excess tissue, and to control bleeding. These units deliver energy in the form of light, with precision focus, and are engineered to perform without damaging surrounding tissues or materials.

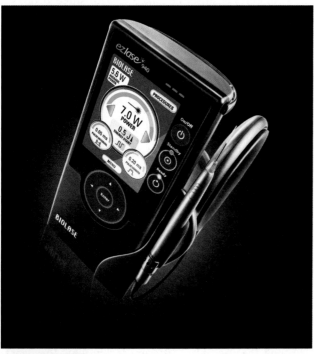

FIGURE 24.38
Dental laser unit.
Courtesy BIOLASE Technology, Inc.

Laser technology is currently being used in five areas of dental care:

- Periodontal therapy and recontouring of gingival tissues
- Whitening teeth with special solutions activated by laser energy
- Curing/hardening of bonding materials
- Curing/polymerization of light-cured restorative materials
- Removing decayed tooth structure

Caution: Dental team members must wear eye protection while using laser technology.

The most recent state-of-the-art uses for lasers involve removing bone with a sapphire tip. This type of handpiece eliminates the vibrations experienced with high-speed handpieces, but there are limitations, such as the inability to remove worn-out metal fillings.

The Electric Handpiece

The electric dental handpiece is often used in dental laboratories for grinding and polishing. Electric dental handpieces use a ball-bearing torque electric motor with a cooling fan. Unit speeds range from 1,500 to 35,000 rpm. Electric handpieces are available with high-speed and slow-speed attachments as well as fiber-optic systems. Some electric handpieces include digital readouts of the bur speeds. Electrical systems are quieter than air-driven systems, so their sound is less irritating for patients. They have a high torque cutting ability, which may not be acceptable for some dental procedures, but will continue to improve as technology develops.

How often should a fiber-optic handpiece be cleaned? What is used to clean it and why? What will happen to dental handpieces if they are not frequently and properly cleaned and lubricated? **?**

Dental Burs

The dental bur is the most important part of the dental handpiece. It is short and highly durable and able to withstand high-speed rotation and the heat that is subsequently generated. Numerous bur shapes are available, each with varying cutting abilities. Burs are made of stainless steel or tungsten carbide and some have diamond cutting edges. All burs have three basic parts: a shank, neck, and head (Figure 24.39):

- *Shank:* the part of the bur that fits into the handpiece
- *Neck:* the part of the bur that tapers to connect the shank with the bur head
- *Head:* the working end of the bur; the part of the bur that cuts or smooths

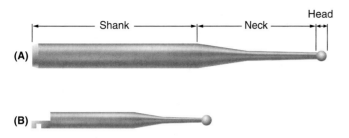
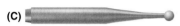

FIGURE 24.39
Main bur shanks: (a) long straight shank, (b) latch-type and (c) friction grip.

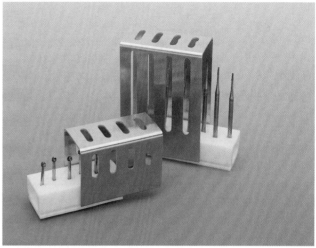

FIGURE 24.40
Bur block.
Courtesy Hu-Friedy

Proper sterilization of dental burs is necessary to prevent cross-contamination of infectious organisms. Debris should be removed by ultrasonic cleaning, brushing with a wire brush, rinsing, and thoroughly patting dry. Burs should be inspected for wear and discarded if damaged. Dry heat sterilization is preferred over steam autoclaving due to the potential for corrosion of the metal. Holders for burs, called bur blocks (Figure 24.40), can be autoclaved and most are magnetic so that these small items are not lost. Burs used for specific procedures can be placed together in the bur block for sterilization.

Bur Shanks

There are three main bur shanks: long straight (HP), latch-type (RA), and friction grip (FG) (see Figure 24.39). The long straight shank is smooth and fits into the straight attachment of the slow-speed handpiece once the prophy-angle or contra-angle has been removed. These burs are usually 40 mm in length and are often utilized for laboratory procedures. The latch-type bur has a notched end that fits into the latch of the contra-angle for use on the slow-speed handpiece. The friction grip fits into the turbine of a high-speed handpiece. The friction grip bur has a smooth shank that is held in place by friction against a metal or plastic chuck that is tightened with a bur tool, a push-button, or latch-type chuck

device. Both the RA and FG burs are normally a standard 20 mm in length, but are available in longer lengths for surgical use and in short-shank lengths for pediatric patients.

Bur Heads

The working end of the bur comes in a wide variety of shapes and sizes (Table 24-1). The basic shapes are round, inverted cone, pear shaped, straight and tapered plain fissure, and straight and tapered fissure cross-cut. Each bur shape has a corresponding number relating to the shape and size of the bur head (Figure 24.41). The dental assistant needs to know four identifying characteristics about dental burs:

- The description of the shape and size of the working end of the bur
- The identifying number describing the bur
- The handpiece attachment into which the bur fits
- The material the bur is made of, such as carbide, stainless steel, or diamond

TABLE 24-1 Dental Bur Names and Shapes, Numbers, and Functions

Bur	Numbers	Function
Round bur	1/4, 1, 2, 4, 6, 8, 10	To remove caries or to open a tooth for root canal treatment
Inverted cone bur	33 1/2, 34, 35, 37, 39, 37L	To establish retention undercuts in a cavity preparation, or to remove caries
Pear shaped	329, 330, 331, 332, 331L	To open a tooth for a restoration or to remove caries
Straight fissure bur	55, 56, 57, 58, 58L	To form walls and place retention grooves in cavity preparations
Plain tapered fissure bur	168, 169, 170, 171, 172, 171L	To form walls and place retention grooves in cavity preparations
Straight fissure cross-cut bur	555, 556, 557, 558, 557L, 557S	To form walls and place retention grooves in cavity preparations
Tapered fissure cross-cut bur	669, 700, 701, 702, 700L	To form walls and place retention grooves in cavity preparations

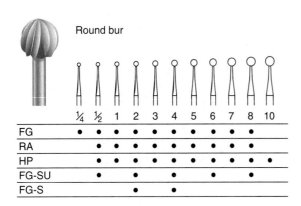

Round bur

	¼	½	1	2	3	4	5	6	7	8	10
FG	•	•	•	•	•	•	•	•	•	•	•
RA		•	•	•	•	•	•	•	•	•	
HP		•	•	•	•	•	•	•	•	•	•
FG-SU		•		•		•		•		•	
FG-S					•		•				

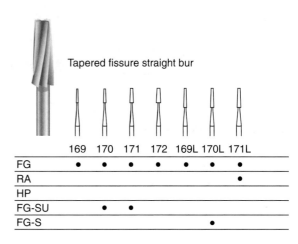

Tapered fissure straight bur

	169	170	171	172	169L	170L	171L
FG	•	•	•	•	•	•	•
RA							•
HP							
FG-SU		•	•				
FG-S						•	

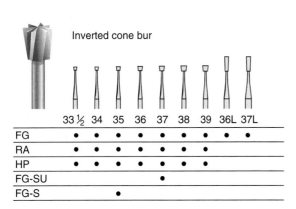

Inverted cone bur

	33½	34	35	36	37	38	39	36L	37L
FG	•	•	•	•	•	•	•	•	•
RA	•	•	•	•	•	•	•		
HP	•	•	•	•	•	•	•		
FG-SU					•				
FG-S			•						

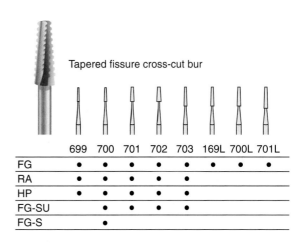

Tapered fissure cross-cut bur

	699	700	701	702	703	169L	700L	701L
FG	•	•	•	•	•	•	•	•
RA	•	•	•	•	•			
HP	•	•	•	•	•			
FG-SU		•	•	•	•			
FG-S	•							

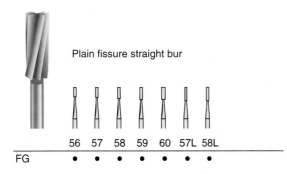

Plain fissure straight bur

	56	57	58	59	60	57L	58L
FG	•	•	•	•	•	•	•

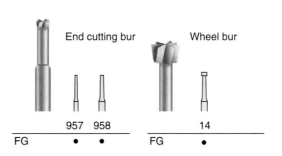

End cutting bur　　Wheel bur

	957	958		14
FG	•	•	FG	•

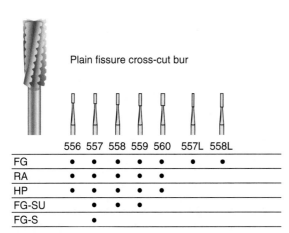

Plain fissure cross-cut bur

	556	557	558	559	560	557L	558L
FG	•	•	•	•	•	•	•
RA	•	•	•	•	•		
HP	•	•	•	•	•		
FG-SU		•	•	•			
FG-S	•						

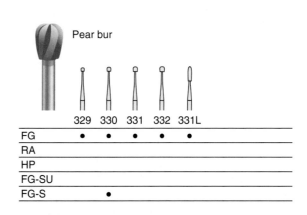

Pear bur

	329	330	331	332	331L
FG	•	•	•	•	
RA					
HP					
FG-SU					
FG-S		•			

FIGURE 24.41
Bur shapes with numbers.

Preparing for Externship

Review general and specialty instruments and burs. The many various burs and their functions are easier to master with knowledge and experience. Pay attention during clinical procedures and practice connecting slow-speed motors, attachments, and burs. Don't be afraid to ask how each piece is connected. Take the time to learn how each part works. Think about the shapes of different burs and visualize how they might be used during dental treatment.

What are the three types of bur shanks? What type of rotary device does each type of bur shank fit into?

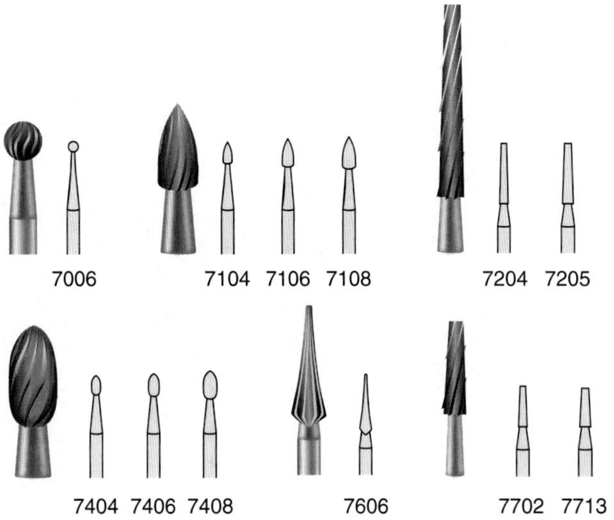

7006
7104 7106 7108
7204 7205
7404 7406 7408
7606
7702 7713

FIGURE 24.43
Finishing burs.

Diamond Rotary Instruments

Diamond dental burs are available in an abundance of different shapes and sizes for friction grip high-speed handpiece application. Diamond bur shapes include round, long and flat cylinder, tapered cylinder, football, flame, and wheel shaped (Figure 24.42). Diamond burs are available in coarse, medium, fine, and ultrafine grit. Coarser grit diamond burs are used for extensive gross reduction of tooth structure during crown and bridge preparation. Coarser grit burs are used carefully by the dentist because they may generate heat and cause damage to the enamel of a tooth. Medium grit may also be used for gross reduction of enamel and dentin. Fine grit diamond burs are used for contouring and shaping restorative materials, and ultrafine grit diamonds are used to smooth and finish composite restorations.

Diamond crystals are permanently bonded to a stainless steel shank, but recent technology has been developed using a chemical vapor depositing technique that physically bonds the diamond crystals to the instrument, which gives longer life to a diamond bur. Diamond burs should be heat sterilized before use and between patients to prevent cross-contamination, which could result in serious illness or even death from infectious organisms.

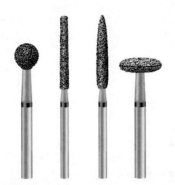

FIGURE 24.42
Round, tapered flat end, flame, and wheel diamond burs.

Contaminated burs should be handled with gloves and eye protection should be used.

Finishing Rotary Instruments

Composite and other tooth-colored restorations must be trimmed and contoured to their proper shape after they have hardened to provide maximum smoothness and aesthetics. Fluted finishing burs, along with fine grit diamonds, are used for this purpose. Finishing burs are available in round, oval, flame, needle, bud, and tapered fissure shapes (Figure 24.43). Finishing burs have 12 or 30 blades called flutes and are designed to be used in a high-speed handpiece. A 12-bladed bur is most often used for finishing composite restorations. The 30-fluted bur may also be used for finer finishing. The dentist may use the finishing bur with or without water.

Abrasive Rotary Instruments

Cutting, grinding, and polishing are other terms for abrading. Abrasive rotary instruments are available in varying degrees of grit from coarse, medium, fine, and extra fine depending on their intended use. Dental abrasive rotary instruments can be used with slow-speed or high-speed handpieces and, like all burs, are available in many shapes and sizes. They come as mounted or unmounted stones and wheels, or impregnated into soft rubber polishing cups, points, and wheels, or as disks designed for use with a mandrel (Figure 24.44). Abrasive strips are also used for cutting, smoothing, or polishing between the teeth. Dental restorations must be smooth and polished to minimize tissue irritation and to make it possible for plaque removal and cleaning.

For ideal wear, amalgam, composite, and gold restorations should be polished. Polishing restores normal contours, smooths margins, creates a shine, and improves the overall appearance and longevity of the restoration.

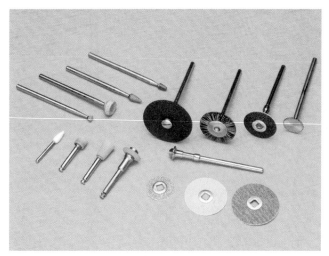

FIGURE 24.44
Various types of stones, points, and wheels.

Polishing creates an abrasion on the tooth or restoration to reduce scratches on smooth surfaces roughened by finishing abrasives. Rotary burs used to polish restorations include cups, points, disks, and powders (Figure 24.45). Each color denotes a different degree of abrasiveness. Brown cups and green cups are used first, followed by polishing points, which are finer. Most amalgam restorations can be polished at least 24 hours after placement, when the material has set. Composite restorations are finished at the time of placement. Aluminum oxide-coated disks are used followed by fine grit polishing cups and points. An aluminum oxide-based polishing paste may be applied with a soft rubber cup to finish polishing a composite. Brown and green polishing points and cups are used on gold with the same points and cups used for amalgam restoration polishing. The final polish for composite may be accomplished

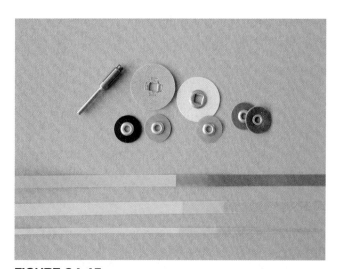

FIGURE 24.45
Sandpaper disks in coarse, medium, fine, and extra fine grits.
Image courtesy Instructional Materials for the Dental Team, Lex., KY

by the use of powders such as silex, tin oxide, or very fine aluminum oxide.

Mandrels

Mandrels are used to hold disks or wheels during their use. Snap-on mandrels are used for sandpaper and linen-backed disks that have a brass center, which snaps onto the mandrel. This is referred to as a Moore's mandrel. Screw-type mandrels are used to mount abrasive disks and unmounted stones. Mandrels may be either the latch type, which fits into a contra-angle head, or have a long straight shank, which fits into the slow-speed straight attachment (Figure 24.46). Screw-on mandrels are used with specific disks and wheels for finishing and polishing items outside of the oral cavity.

Laboratory Rotary Instruments

Laboratory burs are used in a dental office for cutting diagnostic cast models or trimming acrylic dental prostheses such as dentures or temporary crowns (Figure 24.47). They are available in a variety of shapes and sizes, but the most commonly utilized are flame, tapered, or round shaped. Lab burs are larger carbide burs, with

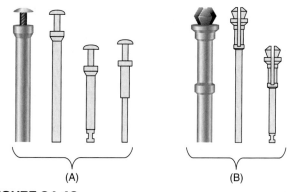

(A)   (B)

FIGURE 24.46
(a) Screw-on and (b) snap-on mandrels for the slow-speed straight attachment and for the contra-angle.

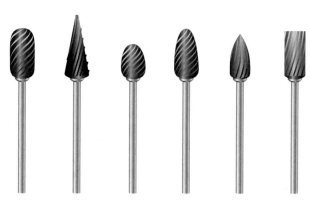

FIGURE 24.47
Laboratory burs.

a normal shank for use in the straight attachment on a slow-speed dental handpiece, or with a wider shank designed for use with a dental lathe.

What are the two types of mandrels? Name some of the various categories and shapes of finishing burs and abrasive rotary instruments used in dental facilities.   **?**

Instrument Systems

Various systems are used to organize dental instruments and accessory supplies. Dental instruments are kept together according to their use in specific dental procedures and are prepared, sterilized, and stored as preset tray or cassette systems. Each procedure in the dental office may have a unique color-coding system to quickly identify the procedure for which the instruments will be used. Some facilities may also use color-coded instruments for certain treatment rooms or specific clinicians. Preset trays and cassettes provide an efficient method of cleaning and organizing instrument setups.

Cassette Systems

Cassette-based dental instrument systems are the best way to manage instruments in any dental facility. Cassette systems provide the safest and most efficient transportation and storage methods for dental instruments and ease of sterilization and organization. The use of cassettes prevents the potential for dental team members to become injured by a contaminated sharp instrument during transportation and cleaning.

Following patient treatment, the cassette holding the instruments and supplies is taken to the sterilization area. Disposable items are discarded and the cassette of instruments is thoroughly cleaned in an ultrasonic unit, then rinsed well, packaged, and placed in the sterilizer. Instruments should be carefully arranged in the cassette and the lock closed before the dental assistant carries the cassette to the sterilization area. Cassettes can be placed directly into an ultrasonic cleaner to remove debris from all instruments. Placing the entire cassette into the ultrasonic unit enables complete cleaning and avoids sharp instrument handling by the dental assistant. After cleaning, the cassette should be rinsed well and dried.

The dental assistant will then prepare the cassette with a sterilization wrap and autoclave tape, which have built-in sterilization indicators to specify whether or not the instrument has been sterilized. The wrapped instrument package should be labeled to identify the procedure for which the instruments are prepared, the date sterilized, and the initials of the person preparing the cassette. Following sterilization, instrument cassettes should be stored for easy access by dental team members.

Tub and Tray Systems

Tub and tray systems are used to arrange supplies for efficient use during dental procedures. They must be kept clean, stocked, and organized. Containers for supplies and trays for dental instruments should be easily disinfected when needed and kept covered at all times to prevent contamination from airborne particles. Expendable items should be dispensed and materials needed for each procedure set out prior to each patient treatment. Instruments must be carefully placed on the tray in their order of use. Tub and tray systems may be color coded to identify particular procedures. Tub and tray systems allow the dental team to perform efficiently.

Contaminated instruments should be cautiously transported to the cleanup area as soon as possible following patient treatment. The dental assistant should use utility gloves and must always be careful not to become stuck by a contaminated sharp instrument. Trays should be disinfected after patient treatment and instruments placed into the ultrasonic cleaner, rinsed, dried, and placed in sterilization bags. Hinged dental instruments may be oiled or soaked in surgical milk to prevent residue buildup and corrosion in the hinged area. Surgical milk is a concentrated preautoclave soak that extends the life of instruments by lubricating them and inhibiting rust.

● SUMMARY

Dental instruments come in a wide variety of sizes and shapes. Each has a particular function. Hand instruments as well as rotary instruments are used during patient care. The treatment to be performed dictates which instruments should be prepared by the dental assistant. Understanding why, where, and how each instrument will be used helps the dental assistant be an effective and efficient member of the dental team.

The assistant and dentist work together as a team. The dental assistant must be able to anticipate the dentist's needs by learning his or her preference as to the proper procedure tray setup with the desired instruments. Dental instruments are expensive and must be cared for properly. Manufacturers' instructions must be diligently consulted to prolong the life of rotary instruments.

KEY TERMS

- **Basic setup:** Instrument setup consisting of a mouth mirror, an explorer, and cotton pliers. p. 359
- **Bevel:** The slanted cutting edge on the blade of a hand instrument that is used to place a distinct beveled angle at the enamel margins of a cavity preparation. p. 357
- **Carvers:** An instrument with sharp cutting edges used to shape tooth anatomy into restorations. p. 363
- **Contra-angle:** The angle at the head of the slow-speed handpiece to which burs attach. p. 369
- **Dental handpiece:** A mechanical device designed for use with rotary instruments. p. 366
- **Fiber-optic system:** A system used with the high-speed handpiece that uses fiber optics to illuminate the oral cavity. p. 368
- **Fulcrum:** The pivotal point or support used to stabilize and control a dental instrument. p. 357
- **Straight attachment:** The nose cone connection for the slow-speed handpiece. p. 368

CHECK YOUR UNDERSTANDING

1. What is the term for the pivotal point used to stabilize and support a dental instrument?
   a. fulcrum
   b. mandrel
   c. rheostat
   d. shank

2. The working end of a dental hand instrument is called a
   a. point.
   b. blade.
   c. nib.
   d. all of the above.

3. The slanted cutting edge of a dental hand instrument is called the
   a. fulcrum.
   b. bevel.
   c. shank.
   d. mono-angle.

4. What instruments are included in the basic setup?
   a. mouth mirror
   b. explorer
   c. cotton pliers
   d. all of the above

5. How are dental instruments arranged on the tray?
   a. does not matter
   b. right to left
   c. left to right
   d. according to their sequence of use
   e. both c and d

6. Uses for a mouth mirror include which of the following?
   a. indirect vision
   b. light reflection
   c. retraction of the tongue, cheek, and lip
   d. all of the above

7. Periodontal probes are
   a. slender, flat, cylindrical instruments with millimeter indentations.
   b. used to determine the depth of the gingival sulcus.
   c. used to determine the outline of soft tissue pockets.
   d. all of the above.

8. What instrument is used to pack amalgam filling material into a tooth preparation?
   a. condenser
   b. hatchet
   c. discoid/cleoid carver
   d. burnisher

9. What is the dental assistant doing while the dentist is using the high-speed handpiece?
   a. evacuating water from the patient's mouth
   b. retracting the tongue, cheek, or lip
   c. looking out the window
   d. a and b only

10. The parts of a dental bur are
    a. the shank.
    b. the neck.
    c. the head.
    d. all of the above.

INTERNET ACTIVITIES

- Go to www.midwestdental.com for information on rotary instruments.
- Go to www.miltex.com and do a search for dental instrument categories in the catalog provided at this website. Read about the various types of dental instruments to learn more about them.

WEB REFERENCES

- Dental Instruments www.watsonent.com/dent.htm
- Dentsply International www.dentsply.com
- DPRWorld.com www.dentalproducts.net
- KAVO Dental Corporation www.kavousa.com/Default.aspx?navid=2&oid=009&lid=Us
- Premier Dental www.premusa.com
- Sweet Haven Publishing Services www.free-ed.net/sweethaven/MedTech/Dental/DentSetups/lessonMain.asp
- webdentistry www.webdentistry.net

25

Ergonomics

Chapter Outline

- Ergonomics in the Dental Office
  —Risk Factors
- Posture
  —The Neutral Position
  —Horizontal Reach
- Injuries Sustained by Dental Assistants
  —Musculoskeletal Disorders
- Muscle-Strengthening Exercises
- Four-Handed Dentistry
  —Practicing Four-Handed Dentistry
- Motion Economy
- Operating Zones
- The Expanded Function Dental Assistant
  —Knowledge and Skills Required of the EFDA

Learning Objectives

After reading this chapter, the student should be able to:

- Identify risk factors for injury in the dental office.
- Describe the most ergonomic ways to deliver dentistry.
- Demonstrate the exercises that can reduce strain and strengthen muscles.
- Identify the basic point of view of four-handed dentistry.
- Define the responsibilities of the dental team to ensure effective four-handed dentistry is practiced.
- Explain the classifications of motion.

Preparing for Certification Exams

- Use the concepts of four-handed dentistry.
- Transfer dental instruments.

Key Terms

Assistant's zone

Carpal tunnel syndrome (CTS)

Cumulative trauma disorder (CTD)

Ergonomics

Expanded function dental assistant (EFDA)

Four-handed dentistry

Fulcrum

Motion economy

Musculoskeletal disorders (MSDs)

Operator's zone

Static zone

Transfer zone

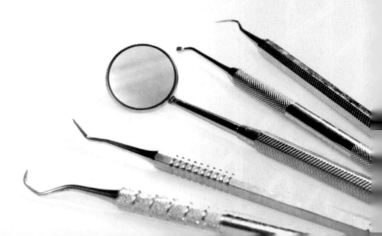

Ergonomics is the study and adaptation of how people work, including the anatomic and physiological characteristics of people in the work environment. In the dental field focusing on the principles of four-handed dentistry and other important ergonomic concepts can result in increased productivity and reduction in stress and strain on the dental team. Range of motion is the manner in which human energy can be conserved while performing a task, such as passing instruments. The objective in the dental office, whether in the clinical, business, or laboratory setting, is to minimize the amount and extent of movement or motions while conserving energy during procedures.

Zones of activity are identified using the patient's face as the face of a clock. This is also known as the clock concept. There are four zones: the operator's zone, assistant's zone, transfer zone, and static zone. To practice efficient four-handed dentistry, every person on the dental team must accept individual roles as well as team responsibilities. The dental assistant who uses the proper techniques while performing his or her job will be successful in avoiding any potential injuries.

Ergonomics in the Dental Office

The delivery of dental care can result in sustained, awkward, and unhealthy postures for the dental team members if poor techniques are practiced. This can lead to chronic pain, injuries, lower productivity, missed work, surgery, or premature retirement. These painful injuries are common in the dental work area and are known as **musculoskeletal disorders (MSDs)**. Numerous risk factors must be addressed to effectively manage and prevent muscle imbalances, decreases in the blood supply to a body organ and tissues, and trigger points that lead to pain and injuries. MSDs can be caused by any of three types of reasons: posture, repetition, and force.

Dental team members are subject to work-related injuries that can cause pain to the back and joints, neck

and shoulders, and wrists and hands. All members of the dental team must be aware of ergonomics and encourage its use in the dental office, including the proper use of equipment and ergonomic instrument design and layout of the workplace. Dental offices are designed so that each work area is efficient for the dental team members.

Four-handed, sit-down dentistry allows the dentist or operator and assistant to work while sitting down. The dental assistant provides a second pair of hands for the operator. When practicing this style of dentistry, the equipment and materials must be within reach of both the operator and assistant, allowing the dental team to function comfortably together while delivering treatment to the patient.

As a dental assistant how can one protect oneself from musculoskeletal disorders caused by job-related responsibilities?

Risk Factors

Dental team members face various risks due to the type of work being performed. Developing repetitive strain injuries is a high risk for dental assistants. A dental assistant who has poor posture and incorrectly uses equipment increases his or her risk for a strain injury. Ergonomic prevention of dental work–related pain and potentially career-ending MSDs is important to both the dental assistant and to the dental office. By decreasing work-related pain and injuries, the dental assistant will not only improve his or her musculoskeletal health but will experience improved productivity in the job.

To decrease risk of injuries while on the job, the dental assistant should adhere to the following ergonomic chairside tips:

• Do not remain in one position for too long.
• Avoid extended, uncomfortable positions.
• Use muscles for balance in easing movement.
• Stay in good physical condition by exercising.
• Stretch neck, back, shoulders, arms, and hands often during short breaks.
• Arrange necessary procedure equipment and materials within easy reach.
• Avoid repetitive and forceful actions during treatment procedures.

Posture

Posture is one of the single most important issues in preventing MSDs, especially lower back pain. Most dentistry is practiced sitting down (Figure 25.1). Although sitting is less stressful than practicing while standing, any position will become strenuous over time. Although posture influences the operator's or dental assistant's ability to reach,

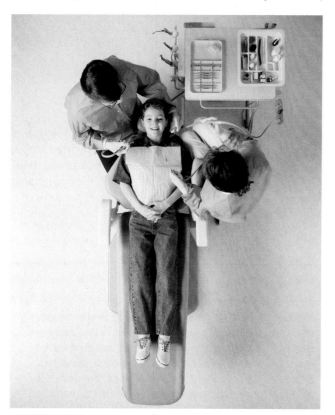

FIGURE 25.1
Correct ergonomic positions for operator and assistant during dental treatment.

hold, and use dental equipment, positioning is what affects how long the operator or dental assistant can perform procedures and tasks without inflicting any injury.

The Neutral Position

The *neutral position* is accomplished by sitting in an upright position with one's weight evenly distributed on the chair. Legs should be slightly separated with both feet on the ring at the base of the chair. Good posture should be practiced with one's back straight up and down rather than twisted or turned. One's thighs should be parallel to the floor, and the front edge of the chair should be even with the patient's mouth. The chair should be positioned close to the side of the patient with one's knees facing toward the patient's head. The height of the chair should be such that the dental assistant's eye level is four to six inches above the operator. This provides the dental assistant a good line of vision into all areas of the patient's mouth.

While assisting the dentist, the dental assistant may perform some tasks that may deviate from the neutral position by reaching, leaning, twisting, or bending. These motions can lead to aches, pains, tingling, and numbness. All of these symptoms of poor posture can lead to strains and sprains. Sprains are typically injuries that occur from sudden movement in the joints that causes stretching or tearing of the ligaments. Strains usually result from overstretching muscles or ligaments. Strains to shoulders are usually caused by repetitively reaching for items that are behind the body.

Horizontal Reach

A horizontal reach occurs when the arm is used to retrieve items within a comfortable distance, never above the shoulders or below the waist. It is the position used when reaching for frequently used items such as the air/water syringe, suction tips, instrument trays, and handpieces. The operatory light and supplies less frequently used may be within reach when the arm is fully extended. All arm reaches should be done from a frontal position. Reaching around the back of the assistant's chair may cause damage to the shoulders and back. Rather than twist one's body to gain access to an item, the dental assistant should use the chair to twist and rotate as needed.

What are the advantages to the dental assistant sitting instead of standing during dental procedures?

Injuries Sustained by Dental Assistants

The common injuries sustained by dental assistants are sprains or strains to the musculoskeletal system. Strain types of injuries can occur to individuals whose body is held in one position for an extended period of time. Repeated performance of a task can increase the risks of injury, especially when the task requires a high amount of force or is being performed with poor posture. Excessive repetition without breaks or pauses can cause development of a variety of **cumulative trauma disorders (CTDs)** such as carpal tunnel syndrome.

Force injuries increase when tasks require a lot of force to be applied during a procedure, causing forceful overextension of any muscle group. At times, the amount of force used can be more harmful than the number of repetitions. Posture can affect the amount of force that is being used. For example, when the hand is flexed or extended, the power grip force is not as effective as when the hand is in a neutral posture. Designs of instruments can also affect force. For example, more force is required to grip a thin-diameter instrument handle than a handle with a larger diameter.

Musculoskeletal Disorders

Dental workers must develop work habits early in their careers to prevent the occurrence of work-related MSDs. Musculoskeletal disorders are caused by daily overuse of certain muscle groups. Daily overuse causes tissue fatigue and inflammation. Prevention and recognizing the symptoms helps to ensure a lifelong, healthy career in the dental profession.

Recognizing Symptoms and Causes

Neck pain is caused by sitting with poor posture for long periods of time and moving the head sideways, twisting the neck, or using awkward positions to look in a patient's mouth. By adjusting one's stance throughout long periods of time and by being conscious about consistently maintaining good posture, the dental assistant can help diminish the chances of experiencing neck pain. Headaches can result from sitting in a poor posture position and using improper head positioning. It is important to change positions and stretch when possible.

Shoulder pain can occur from poor sitting posture for long periods of time where the forearms are not supported. Shoulder fatigue can become worse with poor seating, thus allowing insufficient support for the trunk of the body. Dental procedures usually require long periods of time where a position must be sustained, often with the shoulders and arms held up. With insufficient support for the arms and no place for the arms to rest, the shoulder muscles and tendons can become strained and overused. Some medical terms for the conditions associated with these types of pain include muscle strain, bursitis, and tendonitis.

Elbow, forearm, wrist, and hand pain are caused by a prolonged improper grasp on dental instruments during assisting (mostly during suctioning) procedures. Retracting the lips with the wrist flexed, bent downward and crooked, and bent sideways toward the small finger can cause pain. Wearing gloves during a procedure reduces feeling to the fingertips and the hand, which can result in an instrument being gripped tighter than necessary. Thin instruments and smooth handles also require a tighter grip and can contribute to hand pain. Unbalanced dental instruments force the use of a tighter grip to control the instrument, resulting in muscle strain and inflammation. Some medical terms for these problems include tennis elbow, golfer's elbow, wrist sprain, intersection syndrome, and tendonitis.

Finger numbness results from constriction in the nerves as they progress from the neck, through the shoulder area, down the forearm, and through the wrist. An awkward wrist position, where the wrist is flexed or extended, narrows the wrist space through which these nerves pass. Some medical terms for these more common conditions are carpal tunnel syndrome, Guyon's canal syndrome, cubital tunnel syndrome, and thoracic outlet syndrome.

Carpal Tunnel Syndrome

Carpal tunnel syndrome (CTS) is known as a repetitive stress injury that can cause debilitating pain and tingling in the thumb and first two fingers (Figure 25.2). It is caused by swelling and pressure on the median nerve passing through the wrist. Some symptoms of CTS are painful tingling in the hand(s) that usually occurs at night. The ability to squeeze or make a tight fist can become difficult. The individual may also experience weakened hand muscles, especially in the palm area around the base of the thumb, resulting in a decrease in hand strength.

Adhering to some basic rules can help prevent CTS from occurring. These rules include the following:

- Use a neutral wrist posture when handling dental instruments.
- Alternate the schedule of patients so that a variety of different procedures are done, requiring various hand movements, throughout the day.

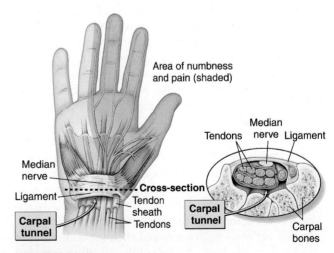

FIGURE 25.2
Anatomy of the carpal tunnel area.

- Take frequent mini stretch breaks.
- Use dental instruments with large, textured handles.
- Alternate the size of one's dental instruments during treatment and switch between instruments frequently.
- Ensure that the dental instruments used are sharp.
- Wear gloves that are made specifically for the left and right hands rather than ambidextrous gloves. Due to the either too tight or too loose fit, ambidextrous gloves can cause stress on the fingers. Good-fitting gloves that are made to fit the right or the left hand are correctly proportioned for the fingers and thumb of each hand.
- Minimize the amount of time that one continuously uses vibrating instruments without stopping.

Muscle-Strengthening Exercises

Dentistry puts dental workers at risk for muscle imbalances. Constant sitting during the day can allow the postural muscles to become weak. These muscles are responsible for holding the operator in the correct posture during the day. Unless stretching, strengthening, and relaxation times are incorporated throughout the day, the postural muscles can become weak, subjecting dental professionals to poor posture, pain, and injury. The muscles responsible for moving the body and head can become tight and painful unilaterally from repeated motions in one direction. These muscle imbalances place unnatural force on the spine and, if ignored, can contribute to MSDs.

Stretching throughout one's day is becoming more common and has shown to help in the prevention of MSDs. Stretching frequently has many benefits. In addition to increasing blood flow, flexibility, and lubrication of the joints, it can reduce pain and injuries by addressing and preventing muscle imbalances. Some examples of exercises for dental assistants include these:

- *Upper back stretches:* These stretches can be performed while standing or seated. To perform these stretches follow these steps: Clasp hands together in front and inhale. Then exhale as arms are extended out in front at chest level. Exhale, stretch forward, sinking the chest inward and rounding the shoulders forward. Hold the stretch for 10 seconds. Breathe slowly and deeply. Inhale, releasing the hands and drawing the shoulders back and down. Repeat two to five times.
- *Shoulders, chest, and elbow stretches:* These stretches can help loosen muscles in the chest and shoulder area. An added benefit of these stretches is the extension of the elbow joint, which helps realign the skeleton. To perform these stretches, follow these steps: Stand and interlace fingers behind the back, with the palms toward the back (Figure 25.3). Straighten the arms and elbows, stretch the arms backward, and then lift them up and away from the back. Perform this stretch slowly and hold for 10 seconds. Relax and breathe slowly and

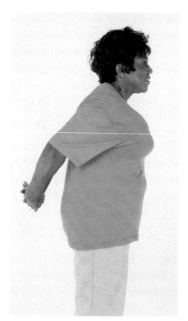

FIGURE 25.3
Dental operator demonstrating back stretches to prevent fatigue.
Andy Crawford © Dorling Kindersley

deeply. Repeat this stretch as often as needed, especially if slumping or rolling shoulders forward is a habit.
- *Hand circles:* To exercise the wrists, rotate each hand five times clockwise and then five times counterclockwise.
- *Fist clenches:* Fist clenches can help relieve tension and pressure in the hand. To perform fist clenches, open and close the fists rapidly five times.
- *Wrist bends:* Wrist bends can be accomplished by bending wrists forward and backward. Hold for four seconds in either position. Use one hand to bend the other at the wrist.
- *Finger bends and rotations:* To flex the fingers, bend the fingers forward and backward, one at a time. Hold for one or two seconds. Use one hand to bend the fingers of the other back and forth from the knuckle. Finger rotations are performed by rotating the fingers clockwise and counterclockwise on the knuckle. Use the fingers of one hand to rotate the fingers of the other.
- *Finger spread:* Finger spreads can help in strengthening and relieving pressure. Spread the fingers wide apart and stretch them outward.
- *Palm rub:* A palm rub can be done to increase circulation. A palm rub involves rubbing the palms together rapidly, then massaging the hands and fingers.

Four-Handed Dentistry

To effectively implement the **four-handed dentistry** concept, each member of the dental team must assume individual as well as team responsibilities. The team must be aware of each other's needs and recognize when to reposition the patient and operating team members to improve access and visibility and reduce repetitive movement. The theory of four-handed dentistry is not production line dentistry. It is based on a set of criteria that define the conditions under which efficiency can be attained. To practice true four-handed dentistry, the following criteria must be met:

- Equipment must be ergonomically designed to minimize repetitive motion.
- The dentist, assistant, and patient should be seated comfortably in ergonomically designed equipment. More ergonomically designed operator and assistant's stools are available nowadays than just a few years ago.
- Motion economy is practiced.
- Moisture control techniques are used to maintain visualization of the work area in the mouth.
- Preset cassettes/trays are utilized when needed.
- All necessary instruments, materials, and supplies are readily available for procedure use.
- Patient treatment is planned in advance in a logical sequence.
- All legal expanded function duties are assigned to qualified auxiliaries based on the state's dental practice guidelines.

Practicing Four-Handed Dentistry

When the dentist and the dental assistant sit down and work together at the dental chair while performing dental procedures on a patient, they are practicing four-handed dentistry. At times, an additional dental assistant may be necessary to aid the first dental assistant or to help with the patient. The use of two dental assistants is known as six-handed dentistry. Although four-handed and six-handed dentistry are both efficient and effective in patient dental care, four-handed dentistry is most commonly practiced. In four-handed dentistry the dentist and the dental team should position themselves to allow access and visibility to all areas of the oral cavity, thus minimizing repetitive motion and maintaining proper posture. The patient's comfort is paramount and is considered in four-handed dentistry.

To practice four-handed dentistry, the dental team members must first review the patient's dental and medical histories. The treatment room should be clean and ready for the dental procedure to be performed. Preparing a treatment room includes having ready a complete setup of equipment, trays, and materials for the scheduled procedure. The dental chair is placed in the upright position ready for the patient. Once the room is ready the dental assistant seats and prepares the patient for treatment. As a review of how to greet and seat a patient as covered in Chapter 22, here is a summary of the general steps to this procedure.

Professionalism

As a dental assistant it is important to treat each patient with the same respect. Treating patients with respect is not only an issue of professionalism but is also an ethical and legal issue. Some of your patients may be hard of hearing. Treating these individuals with respect requires ensuring that these patients are provided methods to ensure that communication occurs. For instance, patients with hearing impairments need to be seated so that they are able to see the lip movements and facial expressions of whoever is trying to communicate with them. Utilizing writing tools to communicate messages may be necessary to ensure that the hearing impaired patient receives clear communication. Be sure to meet your patients' needs by providing them the tools necessary for them to be a part of the decision making process in their dental care. Any consent given by the patient should be documented.

Step 1: Greet the dental patient in the reception area by using the patient's first name, keeping in mind that sometimes patients may not want to be called by their first name (Figure 25.4). Be sensitive to this issue and adjust the greeting to Mr., Ms., or Dr. with the last name as appropriate. Introduce yourself and escort the dental patient into the assigned treatment room.

Step 2: Show the patient a safe place where items such as a purse, sweater, briefcase, or backpack can be stored. Some practices offer a pretreatment antibacterial oral rinse or mouthwash to the patient. This decreases the number of oral microorganisms a great deal and is very beneficial for the operating team because fewer bacteria will be present in the aerosols that are produced during a procedure. It also reduces the chance of cross-contamination.

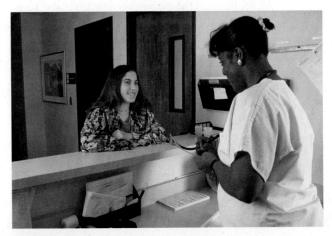

FIGURE 25.4
Dental assistant greeting patient in the reception area.

Life Span Considerations

When treating children, the elderly, or patients who have disabilities, make sure that the patient is seated comfortably and correctly prior to reclining the seat. Depending on the size of the patient, once reclined, it may be important for the patient to move up a bit so that his or her head is positioned correctly at the top of the chair allowing you the ability to use the correct ergonomic position.

Step 3: Have a conversation with the patient about things other than the dental treatment the patient is scheduled for. This can help the patient feel more comfortable and relaxed. Patients may ask questions concerning the treatment for that day or questions concerning future treatments that they may not feel comfortable in asking the dentist. If this occurs and the answers are unclear, reassure the patient that the dentist will discuss the questions with the patient.

Step 4: Seat the patient in the dental chair. For patients who may have lipstick on, offer a tissue and ask the patient to remove the lipstick. Offer lip lubricant.

Step 5: Lower the chair arm. Ask the patient to sit up straight in the dental chair.

Step 6: Place the dental napkin on the patient and give the patient safety glasses to use during the dental procedure.

Step 7: Review the patient's medical history and note any new changes that may have occurred since the patient's last visit. Review dental history and procedures scheduled for that day. Place radiographs on the view box.

Step 8: Inform the patient before adjusting the chair. Recline the patient into the treatment position, usually the supine position, in which the patient is in the reclined position with the patient's knees and nose at about the same level (Figure 25.5). Instruct the patient to slide up in the chair until the patient's head rests comfortably in the headrest at the top of the chair.

Step 9: Position the operatory light about three to five feet over the patient's mouth and tilt it down toward the patient's chest. Turn on the operatory light, being careful not to shine the light into the patient's eyes. Once the light is on, slowly raise the light into the treatment area of the mouth.
- *Maxillary arch:* The light is lowered toward the patient's chest and then the light is tilted, directed upward (Figure 25.6).
- *Mandibular arch:* The light is raised away from the patient's chest and then the light is tilted, directed downward.

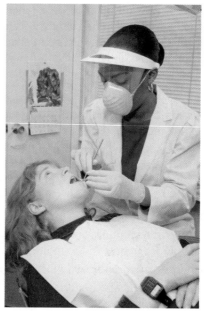

FIGURE 25.5
A patient receiving treatment in the supine position.

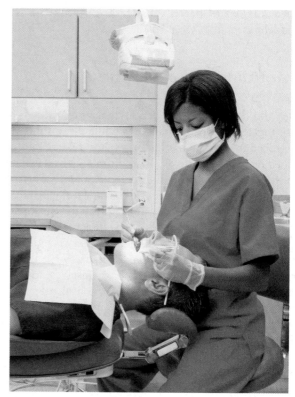

FIGURE 25.6
Positioning the light on the maxillary arch.

Once the light is in place the assistant turns off the light until the procedure is ready to start.

Step 10: Position the operator's chair and the rheostat.

Step 11: Position the dental assistant's chair.

Step 12: Review the treatment room to ensure it is prepared and organized for the dental procedure.

Step 13: Wash hands, put on personal protective equipment (gloves last), and position yourself for the procedure to begin.

Correct Operator Positioning for Procedures

The dental operator's position affects how the patient, dental assistant, and equipment is positioned. Being seated comfortably to perform procedures with easy access to the oral cavity and good visibility into the operating field is important to achieve. The following strategies on the part of the operator will help ensure correct positioning for procedures:

- The operator distributes his or her weight evenly and sits squarely back as far as possible on the seat of the dental stool so that the front edge of the stool touches just behind the knees.
- The operator's thighs are parallel to the floor or slightly lower than the hips.
- Feet are flat on the floor and not crossed. The operator's stool can be adjusted for various heights.
- The operator's lower back area is supported by the lumbar region of the operator's chair. His or her back and neck are straight with the backrest of the chair, and his or her shoulders are parallel with the floor.
- The operator's elbows are kept close to the operator's body.
- The patient's chair should be lowered to allow the operator's forearms to be parallel to the floor when the elbows are bent.
- The distance between the patient's face and the operator's face is approximately 12 to 14 inches.
- When working in the mandibular area, the back of the patient's chair should be raised up slightly for a clearer view into the mouth.

Correct Dental Assistant Positioning for Procedures

The dental assistant needs to develop a thorough understanding of each dental procedure, recognize patient needs, anticipate movements of the operator, and recognize any changes in a procedure. The following strategies for the dental assistant will help ensure correct positioning for procedures:

- The assistant's stool should be positioned four to six inches above the operator for good vision into the work area in the oral cavity.
- The assistant distributes his or her weight evenly and sits as far back as possible on the seat.
- The front edge of the assistant's chair should be about even with the patient's mouth, or the assistant's legs should be parallel to the dental chair, depending on the position of the patient.

- The assistant's feet should be resting on the base or foot ring of the assistant's chair.
- The assistant positions himself or herself as close to the side of the patient as possible.

Motion Economy

Motion economy refers to the manner in which a person can conserve energy while performing a task. Motion economy should be the primary consideration when completing clinical procedures since this concept reduces or eliminates the number and length of motions used during basic treatment procedures. Motions can be classified into five categories:

- Class 1: Finger movements (i.e., when transferring instruments)
- Class 2: Movements of the fingers and wrists or hands (i.e., placing a Tofflemire)
- Class 3: Movements of the fingers, wrists, or hands and the elbows (i.e., suctioning position)
- Class 4: Movements of the arms and shoulders (i.e., making adjustments to the operatory light)
- Class 5: Movements of the entire arm and torso of the body (i.e., taking radiographs)

Understanding the different motions of economy allows the dental assistant to effectively utilize the correct motions and preserve the health of his or her body for many years of painless chairside assisting.

Operating Zones

All treatment activity occurs around the patient. Being familiar with the operating zones is important because these zones serve as guides for the dental team and positioning of the patient to facilitate access to the operative field and improve visibility in the oral cavity.

The work area around the patient is divided into four "zones of activity." Operating zones are identified by viewing the patient's face as the face of a clock, with the forehead being at 12 o'clock. The four zones are the operator's zone, assistant's zone, transfer zone, and static zone.

The **operator's zone** for a right-handed operator is between 7 and 12 o'clock. The **assistant's zone** is in the

Cultural Considerations

When dealing with cultural diversity, always remember to "inform before you perform." Ensure that the patient has full understanding of the procedure and that you do not build up anxiety in the patient by moving too quickly. Allow time for the patient to ask questions. This will make each patient's dental experience positive and successful.

area of 2 to 4 o'clock, the **transfer zone** is in the area of 4 to 7 o'clock, and the **static zone** is in the area of 12 to 2 o'clock (Figure 25.7).

The zones are reversed for the left-handed operator: the operator's zone is between 12 and 5 o'clock, the assistant's zone is in the area of 8 to 10 o'clock, the transfer zone is in the area of 5 to 8 o'clock, and the static zone is in the area of 10 to 12 o'clock (Figure 25.8).

The operator changes position dependent on the dental arch and tooth being treated. The dentist is usually the operator. However, hygienists and dental assistants can also be in the operator's zone when they deliver dental care directly inside the oral cavity. The assistant seldom moves much in the zone of activity, but may find it necessary to raise the operating stool when working on the mandibular arch to improve the line of sight into the oral cavity. The assistant's mobile cabinet or delivery shelves are positioned inside the assistant's zone. They hold instrument trays, dental materials, air/water syringes, and suctioning equipment.

The transfer zone is where the instrument and dental materials are passed from the assistant to the operator and back. This is done in the area below the patient's chin and across the chest where the patient napkin is placed as a protective barrier. Instrument transfers are not made over the patient's face. During transfers, the patient is not touched nor can the patient see movement. The static zone is the zone of least activity. Instruments that can be stored in this area include the curing light, impression materials, and trays or the mobile cabinet when not in use.

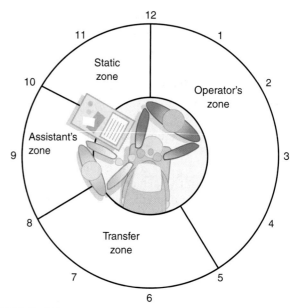

FIGURE 25.8
Zones of activity for a left-handed operator.

The Expanded Function Dental Assistant

The **expanded function dental assistant (EFDA)** is one who has been trained in specific intraoral skills. Utilizing the skills of an EFDA allows the dentist to use his or her time more wisely and efficiently. Because the EFDA can perform a wider range of tasks than a DA, the dentist's time is freed up to see more patients.

Many states require the EFDA to receive formal training before the individual can legally perform specific tasks delegated by the dentist. Even after receiving formal training from an accredited agency, the state dental practice act directs dentists as to which procedures the dentist can legally delegate to the EFDA. The dental practice act for each state also dictates which procedures the EFDA can perform under direct or indirect supervision. Direct supervision means that the dentist must be in the same treatment area while the EFDA performs the delegated duties. Indirect supervision states that the dentist must be in the office but not in the treatment area where the EFDA is performing the procedure. The dentist, however, must be available to evaluate the EFDA's work after completion.

Knowledge and Skills Required of the EFDA

While performing expanded function procedures, the dental assistant assumes the role of operator. The dental assistant sits in the operator's chair and utilizes the operator's activity zone. Knowledge of anatomy, use of a ful-

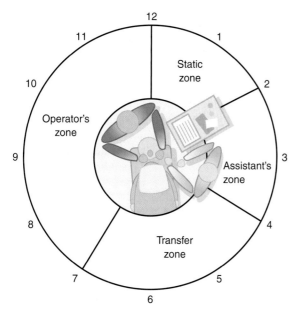

FIGURE 25.7
Zones of activity for a right-handed operator.

Legal and Ethical Issues

Depending on the state in which one works, the dental assistant will only be allowed to do certain tasks as a CDA or EFDA. Once employed be sure to check with the Dental Practice Act in the state in which one works to clarify what duties are acceptable.

crum, mirror skills, cavity preparations, instrumentation, and dental materials application is necessary for the EFDA. Understanding dental anatomy is necessary when performing an expanded function. The EFDA must have knowledge of proper form and function of the teeth and bite (occlusion), structures of the teeth, contours of the teeth, maintenance of contacts for the teeth, pits and fissures in the teeth, and the periodontium.

The mouth mirror is an important instrument when performing expanded functions procedures. The mirror provides indirect vision to areas inside the mouth. When using an instrument intraorally, the operator needs more than the proper grasp when stabilizing the dental instrument. Establishing a **fulcrum**, known as a finger rest, helps in stabilizing the hand. Stabilizing the hand with the fulcrum helps prevent slipping and/or tissue trauma in the mouth. When applying dental materials, knowing the application of the material will depend widely on the material itself. Skills for mixing and applying materials are discussed in Chapter 34.

SUMMARY

Understanding and applying the basic principles of ergonomics and four-handed dentistry allow the staff of the dental practice to function more efficiently. Dental workers must have an understanding of the principles of good body posture and positioning, the occupational risks for repetitive strain injuries, and how instrument design and selection can prevent painful disabling disorders. The body's well-being begins with learning how to take care of it. A daily program of self-care and regular visits to a health support team can help prevent CTS and other musculoskeletal disorders that can damage dental health care workers' quality of life and shorten their careers.

KEY TERMS

- **Assistant's zone:** Positioning zone that is based on the clock concept. For a right-handed operator, the dental assistant is positioned in the zone of 2 to 4 o'clock; for a left-handed operator, the dental assistant is positioned in the zone of 8 to 10 o'clock. p. 385
- **Carpal tunnel syndrome (CTS):** An injury associated with repetitive or continuous flexing and extending of the wrist. p. 381
- **Cumulative trauma disorder (CTD):** An injury associated with ongoing stresses to the joints, muscles, nerve, and tendons. p. 381
- **Ergonomics:** The study and adaptation of how people work, including the anatomic and physiological characteristics of people in the work environment. p. 379
- **Expanded function dental assistant (EFDA):** Dental assistant who can perform certain intraoral procedures delegated by the dentist after the dental assistant has been specially trained in the expanded functions per the applicable state dental act. p. 386
- **Four-handed dentistry:** Clinical procedures performed by the operator and an assistant in a structured dental environment. p. 382
- **Fulcrum:** A "finger rest" at a point in the mouth that is designed to rest and support the hand while using an instrument or handpiece in the patient's mouth; also helps prevent slipping while providing stabilization for the operator's hand during procedures. p. 387
- **Motion economy:** Refers to the manner in which a person can conserve energy while performing a task. p. 385
- **Musculoskeletal disorders (MSDs):** Painful disorders that affect the muscles and bones of the neck, the shoulders, and back. Carpal tunnel syndrome is an example of this type of disorder. p. 379
- **Operator's zone:** The location the person performing the procedure operates within. Based on the clock concept, the right-handed operator is positioned at and performs in the zone of 7 to12 o'clock; the left-handed operator does so in the zone of 12 to 5 o'clock. p. 385
- **Static zone:** The area above or behind the reclined patient. Based on the clock concept, that would be 12 to 2 o'clock for a right-handed operator and 10 to 12 o'clock for a left-handed operator. p. 386
- **Transfer zone:** The area through which materials and instruments are passed. This area is across the patient's chest. Based on the clock concept, for a right-handed operator this would be in the zone of 4 to 7 o'clock and for a left-handed operator in the zone of 5 to 8 o'clock. p. 386

CHECK YOUR UNDERSTANDING

1. Four-handed dentistry is:
   a. the use of a dental assistant together with the dentist.
   b. a team concept in which highly skilled individuals work together in an ergonomically designed environment to improve productivity of the dental team and improve the quality of care for dental patients while protecting the physical well-being of the operating team.
   c. not production line dentistry.
   d. all of the above.

2. Considering the five categories of motion classification, a Class 3 motion involves
   a. the entire arm and shoulder.
   b. the fingers and wrist.
   c. movement of the fingers only.
   d. the fingers, wrist, and elbow.
   e. the entire torso cabinetry.

3. The zones of activity in four-handed dentistry include all of the following except
   a. static zone.
   b. transfer zone.
   c. patient's zone.
   d. assistant's zone.

4. If one moved the fingers, wrist, and elbow, such as when reaching for a handpiece, this would be a motion classified as
   a. Class 1.
   b. Class 2.
   c. Class 3.
   d. Class 4.

5. The operator's zone for a right-handed operator extends from
   a. 7 to 12 o'clock.
   b. 12 to 3 o'clock.
   c. 4 to 7 o'clock.
   d. 12 to 2 o'clock.

6. Which of the following causes of poor posture can also lead to strains and sprains?
   a. reaching and leaning
   b. twisting and leaning forward
   c. overbending and stretching
   d. all of the above

7. Utilizing an expanded functions dental assistant's skill allows the dentist to use time more wisely and efficiently by
   a. increasing productivity.
   b. freeing up time for the dentist, allowing more patients to be seen.
   c. allowing team members to focus on specific tasks, resulting in increased job satisfaction for the dental assistant.
   d. all of the above.

8. The supine position is when the patient is in a
   a. reclined position with knees and nose at about the same level.
   b. upright position with legs crossed.
   c. reclined position with feet elevated even with the level of the heart.
   d. reclined position with the head slightly above the chest.

9. The operator's position is taken by the
   a. person assisting the dentist.
   b. assistant aiding in six-handed dentistry.
   c. person performing the procedure in the oral cavity.
   d. dentist.

10. The neutral position is accomplished by
    a. sitting in an upright position with one's weight evenly distributed on the chair.
    b. placing one's legs together and both feet on the ring of the base of the chair.
    c. adjusting the chair 6 to 8 inches above the operator.
    d. positioning the chair away from the patient's side.

INTERNET ACTIVITY

- Go to www.crest.com. Pick the continuing education topic titled "Four Handed Dentistry Part 3," and watch the video on how to pass and transfer instruments.

WEB REFERENCES

- DPRWorld.com   www.dentalproducts.net
- Mechanisms Leading to Musculoskeletal Disorders in Dentistry   www.posturedontics.com/jada/PD_JADA_OCT03.pdf

26

Moisture Control

Learning Objectives

After reading this chapter, the student should be able to:

- List the components of the oral evacuation system.
- Describe the two types of oral evacuation systems.
- Explain the rationale for the limited area and complete mouth rinsing procedure.
- Explain the role of the clinical dental assistant in maintaining a dry working field.
- Demonstrate the proper placement of the HVE and saliva ejector.
- Demonstrate the use of the air/water syringe.
- List isolation techniques utilized during dental procedures.
- Explain the purpose of the dental dam.
- Explain the advantages and contraindications of the dental dam.
- Identify the components needed for the dental dam procedure.
- Demonstrate the steps for placing and removing the dental dam.

Preparing for Certification Exams

- Maintain field of operation during dental procedures through the use of retraction, suction, irrigation, drying, placing and removing of cotton rolls, and so forth.
- Place and remove dental dam.

Key Terms

Air/water syringe

Biofilm

Complete mouth rinse

Dental dam

Dry angle

High-volume evacuator (HVE)

Isolation

Limited area mouth rinse

Oral evacuation

Saliva ejector

Chapter Outline

- Oral Evacuation Systems
  - —High-Volume Evacuator
  - —Saliva Ejector
  - —Surgical Suction Tips
  - —Air/Water Syringe
  - —Daily Maintenance of the Evacuation System

- Rinsing the Oral Cavity
  - —Limited Area Mouth Rinsing
  - —Complete Mouth Rinsing

- Isolation of Teeth
  - —Cotton Roll Isolation
  - —Dry-Angle Isolation
  - —Dental Dam Isolation

- The Dental Dam
  - —Dental Dam Frame
  - —Dental Dam Napkin
  - —Dental Dam Lubricants
  - —Dental Dam Stamp and Template
  - —Dental Dam Punch
  - —Dental Dam Forceps
  - —Dental Dam Clamps
  - —Dental Dam Stabilizing Cord

- Dental Dam Placement and Removal
  - —The Quick Dam

- Special Applications of the Dental Dam

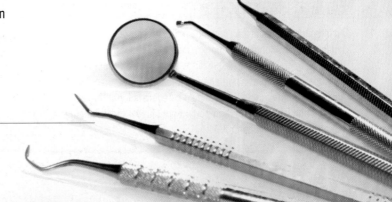

One of the most important duties of the clinical dental assistant is to maintain a clear, dry working field for enhanced visibility. A well-maintained treatment area is essential to the eventual success of the procedure and maximum comfort for the patient. The requirements of maintaining the operating field are determined by the type of procedure, the tooth or teeth being treated, the oral anatomy of the patient, and the preferences of the operator. The dental team uses a variety of components to facilitate and maintain a dry field including a dental dam, cotton rolls, dry angles, high-volume evacuator, saliva ejector, and air/water syringe. These components are used to ensure that:

- Moisture and/or debris do not block the operator's line of vision.
- Saliva, fluids, and moisture do not interfere with the application of dental materials.
- Saliva, fluids, and moisture do not interfere with the use of the dental handpiece.
- Patient comfort is maintained with the removal of saliva, fluids, blood, or debris from the oral cavity.

Oral Evacuation Systems

The term **oral evacuation** is a general term used to describe the process of removing excess fluids, saliva, blood, or debris from the oral cavity during operative dental procedures. The **high-volume evacuator (HVE)** (also called the *high-velocity evacuator*), saliva ejector,

and air/water syringe are utilized together or separately before, during, and after dental procedures to ensure that the dentist has clear visibility of the working field during the process of restorative or surgical procedures and to help ensure that the oral cavity feels fresh, clean, and free of debris for the patient.

The evacuation system is generally referred to as the suction unit and operates with the use of a vacuum unit similar to that of a household vacuum cleaner. The oral evacuation system consists of the HVE, the saliva ejector, and the air/water syringe (three-way syringe; Figure 26.1). The attachment apparatus for the oral evacuation system consists of flexible tubing that is connected to the dental unit and the air/water syringe handle. The handle is the area of the hose where the evacuator tip is inserted and the on/off button is located (Figure 26.2).

Evacuator tips are made of disposable plastic (Figure 26.3). They fit into the handle portion of the oral evacuator hoses. Metal tips are available for use, but have generally been replaced by the disposable or autoclavable

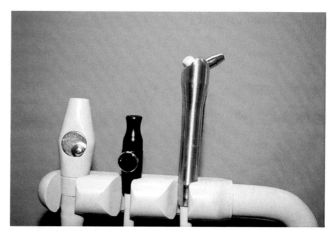
FIGURE 26.1
Oral evacuation system.
Image courtesy Instructional Materials for the Dental Team, Lex., KY

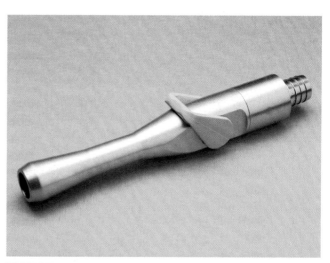
FIGURE 26.2
HVE handle.

plastic tips. These tips are supplied in three basic types and sizes: the HVE, the surgical tip, and the saliva ejector. The type of procedure that is being performed dictates which style and/or size of suction tip is chosen and utilized by the dental assistant.

High-Volume Evacuator

The high-volume evacuator is part of the "dental unit" and is used to remove water, blood, saliva, and debris from the oral cavity and to retract oral tissues such as the tongue and cheek away from the working field. These disposable or autoclavable plastic tips are available in various sizes, lengths, colors, and shapes. They are tubular in shape and may be straight, curved, or angled with slanted vented or unvented openings with beveled ends. This slant allows the tip to be adapted to either the maxillary or the mandibular arch and either the right or left sides of the oral cavity.

The HVE can be placed within the oral cavity utilizing several grasps. The two grasps chosen are based on where the tip will be placed and whether it is used to evacuate fluids or retract tissues or both. The grasps most commonly used are the pen and the thumb-to-nose grasp (Figure 26.4). Generally, the pen grasp is utilized when anterior maxillary or anterior mandibular teeth are being restored or when using the narrow surgical tip during surgical procedures. The thumb-to-nose grasp is used for the maxillary and mandibular posterior teeth or when the assistant needs to utilize the HVE to retract the cheeks or tongue away from the field of operation.

It is important for the assistant to enter the mouth with the HVE tip first in order to establish position before the operator enters with the handpiece and mouth mirror. HVE tips are generally large in circumference and can be straight or slightly bent in design. Each end of the HVE tip is generally beveled so that the tip can be posi-

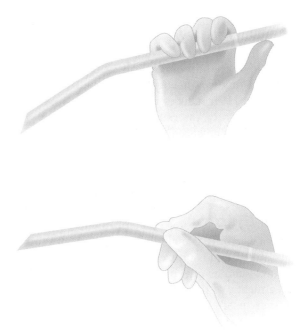

FIGURE 26.4
Two different grasps utilized during HVE placement.

tioned as closely as possible to the treatment area, which is generally distal to the tooth being prepared with the tip placed parallel to the tooth.

When working with a right-handed operator, the dental assistant places the HVE tip parallel to the lingual surface of the right maxillary and mandibular molars. When the right-handed operator is working on the left side of the oral cavity, the dental assistant places the HVE tip on the buccal side of the left maxillary and mandibular molars. When the operator is working on the facial surface of any maxillary or mandibular anterior tooth, the HVE should be placed on the lingual portion of the tooth being worked on. When the operator is working on the lingual surface of any maxillary or mandibular anterior tooth, the HVE tip should be positioned parallel to the facial surface of the tooth being worked on. The HVE tip is positioned by placing the opening of the tip next to the site of treatment while using the side of the tip to retract the tongue or cheek. The assistant must be careful to keep the tip out of the operator's line of vision.

Evacuator tips are also available with a side venting feature. This type of specialized evacuator tip allows the assistant to regulate the power of the suction during procedures. The assistant may place one finger over one side to increase the evacuation power or one finger and thumb over both side venting holes to incorporate maximum evacuation power when needed. In addition, it is essential that the chairside assistant understand the use of the suction tip and become proficient in placement techniques. Improperly placed HVE tips can "catch" and injure the very delicate soft tissues of the mouth or may cause the patient to gag if placed too closely to the soft palate or the posterior region of the patient's tongue.

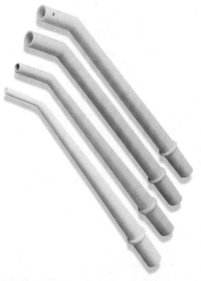

FIGURE 26.3
HVE tips.
Courtesy Young Dental

Table 26-1 lists guidelines for HVE placement, and Procedure 26-1 discusses the various placements for the HVE tip within the patient's mouth.

In addition to the moisture control element, the HVE is an important infection control component of operative dentistry. An HVE reduces the amount of aerosols and contaminants from the patient's saliva and the water sprayed by the high-speed handpieces and the ultrasonic scaler. It reduces the contaminated aerosol for both the patient and the dental team, which is an important infection control consideration.

Saliva Ejector

The **saliva ejector** is a small oral evacuator that is part of the dental unit and is utilized during less invasive dental procedures such as oral prophylaxis, sealants and fluoride treatments, or during the limited area and complete mouth rinse procedures. Saliva ejectors are flexible, plastic straw-shaped devices that are one-third the size of the HVE (Figure 26.5).

Due to the small circumference of the saliva ejector, the main function of this oral evacuator is to remove fluids and liquids from the patient's mouth. The covered tip and the smaller circumference of the saliva ejector pre-

---

TABLE 26-1 Guidelines for High-Volume Evacuator Placement

- Select the appropriate end and place securely into the suction hose to avoid accidental dislodgement.
- When working with a right-handed operator, the assistant operates the HVE with the right hand; with a left-handed operator, the assistant operates the HVE with the left hand.
- Use a thumb-to-nose or pen grasp to hold the HVE.
- Minimize the noise of the HVE by turning the evacuator on completely.
- Place the HVE tip before the operator places the handpiece and/or mirror.
- Angle the HVE with the beveled portion parallel to the tooth and place the tip as close as possible to the tooth surface, avoiding contact with any soft tissue and one tooth distal to the tooth being prepped.
- Keep the edge of the evacuator tip even with or positioned slightly above the occlusal or incisal edge of the tooth.
- Place the tip of the HVE near the tooth surface closest to the assistant.
- When the handpiece is being used on the surface nearest the assistant, place the HVE tip slightly distal to the tooth being treated.
- Avoid contact with the soft palate to eliminate the potential for gagging.
- Avoid contact with sublingual tissues because they can be more susceptible to injury than other oral tissues.
- Remove the tip from the patient's mouth whenever possible to allow the patient to close and swallow.

Preparing for Externship

Learning to manipulate and manage all aspects of moisture control as well as staying out of the operative field of vision can be very intimidating when a dental assistant is first learning to assist the dentist. Regardless of the inexperience of the novice dental assistant, it is important to remember that maintaining a professional attitude through the duration of the procedure creates an atmosphere that is conducive to keeping a patient calm, trusting, and relaxed. Proficiency with the manipulation of the HVE, the saliva ejector, and the air/water syringe comes with practice and perseverance.

---

vent the removal of any solid debris. The flexible, plastic tubing can be bent and shaped for easy placement in the oral cavity. The saliva ejector is utilized during the procedure by (1) holding it throughout the procedure and utilizing it during periodic breaks, (2) performing periodic sweeps of the oral cavity to prevent accumulation of fluids and saliva in the back of the patient's mouth, and (3) positioning the saliva ejector to remain in the mouth during procedures.

It is important to ensure that the saliva ejector is correctly positioned so that it remains in a stationary position in the mouth during a procedure. This is done by bending and forming the tubing into the shape of a candy cane. This shape allows the saliva ejector to be positioned where fluids accumulate in the oral cavity on the opposite side of which the dentist is working (Figure 26.6). This helps to reduce the number of items in the operating field.

The small diameter of the saliva ejector makes this piece of oral evacuation equipment difficult to clean. Due to this fact the saliva ejector is utilized as a single one-time use disposable item. The saliva ejector should be used with a sweeping motion in the corners of the back of the mouth to remove fluids from the patient's oral cavity. Patients should refrain from completely closing around the saliva ejector as research has shown that biofilm from within the interior surface of the saliva ejector tubing can be sucked back into the patient's mouth with the vacuum that is created by the complete closure. Assistants should also be careful not to place the saliva ejector under the patient's tongue to prevent irritation to the soft tissue in that area. Prolonged procedures may increase the possibility of the saliva ejector "sucking" up tissue into the evacuator tip and causing trauma.

The Lingua-Fix

The lingua-fix is utilized to provide retraction while evacuating saliva. This oral evacuator device is a disposable, plastic saliva ejector device that isolates and protects the tongue, evacuates fluids, and maintains a dry work area. The lingua-fix utilizes a locking mechanism, which is

Procedure 26-1 Placing the High-Volume Evacuator Tips

Equipment and Supplies Needed

- High-volume evacuator
- Cotton rolls
- Air/water syringe
- Basic setup
- Dental handpiece

Procedure Steps for HVE Maxillary Right Posterior Tip Placement

1. Place the HVE tip in the holder by pushing the end of the tip into the HVE hose.

2. Position the tip near the lingual surface, just distal to the tooth being worked on.

3. The bevel of the tip should be parallel to the lingual surface of the teeth.

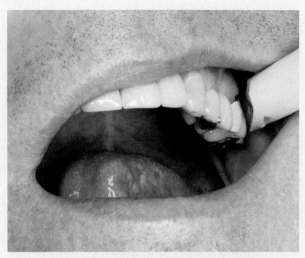

HVE tip placement for maxillary left posterior region.

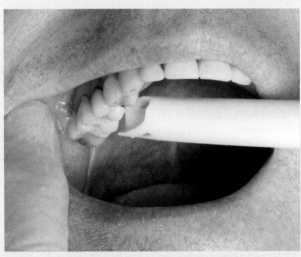

HVE tip placement for maxillary right posterior region.

Procedure Steps for HVE Maxillary Left Posterior Tip Placement

1. Place the HVE tip in the holder by pushing the end of the tip into the HVE hose.

2. Position the tip of the evacuator parallel to the buccal surface of the teeth.

3. To maintain patient comfort, the tip can rest on a cotton roll.

4. The tip may need to be utilized to retract the cheek away from the working area.

Procedure Steps for HVE Mandibular Right Posterior Tip Placement

1. Place the HVE tip in the holder by pushing the end of the tip into the HVE hose.

2. Position the tip across the mandibular left teeth between the lingual surface of the teeth and the tongue.

3. The tip should be parallel to the lingual surface of the teeth.

4. A cotton roll may be utilized to assist in retracting the tongue away from the operator's field of vision.

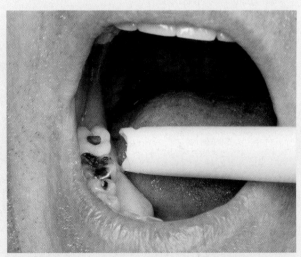

HVE tip placement for mandibular right posterior region.

continued on next page

Procedure 26-1 *continued from previous page*

Procedure Steps for HVE Mandibular Left Posterior Tip Placement

1. Place the HVE tip in the holder by pushing the end of the tip into the HVE hose.

2. The tip of the beveled portion of the HVE tip should be positioned parallel to the buccal surface of the teeth.

3. The tip may need to be utilized to retract the cheek away from the working area.

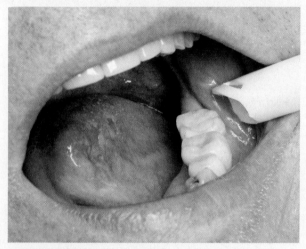

HVE tip placement for mandibular left posterior region.

Procedure Steps for HVE Maxillary Anterior Facial Tip Placement

1. Place the HVE tip in the holder by pushing the end of the tip into the HVE hose.

2. Place the tip parallel to the facial of the anterior teeth when the operator is preparing a tooth from the lingual surface of the tooth.

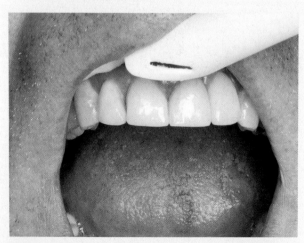

HVE tip placement for maxillary anterior facial when operator is preparing the tooth from the lingual.

Procedure Steps for HVE Maxillary Anterior Lingual Tip Placement

1. Place the HVE tip in the holder by pushing the end of the tip into the HVE hose.

2. The evacuator tip is placed on the lingual surface of the anterior teeth when the operator is preparing a tooth from the facial surface of the tooth.

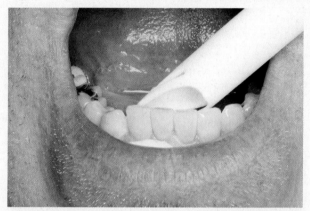

HVE tip placement for maxillary anterior lingual when operator is preparing the tooth from the facial.

Procedure Steps for HVE Mandibular Facial Tip Placement

1. Place the HVE tip in the holder by pushing the end of the tip into the HVE hose.

2. The evacuator tip is positioned on a cotton roll near the facial surface of the mandibular teeth when the operator is preparing a tooth from the lingual side of the tooth.

3. The beveled portion of the tip should retract the lower lip and should be parallel to the facial surface.

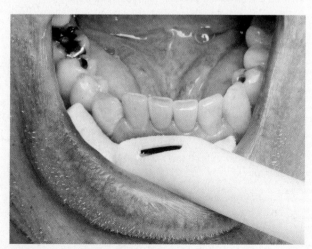

HVE tip placement for mandibular facial when operator is preparing tooth from the lingual.

Procedure 26-1 *continued from previous page*

Procedure Steps for HVE Mandibular Anterior Lingual Tip Placement

1. Place the HVE tip in the holder by pushing the end of the tip into the HVE hose.

2. The evacuator tip is positioned with the bevel parallel to the lingual surface of the teeth when the operator is preparing a tooth from the facial surfaces.

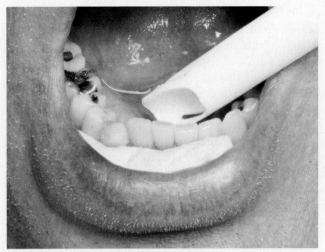

HVE tip placement for mandibular anterior lingual when operator is preparing tooth from the facial.

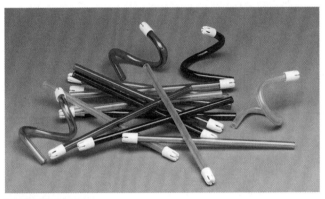

FIGURE 26.5
Saliva ejector.
Courtesy of the Bosworth Company

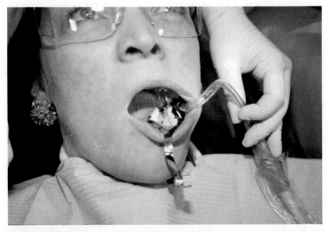

FIGURE 26.6
Saliva ejector placed underneath the tongue.
Image courtesy Instructional Materials for the Dental Team, Lex., KY

placed under the chin to hold the device securely in place (Figure 26.7). The large, soft suction surface firmly but gently retracts the tongue away from the working area while providing suction. The smooth edges and corners ensure patient comfort while maintaining a clear, dry working field. The lingua-fix fits into the saliva ejector hose and is used in place of the saliva ejector for some procedures. The lingua-fix contains a filter trap that traps amalgam and other solid waste material so that it cannot enter the oral evacuator hose.

Surgical Suction Tips

An additional oral evacuator that is only utilized during surgical procedures is the surgical suction tip. Surgical suction tips are designed so that the operative end is

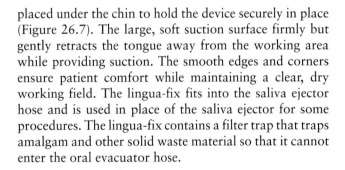

FIGURE 26.7
Lingue-Fix.
Courtesy of David E. Lawler, DDS

much smaller in circumference than the HVE or saliva ejector. The surgical suction tip is placed within the same handle attachment apparatus as the HVE. The smaller tip design ensures that the surgical suction is easily adapted to and placed within oral surgical sites. The smaller tip prevents tissue, bone, and teeth fragments from being "sucked" into the evacuation unit. In addition the smaller tip aids in providing improved vision in very small areas of the working field.

When using this site-specific oral evacuator, the narrow opening may clog frequently when suctioning blood and tissue; thus it may be necessary to clear the tip with sterile water or saline solution. This is done by frequently dipping the surgical suction tip into the solution so that the suctioning action assists in removing any debris that may be lodged in the narrow tip. Surgical tips can be constructed of hard, durable plastic or metal. The plastic tips are typically disposed of after a single use unless the plastic material is autoclavable. Metal tips can be sterilized and reused. Surgical suction tips are part of the surgical setup.

The type of procedure being performed dictates which styles and/or size of suction tips are chosen and utilized by the dental assistant. During most operative procedures, the dental assistant will need to utilize the HVE, the saliva ejector, and the air/water syringe to facilitate an effective and efficient treatment procedure.

Air/Water Syringe

The **air/water syringe**, also referred to as the *three-way syringe*, is part of the dental unit and consists of a syringe with three functions: (1) water spray, (2) air spray, and (3) aerated spray (a combination of both water and air) (Figure 26.8). Syringe tips are attached to the syringe apparatus and are fabricated from either metal, which can be removed and sterilized, or disposable plastic that is discarded after each procedure.

The air/water syringe is primarily used to rinse and dry the oral cavity during and immediately following dental procedures, and as a supplement to oral evacuation procedures. Additionally, the air/water syringe is uti-

lized to keep the mirror clean with air during operative procedures or to facilitate additional retraction of the tongue or cheeks when needed. An operator may use the mouth mirror for indirect vision when preparing a tooth for a restoration. Water from the handpiece can accumulate on the mirror and distort the operator's view. The assistant is expected to keep the mirror surface dry and free from debris by utilizing the air/water syringe without interfering with the operator's line of vision. The air emitted from the air/water syringe removes any water accumulating on the surface of the mirror, which helps provide the operator with an unobstructed view of the operative field.

The air/water syringe is held in the assistant's left hand and the HVE is held in the assistant's right hand when assisting a right-handed clinician. When assisting a left-handed clinician, the air/water syringe is held in the right hand and the HVE is held in the assistant's left hand. For maximum efficiency, when using the air/water syringe, the following should be considered:

- Turn the tip in the direction of the arch: up for the maxilla and down for the mandible.
- To minimize aerosol, keep a close distance between the operative site and the syringe tip.
- To thoroughly cleanse the site, place the tip directly over the opening of the preparation when a cavity preparation is flushed. This will maximize rinsing and evacuating of all debris and water.
- Be assertive when cleansing a site. Do not hold the tip too far away. Place the tip within one-quarter inch of the site to be cleansed and press firmly on the buttons to cleanse the area.
- Quickly move the syringe tip into the area to be cleaned; flush, evacuate, and move the tip out of the area quickly.

The dental assistant needs to be aware of special infection control applications when operating the air/water syringe. The dental unit waterlines that provide the water for the air/water syringes have been shown to contain high concentrations of microscopic bacteria, including microorganisms from patients' saliva. This microscopic bacteria is known as **biofilm**. A biofilm is made up of microorganisms that can accumulate on the inside of dental unit waterlines and can increase a patient's susceptibility to transmittable diseases. The biofilm microorganisms enter the waterlines by retraction up into the syringe as a result of a retraction valve that is designed to prevent dripping. To reduce and prevent the potential of this source of cross-contamination, operators should flush (run water through) the waterlines for at least two minutes at the start of each day and for at least 20 to 30 seconds after each patient appointment during the day. This simple procedure rids the inside of the waterlines of the potentially infectious biofilm, thus protecting the patient. (For more information on dental waterlines, see Chapter 19.)

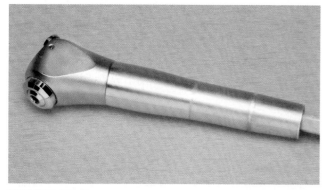

FIGURE 26.8
Air/water, three-way syringe.

Independent or self-contained water reservoirs can be utilized to prevent contaminated biofilm from being introduced into the oral cavity. The self-contained system completely bypasses the dental unit and utilizes sterile or distilled water for irrigation. A water bottle is attached to the dental unit, filled with water, and then pressurized with air from the unit to push the water through the dental unit waterlines. This prevents contaminated backflow from entering the patient's oral cavity. The unit reservoirs and waterlines are purged between each patient and then cleaned and disinfected with commercial-strength detergents at the end of each day. It is important to follow all manufactures guidelines and wear all necessary personal protective equipment (PPE) when disinfecting and purging dental unit waterlines. The water bottle should be cleaned and disinfected at least weekly. Specific cleaning products are manufactured for this procedure.

A new dental assistant has just been hired in the office where you work. You have trained her to correctly flush the dental unit waterlines prior to treating patients at the beginning of each day as well as in between patients. However, you notice that the new dental assistant fails to perform this procedure. How would you address this dental assistant? What facts would you use to instruct this dental assistant on the importance of this critical infection control step?

Daily Maintenance of the Evacuation System

The oral evacuation system requires daily maintenance to maintain the unit in proper working order. Specific guidelines should be followed according to each manufacturer's recommendations; however, the following procedures are basic suggestions:

- Follow all infection control guidelines and wear the necessary PPE when handling contaminated oral evacuation items.
- The Centers for Disease Control and Prevention (CDC) and the Occupational Safety and Health Administration (OSHA) indicate that all hoses should be flushed between patients for 20 to 30 seconds with tap water.
- Flush the HVE and the saliva ejector hoses at the end of the day.
- Check the disposable traps daily and replace when needed.
- Follow the manufacturer's recommendations for maintaining the vacuum pump system.

Rinsing the Oral Cavity

The oral cavity should be rinsed periodically to help maintain a clear working field for the clinician and to maintain patient comfort. Two basic types of rinsing procedures are utilized during patient treatment: limited area rinsing and complete mouth rinsing.

Limited Area Mouth Rinsing

The **limited area mouth rinse** is performed frequently during the operative dental procedure. Limited area rinsing is utilized to remove debris such as water, saliva, tooth fragments, and dental materials that may accumulate during tooth preparation and restorative procedures. It is accomplished quickly and frequently during the procedure to maintain a clear working field and to maintain patient comfort. Limited area rinsing is often performed when the dentist pauses during the procedure and exits the mouth or during periodic breaks while a coronal polishing procedure is being performed (see Procedure 26-2).

Procedure 26-2 Performing a Limited Mouth Rinse

Equipment Needed
- Saliva ejector
- Air/water syringe

Procedure Steps
1. The limited mouth rinse is generally performed by one operator utilizing the saliva ejector and the air/water syringe simultaneously.

2. Turn on the suction and position the tip toward the site for a limited area rinse. The tip of the saliva ejector can be used to retract the cheeks when rinsing on each side of the oral cavity.

3. Spray the combination of air and water (aerated spray) onto the site to be rinsed. The aerated spray provides enough force to thoroughly clean the area.

4. Suction all fluid and debris from the area, being sure to remove all fluids.

Complete Mouth Rinsing

The **complete mouth rinse** is generally performed once all oral procedures have been completed. Sometimes during long dental procedures, when the patient's entire mouth needs refreshing, a complete rinse may be performed. The complete mouth rinse is performed to remove any residual debris and to achieve patient comfort. A complete mouth rinse can be accomplished utilizing the HVE and the air/water syringe, or the saliva ejector and the air/water syringe (see Procedure 26-3). However, if any debris is present in the oral cavity, the HVE must be used to facilitate complete removal of the debris. Rinsing the oral cavity utilizing the air/water aerated spray is not recommended by the CDC.

Why is it important to wear all necessary PPE when flushing dental unit waterlines? **?**

Isolation of Teeth

Isolation is the act of keeping a tooth or an area separate or dry. Certain dental procedures dictate that a tooth, quadrant, or even the entire arch be kept dry and isolated from the moist environment of the oral cavity. The primary objectives for oral isolation include the following:

- Maintain a dry working field within the oral cavity.
- Retract the soft tissues of the oral cavity.
- Aid in infection control techniques by decreasing aerosol sprays.
- Reduce potential contamination to the tooth.
- Increase patient comfort.
- Increase success of restorations by providing a dry operative field.

A variety of techniques are available to achieve these listed objectives. It is important to consider all of the following features when choosing an isolation material and/or technique for an operative, preventive, or surgical dental procedure:

- The material should be easy to apply.
- The material should protect the soft and hard tissues of the oral cavity.
- The material should be comfortable for the patient.
- The material should provide retraction of oral tissues for better visualization.
- The material should prevent moisture contamination.
- The material should be able to sufficiently isolate the area of concern.

In addition to utilizing the HVE and saliva ejector for moisture control, other techniques can be utilized to assist with the required isolation for specific areas and procedures within the oral cavity. The three most common methods of isolation are (1) cotton roll isolation, (2) dry angles, and (3) the dental dam.

Cotton Roll Isolation

Cotton roll isolation involves the use of tightly formed, absorbent, preshaped cotton (Figure 26.9). These rolls are positioned close to the salivary gland ducts, within the vestibule or under the tongue. The rolls are used to absorb the flow of saliva. In addition to moisture control, cotton rolls are utilized during dental procedures as a tool for the placement of dental materials, or to serve as something for the patient to bite on.

Cotton rolls are designed to be flexible for easy placement. Dentists or dental assistants generally place

Procedure 26-3 Performing a Complete Mouth Rinse

Equipment Needed
- Saliva ejector or HVE
- Air/water syringe

Procedure Steps
1. When performing a two-person complete mouth rinse procedure, the dentist will operate the air/water syringe and the assistant will operate the HVE. When performing a one-person complete mouth rinse procedure, the operator will hold the air/water syringe in one hand and the saliva ejector in the other.
2. The operator should have the patient turn his or her head toward the operator to allow for the water to pool on one side making it easier for removal.
3. Turn on the HVE and position it carefully in the vestibule so that it does not come into contact with any soft tissue.
4. With the HVE in position, direct the air/water syringe from the patient's maxillary right across to the side closest to the operator, spraying all surfaces.
5. Continue down to the mandibular arch, following the same sequence. This pattern of rinsing forces the debris to the posterior region of the mouth where the suction tip is positioned for easier removal of fluid and debris.

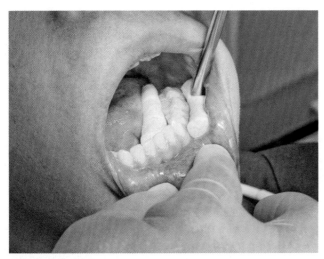

FIGURE 26.9
Cotton roll utilized for moisture control.

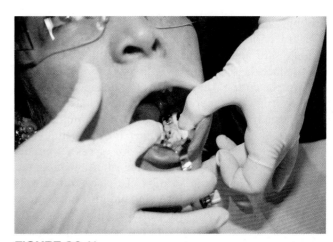

FIGURE 26.11
Cotton roll placement in mandibular arch.
Image courtesy Instructional Materials for the Dental Team, Lex., KY

cotton rolls within the treatment area using cotton pliers or they may place the cotton rolls directly in the patient's mouth with a gloved hand. When utilizing cotton rolls for maxillary isolation, the cotton rolls are placed on the cheek side of the teeth in the muccobuccal fold (Figure 26.10). This area of the vestibule holds the cotton roll securely in place. Secure placement within the mandibular arch is more difficult to obtain because of the movement of the tongue. To place cotton rolls on the lingual side of the mandible, the tongue is gently retracted or raised and the cotton roll is placed between the lingual surfaces of the teeth and the base of the tongue (Figure 26.11). For maximum moisture control, cotton rolls are placed on both the lingual and buccal sides of the mandibular teeth to obtain isolation.

The dentist or the dental assistant can easily remove the cotton rolls following the dental procedure, either with the use of cotton pliers or via direct removal with gloved fingers. When cotton rolls are moist, removal is performed easily. However, it is important to evaluate the cotton rolls prior to removal. If the cotton rolls are dry, it is important to thoroughly saturate the cotton rolls with water from the air/water syringe before removal to prevent pulling on the mucosal tissue and to ensure ease of removal for the patient. Failure to do so can cause tissue irritation. Due to its ease of application, cotton roll isolation is the most common type of isolation utilized during short operative procedures such as simple restorations and sealant application.

There are various advantages and disadvantages to using cotton rolls. Advantages include the fact that they are simple and easy to use, quickly and easily secured, and no additional equipment is needed for placement or removal. Disadvantages to the use of cotton rolls include the fact that these materials do not prevent contamination of the area by the patient's tongue or debris from

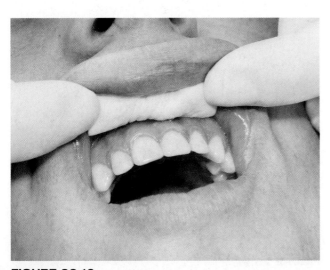

FIGURE 26.10
Cotton roll placement in maxillary arch.

Life Span Considerations

The geriatric population has been the fastest growing patient population in the last several years. In addition, there has been an increase in the incidence of the senior population seeking dental care. With the increase in the number of older patients who are keeping their natural teeth longer, a large percentage of the daily schedule will consist of this patient population. One oral manifestation of older adults is xerostomia, which affects all of the delicate oral tissues. It is important to remember that the use of cotton rolls and dry angles can worsen this condition. It is imperative that the dental assistant thoroughly saturate these moisture control devices before removal to eliminate any undue tissue trauma or irritation.

dropping into the oral cavity. Cotton rolls must also be replaced periodically during the procedure when they become saturated. The dental assistant must remember not to place the tip of the HVE directly over a cotton roll because the cotton roll can easily be suctioned up by the HVE, causing the suction line to become clogged.

Cotton roll holders are designed to hold multiple cotton rolls in a more secure manner for the mandibular quadrant (Figure 26.12). Holders are especially important when the operator is working alone, without an extra hand to maintain isolation. To place cotton rolls utilizing a holder, a metal prong is slid into each cotton roll. The rolls are then seated with one roll positioned on the buccal side of the teeth and the other on the lingual side. After being positioned within the oral cavity, a sliding bar, which is attached to the base of the holder, is slid under and upward toward the chin to secure the cotton roll holder in place (Figure 26.13). Cotton roll holders that are made out of plastic are called isolators. These holders are used once and then discarded.

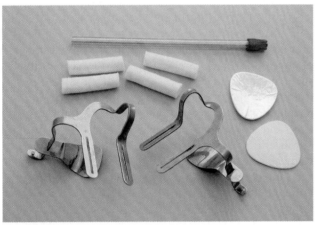

FIGURE 26.12
Moisture control devices: cotton rolls, cotton roll holder, and dry angle.
Image courtesy Instructional Materials for the Dental Team, Lex., KY

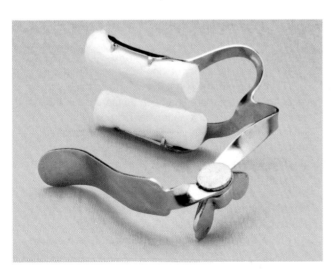

FIGURE 26.13
Cotton roll holder in use.

Dry-Angle Isolation

The dry-angle isolation technique involves the use of a triangular, absorbent pad called a **dry angle** (Figure 26.14). This pad helps isolate posterior areas in both the maxillary and mandibular arches. The pad is placed directly over the Stensen's duct of the parotid gland, which is located directly opposite the maxillary second molar on the buccal mucosa. These pads block the flow of saliva from the Stensen's duct and also protect and retract the tissues of this area.

Dry angles should be periodically replaced when they become saturated and are no longer adequate for moisture control during a procedure. Dry angles can be removed following the dental procedure, either with the use of cotton pliers or via direct removal with gloved fingers. Like cotton rolls, it is essential that these pads be saturated with water from the air/water syringe prior to removal. This prevents pulling in the mucosa and makes removal easier. If the pads are too dry, the surface of the tissues can be damaged when separating the dry angle from the buccal area.

Dental Dam Isolation

The **dental dam** is a thin, stretchable latex or latex-free material that is utilized as the highest level of moisture control during dental procedures. This barrier can be utilized so that a single tooth or a section of teeth within the same quadrant or sextant is visible through the dental dam material. These teeth are referred to as being isolated or exposed. Proper use of a dental dam will aid in achieving greater access to the area of treatment, visibility, and infection control. Other advantages to the use of a dental dam include the following:

• Serves as an important infection control protective barrier and decreases the amount of contaminated aerosol exposure for the patient

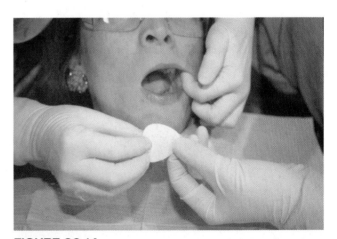

FIGURE 26.14
Dry angle.
Image courtesy Instructional Materials for the Dental Team, Lex., KY

- Protects the patient's oral cavity from contact with debris, irritating dental materials, and infectious material from an infected tooth
- Protects the patient from accidentally inhaling or ingesting small tooth or dental material fragments and other debris
- Protects the tooth from contamination of saliva or debris if accidental pulpal exposure occurs
- Protects the gingival tissues during acid-etching procedures
- Provides the highest level of moisture control
- Improves accessibility to the operating field during treatment by retracting oral tissues
- Provides better visibility because of the contrast between the color of the dam material and the tooth
- Increases dental team efficiency, discourages patient conversation, and may reduce time required for some treatment
- The color of the dental dam material and the isolation assists in shade selection when performing composite or crown/bridge procedures

Reasons for why dental dam isolation may not be performed include the existence of medical or physical conditions such as asthma, respiratory congestion, or oral conditions that may prevent dental clamp placement such as partially erupted teeth or severely misaligned teeth.

Expanded functions dental assistants can efficiently place a dental dam in about three to five minutes by themselves after the dentist has administered the local anesthetic. When working together as a team, the dentist and dental assistant can successfully place the dam in approximately two minutes.

An 8-year-old patient who needs sealants placed on teeth #3, #14, #19, and #30 has been seated in your operatory. Which isolation technique should be utilized during the sealant placement procedure? Why?

The Dental Dam

As noted, the dental dam provides not only moisture control during operative clinical dentistry but also serves as an important infection control protective barrier. The dental dam eliminates exposure to the patient's oral mucosa and saliva. It also helps to reduce the amount of aerosol and spatter created by the contact of the water spray emitted from the high-speed handpiece and the patient's saliva and oral tissues. If not isolated, the spatter created by the use of the high-speed handpiece can become a contaminated airborne aerosol.

Determinants for the type of dental dam chosen include size, color, and thickness (Figure 26.15). Oper-

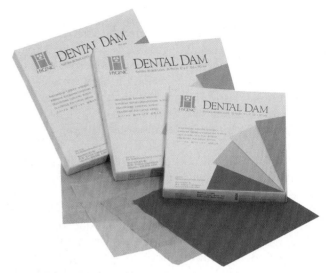

FIGURE 26.15
Dental dam material.
Courtesy Coltene Whaledent

ators generally choose either a latex or latex-free material based on personal preference. The two size varieties include a continuous roll or precut rolls. When using the continuous roll variety, clinicians will dispense the material to the desired length before cutting the material for use. Precut rolls come in various sizes. The 6- × 6-inch size is generally utilized for posterior teeth in the permanent dentition. The 5- × 5-inch size is used for teeth within the primary dentition or anterior teeth in the permanent dentition. Even though the dental dam material is available in a wide range of colors from light to dark, dentists generally prefer to use darker colors for contrast against the white tooth surface and for reduction of glare.

Dental dam gauges (thickness) range from thin/light to medium and heavy. The type of procedure and the dentist preference dictate which gauge is chosen. Endodontists prefer the thin gauges for endodontic procedures because only a single tooth is isolated at a time during endodontic procedures and tearing is less of a problem. The most frequently used thickness for most dental procedures is medium because of its ease of handling and ability to isolate selected teeth. Heavy gauges are chosen when tissue retraction and extra resistance to tearing are important. A heavy-gauge dental dam may be required when working with teeth that have tight contacts or when working with crowns and fixed bridges.

Due to the temperature sensitivity of the latex and latex-free dental dam material, the shelf life of the material can be extended if it is stored in a refrigerator. Dental dam material is also available in flavors such as grape, berry, or mint. The flavored material can facilitate a more positive patient experience and patient compliance with the use of the dental dam.

Dental Dam Frame

The dental dam frame is fabricated of either a durable plastic material or metal (Figure 26.16). The dental dam is stretched and secured around the frame so that it fits tightly around the teeth and is out of the operator's field of operation. Plastic and metal frames are autoclaved in between each patient use.

The Young frame is a stainless steel U-shaped holder with a sharp projection on its outer margin. The Young frame is placed on the outside of the dental dam material (away from the patient's face) and the dam is stretched over the projections of the frame. This technique increases patient comfort because the dam is stretched away from the patient's face. When using the metal Young frame, it is important to remember that the frame will need to be removed prior to exposing any radiographs. This ensures that no metal artifacts appear on the radiograph. When using the plastic U-shaped frame, it is placed under the dam (next to the patient's face). The dam is stretched over the projections, which secures the dam in place and out of the operator's way. Use of the plastic frame is beneficial because the frame is radiolucent and does not need to be removed when radiographs need to be exposed during treatment.

The Ostby frame is a round plastic frame with sharp projections on its outer margin. The Ostby frame is designed so that the frame follows the shape and contour of the lower facial region. The dam material is stretched around the outside of the Ostby frame (away from the patient's face) and secured over the projections.

Dental Dam Napkin

The dental dam napkin is a disposable cloth made from soft, absorbent fabric that is placed between the patient's face and dental dam material (Figure 26.17). The main purpose of the napkin is to absorb any moisture that may accumulate between the material and the patient's face such as saliva, water, or perspiration. The napkin increases patient comfort by protecting the patient's face from contact with the dental dam, reducing the risk of any sensitivity related to the material.

Dental Dam Lubricants

Dental dam lubricants are utilized for two purposes: for patient comfort and to facilitate easier manipulation of the dam material. Zinc oxide ointment or petroleum jelly is generally the lubricant chosen by clinicians. Another type of lubricant is a water-soluble lubricant that is placed on the underside (the side next to the teeth) of the dam material. It is important to note that petroleum jelly should **not** be used for this purpose because it can interfere with the curing of certain dental materials and can cause the integrity of the latex dam material and latex gloves to fail.

Dental Dam Stamp and Template

The dental dam stamp and inkpad are used to mark the dental dam with predetermined markings for the average adult and pediatric size arches (Figure 26.18). A dental dam template, which has holes placed where the teeth

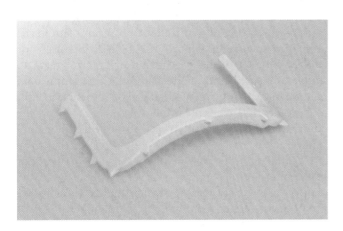

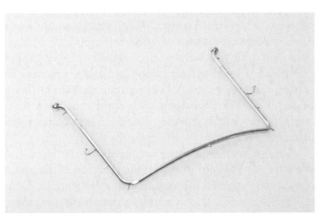

FIGURE 26.16
Plastic and metal dental dam frames.
Courtesy Coltene Whaledent

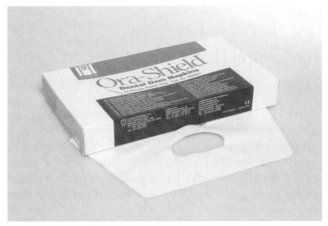

FIGURE 26.17
Dental dam napkin.
Courtesy Coltene Whaledent

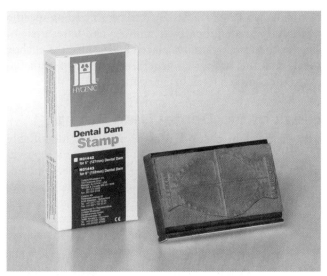

FIGURE 26.18
Dental dam stamp.
Courtesy Coltène Whaledent

should be marked, is utilized as a guide when marking the dental dam material. The template is placed on the dental dam, and a pen is used to mark through the holes of the template and onto the dam material to indicate the position and location of the desired hole(s) to be punched. When using the dental dam stamp, the rubber stamp is "inked" before stamping (marking) the dental dam material. The clinician utilizes the stamped image for punching the desired holes. Clinicians may become proficient in punching the desired holes without having to use the template or the stamp.

Dental Dam Punch

The dental dam punch is similar to a paper punch and is used to create holes in the dental dam material (Figure 26.19). The working end of the punch has an adjustable

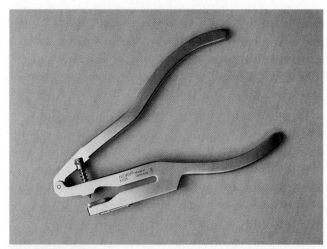

FIGURE 26.19
Dental dam punch.
Courtesy Heraeus Kulzer, Inc.

stylus (cutting tip) that creates the hole as it strikes an opening in the punch plate. The punch plate is a rotary platform with five or six different sized holes. The different sizes of the holes within the face of the punch plate are utilized to create openings within the dental dam material. The holes of the punch plate are approximately 1 mm deep with sharp edges to accommodate the stylus and assist in cutting the material.

The punch plate is rotated according to the size choice corresponding with the teeth to be exposed. Accommodation of the different size teeth determines which hole is selected on the punch plate. The holes on the punch plate are graduated in size and are numbered 1 to 5, with 1 being the smallest size. Each size has a specific recommended use (Table 26-2). Most maxillary molars and the anchor tooth utilize the number 5 hole. The number 4 hole is typically used for mandibular molars. Canines and premolars utilize the number 3 hole. Maxillary incisors need hole number 2 punched, and mandibular incisors utilize hole number 1. Generally mandibular anterior teeth need the smallest hole and maxillary molars need the largest hole.

When the punch plate is rotated, a clicking sound may be heard as the plate falls into position. The click indicates that the stylus is positioned directly over the corresponding hole in the punch plate. It is important to position the stylus directly in line with the holes in the punch plate to prevent the stylus point from becoming dull. When punching the hole within the dental dam material, it is important to carefully inspect the material to ensure that the hole has been punched cleanly without any ragged edges. Material with ragged edges should be discarded because it may tear when the dam is being placed over the crown of a tooth. In addition, material with ragged edges may also irritate the gingiva and allow moisture to leak through the material and contaminate the working field. The anchor tooth holds the dental dam clamp. The key punch hole is punched in the dental dam to cover the clamp and the anchor tooth. The larger, size 5 hole should be utilized when punching for the anchor tooth.

TABLE 26-2 Hole Selection for the Punch Plate

Hole Number	Teeth
1	Mandibular incisors
2	Maxillary incisors
3	Maxillary and mandibular premolars and canines
4	Mandibular molars
5	Maxillary molars and anchor tooth

Dental Dam Forceps

Dental dam forceps (Figure 26.20) are utilized during the placement and removal of the dental dam clamp, which is discussed in the following section. The beaks of the forceps fit into the guide holes on the jaws of the dental dam clamp (Figure 26.21). Once the beaks are securely in the holes, pressure is applied to the handle of the forceps and the clamp jaws are opened slightly.

The handles of the forceps work with a spring action. A sliding bar can be utilized to keep the handles of the forceps in a fixed position while the clamp is being held and positioned on the tooth. The handles are then squeezed to release the clamp. The beaks are positioned so that they are directed toward the arch being treated. This permits the operator to place or remove the clamp without having to rotate the forceps into position.

Dental Dam Clamps

The dental dam clamp is the primary means of anchoring and stabilizing the dental dam around the tooth (Figure 26.22). The clamps are made of chrome or nickel-plated steel and are designed to hold the dental dam secure.

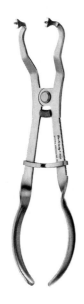

FIGURE 26.20
Dental dam forceps.
Courtesy Hu-Friedy

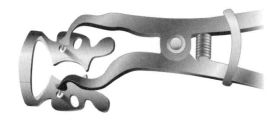

FIGURE 26.21
Correct positioning of the dental dam forceps beaks into the dental dam clamp.

Dental dam clamps are designed to be utilized on specific teeth and are identified by a number and letter system. The tooth that the clamp is placed on is called the anchor tooth. The anchor tooth is generally one or two teeth distal to the tooth or teeth being restored.

Parts of the Dental Dam Clamp

The dental dam clamp has two important identifiable parts that are utilized during the placement and removal of the clamp (Figure 26.23). The bow is the rounded, arched portion of the clamp. This portion is generally placed toward the distal aspect of the tooth and extends through the dental dam when the dam is placed on the tooth prior to treatment. The jaws of the clamp encircle the tooth and are shaped into four prongs. It is important that all four prongs be seated firmly around the gingival and one-third of the tooth to ensure balance and support for the dental dam. The jaws of the clamps are supplied in different sizes for utilization with different teeth within the arch. A hole is located on each side of the jaw of the clamp where the beaks of the dental dam forceps are positioned during placement and removal.

The jaws of the clamp are designed to be winged or wingless. A winged clamp is designed with extra extensions for better retraction. Because the wings are angled toward the gingiva, this type of clamp helps to retain the dental dam. Wingless clamps are identified with names beginning with the letter "W." Wingless clamps do **not** have the extra extensions to assist in retaining the dental dam and are identified with the number of the clamp only.

Some clamps are double bowed. These clamps are called cervical clamps, or butterfly clamps. Cervical clamps are used for Class 5 restorations on anterior teeth and assist with gingival retraction.

Placement of the Dental Dam Clamp

When selecting the clamp, the tooth to be clamped must be evaluated. The mesiodistal width at the cemento-enamel junction (CEJ) of the tooth determines the type and size of clamp to best utilize. The width between the points of the jaws on the clamp should be about the same as the width of the tooth. Proper fit ensures that the points of the jaws are resting securely and safely all around the CEJ of the tooth. Clamps that are too large are inadequate for the needed stabilization. Clamps that are too small are unable to fit across the height of contour of the tooth (the widest point on the facial and lingual aspects of the tooth).

As noted earlier, dental dam clamps are available in many sizes, shapes, and designs that are used to accommodate the different sizes and shapes of teeth within the oral cavity. The jaws of the clamps are designed to fit on the cervical area of the tooth below the height of contour and at, or slightly below, the CEJ. To place the clamp, the jaws are opened wide enough to clear the height of contour. The jaws are then closed slowly on the tooth to fit

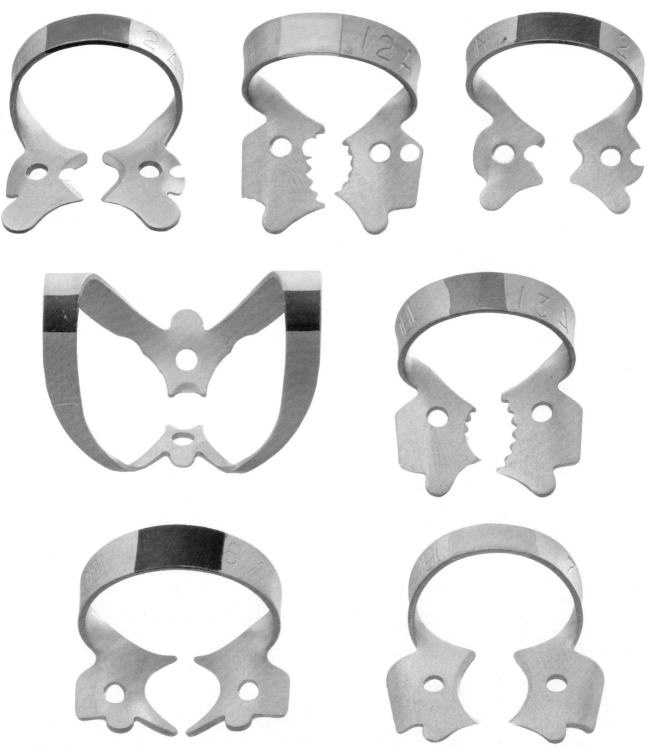

FIGURE 26.22
Various dental dam clamps.
Courtesy Coltene Whaledent

tightly at the CEJ. The clamp must be positioned with all four prongs firmly in place on the tooth before the clamp forceps are removed. If the clamp is not placed properly, it may spring off the tooth and could possibly injure the patient, dentist, or assistant (Figure 26.24). Table 26-3 lists the steps involved in placement of the dental dam clamp.

Posterior dental dam clamps are used on the maxillary and mandibular posterior teeth. These clamps are universal, meaning the same clamp can be placed on the same type of tooth in the opposite quadrant. Anterior dental dam clamps are designed to retract the gingiva on the facial surface, improve visibility for the restoration of cervical Class V restorations, and permit isolation of an

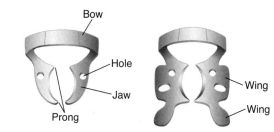

FIGURE 26.23
Parts of the dental dam clamp.

FIGURE 26.24
Placement of the dental dam clamp.

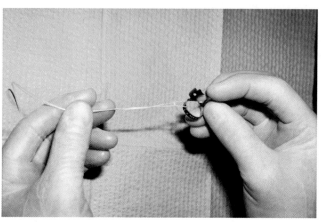

FIGURE 26.25
Ligature tied on a dental dam clamp.
Image courtesy Instructional Materials for the Dental Team, Lex., KY

anterior tooth during endodontic treatment. Pediatric dental dam clamps are utilized for primary teeth and are designed to accommodate the smaller size and shape of primary teeth or partially erupted permanent teeth.

Dental floss or dental tape should always be attached to the bow of the dental dam clamp as a ligature before the clamp is placed in the patient's mouth. This is an important safety step that must not be omitted. The ligature makes it possible to retrieve a clamp should it accidentally become dislodged and then inhaled or swallowed by the patient (Figure 26.25). An 18-inch section of floss is utilized as the ligature. The floss is tied into a slip knot and placed around the clamp. The ends of this ligature are always kept out of the patient's mouth on the outside

of the dental dam material and within easy reach. During treatment, the ligature may be attached to the dam frame to keep it available yet out of the operator's way.

A patient asks you why you are placing dental floss on a dental dam clamp. How would you communicate to the patient the importance of this safety feature? **?**

Dental Dam Stabilizing Cord

The dental dam stabilizing cord is a disposable latex cord that is an alternative to the conventional clamp method of securing the dental dam. The cord is available in three sizes: extra small, small, and large. During insertion, the cord is stretched so that it becomes narrow and then placed interproximally to secure the dental dam material. The cord is used to stabilize the dental dam placement at the opposite end of the clamp or for individual teeth. Once placed and released, the cord resumes its original shape and holds the dam tightly in place. The size of the cord selected depends on the amount of contact space available. The length of the cord depends on the application.

🤝 Professionalism

Patients expect the atmosphere and environment of the dental operatory to reflect a clean, germ-free, sterile quality. It is important that dental personnel mirror the same fresh appearance. To accomplish this, dental assistants should be neatly groomed, which includes a clean and neatly pressed uniform, clean and scuff-free shoes, well-groomed hair, neatly groomed fingernails, makeup that is kept to a minimum, and no jewelry or jewelry that is limited to post earrings only. A well-groomed dental assistant promotes a sense of trust and faith in his or her skills.

TABLE 26-3 Steps for Clamp Placement

1. Determine the anchor tooth and select the appropriate clamp.
2. Tie the floss ligature around the bow of the clamp to permit retrieval if the clamp slips off the tooth.
3. Place the clamp on the dental dam forceps.
4. Squeeze the handles together to open the jaws of the clamp.
5. With the tips of the forceps upward, the locking ring will slide toward the handle of the forceps, holding the jaws of the clamp open.
6. Position the clamp over the tooth.
7. Rotate it lingually to seat the lingual jaw first because vision is more restricted in this area.
8. Rotate the clamp facially to seat the facial jaw. Be certain that the jaws do not drag across the tooth.
9. Squeeze the handles of the forceps to release the locking ring and allow the jaws of the clamp to engage the tooth.

Dental Dam Placement and Removal

Before the dental dam is stamped and punched, the area to be isolated needs to be determined and then examined. Usually, the tooth or two teeth distal to the tooth being restored are chosen as the anchor teeth. The number of teeth to be included in the punch is a personal preference. Some operators like only one or two teeth to be exposed, while others prefer more. To determine the number of teeth to be included in the punch, the operator examines the dimension and shape of the arch. This is to ensure that all aspects of the patient's oral size, anatomy, and prosthetics are duplicated on the dental dam as closely as possible.

After determining which arch is to be treated, the dam is stamped with the dental dam stamp or marked utilizing the dental dam template. The holes are punched according to the tooth being treated and the operator's preference. When punching the holes, it may be necessary to make adjustments to accommodate an extremely narrow or wide arch. Failure to do this will increase the difficulty with inversion of the edges of the holes in the dam. Accommodations may also be necessary for misaligned teeth. If the tooth is lingually malpositioned, the hole-punch size remains the same, but the hole is placed about 1 mm lingually from the natural arch alignment. If the tooth is facially malpositioned, the hole-punch size remains the same, but the hole is placed about 1 mm facially from the normal arch alignment.

Even though there are many places to begin punching the dental dam, usually the key hole punch is punched first. The key punch hole is the largest hole punched in the dental dam. It is the hole that slides over the clamp and onto the anchor tooth. The next holes are punched moving forward, about 3 to 3.5 mm apart. This portion of the dental dam is called the septum and is the portion of the dental dam that fits interproximally between the teeth. The hole spacing should match the space between the patient's teeth. If the holes are too close together, there will not be enough material to seal around each tooth. The dam material will be stretched and the gingival tissue will be exposed to moisture contamination. If the holes are too far apart, there will be excess material between the teeth and the seal will be inadequate. This excess material can get in the operator's way during the procedure. The curve of the arch on the dental dam material should match the curvature of the patient's maxillary or mandibular arch.

Adjustments must be made when punching for patients who have missing or misaligned teeth. Punching for these patients is accomplished by the operator following the patterns of the teeth present in the patient's mouth. Buccal or lingually malpositioned teeth should have holes punched within the dental material either buccal or lingual to the normal alignment pattern. When preparing the dental dam for patients who have missing teeth or edentulous areas, the operator accommodates these areas by leaving space(s) for any of the corresponding missing teeth. For example, if tooth #13 is missing, then a hole would be punched for tooth #12, a space would be skipped for tooth #13, and holes would be punched for teeth #14 and #15.

Dental floss or a plastic filling instrument (PFI) can be used to invert or tuck the edge of the dental dam around the tooth to assist in preventing moisture leakage. Some options of instruments to use include a periodontal probe, spoon excavator, or the flat side of the T-ball burnisher.

Single-tooth isolation is typically used for selected restorative procedures and for endodontic treatments. When isolating two teeth, the second tooth acts as an anchor tooth to hold the clamp. During treatment in the posterior area, this second tooth provides more stability and better visibility. When using multiple tooth isolation, three or four teeth are generally exposed. Generally at least one tooth posterior to the tooth being treated should be isolated (usually the anchor tooth). When maxillary anterior teeth are to be isolated, maximum stability is achieved by isolating the six anterior teeth (canine to canine).

The treatment plan for your patient indicates that endodontic therapy is to be performed on tooth #3. Which dental dam frame would you choose for the dental dam application? Why?

?

There are two methods of dental dam placement. The main differences between the two are the sequencing in the type and placement of the clamp and dental dam. In the one-step method, described in Table 26-4, the dam and a winged clamp are placed at the same time. In the two-step method, first the wingless clamp is placed, and then the dental dam material is stretched

---

TABLE 26-4 The One-Step Dental Dam Placement Procedure

A winged clamp is usually selected for this technique, and the ligature is secured on the bow of the clamp. The bow of the clamp and the forceps holes on the jaws are exposed through the dental dam material. The clamp forceps are placed in the forceps holes and secured. The operator holds the rest of the dam material up and out of the way while placing the clamp and dam on the anchor tooth. After the clamp is secured on the tooth, the wings of the clamp are exposed and placement is completed following the procedure steps. This technique requires less time for placement, yet requires more confidence and practice to master the technique.

Procedure 26-4 Placing a Dental Dam

Equipment and Supplies Needed

- Dental dam stamp or template
- Dental dam material
- Dental dam frame
- Clamp with ligature
- Dental dam punch
- Dental dam forceps
- Dental dam lubricant
- Dental floss

Procedure Steps

1. Following the administration of the local anesthetic, explain the procedure to the patient.

2. Determine which teeth are to be isolated. Examine the patient's oral cavity to determine the anchor tooth, shape of the arch, tooth alignment, missing teeth, and the presence of crowns and bridges.

3. Stamp the rubber dam material with the rubber dam stamp or mark the desired position if using the dental dam template.

4. Use the dental dam punch to punch the holes in the rubber dam. Punch the holes according to the size of the tooth to be restored with the key punch hole being the largest to accommodate the anchor tooth and the clamp.

5. Select the clamp or several clamps to try on the tooth. Clamp design (winged or wingless) and the mesiodistal and faciolingual width of the CEJ should be considered.

6. After choosing the appropriate clamp for the desired tooth, place the floss or waxed tape ligature on the bow of the desired dental dam clamp.

7. Place the clamp on the beaks of the dental dam forceps and lock the forceps into the open position by spreading the jaws of the forceps open.

8. Position the clamp securely on the anchor tooth (one tooth just distal to the tooth being treated). To open the jaws of the clamp, gently squeeze the forceps handle to release the locking bar.

9. Fit the lingual jaws of the clamp on the lingual side of the tooth first. Next, spread the clamp open slightly to fit the buccal jaws of the clamp over the height of contour and fit the buccal jaws onto the buccal side of the tooth. Release the pressure on the clamp but do not release the clamp from the forceps.

10. Check the status of the clamp on the anchor tooth. The jaw points should be placed securely at the CEJ and should not be pinching any gingival tissues. If adjustments are needed, move the wrist to the left and right and by putting more pressure on the distal or mesial of the clamp.

11. Apply the rubber dam lubricant to the underside of the dental dam material.

12. Place the dental dam over the clamp bow by grasping the dam material and placing the index fingers on each side of the key hole punch. Spread the hole wide enough to slip over the clamp. Stretch the hole over the anchor tooth and one side of the clamp, then expose the other clamp jaw so that the entire clamp and anchor tooth are exposed.

13. Pull the dental floss ligature through the dam and drape to the side of the patient's face.

14. Place the dental dam napkin around the patient's mouth and underneath the dental dam material.

15. Stretch the rubber dam material around the projections of the dental dam frame. The frame can be placed either under or over the dental dam material depending on the choice of frame and operator preference.

16. Continue to expose the remaining teeth through each punched hole.

17. Using dental floss, work the dental dam gently between the contacts and below the proximal contacts of each tooth to be isolated.

18. Invert or tuck the dam material until all edges of the dam are sealed.

19. To increase patient comfort, place a saliva ejector under the frame, dam material, and the patient's tongue.

---

over it (see Procedure 26-4). Table 26-5 lists the criteria for determining when the dental dam has been placed correctly.

Regardless of the technique utilized with the placement and removal of the dental dam, dental assistants must be aware of their individual state's practice act with regard to dental dam procedures. Dental assistants assist the dentist in the placement and removal procedures in states where it is not legal for them to place the dental

dam themselves. In states where dental assistants can place the dental dam, the assistants punch the dam, select the clamp, and place and remove the dental dam without the chairside presence of the dentist.

One alternative to the two traditional methods of dental dam placement is the split-dam technique. When utilizing the split-dam technique, the dental dam is secured by stretching a small piece of stabilizing cord through the mesial and distal contacts of the tooth being

TABLE 26-5 Criteria for Clinically Acceptable Dental Dam Placement

- Ligature is placed and visible outside of the oral cavity.
- Dental dam clamp is placed in the correct stable position on the tooth.
- Holes are punched correctly within the dental dam material.
- Anchor tooth is visible through the most distal punched hole.
- Dental dam material is placed without folds or creases.
- Dental dam material is completely inverted around each tooth.
- The oral cavity is free of any soft tissue trauma.
- The dental dam napkin is placed beneath the dental dam material.
- Saliva ejector is in position.

Legal and Ethical Issues

Dental practice acts vary from state to state. Some states require that training, education, and/or certification be completed before direct patient care can be performed by a dental assistant. It is important to remember that a dental assistant may only perform the functions that have been officially delegated to him or her under the dental practice act of the state where the dental assistant is employed. All dental assistants should be adamant about performing only legal functions when complying with dentists' requests when treating patients.

prepared. The disposable latex stabilizing cord is utilized as an alternative to the conventional dental dam clamp and is available in three sizes: extra small, small, and large. The cord is stretched so that it becomes smaller and easily slips between the proximal contacts of the isolated tooth. Once released, the cord resumes its original shape and maintains the placement of the dental dam material.

When removing the dental dam, the HVE should be used to remove all debris from the operating field. To facilitate removal, the dam should be stretched to the facial side, away from the teeth. The operator should place one finger under the stretched material to protect the patient's lips and cheeks while the septum area of the material is cut with the crown and bridge scissors. The

operator should cut the entire septum with one stroke to prevent the material from tearing (see Procedure 26.5).

Which isolation procedure provides the highest level of moisture control? Which isolation procedure is most commonly used by dentists and why?

The Quick Dam

The quick dam is an alternative to full dental dam placement. It is an oval piece of dental dam that has a border of flexible plastic and comes with its own template to mark each tooth (Figure 26.26). Holes are punched in the quick dam material utilizing the same dental dam punch

Procedure 26-5 Removing a Dental Dam

Additional Materials Needed

- In addition to the materials already present for the procedure of placing the dental dam (Procedure 26-4), crown and bridge scissors are required for removal.

Procedure Steps

Following the completion of the restorative procedure, these steps should be performed to facilitate the removal of the dental dam:

1. Explain the procedure to the patient and instruct the patient not to bite down once the dam is removed.

2. Stretch the material facially so that you are stretching the material away from the isolated teeth.

3. Working from posterior to anterior, cut each septum (the area of the dam in between each tooth) with the crown and bridge scissors. To protect the patient, slip the index or middle finger underneath the dam material.

4. Using the dental dam forceps, position the beaks in the holes of the clamp, and open the clamp by squeezing the handle to remove the clamp. Usually, the clamp can be lifted straight off the tooth, but if this is not possible, rotate the clamp facially so the jaws clear the lingual and then rotate the clamp lingually to clear the buccal.

5. Remove the dam, the frame, and the dental dam napkin from the patient's face.

6. Carefully inspect the material to ensure that all pieces are intact. Lay the dental dam material flat and examine to make certain that all the interseptal material is present. If there are any pieces missing, floss interproximally. This should dislodge any missing segment of the dam material.

7. Massage the gingival around the anchor tooth to increase circulation of the area.

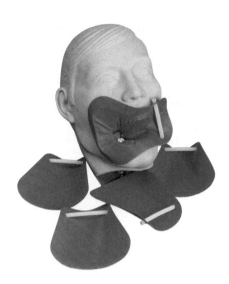

FIGURE 26.26
Alternative to full dental dam placement.
Courtesy Aseptico, Inc.

that is used for the traditional dental dam. After the dam is punched, the dam frame is folded and inserted into the patient's mouth, lying in the vestibular area. A ligature or dental dam clamp may be needed to fully secure the dam in some clinical situations. For placement of the quick dam see Procedure 26-6.

It is important to remember that utilizing the dental dam is essential when excessive saliva flow and an overactive tongue make retraction and consistent maintenance of a dry, clean field impossible. However, the use of a dental dam may not be possible when a tooth that is vital for securing the clamp is missing or not fully erupted.

Patient preparation before implementing the dental dam procedure is imperative. If the patient has never experienced placement of a rubber dam, the clinician should explain the benefits, such as elimination of debris in the mouth and prevention of a contaminated restorative site. Because the patient will not be able to talk with the dam in place, the clinician may suggest signals to be used if the patient should need to communicate.

Special Applications of the Dental Dam

When the dam is to be applied for anterior teeth, the isolation and application procedures change. The isolation of anterior teeth is typically from canine to canine. When isolating the anterior teeth, a dental dam clamp is not required to stabilize the material. However, if one-third of a tooth is being restored, an anterior clamp may be required to retract gingival tissue.

Procedure 26-6 Placing a Quick Dam

Equipment and Supplies Needed

• Quick dam
• Quick dam template
• Dental dam punch
• Dental dam clamps
• Dental dam forceps
• Dental floss
• Tucking instrument

Procedure Steps

1. Examine the patient's dentition to determine the punch pattern. Make note of any misaligned or missing teeth.

2. Use the quick dam template to mark each tooth to be punched and allow for any deviations. Place mark in desired position.

3. Punch the marked teeth according to the corresponding hole size for each tooth.

The quick dam can be used with or without a dental dam clamp.

4. Without a clamp, fold the ends of the quick dam toward each other and press the sides together.

5. Insert the quick dam into the patient's mouth and release the sides. The quick dam fits into the patient's vestibule.

6. Slide the dam over the teeth to be isolated. Use dental floss to tuck the dental dam, and secure the dam with floss ligatures on the distal of the last isolated teeth.

7. Select a clamp and attach a ligature to the bow of the clamp.

8. Secure the clamp in the hole punched for the tooth to be clamped.

9. Apply the clamp forceps, and place the clamp over the tooth.

10. Once the clamp is securely on the tooth, remove the clamp forceps.

11. Place the dam over the teeth to be isolated and tuck the dam.

When utilizing the dental dam in an area where a fixed bridge has been cemented, a hole is not required to be punched for the pontic (fake) tooth within the fixed bridge structure. Holes are punched for the abutments, and spaces are left for the number of pontics present. Slits are cut between the holes with the crown and bridge scissors to allow the bridge to be exposed.

The advantage of the use of the dental dam on pediatric patients becomes important when trying to control the busy tongue and lips of a child. When utilizing the dental dam on children, the basic technique followed is the same as that for adult patients with few modifications. However, one important modification is that a detailed explanation using terminology and language that the child understands should be routine when preparing to place the dental dam on children. This communication can alleviate any fear or anxiety the child may experience. In addition, the dental dam holes are generally punched closer together for children and no holes are punched where teeth are missing or partially erupted.

Why should dental assistants be aware of the state dental practice acts governing the states where they work?

SUMMARY

Moisture control is an integral part of the operative dental procedure. The isolation of a tooth or teeth, the retraction of tissue, and the maintenance of a clean, dry working environment are some of the most important responsibilities a chairside dental assistant performs.

The type of isolation required depends on the duration of the procedure and the degree of dryness necessary. For some procedures, cotton roll isolation and the use of the HVE and saliva ejector may be sufficient. Cotton roll holders may be utilized if additional retraction is required on the mandibular arch. Absorbent dry angles placed over the Stensen's duct of the parotid gland can also be utilized as an adjunct to cotton roll isolation for increased moisture control. This type of isolation offers ease and speed of application. However, risks include contamination of the operating field and limited retraction of soft tissues.

When increased moisture control, retraction, and isolation are required, the dental dam should be utilized.

Regardless of the choice of moisture control procedure, it is imperative that the chairside dental assistant be proficient in maintaining a clear, dry working field. This ensures that the dentist has enhanced visibility for the successful treatment of the operative procedure and enhances patient comfort.

Cultural Considerations

It is important for a dental assistant to have a broad understanding of the cultural diversity of the patients that he or she may treat. The ability to communicate successfully with patients from varying backgrounds and cultural origins depends on the dental assistant using communication skills that encourage attention and cooperation from the patient. Verbal as well as nonverbal behaviors and tone, pitch, rate, and volume are important factors to use when communicating with culturally diverse populations.

KEY TERMS

- **Air/water syringe:** Device that is utilized to emit air, water, and a combination of both in a spray; also known as a *three-way syringe*. p. 396
- **Biofilm:** Microorganisms that accumulate on surfaces inside moist environments such as dental unit waterlines, allowing bacteria, fungi, and viruses to multiply, which can increase a patient's susceptibility to transmissible diseases. p. 396
- **Complete mouth rinse:** A rinse that is generally performed once all oral procedures have been completed; sometimes during long dental procedures, when the patient's entire mouth needs refreshing, a complete rinse may be performed. p. 398
- **Dental dam:** Thin latex or latex-free barrier used to isolate a specific tooth or teeth during treatment. p. 400

- **Dry angle:** Triangular-shaped, absorbent wafer-like pad used for moisture control. p. 400
- **High-volume evacuator (HVE):** Device used to remove saliva, blood, water, and debris from a patient's mouth. p. 390
- **Isolation:** Process of keeping the operative area or teeth separate and dry. p. 398
- **Limited area mouth rinse:** A rinse performed during a clinical procedure when the dentist pauses during treatment. p. 397
- **Oral evacuation:** Process of removing excess fluids, saliva, blood, or debris from the oral cavity during operative dental procedures. p. 390
- **Saliva ejector:** Device used to remove fluids such as small amounts of saliva or water from a patient's mouth; also known as a *low-volume evacuator*. p. 392

CHECK YOUR UNDERSTANDING

1. During the placement of a dental dam, a lubricant is used to
   a. retard the flow of saliva.
   b. help place the clamp on the anchor tooth.
   c. repair the material of a torn dam.
   d. make it easier for the dam to be slipped between the teeth.

2. Removal of the dental dam is accomplished by
   a. cutting the septum prior to removal.
   b. stretching the dam for more efficient removal.
   c. utilizing a quick snap of the material interproximally.
   d. stretching the dam material with the rubber dam forceps.
   e. both a and b.

3. A limited area rinse is one that
   a. is completed at the beginning of the procedure.
   b. is completed at the end of the procedure.
   c. is utilized to rinse the whole mouth.
   d. is utilized to rinse a specific area of the mouth.

4. Why is it important to thoroughly saturate a cotton roll or dry angle prior to removal from the oral cavity?
   a. The cotton roll or dry angle can interfere with the dental materials being used for the restorative procedure.
   b. The cotton roll or dry angle can interfere with the suction of the HVE.
   c. The cotton roll or dry angle can pull on the oral mucosa and cause irritation.
   d. All of the above.

5. The isolation technique that provides a barrier for the highest level of infection control is
   a. cotton rolls.
   b. dental dam.
   c. dry angle.
   d. high-volume evacuator.

6. Tying dental floss around the dental dam clamp
   a. ligates it more securely to the tooth.
   b. keeps the dental dam in place.
   c. prevents accidental swallowing of the clamp.
   d. is really not necessary.

7. Immediately following the removal of the dental dam, the dental assistant
   a. checks the material for missing pieces.
   b. discards the dam material immediately.
   c. sterilizes the dam material for reuse.
   d. all of the above.

8. The color of the dental dam material contrasts with the tooth structure to improve
   a. evacuation.
   b. retraction.
   c. suction.
   d. visibility.

9. Control of saliva from the parotid duct can be accomplished by placing a cotton roll
   a. on the lingual side of the mandibular arch, under the tongue.
   b. in the vestibule, opposite the maxillary second molar.
   c. in the vestibule, opposite the mandibular second molar.
   d. in the vestibule, opposite the maxillary anterior teeth.

10. Which of the following is utilized to increase patient comfort when placing a dental dam?
    a. forceps
    b. clamp
    c. frame
    d. napkin

INTERNET ACTIVITIES

- Go to www.mouthpower.org to view interactive activities on oral hygiene, nutrition, stages of tooth development and exfoliation, and the effects of tobacco on the oral cavity.

- Go to www.atlanticva.org/webandcamsites/dentalhealth.htm to access a variety of dental information and downloadable forms.

WEB REFERENCES

- American Dental Association: Dental Unit Waterlines www.ada.org/prof/resources/topics/waterlines/index.asp
- CDC Guidelines for Infection Control in Dental Health Care Settings www.cdc.gov/OralHealth/infectioncontrol/guidelines/infection_control_guidelines.ppt
- MMWR CDC Guidelines for Infection Control in Dental Health Care Setting www.cdc.gov/mmwr/preview/mmwrhtml/rr5217a1.htm
- Organization for Safety and Asepsis Procedures www.osap.org/displaycommon.cfm?an=1&subarticlebr=25

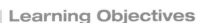

27

Pharmacology

Learning Objectives

After reading this chapter, the student should be able to:

- Define the terminology associated with pharmacology.
- Identify the difference between the chemical, generic, and trade names of drugs.
- Identify parts of a written prescription.
- Define the English meaning for Latin abbreviations used in prescriptions.
- Explain the purpose and use of drug reference materials.
- Explain how drugs are classified.
- Demonstrate an understanding of the drugs used in dentistry.

Preparing for Certification Exams

- Define the study of drugs, the differences in generic and brand names, and regulatory bodies concerned with drugs.
- Discuss drug effects on the human body and how the body processes drugs.
- Describe and explain the different parts of a prescription.
- List and explain the classification of drugs.

Key Terms

Analgesic

Drug interaction

Ethical drug

Generic name

Patent drugs

Pharmacokinetics

Pharmacology

Trade name

Chapter Outline

- Overview of Drugs
  - —Identification and Classification of Drugs
- Categories of Drugs
  - —Prescriptions
  - —Calls Regarding Patient Medications
- Drug Reference Materials
- Drug Administration
- Controlled Substances Act
- Classification of Drugs
- Antibiotic Prophylaxis
- Adverse Drug Effects

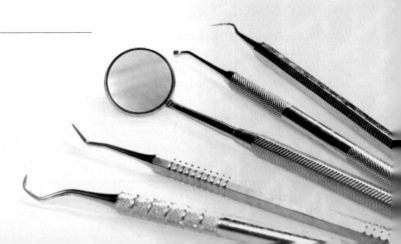

The study of drugs and their effects on the human body is called **pharmacology**. A drug is a substance that affects the function of living cells. Drugs are used for a variety of reasons including curing and/or preventing the occurrence of diseases and disorders and prolonging the life of patients with incurable conditions.

The Food and Drug Administration (FDA), the Drug Enforcement Administration (DEA), and the Federal Trade Commission (FTC) regulate drugs. Several excellent drug reference books and software are available that provide specific information about drugs and medical products such as the *Physicians' Desk Reference* (PDR), *The Pill Book, The Dental Therapeutic Digest*, and *Lexacom*. As a dental assistant it is important to know how to use drug reference books and be familiar with the names of medications and drugs that are used to treat the dental patient.

Overview of Drugs

A drug is defined as any substance used to diagnose, treat, or aid in preventing a disease or create a change to the body's chemical process. Medicines are drugs used in treating diseases. **Pharmacokinetics** is the study of how drugs enter the body, circulate throughout, and exit the body and also how circumstances and conditions can impact the effectiveness of drugs in the body.

The effect that is desired as a result of taking a drug is called the *therapeutic effect*. When a drug causes an unintentional result, the result is called a *side effect*. For

---

Dental Assistant PROFESSIONAL TIP

Endocarditis Prophylaxis Information

If a patient's medical history notes the presence of congenital heart disease, ensure that the patient has been issued a bacterial endocarditis wallet card. If the patient has not received the card from his or her physician, then take an extra step and educate the patient on the prevention of bacterial endocarditis and why endocarditis prophylaxis is important to the patient's dental care. Go to www.americanheart .org/downloadable/heart/1023826501754walletcard.pdf and print out this information to provide to the patient.

Legal and Ethical Issues

Most patients take medications prescribed to them without knowing much about the drugs. They just know that they have been told they need them for a specific problem. More and more patients, however, are taking a more active role in understanding the drugs they are being prescribed. Educating dental patients on what and why they are taking a prescribed medication is important for their health. For years, dentists have relied on drug reference materials such as the *Physicians' Desk Reference* for the latest, most accurate drug information. Now dental patients and their families can better understand their prescriptions through similar resources directed for the layperson such as *The Pill Book*, which is found in most drug stores and *PDRhealth* online at www.pdrhealth.com. Show the dental patient how to use and read about a drug the dentist has prescribed to better understand the potential side effects and interactions.

---

example, if a patient takes a cold medication to help with a runny nose and then experiences an upset stomach from the medicine, the upset stomach is considered a side effect of the cold medication. At times, a patient may need to take more than one drug at a time. If one or more of these drugs changes the effect, either by increasing or decreasing the effect of the other drug, this result is called a **drug interaction**.

Certain drugs can be addicting or habit forming for the patient. Addiction occurs when a person becomes physically dependent on a drug. When a person is physically dependent on a drug, he or she must continue to take the drug to avoid withdrawal symptoms. The person does not necessarily have to be physically dependent; some patients become emotionally and psychologically dependent on drugs, which is termed *habituation*.

Identification and Classification of Drugs

Drugs can be identified in many ways:

- How they are dispensed: over the counter or by prescription
- The substance from which they are derived: plant, mineral, or animal
- The form they take: capsule, liquid, or gas
- The way they are administered: internally (by mouth), rectally, parenterally by injection, inhalation, or direct application to the skin (absorption)

Drugs are classified by their names. All drugs have three names:

1. *Chemical name:* The chemical name describes the exact chemical structure of the drug.

2. *Generic name:* All drugs must have a registered U.S. patent name, which is its **generic name**. The generic name is considered to be a drug's "official" name and starts with a lowercase letter. Generic names are assigned in the United States by the U.S. Adopted Name Council, a group composed of pharmacists and other scientists.

3. *Trade name:* The **trade name** is the name given to a drug by the particular manufacturer that sells the drug. Trade names start with capital letters.

Drugs are also grouped according to other types of classifications, as discussed later in this chapter in the Classification of Drugs section.

What brand name drugs can you think of?

Categories of Drugs

There are two categories of drugs: patent and **ethical drugs. Patent drugs** are drugs that are referred to as over-the-counter (OTC) drugs and can be obtained without a prescription. Prescription drugs (ethical drugs) are any drugs that require a prescription. Prescription drugs always have an inscription on the label that records the name and quantity of the drug supplied. Federal law prohibits dispensing a prescription without a label. A patient taking these drugs must be under the care of the prescribing physician or dentist, and the prescription medications must be dispensed by a pharmacist.

What portion of the prescription includes the name of the drug?

Prescriptions

Prescriptions are a written authorization or an order for a drug. Only individuals such as dentists, physicians, and physician's assistants are legally allowed to write prescriptions. Only when a correctly written prescription is signed by a qualified individual can the pharmacist fill the medication order for the patient. At no time is a dental assistant allowed to prescribe medication or order medications by phone. All prescriptions issued to patients must be recorded in the patient's dental record. For all narcotic orders, the prescription must be written and handed to the patient, rather than being called into the pharmacist, and must contain the physician's DEA number.

By federal law all prescriptions must have the following parts and correct use of abbreviations:

• *Heading:* The heading includes the name, address, and telephone number of the dentist. The superscription includes the patient's name, address, telephone number, age, and the date of when the prescription is written.

• *Body:* The body is identified with the Rx symbol. Included in this area is the inscription, which lists the

name of the drug, dose, and concentration. The subscription tells the pharmacist the amount to be dispensed and the (Sig) that gives directions of how the patient is to take the medication.

• *Closing:* The closing includes the signature of the physician with refill instructions. The DEA number is included on each prescription. Depending on the state, the physician's license number may need to be included.

Figure 27.1 further details the parts of a prescription. Directions that are written on the prescription pad to the pharmacist are usually abbreviated, most often with Latin abbreviations. For example, "Sig: 1 stat 1 qid til gone" is read as "take one tablet now and one four times a day until all medication is completed." Table 27-1 lists some common abbreviations seen on prescriptions.

Calls Regarding Patient Medications

The pharmacist sometimes calls the office with questions regarding a patient's prescription, concerns about the patient's medical history, or to alert the dentist to possible interactions to drugs that a patient is taking. These calls to the office are typically handled by the dentist. If the dentist is not available, the dental assistant can take a detailed message and alert the dentist to the call as soon as possible.

In addition to calls from pharmacists, patients call the office concerning medications or reactions. When these types of phone calls occur, it is important to determine if the dentist needs to be involved. To determine dentist involvement, it is important that the dental assistant ask direct questions and acquire as much information as possible. Based on the acquired information, the dental assistant takes a message so that the dentist can return the call or determines that the dentist's immediate involvement is required. The dental assistant should never diagnose the patient's reaction to the drugs.

Drug Reference Materials

Drug reference materials contain up-to-date information concerning existing drugs or new drugs that have been FDA approved. These books are typically updated on a yearly basis. Every dental office has a few reference books. Some popular reference books include the PDR and other books mentioned earlier, as well as the *Drug Information Handbook for Dentistry*. Online versions of these books are also available for a quick search reference.

These references contain important information sections:

• *Interaction index:* Identifies drugs and foods capable of interfering with some medications.

• *Food interaction cross-reference:* Lists drugs that may interact with certain dietary items.

• *Side effects index:* Pinpoints adverse drug reactions.

Parts of a prescription

1. The dentist's name, telephone number, and registration number.

2. The patient's name, address, and the date on which the prescription is written.

3. The *subscription* that includes the symbol Rx ("take thou").

4. The inscription that states the names and quantities of ingredients to be included in the medication.

5. The subscription that gives directions to the pharmacist for filling the prescription.

6. The signature (Sig) that gives the directions for the patient.

7. The dentist's signature blanks. Where signed, indicates if a generic substitute is allowed or if the medication is to be dispensed as written.

8. REPETATUR 0 1 2 3 p.r.n. This is where the dentist indicates whether or not the prescription can be refilled.

9. ☐ LABEL Direction to the pharmacist to label the medication appropriately.

FIGURE 27.1
Physician's prescription pad with parts identified.

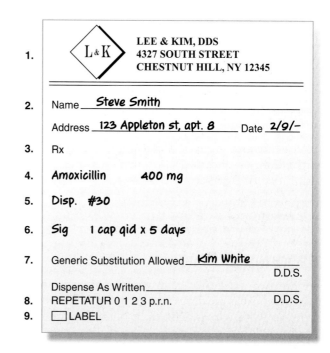

1. LEE & KIM, DDS
   4327 SOUTH STREET
   CHESTNUT HILL, NY 12345

2. Name   Steve Smith
   Address   123 Appleton st, apt. 8   Date 2/9/–

3. Rx

4. Amoxicillin   400 mg

5. Disp. #30

6. Sig   1 cap qid x 5 days

7. Generic Substitution Allowed   Kim White
                                               D.D.S.
   Dispense As Written
8. REPETATUR 0 1 2 3 p.r.n.   D.D.S.
9. ☐ LABEL

TABLE 27-1 Common Prescription Abbreviations

Abbreviation	Meaning
a.a.	of each
a.c.	before meals
a.m.	morning
b.i.d.	twice a day
disp.	dispense
h	hour
h.s.	at bedtime
NPO	nothing by mouth
p.c.	after meals
p.r.n.	as needed
q.	every
q.h.	every hour
q.i.d.	four times a day
q.4.h.	every four hours
q.8.h.	every 8 hours
Sig	take
t.i.d.	three times a day
t, tsp	teaspoon
T, tbs	tablespoon

- *Indications index:* Provides a full range of options for any given diagnosis.
- *Contraindications index:* Lists drugs to avoid when certain medical conditions are present.
- *Generic availability guide:* Shows which forms and strengths of brand name drugs may be available in generic form.

These sections will vary between reference materials. These drug reference materials are typically formatted as *drug monographs*. A monograph provides a description of the drug name, chemical formula, and uniform method for determining the strength and purity of a drug. Some monographs contain the following: generic name, pronunciation, cross-references, dental use, use restrictions, dosage, pregnancy risk factors, and many of the references that may pertain to the drug.

In addition to the drug reference books, many drug reference software programs can be downloaded for use. The Internet also provides a great deal of information and can be utilized as a resource. It is important, though, to be selective and to choose sites that are reputable and credible. For instance, the following website offers credible drug reference information: www.rxlist.com.

Drug Administration

Drugs are administered to patients in a variety of ways. The way a drug is taken depends on how fast or slow the drug will take effect. All doses depend on the size and weight of the patient, the strength and amount of the drug the patient is prescribed to take (also known as the dose), along with how the patient's body system will consume and transform the medication. Once the drug enters the body, the drug undergoes four stages:

1. *Absorption:* The drug is absorbed from the area where the drug is administered. How fast or slow the drug is absorbed into the body systems depends on the method of administration; for example, orally is the slowest method.
2. *Distribution:* When a drug enters the patient's bloodstream, the drug attaches to proteins in the blood and then is released and takes effect as the blood circulates throughout the body.
3. *Metabolism:* Once the drug is released, the drug transforms and is then processed through the liver and kidneys.
4. *Excretion:* The drug leaves the patient's body through the liver, kidneys, saliva, and sweat.

The dentist must determine the drug administration method that will be of most benefit to the patient. The most common routes of administration include:

1. *Oral* (by mouth)
2. *Sublingual* (under the tongue)
3. *Parenteral* (through injection)
4. *Topically* (through tissue)

Other routes, including rectal, inhalation, and vaginal, may be used depending on the type of drug used and its rate of absorption.

Controlled Substances Act

Certain drugs, depending on their potential for addiction and abuse, are controlled by the Controlled Substances Act (CSA). This act was established as the legal foundation for dealing with issues related to abuse of drugs and other substances. This law is a consolidation of numerous laws regulating the manufacture and distribution of narcotics, stimulants, depressants, hallucinogens, anabolic steroids, and chemicals used in the illicit production of controlled substances.

The CSA places all substances that are regulated under existing federal law into one of five schedules, as listed in Table 27-2. This placement is based on the substance's medicinal value, harmfulness, and potential for abuse or addiction. Schedule I is reserved for the most dangerous drugs that have no recognized medical use, whereas Schedule V is the classification used for the least dangerous drugs. Schedule V drugs are available over the counter.

Classification of Drugs

In addition to the classifications discussed earlier in the chapter, drugs are also classified according to chemical content, drug manufacturer, purpose, and effects on the body. A large variety of OTC drugs are available to the dental patient. The dental assistant needs to be familiar with the classifications of drugs in order to understand information presented in a patient chart, to assist with premedicated patients during dental treatment, to assist in dental treatments and pain control, and to aid in

Preparing for Externship

Unfortunately, the use of street drugs has increased during the past few years, making it extremely important to be able to identify signs and symptoms of drug abuse from your patients. Even while on your externship be sure and alert the doctor of any suspicious behavior from patients. Remember to allow the doctor to handle any conversation with the patient regarding potential drug use or abuse.

TABLE 27-2 Schedules of Controlled Substances Act 1970

Schedule	Schedule Drug Description	Abuse	Examples
I	Have no current accepted or medical use. Prescriptions are not usually written for these drugs.	High potential	Heroin, LSD, marijuana, hallucinogenics, depressants, and stimulants
II	Does have acceptable medical use. Requires a written prescription that cannot be renewed or refilled. These drugs can lead to addiction.	High potential	Morphine, opium and opium derivatives, methadone, amphetamines
III	Does have acceptable medical use. Requires a written prescription and can be renewed or refilled. Routinely used in dental offices.	Moderate potential	Stimulants and sedatives combined with brand name drugs such as Tylenol and Motrin (i.e., Tylenol III, Lortab V, Vicodin)
IV	Does have acceptable medical use. Requires a written prescription and can be renewed or refilled. Routinely used in dental offices.	Low potential	Valium, Darvon, Librium
V	Mixtures with limited opiates.	Least potential	Cough syrups, some OTC drugs

medical emergencies as required. Table 27-3 presents a list of drug classifications.

Tobacco, alcohol, and caffeine are drugs that can interact and cause adverse reactions to prescribed drugs. Tobacco and caffeine are habit-forming stimulants. Alcohol is a habit-forming depressant. Not all patients are truthful concerning their use of tobacco, alcohol, and caffeine. It is important for the patient to have a complete understanding regarding all medications being taken and the effects that tobacco, alcohol, and caffeine can have on the patient's health.

Antibiotic Prophylaxis

Antibiotic prophylaxis is a prescribed predental treatment that is designed to prevent bacteria colonization in the heart known as infective endocarditis (IE), previously referred to as bacterial endocarditis. For many years, the American Heart Association (AHA) made recommendations that patients with various heart conditions such as mitral valve prolapse, rheumatic heart disease, calcified aortic stenosis, and congenital heart conditions take antibiotics prior to receiving any dental treatment. As of April 2007, the list of those who need to take antibiotic prophylaxis has significantly decreased due to scientific evidence indicating that the risks of taking preventative antibiotics actually outweigh the benefits for most patients. In addition to the issue of risk, studies indicated that those who took the antibiotics prior to dental treatment were at no greater or lesser risk of contracting IE. According to the American Dental Association (ADA), who participated in developing the new guidelines, the

Professionalism

If you or someone you care for is dependent on alcohol or drugs and needs treatment, it is important to know that no single treatment approach is appropriate for all individuals. Finding the right treatment program involves careful consideration of things such as the setting, length of care, philosophical approach, and individual needs of the person seeking help.

new guidelines are directed toward patients who have the greatest danger of a bad outcome if a heart infection occurred. These individuals include those with

1. artificial heart valves,
2. a history of infective endocarditis,
3. certain specific, serious congenital heart conditions, and/or
4. a cardiac transplant that develops a problem in a heart valve.

If premedications are required and have not been taken by the patient prior to the appointment then the patient may be required to reschedule.

Adverse Drug Effects

An adverse effect is a negative reaction to a drug and involves abnormal, harmful, undesired, and/or unintended side effects. Side effects can be either minor or serious and include appetite changes, blurred vision, dementia, depression, diarrhea, dizziness, drowsiness,

TABLE 27-3 Classification of Drugs

Drug Type	Purpose	Effect	Example of Drugs
Analgesics	Relieve pain.	Reduces sensory function to the brain.	Aspirin, acetaminophen, ibuprofen, codeine, methadone, morphine, oxycodone
Anesthetics	Reduce or obstruct sensation of pain or touch.	Blocks nerve impulses to the brain.	Septocaine, Orajel, procaine, lidocaine, general anesthetics
Antianxiety drugs	Produce a calm/sedating feeling and relax the muscles.	Reduces fear and tension.	Librium, Valium, Xanax
Antibiotics and anti-infectives	Fight infection.	Inhibits or kills the growth of microorganisms.	Penicillin, amoxicillin, Keflex, Ceclor
Cardiovascular drugs	Treat heart diseases and conditions of the blood vessels.	Prevents blood clots, controls high blood pressure, regulates heart rhythm.	Heparin, Coumadin, dicumarol, Lopressor, Procardia, nitroglycerin, Rythmol, Inderal
Anticonvulsants	Treat epileptic seizures.	Reduces stimulation to the brain.	Dilantin, Tegretol, phenobarbital
Allergy drugs	Relieve allergies.	Counteracts histamines.	Benadryl, Dimetane, Claritin
Anti-inflammatories	Treat arthritis and inflammation.	Reduces inflammatory process.	Advil, cortisone, Motrin
Bronchodilators	Treat asthma and bronchospasms.	Relaxes the muscles of the bronchi.	Albuterol, Ventolin
Decongestion drugs	Treat sinus and respiratory conditions.	Reduces congestion in the sinuses.	Sudafed, Afrin

Reviewing all patient medical histories is very important; however, some patients, particularly children and some seniors, may not be aware of the medications they are taking. Updating a patient's medical history is very important at the beginning of each appointment prior to the dental patient receiving dental treatment. If the patient is not able to completely answer questions related to his or her medical history or medications, it is important to acquire this information from another source. For instance, parents or guardians should be consulted about a child's history and a caregiver may need to be consulted to obtain an elderly patient's history.

excitability, headache, hypertension, respiratory difficulties, seizures, and sleeplessness.

An adverse effect that happens when two or more drugs are taken at the same time is called a *drug–drug interaction*. The body processes every drug differently. If two or more drugs are used at the same time, the body can change how the drugs are processed. It can often magnify the level of response, or make the drug ineffective. When this happens, the risk of side effects from each drug increases.

Drugs can also cause problems when they are taken with certain foods or drinks. This is called a *drug–food interaction*. Drug–food interactions can occur with prescription as well as OTC medications, including antacids, vitamins, iron pills, and others. Sometimes the food a person eats affects the ingredients in a medicine and prevents the medicine from working properly. At other times, combining drugs with certain foods or drinks can worsen the side effects. For example, an individual taking certain OTC antihistamines while drinking alcohol may experience an increase in the side effect of drowsiness.

Drug reactions encompass all adverse events related to drug administration, regardless of reasons. The terms *drug allergy, drug hypersensitivity,* and *drug reaction* are often used interchangeably. A drug allergy is an abnormally high sensitivity to certain substances, such as pollens, foods, or microorganisms. Common indications of an allergy may include sneezing, itching, and skin rashes. The best treatment for an allergic reaction is prevention, such as eliminating the substances from the sensitive person's environment. Drug hypersensitivity is defined as an excessive or abnormal sensitivity to a substance. Once a person has identified hypersensitivity to a drug, the individual should avoid taking that drug. If the individual does take the drug, then a more serious allergic reaction may be experienced. Drug intolerance results when a person has a higher threshold than most other people to the normal action of a drug. A drug interaction is a situation in which two or more separate drugs have been absorbed into the body and are affected by each other.

Drug addiction is physical and/or psychological dependency on a drug. When a person is physically dependent on a drug, the person must continue to take the drug to avoid physical withdrawal symptoms. Because the possible adverse effects are different from one drug to another, the dental team must be knowledgeable about drug effects, should have drug reference materials handy, and should carefully read drug labels for any product.

Surprisingly, many people in the United States reach the age of 50 or 60 without having been routinely under a physician's care. Often this lack of care is due to cultural or religious beliefs or sometimes because of economic issues. These individuals' medical conditions are often unknown and some may have never taken medications. For these reasons, these individuals must often be educated on how prescribed medications must be taken and on the adverse drug reactions or medication allergies that could occur. Patients should receive clear instructions on how to communicate with the dental office and their pharmacist if any questionable medication reactions occur.

SUMMARY

As a dental assistant it is important to be informed about the facts related to pharmacology. Whether a drug is prescribed or is an over-the-counter drug, dental assistants must be familiar with the various drugs dental patients may use and the adverse reactions that can occur. Through the use of drug reference materials, the dental assistant can gain significant knowledge. The dental assistant is an important individual in the education of patients about the drugs being prescribed by the dentist for dental treatment. It is important for the dental assistant to communicate with patients about the importance of taking their medications and alerting the office to any adverse effects.

KEY TERMS

- **Analgesic:** A drug that is used to relieve pain (e.g., aspirin, Motrin, morphine). p. 418

- **Drug interaction:** The effect a drug can have when taken with another drug. p. 414

KEY TERMS (continued)

- **Ethical drug:** Any drug that requires a prescription. p. 415
- **Generic name:** Drugs that are sold without a brand name and/or trademark. p. 415
- **Patent drugs:** Drugs that can be obtained without a prescription; referred to as over-the-counter drugs. p. 415
- **Pharmacokinetics:** The study of how drugs enter the body, circulate throughout, and exit the body. p. 414
- **Pharmacology:** The study of drugs. p. 414
- **Trade name:** The name given to a drug by the particular manufacturer that sells the drug. p. 415

● CHECK YOUR UNDERSTANDING

1. Pharmacokinetics is the study of
   a. evidence of past life.
   b. how drugs enter the body, circulate throughout, and exit the body.
   c. how the body functions.
   d. kinetics in the oral cavity.

2. Which popular reference book contains information about drugs used in the dental office?
   a. *Taber's* medical dictionary
   b. *Physicians' Desk Reference*
   c. PDR
   d. Both b and c

3. Which of the following abbreviations is used for "nothing by mouth"?
   a. ID
   b. SC
   c. IH
   d. NPO

4. The signature of the prescriber is placed on which part of a prescription?
   a. heading
   b. salutation
   c. body
   d. closing

5. The drug name, dose, size, and amount to be dispensed are placed on which part of the prescription?
   a. heading
   b. salutation
   c. body
   d. closing

6. The patient's name, address, and birth date are placed on which part of the prescription?
   a. heading
   b. salutation
   c. body
   d. closing

7. If a patient consumes two or more drugs at one time, what type of effect might occur?
   a. side effect
   b. adverse effect
   c. habit forming
   d. none of the above

8. Which drugs are habit-forming stimulants?
   a. alcohol
   b. tobacco
   c. caffeine
   d. both b and c

9. Which schedule of the Controlled Substances Act does morphine, opium and opium derivatives, cocaine, methadone, and amphetamines fall under?
   a. I
   b. II
   c. III
   d. V

10. Which schedule of the Controlled Substances Act does cough syrups and mixtures of opiates fall under?
    a. I
    b. II
    c. III
    d. V

● INTERNET ACTIVITY

- Go to http://library.thinkquest.org/C0115926/drugs/maindrugs.htm and look up drugs by classification, alphabetical order, groups, effects, prevention, treatment, how to get help, and much more. Be knowledgeable on the signs and symptoms of drug abuse.

● WEB REFERENCES

- PDR drug search and information www.pdrhealth.com/drug_info/index.html

28

Anesthesia and Pain Control

Learning Objectives

After reading this chapter, the student should be able to:

- Discuss the commonly used methods to relieve pain.
- Explain the use of topical anesthetics.
- Identify the sites for injection on the maxillary and mandibular arches.
- Describe the complications and precautions related to the use of anesthetic agents.
- Explain how electronic anesthesia is used.
- Explain how inhalation sedation and intravenous sedation are used in dentistry.
- Discuss various types of antianxiety agents used in dentistry.
- Explain the administration process for general anesthesia.

Preparing for Certification Exams

- Assist with and/or apply topical anesthetic to site of injection.
- Prepare carpule hypodermic syringes for injection.
- Select and prepare tray setups and all necessary materials for administration of anesthetics.
- Assist with and/or monitor the administration of nitrous oxide/oxygen analgesia.
- Assist with the administration of anesthetics using the concepts of four-handed dentistry.
- Demonstrate the ability to calm and reassure apprehensive patients.

Key Terms

Analgesic	Induction
Anesthetic	Infiltration
Anxiety	Pain
Duration	Vasoconstrictor

Chapter Outline

- Local and Topical Anesthetic Agents
  - —Topical Anesthesia
  - —Local Anesthesia
  - —Local Anesthetic Solution
  - —Vasoconstrictors
  - —Duration and Action of Anesthetics
- Injection Techniques
  - —Local Infiltration
  - —Block Anesthesia
  - —Intraosseous Anesthesia
  - —Periodontal Ligament Injection
  - —Intrapulpal Injection
  - —Computer-Controlled Local Anesthesia Delivery System
- Local Anesthesia Setup
  - —Tray Setup
  - —Syringes
  - —Needles
  - —Cartridges
  - —Needlestick Reporting
- Complications and Precautions
  - —Paresthesia
  - —Hematoma
  - —Trismus
- Electronic Anesthesia
- Inhalation Sedation
  - —Equipment for Inhalation Sedation
  - —Safety and Precautions: Scavenger Systems
  - —Medical Assessment and Monitoring
  - —N_2O/O_2 Sedation
- Antianxiety Agents
- Intravenous Sedation
- General Anesthesia
- Documentation of Anesthesia and Pain Control

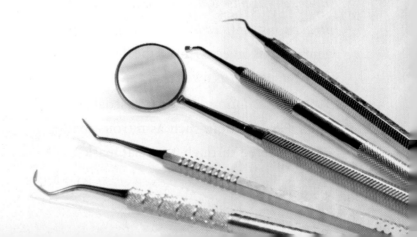

Pain is a subjective experience of an unpleasant sensation that may be described as sharp, throbbing, dull, nauseating, burning, and shooting. Pain can often cause individuals to display various emotions such as anger or depression. In the oral cavity it can occur in teeth, gingiva, roots, palate, tongue, and jaw. Pain perception or interpretation varies with each individual. The ability to withstand pain varies from patient to patient and is known as one's threshold of pain. **Anxiety** is a physiological state characterized by emotions such as fear, apprehension, or worry. The myths about dental pain often outweigh the realities, and the anxiety caused by these myths further intensifies the pain. Pain and fear in dentistry can be controlled by utilizing various anxiety and pain control techniques, including:

- *Anesthetics:* Topically applied, locally injected, or general anesthesia.

- *Analgesics:* Pain relievers including common nonnarcotic medications such as ibuprofen and aspirin. These are typically prescribed by the dentist as premedications or following procedures such as root canals or tooth extractions.

- *Sedatives:* Sedatives are medications designed to help patients relax. These can be prescribed by the dentist when required. Types of sedatives include:

  - *Antianxiety agents:* includes diazepam (Valium)

  - *Intravenous (IV) sedation:* a tranquilizing agent that is injected into the body often while the patient is awake

  - *Inhalation sedation:* a form of sedation in which a medication, such as nitrous oxide, is administered through a special mask.

The control of pain and anxiety has been advanced by the use of new technology that assists in providing less pain while performing dental procedures. Options available for providing this type of dentistry include the use of lasers and the micro air-abrasion unit.

Laser is an acronym standing for light amplified by stimulated emission of radiation. Lasers have been used in dentistry since 1994 to treat a number of dental problems. All lasers work by delivering energy in the form of condensed light, which is delivered through a laser handpiece. When used for surgical procedures, the laser acts as a cutting instrument or a vaporizer of tissue. Use of lasers in dentistry has proven to provide a less painful experience, which in turn has helped in diminishing patient anxieties related to dental procedures.

The micro air-abrasion unit is essentially a tiny sandblaster. It uses a high-pressure stream of aluminum oxide particles to cut away decayed tooth structure. There is no heat, unlike the laser, so it can be used on teeth that already have restorations.

Local and Topical Anesthetic Agents

Local and topical anesthetics are commonly used in dentistry for routine procedures where pain control is needed, such as when seating crowns, matrix band placement, scaling and root planing, and periodontal probing.

Dental Assistant   PROFESSIONAL TIP

Dental assistants must always read the complete history of the patient before preparing for any procedure. The history provides them with information on the patient's current health status, mental condition, and overall feelings or apprehensions. Dental assistants must also make sure that all required tests are done and reports are on file and, further, that the readings of the reports are verified by the dentist as being within normal levels. Dental assistants should make sure that all needed premedications have been used as prescribed.

Topical anesthetics provide surface numbness so that the local anesthetic can be injected with minimal discomfort. Therefore, a topical anesthetic is always applied before injecting a local anesthesia with a needle.

Topical Anesthesia

Topical anesthetics work by numbing the nerve endings in the oral mucosa at the local injection site (Figure 28.1). Application is accomplished with a coated cotton swab (see Procedure 28-1). Maximum effectiveness is obtained by leaving the topical in place at the site for three to five minutes. Topical anesthetics are available in creams, ointments, aerosols, sprays, lotions, patches, and gels. Liquid and spray topical anesthetics can be used to numb a wide area of the local mucosa. Sprays are used for patients with a strong gag reflex. Legally, sprays must be administered by a dentist by spraying the anesthetic directly on the back of the throat. Sprays can be especially useful when taking dental radiographs or impressions.

The topical patch (Figure 28.2) is among a new generation of products that provides anesthesia within 10 seconds. The patch is usually used at injection sites and may also be utilized in areas of inflamed tissue during dental hygiene procedures. The patch can also be used for alleviating discomfort from denture sores and oral ulcers. Some of the commonly used topical anesthetic agents include benzocaine, lidocaine, proparacaine (Alcaine), and tetracaine (also known as amethocaine).

What does absence of the gag reflex mean? **?**

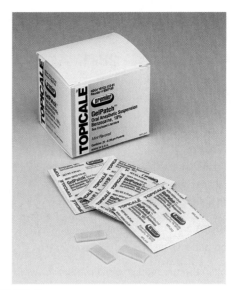

FIGURE 28.2
Topical gel patch.
Courtesy Premier Dental

Local Anesthesia

Local anesthesia, in a strict sense, is anesthesia of a small part of the body such as a tooth or oral mucosa. It is a drug that reversibly inhibits the conduction of signals along nerves, resulting in analgesia and loss of sensation. Historically, the leaves of the coca plant were traditionally used as a stimulant in Peru. Cocaine was discovered in 1860 and first used as a local anesthetic in 1884. The search for a less toxic and less addictive substitute led to the development of the local anesthetic procaine in 1904. Since then, several local anesthetic drugs have been developed and used, notably lidocaine in 1943, bupivacaine in 1957, and prilocaine in 1959.

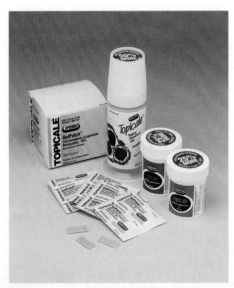

FIGURE 28.1
Topical anesthetic.
Courtesy Premier Dental

Preparing for Externship

Standards for dental assisting program accreditation by the Commission on Dental Accreditation (CODA) require that graduates must be competent in the knowledge and skill required to perform a variety of clinical supportive treatments, including assist with and/or apply topical anesthetic. It is also emphasized that dental assistants learn major causes of pain and anxiety in dentistry. They must be competent in knowledge of the material needed for all types of anesthesia used in dentistry including types of needles, syringes, and anesthetic solutions. They should have knowledge on how much nitrous oxide can be introduced to a particular patient. Knowledge about possible side effects for patients and the dental team resulting from various anesthetic agents is very important for the safety of the dental team and a great help in answering patient concerns.

Procedure 28-1 Applying Topical Anesthetic

Equipment and Supplies Needed

- Basic setup
- Air/water syringe
- Air evacuator
- 2 × 2 sterile gauze squares
- Topical anesthetic gel ointment
- Cotton tip applicator

Procedure Steps

1. Read patient's history.

2. Explain the procedure to the patient to avoid any confusion.

3. Wait for the dentist to do an oral examination and give you permission to apply topical anesthetic.

4. Locate the site of local anesthesia as indicated by the dentist.

5. Dry the area with a 2 × 2 cotton gauze. (*Note:* The site should always be dry so that the topical anesthetic is 100% effective.)

6. Place a small amount of topical anesthetic on the cotton applicator tip, then place on a 2 × 2 cotton gauze. (*Note:* Never reuse applicator tips.)

7. Place the cotton applicator tip with anesthetic at the site of injection.

8. If multiple injections will be needed, then apply the topical application to all injection sites.

9. Keep the material on the site for three to five minutes.

10. Observe and ask patients about the sensation at the site of application.

11. Remove any extra material with the air/water syringe and dispose of the cotton applicator.

12. Use the evacuation system to suction residual topical anesthetic material.

13. Inform the dentist and be prepared to assist in local anesthesia administration.

Local Anesthetic Solution

Drugs used as local anesthetics are approved for use based on nonirritation to the tissues, minimal toxicity, fast and rapid results, complete anesthesia, sufficient duration, complete reversal by leaving the tissue in its original state, and being capable of sterilization without getting deteriorated by heat.

Clinical local anesthetic agents belong to one of two chemical classes: aminoamides (amides) and aminoesters (esters). Amides are the most preferred type of local anesthetic. The main difference between amides and esters is the way they are metabolized in the body. Amide anesthetics are metabolized by the liver. Ester anesthetics are metabolized in the plasma. Commonly used aminoamides for local anesthesia are lidocaine, mepivacaine, and prilocaine. Aminoesters used for local anesthesia include benzocaine and tetracaine.

Local anesthetic agents are selected based on the health of the patient, the procedure to be performed, and the dentist's preference. Esters are prone to producing allergic reactions, so amides are usually selected. Local anesthetics are available in cartridges. The anesthetic agents in the cartridges include sodium chloride and distilled water. The distilled water content of the cartridge is added to increase the volume of the solution to make it injectable.

Vasoconstrictors

A **vasoconstrictor** is any substance that acts to cause vasoconstriction or narrowing of the lumen of blood vessels, resulting in decreased blood loss at the surgical site. They are added in local anesthetics to increase the duration of action and to slow down the intake of the anesthetic agent by prolonging its effect. Vasoconstrictors are added to anesthetic agents typically in ratios of 1:20,000, 1:50,000, 1:100,000, and 1:200,000, which means that 1 part of vasoconstrictor is added, respectively, to 20,000, 50,000, 100,000, or 200,000 parts of anesthetic solutions. The necessary ratio is printed on the label of the carpule, the glass container that holds the anesthetic solution (Figure 28.3). The dental assistant should check with the dentist to determine the desired vasoconstrictor ratio for the patient.

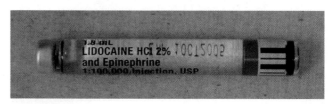

FIGURE 28.3
Local anesthetic cartridge showing vasoconstrictor solution.

It is important to note that vasoconstrictors can cause strain on the heart by increasing the heart rate. Use of vasoconstrictors should be avoided on patients with a history of heart conditions such as unstable angina and recent myocardial infarction. Vasoconstrictors can also interfere with some other drugs. Prior to use, it is important that the dentist review the list of medications the patient is currently taking. A commonly used vasoconstrictor drug is epinephrine.

Duration and Action of Anesthetics

Local anesthetics function mainly by stopping the conduction channel of the nerves after getting diffused along the nerve, thus by blocking the sensation and making the patient feel numbness in the injected sites without loss of patient consciousness. To achieve the maximum local anesthesia effect, a sufficient amount of anesthetic must be injected at the surgical site, because the effects of an anesthetic are diminished when carried through the bloodstream. **Induction** is the length of time from injection until complete anesthesia is achieved. The **duration** is the time from induction to complete reversal of the anesthesia. Based on the duration of action, the local anesthetic agents are classified as follows:

- *Short-acting local anesthetic agents*—duration of less than 30 minutes
- *Intermediate-acting local anesthetics*—duration of about 60 minutes
- *Long-acting anesthetics*—duration of longer than 60 minutes

---

What would be the possible signs of an overdose of local anesthetic?

Injection Techniques

Various injection techniques are used in dentistry for administering anesthetic agents. A technique can be selected based on the location of specific nerve and nerve endings, the type of patient, and the procedure. The dental assistant must know all of the injection sites for effective assisting and application of topical anesthesia prior to local anesthesia injection by the dentist or expanded functions dental hygienist.

Local Infiltration

In the local **infiltration** technique, the local anesthetic agent is infiltrated directly into the oral tissue site. This technique is commonly used for maxillary teeth because the alveolar cancellous bone of maxilla is porous in nature; therefore, the solution diffuses through the bone and reaches the apices of the teeth (Figures 28.4a, b, c).

Infiltration anesthesia is used to numb a single tooth; therefore, every tooth gets a separate infiltration if more than one tooth needs anesthesia. Usually three-quarters of the anesthetic carpule or cartridge is infiltrated at the buccal root tips site and the remaining one-quarter is infiltrated at the single palatal root tip site. Because the soft tissues of the palate are closely attached to the palatal bone, the infiltration at the palatal site is often painful, and topical anesthetic application is always helpful prior to local infiltration. In addition to maxillary infiltration, local infiltration can also be used as a secondary injection to mandibular block injection to numb buccal gingival tissues surrounding the mandibular teeth (Figure 28.5a).

Block Anesthesia

Field block anesthesia, also known as regional anesthesia, is injected around the nerve endings to numb a block of an area, quadrant, or two or three teeth apices. When using nerve block anesthesia, the solution is injected into a nerve bundle to enable diffusion to a wider area, such as the right mandibular quadrant or left mandibular quadrant (Figure 28.5b). This is known as an inferior alveolar nerve block injection because the solution is injected close to the mandibular foramen where the main inferior alveolar nerve is located. This injection is performed because the mandibular bone is very dense and compact, and the anesthetic solution does not diffuse easily through it. Once the solution is diffused along the inferior alveolar nerve, the patient will experience numbness of half of the lower jaw including teeth, tongue, and lip on the affected side.

Another type of block anesthesia is the incisive nerve block, which is given at the site of mental foramen. It is injected to numb the mandibular incisors area as the branch of mental nerve continues on through the mandibular canal to the apices of the anterior teeth. Often this injection is given when only the premolars and/or the incisors need anesthesia (Figure 28.5c).

The nasopalatine nerve block is given by injecting local anesthetic solution into the incisive papilla (Figures 28.5d, e). It numbs the anterior one-third of the hard palate from the right canine to the left canine of the maxillary arch. A maxillary nerve block is performed by injecting local anesthetic solution at the height of the mucobuccal fold above the distal of the maxillary second molar, numbing the buccal, palatal, and pulpal tissues in one quadrant, including the skin of the lower eyelid, side of the nose, upper lip, and cheek.

The lingual tissues and side of the tongue, including the mandibular teeth of the midline, are numbed by injecting the anesthetic solution into the lingual to mandibular ramus and adjacent to the maxillary tuberosity. This is known as a lingual nerve block (Figure 28.5f).

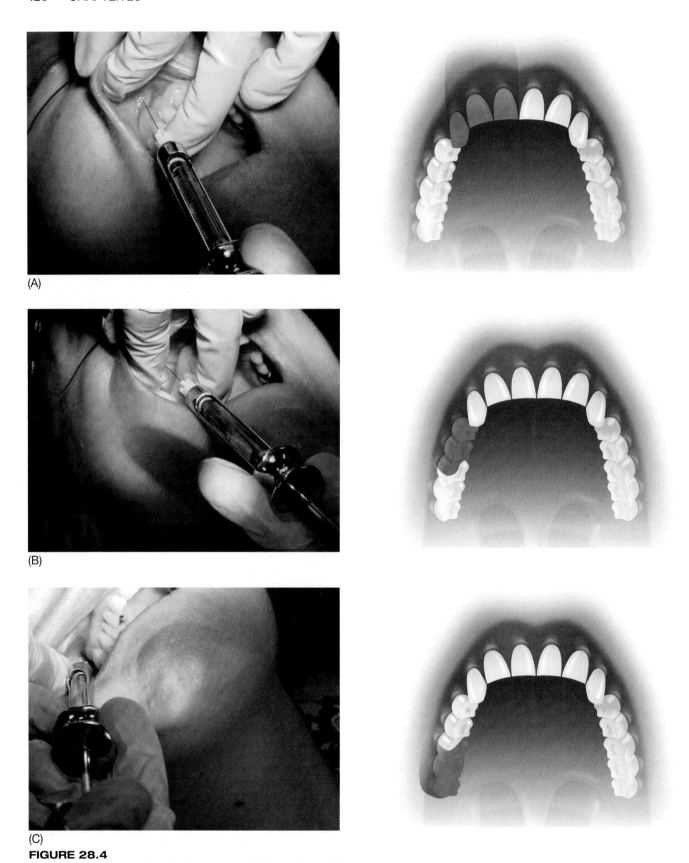

FIGURE 28.4

(a) Maxillary anterior superior alveolar nerve block, (b) maxillary middle superior alveolar nerve block, and (c) maxillary posterior superior alveolar nerve block.

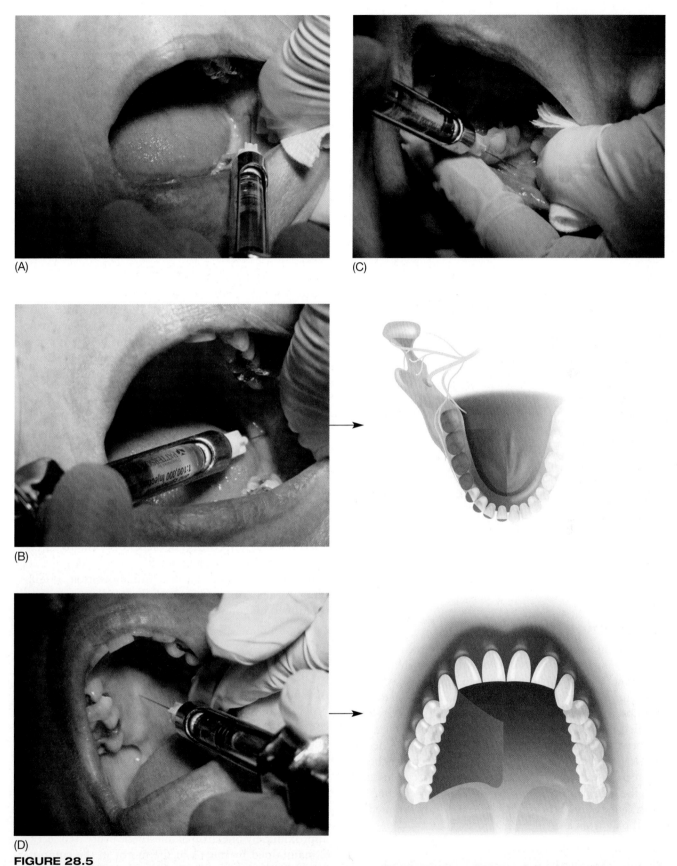

FIGURE 28.5

(a) Long buccal nerve block, (b) inferior alveolar nerve block with illustration showing location of injection, (c) mental nerve block, (d) maxillary greater palatine nerve block with illustration showing location of injection,

(continued)

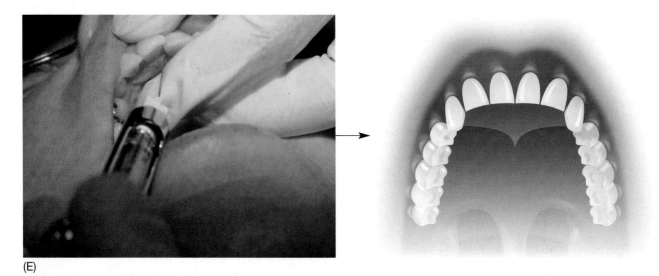

(E)

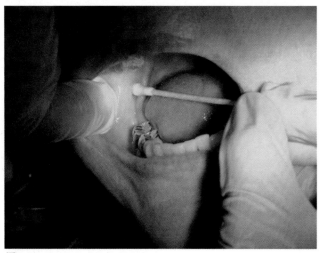

(F)

FIGURE 28.5 (continued)
(e) maxillary nasopalatine nerve block, and (f) lingual nerve block.

Intraosseous Anesthesia

Intraosseous anesthesia injections are given directly into the spongy bone for a single tooth or multiple teeth in the same quadrant. This technique can be used on patients who are not comfortable with the loss of feeling in a numbed tongue and lips. This injection is performed by using an 8-mm-long needle with a 27-gauge size needle (gauge is the diameter of the needle). A perforator is a solid needle that is attached to the slow-speed handpiece that perforates the cortical bone. Then the 8-mm-long, 27-gauge needle is directly inserted into the predrilled hole in the cortical bone for injecting the anesthetic solution. Topical anesthesia is always used to avoid pain from a needlestick.

Periodontal Ligament Injection

A periodontal ligament injection is an alternative technique that involves injection of the anesthetic solution under pressure directly into the periodontal ligament space and surrounding tissues by insertion of the needle into the gingival sulcus along the long axis of the tooth. This injection can be accomplished with either a traditional syringe or a special periodontal ligament syringe known as Lig-a-jet. This technique is used for numbing the pulp of one or more teeth in a quadrant. This technique can also be used as an adjunct to another injection where the surgical site is partially anesthetized.

Intrapulpal Injection

An intrapulpal injection is given directly into the pulp chamber using a 25- or 27-gauge short or long needle. It is commonly used during root canal treatment when some of the nerve endings are not sufficiently numbed by traditional anesthesia. To ease access of the needle to the injection site, sometimes the needle is bent to directly inject the solution in the pulpal chamber. Per the Occupational Safety and Health Administration (OSHA) Bloodborne Pathogen standard, the bending of needles is prohibited on contaminated needles.

Computer-Controlled Local Anesthesia Delivery System

A computer-controlled local anesthesia delivery system provides an almost painless experience. The computer-controlled system uses a microprocessor that is programmed to adjust the pressure of the injection solution depending on the resistance of the tissues (low resistance or high resistance) at the injection site.

The device functions by injecting anesthetic at a constant, slow rate and controlled pressure, regardless of the type and resistance of the tissue. Slow injection of approximately one drop of anesthetic every two seconds is maintained by means of the motor in the computer-controlled local anesthesia apparatus, also known as the WAND. The appliance also enables electronic control of the rate of injection during the entire procedure. Administration of the anesthetic into the surgical site is performed very slowly so as to enable the anesthetic to enter the tissue slowly and under pressure by making passage for the needle, so the stick of the needle is not felt by the patient. It is believed that the maintenance of constant pressure and passage of the anesthetic, with an ideal rate of injection of the anesthetic, are the main reasons for achievement of pleasant and almost painless injections with this system.

Note that the appearance of the system for administering anesthesia has an important role in the patient's total perception of and attitude toward anesthesia. The WAND handpiece with the needle looks like a stick—not a regular syringe with a needle. The system is often called "anesthesia with a stick." It can be presented to children as "anesthesia with a magic stick" and not an injection, which children are far more willing to accept. Some recent studies show that computer-controlled anesthesia for children, particularly those of preschool age, provides two to three times less sensation of pain than in the case of classic local anesthesia.

How does the computer-controlled local anesthesia technique aid in offering painless dentistry to patients?

Local Anesthesia Setup

Dental assistants have the responsibility to stay current with all of the modern equipment and material used for anesthesia in dentistry and for setting up the trays for topical and local anesthetics. In most states, the dental assistant is allowed to apply topical anesthesia prior to application of local anesthesia when indicated by the dentist. Some states also allow dental assistants to assist in inhalation, IV sedation, and general anesthesia procedures. In some states dental nurses are required to obtain credentialing in administrating inhalation anesthesia. These dental nurses typically have extensive training in surgical assisting. Dental assistants should have knowledge of their state's dental practice laws to ensure that the functions performed are allowed.

Tray Setup

The tray setup for local anesthesia includes aspirating syringe, needles, and cotton applicator with topical anesthetic agent, needle recapper, 2 × 2 gauze pieces, and anesthetic cartridges or carpules (see Procedure 28-2). Other equipment and supplies needed are the patient's current medical and dental history and all basic examination instruments including, mouth mirror, explorer, and cotton pliers.

Procedure 28-2 Assembling the Local Anesthetic Syringe

Equipment and Supplies Needed

- Sterile anesthetic syringe
- Sterile disposable needles
- Sterile anesthetic cartridge
- 2 × 2 sterile gauze sponge

Procedure Steps

A. SETTING UP THE TRAY

1. Wash hands and don gloves before preparing the anesthetic syringe.

2. Prepare the type of anesthesia based on the dentist's choice. The dentist will determine the type of anesthetic solution needed according to the patient's health history.

3. Arrange all supplies on a tray at chairside away from the patient's view.

B. THREADING THE NEEDLE

1. Select the right size of needle based on infiltration or block anesthesia.

2. Remove the plastic cap of the needle from the hub end.

3. Screw the needle on the needle end of the syringe, taking care that the end of the needle going inside the syringe does not bend. If the needle bends, retrieve another needle and begin again.

4. Make sure the needle is tightly attached to the syringe. Placing the needle before the cartridge eliminates the possibility of a broken or bent needle.

C. LOADING THE ANESTHETIC CARTRIDGE INTO THE SYRINGE

1. Hold the syringe in one hand and use the thumb ring to pull back the plunger.

2. Use the other hand to place the cartridge into the syringe with the stopper end toward the plunger.

3. Allow the harpoon to engage the stopper by releasing the plunger.

4. Make sure that the harpoon is engaged in the stopper by pulling back the thumb ring. (*Note:* This action should be done gently to avoid breaking of the glass cartridge.)

D. GETTING THE LOCAL ANESTHETIC TRAY READY

1. Place the loaded syringe on the tray out of the patient's sight.

2. Inform the dentist that the setup is ready.

Syringes

The word *syringe* comes from the Greek, meaning "tube." In the ninth century, Ammar ibn Ali al-Mawsili invented the first syringe using a hollow glass tube. Charles Gabriel Pravaz and Alexander Wood were the first to develop a syringe with a needle fine enough to pierce the skin in 1853.

Two types of local anesthetic syringes are available: plain and aspirating. Aspirating syringes are the most commonly used (Figure 28.6). The parts of an aspirating syringe consist of a threaded tip on the needle adapter where the needle attaches, a barrel where the carpule is placed, a piston rod (plunger) with a harpoon attached that embeds itself into the rubber stopper of the carpule, a finger grip, and a thumb ring.

Before injecting the local anesthetic solution, the dentist makes sure that the flow of solution from the needle is even and comes out in a clear stream. This is done by expressing the solution by holding the tip of the needle straight up and gently pushing in the plunger until a continuous stream is seen. Expressing the solution is important because it gets rid of air bubbles from the needle lumen so that no air is introduced in the injection site. Injected air can cause an air embolism. The lumen of the needle is the hole in the shaft of the needle through which the anesthetic solution is passed. Air embolism is a medical condition in which air bubbles are caught in the bloodstream. Usually, small air bubbles are stopped at the lungs, but big air bubbles can be very dangerous and can result in death if they lodge in the heart.

Here are some details about the parts of the syringe (refer to Figure 28.6):

- The thumb ring, finger grip, and finger bar allow the dentist to control the syringe firmly. The thumb ring assists in the aspiration procedure. The thumb is inside the ring

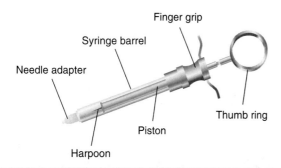

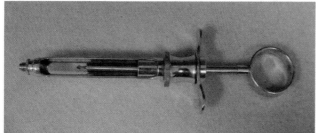

FIGURE 28.6
An aspirating syringe with parts labeled.

while injecting. The fingers hold the finger grip, thus making it easy to pull the syringe back quickly. This may be necessary if an emergency happens, such as a sudden movement from a patient, resulting in breakage of the needle.

- The harpoon is a simple thumb powered-piston pump consisting of a plunger. The plunger can be pulled and pushed along the inside of a cylindrical tube (the barrel), which has a small hole on one end so it can draw liquid in and/or out by the same hole. The harpoon allows the dentist to aspirate (draw back) the injection site to see if the needle tip is located within a blood vessel before injecting the anesthetic solution.

Once the harpoon is engaged in the rubber stopper of the anesthetic carpule, the dentist can apply inward or outward pressure on the stopper by exerting pressure on the thumb ring. Pulling the thumb ring outward also pulls the plunger outward, producing an aspirating effect; whereas pushing inward forces the anesthetic solution through the needle. If by producing the aspirating effect, some blood is noticed entering the carpule, the dentist would immediately retract the syringe and reinject in another area where the blood vessel can be avoided. If by mistake, the anesthetic agent is entered into a vein, it will quickly travel to the heart and may result in constriction of coronary arteries and relaxation of the cardiac muscles, resulting in fainting of the patient. The anatomic arrangement of the veins is that they are always on top of the arteries and nerves.

- The piston rod pushes in the rubber stopper of the anesthetic cartridge by forcing the anesthetic solution through the needle.

- The barrel of the syringe is shaped like a cylindrical tube and holds the anesthetic cartridge in place. The cartridge is loaded on the open side of the barrel. There is an open window on the other side of the barrel that allows the operator to watch for blood during aspiration.

- The threaded tip of the needle adapter is where the needle is attached to the syringe. The cartridge end of the needle passes through the small opening in the center of the threaded tip and punctures the rubber diaphragm of the anesthetic cartridge to ensure passage of fluid from the cartridge to the needle. It is recommended to thread the needle first before loading the cartridge in the barrel because the operator can make sure the cartridge end of the needle is not bent but is clearly penetrating into the rubber diaphragm.

Passing and Receiving the Syringe

The dentist will be ready to administer the local anesthetic after the topical anesthetic is applied by the dental assistant. The assistant passes the syringe with the needle cover in place by holding the barrel of the syringe in the hand. The dental assistant places the thumb ring of the syringe over the dentist's thumb and the finger grip between the dentist's index and middle fingers. While holding the syringe by the barrel, the other hand is used to remove the needle cap.

After the dentist gives the injection, the syringe is carefully removed by grasping the barrel and lifting the syringe out of the dentist's hand. Caution must be taken when grasping the barrel of the syringe because the needle is exposed. Dental assistants must not attempt to recap the needle while the syringe is in the dentist's hand. Some dentists may not pass the syringe back to the dental assistant in order to avoid a possible needlestick. If it is necessary to recap the needle, it must be done using some type of mechanical device, such as a needle guard or recapper or the one-handed scoop technique. The one-handed scoop technique is done by placing the needle cover on a flat surface and then holding the syringe in the dominant hand and scooping the needle cap onto the needle. The syringe is tipped vertically to slide the cover over the needle. The dental assistant must not hold onto the needle cap with the nondominant hand while scooping. The needled cap is secured by grasping it near the hub.

After the patient is dismissed, the syringe must be disassembled safely. It is vitally important to prevent needlesticks from the contaminated needle. It is advisable to first remove the carpule with the needle remaining in place. This provides an air vent to prevent the glass carpule from shattering. To unload the carpule, pull the piston rod back as far as possible to disengage the harpoon from the rubber stopper without pulling the stopper from the carpule. The carpule can then be easily removed from the syringe.

Immediately after the dentist administers the local anesthesia, the dental assistant irrigates and suctions the injection site. This is necessary because the anesthetic solution produces a bitter taste in the patient's mouth. Used disposable needles and syringes must be placed in appropriate sharps disposal containers and discarded as regulated waste. If the syringe is made of metal then it should be sterilized and prepared for reuse (Procedure 28-3).

Needles

Sterile aspirating syringe needles used in dental procedures are made of stainless steel. They are designed for a single use and are available in different gauges and lengths (Figure 28.8). The needle cannot be used if the seal is broken. The gauge of a needle refers to the diameter of the hollow shaft of the needle. The larger the gauge the smaller the diameter or lumen of the needle. The most frequently used gauge numbers are 25, 27, and 30. The lengths of the needles vary, and are classified as long (L) or short (S). Usually, a short needle (1 inch in length) is prepared for maxillary injections and is used for infiltration anesthesia. A long needle (1 5/8 inches in length) is used for mandibular injections and block anesthesia.

Each needle has either a plastic or metal hub designed to screw onto the threaded end of the syringe (Figure 28.7). This hub is positioned to permit the needle to extend inward to penetrate the rubber seal portion of a loaded anesthetic carpule. The plastic caps covering the needle are easily removed from both ends. When placing the needle onto the syringe, only the cap that covers the syringe end of the needle should be removed. This maintains the sterility of the needle portion used to inject the patient.

To provide more protection from needlestick injuries, various safety needles have been developed. Monoject Magellan safety needles are one type. This easy one-handed design offers a safety shield to ensure protection against any exposures from sharps injuries.

Cartridges

Through the color-coding system created by the American Dental Association's Council on Scientific Affairs, standardization was established for all injectable local anesthesia products, which are typically supplied in glass carpules. These cartridges have a rubber or silicone stopper at one end and an aluminum cap with a rubber diaphragm at the other end. The local anesthetic cartridges or carpules are color coded to identify different brands of anesthetics and the ratio of vasoconstrictor contained within the solution. The cartridge also includes information on the supply company, the lot or batch number, and expiration date.

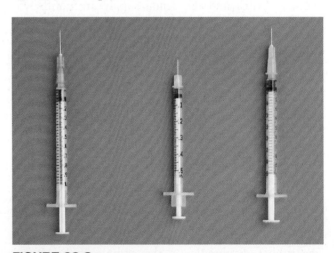

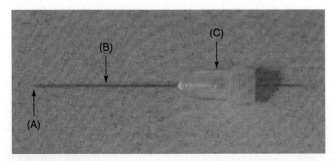

FIGURE 28.7
Needle with parts identified: (a) bevel, (b) shank, (c) hub.

FIGURE 28.8
Syringes with various needle gauges.

Procedure 28-3 Assisting in the Administration of Local Anesthesia

Equipment and Supplies Needed

- Basic setup
- Air/water syringe
- Evacuator
- Topical anesthetic ointment
- 2 × 2 sterile cotton gauze squares
- Cotton rolls
- Cotton applicator tips
- Assembled local anesthetic syringe (see Procedure 28-2)
- Needle recapper
- Sharps disposal jar

Procedure Steps

1. Read patient's history chart.

2. Wash hands and don gloves.

3. Apply the topical anesthetic to the particular injection site as indicated by the dentist, following the guidelines.

4. Dry the area and free it from any saliva.

5. Put cotton rolls for isolation of the injection site.

6. Loosen the needle guard and transfer the loaded syringe with the thumb ring over the operator's thumb.

7. Always transfer the syringe under the patient's chin, so the patient does not see it.

8. Do not release the syringe from your hand until you make sure that the dentist has a firm grip on the thumb ring.

9. As the dentist is giving the injection, monitor the patient for any adverse reactions, making sure you portray a calm and relaxed sense of being.

10. After the injection is completed, replace the needle guard by using a one-handed scoop technique or recapping device.

11. Rinse the patient's mouth with the air/water syringe, and suction with the saliva ejector or high-volume evacuator.

12. Remove the used needle with the guard in place and dispose of the needle in the sharps container.

13. Dispose of the used cartridge in a medical waste receptacle.

14. Prepare the anesthetic syringe for sterilization.

15. Continue monitoring the patient's reaction throughout the procedure.

16. After the surgical procedure is complete, provide patient with postoperative instructions including not to chew on the site for several hours to avoid accidental biting on the cheek or lips.

Specific guidelines are designed for handling anesthetic cartridges. The dental assistant must first check the carpule for cracks or suspended articles floating in the solution. If anything is found, the carpule is discarded and the dentist and the dental supply are notified to ensure that other batches of anesthetic are usable.

Cartridges should be stored at room temperature and protected from direct sunlight. Never use a cartridge that has been frozen and do not use a cartridge if it is cracked, chipped, or damaged in any way. Never use a solution that is discolored or cloudy or has passed the expiration date, and do not leave the syringe preloaded with the needle attached for an extended period of time. The cartridge must only be used on one patient. When storing cartridges on shelves, they should be placed in order based on their expiration date, with the oldest cartridges in front and the newest ones placed behind.

Loading the Cartridge

The rubber diaphragm on the carpule is disinfected before loading it in the syringe. The rubber diaphragm must not be touched after disinfection. Placing the carpule end in the aspirating syringe is fairly easy, using the following steps:

- Break the seal on the needle container and remove only a small portion of the plastic needle cover.
- Insert the needle into the syringe and screw the hub onto the syringe.
- Use the thumb ring to pull the plunger back against the syringe body.
- Place the cartridge into the barrel of the syringe with the rubber stopper end in first, positioned toward the plunger. Gently slide the cartridge toward the needle end of the barrel, so the cartridge end of the needle can be inserted into the rubber without being bent.
- Engage the harpoon into the rubber stopper of the cartridge by holding the body portion of the syringe with one hand while lightly tapping the thumb ring with the other hand.
- Do not tap the thumb ring with too much force; this might cause the glass carpule or cartridge to shatter.

- Make a quarter turn with the thumb ring to ensure that the harpoon is firmly engaged in the rubber stopper.
- If it is, the thumb ring will rotate back to its original position.
- Force a small, but visible amount of anesthesia through the needle to expel air.
- Loosen the needle cap, keeping the plastic needle cover in place until the syringe is passed to the dentist.

Needlestick Reporting

OSHA requires that Engineering and Work Practice Controls must be the primary means used to eliminate or minimize exposure to bloodborne pathogens. Engineering controls reduce employee exposure either by removing, eliminating, or isolating the hazard. Engineering controls are measures such as the use of sharps disposal containers, self-sheathing needles, and safer medical devices such as sharps injury protections and needleless systems that isolate or remove the bloodborne pathogens hazard from the workplace. Work Practice Controls are measures that reduce the likelihood of exposure by altering the manner in which a task is performed, such as prohibiting recapping of needles by a two-handed technique.

Employers must choose to implement the safer medical devices when they are appropriate, commercially available, and effective. Documentation of the implementation of these devices must be recorded annually. Employers must receive input on these devices from those responsible for direct patient care. This input must be documented. Employers must train employees to use new devices and/or procedures and document training in the exposure control plan.

Employers must maintain a log of injuries from contaminated sharps. OSHA's Recordkeeping standard also requires needlestick injuries to be recorded on OSHA Form 300, *Log of Work-Related Injuries and Illnesses*. This includes all work-related needlestick injuries and cuts from sharp objects that are contaminated with another person's blood or other potentially infectious materials (OPIM). If this recorded employee injury is later diagnosed with an infectious bloodborne disease, OSHA Form 300 must be updated.

A dental assistant must immediately inform the dentist as soon as a needlestick occurs and a few drops of blood should be expelled under cold running water in a sink for about a minute. Vigorous mechanical scrubbing with soap and water may prevent viral material from entering tissues. An antiseptic can be applied to prevent possible superinfection due to punctured skin. OSHA Form 300 should then be completed to document the exposure. The dental assistant must follow the clinic's guidelines for obtaining a blood test to test for any diseases that might have entered the body because of exposure resulting from the needlestick. This may require the employer to pay for the tests, or the dental assistant may

have to cover the costs. After the test results arrive, a copy of the original must be attached to the OSHA Form 300 log sheet for future reference. Later tests may be required if exposure to a high-risk disease such as HIV was possible.

How should a dental assistant report an accidental needlestick?

Complications and Precautions

Various complications can occur when local anesthetics are delivered. For instance, if anesthesia is injected into a site that is infected, there is a great risk of spreading the infection. Another complication of anesthesia is an allergic or toxic reaction such as contact dermatitis or, in severe cases, anaphylactic shock. This abnormal body response depends on the type of anesthetic solution used, the amount injected, the rate at which the solution was injected and diffused, interaction with any other medication in the patient's system, and each individual patient's body response.

Local anesthetic drugs are toxic to the heart (where they cause arrhythmia) and brain (where they may cause unconsciousness and seizures). The first evidence of local anesthetic toxicity involves the nervous system, including agitation, confusion, dizziness, blurred vision, tinnitus, a metallic taste in the mouth, and nausea that can quickly progress to seizures and cardiovascular collapse. Direct infiltration of local anesthetic into skeletal muscle will cause temporary paralysis of the muscle. Toxicity can occur with any local anesthetic in terms of an individual reaction by a particular patient. Possible toxicity can be tested with preoperative procedures to avoid toxic reactions during surgery. Table 28-1 lists steps to take in the event of a local anesthetic overdose.

Paresthesia

Paresthesia, or the sensation of feeling numb, is another complication of local anesthesia that can last for hours or days beyond the temporary numbness. Patients should be

---

TABLE 28-1 Management of Local Anesthetic Overdose

1.	Stop dental treatment immediately.
2.	Bring the patient to a supine position.
3.	Supplement oxygen if needed, and clear the airway passage.
4.	Call emergency medical services (EMS).
5.	If seizures occur, protect the patient from injury, but avoid any restraining.
6.	Keep monitoring and recording the vital signs.
7.	Provide cardiopulmonary resuscitation (CPR)/basic life support (BLS), if needed.

advised not to bite their tongue, cheek, or lip while numb. The patient may feel the numb areas as swollen even though they are not, and the patient may complain that the lip feels "fat" or "heavy." The dental assistant can play an important role in educating patients about how the numbness is temporary and will wear off.

Paresthesia can be the result of trauma to the nerve sheath during injection, or hemorrhage into or around the nerve sheath. Paresthesia is usually temporary, but severe damage to the nerve may result in permanent loss of sensation.

Hematoma

Damage to blood vessels around the injection site can result in a hematoma (blood swelling or bruising). It is usually caused by blunt impact, in which the capillaries are damaged, allowing blood to seep into the surrounding tissue. Hematomas often induce pain but are not normally dangerous. Minor bruises are easily recognized by their characteristic blue or purple color in the days following the injury. People also vary in the sturdiness of their capillaries; some people bruise more easily than others. A vitamin C deficiency can make a person more susceptible to bruising.

The treatment for light bruises is minimal. Severe swelling might be reduced by applying ice or by elevating the affected area, if possible.

Trismus

Sudden movement by the patient or use of an incorrect injection technique can sometimes result in damage to the muscles of mastication, which can cause lockjaw, or trismus. The condition usually resolves on its own in 10 to 14 days, during which time eating and oral hygiene are compromised.

The application of heat through a heat bag applied extraorally and gargling with warm saltwater may help ease the severity and duration of the condition.

Why might a dentist decide that a patient needs an extraction?

Electronic Anesthesia

Electronic anesthesia is a noninvasive form of pain control and has low to moderate levels of success. The system blocks pain electronically by using a low current of electricity. Two small sponges or contact pads are placed in the patient's mouth or on the face. These are attached to a control box that the patient uses to select the depth of anesthesia. The sensation felt is a pulsing itch, which can also be described as a mild tingle or twitch. In electronic anesthesia, the patient does not feel the intense numb "fat lip" of local anesthesia. Once the machine is turned on, it takes about two minutes to achieve numbness.

The administration of electronic anesthesia starts with the seating of the patient and positioning of the contact pads on the back of each hand. The site of injection is isolated and dried. A third pad, known as the intraoral receptor, is attached to the lingual side, about 3 to 5 mm from the gingival margin. The patient is instructed to control the activation unit by pressing the control button and gradually increasing the level of the electric current to the level at which the pain is blocked.

Advantages of electronic anesthesia are as follows: the patient receives no injection, the patient controls the level of anesthesia, the patient gets back to normal quickly when the appointment is over, and there is no residual numbness or slurred speech. In addition, there are no risks of an allergic reaction because no chemical is injected and no "shot" is given. Because no needles or cartridges are involved, there is no risk of cross-contamination.

Inhalation Sedation

Inhalation sedation is a type of conscious sedation. Inhalation sedation is also known as laughing gas, relative analgesia (RA), happy gas, gas, nitrous, nitrous oxide, and N_2O/O_2. Inhalation sedation with nitrous oxide (N_2O) and oxygen (O_2) has been described as representing the most nearly "ideal" clinical sedative circumstance. It is colorless, sweet smelling, and nonirritating. It was discovered by Joseph Priestly in 1772. Dr. Horace Wells first used it on his patients in 1884.

Inhalation sedation can be used on patients who are anxious, gagging, or in need of pain relief; for dental procedures where local anesthetic would normally be needed; and for lengthy procedures in a medically compromised patient. Patients who are not good candidates for this type of sedation include patients with respiratory problems, pregnant patients, and those who exhibit psychiatric disorders.

Disadvantages of this type of sedation are the cost of the equipment and chronic exposure complications that can result in problems such as kidney and liver damage.

Cultural Considerations

Dental anxiety is sometimes a shared family experience. Whether it is just an episode of sweaty palms or acute anxiety, the fears and attitudes of parents can easily be passed along to children unintentionally. Sometimes it may be because people grew up without the technical advantages available today. Many times, the most painful part of a procedure is the anxiety a patient endures before even climbing into the chair. As a dental assistant, it is important to allow patients to discuss their fears and anxieties. A good listening ear can often go a long way in calming patient feelings.

To use this type of sedation in a dental office, the dentist, dental assistant, and hygienist must have received special training. An anesthesiologist or another specialist is not required. N_2O/O_2 sedation may be used with patients of all ages.

Equipment for Inhalation Sedation

The equipment needed for N_2O/O_2 inhalation sedation includes compressed gas cylinders, reducing valves (regulators), which are used to control the flow of each gas, pressure gauges, and flow meters. Flow meters indicate the rate and flow of gas and stop the oxygen level from falling below 30% (2.5 to 3.0 liters per minute). The equipment also includes a reservoir bag that combines nitrous oxide and oxygen gases that the patient inhales from the bag. The conducting tubing carries the gases from the reservoir bag to the mask on the nosepiece. Masks are also known as nosepieces and nasal inhalers that allow the patient to inhale the gases (Figure 28.9). Masks are available in adult and children sizes. The masks may be disposable and thrown away after a single use, or they may be made of rubber and can be sterilized or disinfected after every use.

The dental office may have built-in N_2O/O_2 systems in the treatment area (Figure 28.10), or they may have portable units that can be moved from room to room as needed (Figure 28.11). The cylinder stores the nitrous oxide/oxide gas combinations in equilibrium at 650 to 900 pounds per square inch. The cylinders or tanks and the hoses attached to them are color coded blue for nitrous oxide and green for oxygen. (White color coding is used for O_2 in some countries other than the United States.) The cylinders are stored in an upright position, away from heat, and they are chained to the wall (or portable unit) to prevent them from falling on the valve stem, which could cause an explosion (Figure 28.12).

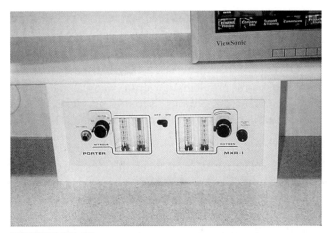

FIGURE 28.10
Nitrous oxide system stabilized as part of the dental system.
Image courtesy Instructional Materials for the Dental Team, Lex., KY

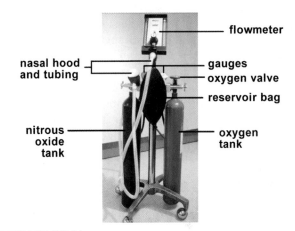

FIGURE 28.11
Portable nitrous oxide system.
Image courtesy Instructional Materials for the Dental Team, Lex., KY

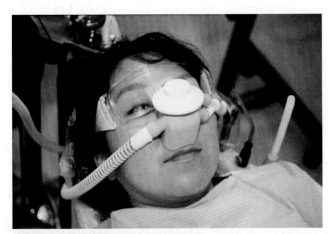

FIGURE 28.9
Nasal mask used for inhalation.
Image courtesy Instructional Materials for the Dental Team, Lex., KY

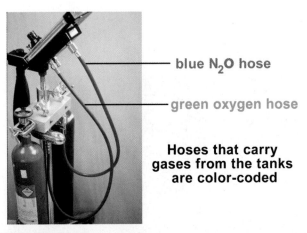

FIGURE 28.12
Nitrous oxide lines are color-coded blue, and oxygen gas lines are color coded green.
Image courtesy Instructional Materials for the Dental Team, Lex., KY

Safety and Precautions: Scavenger Systems

Some of the common complications resulting from N_2O/O_2 inhalation are excessive perspiration, expectoration, behavioral problems, shivering, nausea, and vomiting. Extreme precautions should be taken when administrating N_2O/O_2 inhalation anesthesia. The dental assistant must always make sure that there are no leaks in the hoses or the valves of the cylinders. Patients must be advised not to talk while inhaling the gas mixture because this may make the mask move and some of the gas may escape, which could lessen the effect of the anesthesia. The escaping gas could also be breathed in by the attending dental team.

Where possible, use 100% clean outdoor air for dental operatory ventilation. Supply and exhaust vents should be well separated to allow good mixing and prevent "short-circuiting." A local exhaust hood should be placed near the patient's mouth to capture excess N_2O. An effective anesthetic gas scavenging system can be used because it traps waste gases at the site of overflow from the breathing circuit and disposes these gases to the outside atmosphere (Figure 28.13). The dental team must vent the gas outside the building and use an N_2O monitoring system. An elevation in risk of spontaneous abortion among female dental staff is observed among those who worked with nitrous oxide for three or more hours per week in offices not using scavenging equipment.

While using a scavenging system, the operator must select scavenging masks of proper sizes to fit patients. Prudent use of N_2O to appropriately sedate patients is encouraged. The operator must also monitor the air concentration of N_2O to ensure controls are effective in achieving low levels during dental operations. The scavenger systems should have an evacuation flow rate of 45 liters per minute and incorporate a nasal mask or hood. Another very important point to understand is that nitrous oxide/oxygen should only be used during patient treat-ment and must not be administered unnecessarily or used for recreational purposes that could lead to substance abuse. It is also recommended that N_2O concentration must not be greater than 50% in routine cases so the patient will still be awake and aware of his or her surroundings.

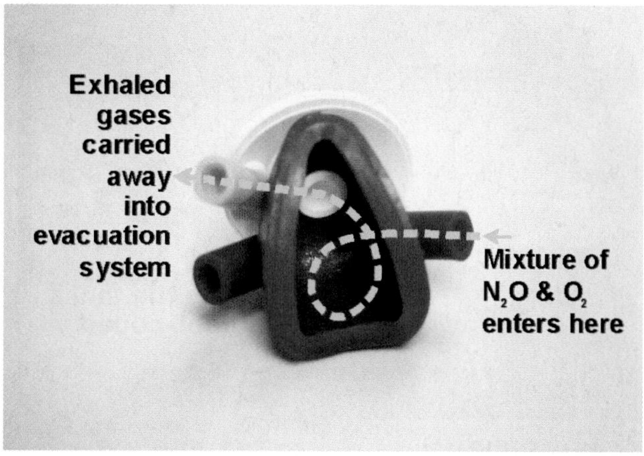

Medical Assessment and Monitoring

The operator must always review the patient's medical history before initiating nitrous oxide analgesia. Patients with chronic pulmonary disease should have a physician consultation prior to N_2O exposure. Because of the expansive nature of nitrous oxide gas, it is not recommended for use in patients with bowel obstructions or middle ear disturbances. In case of retinal reattachment surgery (required to prevent irreversible total loss of vision), modern vitreoretinal techniques are used. These utilize intraocular gases as tamponading (stopping blood) agents. These gases may persist in the eye for up to three months after surgery. During this period, the use of nitrous oxide will cause the intraocular gas bubble to expand, which can result in increases in intraocular pressure. It is suggested that patients who have had retinal reattachment surgery should carry cards giving details of possible complications of intraocular gas. When the N_2O flow is stopped and the gas begins to leave the body, a negative pressure results, possibly leading to complications in the ear, nose, and throat, especially after recent infections or inflammation. The sedative effects of nitrous oxide may enhance medications that produce sleep or lethargy, either directly or indirectly.

The vital signs of blood pressure, pulse, and respiration should be recorded before, during, and after the administration of N_2O/O_2 analgesia. The preoperative readings provide a baseline that can be compared against the intraoperative and postoperative readings. The postoperative readings provide an opportunity to confirm the patient's recovery or identify adverse responses.

It is important to obtain the patient's informed consent before administering N_2O/O_2 analgesia. The patient should be given enough information about the risks, benefits, and alternatives to nitrous oxide to make an informed, reasoned decision about whether or not to proceed with its use. The operator must explain the proper use of the mask as well as proper nasal breathing. The operator must also discuss the process of anesthesia and the sensations of warmth and tingling that the patient may experience. The patient should be reassured that he or she will remain aware, conscious, and in control of his or her actions.

FIGURE 28.13
Scavenger system attached to nitrous oxide mask.
Image courtesy Instructional Materials for the Dental Team, Lex., KY

N_2O/O_2 Sedation

N_2O/O_2 inhalation has rapid onset and rapid peak effect. The administration of gases begins with introducing 100% oxygen and then slowly introducing N_2O until the

Procedure 28-4 Assisting in the Administration and Monitoring of Nitrous Oxide/Oxygen Sedation

Equipment and Supplies Needed

- N_2O/O_2 inhalation system tanks
- Inhalation masks with scavenging system (adult and child sizes)
- Blood pressure cuff
- Pulse rate tester
- Body temperature testing strip

Procedure Steps

A. PREPARING THE EQUIPMENT AND PATIENT

1. Read patient's history.

2. Wash hands and don gloves.

3. Wait for the dentist's permission.

4. Select the size of mask for patient after dentist's consent.

5. Check all parts of the equipment for any leakage and smooth flow.

6. Seat patient, update medical history, and take all vital signs.

7. Explain to the patient the use of nitrous oxide and what to expect. Answer all patient questions in easy and clear English.

8. Have the patient sign an informed consent form.

9. Place the patient in the supine position.

10. Instruct the patient not to talk while inhaling the anesthetic agents because leaks and inadequate anesthesia may result.

11. Place the mask on the patient and adjust accordingly. Tighten the tubing so it is comfortable on the patient.

12. If mask feels uncomfortable to the patient, place a 2×2 gauze square under the edge of the mask.

B. ASSISTING WITH ADMINISTRATION OF NITROUS OXIDE INHALATION

1. When the dentist instructs, adjust the flow meter for the oxygen (O_2) only and release the control knob of the green cylinder with O_2. The patient is given 100% oxygen for one minute.

2. When the dentist instructs, adjust the N_2O flow in increments of 0.5 to 1 L/min, while reducing the O_2 by the same increments.

3. Repeat this process at one-minute intervals until you reach the patient's baseline reading. (*Note:* The patient will start feeling relaxed and slightly sedated.)

4. Record the patient's baseline level, while monitoring the patient's reaction throughout the procedure and also recording all the vital signs.

C. ASSISTING WITH OXYGENATION

1. Toward the end of the procedure, N_2O is reduced in the same increments as it was increased. The goal is to have 100% oxygen at the end of the procedure.

2. Let the patient breathe 100% oxygen for a minimum of five minutes in order to avoid diffusion hypoxia (the feeling of light-headedness).

3. After completion of oxygenation, remove the mask from the patient's nose and place the patient upright slowly because a sudden change of position may cause postural hypotension (fainting).

4. Record the patient's baseline level of N_2O and O_2 and also note the patient's response to the analgesia. (*Note:* This recording acts as a reference for future care and is an important legal document.)

D. DISMISSING THE PATIENT

1. Check the vital signs and do not let the patient leave until all vital signs are within normal range. (*Note:* If possible, the patient should be accompanied by a family member.)

2. To confirm if the patient is fully conscious, the Trieger test can be performed.

3. Record all postanesthesia observations and vital signs in the patient's file.

---

desired mix of N_2O/O_2 is achieved and the patient begins to feel the effects. The administrator must keep an eye on the flow meter and pressure gauges to check on flow of gases.

The desired N_2O/O_2 mix is fed through a tube to which a nasal mask is attached. This mask is put over the nose of the patient and the patient is asked to breathe normally through the nose. The operator may begin with administering 20% N_2O and then increase it by 10% every 60 seconds until the desired effects are observed. The process is completed by administering 100% of oxygen again for three to five minutes near the end of the procedure. This helps to reverse the effects of the nitrous oxide as well as completely remove the gas from the body.

The dental assistant can calculate the concentration of N_2O or O_2 agent simply by dividing the agent flow rate by the total flow rate of both gases added together, and multiplying by 100 to find percentage of either gas. Consider this example: The flow rate of oxygen is 6 liters per minute (L/min); for nitrous oxide it is 3 L/min. So the total flow rate will be 9 L/min. The nitrous oxide concentration will be 3/9 multiplied by 100 = 33% nitrous oxide concentration.

In modern machines there is a type of "double mask" where the outside mask is connected to a vacuum machine to suck away the waste gas. The new masks are available in different colors, designs, and sizes and also come with pleasant fragrances such as vanilla, strawberry, and mint. The twin tubes running to the mask are for "gas in" and "gas out." The "gas out" line is attached to the vacuum machine, and the "gas in" line is attached to the relative analgesia machine. The patient breathes out through a one-way valve in the inner mask, and the exhaust gas is collected inside the outer gray mask and sucked into the vacuum machine.

At the beginning of the sedation, some patients will feel light-headed or dizzy; later a tingling sensation can occur in the arms, legs, or oral cavity. At this tingling stage, some of the dental procedures can be performed. Most of the dental procedures are performed when the patient reaches the feeling of warmth, floating, or heaviness. If the drug is overintroduced, the patient may experience nausea, vomiting, or unconsciousness.

Most patients recover adequately enough to permit their discharge from the office without an escort. Vital signs of the patient at the time of discharge should be confirmed.

Patients using nitrous oxide have been known to experience hallucinations or dreams, including those of a sexual nature. Whether real or imagined, such experiences may induce a patient to file not only a malpractice claim, but also criminal charges. To protect against false accusations of sexual misconduct, a staff member must be in the operatory at all times, including during emergency after-hours visits. Never leave a patient unattended while administering nitrous oxide analgesia (Procedure 28-4).

In which type of patients is nitrous oxide/oxygen anesthesia most beneficial?

Antianxiety Agents

Various drugs, such as diazepam, are useful in the treatment of anxiety and are helpful in reducing anxiety without causing excessive sedation. These agents have no analgesic properties. Antianxiety agents or anxiolytics are used in the management of various forms of anxiety, including generalized anxiety disorder (GAD). Antianxiety

Patient Education

Many people are fearful of dental procedures. This fear may be related to bad dental experiences in the past. Good communication is a strong tool that a dental assistant and dentist can use to ease patients' concerns. Technology, new procedures, and some very sophisticated approaches to dental anesthesia have all contributed to pain-free dentistry, from cleaning to cavity preparations to root canals. The dental team can explain the diagnosis and the procedure to the patient in detail and answer all questions to patients' satisfaction and also discuss information about the latest pain control and antianxiety agents available and how painless dentistry can be performed.

agents can be used as sedatives in many situations including for fearful patients, for a long or difficult procedure, or when patients who are mentally challenged are receiving treatment. They are also used in very young children undergoing extensive treatment. These medications should not be used on women who are pregnant or lactating.

Antianxiety agents can be given orally, intravenously, or by inhalation, but they are generally prescribed as premedication to patients. Patients typically take these medications 30 to 60 minutes prior to treatment. The dental assistant must inform the patient about the possible side effects, which include drowsiness; therefore, the patient must be advised not to drive but instead be escorted by a friend or a family member.

Intravenous Sedation

Intravenous regional anesthesia was first described by August Bier in 1908. This technique is still in use today and is remarkably safe. In dentistry, IV sedation is usually used for extensive oral surgeries and periodontal procedures. Before administration of IV sedation analgesia, a total patient assessment should take place. A physical examination is performed along with updating the patient's medical history. Patients are required to sign an informed consent. A parent or guardian's permission is needed for children up to 18 years of age.

The weight of the patient is determined for dosage calculations. Before surgery, a canula is inserted into a vein of the hand or arm to give fluids, anesthetics, antibiotics, or pain medications. Pain relievers, such as opioids, are usually injected into the IV at regular intervals. Most hospitals offer patient-controlled analgesia (PCA), a system that allows patients to give themselves a fixed dose of a medication by pushing a button. This way the patient does not have to ask the nurse for each dose of pain medicine. Through IV sedation the patient can maintain the ability to keep an open airway and respond to verbal or physical stimulation. After surgery, the doctor may keep the IV catheter in place to deliver pain medications while the patient is in the hospital or outpatient recovery room.

Oral and maxillofacial surgeons and periodontists who have undergone intensive training on its use and operation use this type of anesthesia. General dentists who have gone through an accredited residency program and are approved by their respective state dental boards, based on the regulations, may also use IV sedation in a general dental office. Some specialty offices may have trained nurses who assist in the administering and monitoring of IV sedation. Monitoring includes evaluating the patient's level of consciousness, respiratory function, oximetry, blood pressure, heart rate, and cardiac rhythm throughout the procedure. A defibrillator, supplemental oxygen, and suction are kept available in case they are needed in an emergency.

What should a dental assistant note on the patient's record regarding premedications and IV sedation?

General Anesthesia

In modern health practice, general anesthesia is a state of total unconsciousness resulting from general anesthetic drugs. The anesthetist (anesthesiologist) selects the optimal technique for each patient and procedure. General anesthesia is a complex procedure and involves preanesthetic assessment, administration of general anesthetic drugs, cardiorespiratory monitoring, analgesia, airway management, fluid management, and postoperative pain relief. General anesthesia for dental procedures is typically provided in a hospital operating room.

Documentation of Anesthesia and Pain Control

When an anesthetic agent is administered to a patient, the dental assistant documents the information in the patients chart. The documentation includes preoperative and postoperative vital signs, tidal volume if using inhalation sedation, time when anesthesia began and ended, the type and quantity of anesthetic agent used, number of cartridges used, the peak concentration administered such as "1 × 2% Marcaine with epi 1:100,000," the minutes required by the patient to recover after surgery, and adverse reactions or patient complaints. The dental assistant also records complete details on the patient's condition after recovery. All of these records are maintained in a patient's official file. All information for inhalation anesthesia must be recorded in the progress notes section of the patient record or on a separate nitrous oxide sedation form.

SUMMARY

It is important for the dental team to understand patient concerns and fears related to dental procedures. Effective communication skills are good tools for reducing these fears. A variety of pain control techniques are used in dentistry. Scientists have been doing research for centuries to find better and easier ways of pain control, starting with the use of cocaine and today heading toward the painless dentistry offered by new and improved alternative pain control methods. It is important for a dental assistant to have knowledge about all of the types of anesthesia used in dentistry, the materials used, and how to transfer instruments and operate equipment. It is the responsibility of the dental assistant to use good communication skills and have up-to-date knowledge about the types of anesthetics, their use, and how to avoid complications.

KEY TERMS

- **Analgesic:** Diverse group of drugs used to relieve pain; also known as *painkillers*.   p. 422
- **Anesthetic:** Medication that produces the temporary loss of feeling or sensation.   p. 422
- **Anxiety:** A physiological state characterized by cognitive, somatic, emotional, and behavioral components including fear, apprehension, or worry.   p. 422
- **Duration:** The lasting effect of an anesthetic agent.   p. 425
- **Induction:** The time from injection to the time when complete anesthesia is achieved.   p. 425

- **Infiltration:** A type of local anesthesia in which the anesthetic solution is injected directly into the gingival and alveolar tissue sites to numb the nerve endings in the area.   p. 425
- **Pain:** Defined by the International Association for the Study of Pain as "an unpleasant sensory and emotional experience associated with actual or potential tissue damage, or described in terms of such damage."   p. 422
- **Vasoconstrictor:** Type of drug that constricts blood vessels; used to prolong anesthetic action and to control bleeding.   p. 424

CHECK YOUR UNDERSTANDING

1. Which type of topical anesthetic solution is more likely to be used for an infiltration injection?
   a. spray anesthetic
   b. infiltration anesthetic
   c. patch anesthetic
   d. gel anesthetic

2. Which of the following is an example of a pain reliever that is a nonnarcotic medication?
   a. amides and esters
   b. morphine
   c. ibuprofen
   d. polysaccharides

3. Relaxation and sedation without loss of consciousness is known as
   a. anesthesia.
   b. analgesia.
   c. paresthesia.
   d. hypnosis.

4. Which of the following techniques is used for individual tooth anesthesia?
   a. infiltration
   b. block
   c. intravenous sedation
   d. general anesthesia

5. The ability to withstand pain varies from patient to patient and is known as one's
   a. threshold of pain.
   b. angioplasty.
   c. unstable angina.
   d. hypokinetic.

6. What needle length is typically used when giving infiltration anesthesia?
   a. 0.5 inch
   b. 1 inch
   c. 1½ inches
   d. 1⅝ inches

7. What type of solution do the numbers on the anesthetic cartridge 1:100,000 indicate?
   a. salt
   b. local anesthetic agent
   c. epinephrine
   d. analgesic

8. The higher the number of gauge the _____ the needle.
   a. thicker
   b. thinner
   c. fatter
   d. more useful

9. Vasoconstrictor is a type of drug that
   a. constricts blood vessels.
   b. dilates blood vessels.
   c. reduces blood vessels.
   d. none of the above.

10. Which is the abnormal feeling that can occur after anesthesia has worn off?
    a. pain
    b. allergy
    c. paresthesia
    d. trismus

INTERNET ACTIVITIES

- Learn about painless injection with the WAND II at www.youtube.com/watch?v=w0CqvMvRbsk
- To learn about laser procedures, visit http://video .google.com/videoplay?docid=200084437784450741

5&q=dental+anesthesia&total=68&start=0&num= 10&so=0&type=search&plindex=7

WEB REFERENCES

- American Dental Association: Anesthesia www.ada.org/public/topics/anesthesia_faq.asp
- American Dental Association: Anesthesia for the Dental Visit www.ada.org/prof/resources/pubs/jada/ patient/patient_06.pdf
- American Dental Board of Anesthesiology www.adba.org/index.html
- American Society of Regional Anesthesia and Pain Medicine www.asra.com/
- American Society of Dentist Anesthesiologists www.asdahq.org/
- Dental Sedation Teachers Group: Conscious Sedation www.dstg.co.uk/teaching/conc-sed/
- Ohio State University College of Dentistry www.dent.ohio-state.edu/anesthesiology/faculty.php
- OSHA: Anesthetic Gases: Guidelines for Workplace Exposures www.osha.gov/dts/osta/ anestheticgases/index.html#I
- UCLA: Relief of Pain and Suffering www.library.ucla.edu/biomed/his/painexhibit/panel1.htm

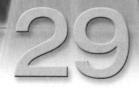

Dental Radiography

Chapter Outline

- Discovery of X-Radiation
  - —Pioneers of Dental Radiography
  - —History of the Cathode Tube

- Radiation Physics
  - —Atomic Structure
  - —Ionization
  - —Electromagnetic Radiation

- The Dental X-Ray Unit
  - —Control Panel
  - —Extension Arm
  - —Tube Head
  - —X-Ray Tube

- Production of X-Rays
  - —Types of Radiation

- Radiation Effects
  - —Somatic and Genetic Effects
  - —Radiation Effects on Critical Organs

- Radiation Measurement
  - —Maximum Permissible Dose

- Radiation Safety
  - —Patient Protection
  - —Operator Protection

- Controlling Radiation
  - —Electricity

- Radiation Image Characteristics
  - —Radiopacity and Radiolucency
  - —Density
  - —Contrast

Learning Objectives

After reading this chapter, the student should be able to:

- Explain how x-radiation was discovered.
- Describe ionization.
- Identify three conditions necessary to produce radiation.
- Recognize the components of the dental x-ray unit and the glass envelope.
- Determine the effects of radiation.
- Define the ALARA concept.
- Relate the protocol for protecting the patient and operator during exposure.
- Explain radiation-controlling factors.
- Describe density and contrast and determine their effects on radiographs.

Preparing for Certification Exams

- Recall electromagnetic radiations.
- List the characteristic properties of x-rays.
- Identify the components of the x-ray tube necessary in the production of x-rays.
- Explain radiation effects and safety.
- Examine radiographic exposure variables.
- Differentiate between primary and secondary radiation.

Key Terms

ALARA concept	Milliampere (mA)
Anode	Photon
Atom	Primary radiation
Cathode	Radiograph
Contrast	Radiolucent areas
Density	Radiopaque areas
Electromagnetic radiation	Scatter radiation
Frequency	Secondary radiation
Ion	Tungsten target
Ionization	Wavelength
Ionizing radiation	X-radiation (X-ray)
Leakage radiation	

One of the primary functions of a dental assistant is to expose, develop, and mount radiographs. A **radiograph** is a recorded image on photographic film. In dentistry the radiograph is vital to diagnosing patients' dental conditions by making it possible for the dentist to view the tissues and surrounding structures that cannot be seen by the human eye. Before dental assistants begin exposing, developing, and mounting radiographs, however, they should understand the history of radiography and the basics of how it works. This information assists dental assistants in understanding how x-rays are produced, risk factors, and techniques for protecting patients as well as themselves.

Discovery of X-Radiation

On November 8, 1895, while experimenting with a glass vacuum tube, Wilhelm Conrad Roentgen (Figure 29.1) discovered **x-radiation.** The glass tube consisted of electrical circuits, a cathode, and an anode. Roentgen, a professor of physics at the University of Wurzburg in Germany, was studying an unusual glow emitted from the glass tube when he made the remarkable discovery that forever changed science and medicine.

During his experiments, Roentgen used screens covered with a material that glowed when exposed to the rays being produced by the cathode tube. He continued to experiment with the mysterious glow and noted that some of the screens that were located beyond where the glow ended were fluorescing. Roentgen realized that something from the tube must be striking the screens. He surmised that the fluorescence was from a mysterious ray coming from the glass tube. He coined this mysterious ray an **x-ray,** with the "x" meaning "unknown." Roentgen contin-

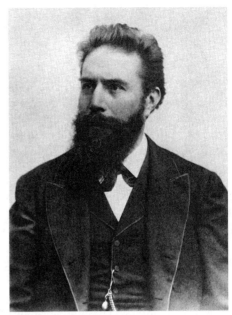

FIGURE 29.1
Wilhelm Conrad Roentgen.

ued experimenting with the unknown ray for several weeks and decided to replace the screens with photographic plates. He would place objects in the ray's path to the photographic plate and then develop the plates. He realized that images could be recorded on photographic plates. Roentgen eventually placed his wife's hand on the photographic plate and exposed it to the rays for 15 minutes. When he developed the plate he could see the image of the bones in her hand (Figure 29.2). This was the first radiograph of the human body. Roentgen later won the Nobel Peace Prize for his discoveries in radiation.

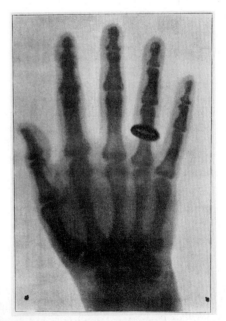

FIGURE 29.2
First human radiograph of hand.
Private Collection/The Bridgeman Art Library

Dental Assistant **PROFESSIONAL TIP**

A large portion of the dental assistant's responsibility is exposing radiographs. It is not only of major importance that dental assistants follow safety protocols during radiation exposure, it is their responsibility. Part of this responsibility requires dental assistants to fully understand the risks involved in this area of their occupation. It is beneficial for all dental professionals to periodically review the safety protocols associated with radiation exposure for the safety of their patients as well as their own.

How does the discovery made by Roentgen affect modern medical and dental practices?

Pioneers of Dental Radiography

The use of x-rays in the dental field quickly became a reality after Roentgen's discovery. The news of his discovery traveled fast, and just two weeks after Roentgen's discovery, the first dental radiograph was taken by Dr. Otto Walkhoff, a German dentist. Walkhoff used a small photographic plate covered in black paper and rubber, and placed it in his own mouth for a 25-minute exposure time. A New York physician, W. J. Morton, produced the first dental x-ray in the United States, on a skull. He also lectured on the usefulness of x-rays in dentistry. Dr. Edmond Kells, a New Orleans dentist, was the first dentist to expose radiographs on a live patient. Dr. Kells, unaware of the adverse affects of overexposure to radiation, used his own hands to determine the adjustment of the primary beam. Initially he experienced pain and redness on his hands, but continued to expose them to radiation. He eventually lost three fingers, his hand, arm, and ultimately his life to overexposure. Dr. William Rollins, a Boston dentist, developed the first dental x-ray unit. During his experimentation with x-rays, Dr. Rollins suffered burns to his hands. This sparked his interest in radiation protection and he eventually published a paper on the dangers associated with radiation.

History of the Cathode Tube

Long before the discovery of radiation, many inventors had experimented with the cathode tube. In 1855 Heinrich Geissler, a German glass blower, developed the first cathode tube. The cathode tube was developed as a way to study luminescence. This was accomplished by using a glass vacuum tube with positive and negative electrodes. When current was passed through the tube, a glow or luminescence appeared.

The cathode tube in which this luminescence was viewed was improved over the years. Johann Hittorf, who used the tube to study fluorescence, realized that the rays that were produced grew in straight lines. He also noted that the rays produced heat and gave off a green glow. Eugen Goldstein of Germany named the rays *cathode rays*.

In 1870 Sir William Crookes and Johann Hittorf redesigned the vacuum tube. Crookes realized that the cathode rays were streams of charged particles. On further study of the streams of charged particles, Joseph Thompson identified the negatively charged particles orbiting an atom as electrons. In 1894 Philip Lenard, while conducting his own experiments, projected cathode rays out of the glass tube. He noted that the cathode rays could penetrate aluminum foil and travel up to one centimeter. When Roentgen later made his discovery in 1895, he was using the Crookes-Hittorf cathode tube. A modern dental x-ray tube is shown in Figure 29.3.

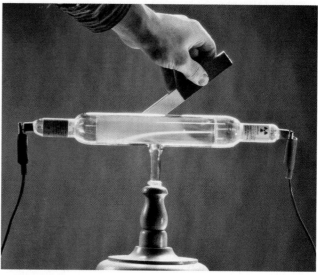

FIGURE 29.3
Crookes tube or cathode ray tube.

Radiation Physics

For the dental radiographer to fully grasp the concepts of x-ray production, it is important to understand basic atomic structure. Our world is composed of matter and energy. Energy results when matter is changed. Matter exists in three states:

- Gas
- Liquid
- Solid

Atomic Structure

The **atom** is the most basic structure of all matter and is composed of two basic parts: the nucleus and electrons (Figure 29.4). The nucleus is the center portion of an atom and is composed of protons that have a positive charge and neutrons that have no charge. As noted previously, electrons are tiny negatively charged particles that orbit the shell of an electron. The number of protons, neutrons, and electrons varies depending on the type of atom. An atom can have as many as seven shells, each containing electrons.

Ionization

Atoms may exist in either a neutral or unstable state. In a neutral state an atom contains the same number of protons as electrons. The gain or loss of electrons from the atom creates an unstable atom known as an **ion**. An unstable atom will attempt to commandeer electrons from nearby atoms. **Ionization** is the process through which electrons are lost from the orbit of an atom, rendering it unstable and thus creating an ion (Figure 29.5). **Ionizing radiation** can be described as radiation that is

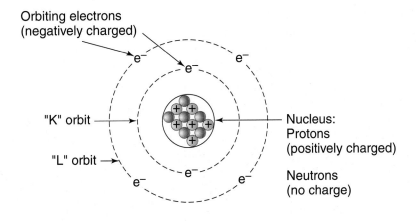

FIGURE 29.4
Diagram of a carbon atom.

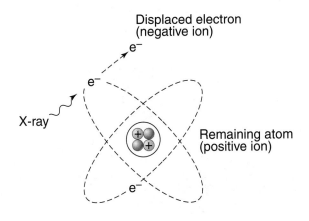

FIGURE 29.5
Ionization occurs when the electron is removed from the atom.

capable of producing ions by adding or removing electrons from the shell of an atom. Ionizing radiation causes adverse biological effects in human cells; therefore, all safety protocols must be followed to keep exposures as low as reasonably achievable.

Electromagnetic Radiation

Electromagnetic radiation is the production of a wavelike energy through space and matter, such as gamma rays, visible light rays, and radio waves. Forms of electromagnetic energy share some similar properties and are groups of energy referred to as photons. **Photons,** also called units of light energy, have no mass or weight and travel in waves at the speed of light (186,000 miles per second) in straight lines.

A **wavelength** is the distance between the crests or high point of the waves. **Frequency** refers to the number of wavelengths passing through a fixed point for a given period of time. Amplitude is the height or size of these waves. The frequency ultimately determines energy: When the frequency is great, wavelengths are short and energy is high. When the frequency is low, wavelengths are long and energy is low. An example of this is radio waves versus x-radiation. Radio waves have low frequency and less energy, and x-radiation waves have high frequency and great energy. Figure 29.6 shows the electromagnetic spectrum for various types of rays as well as a variety of familiar sources of exposure to those rays.

Are people only exposed to radiation in a dental or medical office? Where else might exposure occur?

The Dental X-Ray Unit

The dental x-ray unit used to produce radiation in the dental office is composed of three primary parts: the control panel, the extension arm, and the tube head.

Control Panel

The control panel of the dental x-ray unit contains settings that control the amount of radiation produced, length of time it is produced, and the force that moves the radiation (Figure 29.7). It also contains the exposure button and an indicator light. The details of these control settings are discussed later in this chapter.

Extension Arm

The extension arm is the portion of the dental x-ray unit that supports the tube head and houses the electrical wires that supply the tube head (Figure 29.8).

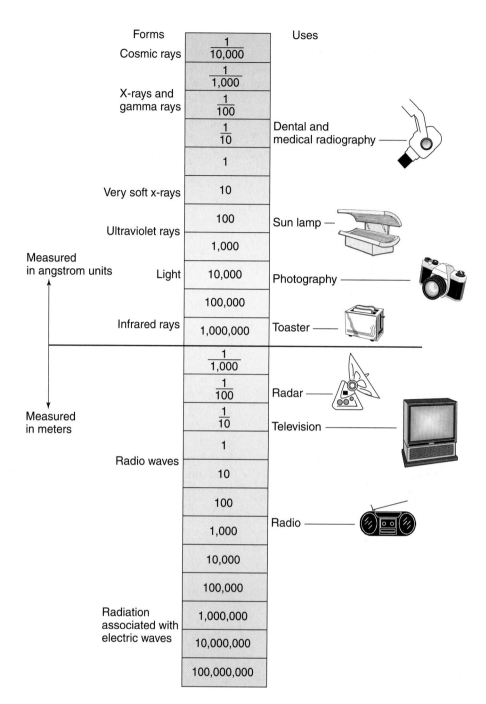

FIGURE 29.6
Electromagnetic spectrum showing where x-rays and other types of rays fall on the spectrum, along with familiar sources of those rays.

Legal and Ethical Issues

Professionals in the dental field must be knowledgeable about their own state dental practice act. The state dental practice act outlines regulations as they pertain to dental professionals in their home state. For example, most states require that personnel taking radiographs must be 18 years of age and that only a dentist may prescribe radiographs for a patient. Knowing the requirements of one's own state will clarify what a dental assistant can legally do or not do as part of his or her job description.

Tube Head

The tube head itself houses the components that make radiation possible and also contains features to ensure the safety of the patient as well as the operator:

- A metal housing makes up the outer portion of the tube head. The metal housing is tightly sealed to prevent radiation leakage. It contains the x-ray tube and transformers, as well as the insulating oil.

- The insulating oil surrounds the x-ray tube and transformers, preventing overheating by neutralizing the heat produced during x-ray production.

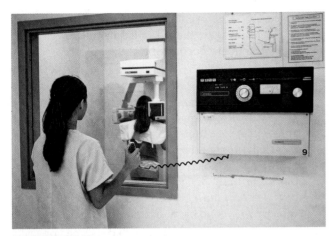

FIGURE 29.7
Control panel.
Jennifer Thomas/Ann Poindexter

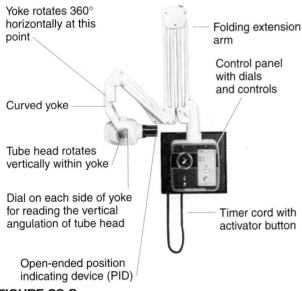

Yoke rotates 360°
horizontally at this
point

Folding extension
arm

Control panel
with dials
and controls

Curved yoke

Tube head rotates
vertically within yoke

Dial on each side of yoke
for reading the vertical
angulation of tube head

Timer cord with
activator button

Open-ended position
indicating device (PID)

FIGURE 29.8
Dental x-ray unit.

- The x-ray tube is the vacuum, sealed glass envelope situated in the metal housing. The glass envelope is the primary component of x-ray production.
- Transformers in the tube head serve to alter the current coming into the x-ray tube head.
- The position-indicating device (PID) is the opening in the tube head that extends away from the body of the tube head itself. The PID is a portal in which x-rays exit the tube head. It is the portion of the tube head that is placed over the area to be exposed. The PID may be round or rectangular. The rectangular PID is preferred because it restricts the primary beam more than the round PID, thus exposing the patient to less radiation.

X-Ray Tube

The x-ray tube or glass envelope houses the necessary components that make the production of x-rays possible. The glass tube is devoid of air, creating a vacuum to pro-

mote the flow of electrons within the tube. This glass itself is leaded to prevent x-rays from exiting the tube except for one small, window area positioned toward the PID. Figure 29.9 illustrates a typical dental x-ray tube.

Cathode

The **cathode** is a negative electrode situated within the glass envelope. The function of the cathode is the production of electrons. The filament portion of the cathode is a coiled wire made of tungsten that serves to produce electrons. The cathode contains a focusing cup made of molybdenum (a hard, heavy metallic substance) that directs the electrons away from the cathode to the opposite electrode, called the anode.

Anode

The **anode** is the positive electrode that sits opposite the cathode. The anode consists of a solid copper stem. Situated at the forefront of the copper stem is a plate of tungsten. The plate of tungsten is referred to as the **tungsten target** or focal spot. Tungsten is used because it has the ability to withstand a great deal of heat without melting. Copper has a low melting point and is not able to withstand the immediate heat created during x-ray production. The focal spot is the area of the anode where electrons are converted to x-rays. The copper stem serves to dissipate the residual heat after the initial production of x-rays.

Production of X-Rays

For x-ray production to occur, three important conditions are necessary:

1. *A source of electrons:* Electrons must be present to create x-rays. The source of electrons in the x-ray tube is the tungsten filament of the cathode. The dental x-ray unit is plugged into an electrical outlet, and the incoming electricity is directed to the filament. The filament then heats up and releases electrons

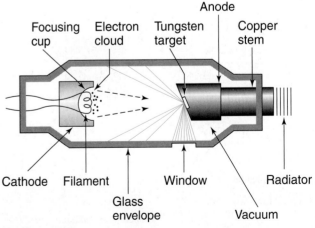

Focusing cup   Electron cloud   Anode   Tungsten target   Copper stem

Cathode   Filament   Window   Radiator

Glass envelope   Vacuum

FIGURE 29.9
Diagram of the tube head depicting x-ray production.

from the atoms of the tungsten filament. This process is known as thermionic emission.

2. *A means to speed up the electrons:* When the electrons are liberated from the tungsten filament, an electron cloud is formed. At this point, high voltage is applied to the cloud, which speeds up the electrons forcing them from the cathode to the anode.

3. *A method to stop the electrons:* When the electrons connect with the tungsten target, they are stopped suddenly. It is at this point that the kinetic energy of the high-speed electrons is converted to heat and x-rays; 99.8% is converted to heat and 0.2% is converted to x-rays. The heat generated is conducted away by the copper stem and the insulating oil of the tube head. Only the x-rays that pass through the unleaded portion of the glass envelope are allowed to leave the tube head.

Does the patient feel heat during radiograph exposure? Why or why not?

Types of Radiation

There are four main types of radiation (Figure 29.10):

1. **Primary radiation** is the initial radiation produced at the tungsten target. It exits the tube head via the window of the glass envelope and the PID. These x-rays are characteristically high-energy waves of great frequency and short wavelengths. These rays travel in straight lines until they collide with matter. Primary radiation is also referred to as the primary beam. This beam is directed to the area of the patient, such as a tooth, that needs to be viewed on a radiograph.

2. **Secondary radiation** occurs when the primary beam comes in contact with and passes through any type of matter. Once the primary beam passes through matter, the beam is weakened, making the wavelengths longer and the frequency of the waves lower.

3. **Scatter radiation** is a form of secondary radiation occurring once the primary beam has interacted with matter. After the primary has connected with matter, it deflects off the matter in different directions in straight lines. Scatter radiation will expose tissues other than those of the primary objective after the initial contact including the operator. Secondary radiation is the most dangerous to the operator. Proper safety protocol must be employed to prevent operator exposure to secondary radiation.

4. **Leakage radiation** is radiation that escapes or leaks out of the tube head. This type of radiation only serves to expose the patient or dental personnel to unnecessary radiation. Dental x-ray units must be inspected on a regular basis to ensure proper functioning without leakage. Each state mandates how often x-ray units should be inspected. The dentist or practice owner is responsible for maintenance and upkeep of x-ray equipment.

Radiation Effects

The cell is the basic structural unit or building block of all living organisms. Cells are complex structures composed of many different atoms and all are susceptible to the damaging effects of x-rays because, as discussed earlier, ionization causes changes in the makeup of atoms. Therefore, damage to a cell's atoms may result in disruption of cell division or death of the cell entirely and, hence, damage to the living organism.

Certain factors are involved when determining the damage incurred as a result of radiation exposure. The dose rate is one of those factors. Dose refers to the actual quantity of x-rays given off by the x-ray tube or the radiation source. The dose rate is the amount of radiation produced and administered during a given period of time and the amount of cell or tissue absorption. A higher dose of radiation causes greater cell damage than does a lower dose.

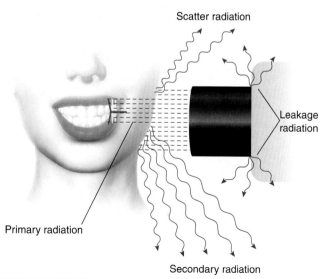

FIGURE 29.10
Types of radiation.

Cultural Considerations

Dental assistants encounter patients who are reluctant to have radiographs taken. A patient's reluctance can be due to any number of reasons and it is important that the dental assistant provide reassurance. Reassurance can come in the form of educating the patient on the necessity and importance of radiographs and on the efforts made to protect the patient from radiation exposure. Identify the safety measures such as use of a lead apron and thyroid collar. Also explain to the patient that the amount of radiation received during dental exposures is minimal.

Another factor is the area or volume of tissue exposed to x-rays. The larger the area exposed to radiation, the more vulnerable the tissues are to damage. Therefore, it is in the best interest of the patient to only expose those tissues under investigation.

Age is another important factor in determining the effects of radiation on living tissues. Children and pregnant women are especially sensitive to the biological effects of radiation.

Tissue sensitivity is a primary factor when considering the effects of radiation on living tissues. This is due to the fact that some tissues in the body are more sensitive to the effects of radiation than others. Cells that have a high threshold against the effects of radiation are referred to as *radioresistant*. Cells that are at greater risk from the effects of radiation are said to be *radiosensitive*. Radioresistant cells include bone, nerve, and muscle cells. Radiosensitive cells include reproductive cells, blood cells, and young bone cells. The cell with the greatest sensitivity to radiation is the lymphocyte, which is a type of white blood cell.

Somatic and Genetic Effects

All cells of the body are either somatic or genetic. Somatic cells are all cells in the body except the reproductive cells. Genetic cells are reproductive cells (sperm and ova). Exposure of the somatic cells to radiation can cause illness, such as cancer, leukemia, or cataracts, directly to the person who is exposed. Radiation trauma that causes changes in a person's genetic cells will not affect the individual exposed, but the individual may pass on genetic anomalies or defects to future generations.

Radiation Effects on Critical Organs

A critical organ is an organ that, if injured, affects the patient's quality of life. Although the risks of exposure during dental radiography are minimal, the fact remains that some tissues and organs are more susceptible to radiation effects than others. Critical organs exposed during dental radiographic procedures include the skin, lining of the gut and mouth, thyroid gland, lens of the eye, and bone marrow.

Radiation Measurement

Radiation is as measurable as weight or distance. Certain units of measure have been assigned to represent the amount or units of radiation administered or received. Currently two systems are used to determine amounts of radiation. The older system is referred to as the traditional system. The newer system is the metric equivalent and is known as the SI or Système International. The dental radiographer should be familiar with both systems:

- The roentgen (R) traditional system unit and the coulombs per kilogram (C/kg) SI unit are the units of

Life Span Considerations

Exposing radiographs on younger children can present difficulties. For example, it can be difficult to gain the child's cooperation when placing the film and having the child remain still during the exposure. The dental assistant must never hold the film or the patient during exposure. If assistance is required, it is the responsibility of the accompanying parent or guardian.

measurement used to define radiation that ionizes one cubic centimeter of air.

- The radiation absorbed dose (rad) traditional system unit and the gray (Gy) SI unit are used to report the amount of radiation absorbed in a substance.
- The roentgen equivalent man (rem) traditional unit and the sievert (Sv) SI unit are used to measure the amount or dose of radiation to which tissues are exposed.

Maximum Permissible Dose

The National Council on Radiation Protection and Measurements establishes radiation protection measurements that determine the maximum amount of radiation that a body is permitted to receive during a given amount of time. The maximum permissible dose (MPD) for occupationally exposed personnel is 5000 millirem(mrem), or 5 rem per year. This amount of radiation to the entire body is associated with minimal risk of injury. The MPD for nonoccupationally exposed persons is 500 mrem, or 5.0 millisieverts (mSv) per year. Occupationally exposed personnel must not exceed an accumulated lifetime dose or maximum accumulated dose (MAD). MAD is determined by means of a formula that uses the worker's age as input. A person must be 18 years of age to work with radiation. Therefore N in the formula refers to the dental professional's present age.

$$MAD = (N - 18) \times 5000 \text{ mrem/year}$$

Radiation Safety

Risk is involved when using radiation; however, the benefits outweigh the risks. When protocol is followed, safety can be provided to both the patient and operator. Due to the biological changes that occur during radiation exposure, precautions must be taken to minimize the risk factors. The operator should use the **ALARA concept** at all times when exposing patients to radiation. *ALARA* means "as low as reasonably achievable." This is a concept of radiation protection that states all radiation exposures must be kept to a minimum.

Patient Protection

Some people may think that patients are protected during exposure to x-rays simply by means of using a lead apron.

Indeed, the lead apron is an important part of patient protection, but protecting the patient actually begins long before the x-rays leave the PID. Patient protection begins by using appropriate and properly functioning equipment.

Collimation

The first factor in reducing patient radiation is collimation. Collimation is the process of restricting the primary beam's output so that only the area of interest is exposed. A collimator (Figure 29.11) is a lead diaphragm disk with an opening in the center that greatly reduces the area of tissue exposed to radiation. Federal regulations mandate that the primary beam not exceed 2.75 inches in diameter.

Reducing the area or volume of tissue exposed to radiation is one major benefit of collimation, but there is also another. Collimation also reduces the amount of secondary radiation generated during exposure. Previously in this chapter it was pointed out that secondary or scatter radiation strikes and exposes tissues outside of the area of interest. By limiting the size of the primary beam, the area or volume of tissue exposed is reduced as well as the amount of secondary radiation produced. This ultimately reduces the amount of radiation the patient receives. Finally, collimation improves diagnostic film quality. Secondary radiation affects the film in an undesirable manner, decreasing the diagnostic value of the film. (See Chapter 30 for more information related to film quality.)

Filtration

Filtration is another method for reducing patient exposure. Filtration is the process through which weak low-energy x-rays are eliminated prior to exiting the tube head. These low-energy rays are too weak to reach the film. Before these weak rays reach the film, they are absorbed in patient tissues, serving only to increase their exposure.

Two types of filtration are used in the dental x-ray unit: inherent filtration and added filtration. Inherent filtration begins as some of the weak x-rays are eliminated

as they exit the window of the glass tube, through the insulating oil and the tube head seal. Any remaining low-energy waves are filtered by added filtration. Added filtration is the placement of an aluminum disk above the collimator in the tube head (see Figure 29.11). The aluminum disk or added filtration serves to eliminate weak low-energy x-rays before they reach the target.

Lead Apron and Thyroid Collar

The lead apron and thyroid collar provide an excellent method for protecting patients against primary and secondary radiation (Figure 29.12). The lead apron covers the patient's vital organs, including the most sensitive ones, such as the reproductive organs, during x-ray exposure. The thyroid collar protects the neck region.

High-Speed Film

The use of high-speed film is another method of reducing patient exposure. As the speed of the film increases, the amount of radiation required to produce a quality radiograph decreases, lowering the amount of radiation to which a patient is exposed.

Film Holding Devices

Film holding devices aid the operator in stabilizing the film, eliminating the need for the patient to hold the x-ray equipment in place, exposing the patient's fingers to

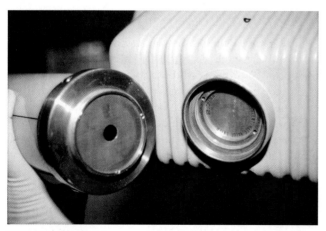

FIGURE 29.11
Collimator and filter.
Image courtesy Instructional Materials for the Dental Team, Lex., KY

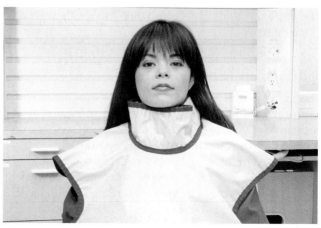

FIGURE 29.12
Protecting the patient with a lead apron and thyroid collar.

unnecessary radiation. Also, properly stabilizing the film with a holder decreases the chance of movement and reduces the possibility of having to retake the x-ray. Examples of film holding devices include the extension cone paralleling (XPC-1 and XCP-II) devices used for periapical radiography, and the Eezee-Grip film holder used for anterior and posterior radiographs. (For more information of film holders see chapter 30).

Proper Techniques

By employing proper techniques, the operator reduces the need to retake films, which in turn lowers the patient's and the operator's exposure to unnecessary radiation. By using proper techniques, the operator produces quality diagnostic radiographs. A radiograph that is not diagnostically acceptable will require a retake.

Operator Protection

The reason for using an established operator protection protocol is to ensure optimum safety during all phases of radiation procedures. It is necessary for the dental radiographer to employ safety measures as soon as training begins. The following is a list of guidelines for the dental radiographer (Figure 29.13):

- Stand at least six feet away or behind a lead barrier if possible.
- Keep away from the primary beam.
- Never hold film during exposure.

Professionalism

Techniques used in radiography are continually being improved to reduce patient exposure to radiation. Both E-speed and Insight film cut exposure times in half and the newer digital x-ray machines also significantly reduce patient exposure. As a member of the dental health team, it is beneficial for the dental assistant to be familiar with these newer techniques. Continuing education in the field of radiography is vital in keeping abreast of the latest technologies used in the dental industry.

- Never hold a patient during exposure.
- A film badge should be worn to monitor possible exposure.

How can the dental assistant safely stabilize a film during x-ray exposures?

Controlling Radiation

Control factors influence the production of x-rays and the diagnostic quality of a radiograph. Controlling factors include the following:

- Milliamperage
- Kilovoltage
- Exposure time

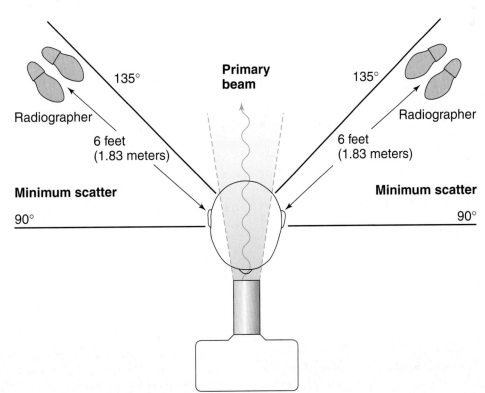

FIGURE 29.13
The radiographer should stand at least six feet from the head of the patient at an angle of 90 to 135 degrees out of the primary beam.

Electricity

To fully understand the production and controlling factors involved in exposing radiation, the dental assistant must first have a basic understanding of electricity. Electricity is the source of energy in the production of x-rays. Electricity can best be described as the flow of electrons through a conductor, referred to as electric current. Direct current is the flow of electrons in only one direction through a conductor. An example of direct current is a battery with a positive and negative pole.

The most common electric current used in home and businesses, however, is AC or alternating current. Alternating current describes the flow of electrons. In AC the electrons move first in one direction, build up to a peak, and then go back down to where they started and build up to a peak in the opposite direction. Two important terms of electrical current are amperage and voltage. *Amperage* is the measurement of electrons moving through a conductor. *Voltage* is the measurement of electrical force that forces electrons to move from the negative to the positive.

Transformers

The x-ray tube head has two electrical transformers that convert incoming voltage from a wall outlet. Most homes and businesses are wired electrically for 110 or 220 volts. The step-down transformer converts the incoming voltage from the 110 or 220 volts down to 3 or 5 volts. The step-up transformer converts incoming voltage from 110 or 220 to 50,000–100,000 volts or 50–100 kilovolts, respectively. One kilovolt (kV) equals 1,000 volts.

Milliamperage

The first stage in x-ray production is the creation of a source of electrons by thermionic emission at the tungsten filament. The milliamperage setting on the control panel regulates the amount of electricity coming into the filament and is measured in **milliampere (mA)** units. Most dental x-ray units have two settings, 10 or 15 mA. Increasing the milliamperage on the control panel increases the amount of electrons boiled off at the filament, which then increases the number of electrons striking the anode. The end result is also an increase in the number of x-rays produced. The milliamperage setting controls the quantity or number of x-rays produced.

Kilovoltage

As already pointed out, great force is used to move the electrons at a high speed from the anode to the cathode. The kilovoltage setting on the control panel regulates the force used to move electrons across the tube gap and is measured in kilovolts (kV).

Increasing the kilovoltage, or the force that causes the electrons to move from the cathode to the anode, causes the electrons to strike the anode with greater energy. This increases the energy of the x-rays produced. Recall that the wavelength of x-rays is determined by energy or penetrating power. X-rays with shorter wavelengths have greater energy or more penetrating power.

Exposure Time

In addition to milliamperage and kilovoltage, another variable in controlling the number of x-rays produced is the exposure time. The exposure time is the length of time electrons are pushed across the tube gap from the cathode to the anode. Most dental x-ray machine exposure times are calculated in fractions of a second, referred to as impulses. An impulse occurs every 1/60 of a second. The exposure button controls the flow of electricity to generate x-rays, and x-rays are only produced while the button is activated.

Radiation Image Characteristics

Radiation image characteristics are influenced by numerous variables that can affect the visual image of the radiograph. It is important for the operator to have a working knowledge of the controlling factors influencing these characteristics so that the operator is able to produce quality diagnostic radiographs.

Radiopacity and Radiolucency

A dental radiograph is a black-and-white image with varying shades of gray. **Radiopaque areas** on a radiograph appear light or white. These represent areas of dense tissue that absorbed the x-rays, not allowing them to pass through. Radiopaque areas on a dental radiograph could include enamel, dentin, bone, and various metal restorations. **Radiolucent areas** are the dark portions of a radiograph. The dark areas represent softer tissues that allow x-rays to pass through. Radiolucent areas on a dental radiograph could include dental pulp and space or air. Figure 29.14 is a bitewing radiograph that shows both radiopaque and radiolucent areas.

Density

Density is described as the overall blackness on a radiograph. Proper density allows images of the teeth and supporting structures to be viewed against a light source. The factors controlling density are milliamperage, kilovoltage, and exposure time.

As discussed, the milliamperage setting controls the number of x-rays produced. Increasing the milliamperage setting will increase the number of x-rays produced, giving the radiograph a darker appearance. Decreasing the

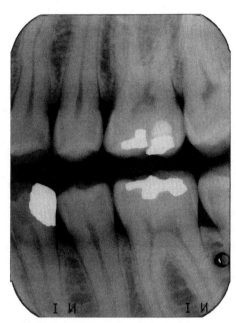

FIGURE 29.14
Bitewing showing radiopacity and radiolucency.

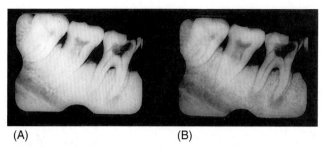

(A)   (B)

FIGURE 29.15
Radiographic contrast: (a) radiograph exposed with high contrast and (b) radiograph exposed with low contrast.

Contrast

Contrast is defined as differences in densities on adjacent areas of a radiograph. At least two different densities are necessary to produce any contrast. There are two types of contrast: low and high. On a high-contrast radiograph (Figure 29.15a), the dark areas are very dark and the light areas are very light, with very little shades of gray between the two. On a low-contrast radiograph (Figure 29.15b), there are gradations of gray between the light and dark areas of the radiograph.

The primary controlling factor for contrast is kilovoltage, which controls the energy of the x-rays. When x-rays are emitted with greater force, they penetrate tissues more evenly, resulting in low contrast. The opposite would be true for a low kilovoltage setting: the energy would also be low and would not penetrate the tissues as evenly, creating high contrast. Thus, kilovoltage controls the quality of the radiograph.

milliamperage setting will decrease the number of x-rays produced, giving the radiograph a lighter appearance. When the exposure time is increased, it increases the length of time x-rays are produced, creating more x-rays. This gives the film a darker appearance. If the exposure time is decreased, the length of time x-rays are produced will decrease, giving the film a lighter appearance.

● SUMMARY

A radiograph is an image recorded on photographic film through the use of x-rays, which penetrate exposed substances and record the image. The x-ray was discovered by Wilhelm Conrad Roentgen in 1895, sparking the invention of radiation procedures used for a variety of purposes.

One of the most important uses of the dental x-ray today is for the detection of disease. The key to safety when using radiation is the ALARA concept: all exposures should be kept "as low as reasonably achievable." The dental radiographer is responsible for safety procedures during the x-ray process for both the patient and the operator. The dentist is responsible for x-ray equipment and its maintenance.

● KEY TERMS

- **ALARA concept:** A radiation protection concept that states all exposures should be kept "as low as reasonably achievable." p. 449
- **Anode:** The positive electrode in the x-ray tube/glass envelope. p. 447
- **Atom:** The basic unit of all matter. p. 444
- **Cathode:** The negative electrode in the x-ray tube/glass envelope. p. 447
- **Contrast:** Differences in densities on adjacent areas of a radiograph. p. 453

- **Density:** The overall blackness on a radiograph. p. 452
- **Electromagnetic radiation:** The production of a wavelike energy through space and matter. p. 445
- **Frequency:** The number of wavelengths passing through a fixed point per given period of time. p. 445
- **Ion:** An electrically charged particle. p. 444
- **Ionization:** The process through which electrons are lost from the shell of an atom. p. 444
- **Ionizing radiation:** Radiation that is capable of producing ions by adding or removing electrons from the shell of an atom. p. 444

KEY TERMS (continued)

- **Leakage radiation:** Radiation that escapes or leaks out of the tube head. p. 448
- **Milliampere (mA):** A unit of measurement used to determine the amount of electrical current; 1 mA is equal to 1/1,000 of an ampere. p. 452
- **Photon:** Small bundle of pure energy that has no mass or weight. p. 445
- **Primary radiation:** Initial radiation produced at the tungsten target that exits the tube head. p. 448
- **Radiograph:** A recorded image on photographic film. p. 443
- **Radiolucent areas:** Dark portions of a radiograph that represent soft tissues (for example, dental pulp) that allow x-rays to pass through; space and air are also radiolucent. p. 452
- **Radiopaque areas:** Light or white portions of a radiograph that represent areas of dense tissue that

absorb x-rays, not allowing them to pass through; examples include enamel, dentin, bone, and various metal restorations. p. 452
- **Scatter radiation:** A form of secondary radiation that occurs once the primary beam has interacted with matter and then is deflected off in a different direction. p. 448
- **Secondary radiation:** Occurs when the primary beam comes in contact with and passes through any type of matter. p. 448
- **Tungsten target:** Portion of the anode struck by electrons (focal spot). p. 447
- **Wavelength:** Distance between the crests or high point of the radiation waves. p. 445
- **X-radiation (X-ray):** High-energy ionizing electromagnetic radiation. p. 443

● CHECK YOUR UNDERSTANDING

1. The production of a wavelike energy through space and matter is called what?
   a. electrons
   b. electromagnetic radiation
   c. ionization
   d. matter

2. Which of the following best describes characteristics of x-rays?
   a. no mass
   b. travel at the speed of light
   c. cannot be detected by the senses
   d. all of the above

3. Which of the following factors limits the size of the primary beam?
   a. collimator
   b. filter
   c. tungsten target
   d. film

4. Which control setting would increase the number or quantity of x-rays produced?
   a. kVp
   b. mA
   c. exposure time
   d. both b and c

5. Scatter radiation is a form of _____ radiation.
   a. collimation
   b. secondary
   c. primary
   d. leakage

6. What type of patient protection eliminates weak, low-energy x-rays before they reach the patient?
   a. filter
   b. collimation
   c. lead apron
   d. high-speed film

7. Which of the following controls the quality and penetrating power of x-rays?
   a. kilovoltage
   b. milliamperage
   c. exposure time
   d. proper technique

8. Which of the following is necessary in order to produce x-rays?
   a. source of electrons
   b. method to speed up electrons
   c. means to stop electrons
   d. all of the above

9. What is the term used to describe an overall blackness on a film?
   a. contrast
   b. density
   c. radiopacity
   d. radiolucency

10. Areas of dense material that cause high absorption of x-rays will appear what color on a radiograph?
   a. black
   b. gray
   c. white
   d. both a and c

INTERNET ACTIVITY

- Go to www.kodakdental.com/documentation/film/ N-414RadSafety.pdf to review radiation safety protocols for dental professionals.

WEB REFERENCES

- History of Radiography   www.ndt-ed.org/EducationResources/CommunityCollege/Radiography/Introduction/ history.htm
- Information on the History of the Cathode Tube   http://library.thinkquest.org/19662/low/eng/cathoderays.html
- National Council on Radiation Protection and Measurements   www.ncrponline.org/

30

Dental Film and Processing of Radiographs

Learning Objectives

After reading this chapter, the student should be able to:

- Recognize the various intraoral film holders and beam alignment devices.
- Describe the composition of a dental film.
- Identify the components of the film packet and determine their functions.
- List the three types of film used in dental radiography.
- Describe intraoral film sizes and the purpose of each.
- Relate the five steps in film processing.
- Explain the steps involved in both manual and automatic dental film processing.
- Describe the components of film processing solutions.
- Recall legal issues pertaining to dental radiography.
- Explain the protocol used for quality control in dental radiography.

Preparing for Certification Exams

- Recall information about film packets: sizes, composition, and speed.
- Identify extraoral film types and uses.
- List steps in film processing.
- Determine infection control used during dental radiography.

Key Terms

Automatic processor	Film processing
Beam alignment device	Film speed
Cassette	Intensifying screen
Cephalometric radiograph	Intraoral film
Dental film holder	Latent image
Duplicating film	Occlusal film
Emulsion	Panoramic radiograph
Extraoral film	Radiograph
Film	

One of the primary functions of a dental assistant is exposing, processing, and mounting radiographs. The dental assistant must understand the proper techniques involved in exposing and processing dental x-ray film to achieve a high-quality diagnostic radiograph and to provide competent infection control during radiographic procedures. The dental assistant should also have the knowledge to troubleshoot problems that can happen during radiographic processing procedures, such as those that arise from technical errors in exposing, processing, or equipment.

Dental Film Holders

Dental film holders are devices used to stabilize dental film in a patient's mouth. The primary benefit of using a dental film holder is a reduction in patient exposure to radiation, preserving the ALARA concept. The ALARA concept refers to keeping the exposure to radiation "as low as reasonably achievable." Employing the use of a film-holding device will reduce patient exposure by:

- Eliminating the need for patients to stabilize the film with their fingers
- Securing the film in place, reducing the possibility of patient movement affecting the final radiograph
- Reducing the need for retakes when used with the alignment devices
- Aligning the position-indicating device (PID) to accurately direct the primary beam

Types of Dental Film Holders

Many different dental film holders are available on the market today. The simplest dental film holder is made of disposable Styrofoam; the bite area contains a slot and a backing plate to stabilize the film while the patient is biting. Other film holders include the Stabe bite block and

---

Dental Assistant   PROFESSIONAL TIP

Sometimes the process of exposing and processing radiographs can become routine, and use of infection control protocols and guidelines can become lax. Therefore, as a dental assistant, it is beneficial to periodically review the protocols associated with infection control during radiographic procedures.

---

the XCP bite block (Figure 30.1). The XCP bite blocks are also available with beam alignment accessories and can be sterilized for reuse. The XCP devices can be used for both periapical and bitewing exposures.

The Eezee-Grip film holder (Figure 30.2) is formerly known as the Snap-a-Ray film holder. The Eezee-Grip is a double-ended instrument that clamps onto the film and locks it in place. Other film-holding devices include the EndoRay, which is used for endodontic x-rays (Figure 30.3), and the Uni-Bite device, which can be used for

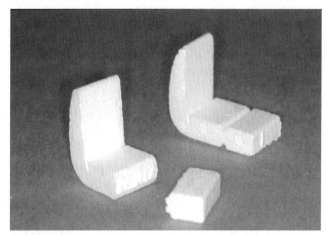

FIGURE 30.1
Disposable bite blocks.

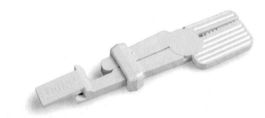

FIGURE 30.2
Eezee-Grip film holder.
Courtesy DENTSPLY Rinn-MPL

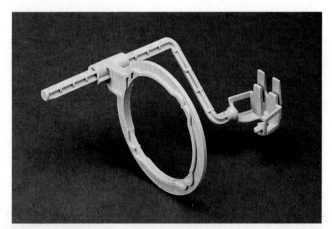

FIGURE 30.3
The EndoRay film holder is designed for use during endodontic procedures.
Courtesy of Dentsply Rinn

bitewing or paralleling techniques. (See Chapter 31 for more information on film stabilizing devices.)

Beam Alignment Devices

Beam alignment devices are used to position the PID to properly direct the primary beam during exposure. By using beam alignment devices, the margin of error during the exposure process is greatly reduced. The Rinn XCP device is an example of a beam alignment device (Figure 30.4). It contains three main components: the plastic bite block, the metal indicator arm, and the plastic aiming ring. Each of these components varies slightly depending on the area of use; for example, a posterior Rinn setup will differ from an anterior Rinn setup. Many of the newer Rinn XCP devices are color coded for easier assembly.

Dental X-Ray Film

The film used for dental radiography is a photographic film that has been modified for dental use. **Film** is the term used to describe the film packet and its components prior to it being developed or processed. A photographic image is made on the film after exposure to radiation. The film is placed behind the area of interest so that the primary beam penetrates those tissues before striking the film. The images of those tissues (also known as the latent images) are then imprinted on the emulsion. **Radiograph** is the term used to describe the film after it has been exposed and developed or processed.

Film Packet

The film must be protected from environmental hazards such as light, chemicals, scatter radiation, moisture, and heat to produce a high-quality diagnostic radiograph. The components of the film packet, including the packet itself, serve to protect it and ultimately aid in the diagnos-

tic quality of the radiograph. Each film packet consists of the following (Figure 30.5):

- A vinyl or paper film covering on the outside of the film packet serves to keep all of the components of the packet together. It also acts as a barrier that prevents moisture, such as saliva, from contacting the film.
- Black paper makes up the second layer of the film packet. It surrounds the film base, protecting it from light.
- The film base, which includes the emulsion on the film, is the film itself, which will become the radiograph.
- A lead foil backing makes up the last layer in the packet. It is situated directly behind the film base in the film packet. The lead foil is composed of a thin, single sheet of lead foil that serves to absorb scatter (secondary) radiation to prevent it from negatively affecting the radiograph. If not absorbed, scatter radiation can produce a fog on the film, reducing its diagnostic quality.

Why does the dental film packet need to be moisture resistant?

Film Composition

The components of the dental film make it sensitive to radiation. During film processing, the chemicals from both the film and the developing solutions react to pro-

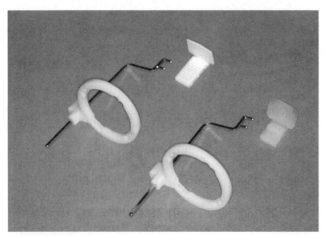

FIGURE 30.4
The Rinn XCP device.

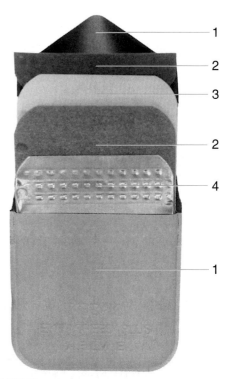

FIGURE 30.5
Film packet displaying contents. (1) Moisture-resistant outer wrap. (2) Black paper. (3) Film. (4) Lead foil backing.

duce an image. The following components, which are shown in Figure 30.6, make up the dental film:

- As noted earlier, the film base is the actual piece of the film packet that will become the radiograph. It is a flexible piece of polyester plastic that has a slightly bluish tint, which enhances the quality of the image. It is designed to withstand moisture and chemical exposure. The primary function of the film base is to provide support for the emulsion.
- The adhesive layer is a thin layer of adhesive material that covers both sides of the film. It functions to attach the emulsion to the film base, and is added prior to the emulsion.
- The film **emulsion** is a coating added to the adhesive that gives the film greater sensitivity to radiation. The film emulsion is composed of a mixture of gelatin and silver halide crystals.
- The gelatin is used as a means to suspend and disperse the silver halide crystals over the surface of the film. The gelatin dissolves during the processing of the film in chemical solutions, allowing the silver halide crystals to react with the developer and fixer.
- The silver halide crystals absorb radiation during exposure and store the energy until processed.
- The protective layer is a thin transparent coating placed over the emulsion. It serves to protect the emulsion during film processing. If no protective layer existed, the emulsion would stick to the rollers of the processor.

Latent Image

The **latent image** refers to the invisible image on film after radiation exposure and prior to developing. The stored image stays in a dormant state and invisible until introduced to chemical agents during film processing.

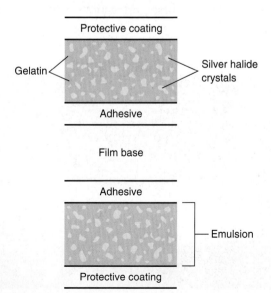

FIGURE 30.6
Composition of x-ray film.

Types of Film

Three types of film are used in dental radiography:

1. Intraoral film
2. Extraoral film
3. Duplicating film

Intraoral Film

Intraoral film is placed directly in the mouth during exposure. It is used to examine the teeth and their supporting structures. **Occlusal films** are intraoral films used to examine large areas of the upper or lower jaws. Intraoral films are available in five sizes:

- Size 0: This is normally used for bitewing or periapical techniques on children under 3 years of age and is the smallest of the intraoral films.
- Size 1: This size of film may be used for periapical techniques used to examine adult anterior teeth or for posterior bitewings on children.
- Size 2: This size of film is used to examine adult teeth using both periapical and bitewing techniques and on children for occlusal radiographs.
- Size 3: This film is used only for the bitewing technique, exposing all posterior teeth on the same side onto one film. It is longer and narrower than size 2 film. This size and technique of film choice are not recommended by the American Dental Association (ADA) for use.
- Size 4: This is the largest of the intraoral films and is used to investigate large areas of the maxilla and mandible bones as well as soft tissue using the occlusal technique. Size 4 film is also called occlusal film.

Extraoral Film

Extraoral film is situated outside of the mouth during x-ray exposures. These types of films are used to investigate large areas of the jaws or skull. Examples of the most

Life Span Considerations

Film placement for radiographic exposures on elderly patients can often present challenges. One of those challenges is shakiness. Elderly people may experience a quivering in the jaw area when occluding on the film holder. If that happens, the film must be stabilized before the exposure. One recommendation is to have the patient help steady the film with his or her own hand during the exposure. This should only be done if there is no other choice because it can cause unnecessary exposure to the fingers and hands. Under no circumstance should the dental assistant stabilize the film during exposures.

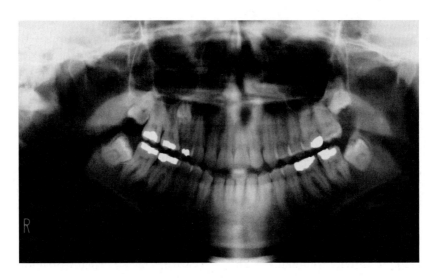

FIGURE 30.7
Panoramic radiograph.

common extraoral films are the panoramic and cephalometric films. The **panoramic radiograph** shows a wide view of both the maxilla and mandible bones on one radiograph (Figure 30.7). The **cephalometric radiograph** shows a profile view of the face and skull (Figure 30.8).

Most extraoral film is screen film that requires the use of an intensifying screen. An **intensifying screen** converts x-rays into visible light, which in turn helps expose the film at a faster rate. Extraoral film is not individually packaged for immediate exposure. It is light sensitive and therefore must be loaded into a **cassette** in a darkroom.

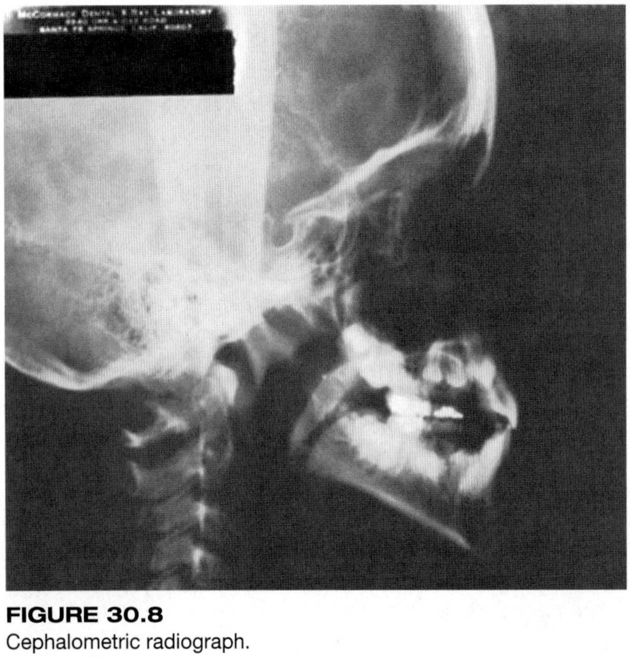

Duplicating Film

Duplicating film is a specialized type of film used to make an identical copy of existing radiographs. This may be required when a patient is moving to another practice, for insurance purposes, or when referring a patient to a specialist. Along with the special film required to duplicate, a duplicating machine is also required (Figure 30.9). Unlike standard film, duplicating film has emulsion on only one side. Like standard film, duplicating film is light sensitive and processing must take place in a darkroom or in a daylight loader.

Film Storage

Like other materials used in the dental office, the dental assistant must follow manufacturer's instructions for use and storage. These instructions usually include

FIGURE 30.8
Cephalometric radiograph.

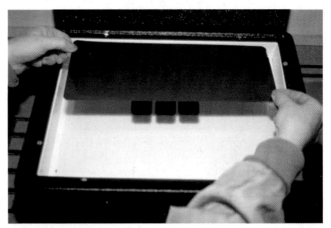

FIGURE 30.9
Example of a film duplicating machine.

optimum storage temperatures (below 70°F), environmental conditions such as low humidity, and storage away from chemical fumes and where radiation is being exposed. The package will also include an expiration date.

Rotation of stored film is very important. Using expired film can result in the reduction of diagnostic quality and film fogging. When new shipments of film arrive, the film with the closest expiration date should be rotated to an area where it will be used first.

Film Speed

Film speed establishes the amount of radiation and exposure time required to create an image on a film. A fast film would require less radiation and exposure time than that of a slower speed film. Film speed is determined by the size of the silver halide crystals, the thickness of the emulsion, and the presence of radiosensitive dyes. The larger the silver halide crystals, which make the film more sensitive to radiation, the faster the film speed.

Film speed is classified using an alphabetical system. A-speed is the smallest grain size of silver halide crystals and the slowest of the intraoral films. F-speed is the largest grain size of silver halide crystals and is, therefore, the fastest of the intraoral films. The American National Standards Institute and the International Organization for Standardization have established standards for film speed. In dental radiography three speeds are available: D-speed, E-speed, and F-speed. D-speed is the slowest and F-speed is the fastest. The faster the speed the less exposure a patient will have to radiation. Any film slower than E-speed is not recommended.

How does using a faster speed film reduce patient radiation?

Film Processing

Film processing refers to the phases the film must progress through to change the film into a radiograph. These phases, which must be done in a certain order, turn the latent image of an exposed film into a visible radiograph. During film processing, careful attention must be placed on the use of proper techniques. The processing techniques are just as critical as the exposure techniques when producing a high-quality radiograph. Poor processing techniques or processing chemicals can lead to retakes, exposing the patient to unnecessary radiation.

What would happen to the radiograph if the film processing did not occur in specific order?

Professionalism

Being a professional dental assistant carries with it heavy responsibilities, not only to your patients but for yourself. These responsibilities include taking the time to perform a task right the first time and using caution. When processing dental radiographs, perform the task correctly the first time and follow protocols. If a procedure has to be done again, it usually involves exposing your patients to unnecessary radiation by having to retake an x-ray. As a dental assistant it is frustrating to have to perform a procedure a second time. Also, from a business standpoint, mistakes can be costly.

The Darkroom

To process high-quality radiographs, a darkroom is required to keep the film safe from light during the processing procedures. Ideally the darkroom should be equipped with hot and cold running water, a manual processing tank, a safelight, racks for film drying, and enough counter space for unwrapping films.

Due to the sensitivity of the films being processed, the darkroom must be well maintained at all times. Opening film in the presence of light overexposes the film, and the resulting image on the film will be too dark or black. The counter working space must be free of any remaining liquids such as chemicals or water to avoid the film's premature contact with any liquids. Premature contact with liquids can result in a radiograph with spots that may interfere with the diagnostic quality. The safelight must be kept at least four feet away from the counter where films are unwrapped. When a safelight is closer than four feet, the radiograph may appear foggy. Other requirements for the darkroom are a timer, floating tank thermometer, door lock, stirring paddles, and film hangers. Additional storage space for chemicals is nice.

Processing Solutions

Film processing solutions are available in a variety of forms:

- Liquid concentrate
- Ready-to-use liquid
- Powder

Both the liquid concentrate and the powder must be mixed with water prior to use. Some manufacturers require the chemicals be mixed with distilled water. Always follow the manufacturer's instructions when preparing, developing, and fixing solutions. Instructions will specify whether tap or distilled water should be used and the ratio of water to chemicals required for mixing.

Composition of Processing Chemicals

Both the developing and fixing solutions are mixtures of several chemicals designed to handle specific functions during the processing phases. Tables 30-1 and 30-2, respectively, list the compositions of the developing and fixing solutions. Water is the vehicle for chemicals in both the developer and fixer. Film processing chemicals are temperature sensitive and close attention to temperature regulation is adhered to. This involves the use of a floating tank thermometer. The optimal temperature for processing is 68°F.

Manual Processing

Manual film processing is a method used to hand process film through the developing, rinsing, fixing, and washing phases. Manual processing requires a processing tank, which consists of a master tank with two one-gallon insert tanks (Figure 30.10 and Procedure 30-1). One insert tank houses the developing solution and the other the fixer. The master tank suspends the two insert tanks so that water can circulate around each of the tanks. The circulating water helps regulate the temperature of the chemicals, so the processing tank must be equipped with a hot and cold water supply. The use of an overflow pipe allows the water in the master tank to reach a specific level before it drains. This keeps the water fresh for rinsing and washing films. The tank must be equipped with a light-tight lid to prevent film from light exposure. The

TABLE 30-1 Developer Composition

Ingredient	Chemical	Function
Developer agent	Hydroquinone	Converts exposed silver halide crystals to black metallic silver. Slowly produces black tones and contrast in the image.
	Elon	Converts exposed silver halide crystals to black metallic silver. Rapidly generates gray tones in the image.
Preservative	Sodium sulfite	Prevents the rapid oxidation of the developing agents.
Accelerator	Sodium carbonate	Activates the developing agent, softens the emulsion, and provides an alkaline environment for the developing agents.
Restrainer	Potassium bromide	Prevents the developer from developing unexposed silver halide crystals.

TABLE 30-2 Fixer Composition

Ingredient	Chemical	Function
Fixer agent	Sodium thiosulfate; ammonium thiosulfate	Removes all unexposed silver halide crystals from the emulsion.
Preservative	Sodium sulfite	Prevents deterioration of the fixing agent.
Hardening agent	Potassium alum	Hardens and shrinks the gelatin in the emulsion.
Acidifier	Acetic acid; sulfuric acid	Neutralizes the alkaline from the developer, preventing further development.

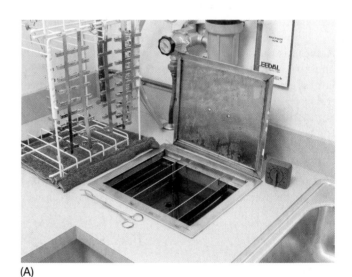

(A)

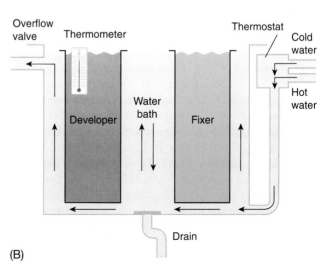

(B)

FIGURE 30.10

(a) Manual processing tank and (b) illustration of how the manual tank functions.

TABLE 30-3 Lengths of Bath Times Based on Processing Temperature

Solution Temperature (°F)	Time in the Developer (minutes)	Rinse Time (seconds)	Time in the Fixer (minutes)	Wash Time (minutes)
65	6.0	30	12	20
68	5.0	30	10	20
70	4.5	30	9	20
72	4.0	30	8	20
75	3.0	30	6	20
80	2.5	30	5	20

lid should also be in place when the tanks are not in use to prevent the oxidation and evaporation of chemicals. Chemicals must be stirred and replenished daily. Intervals for changing chemicals depends on frequency of use in each practice. Manual processing requires the use of film hangers to suspend the film during the processing phases.

A floating thermometer should be used periodically to check the temperature of the developing chemicals. The thermometer is placed in the processing tank. The temperature of the chemicals influences the length of time required to develop a film. The warmer the water, the less developing and fixing time required. Table 30-3 lists the lengths of time for each of the processing steps based on the temperature of the water in the processing tank.

A test film should be taken when fresh chemicals are placed in the tanks to be used as a control film against subsequent films. This quality control step helps the dental assistant determine when the chemicals should be changed. Aging chemicals and the frequency of use diminishes the effectiveness of the chemicals over time. Based on these factors, the time frame for changing chemicals is approximately every three to four weeks.

To process film manually, five steps are performed in the order listed here:

1. Developing is the first phase in film processing. The developer consists of a combination of chemicals designed to reduce the silver halide crystals into black metallic silver, leaving dark areas on the film. Unexposed silver halide crystals are not affected by developing chemicals. Also during the developing stage the film emulsion is softened.

2. Rinsing is the second phase in film processing. This is necessary for two important reasons: first, it stops the developing process, to avoid overdeveloping; and second, rinsing prevents contaminating the fixing solution with the developer.

3. Fixing is the third phase in film processing. During fixation, the chemicals remove the unexposed silver halide crystals from the film. The fixer also hardens the emulsion.

4. Washing is the fourth phase in film processing. Following fixation, the film is placed in a water bath to remove all chemicals from the emulsion.

5. Drying is the fifth and final phase in processing. After washing, the film must be completely dried before handling and mounting. Films may be air-dried or placed in a drying cabinet.

Automatic Processing

Film can be processed automatically using an automatic processing machine or **automatic processor** (Procedure 30-2), which is a machine that automatically processes film through each stage of the developing process.

The automatic processor has openings or feed slots on the outside of the processor where unwrapped films are placed. A roller transporter grabs the film and rapidly carries it through the developing, rinsing, fixing, and drying compartments (Figure 30.12). Not only are the rollers designed to rapidly transport the film through the automatic processor, but they also act as a wringing device by removing the excess chemicals from the emulsion prior to moving the film from one compartment to another.

The chemicals used in automatic processors are not the same as those used for manual processing. The chemicals used in automatic processing are formulated for use at higher temperatures. Processing film at higher temperatures speeds up the developing process.

Automatic processors can be used in a darkroom with a safelight as is done for manual processing (Figure 30.11). Automatic processing can also be used in a room with white light if a daylight loader is employed. A daylight loader is a small compartment attached to the housing of the automatic processor near the feed slot. A daylight loader has a special light shield that protects unwrapped exposed film from white light.

Benefits of automatic processing include the following:

- *Time saving:* Automatic processing takes approximately four to six minutes and even less time for endodontic films. The manual processing method requires about an hour to process and dry.

Procedure 30-1 Processing Dental Film Manually and Performing Infection Control Measures

Equipment and Supplies Needed

- Barriers
- Exposed radiograph
- Safelight
- Master tank
- Thermometer
- Timer
- Stirring paddles
- X-ray rack
- Developer and fixer solutions
- Pen or pencil

Preparation for Film Processing

1. Check developer and fixer solution levels; replenish if low.

2. Stir developer and fixer tanks with appropriate paddles.

3. Establish chemical and water bath temperatures and ensure that the water bath is circulating.

4. Clean counter around the master tank to ensure no chemical solution drops remain. Wash hands.

5. Establish that x-ray racks are clean and in working order and label with patient's name and date.

6. Place barriers on darkroom counter with exposed films (still in the disposable container).

7. Turn off overhead light and turn on safelight.

8. Don gloves.

Procedure Steps for Manual Film Processing

1. Carefully remove wrapper from film, not touching the film but allowing it to fall on the clean barrier.

(Check state guidelines for proper lead foil disposal in your area.)

2. Dispose of contaminated wrapper in the appropriate waste receptacle.

3. Remove gloves. Wash and dry hands, being careful not to get water droplets on film.

4. Carefully attach the film to the rack and check that it is secure. Place film on the rack from the bottom up, alternating sides of the rack.

5. Check the temperature of the developing solution to determine the length of time for developing the films.

6. Place rack in the developing tank and gently agitate to remove any bubbles and then replace the lid on the tank.

7. Set timer for appropriate time (normal developing time is 4½ minutes at 68°F), but always investigate and follow manufacturer's directions.

8. Remove from developer after the appropriate time and rinse in the water bath. Gently agitate for 20 seconds.

9. Place into the fixing solution, then replace the lid on the tank and set the timer. The time required to fix the films is double the developing time, but always investigate and follow manufacturer's directions.

10. Remove from fixer after the appropriate time and place in the water bath for approximately 20 minutes to do a final wash of the films.

11. Remove film from water bath and place film in the film dryer if available or allow to air dry.

12. Remove barriers and clean work areas to prepare for the next film processing.

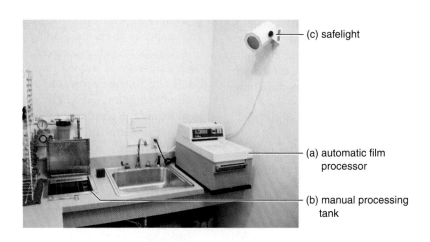

FIGURE 30.11
Darkroom showing (a) automatic film processor, (b) manual processing tank, and (c) safelight.

Procedure 30-2 Processing Dental Film Automatically and Performing Infection Control Measures

Equipment and Supplies Needed

- Automatic processor with daylight loader
- Two disposable containers
- Exposed radiographs
- Paper towel
- Disinfectant
- Gloves

Preparation for Film Processing

1. The automatic processor should be turned on at the start of the workday so the chemicals reach recommended temperatures.

2. Wash and dry hands.

3. Open the top of the daylight loader and place a paper towel on the bottom that will serve as a barrier. Place the disposable containers on the paper towel. One is for the lead foil and the other contains the exposed films but will be used to discard contaminated gloves, paper towel, and film wrapping after the films are loaded into the processor.

Procedure Steps for Automatic Film Processing

1. Don gloves and put hands into the sleeves of the daylight loader.

2. Unwrap film and feed the film into the machine. When processing multiple films, load them slowly to avoid film overlaps during processing. Alternate slots in the processor.

3. Place lead foils in one of the disposable containers and place the film wrappers on the paper towel. (Check state guidelines for proper lead foil disposal in your area.)

4. Continue with steps 2 and 3 until all films have been fed into the processor. Then remove gloves, placing them in the center of the paper towel with the film wrappers.

5. Using only the corners of the paper towel, wrap the paper towel over the gloves and film wrappers and carefully place them in the empty container where the exposed films were.

6. The disposable containers are removed using the lid on the top of the daylight loader. The trash is discarded and the lead foils are taken to the recycling area.

7. Disinfect the daylight loader to prevent cross-contamination.

- *Temperature regulation:* Automatic processors maintain optimal chemical temperatures, which helps with control of the processing times.
- *Less equipment* is needed.
- *Less space* is needed.

Most dental offices currently use automatic processors or digital radiography. Manual processing is not used as frequently as it once was; however, many dental offices still use manual processing as a backup if automatic equipment malfunctions. (For more information on digital radiography, see Chapter 32.)

Processing Errors

Errors during processing may result in low-quality, nondiagnostic radiographs. Eliminating processing errors increases the quality of the radiograph and decreases unnecessary patient exposures that result when retakes are required. Understanding processing errors and their cause along with methods of prevention greatly reduces errors. Many low-quality radiographs can be attributed to the following errors:

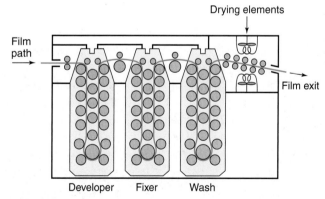

FIGURE 30.12
Inside a typical automatic film processor.

- Time and temperature errors
- Chemical contamination errors
- Film handling errors
- Lighting errors

Tables 30-4, 30-5, 30-6, and 30-7 list these types of errors and offer solutions for fixing them.

TABLE 30-4 Time and Temperature Problems and Solutions

Problem	Appearance	Errors	Solutions
Underdeveloped film	Light	Developing time too short. Developing solution too cold. Developing solution depleted. Thermometer or timer inaccurate.	Check and adjust developing time. Check and adust temperature of developer. Replenish developing solution. Replace thermometer or timer.
Overdeveloped film	Dark	Developing time too long. Developing solution too hot. Developing solution too concentrated. Thermometer or timer inaccurate.	Check and adjust developing time. Check and adjust temperature of developer. Replenish developing water or developer as needed. Replace thermometer or timer.
Reticulation of emulsion	Cracked	Drastic temperature changes occurred between the developer and the water bath.	Check temperatures of the water bath and chemicals.

TABLE 30-5 Chemical Contamination Problems and Solutions

Problem	Appearance	Errors	Solutions
Developer spots	Dark spots	Developer touches the film prior to processing.	Clean work areas in the darkroom between processing.
Fixer spots	White spots	Fixer touches the film prior to processing.	Clean work areas in the darkroom between processing.
Yellow-brown stains	Yellowish-brown color	Fixing time is too short. The fixer is exhausted.	Establish proper fixation time. Monitor and change chemicals as needed.

TABLE 30-6 Film Handling Problems and Solutions

Problem	Appearance	Errors	Solutions
Developer cutoff	Straight white border	Portion of the film was above the low level of the developing solution.	Check and adjust solution levels prior to processing.
Fixer cutoff	Straight black border	Portion of the film was above the low level of the fixing solution.	Check and adjust solution levels prior to processing.
Film overlap	Light or dark areas	Two films contacted each other during processing.	Make sure films are separated prior to processing.
Air bubbles	White spots	Air made contact with film surface during processing.	Gently agitate film racks when placing in processing solutions.
Fingernail mark	Black crescent-shaped marks	Fingernail made contact with film emulsion during processing.	Handle film edges only, in a gentle manner.
Fingerprint mark	Black fingerprint	Contaminated fingers touched film surface.	Use clean hands and handle film edges only.
Static electricity	Black-thin branching lines	Film packets opened too quickly.	Open film packets slowly.
Scratched film	White lines	Soft film emulsion contacted a sharp object.	Handle films, and films on racks, carefully.

Legal Considerations in Dental Radiography

It is the responsibility of all dental assistants to understand the laws pertaining to their position. This is especially true when using equipment that exposes patients to ionizing radiation. Both federal and state governments regulate laws regarding the use of dental radiography equipment. Laws enforcing the certification and training of personnel exposing ionizing radiation are also established. By following the established guidelines, dental assistants can better ensure the safety of the patient as well as the dental team members.

TABLE 30-7 Lighting Problems and Solutions

Problem	Appearance	Errors	Solutions
Light leak	Black exposed area	Film was exposed to light.	Inspect film packets for defects prior to use. Do not expose to light.
Fogged film	All-over grayness with little contrast or detail	Safelight is malfunctioning. Darkroom has light leaks. Expired (old) film used. Film stored improperly. Processing solutions contaminated.	Check safelight bulb and filter. Inspect darkroom for light leaks. Check film expiration date. Store in cool, dry environment. Cover the master tank when not in use.

Legal and Ethical Issues

The dental assistant must be aware of his or her state and local laws pertaining to exposing radiation. For example, in your state, if a patient were to come in with a toothache, do you know if it would be the dental assistant's responsibility or the dentist's responsibility to prescribe an x-ray? Spend some time to make sure you know the laws and ethical codes that guide you in your profession.

Equipment Regulations

The federal government has established laws pertaining to the safety and use of dental x-ray machines manufactured in the United States. Dental equipment made or sold in the United States after 1974 is required to meet federal regulations. These regulations specify safety standards for minimum filtration and x-ray equipment control settings for milliamperage, kilovoltage, and time. State, county, and city laws can also influence x-ray equipment safety regulations, such as requiring periodic equipment safety inspections and x-ray machine registration. When laws or regulations differ among federal, state, and local agencies, the stricter law or regulation applies.

Certification Requirements for Dental Assistants

The Consumer-Patient Radiation Health and Safety Act establishes the protocol for the safe use of x-ray equipment. It also requires individuals that take radiographs to receive training and certification. The amount of training and the certification requirements for individuals exposing radiation are controlled by state law, which varies from state to state. It is the dental assistant's responsibility to comply with his or her own state's laws regarding radiation exposure training and certification. Most states will require that a dental assistant have initial training or become certified prior to exposing radiation.

Quality Assurance in Dental Radiography

The production of high-quality diagnostic radiographs is essential in the diagnosis and treatment of patients; therefore, protocol to ensure this occurs must be followed at all times. Quality assurance refers to following established procedures to ensure that high-quality diagnostic radiographs are produced. A quality assurance plan should be established and implemented to include safety inspections and quality control tests for both equipment and supplies.

Quality Assurance for Dental Equipment

As mentioned earlier in this chapter, state or local agencies require periodic inspections of x-ray equipment. This is done to ensure the safety of the equipment being used for both the patient and the dental assistant. Quality control tests are recommended between inspections to ensure equipment is in good working order. Dental personnel or a representative of the manufacturing company may administer the quality control tests on dental x-ray equipment. For information on effective quality control testing for dental equipment, contact the equipment manufacturer.

Maintaining Film Integrity

Film is temperature sensitive, so careful attention should be given to the environment in which it is stored. Film is also time sensitive and the film with the closest expiration date should be used first. Normally the expiration date is displayed on the box. Always follow the manufacturer's guidelines regarding film storage and care. Though the film may not be expired, it may have been subjected to unfavorable conditions during the shipping process, which could diminish the integrity of the film. Therefore, quality testing is recommended for each new box of film opened. Testing the quality of the film is a simple process that begins by using fresh processing chemicals:

- An unexposed film from the new box is processed (without exposure to radiation).

- After processing, the film should appear clear with a light blue tint; this indicates that the integrity of the film has been maintained and is ready for use.
- After processing, if the film appears foggy the integrity has not been maintained and this film should be discarded.

Maintaining Screens and Cassettes

Extraoral radiography techniques involve the use of cassettes and intensifying screens. The cassettes should be cleaned regularly to remove dirt and debris. Cassettes should also be examined for scratches and defects that can lead to light leakage that would interfere with the diagnostic quality of the radiograph. Cassettes and screens should be cleaned on a regular basis as recommended by the manufacturers and according to their instructions. Commercial cleaners are available for screens and cassettes, but be sure to always follow the specific manufacturer's recommendations for the type and use of cleaning products on screens and cassettes. After cleaning screens an antistatic solution should be applied.

Maintaining View Boxes

View boxes are necessary pieces of equipment used to interpret radiographic images. Light in the view box is provided by a fluorescent bulb inside the box and covered in the front by an opaque plastic or Plexiglas panel. A properly functioning view box will emit a subtle and even light. View boxes must be cleaned after each patient use or covered with a protective material as well as inspected regularly for defects on the opaque panel. Cracked or permanently discolored panels require replacement. Burned-out or constantly flickering bulbs must be replaced as well.

Darkroom Light Leaks

Light leaks in the darkroom will result in radiographs with poor diagnostic quality. The darkroom should be periodically inspected for light leaks. Light leaks can be detected easily by following these steps:

- Enter the darkroom, close the door, and turn off all lights including the safelight.
- Close your eyes for a few moments and then open them and allow your eyes to adjust to the dark.
- After your eyes have adjusted to the dark, look around the room to see if you can detect any light. Focus on areas around the door and handle areas, vents, walls, and ceilings.

If the dental assistant detects a light leak in the darkroom, it should be corrected before films are processed. Fixing a light leak can be as simple as covering the area with black electrical tape or applying weather stripping.

Safelight Testing

Even the safelight must be checked regularly to ensure that the safelight does not interfere with the image on the radiograph. This should be done after the light leak test has been performed in the darkroom, otherwise safelight testing will not be accurate if a light leak exists in the darkroom. The coin test is an easy way to check the safelight (Figure 30.13):

- Enter the darkroom and turn off all lights including the safelight.
- Unwrap an unexposed film and place it on the counter at least four feet from the safelight and put a coin in the center. Then turn the safelight on for three to four minutes.
- Process the film after the allotted time.
- Determine the results: after processing if there is no visible image on the film, the safelight is working well and film processing may continue. If a coin image is visible after processing, the safelight is not working properly. The safelight must be inspected and the problem corrected before film processing continues.

Quality Control for Manual Processing

Quality control measures during manual processing begin with maintaining a clean and organized darkroom. Manufacturer's directions must be followed when mixing the developer and fixer solutions. It is recommended that after fresh solutions are mixed, a control film be developed and kept for comparison with subsequent films. It is recommended that solutions be changed every three to four weeks depending on the frequency of use. When the chemicals become old or worn out, the images on recently developed film will not have the same diagnostic quality as the control film. This signals that it is time to change the solutions. The lid must be kept over the pro-

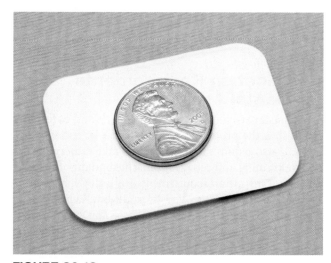

FIGURE 30.13
Coin and film for the safelight test.

cessing tank to prevent contamination from dust, air, and evaporation. Check state guidelines for proper darkroom chemical disposal requirements in your area.

Daily preparations for processing must be attended to before processing can begin. The developer and fixer tanks must be stirred and the solution levels checked. If solutions are low, replenish before processing begins to avoid running into problems with the chemical becoming too old or worn out. The water for the water bath must also be turned on before processing can begin. Ongoing temperature checks of the solutions must be made throughout the day to ensure optimal developing and fixing times.

After processing radiographs, clean the area around the master tank to remove any drops or splatter of chemicals. This will prevent future films from premature contact with processing solutions that will reduce the diagnostic quality of the film.

Maintenance of the Automatic Processor

To ensure that high-quality diagnostic radiographs are produced using the automatic processor, daily upkeep and weekly maintenance are required. Water circulation, chemical levels, and temperatures must be checked on a daily basis. It is also recommended that daily test films be processed to check the integrity of the chemicals and the function of the automatic processor. Perform the following steps to test the automatic processor:

- Enter the darkroom and unwrap two unexposed films. Expose one of the films to light.
- Process both films in the automatic processor.
- Determine the results: if the unexposed film appears clear and dry and the exposed film appears black and dry, the automatic processor and chemicals are functioning properly and film processing may continue. If the test films appear clear or completely black and have not been dried, the processor is not functioning properly. Film processing should not continue until the problems are resolved.

Infection Control in Dental Radiography

In all areas of the dental setting, there are risks involved concerning infectious diseases. In dental radiography there is a greater risk for the spread of disease due to the possibility of cross-contamination. Cross-contamination can occur during the exposure process when the dental assistant places the film in the patient's mouth, leaves the treatment area to activate the exposure button, and then returns to the treatment area to remove the film. Transporting the films after exposure to the darkroom for processing presents more opportunities for cross-contamination. All patient and body fluids are to be

treated as if they are infectious. (For more information on infection control see Chapter 12.)

As a dental assistant you must be proactive regarding infection control during radiation procedures. A protocol must be established and followed for radiographic procedures to reduce possible contamination. For example, a clean barrier must be placed on the exposure button between each patient. Barriers are a great way to minimize the risk of contamination and work especially well for hard-to-disinfect areas such as the exposure button (Figure 30.14 and 30.15). Contaminated areas not covered by a barrier must be disinfected; such areas include counters, the x-ray machine, the lead apron, and dental

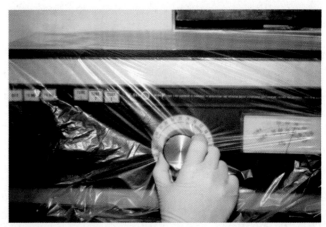

FIGURE 30.14
X-ray control panel with barriers in place.

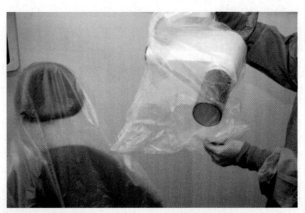

FIGURE 30.15
Operatory with barriers in place for x-ray exposure.

films. Barriers are also available for the film itself (Figure 30.16), which simply require the outer wrapper to be torn away, after which the film is allowed to fall into a noncontaminated container (making sure not to touch the film with contaminated gloves). Film barriers often have sharp edges and can cause discomfort to the patient. Refer to Procedures 30-1 and 30-2, respectively, for infection control protocols for manual and automatic radiographic procedures.

Film-Holding and Alignment Devices

Film-holding devices and alignment devices are classified as semicritical instruments, which means that they come in contact with patient tissues but do not penetrate them. However, semicritical items must be sterilized between each use to prevent cross-contamination. The best method of sterilization for critical and semicritical instruments is to use equipment that provides steam under pressure, such as an autoclave. It is recommended that only instruments capable of withstanding heat sterilization or disposable instruments be used for dental proce-

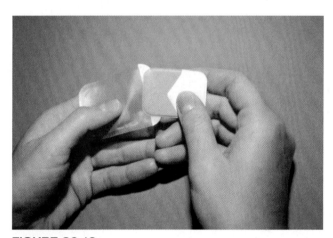

FIGURE 30.16
Film with barriers.

dures. If an item cannot withstand the heat, it must be placed in a cold sterile solution. When using a cold sterile solution, be sure to follow manufacturer's guidelines for use and time.

Handling of Exposed Film

Personal protective equipment must be worn during radiation exposures and when processing radiographs. (See Chapter 12 for a review on personal protective equipment.) After exposure, film is contaminated with the patient's saliva and other potentially infectious material and must be wiped off with gauze or a paper towel. Some manufacturers also allow disinfectant to be lightly sprayed on film packets, but film packets must not be submerged in any type of liquid and must never be placed in a sterilizer.

After wiping/disinfecting the film, it should be placed in a disposable container labeled with the patient's name. The dental assistant must carefully avoid touching the outside portion of the container with contaminated gloves. The outside portion of the disposable container may only be handled after contaminated gloves are removed and hands have been washed. The disposable container must be transported to the darkroom only with clean gloveless hands.

SUMMARY

As a dental assistant you will use film-holding devices to stabilize the film in the patient's mouth along with beam alignment devices to aid in exposing high-quality diagnostic radiographs. Three types of film are used in dental radiography as well as various sizes of intraoral film. The type and size of film depends on the areas to be examined. Special film is also available to duplicate existing radiographs.

Film should be cared for according to the manufacturer's instructions. Films may be processed in a dark-

room using a manual system or an automatic processor. Chemicals used to process the radiographs require daily maintenance. Films must be processed in proper sequence, and care must be taken to maintain infection control protocols during all phases of dental radiation. Equipment and supplies must be maintained, monitored, and tested to ensure quality and function.

KEY TERMS

- **Automatic processor:** Machine that automatically processes film through each stage of the developing process. p. 463
- **Beam alignment device:** Device used to position the primary beam by aligning the position-indicating device. p. 458
- **Cassette:** Used to hold extraoral film during exposure. p. 460
- **Cephalometric radiograph:** Profile of the head and face showing both bone and soft tissue. p. 460
- **Dental film holder:** A device used to stabilize the film in the patient's mouth. p. 457
- **Duplicating film:** Film used specifically for duplicating or copying existing radiographs. p. 460
- **Emulsion:** A coating on the film that gives it greater sensitivity to radiation. p. 459
- **Extraoral film:** Film designed to be used outside of the mouth during x-ray exposure. p. 459
- **Film:** The term used to describe the film packet and its components prior to it being developed or processed. p. 458

- **Film processing:** A series of chemical steps that convert a film into a radiograph. p. 461
- **Film speed:** Establishes the amount of radiation and time needed to expose a film. p. 461
- **Intensifying screen:** A device used in a cassette that converts x-ray energy into light, which causes a decrease in the amount of time needed to expose the film. p. 460
- **Intraoral film:** Film designed to be used in the mouth during x-ray exposure. p. 459
- **Latent image:** An invisible image that is in the emulsion of the film after exposure to radiation and prior to developing. p. 459
- **Occlusal film:** Intraoral film used to examine large areas of the upper or lower jaws. p. 459
- **Panoramic radiograph:** An extraoral film that shows a wide view of both upper and lower jaws on one radiograph. p. 460
- **Radiograph:** A film after it has been exposed to x-rays and developed to show images on a film. p. 458

CHECK YOUR UNDERSTANDING

1. Which of the following can be found in a dental film packet?
   a. bite block
   b. lead foil
   c. PID
   d. radiation

2. An invisible image on film after exposure and prior to processing is called a
   a. visible image.
   b. negative image.
   c. latent image.
   d. all of the above.

3. Which of the following is *not* a film type?
   a. duplicating
   b. intraoral
   c. radiograph
   d. extraoral

4. When storing film it is important to
   a. check the expiration date.
   b. follow manufacturer's instructions.
   c. test the film for each box opened.
   d. all of the above.

5. Which of the following is a vehicle for processing solutions?
   a. silver halide crystals
   b. developer
   c. fixer
   d. water

6. Which of the following processing steps is not included when using an automatic processor?
   a. rinsing
   b. developing
   c. washing
   d. fixing

7. A quality assurance plan should include which of the following?
   a. conducting safety inspections
   b. conducting quality control tests
   c. following manufacturer's guidelines
   d. all of the above

8. The coin test is used to test which of the following?
   a. light leak
   b. temperature
   c. developer
   d. view box

CHECK YOUR UNDERSTANDING (continued)

9. Which of the following are considered to be semi-critical instruments?
   a. film-holding devices
   b. film
   c. alignment devices
   d. both a and c

10. After films have been exposed, how are they transported to the darkroom?
   a. with gloved hands
   b. with clean nongloved hands
   c. in a disposable container
   d. both b and c

INTERNET ACTIVITY

• Research laws regarding dental assistants in your own state by using a search engine such as Google or Metacrawler. Type in the name of your state along with the words "state dental practice act" (e.g., "Colorado State Dental Practice Act") and click on Search. You can also check the Dental Assisting National Board at www.danb.org with regard to specific state requirements.

WEB REFERENCES

• American Dental Association   www.ada.org
• American Dental Association Council on Scientific Affairs: The Use of Dental Radiographs, Update and Recommendations   www.ada.org/prof/resources/pubs/jada/reports/report_radiography.pdf

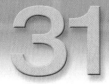

Intraoral Radiographic Procedures

Learning Objectives

After reading this chapter, the student should be able to:

- Describe patient preparation prior to radiograph exposure.

- List three types of intraoral radiograph exposures and the purpose of each.

- List the protocol for using the paralleling technique and the bisecting angle technique to expose periapical radiographs.

- Explain the protocol for exposing bitewing interproximal radiographs.

- Explain the procedure and patient positioning necessary to expose occlusal radiographs.

- Explain techniques for managing radiographs for patients with physical and mental disabilities.

- Describe methods of managing edentulous and pediatric patients or those with a hypersensitive gag reflex.

- Identify technical errors and list methods for correcting them.

- Describe methods for mounting periapical radiographs.

Preparing for Certification Exams

- Expose radiographs.

Key Terms

Ala

Bisecting angle technique

Bitewing radiograph

Cone cut

Elongation

Foreshortening

Horizontal angulation

Interproximal

Long axis of the tooth

Overlapping

Paralleling technique

Periapical radiograph

Perpendicular

Position-indicating device (PID)

Radiograph

Tragus

Vertical angulation

Chapter Outline

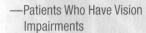

- **Intraoral X-Ray Techniques**
  —Common Vertical and Horizontal Errors
  —Full Mouth Survey
  —Patient Preparation for Intraoral Radiographs
  —Principles for Intraoral Radiography

- **Paralleling Technique**
  —Paralleling Holding Devices
  —Periapical Radiographs Using the Paralleling Technique

- **Bisecting Angle Technique**
  —Periapical Radiographs Using the Bisecting Angle Technique

- **Bitewing Technique**
  —Principles of the Bitewing Technique
  —Bitewing Film Placement
  —Stabilizing the Film During Bitewing Exposures
  —Guidelines for Bitewing Exposures

- **Occlusal Radiographs**
  —Radiograph Exposures Using the Occlusal Technique
  —Maxillary Occlusal Technique
  —Mandibular Occlusal Technique

- **Patients with Special Needs**
  —Patients Who Have Mobility Impairments
  —Patients Who Have Hearing Impairments

- —Patients Who Have Vision Impairments

- **Positioning Difficulties Encountered with Intraoral Radiography**
  —Mandibular Third Molars
  —Endodontic Treatment
  —Edentulous Alveolar Ridges
  —The Gag Reflex
  —Pediatric Patients

- **Technical Errors in Intraoral Radiography**
  —Errors of Angulation and Centering of the PID
  —Film and Digital Receptor Placement Errors
  —Exposure and Film Errors

- **Mounting Intraoral Radiographs**
  —Labial and Lingual Mounting
  —Anatomic Landmarks
  —Intraoral Radiograph Mounting Procedure
  —Radiograph Storage

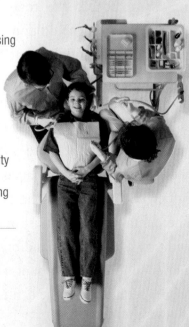

A radiograph is a one-dimensional view of a three-dimensional subject, the patient. Radiographs are also referred to as x-rays or films. Two types of radiographic examinations are used in dentistry: intraoral radiography and extraoral radiography. Intraoral radiography refers to those films that are placed and exposed directly in the patient's mouth. Extraoral radiography refers to films that are placed and exposed outside of the patient's mouth.

Various techniques are used to obtain intraoral radiographs. The purpose of intraoral radiography is to view individual teeth and their supporting structures. Interpretation of dental radiographs by the dentist is essential in the diagnosis and treatment of each patient. The dental assistant has a very important responsibility to ensure proper film exposure, processing, and mounting so that the dentist can accurately view the patient's dental condition. The dental assistant must be confident using the methods required to expose specific radiographs as prescribed by the dentist.

Radiation has a cumulative effect over a person's lifetime, meaning that once an individual is initially exposed, the total radiation amount increases with each additional exposure. For this reason, only essential dental radiographs should be exposed. Every dental assistant must be proficient in the techniques and important skills necessary for exposing dental radiographs for all patients, especially those with special medical needs, and be able to manage positioning difficulties encountered in the dental environment. The dental assistant must also be very familiar with maxillary and mandibular anatomic landmarks in order to mount radiographs in the proper sequence for the dentist to study.

Dental Assistant   PROFESSIONAL TIP

The dental assistant must be gentle with patients during film placement and removal. Remember that film edges are rectangular in shape and the oral cavity is round, especially near the maxillary and mandibular cuspid areas. The tissues of the oral cavity are delicate. The dental assistant must be both accurate and efficient when placing the x-ray film. The patient should not have to keep the film in the mouth any longer than necessary.

The tissues of the oral cavity are delicate especially under the tongue. Wrapping a 2 × 2 gauze square around the mesial corner of the mandibular first premolar x-ray film will make placement of the film more comfortable and make it easier for the patient to hold the film in place. The gauze will not affect the quality of the radiograph but will help with patient compliance.

Intraoral X-Ray Techniques

Two techniques are used for exposing intraoral radiographs: the paralleling technique and the bisecting angle technique. Both techniques require the dental assistant to use the **long axis of the tooth** as a focal point. The long axis of the tooth is an imaginary line passing vertically, or lengthwise, through the center of the tooth.

The bisecting angle technique does not require the use of film holders; however, various film holders are available for this method of exposing intraoral radiographs. In specific cases, such as endodontic treatment, the patient may be asked to hold the film with an instrument such as a hemostat. The American Dental Association (ADA) does not recommend that patients hold x-ray films in their mouth with a finger due to the finger being exposed to radiation.

The American Academy of Oral and Maxillofacial Radiology recommends the paralleling technique for intraoral dental radiographs. This method requires using a film-holding device and eliminates the option of a film being held in place in the mouth by the patient's finger. These devices provide for the x-ray film to be placed parallel to the long axis of the teeth, resulting in a more accurate and less distorted image.

The film holders available incorporate an x-ray beam guiding device that makes PID alignment a simpler task. The **position-indicating device (PID)** is the cylinder (or cone) affixed to the x-ray tube head. It is used to align the x-ray beam with the film in the patient's mouth. The dental assistant often selects the radiographic technique according to his or her preferences and one which will accommodate the patient's specific oral condition.

Common Vertical and Horizontal Errors

Common positioning errors associated especially with the bisecting angle technique of exposing periapical radio-

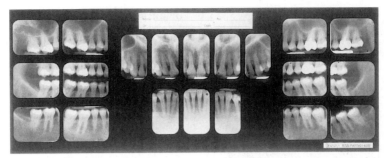

FIGURE 31.1
A mounted full mouth radiograph series.

graphs are vertical errors. Both foreshortening and elongation are vertical angulation errors.

Foreshortening occurs when there is excessive vertical angulation of the PID to the film. **Elongation** takes place when there is insufficient vertical angulation of the PID to the film. The floor-to-ceiling alignment of the PID and central ray establishes an accurate image of the tooth. The dental assistant must make certain that the central ray from the x-ray tube head is directed at a right angle to an imaginary line bisecting the angle between the plane of the film and the long axis of the tooth.

Overlapping is an error in horizontal angulation that occurs when the x-ray beam is not at 90 degrees to the tooth and the film, and images from two adjacent structures are superimposed on top of each other.

Adjusting the PID in a side-to-side direction so that the contacts of the teeth are open allows the radiograph to show the proximal surfaces. Proper horizontal angulation is achieved if the PID is placed in the following ways:

- *Molars:* Direct the central ray between the first and second molars. This should place the PID parallel to the plane of the facial surfaces of the molars.
- *Premolars:* Direct the central ray between the first and second premolars. This should place the PID parallel to the premolar facial plane.
- *Cuspid:* Direct the central ray at the distal surface of the cuspid.
- *Central incisors:* Direct the central ray between the central incisors and the midline of the arch.
- *Central-lateral incisors:* Direct the central ray between the central and lateral incisors.

What are some of the common errors that occur when using the bisecting angle technique and how can they be avoided? **?**

Full Mouth Survey

A full mouth survey (FMS or FMX), also called a complete mouth survey (CMS or CMX), usually consists of 18 to 20 intraoral exposures. When the dental assistant

is exposing radiographs of the teeth, the maxillary and mandibular arches are divided into different segments so that the dentist has a clear view of each individual tooth. The placement of each film is designed to record specific areas and anatomy so that when the views are assembled, such as for an FMX, all teeth are clearly visible and distinguishable from others. The areas needing to be captured for a complete radiographic examination are seen in Figure 31.1.

The full mouth radiographic survey typically includes 16 periapical and 4 bitewing radiographs. Size 2 films are used to record the posterior areas, and the smaller size 1 films are used to record the anterior regions. Size 2 film may be used for the anterior areas depending on the preference of the dentist. If size 2 x-ray film is utilized, then only three maxillary anterior and three mandibular anterior teeth are imaged.

Two types of intraoral radiographic images are used for a dental full mouth radiographic survey:

- Periapical radiographs (Figures 31.2 and 31.3)
- Bitewing/interproximal radiographs (Figure 31.4)

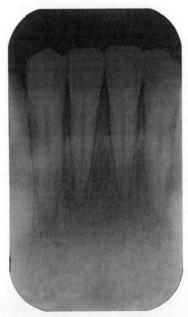

FIGURE 31.2
Anterior periapical radiograph.

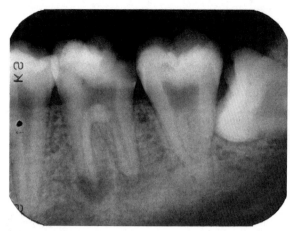

FIGURE 31.3
Posterior periapical radiograph.

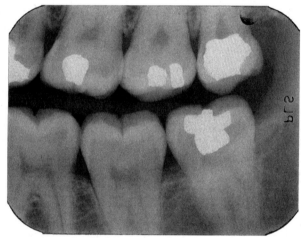

FIGURE 31.4
Horizontal molar bitewing radiograph.

All films must be dimensionally accurate and show diagnostically useful contrast and a sharp distinct image.

A **periapical radiograph** must show the desired teeth and the surrounding areas (including the apices) on the film. The contacts between the teeth should not be overlapped. The contacts should be open and the entire length of the tooth must be shown to include at least one-eighth of an inch past the apices and crowns of the teeth. An ideal periapical radiograph will open the contacts between the neighboring teeth. Periapical radiographic films are used to determine the:

• number, length, and morphology of roots,
• number and shape of root canals,
• condition of the supporting tissues,
• presence of foreign bodies,
• presence of pathological lesions,
• position and relationship of impacted teeth to other structures, and/or
• extent of bone loss.

Bitewing radiographs must open the interproximal contacts between the teeth on the maxillary and mandibular arches. **Interproximal** means between two adjacent surfaces next to each other in the same arch. The tab or wing is placed on the occlusal (biting surfaces) of the teeth during proper film positioning by the dental assistant. Bitewing tabs are most frequently made of cardboard but other materials such as plastic or rubber are available. The Rinn XCP paralleling device has a bitewing apparatus along with the periapical apparatus. The patient closes her mouth gently on the tab to facilitate holding the film in position during exposure of the radiograph. Bitewing radiographs serve to:

• diagnose caries,
• show recurrent caries beneath restorations,
• siscover overhanging restorations,
• show conditions of the alveolar bone, and/or
• show pulpal conditions.

A full mouth radiographic series, which includes periapical and bitewings, is obtained with either the bisecting angle or paralleling techniques and includes the sequence shown in Table 31-1.

When taking radiographs, the dental assistant must be sure to record the date, number of films taken, and any pertinent exposure factors such as kilovoltage and milliamperage used in the patient's record. If the patient has been referred by another dentist, the prescription from the referring dentist and any correspondence regarding

TABLE 31-1 Full Mouth Radiographic Survey

Max Rt Molar (size 2 film)	Max Rt Premolar (size 2 film)	Max Rt Cuspid (size 1 film)	Max Rt Lateral and Central Incisor (size 1 film)	Max Lt Lateral and Central Incisor (size 1 film)	Max Lt Cuspid (size 1 film)	Max Lt Premolar (size 2 film)	Max Lt Molar (size 2 film)
Rt Molar Bitewing	Rt Premolar Bitewing					Lt Premolar Bitewing	Lt molar Bitewing
Mand Rt Molar (size 2 film)	Mand Rt Premolar (size 2 film)	Mand Rt Cuspid (size 1 film)	Mand Rt Lateral and Central Incisors (size 1 film)	Mand Lt Lateral and Central Incisors (size 1 film)	Mand Lt Cuspid (size 1 film)	Mand Lt Premolar (size 2 film)	Mand Lt Molar (size 2 film)

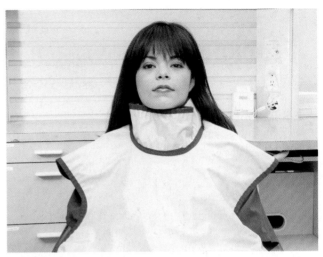

FIGURE 31.5
Patient draped with a lead apron and thyroid collar.

the patient should be filed in the patient's record. All radiographs should be labeled with the patient's name and date of the exposure prior to filing in the patient's treatment chart.

Why are two different types of intraoral radiographic images used for a dental full mouth radiographic survey?

Patient Preparation for Intraoral Radiographs

Regardless of which technique the dentist prefers, a certain protocol must be followed when preparing the patient for intraoral radiographs (see Procedure 31-1). All supplies necessary for the procedure should be set out before seating the patient. Infection control measures must consistently be followed before, during, and after radiograph exposures. A medical and dental history is taken by the dental assistant and reviewed by the dentist prior to obtaining intraoral radiographs.

The patient should be informed of how the procedure will be performed before the dental assistant begins. The patient is seated and positioned comfortably against the back of the chair and headrest, and draped with a lead apron, which includes a thyroid collar (Figure 31.5). All removable items such as eyeglasses, earrings, retainers, jewelry in pierced tongue/lip/nose, and dentures are carefully removed prior to the procedure. The dental assistant should quickly examine the patient's mouth to determine if the patient has any bony protrusions, a shallow palate, a small mouth, or anything that may affect film placement and patient comfort. These may hamper taking radiographs. The dental assistant may need to place the film into the mouth at a different angle than normal for these patients or place a 2 × 2 gauze around the edge of the film for patient comfort.

For those patients with an extremely sensitive gag reflex, having the patient rinse with mouthwash or using distraction techniques will aid the dental assistant in completing quality radiographs. The dental assistant has a responsibility to use techniques that minimize patient discomfort and anxiety such as placing the film gently in the proper position without forcing it or sliding it against delicate tissues. Sliding a film across the patient's sensitive lingual area or palate must be avoided for patient comfort and to avoid stimulating a gag reflex. Confidence and efficiency on the part of the dental assistant will reduce patient apprehension, thereby allowing for cooperation and smooth completion of the procedure. Keeping the fingers between the film packet and sensitive areas ensures that the sharp edges of the film packet will not touch tender areas of the mucosa as the film is placed in the patient's mouth.

The dental assistant should develop a specific routine for exposing a full mouth series of radiographs so that the same teeth are exposed in the same sequence for each patient. Using a systematic approach will ensure that all areas of the mouth are taken and that no films are missed.

Radiation Exposure

Individuals who operate dental x-ray equipment must have basic knowledge of the health risks associated with radiation and must demonstrate familiarity with the basic rules of radiation as discussed in Chapter 29. Both the patient and dental assistant must be kept safe during radiographic exposures. The dental assistant must ensure that the patient is covered with a lead apron and thyroid collar before beginning the procedure. The lead apron should be hung and not folded when stored to avoid unnecessary wear and tear and cracking of the protective lead shielding over time. Recently, nonleaded aprons have been introduced. They are lighter, made of recyclable material, and still protect against harmful radiation.

The acronym ALARA, which refers to "as low as reasonably achievable," is the guiding principle in dental radiography. Dental radiographs are a useful and necessary

Procedure 31-1 Preparing the Patient for Intraoral Radiographs

Equipment and Supplies
- Lead apron and thyroid collar
- Cup or container
- Paper towel

Procedure Steps
1. Explain the procedure to the patient prior to beginning and ask if he has any questions.

2. Seat the patient and adjust the chair in an upright position that is at a comfortable working height for the dental assistant.

3. Adjust the headrest to support and position the patient's head so that the occlusal plane of the maxillary arch is parallel to the floor and the midsagittal plane is perpendicular to the floor.

4. Have the patient remove all dentures, partials, retainers, eyeglasses, and lip, nose, or oral piercing objects. Place them on a paper towel or in a container.

5. Place the lead apron with thyroid collar over the patient.

---

tool in the diagnosis of oral diseases but are only ordered when necessary. The dentist weighs the benefits of radiographs against the consequences of increasing the patient's exposure to ionizing radiation. Only essential radiographs should be exposed and the dental assistant should utilize exposure techniques and processing methods that ensure minimal exposure of radiation to the patient and to the dental assistant.

Radiographs should be exposed and processed accurately the first time to avoid the need for retakes. The dental assistant has an obligation to provide diagnostic quality images without overexposure to the patient and to the dental team member. The essential goal of radiation safety is to prevent injury from exposure to ionizing radiation to patients and dental personnel. Regulations have been established to ensure a maximum permissible dose (MPD) of radiation so that those persons working with radiation are protected. More options for radiation reduction have become available, such as digital radiography.

Principles for Intraoral Radiography

The following guiding principles apply to intraoral radiography whether taking a full mouth series or an individual radiograph:

- *Film placement:* Center the tooth or teeth of interest on the film with the printed side of the film packet facing away from the tooth and PID.

- *Film position:* Position the film and holder toward the center of the oral cavity between the alveolar ridge and the tongue or palate.

- *Vertical angulation:* Properly align the PID in an up-and-down direction to avoid distortion of the image (Figure 31.6). Positive vertical angulation is when the x-ray tube head is positioned above the horizon with

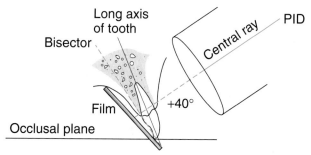

FIGURE 31.6
Vertical projection directed perpendicular to the bisector at approximately +40 degrees with the PID tilted downward.

the PID pointing toward the floor; this position is used for maxillary periapicals and bitewing radiographs. Negative vertical angulation is when the x-ray tube head is positioned below the horizon with the PID pointing toward the ceiling, as is done for mandibular periapical radiographs.

- *Horizontal angulation:* Properly align the PID in a sideways, or right to left direction to aim the central ray of the x-ray beam through the proximal contacts of the teeth (and center of the film) (Figure 31.7). This controls the width of the recorded structures and the ability to see between them.

- *Film exposure:* Use proper exposure time, kilovoltage, and milliamperage settings.

How should the dental assistant place the film packet in the patient's mouth in order to be as gentle as possible and provide for patient comfort? Why should a specific routine be followed when exposing a full mouth set of films?

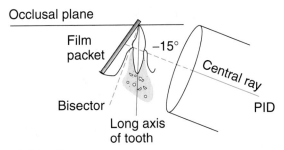

FIGURE 31.7
Horizontal projection directing the central ray through the proximal contacts of the teeth.

Paralleling Technique

The **paralleling technique** for exposing intraoral radiographs is the method recommended by the American Academy of Oral and Maxillofacial Radiology. Fewer operator errors and less image distortion are produced with this technique. When the paralleling technique is used, the x-ray film packet must be placed lingual to the teeth, centered on the tooth and area of interest, with the film extending to cover both the apical and coronal portions of the tooth. The film is placed parallel with the tooth or teeth needing to be radiographed.

When using the paralleling technique the long axis of the tooth and the film are situated parallel with each other. The PID must be guided by the dental assistant so that the central x-ray beam is projected directly **perpendicular**, or at a right angle, to the tooth and the film packet. To properly position the film and PID, a paralleling film-holding device is used. Several varieties of film holders are available from which the dental clinician can choose. Paralleling film holders feature extension rods and a locator ring, which aids in alignment of the PID and x-ray beam. The film usually sits some distance from the tooth in an area of the mouth lingual, or palatal, to the dental arch where there is room to set the film sufficiently to avoid cutting off the apex of the tooth on the radiograph.

Paralleling Holding Devices

Several film holders are available for use with the paralleling technique. They hold the film securely in position to allow the film to sit with its surface parallel to the long axis of the tooth or teeth being radiographed so that the entire image of the tooth is correctly projected on the film. Each paralleling device consists of a bite block, an indicator rod, and an extraoral indicator, usually a locator ring. The indicator rod is a straight line that acts as a visual for the dental assistant to aim between the contacts of the teeth and helps determine horizontal angulations. The bite block holding the film is gently rotated by the dental assistant while it is being placed into the patient's mouth. The bite block is held against the opposing teeth while the patient carefully closes onto it. This allows the

film to be kept in the correct position during exposure of the radiograph.

The patient must be instructed by the dental assistant not to move during the time of film exposure. Any movement by the patient will create a blurred image and the radiograph will need to be retaken. The PID is directed at the center of the film and tooth at a 90-degree angle, or perpendicular, as directed by the locator ring. The most popular paralleling instrument is the Rinn XCP (Extension Cone Paralleling) device or holder (Figure 31.8). Many other types of XCP devices are available on the market that can be selected depending on the dentist's preference.

Assembling the XCP device takes practice and knowledge of the various components (see Procedure 31-2). Once mastered by the dental assistant, paralleling devices are easily manipulated for precise placement of the film in the patient's mouth. The Rinn XCP paralleling apparatus has three distinct methods of assembly:

- Anterior apparatus
- Posterior apparatus
- Bitewing apparatus

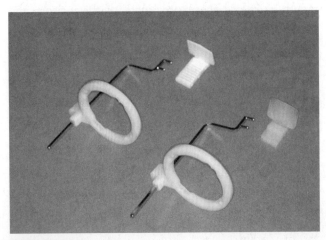

FIGURE 31.8
The Rinn XCP instruments.

Procedure 31-2 Assembling the XCP Paralleling Device

Equipment and Supplies

- Rinn XCP device, anterior and posterior
- Bitewing instruments
- Paper towel

Procedure Steps

1. Wash and dry hands. Lay out paper towels on a disinfected countertop.

2. Gather the sterilized XCP instrument components for the anterior device: the anterior indicator rod, the blue vertical bite block, and the blue locator ring.

3. Insert the two short metal extensions on the anterior indicator rod into the side of the blue bite block.

4. Insert the blue locator ring onto the indicator rod so that the blue bite block is centered within the ring.

5. Gather the components for the posterior XCP device: the posterior indicator rod, the yellow horizontal bite block, and the yellow locator ring.

6. Insert the two short metal extensions on the posterior indicator rod into the side of the yellow bite block.

7. Insert the red locator ring onto the indicator rod so that the yellow bite block is centered within the ring.

8. Gather the components for the bitewing XCP device: the bitewing indicator rod, the red bite block, and the red locator ring.

The film packet is positioned with its long axis vertically for incisors and canines, and horizontally for premolars and molars, with sufficient film extending at least one-eighth of an inch beyond the apices so it records the apical tissues. After assembling the device, the film must be centered when viewed by the dental assistant through the locator ring. If the film is not centered, the device must be reassembled until it is correct. It is imperative to properly position the paralleling device so it is aligned flush with the PID and the tube head cylinder. A Rinn device called the Uni-Grip disposable holder has recently been designed for use with either film or digital sensors.

Anterior Extension Cone Paralleling Device

The anterior portion of the paralleling device is used to record both the maxillary anterior teeth and the mandibular anterior teeth. The bite block and film are placed vertically on the extension rod and in the patient's mouth to record the entire length of the incisors and canines. The Rinn XCP anterior components are color coded blue to differentiate them from the posterior and bitewing devices.

Placing a cotton roll between the bite block and the incisal edges of the anterior teeth aids in keeping the tooth and film parallel with each other. Use of a cotton roll in this manner is optional but it ensures that the incisal edge of the anterior tooth is present in the developed film. Other brands of paralleling devices are color coded as well.

Posterior Extension Cone Paralleling Device

The Rinn XCP posterior components are color coded yellow to differentiate them from the anterior and bitewing devices. The film is placed horizontally into the slot on the yellow posterior bite block. The posterior horizontal portion of the device and the connecting rod must be disassembled and reassembled along with the locator ring depending on which quadrant is being exposed. The maxillary right and the mandibular left quadrants require the same assembly and then must be changed to be used for the maxillary left and the mandibular right quadrants.

After assembling the device, the film must be centered when viewed by the dental assistant through the locator ring. If the film is not centered, the device must be reassembled correctly before placing it into the patient's mouth.

Bitewing Extension Cone Paralleling Device

The bitewing XCP bite block contains a bracket for holding the radiograph film. The bite block is available for horizontal or vertical bitewing films and when properly positioned in the mouth will rest on the opposite side of the mouth being radiographed. When the device is properly assembled with the x-ray film centered in the locator ring and placed in the patient's mouth, the locator ring is moved down the connecting rod until it is almost in contact with the patient's face. This ensures the correct focal spot to film distance. The x-ray tube head, or PID, is then aligned with the locator ring and the exposure made by the dental assistant. The Rinn XCP bitewing components are color coded red to differentiate them from the anterior and posterior devices.

What type of image would occur if the patient moves during exposure of the radiograph? How can the dental assistant prevent this error?

Periapical Radiographs Using the Paralleling Technique

Prior to seating the patient for periapical radiographs, the dental assistant prepares all necessary items, including a cup or disposable container for exposed films. All intraoral films have an embossed dot (a raised spot) to identify right and left. This dot is located on the side of the film facing the x-ray tube and assists in ensuring that the radiograph gets mounted correctly.

When placing the film packet inside the mouth, the dental assistant should hold the instrument by the bite block or ring. For maxillary films the top portion of the film should be tilted toward the center of the mouth making a "V" shape with the bite block. This technique prevents the film packet from scraping across the patient's mucosa on the palate or alveolar ridge. For mandibular films or bitewings, the dental assistant must lift the tongue out of the way with a finger so that the lower border of the film packet can fall into place between the tongue and lingual side of the teeth. The dental assistant should always be extremely gentle with the tender tissues under the tongue. When the film is in place, the dental assistant instructs the patient to gently and slowly close, not bite, his teeth together.

After the film has been placed properly, the dental assistant adjusts the locator ring down the rod near the patient's face. After the film is exposed, the dental assistant should carefully and gently remove the film and device from the patient's mouth.

Methods for Obtaining Periapical Radiographs

Depending on the type of periapical radiograph that needs to be taken, the dental assistant (DA) should follow some standard steps (see Procedure 31-3). If periapical radiographs need to be taken of the maxillary incisor area, the DA should:

1. Set the proper exposure time.
2. Place the film in the anterior paralleling device.
3. Position the device with the film in the patient's mouth.
4. For size 2 film for an 18-film FMX, center the film vertically on the midline so that it is parallel with the long axis of the two central incisors. For size 1 film for a 20-film series, the contact between the lateral and central is centered.
5. Adjust the locator ring down the rod close to the patient's face, align the PID parallel with the locator ring, and quickly expose the film.

When using size 2 film, the central incisors and lateral incisors will be visible. When using size 1 film, only the central incisors will be visible on the patient's radiographs. Figure 31.9 shows how a maxillary incisors exposure is obtained and a radiograph of the final outcome.

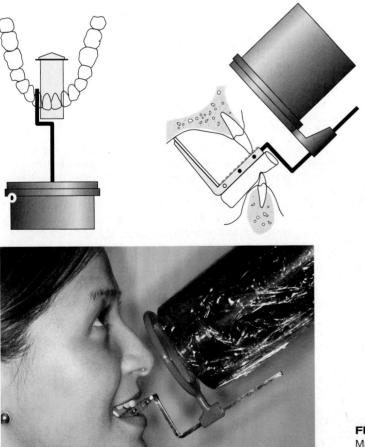

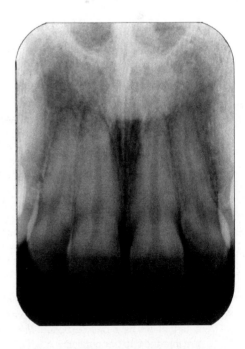

FIGURE 31.9
Maxillary incisors exposure: Diagrams and images showing relationship of film, teeth, XCP® instrument, and PID.

Procedure 31-3 Taking Full Mouth Radiographs Using the Paralleling Technique

Equipment and Supplies

- Rinn XCP device, anterior, posterior, and bitewing
- Periapical film
- Lead apron with thyroid collar
- Cup or container
- Cotton rolls
- 2 × 2 gauze squares
- Paper towel

Procedure Steps

1. Seat the patient comfortably in the chair, explain the procedure, and ask if she has any questions. Drape the lead apron on the patient and assure the patient that the procedure will be completed as quickly as possible. Adjust the control panel settings.

2. Adjust the chair in an upright position to a comfortable working height for the dental assistant. Adjust the headrest to support and position the patient's head so that the occlusal plane of the maxillary arch is parallel to the floor and the midsagittal plane is perpendicular to the floor.

3. Wash and dry hands. Don gloves. Prepare the film-holding devices.

4. Ask the patient to remove any oral prostheses, eyeglasses, earrings, and oral piercings.

5. Look inside the mouth to assess the size and shape of the oral cavity and to identify landmarks such as tori that may cause the patient to be uncomfortable during the radiographic procedure.

6. Begin the full mouth radiograph series in the anterior by inserting a film vertically into the backing plate of the blue bite block by bending it slightly backwards. Make sure that the smooth (white) side of the film packet is facing the locator ring.

7. Place the anterior edge of the bite block on the incisal surface of the maxillary anterior teeth to be radiographed by inserting it at an upward angle for patient comfort. Instruct the patient to close the teeth together slowly but firmly. Slide the locator ring down the indicator rod to near the patient's face, align the PID parallel with the ring, and expose the film. Instruct the patient not to move each time you are ready to expose a radiograph.

8. Remove the film and film-holding device carefully from the patient's mouth. Repeat until all prescribed maxillary anterior films have been exposed. Place each exposed film into the cup or container.

9. Place the anterior edge of the bite block on the incisal surface of the mandibular anterior teeth to be radio-graphed by inserting it at a downward angle for patient comfort. Instruct the patient to close the teeth together slowly but firmly. Slide the locator ring down the rod to near the patient's face, align the PID parallel with the ring, and expose the film. Remove the film and film-holding device carefully from the patient's mouth. Repeat until all prescribed mandibular anterior films have been exposed.

10. Insert a film horizontally into the backing plate of the bite block by bending it slightly backwards. Make sure that the smooth side of the film packet is facing the locator ring.

11. Place the bite block on the occlusal surfaces of the posterior teeth to be radiographed by inserting it into the mouth at an upward angle for maxillary teeth and at a downward angle for mandibular teeth. Gently pull the cheek around the indicator rod where necessary so that the XCP device is inside the mouth and not pulling on the cheek area.

12. Instruct the patient to close the teeth together slowly but firmly. Slide the locator ring down the rod to near the patient's face, align the PID parallel with the ring, and expose the film. Remove the film and film-holding device carefully from the patient's mouth. Repeat until all prescribed posterior films have been exposed.

13. Insert a film into one side of the bracket plate of the bitewing, then slightly flex the film, insert the opposite edge into the other side of the bracket, and center the film. Make sure that the smooth side of the film packet is facing the locator ring.

14. Gently place the bite block on the occlusal surfaces of the premolars aligning the anterior border of the film packet with the distal portion of the mandibular cuspid.

15. Instruct the patient to close firmly to retain the position of the film. Slide the aiming ring down the indicator rod close to the skin surface and align the PID on the ring. Expose the radiograph and then carefully remove the film and XCP device.

16. Repeat for the molar bitewing aligning the anterior border of the film packet with the distal portion of the second premolar.

17. Repeat the premolar and molar bitewing radiographs on the opposite side of the patient's mouth.

18. When all prescribed radiographs have been completed, remove gloves, wash and dry hands, remove the lead apron from the patient, and release the patient. Transport the films to the processing area. Record the radiographs in the patient's record.

Cultural Considerations

If the patient does not speak the same language as the dental assistant, then nonverbal communication may be needed so that the intraoral radiographs will be of proper quality. The dental assistant should always explain to patients how radiographs will be taken. Patients must understand that they are not to move during each exposure. The dental assistant may need to use his or her hands to place the patient's head in the proper position and use hand gestures and facial expressions to illustrate how to hold the radiographic film-holding device by closing the teeth together.

If exposing radiographs of the maxillary cuspid area, the dental assistant follows the same steps centering the film so that it is parallel with the long axis of the cuspid (Figure 31.10).

For radiographs of the maxillary premolar area, the film is centered on the second premolar so that it is parallel with the tooth's long axis and overlapping the distal contact of the cuspid and the mesial contact of the first molar (Figure 31.11).

The device is positioned in the patient's mouth with the film centered on the second molar so that it is parallel with the tooth's long axis and overlapping the distal contact of the second premolar and including the third molar or maxillary tuberosity area (Figure 31.12). The locator ring should then be adjusted, the PID aligned, and the film exposed.

When exposing periapical radiographs of the mandibular incisor area, the film is placed vertically in the anterior paralleling device and the film is centered on the midline so that it is parallel with the long axis of the two mandibular central incisors (Figure 31.13). When using size 1 or 2 film, the central incisors and lateral incisors are visible.

Periapical radiographs of the mandibular cuspid area require that the film be centered on the mandibular cuspid so that it is parallel with the long axis of the cuspid (Figure 31.14). The film should overlap the mesial contact of the lateral incisor and the distal contact of the first premolar.

For radiographs of the mandibular premolar area, the film is placed horizontally in the posterior paralleling device and is then centered on the second premolar so that it is parallel with the tooth's long axis and overlapping the

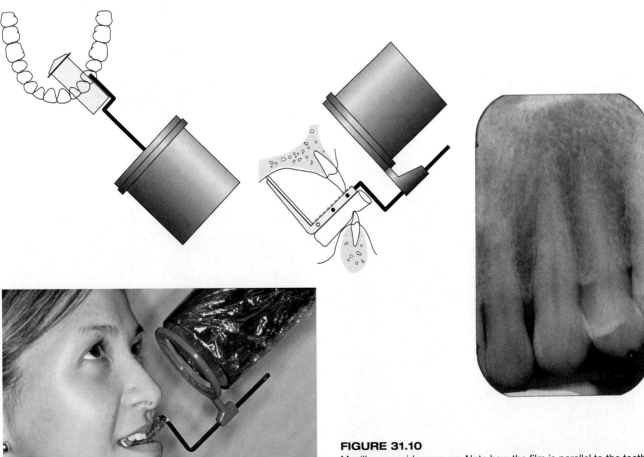

FIGURE 31.10

Maxillary cuspid exposure: Note how the film is parallel to the teeth with the bite block inserted to its full length to position the film up into the midline of the palate to achieve parallelism with the long axis of the canine.

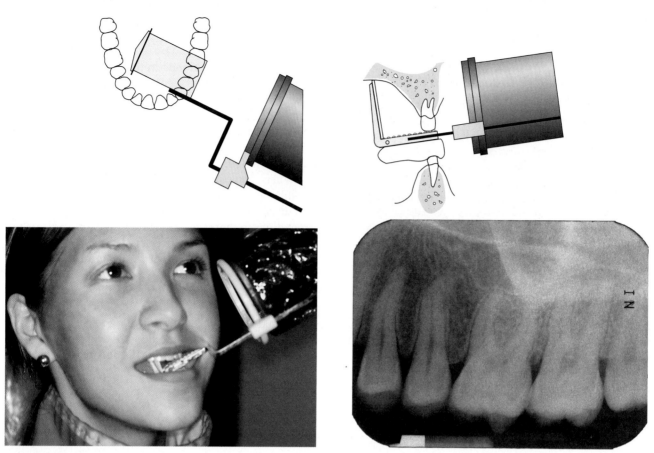

FIGURE 31.11
Maxillary premolar exposure: Note the relationship of film, teeth, XCP® instrument, and PID in the illustrations provided.

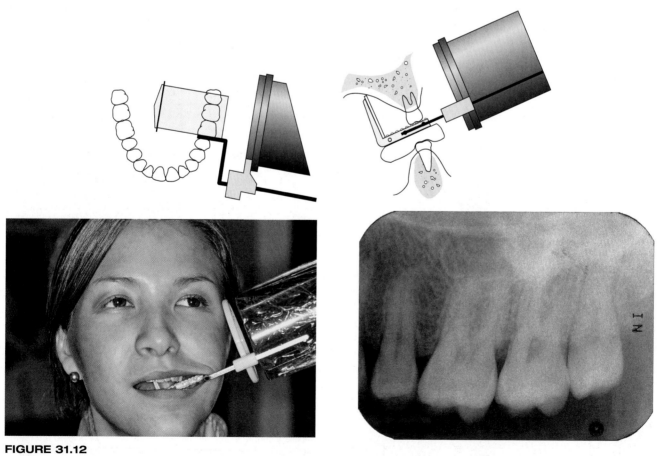

FIGURE 31.12
Maxillary molar exposure: Note in the illustrations how the film is positioned horizontally with the long dimension.

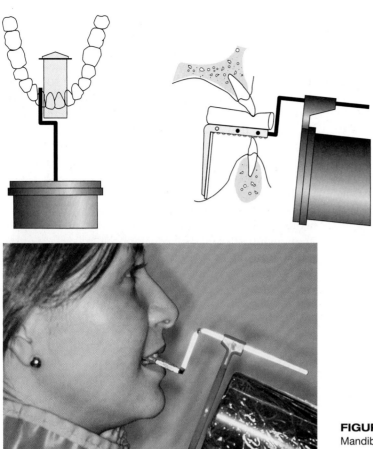

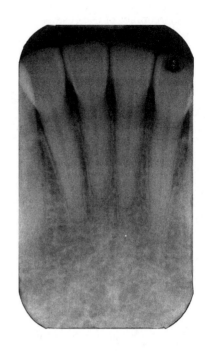

FIGURE 31.13
Mandibular incisors exposure: Note how the film is positioned parallel to the teeth.

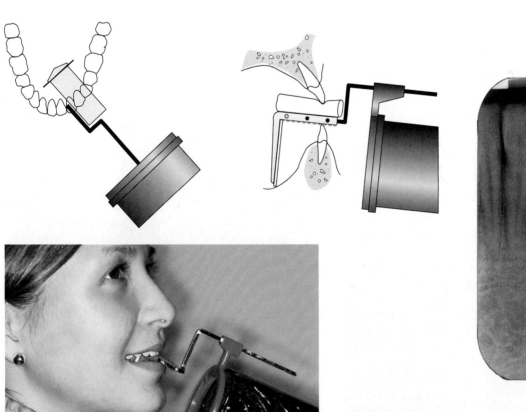

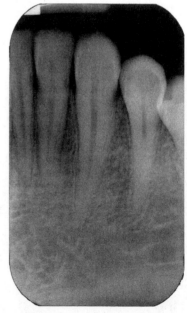

FIGURE 31.14
Mandibular cuspid exposure: Note in the illustrations the relationship of film, teeth, XCP® instrument, and PID. Radiograph provides example of desired outcome.

distal contact of the cuspid and the mesial contact of the first molar (Figure 31.15).

Mandibular molar area films are exposed with the film placed horizontally in the posterior paralleling device (Figure 31.16). The film is then centered on the second molar so that it is parallel with the tooth's long axis and overlapping the distal contact of the second premolar and including the third molar or retromolar pad area. As with the other films, the locator ring must be adjusted and the PID aligned prior to film exposure.

Why must the film and bite block be placed toward the center of the oral cavity when using the paralleling technique for intraoral radiographs?

Bisecting Angle Technique

Another method employed for exposing periapical radiographs is the **bisecting angle technique**. In this technique, the x-ray film is placed at an angle as close as possible to the tooth or teeth being examined (Figure 31.17). To project the proper image of the tooth onto the film, the dental assistant must visualize an imaginary line bisecting the long axis of the tooth and the plane of the film packet. This imaginary line must be seen in the mind's eye midway between the tooth and the film. With the bisecting angle technique, the PID and x-ray beam are directed perpendicular to this imaginary plane that equally bisects a triangle created by the long axis of the tooth and the film. Table 31-2 summarizes the angles used in the bisecting angle technique for various exposures.

The film may be held in place utilizing a bite block or film holder, a bisecting angle instrument (BAI), or a hemostat. The border of the film must extend one-eighth of an inch past the incisal edge or occlusal surface of the tooth. Some of the other types of film holders used for this technique are the Stabe film holder and the Eezee-Grip (formerly Snap-a-Ray) device (Figure 31.18).

Periapical Radiographs Using the Bisecting Angle Technique

Exposing radiographs using the bisecting angle technique requires that the dental assistant recognize certain anatomic landmarks of the face since a locator ring is not used to aim the PID and central x-ray beam. The most important landmarks to be aware of are the ala of the nose, the tragus of the ear, the canthus of the eye, and the border of the mandible. The **ala** is the winged flare of the

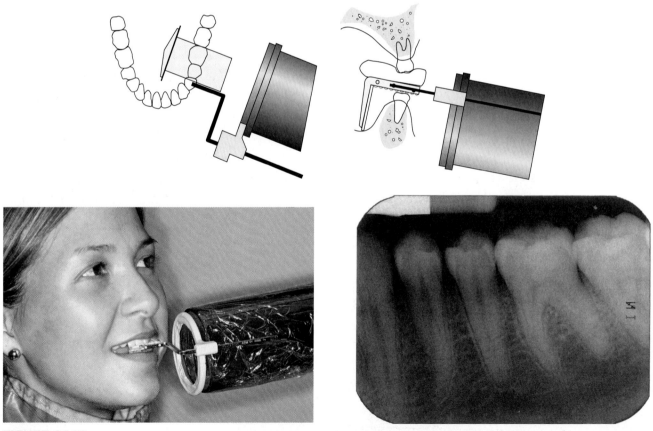

FIGURE 31.15
Mandibular premolar exposure: Note the picture of the patient showing position of the XCP® instrument and PID.

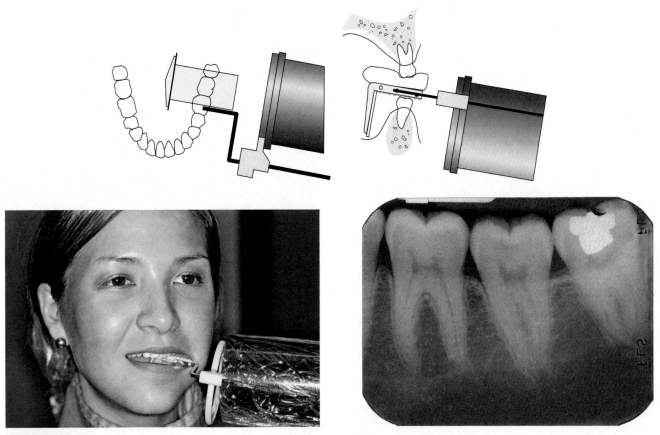

FIGURE 31.16
Mandibular molar exposure: Note how the film is placed horizontally in the posterior paralleling device to obtain an accurate radiograph as shown here.

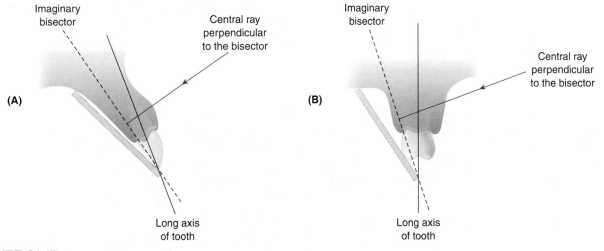

FIGURE 31.17
Bisecting technique using an imaginary line to bisect the long axis of the tooth and the plane of the film packet.

nostril. The **tragus** is the prominence of tissue located toward the middle opening of the ear. The canthus is either corner, or angle, of the eye where the eyelids meet. The inner canthus is closer to the nose, and the outer canthus is closer to the temple. The border of the mandible is the outer portion of the lower jaw.

Knowledge of these landmarks is crucial in order for the dental assistant to have the correct location for the central x-ray beam to expose diagnostic quality radiographs especially when utilizing the bisecting angle technique. (For more information on anatomic landmarks review Chapters 5 and 6.)

Positioning the Patient

When exposing radiographs of the maxillary arch, the dental assistant must position the patient so that the

TABLE 31-2 Bisecting Angle Vertical Angulation

Tooth Area	Maxillary (degrees)	Mandibular (degrees)
Incisor	+40 to +45	−15
Cuspid	+45	−10 to −20
Premolar	+30 to +35	−5 to −10
Molar	+20 to +25	−5 to 0
Bitewings	+5 to +10	+5 to +10

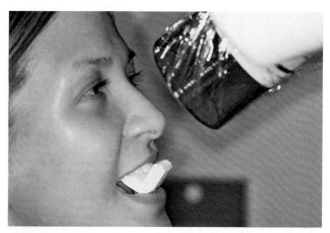

FIGURE 31.19
Patient positioned for maxillary radiographs using the bisecting technique.

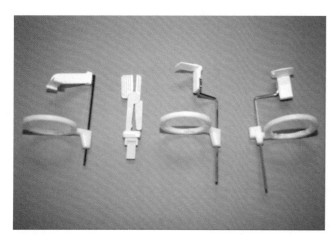

FIGURE 31.18
Film-holding devices.

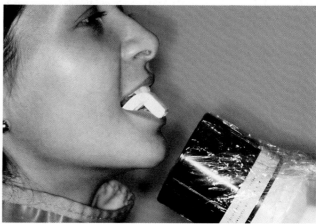

FIGURE 31.20
Patient positioned for mandibular radiographs using the bisecting technique.

ala–tragus line, also called the Frankfort plane, is horizontal and parallel with the floor. This is an imaginary line drawn from the ala of the nose to the tragus of the ear. When exposing radiographs on the mandibular arch, the headrest should be lowered so that an imaginary line running from the corner of the patient's mouth to the tragus of the ear is parallel to the floor. For a proper bisecting angle radiograph, the midsagittal plane, or midline, must be perpendicular to the floor for both the maxillary and the mandibular arches (Figures 31.19 and 31.20).

Positioning the Film and the PID

As with the paralleling technique, the dental assistant should place the film and holder into the patient's mouth gently without irritating oral tissues. Carefully direct the film and holder into position. Center the film packet behind the tooth to be radiographed, with the printed side away from the tooth, and with the dot toward the incisal or occlusal surface. The smooth side of the film must face the tooth and the PID.

The central ray must be centered on the film. If it is not aimed correctly, part of the film will not be exposed and the radiograph will have a **cone cut** error. A cone cut is an error created when only part of the image is

seen on the radiograph due to improper alignment of the PID with the film. The central x-ray beam must be centered on the film and area to be radiographed using the patient's facial anatomic landmarks as follows (Figure 31.21):

- *Maxillary incisor:* at the tip of the nose
- *Maxillary cuspid:* beside the ala of the nose
- *Maxillary premolar:* below the pupil of the eye
- *Maxillary molar:* below the outer canthus of the eye
- *Mandibular incisor:* at the tip of the chin
- *Mandibular cuspid:* directly below the ala of the nose
- *Mandibular premolar:* above the border of the mandible, directly below the pupil of the eye
- *Mandibular molar area:* above the border of the mandible, directly below the outer canthus of the eye

Using the proper angle for the PID and central x-ray beam is mandatory for exposing accurate radiographs when the dental assistant utilizes the bisecting angle technique. The PID must be slanted for correct vertical angulation using the correct bisecting angle relationship of the film to the tooth (Figure 31.22). In addition, the dental assistant should confirm that the correct horizontal angulation is projected through the interproximal contacts of the teeth before exposing the radiograph (Figures 31.23 and 31.24). The dental assistant must also ensure that the PID is centered precisely on the film. Common errors associated with the bisecting method include those discussed earlier: foreshortening, elongation, overlapping, and cone cutting.

Bitewing Technique

Common to both the paralleling and bisecting methods of producing a full mouth radiographic survey is the bitewing technique. **Bitewing radiographs** are the most common radiographic film exposed for diagnosing a patient's oral condition. The bitewing technique produces radiographs that show the coronal portion of the teeth and surrounding alveolar processes of both the maxillary and mandibular arches on one film. Bitewing radiographs are used primarily for interproximal examinations of the teeth. They also show the level of the alveolar bone surrounding the teeth and conditions of other

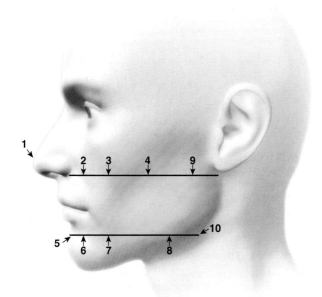

1. Maxillary incisors
2. Maxillary cuspids
3. Maxillary bicuspids
4. Maxillary molars
5. Mandibular incisors
6. Mandibular cuspids
7. Mandibular bicuspids
8. Mandibular molars
9. Tragus of ear to ala of nose
10. Border of mandible

FIGURE 31.21
Landmarks of the face.

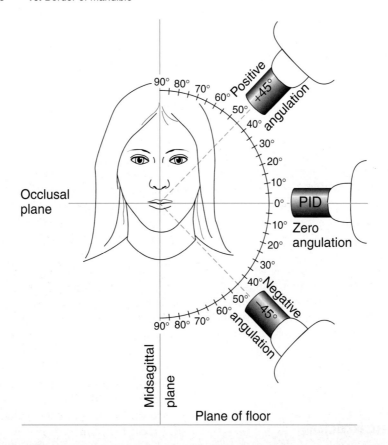

FIGURE 31.22
Positioning of the PID. Angle the maxillary views with positive angulation and the mandibular views with negative angulation. Bitewing radiographs are exposed at almost 0 degrees or at +5 to +10 degrees.

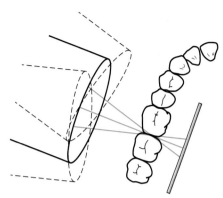

FIGURE 31.23
Correct horizontal angulation.

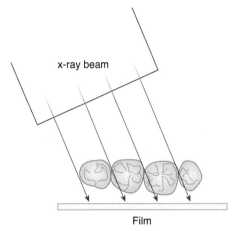

FIGURE 31.24
Incorrect horizontal angulation.

periodontal supporting structures. Interproximal examinations detect:

- interproximal caries
- overhanging restorations
- improperly fitted crowns
- recurrent caries beneath restorations
- certain pulpal conditions
- resorption of the alveolar bone
- destruction of many periodontal tissues
- interproximal calculus

Bitewing x-ray film packets need a tab or wing applied to them. The tab is used to secure the film in the patient's mouth between the arches during exposure. Interproximal radiographs may be exposed of the anterior or posterior teeth but are more often required only for posterior areas depending on the preference of the dentist.

Principles of the Bitewing Technique

For the dentist to perform an interproximal examination with a bitewing radiograph, the central ray of the PID

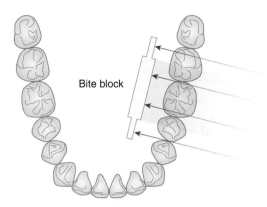

FIGURE 31.25
The radiograph film must be positioned such that it is centered on the premolars so that the central x-ray beam is directed through the proximal contacts of each tooth.

must be aimed horizontally so that it is parallel with and directed through the proximal contacts of the teeth (Figure 31.25). The surface of the tooth crowns cannot overlap each other. If they are overlapped, detection of caries between the teeth is impossible.

Essential to a diagnostic-quality bitewing radiograph are the proper placement and stabilization of the film in the patient's mouth. In addition, the vertical and horizontal angulation of the PID and the central ray of the x-ray tube head must be correct. Adjusting the PID in a side-to-side direction so that the contacts of the teeth are open allows the radiograph to show the proximal surfaces. The primary function of bitewing radiographs is to provide information helpful to the dentist in diagnosing caries and the early stages of periodontal disease.

Bitewing Film Placement

The bitewing film is placed parallel to the teeth. Positioning the film more to the lingual of the teeth may be best depending on the patient's anatomy and comfort. The tab of the film is centered with the line of the tab parallel to the occlusal plane of the teeth. The premolar bitewing film should extend from the distal of the canine to the mesial of the first molar. The molar bitewing should extend from the distal of the second premolar to the distal of the third molar area.

The dental assistant should gently rotate the corner of the premolar film to fit within the lingual area between the tongue and teeth as well as the palatal area. The dental assistant must hold the tab on the occlusal surfaces of the mandibular teeth to provide an equal distribution of the maxillary and mandibular teeth as the patient is asked to close her teeth together. The dental assistant should not use the word *bite* when asking the patient to close her mouth. The bitewing tab should gently be closed on for the patient's comfort and so the tab is not pulled off the film.

For adults, posterior bitewings are taken in two views on each side of the mouth. One view will consist of the premolars and the other view will contain the molars. For children either one or two views will be taken on each side of the mouth depending on the age of the patient and the preference of the examining dentist. When the first permanent molars have erupted into the oral cavity, the dentist often prefers four bitewings to be taken. Until then two bitewings, one on each side of the mouth, are usually sufficient for the dentist to perform an interproximal examination.

Stabilizing the Film During Bitewing Exposures

Bitewing radiographs are taken or exposed using the paralleling technique. The interproximal paralleling device is used to secure the film and to aim the PID for the paralleling technique. The film must be centered within the locator ring. When using a film holding device or any beam alignment device, the primary beam is automatically directed in a parallel position to the film. A bitewing tab can be placed on the film to allow it to be held in place by the occluding teeth (Figure 31.26).

With the paralleling technique there is no locator ring and the dental assistant must ensure that the primary beam is directed toward the center of the tab and therefore directly on the film as well as angled between the contacts of the teeth. The patient is positioned so that the ala–tragus line is parallel with the floor and the midsagittal plane is perpendicular to the floor. As noted earlier, the ala–tragus line is an imaginary straight line drawn from the ala of the nose to the tragus of the ear. The midsagittal plane is the midline down the center of the body in anatomic position. To ensure the film is held in position, the dental assistant must be sure that the patient closes gently but firmly on the bite wing tab or film holder.

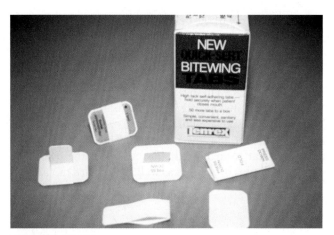

FIGURE 31.26
Bitewing tabs.

PID Placement

The central x-ray beam should be aimed toward the film at a slight positive vertical angle for bitewing radiograph exposure because the teeth are not absolutely vertical but are at about a 10-degree slant. This means that the PID is directed downward toward the floor at a +5- to +10-degree angle in order to produce a quality bitewing radiograph.

The central ray of the x-ray tube head should strike the film at a right angle while passing through the interproximal spaces of the teeth being radiographed. The dental assistant must imagine a horizontal line coming from the tube head and aim it directly between the contacts of the teeth. The angle necessary to aim between the premolars is slightly different than the angle required to open the contacts between the molars. The PID must be directed at an angle more from the front of the jaw in order to open the contacts between the premolars. The PID is directed more to the side of the face and directly on the molar area to view the contacts between the molars.

The dental assistant should always look at the contact areas prior to exposing the radiograph in order to visualize opening the contacts between the teeth to be radiographed. The patient should be told to keep holding his teeth together but to separate the lips so the contact areas can be seen by the dental assistant.

Guidelines for Bitewing Exposures

Regardless of the type of device used for stabilization of bitewing radiographs, the film is always situated parallel to the crowns of the upper and lower teeth. Bitewing radiographs have these requirements:

- The film must be placed in the mouth parallel to the tooth crowns of both the upper and lower arches.
- The film must be stabilized when the patient bites on the tab or the film holder.

- The central ray of the beam is directed through the contact areas of the teeth using a +5- to +10-degree vertical angulation.

For proper exposure of the premolar areas, the x-ray film must be placed in the patient's mouth centered on the premolars and include the distal half of the maxillary and mandibular cuspids (Figure 31.27).For a bitewing radiograph of the molars, the film should be centered on the second molar to include the distal half of the maxillary and mandibular premolars as well as the third molar area (Figure 31.28).

Unlike periapical radiograph views when the clinician must cover all of the tooth apices, in bitewing radiographs the dental assistant only needs to move the film backward from the premolar position to the molar position. The film is moved enough to ensure an examination of the last interproximal contact. Due to the curvature of the arch, the horizontal angles are different on the premolar areas than on the molar areas. This allows the central x-ray beam to open the contacts between all of the interproximal surfaces of the teeth.

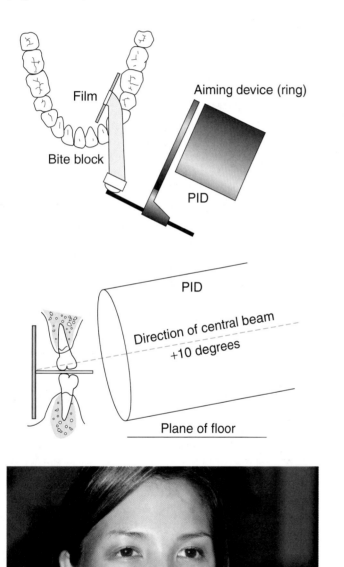

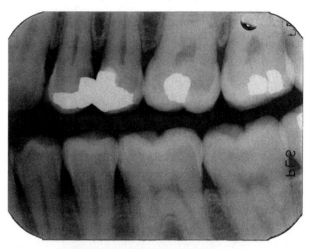

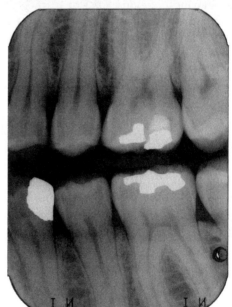

FIGURE 31.27
Premolar bitewing radiograph using a bitewing tab: Note the horizontal projection is through the 1st and 2nd premolar. The vertical projection is directed perpendicular to the film at about 10 degrees with the PID titled downward.

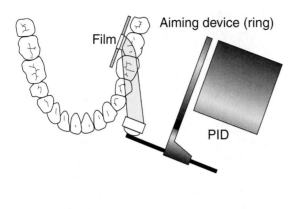

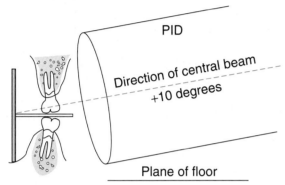

FIGURE 31.28
Illustration showing placement of Rinn XCP device for obtaining molar rightwing radiograph (for example of radiograph please see Figure 31-4).

What is the primary use for bitewing radiographs? What will happen if the central x-ray beam is not directed correctly for bitewing exposures? **?**

Occlusal Radiographs

Occlusal radiographs provide a means to diagnose and examine larger areas of the maxillary or mandibular arches than is possible with other intraoral methods. The occlusal technique is used to supplement periapical and bitewing radiographs. Occlusal radiographs are utilized less often than other radiographs, but are taken more frequently for pediatric patients. Depending on the preference of the dentist, this method can be used in cases where it is difficult for the patient to open his or her mouth wide enough for periapical films to be placed. Occlusal films may also be appropriate for patients who are edentulous (without teeth) or patients with trismus (contractions of the muscles of mastication).

This technique gets its name from the placement of the film between the occlusal surfaces of the teeth for exposure. During this invaluable method of intraoral radiography, the patient closes down or occludes onto the x-ray film packet. The dental assistant may even tell the patient to close her teeth together on the film as if biting on a sandwich. Occlusal films are used to:

- locate pathological lesions
- discover the presence of impacted teeth
- determine if fractures of the jaw exist
- locate root fragments of extracted teeth
- determine if supernumerary unerupted teeth are present
- locate stones in salivary ducts
- examine cleft palates

Occlusal radiographs may be used by the dentist as part of a pediatric full mouth series (Figure 31.29).

Radiograph Exposures Using the Occlusal Technique

The occlusal technique uses larger size 4 films, also called occlusal films, but size 2 films may be used for a smaller child's mouth. (Review Chapter 30 for a discussion of film sizes.) The film is situated in the mouth between the occlusal surfaces of the maxillary and mandibular teeth. It must be positioned with the "dot up" side toward the arch to be examined—toward either the maxillary or the mandibular teeth. The film is stabilized when the patient gently occludes on the film packet. No film-holding devices or beam alignment devices are necessary. This technique uses the patient's teeth to hold the film in place during exposure of the film.

Maxillary Occlusal Technique

To make a radiograph of the entire maxillary arch using the occlusal technique, the dental assistant must do these tasks:

1. Prepare the x-ray unit with the proper settings. Ask patient to remove eyeglasses or any removable objects or appliances from her mouth.

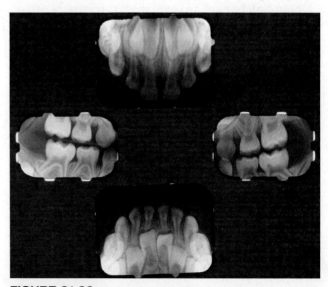

FIGURE 31.29
Radiographic survey of primary dentition.

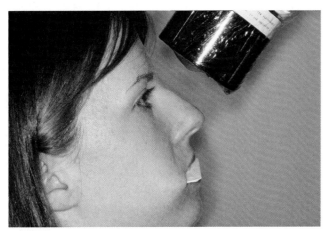

FIGURE 31.30
Position of the tube head for taking a maxillary occlusal radiograph.

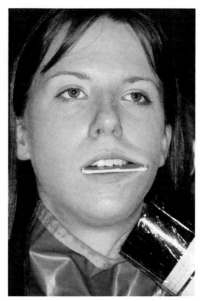

FIGURE 31.31
Positioning of a patient for taking a maxillary occlusal radiograph (anterior).

2. Position the patient so that the ala–tragus line is parallel with the floor and the midsagittal plane is perpendicular to the floor.

3. Place the film in the patient's mouth. Ask the patient to relax the muscles of the mouth and cheek as much as possible. To place the film packet, retract one corner of the patient's mouth until the film packet can be inserted. Position the packet far enough into the mouth so that it covers all of the teeth and with the narrow sides touching the cheeks. If the patient has wide arches the film may be placed with the wide sides touching the cheeks in order to ensure that the entire arch is radiographed. Care must be taken to avoid gagging the patient.

4. Have the patient close gently but firmly onto the film packet to hold it in place.

5. Position the tube head. For maxillary anterior occlusal radiographs, set the vertical angulation of the PID at +65 degrees. Center the tube head cylinder on the bridge of the patient's nose so that the central x-ray beam will be projected onto the film (Figure 31.30).

6. For maxillary posterior occlusal radiographs, set the vertical angulation of the PID at +75 degrees.

7. Make the exposure.

Mandibular Occlusal Technique

The mandibular occlusal technique (Figure 31.31) is similar to the maxillary method except the patient is positioned in a more reclined position in the dental chair and the angulation of the PID is set at a much different angle. The dental assistant performs the following tasks:

1. Prepare the x-ray unit with the proper settings. Reduce the kilovoltage setting for edentulous patients and children.

2. For mandibular anterior occlusal radiographs, position the patient so that the ala–tragus line is at a 45-degree angle with the floor, and the midsagittal plane is perpendicular to the floor.

3. Place the film in the patient's mouth with the dot side toward the occlusal surfaces of the mandibular teeth and the short side of the film packet toward the patient's cheeks. If the patient has a large mandibular arch, the film should be placed with the long side of the film toward the cheeks. Ask the patient to close gently on the packet to hold it in place.

4. Position the tube head. Locate the PID under the patient's chin so that the central ray is centered on the film packet and angled 90 degrees perpendicular to the film.

Occlusal Radiographs for Specific Views

The dentist may request that the dental assistant place the occlusal film on the right or left side of the patient's maxillary or mandibular jaw rather than centered on one jaw or the other. This is done when the dentist must determine the location of an object in a specific area that was

Legal and Ethical Issues

Radiographs are part of the patient's permanent and legal dental record. The dental assistant must ensure that they are labeled with the patient's name and date of exposure. The dental assistant should also document in the patient's record the date and how many exposures were taken of the patient. This documentation must include any exposures that were retaken. When films are duplicated to send to insurance companies or for use by another dental office, they must be labeled accurately.

viewed on another radiograph. A variety of angles will aid the dentist in determining the buccal and lingual aspects of the mandible or the buccal and palatal aspects of the maxillary arch. These various radiographs give the dentist a view from different angles of the same objects in the oral cavity and contribute to an overall inspection of the patient's anatomy.

What is the purpose of occlusal radiographs? What technique will the dental assistant use when aligning the PID before exposing an occlusal radiograph?

Patients with Special Needs

All dental offices should be able to treat patients who have special medical needs and disabilities. Disabilities can range from developmental disabilities to mental or physical disabilities. Special needs patients include those with autism, cerebral palsy, Down syndrome, hearing and visual impairments, and mobility impairments. Dental facilities must have easy access for patients with wheelchairs or walkers. Patients with cerebral palsy may have a severe gag reflex making it difficult to expose dental radiographs. Dental assistants have an obligation to learn to serve patients with disabilities.

Dental assistants must also be sensitive to those patients with dental fears and know how to encourage those individuals to obtain and agree to treatment. There are many ways to encourage a reluctant or frightened patient who might otherwise have to go to a hospital and be put under sedation for oral care. The best way to help a patient through an uncomfortable procedure is to use distraction techniques such as having patients breathe through their nose or asking them to wiggle their toes. Encouraging the patient to engage in deep and slow breathing patterns can help, as can just talking calmly to the patient.

Due to some patients' fears and apprehension regarding dental treatment, the dental assistant must develop methods to keep a patient's mind off the radiographic procedure. Methods can include use of diversion or something as simple as asking the patient to count each tooth. Depending on the patient's situation the dentist may need to use sedation techniques to calm the patient; however, some patients can only be treated under general anesthesia.

Patients Who Have Mobility Impairments

Positioning difficulties during the procedure of exposing of radiographs could exist if a dental patient uses a wheelchair. The patient's needs must be accommodated. Some patients can be moved from the wheelchair into the dental chair for treatment, whereas others will need to have radiographs exposed and be treated while in their own chair. The area for exposing radiographs must be physically accessible by wheelchair and the tube head must be able to reach a seated patient (Figure 31.32). Due to the accumulative effects of radiation exposure, the dental assistant should never hold the film stable in a patient's mouth. The patient's caregiver or guardian may help hold the film in place when necessary. The caregiver and the patient must wear a lead apron.

Patients Who Have Hearing Impairments

Federal laws require dentists to ensure that their services and facilities are equally accessible to those who have disabilities and those who do not. Under the law dentists must provide effective communication, including supplying auxiliary aids and services when necessary. For those who have hearing impairments, the dentist can request an interpreter if needed. The need will vary depending on the patient's requirements, the procedure involved, and the current situation with the patient. Often patients with hearing impairments bring an interpreter with them to dental appointments. Some individuals with hearing impairments read lips. For this reason it is important for the dental assistant to maintain eye contact with the patient and avoid walking around the operatory while speaking.

Patients Who Have Vision Impairments

Providing comprehensive dental care to people with vision impairments is not only rewarding but an obligation for health care providers. People with vision impairments should be communicated with just like anyone

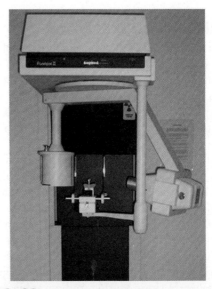

FIGURE 31.32
Panoramic unit that accommodates patients in wheelchairs. Image courtesy Instructional Materials for the Dental Team, Lex., KY

else. The dental environment should be relaxed and casual. Young patients with vision impairments should be allowed and encouraged to touch some of the dental equipment and instruments. Each patient should be informed specifically of what to expect during the radiograph procedure and be told when something such as a dental x-ray film is going to be placed into or removed from his or her mouth.

Why would the dental assistant need to explain clearly to a patient with a vision impairment what to expect during a radiographic exposure?

Positioning Difficulties Encountered with Intraoral Radiography

Radiography techniques may need to be modified based on the needs of the patient. The main difficulties encountered with obtaining intraoral radiographs involve issues such as capturing x-rays of mandibular third molars. Taking films of teeth that have been endodontically treated requires that the film be exposed with the file still in the root canal. The dental assistant needs to place the films in a different manner for patients with edentulous alveolar ridges and use distraction techniques for individuals who have strong gag reflexes. Other special conditions that should be considered when positioning patients for intraoral radiographs include a shallow palate or shallow floor of the mouth, maxillary or mandibular tori, excessive root length, and trismus, in which the muscles spasm and the patient cannot open the mouth very wide.

Mandibular Third Molars

The main difficulty for mandibular third molar radiographs is in the placement of the film packet. When an entire mandibular third molar must be radiographed, the film packet must be placed far enough into the posterior area to capture the apex of the tooth. This is particularly important when the molar is horizontally impacted. To determine the condition of the mandibular third molar, the dentist must be able to view the entire tooth and surrounding tissues, including the inferior vascular canal. The dental assistant must ensure that the edge of the periapical radiograph film is posterior enough so that it is mesial (toward the midline) of the first molar and extending as far beyond the second molar as can be tolerated by the patient. Distraction techniques, such as those mentioned earlier, work well to help the patient keep the film in the proper position during radiographic exposure. Extraoral panoral radiographs are often used to examine third molar areas.

Endodontic Treatment

When a patient is to receive endodontic care, it is important for the dentist to be able to determine the length of the root canals of each tooth. To do so, the dentist relies on good periapical radiographs.

Challenges encountered when exposing radiographs during endodontic treatment include film packet placement and stabilization. This is due to the presence of endodontic instruments in the patient's mouth such as the dental dam and dental dam clamps. Identification and separation of the root canals of multirooted teeth aid the dentist during endodontic treatment. Assessing root canal lengths from distorted foreshortened or elongated radiographs is impossible for the dentist.

When taking an intraoral radiograph on a patient receiving endodontic care, it may be necessary to ask the patient to hold the film packet. This can be done by use of a hemostat or other type of film packet holder. Some manufacturers incorporate a small basket on the platform area to accommodate the handles of endodontic files while still allowing the film packet to be parallel. The Rinn Company's EndoRay device accommodates endodontic files (Figure 31.33).

The dental assistant may be asked to take two different radiographs of a tooth undergoing endodontic treatment. This may need to be done using different horizontal x-ray tube head positions in order to view different root canals normally superimposed over each other. This is especially true for maxillary molars.

Edentulous Alveolar Ridges

Placing a radiograph film packet for a patient who is edentulous (without teeth) or partially edentulous is difficult. In edentulous patients the lack of height in the palate or loss of the alveolar ridge depth contraindicates the paralleling technique; therefore, all periapical radiographs should be taken on edentulous patients using a modified bisected angle technique.

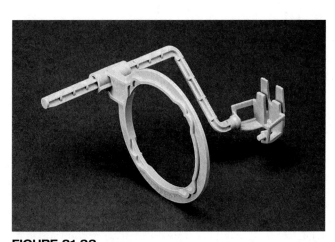

FIGURE 31.33
Paralleling device used for endodontic procedures.
Courtesy of Dentsply Rinn.

The dental assistant will need to assess the long axis of the film packet and the alveolar ridge and adjust the PID as necessary. In partially edentulous patients, the paralleling technique can be used and a cotton roll placed in the area of the missing teeth so the film holder is not displaced when the patient closes his mouth (Figure 31.34). Panoramic and occlusal films may also be used to assess the alveolar ridges of edentulous patients.

The Gag Reflex

Patients with strong gag reflexes can be challenging and require patience and reassurance from the dental assistant. The dental assistant can provide reassurance to the patient by demonstrating the ability to perform the tasks successfully. The dental assistant should be sure to preset the exposure time before placing the film in the patient's mouth, prealign the PID, and be ready to act quickly. The most common area to elicit the gag response is the maxillary molar periapical view. Those films should be taken last. Placement of the x-ray film toward the midline and away from the soft palate will reduce the tendency for gagging.

A variety of strategies can be used on patients who have a strong gag reflex:

1. Have patients breathe through their noses to take away some of the sensitivities of the soft palate as well as distract them.
2. Ask patients to wiggle their toes or hold a foot up off the dental chair.
3. Apply topical anesthetic sprays into the mouth to temporarily numb the area. Note that only dentists are legally allowed to apply topical anesthetic sprays.
4. Hum to patients.
5. Place salt on the tip of patients' tongues if they are not hypertensive.
6. Ask patients to rinse with mouthwash.
7. Provide patients with positive reinforcement.

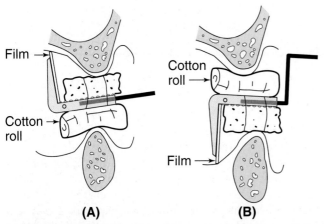

FIGURE 31.34
Using cotton rolls to aid in positioning the paralleling device for a radiograph of a partially edentulous patient.

Pediatric Patients

The main technical problem with children, other than patient management issues, is the size of their mouth and the difficulty of placing the film packet intraorally. Size 0 film may be used for the pediatric patient, and the dentist may request a combination of bitewing radiographs and occlusal radiographs using a modified bisecting technique.

When working with pediatric patients the dental assistant should develop methods to distract patients during radiograph procedures. Using diversion methods, such as asking the patient to count each tooth, may be useful. The dental assistant may count the pediatric patient's teeth beginning in any area just to take the patient's mind off of what is being placed and held in his mouth. The patient's caregiver or guardian may need to help hold the film or film-holding device in place. This is only done with very young and uncooperative patients and if the parent or caregiver is willing. In these cases both the caregiver and the patient must wear a lead apron.

Using language appropriate for a child and showing a sample of radiographs to an uncooperative pediatric patient may be helpful. Because of the smaller size of the pediatric patient, exposure factors such as exposure time, kilovoltage, and milliamperage are reduced.

What are some special dental needs that may create positioning difficulties for the dental assistant?

Technical Errors in Intraoral Radiography

Only essential radiographs should be taken of patients. Keeping the total number of radiographs to a minimum requires an assessment of their necessity each time a patient visits the dental office. Proper techniques must be used by the dental assistant to avoid retakes. Retaking a radiograph on a patient because of an unnecessary technical error results in increased radiation exposure to that patient.

To recognize technique errors and correct them, the dental assistant must know what an ideal radiograph looks like, then compare the radiograph with the error to the "ideal" film. Critical factors to consider when exposing a radiograph include accurate film or digital receptor placement, proper angulation and centering of the PID, effective patient management, and correct exposure time. It is important for the dental assistant to recognize technical errors, determine their cause, and follow the appropriate steps to correct the error(s), as discussed next and summarized in Table 31-3.

TABLE 31-3 Technical Errors, Their Cause, and How to Prevent Them

TECHNICAL ERROR	CAUSED BY	PREVENTED BY
Foreshortening	Excessive vertical angulation	Make sure the film is parallel to the long axis of the tooth and that the central ray is directed perpendicular to the film.
Elongation	Not enough vertical angulation	Make sure the film is parallel to the long axis of the tooth and that the central ray is directed perpendicular to the film.
Overlapping	Improper alignment of the central ray to interproximal spaces	Make sure the central ray is directed between the tooth contacts.
Cone cut	Failure to center the PID over the film	Make sure the PID is centered on the film and within the rectangular marks on the paralleling device.
Backward film	Placing the film with the lead foil side facing the PID, which results in lighter than normal film and a "herringbone" or "tire-track" pattern on the film	Make sure the film is placed with the white or plain surface facing the PID.
Double exposure	Film has two images exposed on one film.	Make sure exposed and unexposed films are kept separate from each other.
Blurred image	Patient movement	Make sure the patient is told not to move during the exposure.
Unexposed	Film not exposed to radiation and is clear	Make sure exposed and unexposed films are kept separate from each other.
Dark image	Overexposed	Use proper exposure settings for the patient and type of film.
Light image	Underexposed	Use proper exposure settings for the patient and type of film.
Artifact on film	Radiopaque objects on film caused by jewelry, eyeglasses, or a prosthesis	Make sure patients have removed eyeglasses, piercings, and removable prostheses before exposure.
Missed apices of teeth	*Bisecting angle technique:* film placed too far above or below the incisal edges *Paralleling technique:* film placed too close to teeth	*Bisecting:* Make sure only one-eighth inch of film extends from incisal edge. *Paralleling:* Make sure film is placed at the middle of the palate parallel to lingual surfaces of teeth and make sure the bite block is seated correctly.
Film too far mesial	Cuts off apices of premolars or third molars	Make sure film is placed to include more than one-half of the distal of the canine or mesial of first molar.
Film too far distal	Fails to include distal of canine or mesial of premolar	Make sure film is centered on the proper area to be exposed.
Bent film	Excessive pressure on one area of the film causes distortion of tooth and bone	Do not excessively bend film, and ask the patient to gently close on the film.

Errors of Angulation and Centering of the PID

For successful intraoral radiographs, proper angulation and centering of the PID is essential. Foreshortening, elongation, overlapping, and cone cutting are all errors in PID alignment. For example, not enough vertical angulation causes elongation of the tooth (Figure 31.35). Excessive vertical angulation causes foreshortening of the tooth on the film (Figure 31.36). Excessive vertical angulation may also cause the cusp tips or apex to be cut off of the film. The dental assistant must make sure that the film is parallel to the long axis of the tooth and that the central ray is directed perpendicular to the film.

Incorrect horizontal alignment of the PID will result in overlapping of teeth on the x-ray (Figure 31.37). Make sure the central ray is directed between the tooth contacts. When part of the film is not exposed, a cone cut error results (Figure 31.38). The dental assistant must make sure the PID is centered on the film and within the ring on the paralleling device.

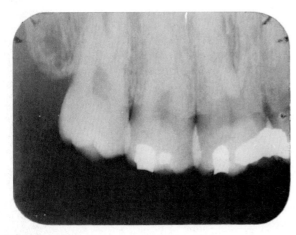

FIGURE 31.35
Problems with inadequate vertical angulation cause elongation.

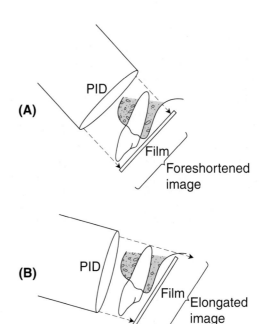

Film and Digital Receptor Placement Errors

Problems with intraoral radiographs can occur due to errors in film or digital placement. If the film was placed in the patient's mouth backward, this would result in a herringbone or tire-track pattern being seen on the film. The film exposure would also be lighter than normal. The dental assistant can ensure this error does not happen by placing the film with the white or plain surface facing the PID (tube head).

When exposing intraoral radiographs, film placement is critical for successful radiographs. The film packet should be located in the proper position in the patient's mouth so that the dentist will have a diagnostic view of the apex and surrounding areas of the tooth or teeth in question. If the film has the apices cut off during the bisecting angle technique, the film was placed too far above or below the incisal edges. The dental assistant must make sure only one-eighth inch of film extends past the incisal or occlusal edge so that at least one-eighth inch past the bone around the apex is visible on the x-ray. If the apices were cut off during the paralleling technique the film was placed too close to the teeth.

During the paralleling technique the dental assistant must place the film at the middle of the palate parallel to lingual surfaces of teeth and make sure the bite block is seated correctly. If the film is placed too far forward in the mouth, the apices of the premolar teeth may be cut off. The premolar film should include the distal one-half of the canine. If the film is placed too far back in the mouth, the film will not include the distal of the canine nor the mesial of the premolar area. When exposing periapical radiographs on a third molar, the film must be placed just mesial of the first molar, or center the film and PID on the second molar to ensure a view of the third molar area.

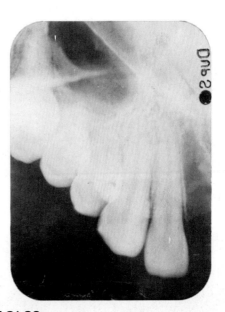

FIGURE 31.36
(a) Illustration of vertical angulation resulting in foreshortening of the image and elongation of the image. (b) Foreshortening caused by both an excessive vertical angulation and incorrect film positioning.

Exposure and Film Errors

When obtaining intraoral radiographs, the dental assistant must pay close attention to issues related to film exposure. For instance, if two images are exposed on one film, a double image will result. Another film may not have been exposed to radiation at all and will be clear. Figures 31.39 and 31.40, respectively, shows examples of overexposed and underexposed film.

The dental assistant should follow a specific routine every time radiographs are taken to be certain no areas are missed and keep exposed and unexposed films separate from each other to be sure only one exposure is taken

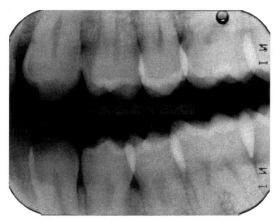

FIGURE 31.37
Overlapping.

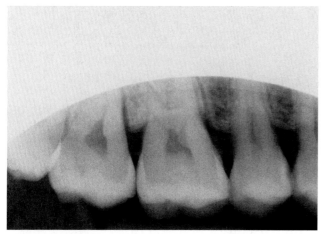

FIGURE 31.38
Cone cut error.

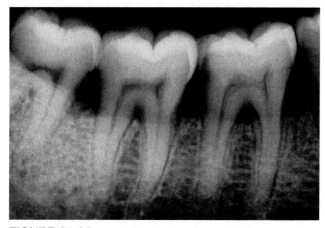

FIGURE 31.39
Overexposed and overdeveloped film.

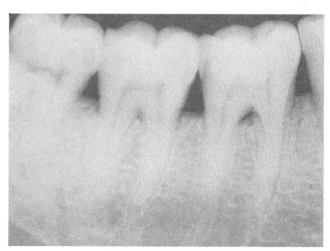

FIGURE 31.40
Underexposed film.

aligns the PID, the patient must be instructed not to move. The patient must understand how important it is not to move during the exposure. The dental assistant should recheck the patient and the tube head before pressing the exposure button.

During film exposure a light or dark image technical error may occur. The film image may be too light or too dark for the dentist to interpret. These types of errors are caused by either the x-ray operator taking her finger off the exposure button too soon, the exposure time being set too short, or the exposure time and film speed being incompatible. These would create a light image technical error. A dark image technical error is produced when the exposure lasts too long or the kilovoltage or milliamperage setting is too high. To avoid these types of errors, the dental assistant must use the proper exposure time and keep a finger on the switch until the audible indicator stops. Manufacturer's directions should be followed to ensure film speed and exposure time matchups. The proper kilovoltage and the film speed must be compatible with the amount of time for which the film is to be exposed.

The presence of an artifact on film is an error that will occur if the patient has not been instructed to remove personal items such as jewelry, eyeglasses, piercings, or a removable partial or complete prosthesis. Artifacts on film appear as radiopaque objects. The dental assistant must ensure that patients have removed these items prior to beginning the exposures.

Bending of film can cause distortions on exposed radiographs and can crack the emulsion on the film creating a radiolucent line (Figure 31.41). Blurring of the tooth and distortion of the bone pattern will occur with bent film. Excessive pressure on one area of a film can cause bending of the film. The dental assistant must ensure that he or she does not bend the radiograph film. Bending the film can be avoided by placing the film in the patient's mouth carefully and having the patient gently close her mouth on the film.

on each film. The exposed films should be placed in a cup or on a paper towel to promote infection control.

Another issue that can affect film exposure is when the patient moves during exposure of the film. This can result in a blurred and undiagnostic image. After the dental assistant places the film in the proper location and

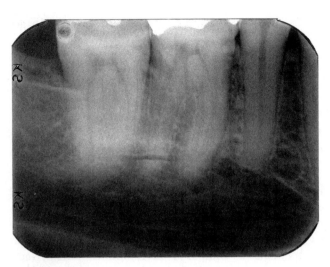

FIGURE 31.41
A black crease present on a film that has been bent.

How will the dental assistant know that the film was placed backwards in the patient's mouth?

Mounting Intraoral Radiographs

Mounting radiographs makes viewing easier. By mounting the radiographs, the films can be placed in order to provide a clear visual of how the teeth appear in the patient's mouth. Placing films on a mount also reduces the need to handle each film individually, protects the film from damage, and provides a permanent record of the patient's films.

Proper film mounting techniques are essential in order for the dentist to interpret and diagnose patients' dental conditions. Improperly mounted radiographs could cause the patient considerable discomfort and create legal issues for the dentist and the dental facility, for instance, if a tooth is mistakenly treated due to improperly mounted film.

A wide variety of x-ray mounts are available from which the dentist can choose. They can be made from cardboard or plastic and contain openings, or windows, for individual films to be placed. Mounts are available for individual films, for 2 to 4 bitewing exposures, or for 18 to 20 intraoral exposures. Films must be mounted correctly and identified with the patient's name, date of the exposure(s), and prescribing dentist. Mounting a full set of radiographs requires that the dental assistant recognize the normal anatomic landmarks of the maxilla and mandible. An illuminator or view box provides an ideal location for the dental assistant to mount the films. The illuminator makes it possible for the dentist to accurately interpret the radiographs.

Radiographs should be mounted with clean dry hands to avoid scratching or smearing the film surface. Films should be handled by the edges only. There are only two ways an x-ray film can be placed in the mount and both depend on the embossed dot for identification of the patient's right and left sides. The embossed dot is part of the manufacturing process and placed so that dental personnel can differentiate the right and left side of the patient when mounting the radiographs. The dental assistant must follow the method established by the dental office for mounting patient films. Mounting radiographs is done by using either the labial or lingual mounting method.

Labial and Lingual Mounting

Labial mounting is the most common method for mounting full mouth radiographs. This system requires that the x-ray films be placed in the mount with the embossed dot convex, facing up or toward the dental assistant, which provides a normal right to left view of the patient's dentition. When looking at the FMX series of radiographs mounted in the labial method, it is as if the dental assistant is seeing the patient's mouth directly, that is, looking at the patient's right and left sides. Therefore, the right side of the patient's mouth is on the dental assistant's left and the left side of the patient's mouth is on the dental assistant's right.

When the embossed dot is placed concave or away from the viewer, this is known as lingual mounting. With this technique the radiographs are viewed as if from the patient's point of view of right and left. Preference by the dentist determines how the dental assistant is to mount the radiographs. Regardless of the mounting method, the dental assistant must ensure that all dots on the films are consistent and all film exposures are located correctly in each window of the mount.

Anatomic Landmarks

By recognizing the normal anatomic landmarks of the maxilla and mandible, the dental assistant is able to properly place the films in the correct location on the x-ray mount. The following is a description of the landmarks that are seen on each radiograph of a full mouth series:

- *Maxillary incisor area:* Incisors are wider mesially/distally and are bigger than the mandibular incisors and there is a large radiopaque region caused by the bone of the nasal septum.
- *Mandibular incisor area:* These are smaller incisors than the maxillary incisors and there is a circular network of tiny radiopaque lines in the center below the roots caused by the genial tubercles.
- *Maxillary cuspid area:* These are the longest teeth in the mouth and much larger than the mandibular cuspids

that usually show a distinct wavy radiopaque line above or near the apices of the teeth caused by the floor of the maxillary sinus.

- *Maxillary bicuspid area:* These should show the distinct wavy radiopaque line of the maxillary sinus above the apices (will not be seen on a mandibular film).
- *Mandibular cuspid area:* These are smaller than the maxillary cuspids.
- *Mandibular bicuspid area:* This is a dark area (radiolucent) below the root apices representing the mental foramen.
- *Maxillary molar area:* These are made up of three roots curving toward the posterior that may be indistinct and there will usually be a distinct wavy radiopaque line above or near the apices of the teeth.
- *Mandibular molar area:* These will show two distinct roots curving toward the distal. The mandibular nerve canal frequently shows as a radiolucent narrow band running horizontally under the apices.

In general, the roots of the teeth curve toward the distal of the mouth, which aids the dental assistant in recognizing how to orient a full set of radiographs when mounting them. The bone of the mandible curves up at the posterior of the mouth as in a smile.

Intraoral Radiograph Mounting Procedure

Before beginning the procedure of mounting radiographs, the dental assistant needs to wash and dry the hands and label the mount with the patient's name, date of exposure, and prescribing dentist's name. All films should be placed on a clean, dry, flat working surface with the dot side placed according to the dentist's preference. Using the appearance of the anatomic landmarks and shape of the teeth the films should be divided into the following groups:

- maxillary periapicals
- bitewings
- mandibular periapicals

The films should be laid out in the order indicated by the pattern on the mount following either the labial or lingual mounting method. Many dental assistants prefer to mount the bitewing films first so that restorative materials, anatomic landmarks, and the shape of the teeth can be compared when mounting the periapical radiographs. The dental assistant should place each radiograph in the proper position in the mount using the natural progression and arrangement of teeth. Once the radiographs are mounted, the dental assistant should evaluate them for accuracy of placement and to ensure that placement of all of the embossed dots is consistent (Procedure 31-4).

Radiograph Storage

Radiographs should always be labeled with the patient's name and date of exposure and stored in the patient's dental record. Individual films may be placed in a mount or in a small coin envelope labeled with the patient's name and date of exposure. These should be stored in the patient's record. Radiographs are a legal record of the patient's condition and must be protected from loss, fire, or other damage.

Procedure 31-4 Mounting Intraoral Radiographs

Supplies

- Processed radiographs
- X-ray mount
- Pen or pencil
- Patient chart
- X-ray view box
- White paper

Procedure Steps

1. Gather all necessary supplies. Wash and thoroughly dry hands. Select the appropriate size mount and label it with the patient's name and date of exposure.

2. On the piece of white paper, identify the maxillary and mandibular anterior, maxillary and mandibular posterior, and bitewing views. Group them together with the embossed dot facing up. Handle films by the edges only, never on the front or back.

3. Once the films are arranged properly place them into the mount in their correct location. Slide each radiograph completely into the appropriate window on the mount. Mount the bitewing radiographs first. Use them to identify restorations and missing teeth which will assist in mounting the other radiographs.

4. Use anatomic landmarks as clues to mount the remaining periapical radiographs.

5. After mounting the films, either put them in the patient's chart, or on the view box for the dentist to view.

Radiographs are the property of the dentist and the originals are maintained at the dental facility. When patients need to take radiographs with them, the dental office will provide duplicates. Dental radiographs are used by forensic scientists to identify victims of accidents and during criminal investigations.

What is used to determine if a radiograph was taken on the right or left side of the patient's mouth?

SUMMARY

Various techniques and equipment are used along with radiograph film to produce a full mouth radiographic survey. The dental assistant must accurately capture each intraoral view of the patient's dentition. The paralleling technique is preferred over the bisecting angle technique because the former produces the most accurate representations of the desired oral structures. Once mastered by the dental assistant, paralleling devices are easily manipulated for precise placement of the film in the patient's mouth. It is the dental assistant's responsibility to provide radiographs with high diagnostic value for the dentist to interpret. Preventing trauma to the sensitive intraoral tissues and patient comfort during exposure of radiographs must be the focus of the dental assistant. This will enhance patient compliance for the procedure.

Once the film is properly placed in the patient's mouth for each view, the PID is aligned outside the mouth and positioned to match the vertical and horizontal planes of the teeth and must cover the entire film packet. Improper alignment of the vertical angle or horizontal angle will result in image errors. It may be necessary to retake the film in order to correct the problem and produce a diagnostic radiograph.

The dental assistant must have an established order or routine for film exposures, especially when it involves exposing multiple radiographs such as a full mouth series. Using an established routine for film exposures will reduce the chance of forgetting an exposure or reexposing the same area multiple times. Also by establishing a specific order, the dental assistant will increase efficiency and therefore decrease the time required to expose a full mouth series of radiographs.

Once all films have been developed, the dental assistant places the films in the proper sequence in a mount that is labeled with the patient's name and date of exposure. Radiographs are part of the patient's legal record.

KEY TERMS

- **Ala:** The winged flare of the nostril. p. 486
- **Bisecting angle technique:** Method of exposing radiographs in which the position-indicating device (PID) and x-ray beam are directed perpendicular (at 90 degrees) to an imaginary line that equally bisects a triangle created by the long axis of the tooth and the film. p. 486
- **Bitewing radiograph:** Radiograph used primarily to examine the interproximal surfaces of the teeth. p. 489
- **Cone cut:** An error created when only part of an image is seen on a radiograph due to improper alignment of the PID with the film. p. 488
- **Elongation:** A vertical angulation error that occurs when there is insufficient vertical angulation of the PID to the film. p. 475
- **Foreshortening:** A vertical angulation error that occurs when there is excessive vertical angulation of the PID to the film. p. 475
- **Horizontal angulation:** Proper alignment of the PID in a side-to-side or back-and-forth direction. p. 478
- **Interproximal:** Between two adjacent surfaces next to each other in the same arch. p. 476

- **Long axis of the tooth:** An imaginary line passing vertically, or lengthwise, through the tooth that divides the tooth in half. p. 474
- **Overlapping:** A horizontal angulation error that occurs when the x-ray beam is not at 90 degrees to the tooth and film, and images from two adjacent structures are superimposed on top of each other. p. 475
- **Paralleling technique:** Method of exposing periapical radiographs in which the long axis of the tooth and the film are situated parallel with each other and the PID is directed at the center of the film and tooth at a 90-degree angle, or perpendicular, as directed by the locator ring. p. 479
- **Periapical radiograph:** Radiograph that shows the desired teeth and the surrounding areas including the apices. p. 476
- **Perpendicular:** Intersecting at or forming a right angle, or a 90-degree angle, to the tooth and film packet, creating a corner (the opposite of parallel). p. 479
- **Position-indicating device (PID):** A cylinder (or cone) affixed to the tube head that is used to align the x-ray with the film in the patient's mouth. p. 474

KEY TERMS (continued)

- **Radiograph:** A one-dimensional view of a three-dimensional subject, the patient; also known as x-ray or film.   p. 474
- **Tragus:** The prominence of tissue located toward the middle opening of the ear.   p. 487

- **Vertical angulation:** Proper alignment of the PID in an up-and-down direction.   p. 478

CHECK YOUR UNDERSTANDING

1. Which of the following is a type of intraoral radiography?
   a. periapical
   b. panoramic
   c. bitewing
   d. both a and c

2. Which of the following techniques are used to expose periapical radiographs?
   a. occlusal technique
   b. bisecting angle technique
   c. paralleling technique
   d. both b and c

3. Which of the following would need to be corrected to prevent overlapping contacts on a radiograph?
   a. vertical angulation
   b. horizontal angulation
   c. film size
   d. film-holding device

4. Periapical radiographic films are used by the dentist to determine
   a. the length of the tooth root.
   b. the number and shape of root canals.
   c. the condition of the supporting bone and gingiva.
   d. the presence of pathological lesions.
   e. all of the above.

5. What type of intraoral film exposure is used by dentists to examine large areas of the maxilla or mandible?
   a. occlusal radiograph
   b. periapical radiograph
   c. bitewing radiograph
   d. panoramic radiograph

6. What are the most common radiographic films exposed for diagnosing a patient's oral condition?
   a. occlusal radiograph
   b. periapical radiograph
   c. bitewing radiograph
   d. panoramic radiograph

7. What might help the dental assistant expose radiographs for a patient who has a gag reflex?
   a. Ask patient to breathe through nose.
   b. Ask patient to wiggle toes.
   c. Use a topical anesthetic spray.
   d. Act confident.
   e. All of the above.

8. What error took place if the film has a herringbone or tire-track design on it?
   a. patient movement
   b. bent film
   c. backward film
   d. overlapping

9. What errors are caused by improper vertical alignment of the PID?
   a. foreshortening
   b. overlapping
   c. elongation
   d. both a and c

10. How is the embossed dot on the radiograph placed when using the labial mounting technique?
    a. convex
    b. concave
    c. toward the operator
    d. a and c

INTERNET ACTIVITIES

- For additional information on film placement using the paralleling technique, visit www.fleshandbones.com/readingroom/pdf/229.pdf
- Research mounting of a full mouth survey at www.waybuilder.net/sweethaven/MedTech/Dental/DentalRad/lessonMain.asp?iNum=fra0304

WEB REFERENCES

- American Academy of Pediatric Dentistry: Dental Care for Special Child   www.aapd.org/publications/brochures/specialcare.asp
- Clinical Practice: Introducing Digital Radiography in the Dental Office: An Overview   www.cda-adc.ca/jcda/vol-71/issue-9/651.pdf
- Free Education on the Internet: Fundamentals of Dental Radiography   http://free-ed.net/free-ed/MedArts/DentalRad01.asp
- Indiana State Department of Health: Dental Radiography Study Guide   www.in.gov/isdh/regsvcs/radhealth/pdfs/dental_study_guide.pdf
- Journal of the American Dental Association: The Use of Dental Radiographs   http://jada.ada.org/cgi/content/full/137/9/1304

Extraoral and Digital Radiographic Procedures

Chapter Outline

Learning Objectives

After reading this chapter, the student should be able to:

- Explain how to load film in an extraoral radiograph cassette.

- Discuss how to prepare a patient for extraoral and digital radiograph exposure.

- Describe patient positioning and extraoral radiograph exposure techniques.

- Identify landmarks in a panoramic radiograph.

- List common panoramic radiograph technique errors and how to correct them.

- Describe how cephalometric, Towne's, and Waters view extraoral radiographs are exposed.

- Discuss digital radiograph technology and the three methods used for obtaining digital radiographs.

Preparing for Certification Exams

- Expose and process panoramic, extraoral, and digital radiographs.

Key Terms

Ala–tragus line	Frankfort plane
Anterioposterior plane	Intensifying screens
Cassette	Lateral
Edentulous	Midsagittal plane
Extraoral radiographs	Panoramic radiography

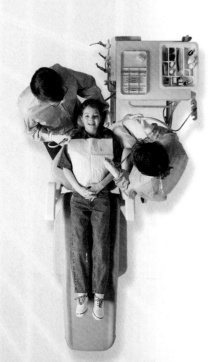

Extraoral radiographs

are those taken outside of the mouth. These x-ray films are taken with sheet film placed inside a protective film-holding container called a **cassette**. A cassette can be soft or rigid. Cassettes serve as light-tight film holders and are equipped with two **intensifying screens** that convert x-ray energy into light energy. The sheet of film is placed between the two screens. When activated by radiation, a fluorescent glow from the intensifying screens exposes the film. Extraoral radiographs include panoramic and cephalometric radiographs as well as several other views of the neck and skull that may be used to diagnose certain patient conditions. Newer panoramic and extraoral radiography machines are capable of producing digital radiographs on a computer screen. Both intraoral and extraoral images can be created with digital imaging systems.

Panoramic Radiography

Panoramic radiography is a radiographic technique for producing an image of the facial structures that includes both the maxillary and mandibular arches (Figure 32.1). The image includes supporting structures such as the maxillary sinus, nasal fossa, temporomandibular joint, styloid process, and hyoid bone. The image is obtained by rotation of the x-ray source and the film cassette at the same speed in opposite directions around the sides and back of the head (Figure 32.2). Panoramic radiography is the most commonly used extraoral imaging in dentistry.

Panoramic radiograph machines have many components, each of which has a specific function as described in Table 32-1.

Dental Assistant PROFESSIONAL TIP

As a dental assistant it is important to pay attention to your patient's level of comfort. The thickness of current corded digital radiograph sensors may make placement in the mouth more difficult for the dental assistant; however, proper positioning techniques, confidence, and efficiency during the procedure will minimize problems. Often, positioning sensors farther away from the teeth, more toward the center of the mouth, makes the patient more comfortable.

Preparing for Externship

Proper care and cleaning of film cassettes and intensifying screens is very important. The dental assistant must take care not to scratch or stain the screens with chemicals because these will seriously affect emission of the screen. The film cassettes and screens should be cleaned with the appropriate cleaning and antistatic solution supplied by the manufacturer. Wipe one screen at a time and wipe in one direction only. After cleaning, the dental assistant should wipe each screen with a dry gauze square or lint-free cloth and leave open until thoroughly dried.

Panoramic Image Receptors

Film used for panoramic radiography is more sensitive to light and packaged differently than intraoral film. It is 5 × 12 inches, 6 × 12 inches, or 15 × 30 cm in size. Panoramic film holders may be rigid or flexible with intensifying screens on each side of the internal walls. The screens have a crystalline phosphor layer that produces visible light when exposed to x-rays and reflects that light back to the film, reducing the exposure time to the patient. Rare earth elements are used as intensifying screen material, and film is manufactured for use with certain screens. For instance, Kodak film is packaged as green-sensitive film to be used with rare earth screens and blue-sensitive film with X-Omat screens.

Screen film is packaged in boxes containing 50 to 100 films and must be handled in a darkroom. Extraoral sheet film is extremely sensitive to light; sometimes even the light from a red safelight is enough to affect the film if exposed to it long enough. The dental team must ensure that the film is used in complete darkness and only with safelight filters that are compatible with the particular type of film. The film manufacturer should be consulted to make certain the specific film is compatible with a particular type of safelight.

A single film is loaded between the screens, the cassette latch is closed prior to leaving the darkroom, and

Cultural Considerations

Nonverbal communication may be needed if the patient does not speak the same language as you. All patients must be informed about how the radiograph will be taken; for instance, whether it is a panoramic image, another extraoral film, or through use of a digital sensor. They must understand that they are not to move during the exposure and to follow other instructions given. The dental assistant may need to use his or her hands to put the patient's head in the proper position so that the patient realizes what is needed.

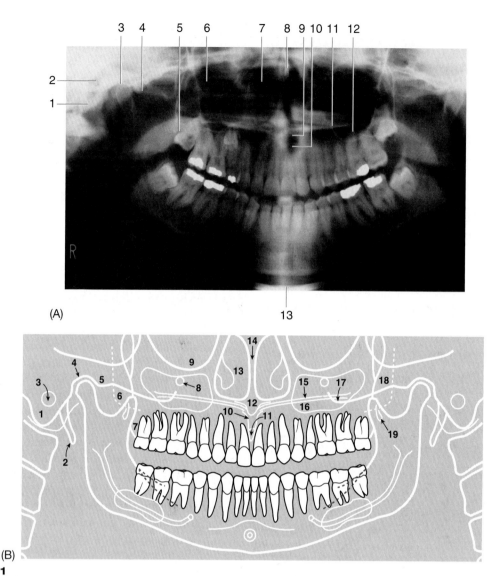

FIGURE 32.1

(a) Panoramic radiograph showing the maxilla and surrounding normal anatomic landmarks: (1) mastoid process, (2) external auditory process, (3) glenoid fossa, (4) articular eminence, (5) maxillary tuberosity, (6) orbit of the eye, (7) nasal cavity, (8) nasal septum, (9) incisive canal, (10) incisive foramen, (11) hard palate, (12) maxillary sinus, and (13) chin rest (machine part artifact).

(b) Drawing of panoramic radiograph showing the maxilla and surrounding normal anatomic landmarks: (1) mastoid process, (2) styloid process, (3) external auditory meatus, (4) glenoid fossa, (5) articular eminence, (6) lateral pterygoid plate, (7) maxillary tuberosity, (8) infraorbital foramen, (9) orbit of the eye, (10) incisive canal, (11) incisive foramen, (12) anterior nasal spine, (13) nasal cavity, (14) nasal septum, (15) hard palate, (16) maxillary sinus, (17) zygomatic process of the zygoma, (18) zygoma, and (19) hamulus.

the cassette is then placed into the cassette holder on the panoramic machine (Figure 32.3). The dental assistant must be sure to secure the cover on the film box while in the darkroom so that the other sheet film in the box is not destroyed by being exposed to white light.

Panoramic Radiograph Positioning

Positioning of the patient should be done according to the manufacturer's recommendations. Head positioning devices and chin rests are important for accurate placement. The dental assistant must take the time to position the patient correctly and to explain the purpose and operation of the equipment. The patient should be informed that the panoramic x-ray unit goes around the back of the head and that the patient must not move during the entire time of the exposure. Four anatomic planes are used to position patients in the panoramic unit:

- Midsagittal plane
- Ala–tragus line
- Frankfort plane
- Anteroposterior plane

The **midsagittal plane** is a horizontal line perpendicular (at a right angle) to the floor, or the line that divides

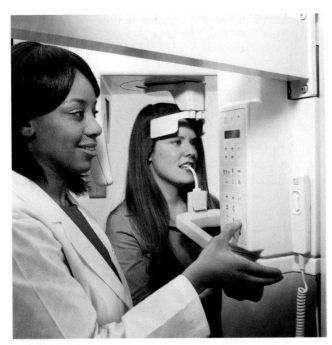

FIGURE 32.2
Panoramic radiograph machine with patient positioned for exposure.
Courtesy Gendex Dental Systems

TABLE 32-1 Panoramic and Extraoral Unit Components and Their Function

Panoramic and Extraoral Unit Component	Component Function
X-ray tube head	Houses the x-ray generator and beam limiter. X-rays are emitted from the tube head during an exposure.
Rotating arm	Supports the x-ray tube head and film cassette holder, rotating them around the patient's head when an exposure is made.
Temple supports	Supports stabilization of the patient's head to maintain correct positioning.
Forehead support	Stabilizes the forehead of the patient.
Film cassette holder	Holds film cassette in correct position.
Mirror	Used by the operator to assist in patient positioning and to check the position of the patient's head.
Chin rest	The chin rest and bite block rod are used to properly position the patient.
Chin rest arm	Supports the chin rest base and may be raised or lowered as needed.
Hand grips	Held by the patient during positioning and exposure, for stability and image clarity.
Superstructure	Supports the drive, rotating arm, and chin rest arm. The height is adjusted electrically by the operator during positioning.

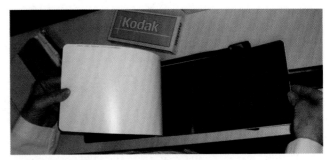

FIGURE 32.3
Flexible cassette used for panoramic and extraoral imaging.
Image courtesy Instructional Materials for the Dental Team, Lex., KY

the body into right and left halves (Figure 32.4). Many machines display a vertical alignment light or mirror so that the right and left sides of the dental arches are shown equally.

The plane of occlusion is a horizontal line parallel to the floor. This plane includes the **Frankfort plane**, which is a horizontal line from the upper margin of the ear to the lower margin of the eye orbit (Figure 32.5), and the **ala–tragus line**, which runs from the winged flare of the nostril (ala) to the opening of the ear (tragus).

These landmarks are used to align the vertical position of the patient's head. Some machines provide a horizontal alignment light to obtain a proper vertical position. The **anterioposterior plane** is a forward–backward plane aligned with a specific landmark that varies among panoramic units (Figure 32.6). It is often aligned between the maxillary lateral incisor and cuspid contact.

When positioning a patient, the individual should be asked to remove any glasses, jewelry, piercings, and other metallic devices on and around the head and neck areas. Full or partial dentures should also be removed. Several

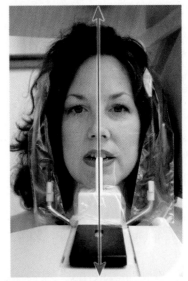

FIGURE 32.4
Midsagittal plane.
Courtesy Gail Williamson, RDHMS, Professor of Dental Diagnostic Sciences, Indiana University School of Dentistry

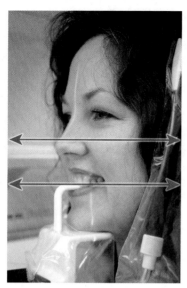

FIGURE 32.5
Ala–tragus line.
Courtesy Gail Williamson, RDHMS, Professor of Dental Diagnostic Sciences, Indiana University School of Dentistry

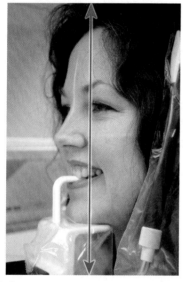

FIGURE 32.6
Anterioposterior plane.
Courtesy Gail Williamson, RDHMS, Professor of Dental Diagnostic Sciences, Indiana University School of Dentistry

additional instructions must be given to the patient, including:

- How to bite on the bite block
- To close the lips
- To place the tongue against the roof of the mouth
- To keep completely still during the entire cycle of the exposure

Panoramic lead aprons that cover the shoulders should be used. Some designs are double sided to cover both the patient's front and back. The lead collar should not be used for panoramic radiography because it blocks the image of the patient's neck and possibly part of the lower jaw.

Common Panoramic Technical Errors

Not taking patient factors into consideration is a common panoramic technical error. Patient factors with regard to exposure settings must be considered before exposing a panoramic radiograph. Exposure settings that the dental assistant must understand are the milliamperage (mA), which determines the quantity of radiation electrons produced, and kilovoltage (kV), which determines the quality and penetrating power of the electrons. Patient factors must be taken into consideration when determining the exposure setting. Factors include if the patient is obese, has a large bone structure, or has a small bone structure. It is important to select the appropriate kV and mA for each patient. Manufacturers typically provide exposure setting recommendations.

Exposure factor problems occur when the film is underexposed or overexposed. A light pale film has had too little exposure. If this occurs, the dental assistant should increase the kilovoltage or milliamperage setting or use the next higher setting.

Another technical error is that of improper positioning of the patient. Improper positioning can cause various errors to occur. The patient must be positioned correctly in the panoramic unit. Table 32-2 lists common panoramic radiograph errors and how they can be corrected. If the patient's head is positioned too far forward, positioned too far back, or tilted to one side the panoramic radiograph will not be of diagnostic quality. Ghost images occur when an object is imaged twice, once on the normal side of the x-ray beam and again on the opposite side (Figure 32.7).

Artifacts are unwanted objects or unreadable areas on a radiograph. The chin rest, bite piece, and alignment devices aid in exposing the best possible panoral film. Manufacturer's directions should always be consulted when using any equipment. The lead apron is placed on the back of the patient for exposure with a panoramic radiography unit, and the dental assistant must ensure that the patient's shoulders holding the lead apron are

Patient Education

The dental assistant can avoid many radiographic exposure errors by ensuring that patients understand what is expected of them during x-ray exposure. Patients must be instructed to remain still while the panoramic machine rotates around their heads. Good communication between the dental assistant and the patient should help the patient feel more at ease and comfortable during this process.

TABLE 32-2 Common Panoramic Film Errors and Corrections

Problem	Cause	How to Correct	Hints
Anterior teeth in both arches are out of focus; they are blurred and narrow in appearance; premolars are slightly overlapped.	Patient positioned too far forward.	Be sure the patient's teeth are correctly biting the bite block and the chin is resting properly in the chin rest. The anterior incisors must be in the groove on the bite block.	This problem often occurs when the anterior teeth are missing. A cotton roll could be used to raise the alveolar ridge.
Anterior teeth of both arches are out of focus; they are blurred and wide in appearance; excessive ghosting of mandible and spine.	Patient positioned too far back.	Check placement of patient's chin in the chin rest and position the incisors in the bite block groove.	The dental assistant may need to purposely move the patient further forward to obtain a proper image.
Apices of lower incisors are out of focus and blurred; shadow of hyoid bone is superimposed on the anterior mandible; condyles may be cut off at the top of the radiograph and premolars are severely overlapped.	Patient's head is tilted downward; chin is positioned back while forehead is positioned forward.	Use the reference lines on the panoramic unit to align the planes of the face properly.	Each panoramic unit has different instructions on how to align anatomic structures with specific lines on the machine. It is better to err with the chin too far down than too far up.
One condyle is larger than the opposing one; image appears to be tilted; one angle of mandible is higher than the other.	Patient's head is tilted to one side; film is crooked in cassette.	If the panoramic unit is equipped with a positioning light, adjust the patient's head until the vertical positioning light aligns with the midsagittal line of the patient. If there is no light, align the midsagittal plane visually so that it is perpendicular to the floor.	There may be an anatomic or pathological reason for the difference in the right and left condyle sizes. If the occlusal plane is parallel to the bottom edge of the film, the difference is probably anatomic or pathological. On units with mirrors, you can tape a vertical line on the mirror that the patient can use as a reference point.
Dark shadows appear in the maxilla below the palate; maxillary apices are obscured.	Patient's tongue was not fully placed against the roof of the mouth.	Ask the patient to place the tongue fully against the roof of the mouth and hold it there during the exposure.	To help patients understand about placing the tongue, ask them to swallow and note how the tongue feels against the palate, and then ask them to hold that position for the duration of the exposure.
Portion of the image is blurred; lacks sharpness.	Blurred images on radiographs are the result of motion during exposure.	Remind the patient to remain perfectly still during the exposure.	Take time to explain to the patient how the equipment moves prior to taking a panoramic x-ray. The patient will have a better idea about how long he or she will have to remain motionless. If the patient has a very wide head or protruding ears, these structures may touch the receptor during machine rotation and the patient may unintentionally move.
Pyramid-shaped opacity appears in the middle of the image.	Patient was slumped; spinal column was not erect, causing a ghost image of the spine to be superimposed in the center of the film.	Keep spine erect. Do not allow patients to reach their chin to the chin rest. Ask them to drop, or lower, their shoulders.	Patients with short, thick necks or those with arthritis may not be positioned in such a way as to eliminate this artifact.

(continued)

TABLE 32-2 Common Panoramic Film Errors and Corrections *(continued)*

Problem	Cause	How to Correct	Hints
White radiopaque artifact (image) appears on film.	Common objects should have been removed before the radiograph exposure.	Remember to ask the patient to remove eyeglasses, earrings, necklaces, hair pins, hearing aids, ornamental hair pieces, etc.	Do not forget to ask the patient to remove tongue piercings as they will interfere with a quality panoramic image.
Random white artifacts are seen on the film.	Lint or small pieces of debris have gotten between the film and screens; intensifying screen was scratched or splashed with x-ray chemicals.	Clean intensifying screens to remove dirt; check them for scratches or contact with chemical solutions.	The phosphor layer of the intensifying screens absorbs the x-rays, then converts them to light in the form of a fluorescent glow, which exposes the film. If the screen is scratched or dirty there will be an unexposed area.
Dark artifacts or black tree-like marks appear on the film.	Film is bent or creased; processing chemicals splashed, or static electricity.	Handle film with caution. Static is normally caused by low humidity or static-producing objects. Carefully remove exposed film from the cassette.	Avoid rapidly pulling the film from the package and hold it only at the corners. Increase humidity in the room where the film is stored. Place rubber mats on the floor where the film is unboxed and placed in the cassette.
Film is fogged; overall darkening of film.	Film is old or improperly stored; film was exposed to white light; safelight was too close to work area or wrong wattage or color.	Check the expiration date on film. Check for light leaks, possible other light sources. Check the safelight bulb wattage and distance from working surface.	Special care is needed to protect film. Film will fog if exposed to humidity, chemical fumes, or x-radiation. Keep unused film in sealed boxes and store below 70°F.

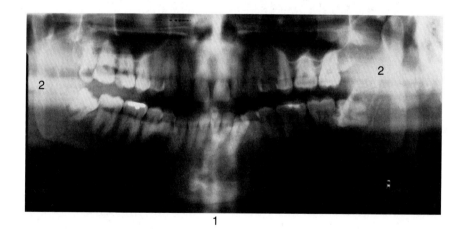

FIGURE 32.7
Panoramic radiograph showing ghost images. (1) Ghost image of the spinal column (cervical vertebrae), and (2) ghost image of the opposite side of the mandible.

held low enough so they do not interfere with rotation of the unit or a proper image. A lead apron can also create an unwanted artifact on the radiograph.

The dental assistant must always prepare the patient for radiography. The dental assistant should first look in the patient's mouth to determine basic oral anatomy and ask the patient to remove eyeglasses, hairpins or clips, earrings, any piercings, and removable prostheses. Kodak, a leading manufacturer of panoramic films, sug-

gests dental assistants follow these 10 steps to obtain panoramic radiographs:

1. Load cassette.
2. Set exposure factors.
3. Have patient remove jewelry; place lead apron on patient.
4. Have patient bite on bite rod.
5. Adjust the chin tilt.

6. Position the side guides.
7. Have the patient stand up straight.
8. Have patient swallow, hold tongue to roof of mouth, and hold still.
9. Expose the film.
10. Process the radiograph.

Errors in exposure factors, in technique, and during processing of the film can cause undesirable results and possibly an unreadable image (Figures 32.8 and 32.9).

As a dental assistant how can you ensure that exposure errors do not occur? **?**

Other Extraoral Radiography

Extraoral radiographs are used to confirm the dentist's suspected clinical diagnosis (Figure 32.10). Although they do not provide an image as detailed and clear as an intraoral radiograph, they can be used to assist with the diagnosis of facial trauma, tumors or cysts, or to assess skeletal growth.

Large x-ray units are designed specifically for extraoral radiographs although some types of panoramic machines can be converted for use in extraoral radiography. Extraoral film sizes are 5 × 7 or 8 × 10 inches and

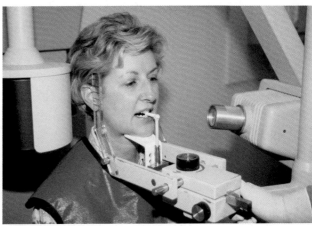

FIGURE 32.10
Patient being positioned by the dental assistant for an extraoral radiograph.
Image courtesy Instructional Materials for the Dental Team, Lex., KY

are processed best in an automatic processor. The primary skeletal landmark used for positioning the patient and the central x-ray beam for extraoral radiography is the canthomeatal line, which runs from the outer canthus of the eye to the middle of the ear opening (auditory meatus). Extraoral radiographs are most commonly used by oral surgeons and orthodontists.

Cephalometric Skull View

A cephalometric radiograph is a **lateral** view of the skull that is taken from the side of the patient (Figure 32.11). It is used to measure facial relationships and to predict growth patterns for orthodontic treatment. An orthodontic dental assistant uses the radiograph to create tracings for the orthodontist in order to analyze the patient's

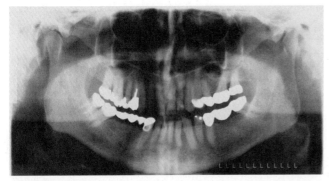

FIGURE 32.8
Positioning error: Patient's chin is too low, resulting in an exaggerated "smile" appearance and a pronounced radiolucent air space.

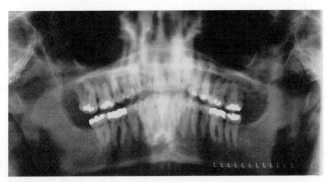

FIGURE 32.9
Positioning error: Patient's chin is too high, resulting in a "frown" appearance and a widened appearance of the hard palate.

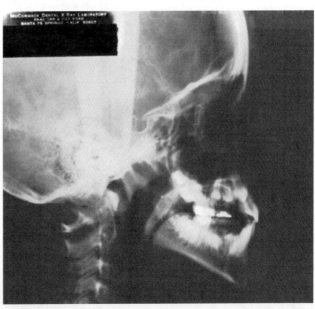

FIGURE 32.11
Cephalometric radiograph.

skeletal growth. The patient's head is held in the extra-oral radiograph machine in relationship to the x-ray beam and the Frankfort plane. The cassette is held vertically by a holding device during exposure and positioned as low as possible on the patient's shoulder. The patient stands or sits upright with teeth closed and shoulders low.

Towne's Skull View

The Towne's view is an anterior/posterior (AP) film projection. The x-ray beam is directed at the anterior, or front, of the skull and through to the posterior. This radiograph is used to assess the mandibular condyles. It is especially useful in cases of suspected fractures of the mandible, but may also be used for detailed images of the middle ear and the floor of the eye orbits.

The reverse-Towne's radiograph is taken with the patient facing the film cassette with the midsagittal plane perpendicular to the floor (Figure 32.12). The patient is asked to hold his or her mouth wide open with the chin tucked down until touching the chest. The top of the patient's forehead should be resting against the cassette. This view is useful when examining the condylar neck of the mandible for fractures.

Waters Skull View

The Waters view is a variation of the posterior/anterior (PA) film projection. It is the best view for evaluating facial fractures, the maxilla, the sinuses, zygomatic arches, eye orbits, and the coronoid process. To obtain this view, the patient's chin should touch the cassette and the nose should be positioned at about 0.75 inch from the film cassette (Figure 32.13).

Additional Extraoral Radiograph Techniques

Extraoral radiographs may be exposed in order to diagnose specific conditions for patients. Transcranial radiographs

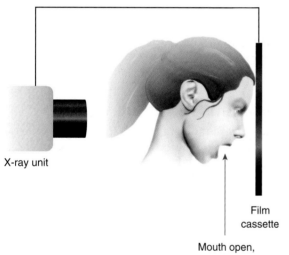
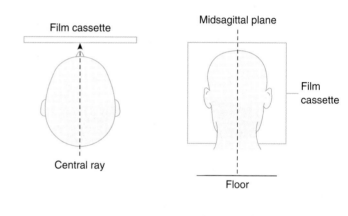

FIGURE 32.12
Technique for taking a reverse-Towne's radiograph.

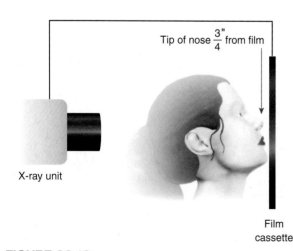
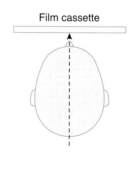
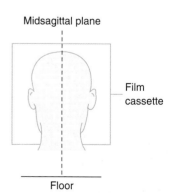

FIGURE 32.13
Technique for taking a Waters radiograph.

may be exposed with 5 × 7 or 8 × 10 screen film to provide a view of the long axis of the mandibular condyle in relationship with the maxillary fossa for patients with temporomandibular joint (TMJ) dysfunction. The submentovertex view is used to evaluate fractures or displacement of the zygomatic arch. A lateral oblique view is excellent for viewing the body and ramus of the mandible. The Caldwell view is best for seeing the eye orbits and ethmoid sinuses.

Some radiographic techniques will require referral to a specialist. Computed tomography (CT) is a technique of exposing radiographs from any part of the body by scanning it in layers of digital data that are sent to a computer monitor. Magnetic resonance imaging (MRI) is often used to diagnose soft tissue conditions of the TMJ and does not involve exposure to radiation.

Which dental specialists most often use extraoral radiographs?

Digital Radiography

Digital radiography has been around in dentistry for a long time and has improved significantly from the early days of its use. Although conventional radiography is still in use by most dental offices, technological advances in digital radiography are making the transition to film-less dental offices easier.

Digital radiography systems have many advantages:

- Radiographic images can be immediately displayed on the computer monitor.
- Images can be enhanced by changing the contrast to lighten or darken the image, by enlarging the image, or by adding color to a specific area to bring out greater detail.
- Chemicals are not used in the development process.
- Images are stored electronically.
- Images can be sent electronically to the patient, other clinicians, and insurance companies.
- Photo quality hard copies can be produced whenever desired.
- Radiation is reduced 70% to 80% compared to conventional radiographic film techniques.
- Image sensors can be reused many times.

A disadvantage of digital sensors is their bulkiness compared to thinner conventional radiograph film. The dental assistant must be extremely gentle and aware of how the sensor is being placed in the patient's mouth. Sensors must be disinfected between patients. They cannot be autoclaved or soaked in a disinfectant solution. They should be wiped with a disinfectant between patients and covered with a clean plastic sheath for each new patient.

Digital radiographic imaging is quicker than conventional x-ray film exposure and processing techniques.

Digital radiographs are available for immediate viewing on the computer monitor, and the dentist can adjust the image to facilitate an easier diagnostic reading. By placing a large image of a radiograph on a computer monitor, the patient can view the image and be included in the diagnosis. This can help to improve patient acceptance of the treatment plan.

Digital radiography systems have two main components: the device that captures the image and the computer software that stores, retrieves, displays, and enhances the image. Various software programs have been developed for digital radiography. Three styles of digital radiography are currently being used: direct sensors, phosphor plates, and digital scanners.

Direct Sensors

There are two types of direct sensors. They are either corded sensors, which capture the image directly, or noncorded wireless sensors, which capture the image indirectly and then digitalize it with a scanner. Direct sensors are the most popular digital radiography systems. They utilize either a charge-coupled device (CCD) sensor that is hooked up directly to a video capture card on the operator computer or complementary metal-oxide semiconductor (CMOS) chips with active pixel sensors (APS). (These technologies are the same ones used in everyday digital cameras.)

Both types of sensors provide for immediate viewing of the image, which is especially important in endodontic treatment and implant surgery procedures. The sensor itself is about the same size as traditional x-ray film but thicker. The sensor is 3 to 5 mm thick and is placed in the patient's mouth just as conventional film is placed. Film holders and aiming rings are available to enhance sensor placement accuracy (Figure 32.14).

The hard sensor must be covered with a disposable plastic barrier and can be used thousands of times before needing to be replaced. The sensors are expensive and fragile, so care must be taken by the dental assistant

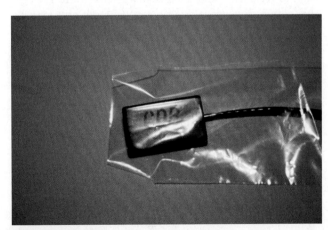

FIGURE 32.14
Wired digital sensor being placed into a special film holder.

when using this technology. When using a corded sensor, the dental assistant must work around the wire attached to the sensor so as not to break it. There are many sensor designs including wireless sensors that use radio-frequency transmission and microwave technology to eliminate the wired connection.

Phosphor Plate Technology

The newer cordless digital radiography systems use storage phosphor technology. This system utilizes sensors made from a plastic plate coated with phosphor material that is sensitive to x-rays. The plate is called a PSP (photo-stimulable phosphor plate) and is similar in size and thickness to x-ray film; some plates are even thinner than film. When the PSP sensor is exposed to an x-ray, a latent image is created and stored on the plate.

After the individual films have been taken like traditional radiographs, they are placed in a drum that can hold a full mouth series of radiographs. The drum is placed in a laser scanner. The film images are visible on the computer screen within 90 seconds to 4 minutes, depending on the number of films being processed.

The sensors can be reused many times by exposing them to white light on a view box for at least 2 minutes in order to erase the previous images. The thinner intraoral sensors come in the same sizes as film and are more easily tolerated by patients. Panoramic and cephalometric imaging plates are also available. The dental assistant must be careful not to damage the expensive imaging plate by scratching or creasing it.

Digital Scanners

Direct scanning of existing radiographic film can be accomplished with scanning software. This requires a high-quality scanner with a transparency adapter. The radiographs are placed on the scanner and can then be seen on the computer monitor. Direct scanning is currently the only system available for digitalizing existing radiographs. These systems can be utilized to convert existing records to digital format for electronic storage. This conversion process is time consuming and may be delegated to the dental assistant.

Extraoral Digital Radiography

Digital radiograph systems are increasingly being utilized for extraoral as well as intraoral views of patients (Figure 32.15). They quickly capture panoramic images using a digitally controlled high-frequency generator that mini-

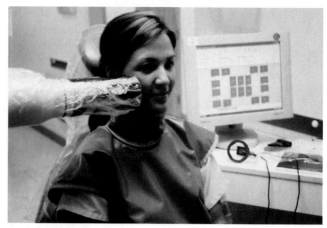

FIGURE 32.15
Digital radiography system.

mizes patient radiation compared to conventional film techniques. The image programming takes place with the computer rather than the panoramic radiography unit.

Some digital panoramic systems have dual technology that adds cephalometric options. All panoramic and cephalometric units include patient positioning features that include a chin rest, bite piece, ear supports, adjustable forehead and nose support, and Frankfort plane positioning light beams. Digital panoramic machines use an electronic detector that is either a CCD similar to that used in a digital camera or a PSP. Digital panoramic systems include designs accessible for children and patients with disabilities.

For which specific specialty procedures would immediate viewing of digital radiographs be a benefit?

Life Span Considerations

For children and the elderly, radiation exposure should be reduced by one-fourth. Young children are still growing and their bone is less dense. For elderly patients and those who are **edentulous**, the bone is also less dense, needing less radiation. Manufacturer's instructions must be consulted for each radiographic unit in order to set the machine for the proper amount of reduced radiation.

SUMMARY

The benefits of radiographs in dentistry far outweigh the risks of exposure to radiation when proper safety procedures are followed. The dentist is responsible for all aspects of safe radiation exposure in the dental office. The dentist determines which patients need radiographs, determines which radiographs are needed, supervises exposure of the films, and interprets the images.

Extraoral radiographs such as panoramic and cephalometric radiographs use less radiation than intraoral films due to use of a cassette containing intensifying screens. The dental assistant must understand the manufacturer's instructions for use with each particular x-ray machine. Proper positioning principles include machine preparation, patient preparation, and patient positioning. Darkroom procedures must also be strictly followed so that unnecessary exposure to radiation is avoided.

With digital radiography the need for darkroom chemicals is eliminated because the images appear on a computer monitor. State-of-the-art digital radiography systems are becoming more popular. Digital radiographic images can be stored, sent electronically, or printed for inclusion in a patient's record. The key to proper printing is to use quality photographic paper and a printer that is compatible with the digital technology software and computer system. Manufacturers of digital radiographic systems should be consulted to ensure successful images are created. The initial cost of the digital software system and equipment is more than that of conventional radiography; however, it is an investment in the future. Improvements in digital radiography will encourage its use, and the cost of the devices will slowly decline.

Professionalism

Unnecessary radiation exposure to patients results when films need to be reexposed due to faulty radiographic or processing techniques. Dental assistants must take the time to understand proper procedures during film exposure and throughout darkroom procedures to ensure retakes of films are kept to a minimum. The dental assistant must also label and store radiographs correctly to avoid the need for retakes.

KEY TERMS

- **Ala–tragus line:** Line that runs from the winged flare of the nostril (ala) to the opening of the ear (tragus). p. 509
- **Anterioposterior plane:** A forward–backward plane that is aligned with a specific landmark. p. 509
- **Cassette:** A protective film-holding container with two intensifying screens. p. 507
- **Edentulous:** Without teeth. p. 516
- **Extraoral radiographs:** X-rays taken outside of the mouth. p. 507

- **Frankfort plane:** A horizontal line from the upper margin of the ear to the lower margin of the eye orbit. p. 509
- **Intensifying screens:** Screens used to expose sheet film to light when activated by radiation. p. 507
- **Lateral:** From the side. p. 513
- **Midsagittal plane:** A horizontal line perpendicular (at a right angle) to the floor. This line divides the body into two equal parts: right and left halves. p. 508
- **Panoramic radiography:** An image of both the maxillary and mandibular arches. p. 507

CHECK YOUR UNDERSTANDING

1. What is the function of intensifying screens in extraoral radiography?
   a. to produce visible light when exposed to x-rays
   b. to reflect light back to the film
   c. to reduce exposure time to the patient
   d. all of the above

2. What are intensifying screens made of?
   a. rare earth elements
   b. crystalline phosphor layer
   c. both of the above
   d. none of the above

3. Which of the following is important for accurate patient placement in a panoramic machine?
   a. head positioning devices
   b. chin rests
   c. bite block
   d. hand grips
   e. all of the above

4. What will the dental assistant ask the patient to remove before exposing radiographs?
   a. jewelry
   b. metallic devices on or around head and neck
   c. removable prostheses
   d. all of the above

CHECK YOUR UNDERSTANDING (continued)

5. When using a lead apron for a panoramic radiograph, it is important to not use one
   a. that covers both the shoulders and back.
   b. with a lead collar.
   c. that provides radiation protection to the patient.
   d. that is grey.

6. What instructions will the dental assistant give the patient prior to panoramic exposure?
   a. how to bite on the bite block
   b. to close his or her lips
   c. to place the tongue against the roof of the mouth
   d. to keep completely still during the entire cycle of the exposure
   e. all of the above

7. What is a cephalometric radiograph?
   a. a lateral view of the skull that is taken from the side of the patient
   b. a parallel view of the skull that is taken from the side of the patient
   c. used to measure facial relationships
   d. Both a and c

8. Which dental specialists most often uses extraoral radiographs?
   a. oral surgeons
   b. orthodontists
   c. endodontists
   d. both a and b

9. What size does extraoral film come in?
   a. 5 × 7 inches
   b. 8 × 10 inches
   c. both of the above
   d. none of the above

10. What types of digital radiography are currently being used?
    a. direct sensors
    b. phosphor plates
    c. digital scanners
    d. all of the above

● INTERNET ACTIVITY

- Go to www.learningdigital.net to learn more about digital radiography.

● WEB REFERENCES

- The Digital Dentist   www.thedigitaldentist.com
- Journal of the American Dental Association: Panoramic and Cephalometric Extraoral Dental Radiograph Systems   http://jada.ada.org/cgi/content/full/133/12/1696
- Journal of the American Dental Association: Why Switch to Digital Radiography   http://jada.ada.org/cgi/content/full/135/10/1437
- Kodak Dental Radiography Series: Successful Panoramic Radiography   www.kodakdental.com/documentation/film/N-406SuccPanRad.pdf
- Signet: The Best of Digital Dental X-Ray Panoramic Technology   http://www.dxis-net.com

33

Restorative and Aesthetic Dental Materials

Learning Objectives

After reading this chapter, the student should be able to:

- Discuss the criteria that must be met for acceptance of a new dental material.

- List and explain the various properties considered when selecting a dental material.

- Compare and contrast direct and indirect restorations.

- List the elements in dental amalgam and their properties.

- Explain the indicators for the use of dental amalgam.

- Describe the procedure for mixing and delivering dental amalgam.

- Explain the indications for use of dental composite resin.

- Explain the indications for use of glass ionomers.

- Describe the uses for temporary dental materials.

- Compare and contrast gold and ceramic restorations.

Chapter Outline

- Standardization of Dental Materials

- Properties of Dental Materials
  —Mechanical Properties
  —Thermal Properties
  —Electrical Properties
  —Solubility
  —Application Properties

- Restorations
  —Direct Restorations
  —Indirect Restorations

Preparing for Certification Exams

- Assist with basic restorative procedures.
- Mix, place, and carve amalgam.
- Place, cure, and finish composite restorations.
- Place intermediate restorative material.

Key Terms

Alloy

Amalgam

Bonding

Composite resin

Curing

Filler

Galvanic

Inlay

Malleability

Matrix

Onlay

Palladium (Pd)

Platinum (Pt)

Trituration

Viscosity

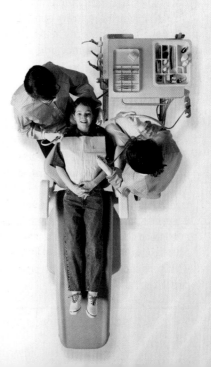

The study of dental materials is complex because of the constant changes and improvements made each year in the various areas of dentistry. The evolution of cosmetic dentistry in the last 20 years has spawned a new era of dental materials designed to withstand the forces of the oral environment while reestablishing and maintaining aesthetic beauty. Still, traditional materials such as amalgam and gold have their place among the composite resins and ceramic restorations. It is important for dental assistants to know how dental materials are evaluated, what properties these materials possess or lack, and in what situation each material is appropriate.

Standardization of Dental Materials

Since 1920, the National Institute of Standards and Technology (NIST) has researched dental materials to ensure they provide safe, efficient, and economical benefits for the public and dental care professionals. In 1928, the American Dental Association (ADA) joined the NIST in dental materials research. Then in 1948, the U.S. Congress established the National Institute of Dental Research (NIDR), one of three branches of the National Institutes of Health (NIH). The NIDR is now the primary sponsor of dental research.

The ADA's Council on Dental Materials, Instruments, and Equipment has 55 specifications for dental materials. Manufacturers send their research and samples of their products to the ADA to determine if the specifications have been met and if the product will receive

---

Dental Assistant PROFESSIONAL TIP

Numerous dental journals arrive at the dental office every month. To stay educated on the latest developments in dental materials, the dental assistant should take the initiative to read one or two of the dental products and research journals every month. The dentist is often overwhelmed by the amount of journals he or she is expected to read. It is extremely helpful to be aware of a new material and present the information to the dentist. Some offices even hold staff meetings to discuss articles read for the betterment of the office and patients. Also, the assistant should try to attend continuing education workshops or dental meetings that provide opportunities to see new dental materials.

---

the ADA Seal of Acceptance. Criteria for a new dental material include the following:

- Must not be poisonous or harmful to the body
- Must not be harmful or irritating to the tissues of the oral cavity
- Must protect the tooth and tissues of the oral cavity
- Must resemble the natural dentition as closely as possible so as to be aesthetically pleasing
- Must be easily formed and placed in the mouth to restore the mouth's natural contour
- Must conform and function properly for the intended purpose

The Food and Drug Administration (FDA) is the regulatory agency for all dental and medical materials intended for human use. Once a product has been evaluated and approved by both the FDA and ADA it can be marketed to the dental profession.

Properties of Dental Materials

The oral cavity is a harsh environment. Restorative materials must withstand the conditions of extreme pressure, thermal changes, possible acidity, and other potentially destructive forces. When choosing a dental material, the dentist must consider what material is best for treating the patient's tooth. The dentist and the dental assistant must understand the properties of the materials to be able to select the best material for each clinical situation.

Mechanical Properties

The average adult with natural teeth can bite at a force of approximately 200 pounds per square inch with the posterior teeth and 55 pounds per square inch using the anterior teeth. Dental materials must be able to withstand these extreme mechanical forces of biting and chewing.

Preparing for Externship

Prior to and during an externship, the dental assistant should take the time to review the categories of dental materials. Each office will have different materials and ways to store each type of material. Ask the dentist what the working time is for each hand-mixed material as well as the curing time. Be familiar with the curing light and triturator. Always double-check the settings to make sure they have not been changed from the manufacturer's recommendations, unless the doctor has requested a different setting. Know who orders the dental supplies and how the supplies are organized. If this system is not explained and understood, an important material may be used up without backups being ordered. Work in a dental office can quickly come to a halt if supplies become depleted.

Mechanical properties are the properties of a material that reveal the elastic and inelastic reaction when a force is applied. Force is defined as any push or pull acting on an object. Force creates a stress and strain on a material (Figure 33.1). Stress is the force applied to deform or strain a material. Strain is the actual deformation of the material. Examples of mechanical properties include:

- *Tensile stress:* pulling and stretching of a material
- *Compressive stress:* squeezing of a material without crushing
- *Shear stress:* parallel forces created by sliding in opposite directions

Thermal Properties

Humans eat and drink items of varying thermal degrees. For example, eating hot pizza and drinking a cold soda quickly changes the temperature of the oral cavity. Thermal change is important to understand for expansion and contraction reasons and because of the need to protect the pulp of the teeth.

The expansion and contraction abilities of a dental restorative material must be the same as, or close to the same as, the expansion and contraction abilities of the natural tooth structure. Significantly different rates of expansion and contraction can result in fractured teeth or small leaks between the restoration and the natural tooth structure known as microleakage. Microleakage allows for bacteria to flourish between the tooth and restoration, causing recurrent caries. Materials also should not conduct extreme heat or cold to prevent damage to the pulp.

Electrical Properties

Different restorative metals have different electrical properties. When two dissimilar metals come in contact with each other, an electrical current can occur. This is equivalent to the mouth acting as a battery. Patients often report feeling a small shock or dull ache in a tooth. This is known as **galvanic** shock. Conditions in the oral cavity for galvanic action to occur require:

- Salts found in saliva, which are a good conductor of electricity
- Two dissimilar metals acting as a battery such as a piece of aluminum foil coming in contact with an amalgam filling

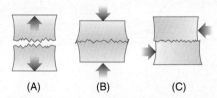

(A)   (B)   (C)

FIGURE 33.1

Examples of stress and strain: (a) tensile stress, (b) compressive stress, and (c) shear stress.

Galvanic action can lead to the corrosion of either one or both of the contacting metals.

Corrosion or deterioration of the metal restoration can occur due to galvanic action with another dissimilar metal restoration or foods containing metallic forms. Tarnish is surface discoloration that occurs over time and can be polished away. Corrosion and tarnish both occur by oxidation.

Solubility

Solubility is the measure of how much a material will dissolve in a liquid. Certain dental materials are highly soluble. These materials are not meant to be long-lasting restorative materials. If a highly soluble material is used, the patient must be told to return for a more long-term restoration; otherwise, the natural tooth structure will eventually be exposed and become highly susceptible to caries. Most dental restorative materials have low solubility, will not wash away, and can be used as long-term restorations.

Application Properties

For a dental material to be successful, it needs to exhibit certain properties, known as application properties, at the time of placement. These properties allow the material to be manipulated until its final form is achieved. Flow is the ability of a material to be pliable enough to be molded and manipulated into the preparation of the tooth. Once caries have been removed from a tooth, a cavity or hole with rounded, square, or irregular walls and floor exists. The material must be designed to adapt to the contour of the preparation without voids or gaps.

Adhesion

Adhesion is the ability of a material to adhere or stick to a dissimilar material. The adhesion of a dental restorative material to a tooth structure is a major concern. If adhesion fails, microleakage will occur and the restoration is considered a failure. For adhesion to be successful, the dental material must have certain characteristics including these:

- *Wetting* is the soaking of an object with a liquid. Some dental materials need the ability to easily flow over small irregular surfaces. For example, water has high wetting ability due to its ability to flow easily and cover a surface.
- *Viscosity* is the resistance of a material to flow. It is important for some dental materials to be less fluid or more viscous. Corn syrup is a good example of a viscous liquid. Viscous materials are not good wetting agents.
- *Surface characteristics* of the tooth wall affect the wetting ability of a dental material. If the wall surface is rough, a wetting agent will flow more readily than if the wall is smooth. Liquids tend to bead up on a smooth surface, making wetting difficult.
- *Thin film thickness* is a must for proper adhesion to occur. Film thickness is measured in micrometers. Generally, the thinner the film, the stronger the adhesive interface. If the adhesive interface is too thick, the likelihood of the materials failing is increased.

Retention

Retention is the ability to keep a restoration from displacement or to hold two objects firmly together. Two forms of retention are important in dentistry: mechanical and chemical retention. The dentist must prepare teeth to allow for the most mechanical retention possible per the dental restorative material to be used. For example, a simple occlusal amalgam requires a preparation where the floor of the cavity is wider than the opening of the preparation so the hardened amalgam will not fall out and is locked into the tooth by mechanical retention. This is known as an undercut. (This will be reviewed further in Chapter 38.) Chemical retention occurs when two materials have a chemical reaction to create retention. Some composites will actually chemically attach to some metals. Retention is extremely important in dentistry so the restorations will not fall out of the teeth.

Curing

Curing of a dental material is the process by which the material hardens to perform its function. Most dental materials requiring curing are pliable and molded to their final shape prior to auto-curing or dual curing. An auto-cured material undergoes a chemical reaction, which is the curing process. Once mixed, the material has a limited working time. If not placed in the tooth in a set amount of time, the material will harden in an inappropriate shape. Some materials are known as light-cured materials due to curing by use of ultraviolet light or more

commonly a high-energy or blue spectrum curing light. Many aesthetic dental restorative materials are pliable until the curing light is shined directly on the material, initiating the chemical reaction to harden the material (Figure 33.2).

Other dental materials are dual cured. Some of the dual-cured materials begin their hardening process once mixed but do not finalize their cure until the curing light is placed on the restoration. Other dual-cured materials are designed to finalize their curing reaction after the use of the light. For example, if a large cavity is filled with this type of dual-cured material, the final cure occurs deep in the restoration after the use of the light where the light cannot possibly have penetrated.

What other properties should a dental restorative material possess to survive in the oral environment?

Restorations

For thousands of years, numerous items have been used to fill cavities in teeth including stone chips, lead, tin, platinum, silver, gold leaf, aluminum, and even asbestos. Some of these materials came from ordinary metals used for other applications such as shotgun pellets. Today, dentistry still uses some of these same materials, but due to advanced technology, the metal mixtures have been researched and developed to be safe and effective for restoring the human dentition. Restorations are divided into two distinguished groups, direct restorations and indirect restorations.

Direct Restorations

Direct restorations are the materials by which cavities are restored in the mouth with pliable, workable, adaptable materials. These materials are carved, shaped, and finished within the oral cavity. Some of these materials

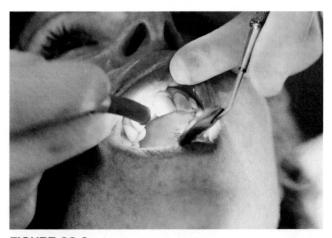

FIGURE 33.2
Light curing of an aesthetic composite resin.

include amalgam, composite resins, glass ionomers, and intermediate restorative materials. The majority of dental restorations are direct restorations.

Amalgam

In 1832, a new dental restorative material was brought to the United States from France. This material is known as amalgam. **Amalgam** is a soft metal made of alloy mixed with mercury to restore form and function to teeth. An **alloy** is a mixture of two or more metals. Amalgam has proven to be an effective, long-lasting, and rather inexpensive dental restorative material. According to the Centers for Disease Control and Prevention, less than 100 million amalgam restorations are placed in the United States annually.

As a direct restorative material, amalgam is placed by pressing (condensing) it into the cavity preparation initially with an amalgam carrier followed by a plugger or condenser and finally finished and carved by numerous other instruments. When working for a dentist it is important for dental assistants to know which amalgam instruments are preferred by the dentist and the order in which he or she prefers to use them. In some states, dental assistants are legally allowed to place dental amalgams.

The composition of dental amalgam is regulated by the ADA. It consists of 43% to 54% mercury and 46% to 57% alloy. Each component of the alloy serves a purpose:

- Silver provides strength.
- Tin provides workability and strength.
- Copper provides strength and resistance to corrosion.
- Zinc suppresses oxidation.

Classifications of Dental Amalgam   There are several classifications of dental amalgam based on different combinations of the four metals used in the alloy and the particle sizes of the alloy. The powder forms of the metals may be spherical, irregular, or a combination of spherical and irregular. Particle shape affects the working ability of the material. Spherical particles have smoother surfaces and require less mercury when mixed and are also easier to condense into the preparation and to polish. Alloys containing both spherical and irregularly shaped particles adapt well to the prepared tooth wall and to the adjacent tooth, creating a good contact.

Alloys may also vary in copper content and zinc content. The increased percentage of copper in high-copper alloys increases the alloy's strength and corrosion resistance. High-copper mixtures are very commonly used in dentistry.

Mercury is the other component of most dental amalgam. It is important to mix the appropriate amount of mercury with the appropriate amount of alloy. The ratio is most often 1:1, mercury to alloy. This mix allows for good workability. There are nonmercury alloys known as Galloy. Galloy is composed of gallium, indium,

and tin. This direct filling material is approved by the ADA, but is recommended for very limited use only in small fillings, due to sensitivity caused by moisture, which can result in increased corrosive and expansive properties. If Galloy is used, the cavity should be lined prior to placement of Galloy and the tooth sealed after placement.

It has long been known that mercury is very hazardous. This fact has created a great two-tier controversy: whether mercury in dental restorations is safe or harmful to patients and whether mercury vapor toxicity affects dental personnel over time. It has been proven that dental restorations release minor amounts of mercury vapor. The amount of mercury vapor released has been shown not to cause any adverse health effects. Studies show that individuals with a mouth full of amalgam restorations have a mercury level well below the necessary amount to have toxic effects. In fact, the public is exposed to higher levels of mercury in foods, air, and water. When mercury is mixed with alloy, **bonding** to the other metals alters it. Even chewing and grinding pressure on amalgam restorations has been shown to release very little vapor at a level well below the danger level. The ADA, the FDI World Dental Federation, and the World Health Organization all support the safety and efficacy of dental amalgam.

As for the safety of the dental team, guidelines must be followed to avoid possible toxicity to mercury (Table 33-1). Symptoms of mercury poisoning include tremors, kidney dysfunction, central nervous system disorders, and dementia. Many years ago, alloy was mixed with mercury by hand and squeezed in cheesecloth to remove the excess mercury. As a result, many dental professionals became ill with mercury poisoning. This process of handling amalgam is no longer in use.

Legal and Ethical Issues

Because some patients will question the use of various dental materials such as amalgam, it is important for the dental assistant to stay educated on the materials used in the dental office. If a patient expresses concern regarding the use of amalgam, the dental assistant can discuss the opinion of the American Dental Association. The ADA supports the use of dental amalgam. It is considered unlawful for a dentist to recommend the removal of dental amalgam, strictly for monetary gain due to the potentially harmful effects of the material. The amalgam restorations must be declared defective. If a patient requests the removal of a nondefective restoration, a consent form should be signed dually informing the patient of the pros and cons of removing the material. With the development of aesthetic dental materials, patients often want the dark amalgams or gold restorations removed based purely on aesthetics. Patients have a right to choose for themselves the best treatment option or materials.

TABLE 33-1 Guidelines for Working with Amalgam

1. Always wear protective clothing including disposable gloves, mask, and glasses.
2. Use a no-touch technique, which utilizes only instruments to handle amalgam.
3. Use the cover on the amalgamator or triturator to prevent escape of mercury vapor.
4. Discard and store scraps of amalgam and mercury in an unbreakable, closed jar filled with x-ray fixer.
5. When removing amalgam, use water spray and high-volume evacuation to remove particles.
6. Use a dental tray with a lip to retain spillage.
7. Keep a mercury spill kit in the office and make all personnel aware of its use.

Amalgam Capsules   Amalgam suppliers deliver the ingredients of amalgam in a premeasured and self-contained capsule. This capsule prevents handling of mercury before it is mixed with the alloy. Within the capsule, a membrane separates the alloy from the mercury (Figure 33.3). Capsules are available in 600 and 800 mg. The 600-mg capsule is approximately the appropriate amount of amalgam for a small restoration, whereas the 800-mg capsule is more appropriate for a larger restoration. If more material is necessary, the dental assistant may mix more capsules as needed.

The mixing of alloy with mercury to form the amalgam for dental restorations is known as **trituration** or amalgamation. Prior to trituration, some capsules require the use of an activator (Procedure 33-1). This instrument presses the two ends of the capsule together, breaking the separator and allowing the alloy and mercury to come into contact. Most amalgam capsules are now self-activating and do not require the use of an activator. The capsule is then placed in the amalgamator or triturator, which has a preset timer per the manufacturer of the amalgam. The lid must be closed before activating the triturator. (Procedure 33-1)

After the triturator or amalgamator completes the cycle, the capsule is removed and the two halves of the capsule are separated, allowing the amalgam to fall into an amalgam well. The dental assistant fills the amalgam carrier with the amalgam by pressing the carrier into the soft pliable amalgam and filling the appropriate end of the carrier per the size of the preparation or per the dentist's specifications.

The amalgam carrier is handed to the dentist to deliver the amalgam to the preparation and then is handed back to the assistant for more material. The amalgam is pressed into the preparation in increments with a condenser to ensure good condensation or fit to the cavity preparation walls and to help release excess mercury. The restoration is overfilled slightly with amalgam to allow for carving and finishing. The dentist can now form the amalgam to represent the natural anatomy of the tooth. Numerous instruments are available for carving and finishing. Finally, the margins are burnished to close any possible open areas and to remove flash or excess amalgam. The dentist must check the patient's occlusion and adjust the restoration accordingly.

The dental assistant should provide the patient with postoperative care instructions:

1. Do not chew any hard foods for 24 hours. The amalgam continues to harden for this period of time.
2. Do not chew gum for 24 hours.
3. Wait to chew anything until the anesthetic is gone. If the patient chews before the numbness from the anesthetic is gone, he may bite his cheek and tongue, creating sore soft tissue.
4. If the amalgam is a two-surface restoration with a contact to another tooth, the patient should not floss that area for 24 hours.
5. If the restoration feels high or the other teeth are not occluding, the patient should call the office for a check and adjustment of the occlusion.

Composite Resins

Composite resin is tooth-colored restorative material made of silica or porcelain fillers or particles interlaced with liquid resin that binds the particles together to form a hard restorative material. Introduced in the 1960s, composite resin has become the dental material of choice to restore caries, deformities, and minor traumatic fractures or chips in the anterior teeth. Since that time, the composites have been greatly improved to withstand the pressures and stresses of the posterior teeth. Many dentists and patients want the posterior teeth to look just as natural as the anterior teeth. Therefore, composite resin materials are used throughout the mouth to repair and visually improve teeth to appear as natural tooth structure.

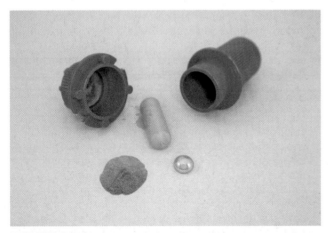

FIGURE 33.3
Ingredients of an amalgam capsule: alloy, separating membrane, and mercury.
Image courtesy Instructional Materials for the Dental Team, Lex., KY

Procedure 33-1 Mixing, Placing, and Carving of Dental Amalgam

Dental assistants should be sure to check with their state practice laws to determine what tasks they are allowed to perform versus the tasks that are to be accomplished by the dentist.

Materials and Instruments

- Amalgam capsule
- Amalgam well
- Activator
- Amalgam carrier
- Pluggers/condensers
- Carving and finishing instruments
- Occlusal paper
- Dental floss

Procedure Steps

1. Activate the amalgam capsule with the activator.

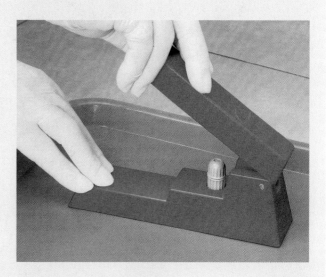

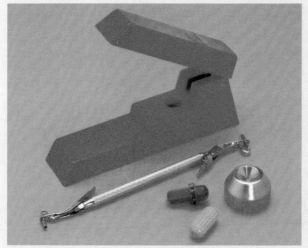

Basic tray setup containing amalgam capsule, amalgam well, activator, and amalgam carrier.

2. Place the capsule into the triturator, close the lid, check for the appropriate settings, and begin trituration.

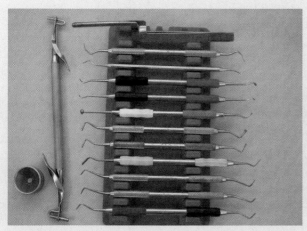

Extended assistant tray setup containing additional instruments such as pluggers, carves, and fnisheers.
Images courtesy Instructional Materials for the Dental Team, Lex., KY

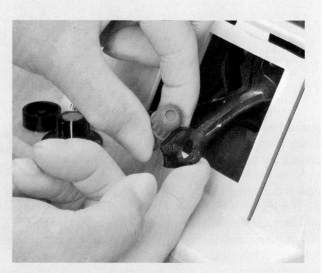

continued on next page

Procedure 33-1 *continued from previous page*

3. Remove the capsule from the triturator, open the capsule, and spill the amalgam into the amalgam well.

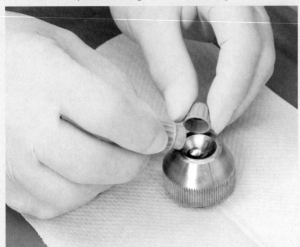

4. Fill the amalgam carrier by pressing the end of the carrier into the soft amalgam so as to pack the carrier to the top with amalgam. (The dentist may request the small end or the large end of the carrier first.)

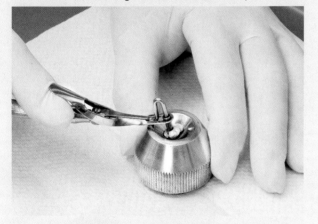

5. Transfer the carrier to the dentist with the filled end on the carrier toward the preparation to be filled.

6. Continue the handoff of the amalgam carrier to and from the assistant to the dentist until the preparation is overfilled.

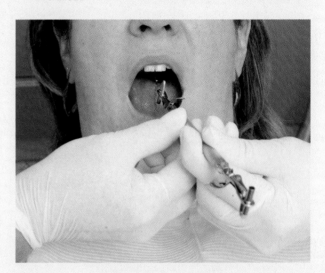

Studies have shown that composite restorations may last just as long as amalgam restorations. Because the use of composite resin materials in the posterior teeth is still considered relatively new, studies of all of the new generations of materials are ongoing. Failure of composite resins occurs due to secondary caries, fracture, and loss of marginal integrity. Other disadvantages include occasional postoperative sensitivity and discoloration of the composite material over time due to tea, coffee, and other staining foods (Figure 33.4). Materials research and development is continuous, and new and improved generations of composite resins are placed on the market annually. Studies and comparisons of composite resins and amalgam will continue.

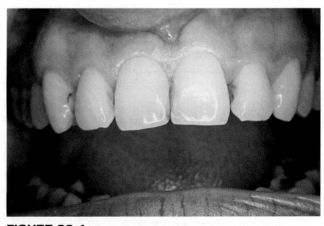

FIGURE 33.4
Example of a stained anterior composite.
Image courtesy Instructional Materials for the Dental Team, Lex., KY

A composite restoration has these advantages:

- Improves aesthetics by restoring the natural appearance of the teeth and smile
- Bonds to tooth structure to support remaining natural tooth
- Conserves natural tooth structure
- Helps to prevent breakage of remaining natural tooth structure
- Insulates tooth structure from extreme temperature changes

A composite resin restorative material has three major components:

1. Inorganic fillers
2. Organic resin matrix
3. Coupling agent

Fillers Fillers are rocklike particles that add strength to the composite resins. This component may be made of quartz, glass or porcelain, and silica. A colorant is added to provide numerous shades of composite resin. A requirement of the filler is to reflect light allowing for the aesthetic appearance of the material. Numerous factors are taken into consideration when choosing a composite restoration, including the amount of filler, particle size of the filler, and the types of filler. Varying combinations of these factors provide the strength, wear resistance, and finish and polish of the composite.

As with amalgams, the composites are classified by particle size: megafill, macrofill, midifill, minifill, microfill, and nanofill. A combination of different particle sizes is referred to as a hybrid filled composite. The macrofilled composites contain the largest of the fillers. These are the traditional restorative composites of the posterior teeth providing the greatest strength and wear resistance but have poor polishing ability, leaving a duller, coarser surface. Microfilled composites have much smaller filler particles to allow for higher polish, smoothness, and aesthetics. This material is primarily used for the anterior teeth where great strength is not required. Hybrid composites are composed of numerous particle sizes allowing for higher polish than the macrofilled composites yet greater strength and wear resistance than the microfilled composites.

Resin Matrix Resin **matrix** is the binding substance holding the filler particles together, the foundation of the composite. This liquid-like monomer material is known as bisphenol-A-glycidyl dimethacrylate or BIS-GMA. Alone, it is not strong enough to be used as a restorative material, but with the addition of the fillers and the coupling agent, the reaction can take place to create a filled resin composite suitable for a dental restorative material.

Coupling Agent The coupling agent is an organosilane compound that coats the filler particles. The silane portion of this compound is attached to the particles, and the organic portion reacts with the resin to chemically bond the filler particles to the resin matrix. Other ingredients required for the reaction to occur include initiators, accelerators, retarders, and ultraviolet light stabilizers.

Forms of Composite Resin Manufacturers supply composite resins in various delivery systems. Some are supplied in premeasured individual lightproof carpules that are loaded into a delivery gun for application into the prepared tooth. Others are supplied in a long tube for multiple uses by syringing the appropriate amount of material into a lightproof container (Figure 33.5a). All of the composite resin ingredients are premixed and ready for use in either delivery system.

The materials vary in the viscosity or ability to flow. The macrofill composites tend to be more viscous and easily condensable with the appropriate instrument, whereas the composites with very few filler particles tend to be less viscous and flow more easily. The dental assistant should know the different composite resins and the materials the doctor uses for each type of restoration. Some doctors may use a variety of composite materials in a single restoration.

Most composite resins are supplied in kits (Figure 33.5b) with various colors and viscosities along with a shade guide (Figure 33.6a). Selecting the best shade for the restoration is extremely important and the dental assistant is often responsible for doing the choosing. This task takes time and practice. A clinical tip is to try small amounts of numerous shades of the composite directly on the tooth surface to be restored prior to the restoration (Figure 33.6b). These small amounts of material should be light cured because the true shade of the material is not accurate until cured. Once the shade is chosen, the sample composites are easily removed with slight pressure. Remember, the goal is not only to restore the tooth but also to obtain the best aesthetic outcome possible when using composite resin.

The kit also may contain the acid etch and bonding system. In the past, the manufacturers suggested their composite resin be bonded by their brand of etch and bond. Now, most composites are compatible with most bonding systems and may be mixed and matched as the dentist deems necessary.

Composite Resin Procedure (Procedure 33-2) The tooth structure must be prepared prior to receiving the composite resin. The tooth has a layer called the smear layer, which must be removed to expose the prisms of the enamel. The smear layer is a thin layer of tooth debris created by rotary action of the dental handpiece. A chemical of 30% to 50% phosphoric acid is syringed onto the surface of the preparation to remove the smear layer and open the prisms of the enamel. Once the enamel and dentin have been prepared, the bonding agent is applied. The bonding agent is a low-viscosity resin adhesive. This adhesive is applied very thinly and then light cured. The tooth is now ready to receive the composite resin restorative material.

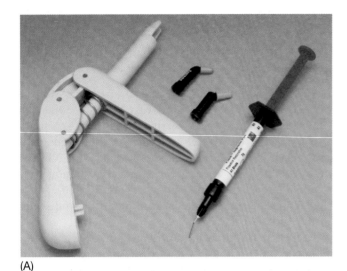

(A)

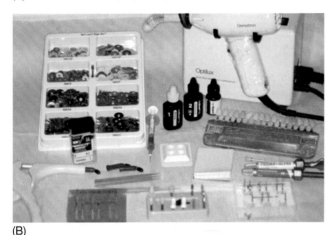

(B)

FIGURE 33.5
(a) Delivery systems for composite resin: individual carpules with composite delivery gun and multiple-use syringes. (b) Example of a composite resin kit.
Images courtesy Instructional Materials for the Dental Team, Lex., KY

CURING LIGHTS The resin bonding material and the composite resin require the use of a blue spectrum light source to activate the chemical reaction for bonding, known as polymerization. This light is a combination of tungsten and halogen lighting. Numerous manufacturers make the various types of curing lights.

The dental assistant must be familiar with the type of light and the specifications for its optimal use. Some lights require only 5 seconds to cure 2 mm of composite resin material, whereas others, especially older generations of curing lights, may require up to 60 seconds of exposure to cure 2 mm of material. Other issues to consider when deciding length of curing time include manufacturer's instructions, the thickness of the material being cured, and the shade of the material being placed.

Note that the overhead dental lamp and the ceiling lights emit white light. White light is all the colors of the rainbow including the blue spectrum light. These light sources will cause polymerization or curing of the composite resin. This is the reason the composite resin mate-

rial is supplied in lightproof delivery systems and must be protected from any light source prior to placement and final curing.

FINISHING AND POLISHING COMPOSITES Composites have a completely different means of finishing and polishing than do amalgam restorations. Prior to polymerization, the pliable composite resin may be sculpted and manipulated to emulate the natural form of tooth anatomy. Once polymerization has occurred, the composite resin must be finished and polished using rotary instruments and burs. If the occlusion needs to be adjusted, rotary instruments must be used.

After completion of the procedure, the dental assistant should provide the patient with postoperative care instructions:

1. The composite restoration is fully cured to the maximum prior to the patient leaving the office. Due to this fact, the patient does not need to wait to eat or drink.
2. To avoid causing any harm to the cheeks and tongue, the patient should wait to chew anything until the anesthetic has metabolized.

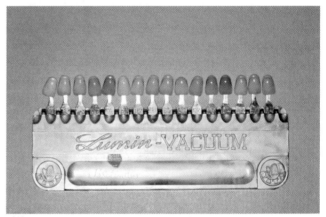

(A)

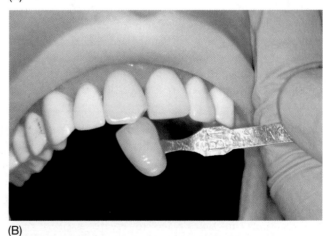

(B)

FIGURE 33.6
Shade matching (a) using an extensive shade guide and (b) using small samples of various colors of composite placed directly on the tooth to be restored.
Images courtesy Instructional Materials for the Dental Team, Lex., KY

Procedure 33-2 Chemically Preparing, Placing, Curing, and Finishing Composite Resins

Dental assistants should be sure to check with their state practice laws to determine what tasks they are allowed to perform versus the tasks that are to be accomplished by the dentist.

Materials and Instruments

- Composite resin carpules and delivery gun or syringes
- Mixing wells with lightproof shield
- Brushes
- Acid-etch syringe with tips
- Bonding system
- Curing light
- Pluggers/condensers
- Plastic instruments
- Carving instruments
- Rotary instruments with carbide burs and finishing points, discs, and/or cups
- Sanding strips
- Matrix system
- Occlusal paper
- Dental floss

(See Chapter 24 for description of hand rotary instruments and burs.)

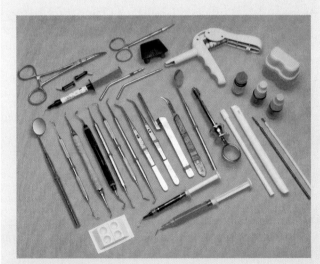

Composite resin tray setup.

Procedure Steps

1. Select the shade of the tooth to be restored. Use natural light. Fluorescent light will alter the shade selection.

2. Confirm moisture control that is necessary for the bonding procedure to occur.

3. Place carpule of proper shade into the delivery gun, or syringe the proper shade into a mixing well. Dispense adhesive into well and cover with the lightproof shield.

4. Pass the syringe of phosphoric acid to the dentist.

5. Rinse and suction etch from the preparation. Dry with air.

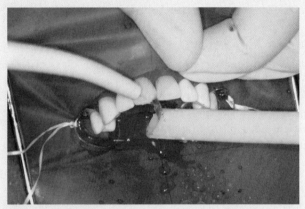

Acid etch being rinsed off the tooth and suctioned away.
Image courtesy Instructional Materials for the Dental Team, Lex., KY

6. Pass brush with bonding agent to dentist. Thin the adhesive with air from the air/water syringe.

7. Light cure adhesive as necessary.

8. Pass composite resin material to dentist.

9. Pass necessary instruments for material manipulation to dentist.

10. Light cure material as necessary during material placement.

11. Have carbide burs and polishing items ready and available.

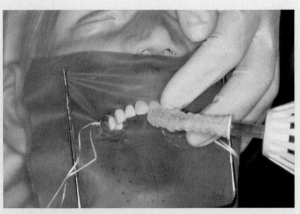

Light curing of composite material.
Image courtesy Instructional Materials for the Dental Team, Lex., KY

3. The tooth may be sensitive to cold for a short period of time. If this sensitivity persists for more than a few days or progresses, the patient should call the office to have the restoration and the occlusion checked. This is usually a sign of an occlusion problem.

4. If the restoration feels high or the other teeth are not occluding, the patient should call the office for a check and adjustment of the occlusion or bite.

How do amalgam materials differ from composite materials in structure and tooth preparation requirements?

Glass Ionomers

Glass ionomers are composed of silicate glass powder and a liquid solution of polyacrylic acid. The most unique and beneficial advantage of glass ionomers is the release of fluoride into the tooth structure, allowing for this auto-cured, tooth-colored material to exhibit a low rate of leakage and recurrent decay. Glass ionomers also have the ability to chemically bond to enamel and dentin.

This group of materials has numerous applications in dentistry. The primary uses of glass ionomers include the following:

1. Non–load-bearing restorations
2. Cavity liners (For more information on cavity liners, see Chapter 34.)
3. Bonding agents
4. Core material for buildup prior to a final restoration
5. Cements for permanent crowns and bridges (For more information on crowns and bridges, see Chapter 40.)
6. Restorations for patients with high risk of recurrent decay

Glass ionomers can be blended with an alloy to create a very strong, wear-resistant dental material. The combination of glass and metal provides for hardness, toughness, and a level of radiopacity. Metal-reinforced glass ionomers are best applied for core buildups and repair of fractured cusps.

Another restorative material known as a compomer or resin-ionomer is a combination of glass ionomer and a resin component. Resin-ionomers are auto- or light-cured, tooth-colored restorative materials with the ability to release fluoride. These materials offer improved properties such as greater compressive strength and resistance to dehydration. They are also easier to place than other glass ionomers. Resin-ionomers are used for small non–load-bearing restorations, cavity liners, and cements for crowns and bridges.

Glass ionomers are supplied in several different delivery systems from the manufacturers (Figure 33.7). When supplied as a powder and a separate liquid, the

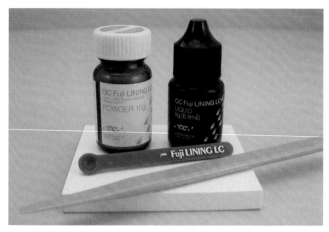

FIGURE 33.7
Glass ionomers are supplied in numerous forms.
Image courtesy Instructional Materials for the Dental Team, Lex., KY

two parts of the material must be carefully measured and dispensed on a glass mixing slab or a treated mixing pad. The powder is incorporated into the liquid in small increments but rather quickly. The working time is less than 45 seconds.

Glass ionomer may also be supplied in a capsule similar to amalgam. This system ensures delivery of the proper amount of each ingredient and correct working time due to the use of a triturator. Other systems include ones in which two pastes are mixed and the new mixture is then placed into a compule and from there to a delivery gun, single syringe, cartridge, or single-use compule.

Temporary Restorative Material

In most dental offices, placement of temporary restorations is a daily occurrence. Numerous situations arise that require a temporary restoration, and numerous materials may be utilized for such restorations. The purposes of a temporary dental restoration include the following:

1. To stabilize a tooth or to restore function for a limited period of time
2. To provide the patient relief of discomfort until a diagnosis can be determined
3. To provide aesthetics to the patient until a permanent restoration can be placed
4. To maintain the position of a prepared tooth as well as the surrounding teeth until a permanent restoration is placed
5. To protect a prepared tooth against temperature changes and food particles

Temporary restorative materials include both intermediate restorative and provisional restorative materials. The dental assistant should help the patient understand the purposes of the restoration that he or she will be receiving. These restorations are not meant to be permanent, although these transitional materials are meant to last one to three years.

The selection of the temporary material is based on the condition and the location of the tooth in need of the restoration. For example, a patient presents to the dental office with a broken cusp of a molar. If there is not enough time in the dentist's schedule to prepare the tooth for a permanent restoration, a composite resin or other material may be used as a temporary restoration to help protect the area until the patient can return for the final preparation and restoration of the broken tooth. If a patient presents to the dentist with undetermined discomfort in a tooth, the dentist will remove the decay or failing restoration and place an intermediate restorative material to allow the tooth to calm before deciding on the type of final restoration required. (Procedure 33-3)

One of the best soothing materials used in temporary situations is intermediate restorative material, better

Procedure 33-3 Preparing and Delivering Intermediate Restorative Material

Dental assistants should be sure to check with their state practice laws to determine what tasks they are allowed to perform versus the tasks that are to be accomplished by the dentist.

Materials and Instruments

- Liquid and powder container of IRM with measuring scoop
- Mixing pad
- Spatula

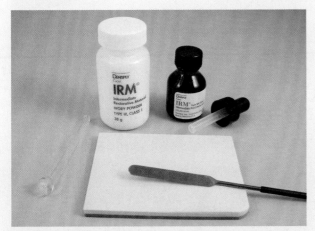

Tray setup for IRM including powder, liquid, scoop, mixing pad, and spatula.
Image courtesy Instructional Materials for the Dental Team, Lex., KY

Procedure Steps

1. Shake the powder prior to dispensing.

2. Dispense powder using the provided measuring scoop onto the mixing pad.

3. Dispense liquid onto the mixing pad. (IRM is made in a 1:1 ratio, meaning one scoop of powder to one drop of liquid.)

4. Mix powder into liquid in increments to form a stiff paste. Mixing time should be less than one minute.

5. Roll the IRM into a ball for easy delivery into tooth.

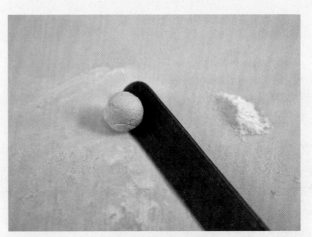

Image courtesy Instructional Materials for the Dental Team, Lex., KY

6. Wipe the spatula clean before material sets.

7. Set IRM in the restored tooth.

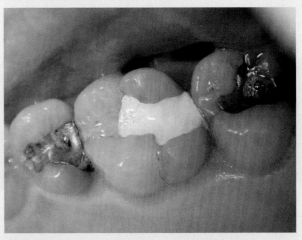

Image courtesy Instructional Materials for the Dental Team, Lex., KY

known as IRM. IRM is composed of zinc oxide-eugenol. The sedative effect is supplied by the eugenol. This material may be placed in a tooth with very deep caries while awaiting another restorative or endodontic procedure. IRM is used in primary teeth with caries just prior to exfoliation instead of permanently restoring such a

tooth. IRM is provided as a powder and liquid, to be mixed on a treated pad or glass slab. It is also provided in a premeasured capsule, activated, triturated, and extruded. Because IRM is a temporary material, the dental assistant may prepare and place IRM on the patient's tooth, depending on individual state practice acts.

Procedure 33-4 Preparing and Delivering Provisional Restorative Material

Dental assistants should be sure to check with their state practice laws to determine what tasks they are allowed to perform versus the tasks that are to be accomplished by the dentist.

Materials and Instruments

• Stint
• Spatula
• Delivery gun with material cartridge and tip
• Mixing pad
• Tubes of temporary cement

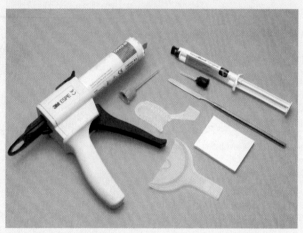

Provisional tray setup.

Procedure Steps

1. Fill stint with provisional material.

2. Place stint over prepared tooth or teeth. Allow material to cure per manufacturer recommendations.

3. Remove stint from the mouth and then remove the provisional material from the stint.

4. Trim, finish, and polish the stint so no rough edges are felt.

5. Mix temporary cement and fill the provisional.

6. Seat provisional onto prepared tooth. Allow cement to cure.

7. Remove excess cured cement from around the tooth or teeth.

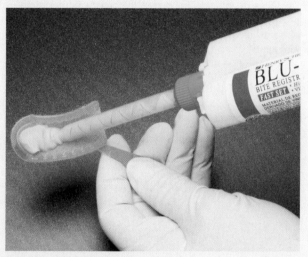

Filling the stint with provisional material.

8. Check and adjust the occlusion.

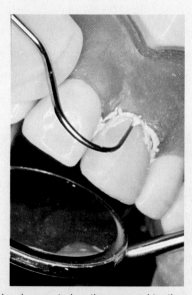

Final provisional cemented on the prepared tooth.
Image courtesy Instructional Materials for the Dental Team, Lex., KY

Provisional Restorative Materials Provisional restorations are meant to cover the entire tooth or the majority of the tooth structure. A provisional restoration may span numerous teeth as for a bridge. Even provisional dentures are occasionally necessary to allow a patient to heal prior to making a final set of dentures. Provisional restorations are necessary to protect the prepared tooth or teeth and soft tissue for a short period of time until the final restoration has been returned from the laboratory. Due to the coverage of tooth structure, the material chosen must be able to withstand chewing forces and other oral conditions. (Procedure 33-4)

Temporary Restorative Procedure Prior to preparation of the tooth, a thermoplastic stint or impression is made to imitate the original tooth structure. Occasionally, a wax model of the patient's teeth created by the laboratory or by the dentist may be used to make the stint. After the preparation of the tooth or teeth, the stint is filled with the provisional material. This material is usually an auto-cured acrylic or light-cured composite resin. The provisional version of the composite resin has different properties than the restorative version.

Once the stint is filled, it is then placed over the prepared tooth and allowed to cure. After curing, the provisional form is removed from the stint and finished, polished, and cemented to the prepared tooth with temporary cement. (See Chapter 35 for information on dental cements.) The occlusion is then checked and adjusted.

Most states allow the dental assistant to make and deliver provisional restorations due to the ability to reverse the procedure. It is appropriate for the dentist to check and adjust the occlusion. (See Chapter 41 for a more extensive discussion on provisional restorations.)

Indirect Restorations

Indirect restorations or castings are restorations created in the office by a laboratory technician or they can come from an outside dental lab source. An indirect restoration is made from a cast of the patient's tooth. When the casting is ready for use, the dentist places the restoration on the appropriate tooth to ensure fit prior to bonding. The dentist then bonds or cements the restoration such as a crown, **inlay**, **onlay**, or veneer onto the tooth followed by minor adjustments and finishing and polishing.

Alloys

A traditional casting is made of a gold alloy. In modern aesthetic dentistry, the casting is a milled ceramic core stacked with porcelain. Pure gold is extremely soft and malleable like gold jewelry. Therefore, pure gold is not a good restorative material to withstand the extreme forces of the chewing muscles. A dental restoration of pure gold would be crushed. Some positive aspects of using gold in the oral cavity are its biocompatibility and ability to resist tarnishing or discoloring. The human body accepts

gold as a foreign object, but because pure gold is too soft for restoring a tooth, it must be mixed with other metals to form an alloy with more acceptable properties to be used as a restorative material (Figure 33.8).

The metals used to create indirect restorative alloys are noble metals and base metals. The noble metals, those resistant to corrosion or oxidation, that are utilized in dentistry are gold (Au), palladium (Pd), platinum (Pt), and silver (Ag). **Palladium** is a white-silver tarnish-resistant metal. **Platinum** is also a white-silver metal that does not corrode in air.

The other group of metals, known as base metals, used for indirect restorations includes copper and zinc. Copper increases the hardness of the alloy, and zinc scavenges oxygen during processing. Gold alloys are characterized by hardness and **malleability**. They are divided into four types:

1. Type I alloys are soft and used for casting inlays in low stress areas.
2. Type II alloys are medium in hardness and used in casting of all other inlays of greater stress and some bridge abutments.
3. Type III alloys are considered hard in comparison to Type I and Type II alloys. They are utilized for inlays, crowns, three-quarter crowns, and bridge abutments.

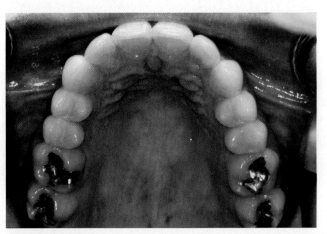

FIGURE 33.8
Gold crown.
Image courtesy Instructional Materials for the Dental Team, Lex., KY

4. Type IV alloys are the hardest of the gold alloys. This alloy is the most appropriate material for removable partial dentures.

Ceramics

Ceramic is an extremely hard, heat- and corrosive-resistant material that is clay fired at a very high temperature. Dental ceramics are compounds of metallic and nonmetallic elements. The metallic component provides durability and resistance to temperature change. The nonmetallic element of ceramic provides the aesthetic value of the restoration. Examples of dental ceramics include porcelain, alumina, and zirconia.

Porcelain is the most common type of ceramic used in dentistry. It provides for the aesthetic translucency that matches natural tooth structure. Restorations made of porcelain fused to metal restorations are commonly used throughout the mouth. The gold alloy casting provides the strength, while the very hard porcelain fused to the casting also provides strength as well as aesthetics. Porcelain may be stained to many different colors to match natural tooth structure. The laboratory must have a good depiction of an adjacent tooth to be able to match the porcelain of a crown to that natural tooth. Porcelain is created with great heat and pressure making it much stronger than a direct composite resin restoration.

The most natural of all dental restorations are the all-ceramic restorations. Rather new to dentistry, these restorations can provide great strength while providing the best aesthetics. In the last two decades, the all-ceramic crowns and veneers were most commonly used in the anterior. But with new improvements in ceramic technology, dentists are able to place all-ceramic crowns in the posterior that will withstand chewing forces. This new material, developed in Germany, is known as zirconium oxide. In the past, the ceramic substructures for crowns and bridges were brittle and not strong enough to

Professionalism

It is the responsibility of the dental team to provide all necessary information to a patient concerning his dental health and to educate the patient as to his options of dental materials. It is the patient's right to choose what dental material is best for his oral health and personal finances. As a member of the dental team, the dental assistant should not persuade a patient to choose one material over another but only provide the facts or advantages and disadvantages of each available material.

withstand the forces associated with chewing. Research has shown zirconium oxide to have excellent mechanical properties, aesthetic appearance, and biocompatibility. Studies in the United States have preliminarily predicted zirconium oxide to have a failure rate of 2% over a five-year period. For these reasons, zirconium oxide is a very promising dental material.

The final restoration or the substructure of an all-ceramic restoration is machined or milled using technology known as CAD/CAM, which scans the preparation of the tooth and digitally mills a pore-free block of alumina or zirconia ceramic. Most often the core is created mechanically and then a laboratory technician hand sculpts fine porcelain to the exterior and fires it to emulate the natural tooth structure.

To summarize, the advantages of ceramic restorations include:

- Superior aesthetics
- Strength
- Provides insulation to the underlying tooth structure
- Extremely low rates of expansion and contraction with temperature changes

SUMMARY

Numerous dental materials are available for treating dental restorations, and materials are constantly improving. Each clinical situation may utilize one or more of a number of materials. Dentists must choose which material is best suited for each situation. The dental assistant needs to recognize which material the dentist will select for a particular procedure and be able to assist the dentist efficiently.

To provide the best care possible to the patient, the dental team should work on being familiar with the latest materials and their applications. Amalgam is a controversial dental product and each dentist will have a policy concerning its use. Composite resin is continually improving, and studies show they may last just as long as amalgam in the proper environment. As with all evolving materials, more research is necessary. Indirect restorations are increasingly gaining popularity for their superior properties and aesthetics. As research continues and the properties of dental materials improve, the days of black or yellowed, fractured or worn restorations will be a thing of the past.

KEY TERMS

- **Alloy:** A mixture of metals.   p. 523
- **Amalgam:** A soft metal made of alloy mixed with mercury to restore form and function to teeth.   p. 523
- **Bonding:** *Verb:* Adhering tooth-colored resin composite to a tooth surface to create a bond. *Noun:* Process by which tooth-colored resin composite is bonded, sculpted, hardened, and polished to tooth surfaces, usually for aesthetic purposes.   p. 523
- **Composite resin:** Tooth-colored filling material made of silica or porcelain particles interlaced with liquid resin.   p. 524
- **Curing:** Chemical or physical process that improves the properties of a dental material, such as hardness and strength.   p. 522
- **Filler:** Silica or porcelain particles that add strength to composite resins.   p. 527
- **Galvanic:** Relating to an electric shock due to two different metals coming in contact.   p. 521
- **Inlay:** A gold, porcelain, or resin filling made to fit a prepared cavity cemented or bonded in place to restore a decayed or broken tooth.   p. 533
- **Malleability:** The property of being shaped or formed under pressure without breaking.   p. 533
- **Matrix:** The binding substance that holds filler particles together, especially in a composite resin.   p. 527
- **Onlay:** A gold, porcelain, or resin filling that also covers one or more cusps of a tooth; used to restore a decayed or broken tooth.   p. 533
- **Palladium (Pd):** A soft, silver-white, tarnish-resistant, naturally occurring metal related to platinum; considered a precious metal.   p. 533
- **Platinum (Pt):** A silver-white precious metal that does not corrode in air.   p. 533
- **Trituration:** The mixing of alloy with mercury to form amalgam.   p. 524
- **Viscosity:** The resistance of a material to flow.   p. 522

CHECK YOUR UNDERSTANDING

1. Which regulatory agency is responsible for all dental and medical materials intended for human use?
   a. American Dental Association
   b. Food and Drug Administration
   c. United States Dietary Association
   d. National Institutes of Health

2. Galvanic shock occurs when
   a. two dissimilar metals come in contact, creating a minor electrical current.
   b. two similar metals come in contact, creating a minor electrical current.
   c. three metals and calcium come into contact and generate a major shock.
   d. saliva conducts a current to a tooth with a metal filling.

3. Properties to consider when selecting a dental material include
   a. mechanical properties.
   b. thermal properties.
   c. electrical properties.
   d. corrosive properties.
   e. all of the above.

4. Which metal is not found in dental amalgam?
   a. silver
   b. tin
   c. copper
   d. mercury
   e. none of the above

5. A patient who received an amalgam restoration can eat right away because the restoration is as hard as it is going to be immediately after placement.
   a. true
   b. false

6. Which is not an advantage to placing composite restorations?
   a. improves aesthetics by restoring the natural appearance of the teeth and smile
   b. bonds to tooth structure to support remaining natural tooth
   c. conserves natural tooth structure
   d. releases fluoride into the tooth to protect the pulp

7. Fluoride-releasing glass ionomers are most often applied to
   a. large restorations.
   b. cavity liners and bases.
   c. core builds prior to an indirect restoration.
   d. indirect restoration cement.
   e. a, b, and c.

8. Intermediate restorative material (IRM) is primarily used to
   a. fill a cavity preparation for a short period of time while providing pain relief.
   b. provide long-term support to the remaining tooth structure.
   c. fill small cavity preparations as a permanent restoration.
   d. cement indirect restorations.

CHECK YOUR UNDERSTANDING (continued)

9. Dental gold is an alloy containing
   a. gold.
   b. platinum.
   c. palladium.
   d. copper.
   e. all of the above.

10. All-ceramic restorations are
   a. created by the dentist in the oral cavity.
   b. poor aesthetic restorations.
   c. created by the laboratory technician or in the office by a milling machine.
   d. not able to be used under any circumstance in the posterior.

INTERNET ACTIVITY

- Because of the controversy concerning the use of dental amalgam containing mercury, it is important to be well informed about the issue. Visit www.fda.gov/cdrh/consumer/amalgams to see the latest information from the Food and Drug Administration. The FDA is the regulatory agency that is tasked with evaluating the medical risk to patients and the public of any dental material.

WEB REFERENCES

- Academy of General Dentistry   www.agd.org
- American Dental Association   www.ada.org
- Centers for Disease Control and Prevention   www.cdc.gov
- Pierre Fauchard Academy   www.fauchard.org
- U.S. Food and Drug Administration   www.fda.gov

34

Dental Liners, Bases, and Bonding Systems

Learning Objectives

After reading this chapter, the student should be able to:

- List levels of tooth sensitivity to determine what type of dental preparation materials should be selected prior to the final restoration procedure.

- Identify the proper cavity liner and varnish to be used in restoring tooth structure prior to the final restoration procedure.

- Discuss how and why dentinal sealers are used in restoring tooth structure prior to the final restoration procedure.

- Explain how dental bases are used in restoring tooth structure prior to the final restoration procedure.

- Explain the difference between cavity liners, cavity varnishes, dentinal sealers, and dental bases.

- Discuss the bonding and etching processes and the importance of the setting process to the bonding of material to a tooth.

Preparing for Certification Exams

- Receive and prepare patients for treatment, including seating the patient and positioning the chair.

- Perform coronal polishing (according to the applicable state dental practice act).

- Mix dental materials.

- Perform sterilization and disinfection procedures.

- Using the concepts of four-handed dentistry, assist with basic restorative procedures.

- Place, cure, and finish composite resin restorations (according to the applicable state dental practice act).

- Place liners and bases.

Key Terms

Acid etchant

Desiccation

Eugenol

Sedative

Smear layer

Traumatic occlusion

Chapter Outline

- Cavity Preparations
- Supplementary Dental Materials and Their Application
- Pulpal Stimuli and Responses
- Dental Liners
  —Types of Dental Liners
  —Application of Dental Liners
- Varnishes
  —Types of Varnishes
  —Application of Varnishes
- Dentin Sealers
  —Types of Dentin Sealers
  —Application of Dentin Sealers
- Dental Bases
  —Types of Dental Bases
  —Application of Dental Bases
- Dental Bonding
  —Types of Dental Bonding
  —Acid Etchants
- Dentin Bonding
- Enamel Bonding
  —Application of Dental Bonding

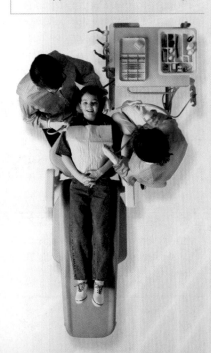

Dental material used to restore

teeth can be placed into two categories: (1) intermediary, which includes liners, bases, and cements, and (2) supplementary, which includes bonding agents and restorative materials. All materials used in the restoration of a tooth prior to the placement of the final restorative material are known as intermediary, because they occupy the place between the tooth and the restoration. These materials are used for specific purposes such as minimizing sensitivity and offering a therapeutic effect to the tooth.

Each dental material is chosen for its unique characteristics. Intermediary or supplemental materials provide added protection to the pulp and surrounding structures. Material selection is determined by preparation site, involvement, and physical makeup of the tooth. It is the dental assistant's responsibility to maintain the materials, follow proper mixing procedures, and know when and where the materials are used.

Cavity Preparations

The methods of cavity preparation depend on the location and type of restorative problem such as tooth decay or a fracture involving the enamel and/or dentin. How much of the tooth structure is cut depends on the extent, location, amount of tooth loss due to the decay or fracture, and the type of restorative materials that will be used. The dental assistant's knowledge of the step-by-step procedure in cavity preparation helps to ensure a successful outcome.

Supplementary Dental Materials and Their Application

After a cavity preparation is completed, supplementary materials are placed prior to the final restorative mater-

---

Dental Assistant PROFESSIONAL TIP

Make a folder small enough to keep chairside that holds manufacturers' directions for dental materials. This information can then be quickly referenced when needed.

Life Span Considerations

As we get older our teeth change. The pulp in the teeth recedes and the teeth become much less sensitive to dental materials. At this point, liners, varnishes, and bases are no longer needed in the restoration process.

---

ial. The dentist selects the material to be used depending on the extent of the remaining tooth structure, how far the preparation extends into the dentin, and how close to the pulp the final preparation will be.

A liner, varnish, sealer, base, bonding agent, sedative base, or a combination will be used when the preparation is moderate to deep. The order of application depends on the type of restorative material being used, as listed in Table 34-1.

Pulpal Stimuli and Responses

When the enamel is compromised by decay, the patient will typically experience sensitivity and discomfort. After the tooth is restored, that sensitivity may take weeks or even months to subside. During the excavation (removal of decay) of caries, the dentist decides if any supplemental material should be placed to help prevent pulpal sensitivity. Depending on the depth of the decay, pulpal sensitivity may be apparent after the restorative material has been placed. The pulp can respond differently to various types of stimuli. Types of pulpal stimuli and examples include:

- *Biological* (e.g., saliva in contact with the pulp)
- *Chemical* (e.g., acidic materials in contact with the pulp)
- *Mechanical* (e.g., result of **traumatic occlusion** or vibration of the handpiece)
- *Physical* (e.g., thermal changes or a galvanic or electrical reaction from metals in contact with the tooth)

Dental Liners

Dental liners are used to seal tooth structure in the deepest portion of the dental preparation (Figure 34.1 and Figure 34.2). Liners protect the pulp against microleakage and protect the pulp in deep cavities. An indirect pulp

---

Preparing for Externship

As a dental assistant it is important to be knowledgeable about the how, when, and why of mixing all types of supplementary materials. Be sure to spend extra time studying these areas to ensure a solid knowledge base about dental materials.

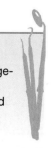

TABLE 34-1 Order of Application of Supplementary Dental Materials

Restorative Material Type	Cavity Preparation Depth		
	Shallow	Moderately Deep	Deep
Amalgam	1st: Dentin sealer 2nd: Bonding system	1st: Base 2nd: Dentin sealer 3rd: Bonding system	1st: Liner (sedative) 2nd: Base 3rd: Dentin sealer 4th: Bonding system
Composite resin	1st: Bonding system	1st: Bonding system	1st: Liner (sedative) 2nd: Bonding system
Precious metal (gold) inlays or onlays		1st: Base	1st: Liner (sedative) 2nd: Base
Porcelain or ceramic	1st: Bonding system	1st: Bonding system	1st: Liner (sedative) 2nd: Bonding system

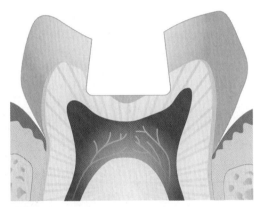

FIGURE 34.1
Area of placement of cavity liner in a preparation.

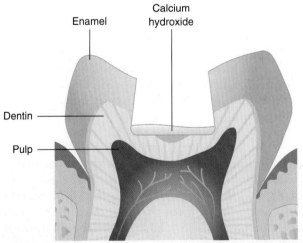

FIGURE 34.2
Placement of a cavity liner.

cap liner is placed when there is a possibility of pulp exposure or if the potential exists to come too close to the pulp. When the pulp is exposed during a caries excavation, the dentist places a pulp cap directly onto the pulp nerve to protect the exposure.

Not all liners are pulp friendly and the determination of which liner, if any, should be used is made by the dentist during the final restorative process. Common commercial liners include Cavitec, Dycal, Hydrex, Life, Pulprotex, Temres, Timeline, Ultraband, and ZOE.

Types of Dental Liners
Three types of dental liners are used in cavity preparations (Figure 34.3): (1) calcium hydroxide, (2) glass ionomers, and (3) zinc oxide eugenol cement.

Calcium hydroxide, known by the manufacturer's name of "Dycal," is a common type of dental liner used during the restorative process of preparing the tooth for a filling. Initially, calcium hydroxide was used to protect the pulp and aid in the formation of secondary dentin. However, studies have shown that calcium hydroxide alone does not promote the formation of secondary dentin. The use of a mild irritant stimulates the promotion of dentin growth. By using a sealer such as ZOE over the pulp portion of the cavity prepared area and then placing calcium hydroxide, secondary dentin was generated.

The dental assistant must understand that saliva will contaminate the process and break down the calcium hydroxide, which interferes with its protective qualities. A characteristic of calcium hydroxide is that it will dissolve when subjected to water, such that over time it will break down and further dissolve under a deteriorating restoration. Calcium hydroxide does not bond to the tooth, but does have an antibacterial property that stimulates the tooth to begin producing secondary dentin.

Calcium glass ionomers are used both as a restorative material and as a dentin liner. They are ideal for sealing dentin under different types of restorative materials, such as composite resin bonding and amalgam restorations. Some qualities of calcium glass ionomers are the ability to release fluoride, ability to bond, and their strength.

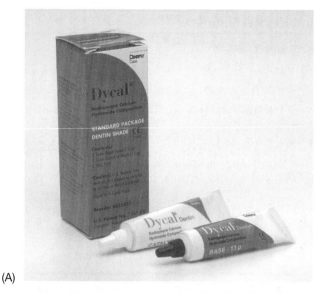

(A)

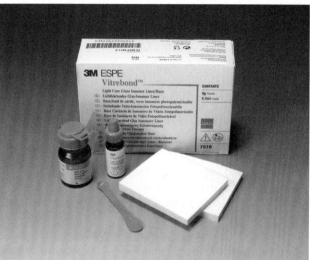

(B)

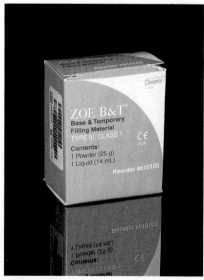

(C)

FIGURE 34.3
Various brand name liners: (a) Dycal, a calcium hydroxide liner;
(b) Vitrebond, a glass ionomer liner; and (c) ZOE cement.
Courtesy 3M ESPE

Zinc oxide eugenol cement, commonly known as ZOE, is used as a temporary restorative material and liner to provide a sedative base. **Eugenol** provides a **sedative** (soothing) effect to the pulpal tissue, but should not be applied directly onto a vital pulp because of the number of impurities it contains and the irritation it can cause to the pulp chamber. ZOE is very weak; therefore, the dentist will first place calcium hydroxide and then a layer of ZOE. Taken together, these steps encourage a sedative effect and creation of secondary dentin. The dental assistant must be proficient in the mixing and application of ZOE.

Application of Dental Liners

The dental assistant must have thorough knowledge of how to mix, store, and apply all types of dental liners. (See Procedures 34-1 through 34-3.) Always read the manufacturer's directions on mixing and storing procedures to ensure the success of the material.

Two types of delivery systems are available for mixing dental liners: a two-paste system and a one-paste or one-step light-cured system. The two-paste systems are mixed manually with a spatula on an oil-impermeable paper pad or clean glass slab. The use of an oil-impermeable pad prevents absorption of the material into the remainder of the mixing pad. Light-cured liner materials require no mixing because they are premixed and ready for use. They are set by light curing.

If you do not have a treated pad on which to mix ZOE, what do you mix it on?

Varnishes

Varnishes are used to protect the tooth from the damaging effects of moisture. Liquid varnishes protect and seal the dental tubules, thus providing insulation to the pulpal tissue. Dental varnishes are classified as liners when used under the cavity preparation for dental amalgam restorations.

Amalgam restorations shrink once they are completely set. Over time the shrinkage gap between the prepared tooth and amalgam fills in with corrosion that prevents marginal leakage. Varnishes seal these areas until the complete set is obtained. They also prevent metallic ions from migrating from the metal of the amalgam to the tooth by providing a barrier for the dentinal tubules to prevent sensitivity.

Types of Varnishes

Dental varnishes are liquids composed of resins. They are made of polyurethane polymers that are suspended in an organic solvent, such as acetone, ether, or chloroform. Dental varnishes are known as copal varnishes, which are

Procedure 34-1 Applying a Calcium Hydroxide Liner

Dental assistants should check their state dental practice laws to determine their role in this application.

Equipment and Supplies

- Tubes of calcium hydroxide "catalyst" and "base" (from same manufacturer)
- Small mixing pad (provided by the manufacturer)
- Small spatula
- Calcium hydroxide applicator instrument
- 2 × 2 gauze pads

Procedure Steps

1. Dispense small equal portions of the catalyst and base onto the special mixing pad.

2. Quickly mix the two pastes in a circular motion over a small area with the spatula.

3. After a homogenous mixture has been achieved, use a 2 × 2 gauze pad to wipe clean the spatula.

4. Using the ball tip of the applicator, pick up a small amount of material and apply in a thin layer directly over the pulp.

5. Use the explorer to remove any material that may have gotten onto the enamel.

6. Clean and disinfect all equipment.

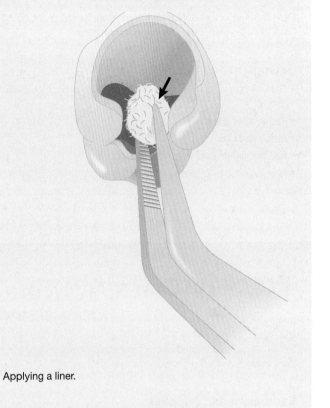

Applying a liner.

---

available with or without fluoride. Because of the organic solvent, dental varnishes cannot be used under resin or composite restorations. However, universal varnish can be used under all types of restorations.

Varnishes are highly effective as a dentin sealer, providing fluoride release to the enamel, root structure, and dentin. Fluoride-releasing varnishes are also used for hypersensitivity of the cervical areas. Common commercial dental varnishes include Caulk, Cavaseal, Chembar, Copalite, Handiliner, hydroxyline, Repelac, and Varnall.

Application of Varnishes

The type of varnish used determines the application process. For example, the use of a dental varnish is contraindicated when using composite resins and glass ionomer restorations due to their staining capabilities. When applying varnish the use of a cotton pellet or microbrush/sponge is most common. (See Procedure 34-4.) Another way to apply varnishes is by the use of direct adhesion. An example of that would be the placement of a primer prior to the restoration.

What types of dental varnish would you find in a prosthodontic office for use under composite resin bonding restorations? **?**

Dentin Sealers

Dentin sealers are used to assist the treatment of hypersensitivity that may occur after a new restoration has been placed. Dentin sealers are commonly known as *desensitizers*, and are used instead of dental varnishes. The desensitizer is intended to seal the dentinal tubules that prevent oral fluids and bacteria from seeping between the tooth and the restorative material over time. Dentin sealers do not form a surface layer, a quality that is desired and can be used under all restorations.

Types of Dentin Sealers

Some dental sealers seal the outer edge of the tubules, and others leave salts or proteins within the tubules. However, occluding or covering up the tubules can be accomplished

Procedure 34-2 Applying a Glass Ionomer Liner

Dental assistants should check their state dental practice laws to determine their role in this application.

Equipment and Supplies

- Glass ionomer cement powder/liquid, with manufacturer's scoop
- Paper mixing pad
- Small spatula
- Ball burnisher applicator instrument
- Moistened 2 × 2 gauze pads

Procedure Steps

1. Dispense material per manufacturer's directions.

2. Dispense the powder on the other half of the pad.

3. Incorporate the powder and liquid according to the manufacturer's directions.

4. Use a 2 × 2 gauze pad to wipe clean the spatula.

5. Apply liner (see Procedure 34-1, step 4).

6. Clean and disinfect all equipment.

Procedure 34-3 Applying a Zinc Oxide Eugenol Cement Liner Using the Two-Paste System

Dental assistants should check their state dental practice laws to determine their role in this application.

Equipment and Supplies

- Two-paste ZOE cement liner "accelerator" and "base" (from same manufacturer)
- Small mixing pad (provided by the manufacturer)
- Small cement spatula
- Small ball burnisher applicator instrument or a plastic instrument
- Moist 2 × 2 gauze pads

Procedure Steps

1. Dispense material per manufacturer's directions.

2. Quickly gather the materials and mix the two pastes.

3. Use a moistened 2 × 2 gauze pad to wipe clean the spatula.

4. Apply liner (see Procedure 34-1, step 4).

5. Clean and disinfect all equipment.

Procedure 34-4 Applying Dental Varnishes

Dental assistants should check their state dental practice laws to determine their role in this application.

Equipment and Supplies

- Dental varnish
- Cotton pliers, cotton pellets, or microbrush applicators

Procedure Steps

1. Open bottle of varnish and saturate the cotton pellet or applicator.

2. Apply to walls and margins of cavity preparation.

3. Allow the varnish to air dry.

4. Prepare a second varnish. Saturate the cotton pellet with second varnish if the second varnish is needed.

5. Apply second varnish if needed.

6. Clean and disinfect all equipment.

using many products. The end result is that the tubules are blocked, which prevents fluid movement within them.

One dentin sealer product that is designed to cut off the flow of the tubule fluids by sealing tubules is Gluma. Gluma contains glutaraldehyde. Glutaraldehydes precipitate and coagulate proteins/amino acids within the tubule. Gluma also contains a methyl methacrylate, which seals the tubules.

Other bonding/sealing agents containing methyl methacrylate or some type of surface precipitant have been recommended for chairside treatment of dentinal sensitivity. Examples include All-Bond DS Desensitizer, Confi-Dental, Micro Prime, Hurriseal, and Microjoin. Dentin sealer desensitizers should be used sparingly and not come in contact with soft tissue due to the 2-hydroxyethyl methacrylate (HEMA) and glutaraldehyde within the sealer.

Application of Dentin Sealers

When a dentin sealer is to be placed on a tooth, a dry and clean preparation is required. This task can be accomplished by using a saturated applicator to place the sealer on the floor of the cavity preparation. After placing the sealer on the tooth, wait 30 seconds and then air dry. (See Procedure 34-5.) Overdrying should be avoided.

What are the common reasons a tooth will become sensitive under a newly placed restoration?

Dental Bases

When performing a cavity preparation, the dentist makes a conscious effort to keep the cavity preparation as small as possible. Caries, though, can go deep into the grooves of the tooth structure. As the dentist opens the preparation, he or she may find a much larger involved carious area than anticipated. Should the preparation become moderately deep or too close to the pulp, the dentist will most likely place a base under the final restoration. The base is another product placed between the liner and permanent restoration to help protect the pulp. Most dental cements can be used as a base and are applied over a liner in a thick layer. The pulp can be protected with a base by using it as an insulator, as a protective covering, or as a sedative.

Types of Dental Bases

There are three types of bases: insulating, sedative, and protective:

1. Zinc oxide eugenol is best used as an *insulating or sedative base*. The eugenol (oil from cloves) can provide a soothing effect on the pulp.
2. Zinc phosphate cement may be used depending on the preference of the dentist. Due though to the phosphoric acid found in this type of cement, it is not used as often as polycarboxylate. If used, a liner is placed between the cement and the restoration in order to protect the pulp.
3. Polycarboxylate cement is ideal for use as a *protective or insulating base*. Any dental cement can be used as a

---

Procedure 34-5 Applying Dentin Sealers

Dental assistants should check their state dental practice laws to determine their role in this application.

Equipment and Supplies
- Dental sealer material
- Microbrush applicators

Procedure Steps
1. Perform moisture control. Tooth should be dry and clean.
2. Apply saturated applicator to the cavity preparation.
3. Wait 30 seconds. Air dry.
4. Repeat a second application if patient has had sensitivity history.
5. Clean and disinfect all equipment.

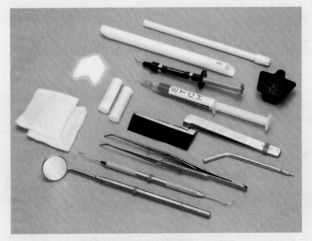

Equipment for applying dental sealants.

TABLE 34-2 Examples of Common Commercial Dental Bases

Glass Ionomers	Resin-Type Glass Ionomers	Polycarboxylate	Zinc Oxide Eugenol	Zinc Phosphate
• ASPA	• Fuji Duet	• Carboxylon	• IRM	• Dropsin
• ChemBond	• Vitremer cement	• Durelon	• ZOE	• Fleck's Extraordinary
• Dentine cement Fuji Bond		• Hy-Bond	• ZOE 2200	• Hy-Bond SP
• Ketac-Bond		• PC Cement		• Modern Tenacin
• Vitrebond		• Polybond		• Zinc Cement Improved
• Zionomer		• Poly-FPlus		
		• Tylok Plus		

base; however, only some types of bases can be used under certain types of permanent restorations. All cements have similar insulating and thermal conductivity features. Resin-type bases and glass ionomers are commonly used because of their ability to bond to the dentin for retention. Table 34-2 provides examples of commonly used commercial dental bases.

Application of Dental Bases

Dental bases are used to provide a buffer between the pulp and the final restoration. A dental base is much thicker than a liner, varnish, or sealer and covers the pulp and floor of the cavity preparation (Figure 34.4). Dental bases may be applied by an expanded functions dental assistant when delegated by the dentist according to each state's dental practice act. (See Procedures 34-6 through 34-8.) The type of base to be applied will determine the procedure to be followed.

How might the application of a dental base be explained to a patient?

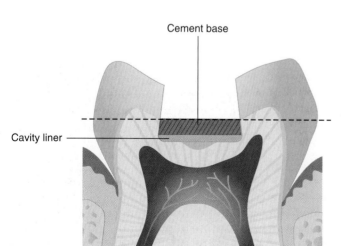

Cement base

Cavity liner

FIGURE 34.4
Placement of a base in the cavity preparation.

Professionalism

In Chapter 3, the discussion of dental ethics and the law advises dental assistants to be knowledgeable about the laws of their individual state's dental practice act. Depending on your particular state's dental practice act, the expanded functions dental assistant may place, apply, mix, and assist with dental materials.

Dental Bonding

Dental bonding agents are referred to as dental adhesives and bonding resins. Dental bonding is a procedure in which a tooth-colored resin material is applied to the tooth and set with a curing light. Bonding agents are used to improve retention between the prepared tooth and contact of material. Bonding resins bond with enamel and dentin to amalgam, composites, nonprecious metals, and porcelain. Bonding materials can be purchased as a complete kit.

Types of Dental Bonding

Bonding agents are low-viscosity resins that are used to improve retention between enamel and a restoration or dentin and a restoration. They can also contain fluoride, which aids in the prevention of caries. In dentistry, bonding agents are used for sealing dental tubules, bonding enamel to repair fractured teeth, and bonding amalgam to dentin for a restoration. They can be dual cured chemically (catalyst and base) or light cured. The dental assistant should be familiar with bonding materials.

Acid Etchants

The application of **acid etchants** is essential in preparing enamel and dentin for bonding resin materials to the tooth structure. (See procedure 34-9.) The etchant product is usually maleic acid etchant or phosphoric acid etchant, and it is used to remove the **smear layer**. Acid etchants are supplied in liquid or gel form for easy appli-

Procedure 34-6 Applying Zinc Oxide Eugenol Cement Base

Dental assistants should check their state dental practice laws to determine their role in this application.

Equipment and Supplies

- Zinc oxide powder and scoop dispenser
- Eugenol liquid and dropper
- Small mixing pad (provided by the manufacturer)
- Small cement spatula
- Plastic instrument
- Amalgam condenser
- 2 × 2 gauze pads

Procedure Steps

1. Dispense the powder and liquid per manufacturer's instruction onto a special mixing pad.

2. Using the spatula, combine half the powder into the liquid and mix thoroughly for about 20 to 30 seconds.

3. Then pull the remaining powder into the mixture, mixing for another 20 to 30 seconds until the material becomes putty-like.

4. Place portion needed in the cavity preparation.

5. Use a moistened 2 × 2 gauze to wipe clean the spatula and condenser.

6. Clean and disinfect all equipment.

Procedure 34-7 Applying Zinc Phosphate

Dental assistants should check their state dental practice laws to determine their role in this application.

Equipment and Supplies

- Zinc phosphate powder and liquid with scoop dispenser
- Glass slab, chilled
- Small cement spatula
- Amalgam condenser
- Plastic instrument
- 2 × 2 gauze pads

Procedure Steps

1. Dispense the powder and liquid per manufacturer's directions onto a chilled glass slab.

2. Using the spatula, mix small increments of powder into the liquid until the material is a thick or putty consistency. Allow for dissipation of heat.

3. Use a moistened 2 × 2 gauze to wipe clean the spatula and condenser.

4. Using the condenser, place the putty on the end and carry to the dentist for placement.

5. Use a moistened 2 × 2 gauze to wipe the condenser tip if necessary.

6. Clean and disinfect all equipment.

---

cation and management inside the cavity prepared area. The preparation of the tooth with dental burs creates a smear layer of debris. The smear layer is burnished into the underlying dentin and dentin tubules. When the smear layer is removed a mechanical retention is established and the resin bonds.

Strict guidelines should be maintained during application of an acid etchant. Acid should not come in contact with soft tissue or adjacent teeth. It is important to be careful that the etched teeth are not contaminated with saliva. If etched teeth are contaminated, reapply etchant according to the manufacturer's directions. Contamination can be avoided by using cotton roll isolation or a rubber dam. Should the etchant touch oral tissue, it may cause an acid burn. The dental assistant should take precautions to ensure that the etchant does not come in contact with the skin or eyes. If this does occur, cold water should be used to wash the area or an emergency eye wash station may be utilized.

Dentin Bonding

Dentin bonding is used as an adhesive when the dentist restores the tooth with dental resin material. The bonding adhesive is used to form mechanical retention to dentin after etching. This procedure helps to

Procedure 34-8 Applying a Polycarboxylate Cement Base

Dental assistants should check their state dental practice laws to determine their role in this application.

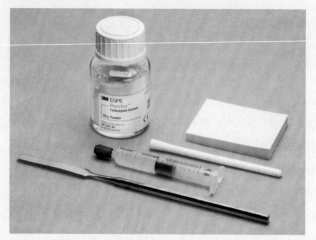

Equipment used for applying polycarboxylate cement base.

Equipment and Supplies

- Polycarboxylate powder and scoop dispenser
- Polycarboxylate liquid and dropper
- Mixing pad (provided by the manufacturer)
- Small cement spatula
- Plastic instrument
- Amalgam condenser
- 2 × 2 gauze pads

Procedure Steps

1. Dispense powder and liquid per manufacturer's directions. Keep in mind that when mixing polycarboxylate the mixture is thicker for a base than when used as a liner or cement.

2. Using the spatula, combine all the powder into the liquid and mix thoroughly and all at once within 30 seconds.

3. Roll material into a ball.

4. Using the condenser, place the putty onto the end and place into the preparation.

5. Clean and disinfect all equipment.

Procedure 34-9 Applying a Dental Acid Etchant

Dental assistants should check their state dental practice laws to determine their role in this application.

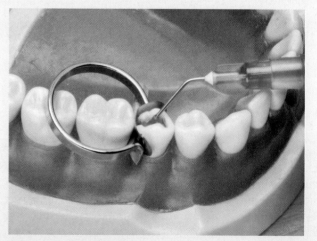

Applying an etchant material.

Equipment and Supplies

- Rubber dam or cotton rolls (for isolation)
- Dental acid etchant
- Applicators: syringe, cotton pellets, small applicator tips or microbrush applicators
- Dappen dish
- Timer

Procedure Steps

1. Use rubber dam or cotton rolls to isolate the area if necessary.

2. Clean the surface thoroughly.

3. Etch the surface following manufacturer's directions.

4. Go to next procedure in bonding restoration process.

5. Clean and disinfect all equipment.

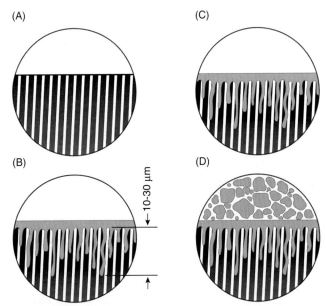

FIGURE 34.5
Process of bonding: (a) enamel rods unetched, (b) enamel rods etched, (c) bonding agent mechanically bonding to tooth, and (d) resin chemically bonding to bonding agent.

ensure a chemical and mechanical bond to secure the restoration (Figure 34.5).

When applying dentin bonding resin material, it is important to air dry the tooth. However, keep in mind that overdrying the dentin or causing **desiccation** will cause damage to the tooth structure and should be avoided during the deepest cavity preparation procedure.

Enamel Bonding

There are various reasons to bond directly to the enamel:

- *Orthodontics:* Orthodontists bond brackets directly to the tooth enamel.
- *Dental sealant:* Sealants are placed to protect the tooth from decay.
- *Resin-bonded veneers and bridges:* These are directly bonded to the enamel surface.

Resin materials such as sealants, cements, or resin restorative materials flow into and surround enamel

Patient Education

Patients may complain about one or more teeth that are occasionally painful. The pain may be invariably triggered by thermal changes or dental manipulations. This problem may be due to a condition known as dentinal hypersensitivity, which is a relatively simple condition to treat. Hypersensitivity can sometimes be treated by applying either a fluoride paste, bonding agent, or dentin sealer.

Procedure 34-10 Applying Dental Bonding

Equipment and Supplies

- Rubber dam or cotton rolls (for isolation)
- Bonding system with primer or conditioner/adhesive material

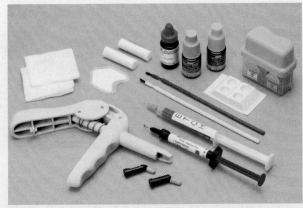

Equipment used for applying a dental bond.

- Applicators: syringe, cotton pellets, small applicator tips or microbrush applicators
- Dappen dish
- Air/water syringe
- Curing light and shield
- Timer

Procedure Steps

1. Etching has been completed. Move quickly to prevent bacterial contamination of the dentin.

2. Apply primer if indicated.

3. Apply bonding resin or composite restoration material. Set with curing light.

4. Place small increments of bonding resin into the cavity preparation and set in layers until preparation is completely filled.

5. Clean and disinfect all equipment.

rods. As the material hardens around these areas, it creates a strong mechanical bond between the restoration and the enamel.

Application of Dental Bonding

Steps in the application of bonding agents vary with manufacturers, so be sure to always refer to the specific manufacturer's directions for each product to be used. The dental assistant prepares the materials for each step and keeps the area isolated, dry, and free of debris, while also maintaining patient comfort. (See Procedure 34-10.)

If an area not to be etched becomes wet or contaminated during the etchant process, what should be done?

SUMMARY

The dental assistant can complete many procedures that involve the use of dental materials. Having a thorough understanding of equipment, materials, preparation, and mixing is essential. It is the dental assistant's management, usage, and storage of the material that helps to ensure a successful restoration. Having a knowledge base of the materials and requirements allows the dental assistant to anticipate the next step. Depending on one's state dental practice act, various procedures may be performed and accomplished.

Cultural Considerations

Listening to your patients is always important. An individual's culture may mean that his or her native language may be something other than English. This can make communication sometimes challenging. It is up to each dental team member to ensure that the patient feels heard and that the patient's issues get addressed. Patience, care, and understanding can go a long way in ensuring patient satisfaction.

KEY TERMS

- **Acid etchant:** A bonding technique in which tooth structure is etched with phosphoric acid to create the rough surface necessary for mechanical and micromechanical bonding. p. 544
- **Desiccation:** The removal of all moisture from an area; the process of drying out. p. 547
- **Eugenol:** A clear to pale yellow, oily aromatic liquid made from clove oil that is sometimes used in dentistry as an anti-inflammatory and antimicrobial. Contains soothing qualities and has a pleasant, spicy, clove-like taste. p. 540

- **Sedative:** A material that has a soothing effect on the patient. p. 540
- **Smear layer:** A very thin layer of debris on newly prepared dentin. p. 544
- **Traumatic occlusion:** An occlusion that does not properly articulate, causing additional pressure to a specific area of a tooth and causing the pulp to feel "bruised." p. 538

CHECK YOUR UNDERSTANDING

1. Which one of the following chemicals is used for etching enamel?
   a. eugenol
   b. zinc oxide
   c. phosphoric acid
   d. resin

2. Calcium hydroxide is used as a liner to
   a. promote secondary dentin.
   b. insulate the pulp thermally.
   c. protect the pulp from bacteria.
   d. insulate the pulp chemically.

3. Which of the following is true about varnishes?
   a. They are used as a base.
   b. They can be used to seal the dentin tubules.
   c. They can be used with all types of restorations.
   d. They are placed under sealant material as an adhesive.

4. What is another name for a dentin sealer?
   a. varnish
   b. temporary filling
   c. permanent luting
   d. desensitizer

CHECK YOUR UNDERSTANDING (continued)

5. Which of the following is used in enamel bonding?
   a. sealants
   b. orthodontic brackets
   c. dentinal tubules
   d. both a and b

6. What does etching do in terms of preparing a tooth for a final restoration?
   a. cleans the plaque off the enamel
   b. removes the smear layer
   c. allows moisture to be present during bonding
   d. is an adhesive

7. A base is placed _____ of the cavity preparation.
   a. along the enamel margins
   b. in the pulpal floor
   c. in the enamel floor
   d. in the dentin floor

8. Which of the following is the correct sequence for applying supplementary materials when a deep cavity preparation is being restored?
   a. dentin sealer, base, bonding, liner
   b. bonding, base, liner, dentin sealer
   c. liner, base, dentin sealer, bonding
   d. base, liner, dentin sealer, bonding

9. Bonding agents can be used for
   a. bonding dentin.
   b. bonding enamel.
   c. providing a shiny surface.
   d. both a and b.

10. Acid etchant is usually
    a. maleic acid.
    b. citric acid.
    c. phosphoric acid.
    d. both a and c.

INTERNET ACTIVITY

- Go to "Ask Dr. Spiller" at www.doctorspiller.com/dental_materials.htm to learn about hybrids and types of composites and how they are made.

WEB REFERENCES

- The Academy of Dental Materials   www.academydentalmaterials.org

Dental Cements

Chapter Outline

- Classification of Dental Cements
- Types of Cements
  —Zinc Oxide Eugenol Cement
  —Zinc Phosphate Cement
  —Polycarboxylate Cement
  —Glass Ionomer Cement
  —Composite Resin Cement
- Removing Excess Cement

Learning Objectives

After reading this chapter, the student should be able to:

- Classify dental cements.
- Recognize the benefits of using dental cements.
- Explain the difference between temporary and permanent cements.
- Discuss factors that determine the type of cement to be used.
- Describe how to remove excess dental cement.

Preparing for Certification Exams

- Prepare procedural trays/armamentaria setups.
- Complete laboratory authorization forms.
- Transfer dental instruments.
- Demonstrate knowledge of ethics, jurisprudence, and patient confidentiality.
- Mix dental materials.
- Provide patient education.
- Remove excess cement.
- Place, cure, and finish composite restorations.

Key Terms

Chemically cured

Exothermic reaction

Homogenous

Light cured

Luting agent

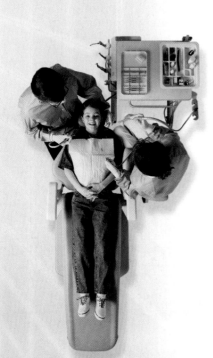

Using cements correctly for the treatment of various procedures is an important task that must be accomplished by the dental assistant. The dental assistant must not only know how to accurately mix the materials, but must also be familiar with proper storage techniques to ensure an adequate life span for the cements being used. Following the manufacturer's directions is critical for the strength and long-term success of the restoration provided to the dental patient.

Classification of Dental Cements

Dental cements are used for a variety of purposes. The International Standards Organization (ISO) and American Dental Association (ADA) have classified cements into three specific categories of use: (1) **luting agent** applications, (2) restorative applications, and (3) liner or base applications.

The selection of cements for a particular application requires knowledge of the chemistry and physical property of the cement type. For instance, for a restorative application, a high-strength base such as zinc polycarboxylate would be used, whereas for a temporary restoration, a low-strength base such as zinc oxide eugenol would be selected for its sedative qualities prior to placing a permanent restoration.

Table 35-1 lists some of the various dental cements commonly used in dentistry.

Dental Assistant PROFESSIONAL TIP

Maintaining the latest information on dental cements and how they are used help ensure accurate time management during chairside procedures. Be sure to stay current by joining your local dental assisting association and attending continuing education seminars.

Types of Cements

A wide variety of cements are used in dental restorations. Most have versatile properties, uses, and mixing techniques. The distinguishing characteristics of cements, such as whether they release fluoride or have low solubility, make these materials incredibly useful to dentists when performing restorations. As a dental assistant, it is important to stay current on the various types of dental cements available.

Cultural Considerations

Help to make patients feel comfortable during dental procedures by using kind words of reassurance, providing a gentle pat on the shoulder, and informing the patient of what is occurring. Pay attention to your patient's body language. This can tell you more than words. For instance, if you notice that your patient is grasping the arm rest of the chair with a tight grip, stop the procedure for a moment and inquire as to the patient's concern. If you sense the patient is feeling uncomfortable or nervous, try to provide comfort. Keeping a multiple-language dictionary in the office will provide assistance in speaking with patients whose first language is not English.

TABLE 35-1 Trade Names and Uses of Various Dental Cements Commonly Used in Dentistry

	Glass Ionomer	Resin Modified Ionomer	Chemically Cured Resin Cement	Dual-Cured Resin Cement	Zinc Phosphate	Zinc Poly-carboxylate	Zinc Oxide Eugenol
	Fuji (GC)	Advance (Caulk)	Panavia 21 (J. Morita)	Resinomer (Bisco)	Tenacin (Caulk)	Durelon (ESPE)	Temp-Bond (Kerr)
	Ketac Cem (ESPE)	Vitremer Luting (3M)	Clearfil CR Inlay (J. Morita)	Enforce (Dentsply)	Fleck's (Mizzy)	Tylok Plus (Caulk)	Fynal (Caulk)
Selected Uses	High-strength base, low-strength liner, permanent cement for cast restorations	Permanent cement for cast restorations	Permanent cement for cast restorations	Permanent cement for cast restorations	Insulating base and permanent cement for cast restorations	High-strength base, used as a temporary restoration. Also, permanent cement for cast restorations	Temporary restoration, sedative dressing has low strength as a base

How are cements selected for an individual restoration?

Zinc Oxide Eugenol Cement

Zinc oxide eugenol cement, also known as ZOE, is the most multipurpose cement used. ZOE is soothing to the pulp and assists in the generation of secondary dentin. Type I ZOE cement has low strength and great antimicrobial properties and, therefore, is ideal as a temporary restoration. Type II ZOE is used as a permanent cement for cast restorations. Type II is strong because it has reinforcing agents such as alumina and polymers (resins)

added to the powder. In addition, ethoxybenzoic acid is added to the eugenol, which offers strength along with antimicrobial properties.

ZOE is available in several forms: powder/liquid, two-paste systems, capsules, and syringes. The powder is a combination of zinc oxide resin, zinc acetate, and an accelerator. The liquid portion consists of eugenol and is sometimes mixed with clove oil. Mixing these types of cements requires an understanding of how they will be used. The ZOE cements can be mixed to a luting consistency or putty-like consistency. The dental assistant should be knowledgeable about mixing ZOE cements.

Zinc Phosphate Cement

Zinc phosphate cement is classified into two types. Type I is a fine grit that is used for permanent cast restorations. Type II is a medium grit that is used as an insulating base in deep cavity preparations. The liquid solution is phosphoric acid in water buffered by agents that slow down the setting reaction. Because the liquid contains acid, it is irritating to the pulpal tissue. Prior to placing zinc phosphate, a liner or sealer is used to eliminate pulpal irritation.

The powder in zinc phosphate is primarily zinc oxide with a small amount of magnesium oxide and pig-

---

Procedure 35-1 Mixing ZOE Type I Temporary Cement

Equipment and Supplies

- Cotton rolls (for isolation)
- ZOE two-paste system (temporary bond)
- Treated paper mixing pad
- Spatula

Procedure Steps

1. Dispense equal lengths of accelerator and base on treated pad.

2. Spatulate until homogenous.

3. Place in temporary crown and seat.

4. Clean and disinfect all equipment.

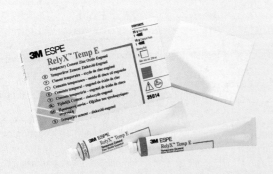

Temporary bonding cement.
Courtesy 3M ESPE

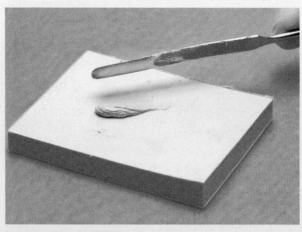

Homogenous mix of ZOE.

Procedure 35-2 Mixing ZOE Type II Cement for Permanent Cementation

Equipment and Supplies

- ZOE powder/liquid
- Treated paper pad or glass slab
- Small spatula
- 2 × 2 gauze pads

Procedure Steps

1. Dispense powder and liquid according to manufacturer's directions.

2. Divide the powder into increments.

3. Dispense the liquid near the powder on the mixing pad.

4. Blend the powder and liquid all at once.

5. Check to ensure that the mix has a **homogenous** color.

6. Be sure cavity preparation is dry and clean.

7. The inside of the indirect restoration should be loaded and handed to the dentist.

8. Clean and disinfect all equipment.

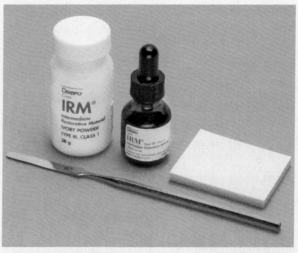

ZOE in powder and liquid form.

ments. The powder can be purchased in a variety of shades of white, yellow, and gray. During the setting process, zinc phosphate undergoes a chemical **exothermic reaction** (releases heat). To slow the setting time, zinc phosphate should be mixed on a cooled glass slab, placing the liquid last to prevent condensation from contaminating the liquid. (See Procedures 35-1 through 35-3.)

Polycarboxylate Cement

Polycarboxylate cement (also known as zinc polycarboxylate) can be used as permanent cement for cast restorations (fixed prostheses) or as an intermediate restoration or insulating base under amalgam and composite restoration (Figure 35.1). Polycarboxylate cement is less irritating to the pulp than zinc phosphate cement, and the pulpal reaction is similar to that of ZOE cement. It is also the first cement that had the ability to chemically bond to the tooth structure.

Polycarboxylate cement is a mixture of powder and liquid form and capsules that must be mixed prior to use in a restoration. (See Procedure 35-4.)

Glass Ionomer Cement

Glass ionomer powder is silicate glass containing calcium, aluminum, and fluoride. The liquid is an aqueous solution (contains water) of polyacrylic acid. Glass

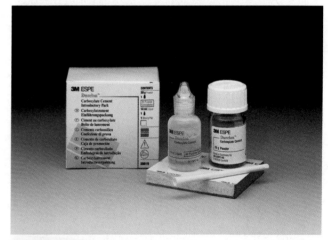

FIGURE 35.1
Polycarboxylate cement.
Courtesy 3M ESPE

ionomer cement mechanically and chemically bonds to enamel, dentin, and metallic materials. Type I is used for cementing metal restorations and orthodontic brackets, Type II for restoring areas of erosion near the gingiva, and Type III for liners and dentin bonding agents.

Glass ionomer cements are fluoride releasing, which helps to prevent recurrent decay under the restoration. These cements come packaged as self-cured, **light cured**, or premeasured capsules. To properly mix these cements,

Procedure 35-3 Mixing Zinc Phosphate for Permanent Cementation

Equipment and Supplies

- Zinc phosphate powder and liquid with dispenser
- Glass slab
- Small spatula
- 2 × 2 gauze pads

Procedure Steps

1. Measure powder according to manufacturer's directions and dispense the powder at one end of the slab and the liquid at the other end.

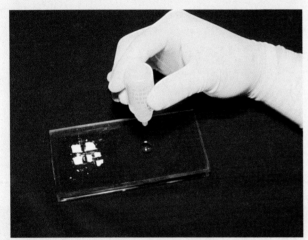

Position of bottle for dispensing cement liquid.
Image courtesy Instructional Materials for the Dental Team, Lex., KY

2. Divide the powder into increments.

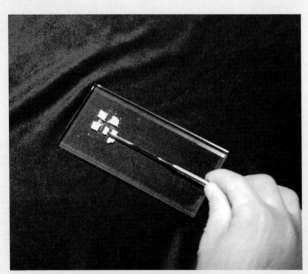

Zinc phosphate powder divided into sections to be mixed into the liquid cement.
Image courtesy Instructional Materials for the Dental Team, Lex., KY

3. Incorporate each powder increment into the liquid.

4. Using the spatula, mix thoroughly, using large figure 8 type strokes over entire glass slab ensuring that each increment of powder is mixed thoroughly before adding another increment of powder.

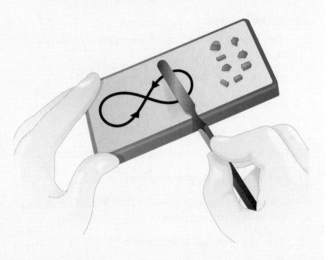

5. Test mix for correct cementation consistency. The cement should string up and break about one inch from the slab.

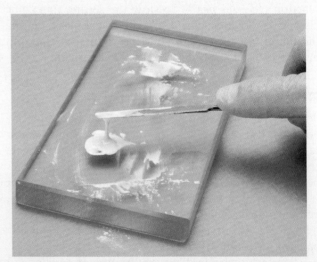

Homogenous mix of zinc phosphate cement with a one-inch draw.

6. Fill the casting by gathering cement mix onto the spatula.

7. Slide the edge of the spatula along the margin, allowing the cement to flow from the spatula into the casting, or use a Woodson for lining smaller castings.

continued on next page

Procedure 35-3 *continued from previous page*

8. Place the tip of the spatula or Woodson into the restoration and move the mixture so that it completely covers all the inside walls.

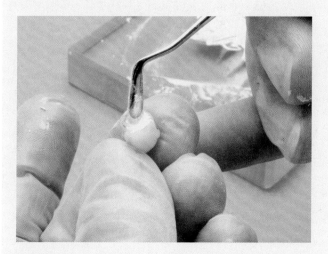

9. Turn the casting over in your palm and transfer to the dentist.

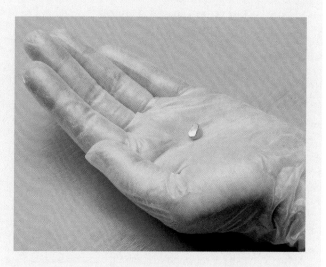

10. Clean and disinfect all equipment.

Procedure 35-4 Mixing Polycarboxylate Cement

Equipment and Supplies

- Polycarboxylate powder/liquid and dispenser
- Treated oil-resistant paper pad or glass slab
- Small spatula
- 2 × 2 gauze pads

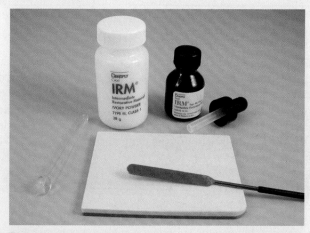

Treated mixing pad, polycarboxylate powder, liquid, and measuring scoop with a metal spatula.
Image courtesy Instructional Materials for the Dental Team, Lex., KY

Procedure Steps

1. Dispense powder and liquid according to the manufacturer's directions.

2. Mix the powder into the liquid quickly with the flat side of the spatula, all at one time, to a homogenous consistency.

3. Check to ensure that the consistency of the cement is correct. It should be somewhat thick and have a shiny, glossy surface.

4. With the casting inner opening facing upward, gather cement mix onto the spatula and slide the edge of the spatula along the margin, allowing the cement to flow into the casting.

5. Place the tip of the spatula or a Woodson to move the mixture so that it completely covers all inside walls of the casting with a thin lining of cement.

6. Turn the casting over in your palm and transfer it to the dentist.

7. Transfer a cotton roll to the dentist for the patient to bite down on to help seat the casting and disperse the excess cement.

8. Clean and disinfect all equipment.

Procedure 35-5 Mixing Glass Ionomer Cement

Equipment and Supplies

- Glass ionomer cement powder and dispenser
- Glass ionomer cement liquid and dropper
- Treated oil-resistant paper pad or glass slab
- Small spatula
- 2 × 2 gauze pads

Procedure Steps

1. Dispense the powder and liquid according to manufacturer's directions.

2. Mix the powder into the liquid one increment at a time until all is mixed.

3. Check to ensure that the consistency of the cement is correct. It should be somewhat thick and have a shiny, glossy surface.

4. Place cement into the restoration.

5. Clean and disinfect all equipment.

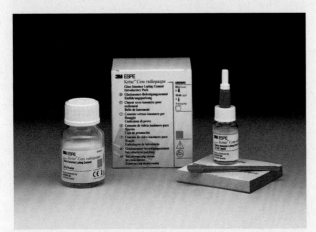

Ketac Cem bottle of liquid, powder, mixing pad, and scoop.
Courtesy 3M EPSE

the dental assistant must pay strict attention to ensure that the manufacturer's directions are closely followed. (See Procedure 35-5.)

Composite Resin Cement

Composite resin cements have many uses in a large variety of procedures, such as cementation of cast metal restorations, porcelain/resin restorations, veneers, orthodontic brackets, and endodontic posts (Figure 35.2). They have a thin film thickness and are not easily dissolved by oral fluids in the mouth. A key factor in using composite resin cements is that the tooth must be plaque and debris free. The tooth must also be prepared by etching or treated with a bonding system prior to cementing.

Composite resin cements come in powder/liquid, syringe-type, **chemically cured**, and light-cured versions. As with all cement mixing, it is important for the dental assistant to understand the variety of composite resins and how they are used. (See Procedure 35-6.) The classification of and uses for dental cements are summarized in Table 35-2.

If a liner is not used under zinc phosphate cement, what would the patient experience?

Removing Excess Cement

After cement has been placed in a cast restoration (fixed prosthesis), the excess cement is removed. The timing of removing the excess cement is determined by the type of material used. In most states, expanded functions dental assistants are allowed to perform this procedure under the direct supervision of the dentist.

Patient Education

Postoperative instructions for crown cementation must be made clear to the patient. Understanding the importance of keeping the margins of the crown clean to avoid caries around the crown must be stressed.

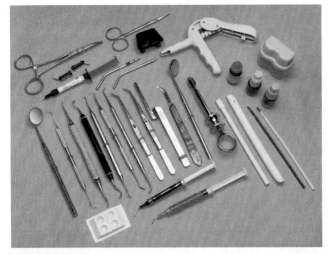

FIGURE 35.2
Composite resin cement kit.

TABLE 35-2 Classification of and Uses for Dental Cements

Generic Name	Mixing Spatula (Metal/Teflon)	Mixing Table (Coated/ Noncoated or Glass Slab)	Type I or Type II	Consistency of Cement for Use	Base/ Liner/ Permanent	Name Brand
Zinc Oxide Eugenol	Stainless steel metal *(Note: Instrument should not be used with any other cement.)*	Coated paper tablet or glass slab	Type I	Luting	Base or liner	Temp-Bond (Kerr)
			Type II	Putty; dough ball	Temporary restoration	IRM
Zinc Phosphate	Stainless steel metal	Cooled glass slab	Type II	Thick; can draw spatula one inch high from tablet	Insulating base	Fleck's (Mizzy)
			Type I		Permanent for cast restorations	
Polycarboxylate	Stainless steel metal	Coated paper tablet or glass slab		Thick; can draw spatula one inch high from tablet	Temporary restoration and permanent for cast restorations	Durelon
Glass Ionomer	Teflon spatula (autoclavable)	Auto mix (premeasured capsules); noncoated or coated tablet	Type I	Luting	Permanent cement metal restorations	Ketac Cem
			Type II	Thick putty type	Gingival erosion	Ketac Bond
			Type III	Luting	Liner for dentin bonding	Fuji
Composite Resin	Direct bond; auto mix syringe	Coated paper tablet		Putty-like ball	Permanent bond; direct restorative material; cement cast restoration	Lumineers Acrytemp

Procedure 35-6 Mixing Commercial Resin Cements

Equipment and Supplies

- Resin cement powder/liquid or syringe type
- Etching system and bonding system
- Applicators; syringe, cotton pellets, small applicator tips or microbrush applicators
- Plastic instrument and small spatula
- Treated oil-resistant paper pad
- 2 × 2 gauze pads

Procedure Steps

1. Apply etchant to enamel and dentin, rinse, air dry.

2. Apply a bonding adhesive to enamel and dentin, and dry gently.

3. Light cure each surface for 10 seconds.

4. Apply primer to etched porcelain.

5. Dispense ratio of powder-to-liquid onto a mixing pad and mix. Apply a thin layer of mixture into the prepared surface of the restoration.

6. Seat crown, light cure margins for 40 seconds. (Be sure to check your state practice act to ensure that you are able to perform this step.)

7. Clean and disinfect all equipment.

Procedure 35-7 Removing Excess Cement

Equipment and Supplies
- Mirror
- Explorer
- Dental floss

Procedure Steps

1. Use the explorer to examine remaining cement to ensure it has properly set.

2. Carefully run the edge of the explorer in a horizontal direction just under the cement's edge, pulling the excessive material away from the tooth and casting.

3. Tie a knot in the middle of the dental floss, and floss the contacts by passing the knot through both the mesial and distal contacts. This helps remove excess cement from the interproximal area.

4. Clean and disinfect all equipment.

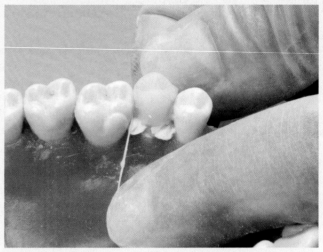

Knotted dental floss between contacts can be used to remove interproximal cement.

The use of a fulcrum is critical when removing cement from around the margins, interproximal areas, and adjacent teeth where excess cement is attached. It is important to remove the excess cement because cement left behind can cause irritation, inflammation, and ultimately bone loss—most often due to buildup of plaque or the size of the excess cement remaining. Any cement remaining in the contact area can set too rapidly or too slowly or can produce tooth sensitivity.

To remove cement, double knot a piece of floss and run it through the interproximal areas. (See Procedure 35-7.) This assists in removing cement that may be lodged without disturbing the area. The two most popular cements that cause this problem are resin reinforced glass ionomer and resin.

After gross supragingival set cement has been removed, use an instrument to retract the gingiva to provide clear vision to the marginal area. Cement can usually be removed without difficulty from the "gingival crevice."

After application of a restoration has been completed, the patient should be given specific instructions to follow. These instructions should be given both verbally and in writing. The instructions may suggest that the patient avoid anything sticky or extreme temperature changes such as hot to cold for the first 24 hours. This is due to the thermal changes of expansion and contraction of the cement during the setting process. If instructions are not followed, the patient may experience sensitivity.

Preparing for Externship

With any procedure, the dental assistant must be familiar with the procedure prior to seating the patient. Confidence in one's abilities is gained through knowledge. Patients' fears are minimized when they see that the dental assistant is proficient in performing the required tasks. Do not be afraid to ask another dental assistant or the dentist questions if you are unsure of what is entailed with a scheduled procedure.

Life Span Considerations

When dealing with children, using words they can easily relate to may make procedures easier. For example, if your patient is a young child who is receiving a crown, use words like *glue* rather than *cement* or *cap* instead of *crown*. Use of simple words will help the child understand the procedure more clearly.

SUMMARY

The dental assistant's role in mixing dental cements is very important. Exact mixing is critical for proper setting times, seating of the restoration, and stability of the cement. Being knowledgeable about how restorative procedures are accomplished, the types of cement used, and how cements are mixed helps to ensure that these treatments are accomplished smoothly and efficiently.

KEY TERMS

- **Chemically cured:** Process of mixing two materials together to create a chemical reaction that makes a material harden (set).   p. 556
- **Exothermic reaction:** A chemical reaction that gives off heat.   p. 553
- **Homogenous:** The characteristic of having a uniform structure or composition throughout.   p. 553
- **Light cured:** Process of using a high-intensity light to make a material harden (set).   p. 553
- **Luting agent:** A viscous material placed into a dental prosthesis that attaches the prosthesis firmly to the tooth by means of a chemical reaction.   p. 551

CHECK YOUR UNDERSTANDING

1. Which of the following are advantages of glass ionomer cements?
   a. used for permanent restorations
   b. highly adhesive
   c. reduce caries by fluoride release postrestoration
   d. all of the above

2. Mixing times should be determined by
   a. observing the consistency of the cement.
   b. following the manufacturer's instructions.
   c. the amount of powder used.
   d. the amount of time available.

3. If the operatory is warm, dispensing the liquid last will
   a. save time.
   b. make the mixing go faster.
   c. prevent condensation from contaminating the liquid.
   d. speed up the setting time.

4. Zinc oxide eugenol is
   a. the cheapest cement available.
   b. the fastest setting cement.
   c. the hardest to mix.
   d. one of the most multipurpose cements used.

5. When mixing cements, the mix should
   a. be homogenous in color.
   b. be grainy.
   c. *never* be mixed all at once.
   d. have streaks.

6. Zinc phosphate cement
   a. creates an exothermic reaction when it is mixed.
   b. should be mixed on a glass slab.
   c. should string about an inch when ready to use.
   d. all of the above.

7. Glass ionomer cements can be used to
   a. cement orthodontic brackets.
   b. cement permanent fillings.
   c. restore areas of erosion near the gingiva.
   d. both a and c.

8. Which key factors must happen prior to using a composite resin cement?
   a. Tooth must be free of plaque and debris.
   b. Area needs to be prepared with acid etching.
   c. Area may be treated with a bonding system.
   d. All of the above.

9. It is critical to remove excess cement from around a crown because
   a. it can cause gingival irritation.
   b. it can cause bone loss.
   c. it's not important; the cement will come off on its own.
   d. both a and c.

10. Glass ionomer cements release _____ to help prevent caries.
    a. heat
    b. water
    c. dentin
    d. fluoride

INTERNET ACTIVITY

- Go to the Crest website at www.dentalcare.com/drn.htm. See numerous patient instructions in a variety of languages. Take a look at the patient education link, then click on the "Chairside Communication" link for a quick glance at a language guide. Download the sheet and keep it chairside to assist you in communicating with patients whose native language is not English.

WEB REFERENCES

- DentalCements.com   www.dentalcements.com
- DoctorSpiller.com   www.doctorspiller.com

36

Impression Materials

Learning Objectives

After reading this chapter, the student should be able to:

- Describe the various purposes for which dental impressions are necessary.

- Discuss the differences between preliminary and final impressions.

- Identify the impression materials required for preliminary and final impressions.

- Describe impression tray choices.

- Demonstrate the ability to choose the proper size impression tray.

- Demonstrate preparing alginate impression materials, recording an impression, inspecting the impression for defects, and disinfecting the impression.

Chapter Outline

- Types of Impressions

- Impression Materials
  - —Impression Trays
  - —Hydrocolloid Impression Materials
  - —Elastomeric Impression Materials

- Problem-Solving Impression Techniques

- Bite Registration
  - —Wax Bite Registration
  - —Elastomeric Bite Registration

Preparing for Certification Exams

- Fabricate preliminary impressions.
- Fabricate final impressions.
- Demonstrate understanding of the OSHA Bloodborne Pathogens standard.
- Demonstrate understanding of the Centers for Disease Control and Prevention guidelines.

Key Terms

Bite registration	Impression
Cast model	Polymerization
Frenula	Sol
Hydrophilic	Syneresis
Hydrophobic	Viscosity
Imbibition	Wettability

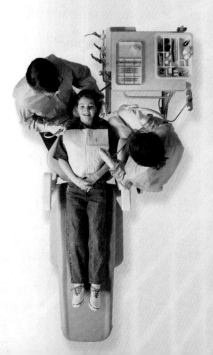

A cast model is a gypsum replica of

the mouth. It is made by using impression materials. An **impression** taken of a person's teeth and surrounding tissues is a negative representation of the oral structures into which dental gypsum material is placed in order to make an accurate positive copy of the patient's dentition. The area reproduced may be composed of either hard or soft tissues or both. The impression material must be inserted into the mouth while it is still soft enough to shape, kept in the mouth during the specified setting time, and quickly but gently removed when set.

Impressions are made for diagnostic reasons and to construct various types of dental appliances. Cast models made from quality impressions are necessary for fabrication of crowns, bridges, veneers, partial dentures, and complete dentures. Models are used during prosthodontic and orthodontic treatment and to fabricate athletic mouth guards, bleaching trays, and custom trays.

The dental assistant, under supervision of the dentist, or the dentist makes the impressions and bite registration and pours gypsum into the models. It is important for the dental assistant to acquire good techniques for making impressions and to pour quality diagnostic cast models. Trays used to hold impression materials must be the proper size and fit for the patient. Tray adhesives, if needed, must be compatible with the specific type of impression material utilized.

Types of Impressions

Dentists, dental assistants, and dental laboratory technicians work as a team to create and maintain dental casts. The dentist diagnoses a particular problem in a patient's mouth and presents solutions. These solutions are dependent on the specific nature of the case and the patient's comfort and budget. A clear diagnosis of the patient's

---

Dental Assistant   PROFESSIONAL TIP

Well-fitting indirect restorations can only be made if accurate models of the oral tissues are made from high-quality impressions. Choose the appropriate tray size. Measure the impression materials correctly. When inserting the tray into the patient's mouth, the tray must be pushed with enough pressure to seat the impression completely onto the area—push down on the mandibular arch and use upward pressure to seat the maxillary tray. Hold the tray gently in position until the impression material has thoroughly set.

---

condition is often made through the use of dental cast models. These casts allow the dentist to examine how the teeth fit together and what may be hampering the patient from chewing or speaking well. Sometimes the exact solution is not fully determined until impressions of the patient's mouth are made and the dentist consults with the dental technician.

Most often it is the dental assistant who makes the impression of the patient's teeth and mouth structures and pours a preliminary hardened cast. (Note, however, that in some states only the dentist is allowed to take impressions.) The dentist examines this cast and sends it to the dental technician with recommendations for the creation of dental restorations. Often the dentist recommends replacement prosthetic devices for missing teeth or the dentist may urge the patient to have the teeth realigned through braces or other orthodontic appliances. Dental technicians make wax diagnostic representations from the cast for various restorations such as crowns, bridges, partial dentures, and implants. These models are used by technicians to create metal frameworks and tooth structures.

Types of dental impressions fall into two categories: preliminary impressions and final impressions. Preliminary impressions are used for:

- Study models
- Matrix for provisional/temporary crowns or bridges
- Orthodontic models
- Bleach trays

Life Span Considerations

Dentists are increasingly sensitive to the special needs and the importance of dental health in the older patient. For seniors who have lost some or all of their natural teeth, dentures, partial dentures, implants, or fixed crowns and bridges can replace missing teeth and significantly improve patients' overall health as well as their smiles. To replace missing teeth, impressions of the patient's mouth are necessary. Informing the patient about the process before taking the impressions helps patients understand how to tolerate the procedure.

- Athletic mouth guards
- Orthotic splints
- Working models for design and fabrication of appliances or space maintainers

Final impressions are used for:

- Crowns
- Bridges
- Veneers
- Implants
- Partial dentures
- Complete dentures

An impression of how the patient's maxillary and mandibular arches come together, or occlude, has numerous indications in prosthodontics, conservative restorative dentistry, implant dentistry, and orthodontics. An accurate and stable occlusal registration is essential for achieving proper function when placing restorations. **Bite registration** materials are used to record and simulate how the patient's arches occlude. Bite registration materials vary from wax to extremely accurate elastomeric or silicone materials, which ensure that restorations fit precisely.

Why is the ability to make dental impressions so important to the treatment of certain dental conditions?

Impression Materials

The American Dental Association sets forth standards and specification requirements for the safety and effectiveness of all dental products. These specifications apply to materials used in dentistry to make impressions of teeth and other tissues in the oral cavity.

In the moist environment of the patient's mouth, the only way to ensure that the fine details of real dental anatomy are recorded is by using impression materials that are not hindered by the moisture present in the mouth. Impression materials may be **hydrophilic** with a tendency toward complete wetting and work well in a moist environment, or **hydrophobic** with an aversion for water and with less wetting ability.

Other requirements for impression materials are dimensional stability for accuracy, tear strength, elastic recovery, and wettability. The materials must not expand, contract, or become deformed in any way. Tear strength and elastic recovery refer to the ability of the material to retain its shape and not become deformed when removed. **Wettability** is the capacity of a material to flow over a surface and capture all irregularities. The **viscosity** of dental materials refers to their ability to flow or not flow. Impression materials are available in different viscosities: low, medium, and high. Low-viscosity materials flow into

the gingival sulcus more easily than high-viscosity materials. They are used in a syringe and extruded into the area around the gingiva. Medium viscosity is also called monophasic viscosity because it may be used in the tray or injected through a syringe tip. High-viscosity materials are only to be used in an impression tray. Impression materials must also be able to be disinfected without being distorted by the disinfecting solution.

An impression material must meet a wide range of requirements in order to provide an accurate impression of the different tissues in the mouth. In addition to the requirements already mentioned, some of the more important requirements of dental impression materials include these:

- The material should flow or be pliable at a temperature that will not injure the oral tissues.
- It should set quickly, preferably within two to four minutes, at body temperature.
- It should unite into a solid mass without adhering to the oral tissues or to the materials used for the cast model.
- It should fall into all irregularities and fine lines in the area to be reproduced without displacing soft tissue.
- It must retain an accurate reproduction of surface detail when it solidifies and is withdrawn from the mouth.
- It must have dimensional stability; that is, it must not expand, contract, or become deformed in any way because of temperature changes, atmospheric conditions, or pouring of the cast.
- It must not be too unpleasant for the patient in terms of its taste and smell.

Impression materials are available as nonelastic and elastic. Nonelastic impression materials used in dentistry are compounds, waxes, and zinc oxide eugenols. The elastic group includes the aqueous hydrocolloids agar and alginate and four types of nonaqueous elastomers: polysulfide, polyether, silicone, and polysiloxane. Aqueous materials are mixed with or contain water and nonaqueous do not.

Manufacturers do not guarantee that their products have the proper physical properties of accuracy and appropriateness of setting and working times necessary for clinical success if they are used after their expiration dates. Setting time is defined as the transitional time in which plastic properties permit molding of the area. Working time includes the length of time required to mix the material, to place it into the tray or around the tooth and into the tray, and to seat it in a patient's mouth. Manufacturers also stipulate the minimum time before a material should be removed from the mouth. As always, read the manufacturer's instructions fully.

Why would it be important for impression materials to not be too unpleasant for the patient?

Impression Trays

A tray is needed to carry impression material to the mouth and hold it against tissues while it hardens. A variety of trays are available for this purpose (Figure 36.1). Impression trays are shaped to match the contour of the dental arches. Stock dental impression trays are available in stainless steel, nickel or chrome-plated brass, aluminum, or as disposable plastic. They come in stock sizes or are made in the dental office or lab as custom-fit trays.

Trays are chosen specifically for the purpose of obtaining full arch, partial arch, edentulous, or partially edentulous impressions. Another type of tray used for dental impressions is the triple tray or dual-arch tray. This an economical, disposable, one-piece plastic frame with gauze inserts where impressions of the maxillary and mandibular arches as well as the patient's occlusion are made simultaneously. The area being reproduced, the opposing arch, as well as the patient's bite are recorded using the triple tray or dual-arch technique.

Stock Impression Trays

Stock impression trays are shaped to fit over the average maxillary and mandibular arches. Stock trays come in many sizes for both the maxillary and mandibular arches and are made to fit everyone moderately well. Stock trays may be rim-lock, mesh metal, or plastic. Rim-lock trays have a metal border to hold impression material in the tray. Metal mesh trays allow impression material to flow into the perforations, which helps the impression to stay in the tray. Tray adhesive may be used if necessary and is often used with disposable plastic and custom trays, with or without perforations.

The size of the stock tray is identified on the handle. Some stock trays can be bent to the requirements of an individual patient. Disposable stock trays and custom trays can be cut and trimmed with acrylic burs to better fit a patient's mouth. Some considerations for choosing a

tray include whether the patient has third molars or if the patient has a maxillary torus or mandibular tori. A torus (plural: tori) is a bony growth that makes taking impressions especially uncomfortable for the patient. Mandibular tori are located bilaterally on the lingual sides of the arch in the premolar area. A custom tray may be indicated for use during an impression of a patient with mandibular tori. Depending on the individual patient needs and preferences of the dentist, the custom tray may be fabricated with or without a handle. Wax can be used to extend any tray, create better peripheral borders (called border molding), and make a stock tray more comfortable for a patient (Figure 36.2).

Custom Impression Trays

A custom tray is constructed on a diagnostic cast model from a preliminary impression and made exclusively for one individual patient. Custom trays can be constructed from visible light-cured resins, acrylic resins, or thermoplastic or they can be vacuum formed. (Chapter 37 provides more information on making custom trays.)

A custom tray must fit properly on the peripheral border areas in the vestibules of the patient's mouth in order for accurate construction of partial and complete dentures. A custom tray must not impinge on the patient's **frenula** (singular: frenulum), the folds of tissue connecting the cheeks and lips to the alveolar mucosa. The periphery, or the outer border portion of the tray surface, cannot distort these soft tissues when placed in the mouth. Impressions of these areas are mandatory for fabrication of removable prosthodontics by the laboratory technician.

What types of custom trays may be fabricated by the dental assistant?

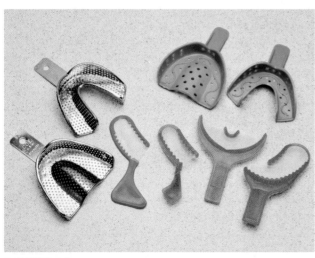

FIGURE 36.1
Various types of dental impression trays.

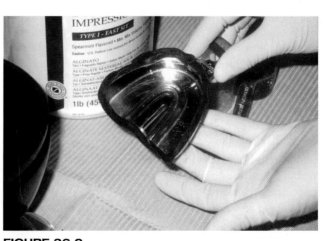

FIGURE 36.2
Utility wax that can be used to extend the edges of impression trays.
Image courtesy Instructional Materials for the Dental Team, Lex., KY

Hydrocolloid Impression Materials

Hydrocolloid impression materials are used for the fabrication of fixed and removable prostheses. Understanding what the term *hydrocolloid* means can help to further one's knowledge about this type of impression material. *Hydro* means "water" and *colloid* is a state in which particles of one substance are uniformly distributed and dispersed in the medium of another substance.

A **sol** is a viscous liquid whose particles become attached to each other, forming a loose network. The colloid becomes viscous, thickened, and hardened, into a gel, an elastic solid. A viscous liquid sol can be converted into an elastic solid gel in one of two ways:

1. Via a chemical reaction, which is irreversible (alginate)
2. Via a reduction in temperature, which is reversible because the sol is formed again on heating (agar)

Hydrocolloids are placed in the mouth in the sol state where they can record sufficient detail, then are removed when the sol has reached the gel state. The basic component of hydrocolloids is a product extracted from certain types of marine kelp. The exact composition of materials varies with manufacturers. Hydrocolloid materials change from one state to another because of thermal changes.

The two types of hydrocolloids used in dental impressions are alginate and agar. Impression materials that are altered through a chemical change are known as irreversible hydrocolloids. Alginate impression materials, once converted to the gel form, cannot be converted back; hence, alginate is an irreversible hydrocolloid. That is, once the chemical change has taken place, it cannot be reversed to return to its previous state. Agar is a reversible hydrocolloid because it can pass repeatedly between a highly viscous gel state and a low-viscosity sol state simply through heating and cooling. Both forms of hydrocolloid must be stored in airtight containers at room temperature.

Hydrocolloids are adversely affected by these two processes:

- **Syneresis:** The process of contracting and shrinking with time as water is lost, which causes the impression to dry out and not be accurate
- **Imbibition:** The process of absorbing water, which causes swelling, creating a distorted impression

Irreversible Hydrocolloid: Alginate

Alginate is the most widely used impression material. Alginate is available as a fast-setting or regular setting material. It is designed for making impressions for case study models, orthodontic models, and opposing models during fabrication of fixed and removable prostheses, or to construct bleaching trays, custom trays, and occlusal splints.

The primary components of alginate are sodium alginate (seaweed extract), calcium sulfate, sodium phosphate, and potassium fluoride. Alginate material is available in bulk, single-canister containers (Figure 36.3), or single-use pouches. Alginate is indicated for making dental impressions for fabrication of cast models.

Alginate should not be used on patients with a history of severe allergic reaction to any of the components of alginate. Dental professionals should wear protective eyewear, mask, gloves, and clothing while using these materials. Patients should also wear protective eyewear. Prolonged exposure to the eyes should be avoided. The airborne powder particles should not be inhaled, and alginate should not be swallowed. If accidental swallowing occurs, the person should drink lots of water. The material is not hazardous if ingested in small quantities. Alginate should be prepared in a well-ventilated area. The canister lid should be replaced immediately after dispensing. Alginate impressions should be poured with gypsum material right away so that the impression does not distort by drying out or absorbing water (Procedure 36-1).

Alginate impression material should be stored out of direct sunlight at room temperature. Prolonged heat makes the product unstable as does excessive humidity. Expiration dates should always be checked when using dental materials. The alginate canister should be gently tumbled to fluff the powder prior to each use and the lid tightly closed. Upon mixing the powder with water, a chemical reaction takes place and a gel is formed. This reaction occurs quickly. The dental assistant must move efficiently during mixing and when loading the tray. The powder should be measured to the manufacturer's instructions. It is manipulated by separately measuring the powder and the water and then adding the measured powder to the measured water in a clean flexible rubber bowl or vacuum mixer. Figure 36.4 shows two increments of alginate prepared for an impression procedure.

Alginate materials have a well-defined working time. Alginate must be spatulated well for 45 seconds for a fast set and one minute for a regular set, placed in a tray, and carefully inserted into the patient's mouth. Immediately

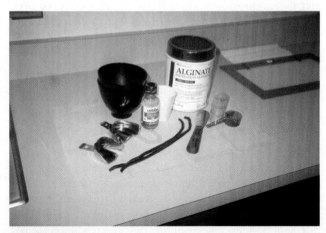

FIGURE 36.3
Alginate impression materials.
Image courtesy Instructional Materials for the Dental Team, Lex., KY

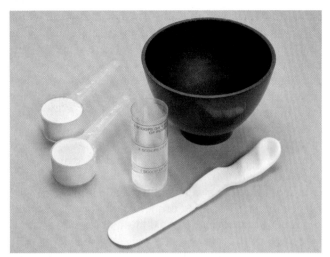

FIGURE 36.4
Two increments of alginate prepared for an impression procedure.

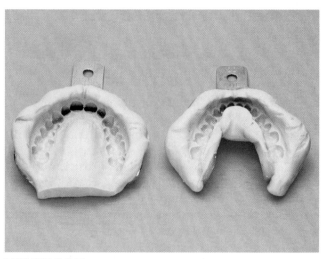

FIGURE 36.5
Maxillary and mandibular alginate impressions.

prior to inserting the alginate impression into the patient's mouth, the surface of the alginate material in the tray should be smoothed with a wet finger. This has been shown to reduce the possibility of trapping air against the teeth and tissues.

The impression should be removed from the mouth two to three minutes following gelation (Figure 36.5). It should be removed quickly with a gentle snapping motion. This maximizes tear strength and minimizes permanent deformation of alginate material. The dental assistant should keep a finger between the impression and the opposing arch to ensure that the tray is not removed so forcefully that it causes damage to other teeth. The impression should be poured immediately with gypsum material to prevent dimensional changes.

Properties of alginate include the following:

- It provides good surface detail.
- The reaction sets faster at higher temperatures.
- It is elastic enough to be drawn over the undercuts, but tears over deep undercuts.
- It is not dimensionally stable when storing over long periods due to evaporation.
- It is nontoxic and nonirritant for the majority of patients.
- The setting time depends on the technique and type of impression material chosen.
- Alginate powder is unstable during storage in the presence of moisture or warm temperatures.

When mixed with water, the process of gelation of the impression material occurs; that is, the powder and water become a gel. When mixing the impression material with water, the water and powder ratio should not be altered as a means of manipulating setting time. If done this will reduce gel strength and change dimensional accuracy. Room temperature water should be used to ensure a sufficient amount of time is provided to mix and

set the impression. Faster or slower setting times can be achieved by using warm or cold water.

Alginate impression material has these advantages:

- Low cost
- High degree of wettability
- Pleasant taste
- Nontoxic
- Easy to use
- Good surface detail

Disadvantages of alginate are:

- Poor dimensional stability
- Inability to produce fine detail
- Incompatibility with some gypsum materials
- Difficult to disinfect
- Poor tear strength
- Must be poured immediately
- Setting time dependent on operator handling

Disinfecting Alginate Impressions

It is important to disinfect the alginate impression as soon as the tray has been removed from the patient's mouth. The impression should be rinsed with cold water to remove any saliva or blood. It should be covered with a damp napkin to prevent syneresis. Alginate impressions should be disinfected with a hospital-level disinfectant. Acceptable disinfectants are those that are registered with the Environmental Protection Agency (EPA) as tuberculocidal. The impression should be in contact with the disinfectant for no longer than 10 minutes to avoid imbibition. Iodophors, sodium hypochlorite, chlorine dioxide, and quaternary ammonium compounds are all approved as disinfectants for alginate impression materials.

To disinfect an alginate impression, thoroughly soak it by spraying with a recommended disinfectant and then place it in a plastic bag for the contact time recommended

Procedure 36-1 Obtaining an Alginate Impression

Equipment and Supplies

- Alginate canister
- Plastic measuring cup for powder
- Plastic measuring cup for water
- Flexible rubber bowl
- Flexible broad blade lab spatula
- Paper towels
- Proper size sterile trays
- Water
- Small plastic bag
- Utility wax (if necessary)

Procedure Steps

1. Tumble the container to gently fluff powder. Explain the procedure to the patient.

2. Select and/or prepare suitable impression tray. Rigid rim-lock or perforated trays are recommended. Try the mandibular and maxillary trays in the patient's mouth to ensure proper fit and comfort.

3. Dip supplied scoop lightly into powder until scoop is full. Do not pack scoop. Tap scoop against rim to ensure that a full measure without voids has been scooped out. Scrape excess off with spatula to achieve level scoop.

4. Empty two scoops of powder into a clean dry mixing bowl for the mandibular impression and three scoops of powder for a maxillary impression. For a single-use pouch, tear open and empty its contents into the bowl.

5. For two scoops, add two-thirds measurement of the alginate powder measuring cup of room temperature water. For each three scoops of powder, add one full measure of water so that all three increments on the water measuring cup are used. Note that cooler water retards setting, and warmer water accelerates setting.

6. Mix water and powder carefully until all powder is wet. Once all powder is incorporated, continue to spatulate in a vigorous fashion. Do not whip or stir the alginate material. The spatula should be flattened using pressure against the bowl to reduce incorporating air. Spatulate regular set material for one minute and fast set material for 45 seconds.

7. Once the alginate appears homogenous and creamy (i.e., without lumps), put it into the tray. To minimize the trapping of air, wipe the loaded spatula against the tray rim, allowing material to flow from the spatula into the tray. Load the mandibular tray from the lingual sides and use the flat side of the blade to condense the material firmly in the tray. Place the majority of the alginate in the anterior portion of the tray.

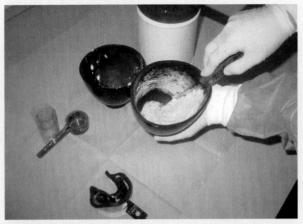

Mixing the alginate.
Image courtesy Instructional Materials for the Dental Team, Lex., KY

8. Use a wet finger to smooth the alginate surface, to eliminate any air pockets trapped near the surface, and to remove excess material from posterior areas. Ask the patient to relax and take a deep breath through the nose and to keep breathing through the nose during the entire procedure. An optional method is to use a finger to place some alginate material on the occlusal surfaces of the teeth first.

9. Insert filled tray into the mouth. Use the side of the tray to push one side of the cheek out of the way and a finger on the other side to do the same thing, and then slide the tray into the mouth. For an impression of the mandibular arch, ask the patient to lift the tongue as the tray is inserted. Press the tray gently into position centered over the arch, placing the posterior portion first to form a seal so the material flows forward and not down the throat.

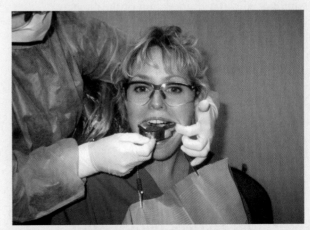

Placing the maxillary tray into the patient's mouth.
Image courtesy Instructional Materials for the Dental Team, Lex., KY

continued on next page

Procedure 36-1 *continued from previous page*

10. Push firmly up when seating the maxillary tray and press firmly down when seating the mandibular tray. Do not overseat or press the tray to touch the teeth. Immediately lift the patient's lips loosely over the tray so impressions of the oral vestibule and frenula will be captured. Hold the seated tray immovable for one minute or until alginate is no longer sticky.

11. Once the material has set, gently break the seal by moving the tray up and down or using the side of a finger at the periphery. Snap the tray loose from the arch and remove the impression tray from the patient's mouth, protecting the opposite arch with a finger.

12. Check for and remove any residual material from the mouth, between the teeth, or from around the patient's face. Give the patient a damp tissue and have her or him rinse with warm water.

13. Rinse impression thoroughly under running water. Spray with disinfectant solution, wrap in a wet paper towel, and place in a labeled plastic bag before pouring. Do not store impression submerged in water.

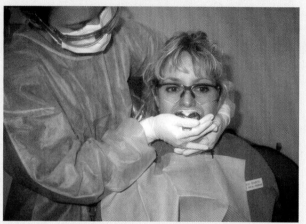

Removing the maxillary tray.
Image courtesy Instructional Materials for the Dental Team, Lex., KY

---

by the disinfectant manufacturer, but not longer than 10 minutes. Spraying with glutaraldehyde is not recommended. Water-based disinfectant solutions are preferred.

Following disinfection, the impression should be rinsed thoroughly with water and lightly air dried. The impression should be poured with gypsum as soon as possible. If pouring is delayed, the impression should be wrapped in a wet towel. The amount of distortion in an impression is proportional to the delay in pouring and the amount of water evaporation of the alginate.

Several alginates that contain disinfectant are available, and some manufacturers also make an antimicrobial and dustless alginate so that fewer particles of impression material powder become airborne. Some dentists also offer flavorings to make the impression process more tolerable and to distract patients from the discomfort.

What role does the dental assistant have when it comes to making dental impressions? **?**

Reversible Hydrocolloid: Agar

When performing crown and bridge restorative procedures, reversible hydrocolloid impression materials are often used. Reversible hydrocolloids are composed of agar (derived from seaweed), potassium sulfate, borax,

and water. These impression materials are supplied in tubes and are heated in a conditioning unit with three compartments:

- The first compartment is a boiling bath, or conditioning bath, used to boil the tubes in 212°F water for 8 to 12 minutes to create a change from sol to gel.
- The second compartment is a storage bath. The tubes can be stored in the second compartment at 151°F for a minimum of 10 minutes, but can be stored up to 8 hours.
- The third compartment is a tempering bath in which the material is kept for 10 minutes at 110°F to lower the temperature of the material.

Once the tubes have been heated in the three compartments, the process for using reversible hydrocolloid impression materials involves these steps:

- Place the impression material in the tray.
- Eject the syringe material around the treatment area in the patient's mouth.
- Seat the tray in the patient's mouth.
- Cool the tray with 60° to 70°F water routed through tubes for three to five minutes.
- Remove the tray from the patient's mouth and pour gypsum into it.

Reversible hydrocolloids exhibit syneresis and imbibition, meaning that the material contracts with time and exudes water, which has the result of causing the impression to shrink. These materials are also prone to water absorption when exposed to water or high humidity causing improper setting of the impression. Both syneresis and imbibition have the potential to cause poor dimensional stability in the impression.

When inserting reversible hydrocolloid into the mouth a rim-lock, water-cooled tray is used. After gelation, the impression should be removed quickly with a gentle snap, to minimize tearing and permanent deformation. The impression should be poured immediately to prevent changes in its dimensions due to syneresis or imbibition.

Hydrocolloid tubes can be boiled a total of three times. Unused materials that have already been boiled should be allowed to return to room temperature and may be reboiled with the next batch. The primary advantage of hydrocolloid materials is that a week's worth of impression material may be processed at once and maintained for immediate use during the entire work week. Setting time in the mouth is between 5 and 10 minutes.

Advantages of reversible hydrocolloids include:

- Low cost of material
- High degree of wettability
- Nontoxic
- Nonstaining
- Require no mixing

Disadvantages of reversible hydrocolloids include:

- Difficult to disinfect
- High cost of equipment
- Low tear strength
- Poor dimensional stability
- Must be poured immediately

Why would you choose one type of impression material over another? What factors would affect your decision?

Professionalism

The impression tray must fit the patient's arch properly whether a stock, custom, or dual-arch impression tray is used. Dual-arch impression trays are very popular but must be used correctly. Sufficient impression material must be used on both sides of these trays. The posterior cross-bar must clear the patient's third molars or it will flex and cause distortion of the impression. Ask the patient to open the mouth. If the tray is difficult to remove, use your finger and thumb between the upper and lower periphery in the mucobuccal fold area for removal. Do not exert excess force on the handle. Examine the impression for accuracy of detail.

Elastomeric Impression Materials

Elastomeric materials are used to create impressions for diagnostic casts of both the maxillary and mandibular arches. The impressions may be used for preliminary study models or for the purpose of constructing fixed and removable prostheses. Bite registrations are also made with elastomeric impression materials. The physical properties of elastomeric materials vary as do their indications for use, contraindications, storage, and mixing instructions.

Elastomeric impression materials are also known as nonaqueous elastomers because they are not used with water. Nonaqueous elastomers include synthetic rubber materials that have existed for many years. They come in various viscosities as low, medium, and high and also in putty formulations. These materials are supplied as a base and a catalyst material that, once mixed, generate a chemical reaction that causes the two materials to solidify. The setting of the base and catalyst is the **polymerization** process, a chemical reaction that causes two materials to harden together. Elastomeric impression materials may be mixed by hand or through a dispenser and cartridge self-mixing delivery system.

Polysulfide Impression Materials

Polysulfide materials were the first elastomers. They are indicated for removable and fixed prosthodontic impressions due to their good reproduction of detail. These rubber elastic materials are hydrophilic and they duplicate oral tissues well. Polysulfide impression material is composed of a base and a catalyst.

The most ideal technique for use with this material is to apply adhesive in a uniform layer on a custom tray (Figure 36.6). Equal lengths of the base and catalyst pastes should be extruded. The material should be manipulated with a spatula and uniformly mixed within one minute (Figure 36.7). It must be placed into the tray

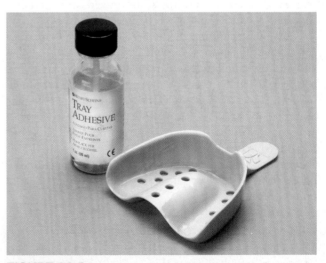

FIGURE 36.6
Impression tray with adhesive agent.

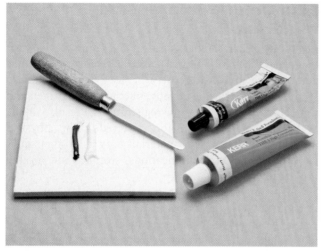

FIGURE 36.7
Polysulfide impression materials prepared to be mixed.

and seated in the patient's mouth. Setting time for polysulfide impression materials is 8 to 12 minutes. The cast must be poured within one hour.

Advantages of polysulfide impression materials include lower cost compared to silicones and polyethers, long working time, and high tear strength and flexibility. The primary disadvantage of polysulfide material is its poor dimensional stability. These impressions must be poured within one hour and may only be used for one pour. Custom trays must be used for polysulfide impressions. Mixing these materials can be messy and can stain clothing, and they have an unpleasant odor. The material must stay in the patient's mouth for a long setting time.

Polyether Impression Materials

Polyether impression materials are indicated for use in crown and bridge restorations and for bite registrations. They are available in three viscosities. Polyether requires that an adhesive be applied to a stock or custom tray. These materials are extruded in equal lengths from tubes and hand mixed or automatically mixed and extruded from handheld devices or mechanical dispensers.

Advantages of polyether impression materials are their good flow, dimensional stability, highly accurate details, and good wettability. They are relatively hydrophilic and perform well in the presence of some moisture. They can be used with stock or dual-arch trays. Disadvantages are that polyether materials are expensive, have a short working time, are rigid and difficult to remove from undercuts, and taste bitter to patients. They have low tear strength and change dimensions as water is absorbed. They can be poured only once within 48 hours due to possible distortion of the impression.

Silicone Impression Materials

The silicone group includes condensation silicones and addition reaction silicones (Figure 36.8). They are classified according to their method of polymerization or setting. There are condensation curing silicones, called Type I, and addition curing silicones, called Type II. Silicone rubbers are available in light, medium, and heavy bodies as well as a very high viscosity putty material. The putty is commonly combined with a low-viscosity silicone when recording impressions. This procedure is known as the putty-wash technique.

Condensation Silicone Impression Materials Condensation silicone impression materials are indicated for complete dentures and for fabrication of crowns and bridges. These materials are used as a base paste, a catalyst paste, or base paste and putty mixed with a liquid catalyst. Condensation silicones are often used with a putty-wash technique. This reduces shrinkage during the polymerization process. Condensation silicones are used with stock trays. The putty is placed in the tray as a preliminary impression, then removed, and the wash material is ejected around the teeth and the tray reseated in the mouth.

The advantages of condensation silicone materials are that they are elastic, taste clean and pleasant to the patient, are used with stock trays, and have good working and setting times. Disadvantages include poor dimensional stability and the possibility of shrinkage during polymerization. Condensation silicone impressions must be poured within six hours due to their low wettability. Silicone rubber impression materials are very hydrophobic so unless the teeth are properly rinsed and dried the impression may not be accurate.

PUTTY-WASH TECHNIQUE The putty-wash technique is commonly used in dental practices. There are three ways of recording a putty-wash impression:

- *One-stage impression:* Putty and wash are recorded simultaneously.
- *Two-stage unspaced:* Putty is recorded first and then setting is relined with a thin layer of wash and replaced back into the mouth.

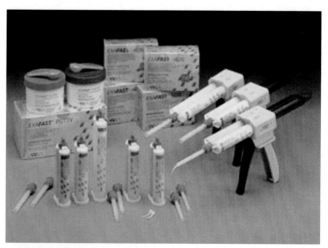

FIGURE 36.8
Silicone impression materials.
Courtesy of GC America

• *Two-stage spaced:* Putty is recorded first and after the setting a space is created for the wash.

Problems with the putty-wash technique include possible distortion caused by tray recoil. Considerable force is needed to seat a putty impression, which may cause outward flexing of the tray wall or the material. Upon removing the tray from the mouth, the tray walls may rebound (hence, the term *tray recoil*), causing inaccuracies in the poured cast model. The most convenient and reliable way of recording a putty-wash impression is to use the one-stage technique with silicone putty in a rigid metal tray and a light-bodied wash extruded around the tooth preparation with a syringe (Figure 36.9). This technique requires the dentist and dental assistant to work efficiently as a team.

Polysiloxane Impression Materials Polysiloxane or vinyl polysiloxane (VPS) impression materials are also called addition reaction silicones. They are the most dimensionally stable impression materials and are used for crowns, bridges, implants, dentures, partial dentures, and bite registrations. They are available as two pastes, a base and a catalyst, and they come in low-, medium-, and high-viscosity consistencies. These materials are most commonly used as a base and catalyst with a cartridge delivery system but are also available in tubes or unit dose cartridge applicators. The appropriate adhesive should be applied to a custom tray. Heavy-body material should be used in the tray and a lighter-body material extruded around the tooth preparations. Putty-wash techniques can be used with stock trays.

Advantages of addition reaction silicones are their high degree of accuracy, excellent dimensional stability, high recovery from deformation, and adequate tear strength and working time. In addition to a pleasant smell, other advantages of these impression materials include the ability of the impression materials to be:

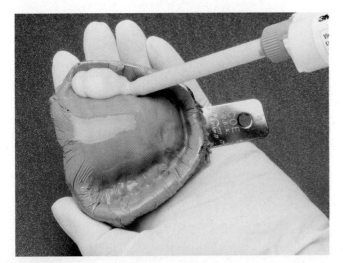

FIGURE 36.9
Putty impression and light body material being extruded into the tray for a second impression.

• Poured up with gypsum material within one week
• Used with stock or custom trays
• Poured for multiple casts
• Easily mixed

Note, however, that polysiloxane materials are very expensive and that latex glove powder inhibits the setting of these materials. The patient's health history should always be checked to confirm that the patient does not have an allergy to latex. In fact, it is important to review the patient's health history before any treatment is begun, including the taking of impressions. Due to glove powder inhibiting the setting of some materials, retraction cords should be handled with cotton pliers and nonlatex gloves worn during mixing. For the best quality impression, the teeth should be polished with pumice or treated with hydrogen peroxide and rinsed well prior to inserting the impression material.

The dentist and dental assistant must work quickly and coordinate as a team when working with these materials. While the dentist extrudes the light-body material from the cartridge or syringe around the treatment area, the dental assistant loads the impression tray with the heavier material. Vinyl polysiloxane is a hydrophilic impression material that is not affected by moisture. Techniques designed for use with these materials include dual–phase, one-step, full-arch or quadrant impressions and dual–phase, one-step, double-arch impressions designed to capture an impression of one tooth (Procedure 36-2). Addition reaction silicone materials cannot be intermixed with materials from other manufacturers such as polyether, polysulfide, or condensation cured silicones. Manufacturer's instructions should be read to understand precautions necessary when using all dental materials.

Vinyl-Polyether Hybrid Impression Materials

The newest class of elastomeric impression materials is a vinyl-polyether hybrid material called SENN. SENN is a new hybrid polyether/polysiloxane impression material that combines the properties of polyether and vinyl polysiloxane impression materials. It is an odor-free, pleasant-tasting hybrid impression material with hydrophilic properties, high tear strength, excellent dimensional accuracy, and resistance to deformation. This vinyl-polyether is available in two setting times (fast and regular) and four viscosities (putty, heavy body, monophase, and light body). If powdered gloves are used to mix the material the setting reaction can be contaminated and it will not polymerize.

If impression materials are so greatly impacted by the powders in latex gloves, why would a dental assistant prefer to wear a powdered versus nonpowdered glove?

Procedure 36-2 Obtaining a Vinyl Polysiloxane Cartridge Single-Phase Impression

Equipment and Supplies

- Metal tray, a firm disposable tray, or custom tray
- Adhesive
- Low-viscosity cartridge material
- High-viscosity cartridge material
- Two cartridge dispensing guns
- Two cartridge syringe tips
- One intraoral tip
- 2 × 2 gauze squares

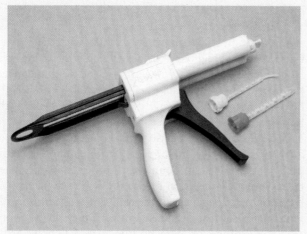

Polysiloxane dispensing gun, body cartridge, mixing tip, and syringe tip.

Procedure Steps

1. Select and prepare suitable tray. Use rigid trays of sufficient size to provide at least a 2- to 3-mm thickness of impression material. Dual-arch trays may be used to record the opposing dentition and bite registration of the two arches.

2. Brush a thin lay of tray adhesive onto the rigid tray following manufacturer's instructions.

3. Raise the release lever vertically upward on the cartridge dispensing gun, while simultaneously pulling the plunger all the way back in the dispenser handle.

4. Load the cartridge by opening the cartridge lock using the top clasp. Orient and insert the cartridge with notches aligned as necessary. Close the top clasp to lock the cartridge into the dispenser gun.

5. Remove the cartridge cap by turning it 90 degrees in the counterclockwise direction. The cap can be replaced on the cartridge when storing after initial use, or the used mixing tip can be left in place until the next use after disinfection to serve as a self-sealing cap.

6. Dispense a small amount of base and catalyst material onto a 2 × 2 gauze square before installing the mixing tip to ensure an even flow from the cartridge. Use gentle pressure. Be sure a mixed material plug does not exist. If a plug exists, clear it away with an instrument. Wipe away excess material from the cartridge carefully so the base and catalyst do not cross-contaminate each other and cause obstruction of the nozzle.

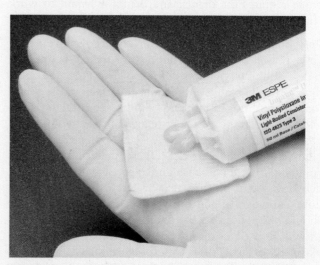

Extrude a small amount of cartridge material before attaching mixing tip.

7. Install a mixing tip in both the light-body and heavy-body cartridge by lining up the notch on the outside rim of the mixing tip with the notch on the cartridge flange. Ensure the holes are aligned properly. Turn the tip to align it in the cap.

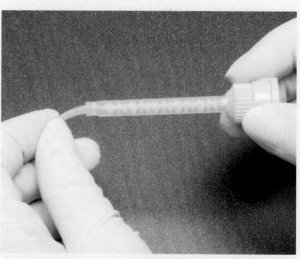

Attach the syringe tip to the light body material cartridge.

continued on next page

Procedure 36-2 *continued from previous page*

8. When notches are aligned, turn the mixing cap 90 degrees in the clockwise direction to lock it in place. Attach the intraoral tip to the end of the light-body mixing tip for direct intraoral syringing around the gingival sulcus.

9. Clean the tooth with an air/water spray. Remove excess water with suction. Do not desiccate or overdry the tooth.

10. The assistant should pass the dispensing gun with the wash material and intraoral tip to the dentist and receive the cotton rolls that were used to keep the working area dry.

11. The assistant dispenses tray material into the tray, ensuring that the least amount of air has been incorporated into the material. For best results the dispensing tip should be submerged in the impression material during extrusion to prevent introducing air bubbles into the mix. The tray must be loaded within 35 seconds from the time of first syringing the wash material.

12. At the same time as the assistant is loading the tray, the dentist injects syringe material into any existing anatomy and continue syringing around the preparation until it is completely covered with syringe material.

13. The assistant passes the loaded tray to the dentist and receives the cartridge gun. The dentist or assistant holds the tray in position in the patient's mouth until the

material is firmly set. The minimum removal time for fast set is three minutes from the start of the mix. Higher temperatures reduce work times, and lower temperatures increase the time.

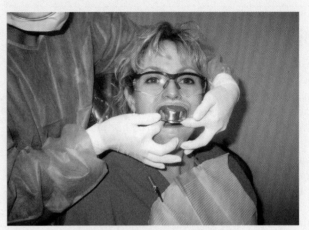

The dentist or dental assistant holding the impression tray in place until the material is hardened.
Image courtesy Instructional Materials for the Dental Team, Lex., KY

14. The impression should be removed from the mouth by pulling slowly to break the seal, and then snapped out along the long axis of the tooth. The patient's mouth should be rinsed and the impression should be rinsed under cold water and disinfected according to manufacturer's instructions.

Problem-Solving Impression Techniques

Making a highly accurate impression is the first and most important step in creating a superior crown and bridge restoration. Even the most experienced clinician using the best materials can encounter problems when making an impression. Upon removing the impression from the mouth and rinsing it, the impression should be inspected for flaws. Common visible flaws related to impression techniques include:

- Lack of impression detail
- Finish line not visible
- Voids or tearing on margins
- Air bubbles in critical places
- Unset impression material on surface of impression and cast
- Improper tray seating
- Tooth contacting tray
- Poor bond of impression material to the tray
- Cast model discrepancies

To avoid these problems, the tooth preparation area should be rinsed and dried just prior to making the impression. Good retraction technique with proper moisture control and proper tissue retraction provides the best method for creating a detailed impression. Manufacturer's working time specifications should be followed. Voids are prevented by keeping the syringe tip of elastomeric materials directly immersed in the material while filling the tray to avoid trapping air. Voids are also created by a poor bond between syringed and tray material or salivary contamination of the syringed material.

Air bubbles may occur as a result of mixing, tray loading, or tray seating. Air can easily become trapped at the gingival sulcus as the syringe tip extrudes material around the area. Excellent syringing techniques prevent trapped air in this critical area. Prior to placing the cartridge mixing tip, a small amount of material should be extruded to prevent blockage of mixed base and catalyst material. A partial blockage makes extrusion difficult and may alter the base and catalyst ratio.

The tray must be the proper size for the patient. It must be seated slowly into position in the patient's mouth and held in place with passive pressure. Unnecessary pressure will cause improper seating of the tray and may cause a tooth to contact the tray. Weaker plastic trays can allow flexing of the tray, which creates inaccurate impressions. Stiffer, more rigid trays are ideal.

What are some problems that may be encountered when taking dental impressions? How can these be prevented?

Bite Registration

A bite registration is necessary to determine the accurate occlusal relationship between the maxillary and mandibular arches. This is essential for the dental laboratory technician to mount the cast models for construction of fixed and removable prosthodontics.

A bite registration can be done in many different ways. The most common method of taking a bite registration has been to use wax, but more recently elastomeric impression materials have been utilized because they provide more accurate results with less distortion. Bite registration may be accomplished with wax, zinc oxide eugenol paste, acrylic, polyether, and vinyl polysiloxane materials (Proceducre 36-3).

It is helpful to ask the patient to close her teeth together to observe the occlusion on both sides of the mouth prior to placing the bite registration material between the teeth. The patient must understand what is being asked of her in order for the prostheses to fit properly when being seated in place. Any deformation when removing the bite registration from the mouth will result in inaccurate articulation of the casts and ultimately faulty restorations.

Wax Bite Registration

Waxes for bite registration come in wafers and sheets. Bite wafers may have foil in between wax layers to prevent the teeth from biting through. Sheet wax is folded into layers and bent to the rounded shape of the patient's arches. Both wafer and sheet wax are softened by running the wax under hot water, by using a hot water bath, or by using a lab torch. The bite registration material is placed in the patient's mouth while it is still warm, and the patient is asked to close his or her teeth together completely.

Why do you think elastomeric material might be better than wax for recording a patient's bite relationship?

Elastomeric Bite Registration

Elastomeric materials have proven to be superior to wax for registration of the patient's occlusal relationship. Polyether and vinyl polysiloxane are most commonly

Cultural Considerations

It may be necessary to use hand signals and facial expressions to communicate with patients who speak a language other than English or for those that who are hard of hearing. The dental assistant may suggest that the patient seek out someone who can translate for him or her such as a family member of the patient or a coworker. Show the patient a cast model. Explain the impression procedure as best you can by showing the patient that the tray must fit into the mouth while it is empty. Demonstrate lifting the tongue when seating the mandibular tray and taking a deep breath before inserting the maxillary impression into the mouth. This will help patients understand what you need them to do during the procedure.

used for this purpose. The bite may be recorded with or without a tray. The cartridge dispenser may be applied directly on the occlusal and incisal surfaces of the teeth on the lower jaw. The elastomeric material is then extruded and the patient is asked to close his mouth. Another alternative is to extrude the impression material onto both sides of a bite registration tray and then ask the patient to close his mouth onto it.

Elastomeric bite registration materials set within 30 seconds to two minutes, depending on the material used. For this reason it is important for the dental assistant to work quickly to achieve a bite registration. The patient should be informed as to what to do and the correct occlusion observed before the bite registration material is placed. The dental assistant should retract the cheek to ensure the patient's teeth are occluding together properly. The cheek should be retracted enough to expose the first molar to be sure the correct relationship of the bite is recorded.

Patient Education

When preparing a patient for dental impressions, the dental assistant can improve patient comfort and decrease patient anxiety by taking time to explain the procedure to the patient and why it must be done. Try the impression trays in the mouth before mixing the impression material so the patient knows what to expect. Remove any excess material that may sit in the back of the mouth on the soft palate. Have the patient swallow and take a deep breath before placing the maxillary impression into the mouth. Confidence on the part of the dental assistant will eliminate patient discomfort as will working quickly and efficiently. Talk with your patients while the material sets to help get their minds on something other than the procedure.

Procedure 36-3 Obtaining a Vinyl Polysiloxane Bite Registration

Equipment and Supplies

- Bite registration cartridge material
- Cartridge dispensing gun
- One cartridge syringe tip
- One intraoral tip

Procedure Steps

1. Ensure the patient is sitting in an upright position. Ask the patient to close her back teeth together. Tell the patient that this is how you need her to close with the bite registration material in place. Observe how both sides of the arches occlude.

2. Place the bite registration material cartridge into the dispensing gun.

3. Dispense material onto the occlusal surface of the patient's arch starting in the posterior molars on one side and continuing to syringe the material onto the anterior teeth and around to the molars on the opposite side. A full-arch bite registration will ensure an accurate occlusal record.

4. Have the patient close her mouth, or guide the patient's jaw into the proper position.

5. Most vinyl polysiloxane bite registration materials will set in 20 to 30 seconds.

6. Remove the bite registration from the mouth. Rinse the material, dry, and disinfect according to manufacturer's instructions.

7. Be sure to avoid contact with any chemicals known to inhibit setting of vinyl polysiloxane such as latex gloves and acrylic residues. Wear vinyl gloves during this procedure.

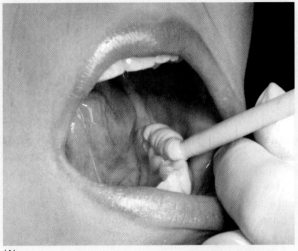

(A)

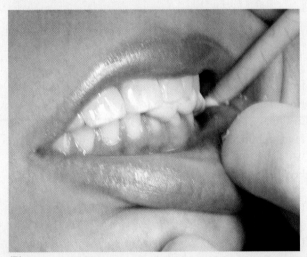

(B)

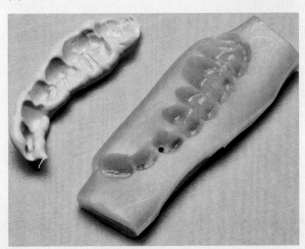

(C)

(a) Bite registration material being extruded onto the occlusal surfaces, (b) patient in accurate occlusion for the impression, and (c) vinyl polysiloxane and wax bite registrations.

SUMMARY

Various impression materials are placed on preformed impression trays and used to reproduce the structure of a patient's teeth and other oral structures. These impressions provide the negative into which gypsum material will be poured in order to create the positive cast study models. The casts are used for creation of prosthetic devices such as crowns, bridges, veneers, implants, partial dentures, and complete dentures.

Each impression material has properties indicated for specific purposes, and manufacturer's directions must be followed to ensure proper results. Once placed in the patient's oral cavity as a sol, impression materials are converted to gels through thermal or chemical processes. The ability to record consistently good impressions and create diagnostic cast models is both a science and an art.

Many factors contribute to inaccurate articulation of cast models including inaccuracy in dental materials or bite registrations, alginate impressions not being poured in a timely manner, or teeth being contaminated with preparation materials used prior to the impression or bite registration. Perfection cannot be achieved each and every time, but with proper attention to detail and practice the dental assistant will achieve the experience and skills necessary to accomplish successful impressions.

Preparing for Externship

Making a quality impression the first time takes experience. Before attending an externship, practice making impressions as often as possible on fellow classmates or even on yourself. When using yourself for a patient, think about good impression techniques and how efficiently a quality impression can be made the first time with consistent results.

KEY TERMS

- **Bite registration:** A record of how the patient's maxillary and mandibular arches occlude.   p. 563
- **Cast model:** A gypsum replica of the mouth made from an impression of a patient's mouth.   p. 562
- **Frenula:** Folds of tissue connecting the cheeks and lips to the alveolar mucosa.   p. 564
- **Hydrophilic:** A tendency toward compatibility with water or complete wetting ability.   p. 563
- **Hydrophobic:** A tendency away from water, an aversion to it, and less wetting ability.   p. 563
- **Imbibition:** The process of absorbing water, causing swelling.   p. 565
- **Impression:** A negative replica of a person's teeth and oral structures into which dental plaster or stone is placed in order to make an accurate copy or positive replica of the patient's dentition.   p. 562
- **Polymerization:** A chemical process that causes two materials to harden together.   p. 569
- **Sol:** A viscous liquid whose particles become attached to each other, forming a loose mass.   p. 565
- **Syneresis:** The process of contracting and shrinking with time as a result of losing water.   p. 565
- **Viscosity:** The property of a material that causes it to flow or not flow easily.   p. 563
- **Wettability:** The capacity of a material to flow over a surface and capture all irregularities.   p. 563

CHECK YOUR UNDERSTANDING

1. Models made from dental impressions are used for which of the following dental procedures?
   a. prosthodontics
   b. orthodontics
   c. athletic mouth guards
   d. bleach trays
   e. all of the above

2. What types of dental impressions are made in the dental facility?
   a. preliminary impressions
   b. final impressions
   c. bite registration
   d. all of the above

3. Which of the following terms refers to the ability of a material to flow or not flow easily?
   a. wettability
   b. hydrophobic
   c. hydrophilic
   d. viscosity

4. Which of the following materials is used for stock impression trays?
   a. stainless steel
   b. aluminum
   c. chrome-plated brass
   d. disposable plastic
   e. all of the above

CHECK YOUR UNDERSTANDING (continued)

5. What are the main types of custom trays?
   a. methyl methacrylate
   b. visible light-cured
   c. thermoplastic
   d. all of the above

6. What should the dental assistant do immediately prior to inserting an alginate impression into the patient's mouth?
   a. Disinfect the impression material.
   b. Dry the patient's teeth.
   c. Smooth the surface of the alginate with a wet finger.
   d. Do nothing but insert the impression into the mouth.

7. In which of the following viscosities are elastomeric impression materials available?
   a. low
   b. medium
   c. high
   d. putty
   e. all of the above

8. Which of the following are used in elastomeric impression materials?
   a. polysulfide
   b. polyether
   c. silicone
   d. polysiloxane
   e. all of the above

9. What viscosity is the syringe material that is extruded around the tooth into the gingival sulcus?
   a. low
   b. medium
   c. high
   d. putty

10. What will happen if powder from gloves touches nonaqueous elastomeric impression materials?
    a. Nothing will happen.
    b. The impression will be distorted.
    c. The impression will not have good detail.
    d. The impression material will not set.

INTERNET ACTIVITY

- Go to www.dentrek.com/docViewer.asp?x_documentID=121 for an impression troubleshooting guide.

WEB REFERENCES

- British Dental Journal: Crowns and other extra-coronal restorations: Impression materials and technique
  www.nature.com/bdj/journal/v192/n12/full/4801456a.html
- DENTSPLY International   www.dentsply.com
- enotes.com: Encyclopedia of Nursing and Allied Health   http://health.enotes.com/nursing-encyclopedia/dental-casts
- GC America, Inc.   www.gcamerica.com
- Heraeus Kulzer   www.heraeus-kulzer-us.com
- Premier Dental   www.premusa.com/dental/prosthetic.asp

37

Laboratory Materials and Procedures

Chapter Outline

Learning Objectives

After reading this chapter, the student should be able to:

- Explain safety and infection control procedures required in a dental laboratory.
- Identify how to care for dental laboratory supplies and equipment.
- State the properties of dental gypsum materials.
- Demonstrate pouring a gypsum model from an alginate impression.
- Demonstrate trimming maxillary and mandibular dental models with a model trimmer.
- Describe various methods of constructing custom trays and demonstrate creating a light-cured custom tray.
- Describe manipulating dental waxes and compounds and their uses.
- Demonstrate the ability to construct an acrylic custom tray.

Preparing for Certification Exams

- Pour, trim, and evaluate the quality of diagnostic casts.
- Fabricate custom trays to include impression and bleaching trays, and athletic mouth guards.
- Demonstrate understanding of the OSHA Bloodborne Pathogens standard.

Key Terms

Anatomic portion	Gypsum
Articulator	Lathe
Aseptic	Model trimmer
Centric occlusion	Prostheses
Facebow	Unit dose concept

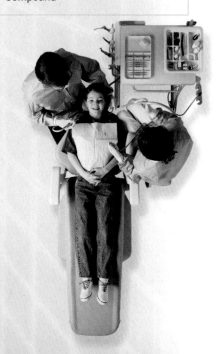

Many procedures in dentistry require laboratory techniques and equipment. Some procedures will be accomplished in the dental facility and others will be completed at a dental laboratory. The extent of laboratory diagnostics done in the dental office varies. The dental assistant is involved with the patient at chairside as well as during certain aspects of lab procedures, including the creation of diagnostic cast models from impressions taken of the patient's dentition. Another of the dental assistant's tasks involves pouring preliminary alginate impressions.

Some offices may have a dental laboratory technician at an on-site laboratory who fabricates various dental **prostheses**. Dental prostheses are artificial replacements for teeth and other oral structures such as crowns, bridges, implants, dentures, and partial dentures. Prostheses are fabricated outside of the patient's mouth and require an assortment of materials and techniques.

The dental assistant must understand the properties of dental lab materials and how to use them in order to carry out steps necessary to assist the dentist in quality patient treatment. Standard precautions to avoid cross-contamination of infectious diseases should be observed in the dental laboratory at all times. Laboratory safety and infection control must be followed to protect the patient and all dental personnel.

Dental Assistant **PROFESSIONAL TIP**

When mixing gypsum always start with a clean bowl and clean the bowl immediately after use. Particles of old mix left in the bowl can accelerate the set of future mixes. Reseal any gypsum material package tightly to avoid contamination.

Patient Education

Part of patient education should be to explain to patients why models are needed and how they will be used. Before any dental treatment begins, the dental assistant should inform the patient about what to expect. Be brief and to the point. Think about what you would want to know about impressions and models if you were the patient. Be proud of your work and show the patient his models when the models are complete. Note, however, that you should ask your dentist for permission first before showing the patient the models.

Safety in the Dental Laboratory

Each dental laboratory must have written policies and general rules to protect all employees of and visitors to the facility. It is the responsibility of the health care provider, the dental technician, and the dental laboratory to ensure the safety of patients, the dental team, and the dental lab technician. The Occupational Safety and Health Administration (OSHA) Bloodborne Pathogens standard guidelines to be followed in a dental laboratory environment include:

- Wearing eye protection and masks whenever indicated by risk involved
- Wearing appropriate clothing such as lab coats and closed-toe shoes, and not wearing neck ties or long, dangling earrings; lab coats worn in the lab should not be worn outside the lab
- Not allowing any food, drink, or cosmetics in the lab
- Tying long hair back and away from the face
- Following manufacturer's instructions when operating equipment
- Venting fume hoods used whenever there is a possibility of exposure by inhalation
- Reading labels carefully when handling chemicals
- Donning gloves whenever blood or any potentially infectious material is handled
- Disinfecting countertops after work is completed
- Washing hands with antimicrobial agent
- Notifying the dentist in case of accidental exposure to infectious material
- Knowing the location of the Material Safety Data Sheets, the eye wash station, the first aid kit, and fire extinguisher in case of emergency

See Chapter 12 for more information about the OSHA standard and infection control.

Health and safety concerns vary depending on the type of lab environment. Cutting corners—whether to save time or money—can have serious health consequences. It is important for the dental assistant to take the time to learn how to use and maintain the equipment and materials used in the dental lab. Alcohol torches, dental handpieces, lab burs, and lathes are a few of the common types of equipment found in a lab. Proper ventilation equipment should be utilized. Knives, spatulas, and a variety of hand instruments are also used. Cuts, burns, and puncture wounds are the most common types of injuries sustained in the dental laboratory.

It is important to know how to use and maintain equipment and tools to help avoid accidents and to be familiar with the location of fire extinguishers, emergency exits, the eye wash station, and the first aid kit. Rubber gloves should always be worn to clean up chemical spills. Chemicals should be disposed of according to manufacturer's directions. The dental assistant should always wear personal protective equipment when there is a potential of exposure to pathogens. Eye protection is especially important when operating rotating dental equipment. Gloves must be worn when handling contaminated objects such as patient prostheses.

Infection Control in the Dental Laboratory

It is important to maintain excellent communication between the dental office and each dental laboratory where patient materials such as impressions and models are sent for processing (Figure 37.1). It is the responsibility of the dental office and the dental laboratory to protect patients and the clinical dental staff. Dental labs, whether in-house or off-site, should be isolated from possible transmission of pathogens and be prepared to prevent cross-contamination between patients and dental health care workers.

Disinfecting Impressions

Dental impressions should be disinfected according to manufacturer's directions. When preparing hydrocolloid and vinyl polysiloxane materials, the impression should be gently rinsed to remove blood and other debris. The

impression should be thoroughly soaked by spraying it with hospital disinfectant. Some commonly used disinfectants include glutaraldehyde, iodophors, sodium hypochlorite (1:10), complex phenolics, chlorine dioxide, and dual or synergized quaternary ammoniums. The product with the shortest contact time will cause less distortion during this process. Impressions should be loosely wrapped in a plastic bag to prevent evaporation of the disinfectant. The manufacturer's recommendations should be followed on how long to disinfect. Note that polyether impressions cannot be immersed in a disinfectant solution because they are hydrophilic and have a tendency to distort when placed in liquid solutions. Table 37-1 lists acceptable disinfecting methods for the various types of impression materials, and Table 37-2 provides information on proper sterilization methods for impression trays. Trays that are disposable should be discarded and should be used for only one patient. The dental assis-

TABLE 37-1 Disinfecting Methods for Impression Materials

Impression Material	Disinfecting Methods
Alginate	Iodophors, sodium hypochlorite
Polysulfide	Glutaraldehyde, iodophors, sodium hypochlorite, complex phenolics
Silicone	Glutaraldehyde, iodophors, sodium hypochlorite, complex phenolics
Polyether	Iodophors, sodium hypochlorite, complex phenolics (use spray rather than immersion)
Vinyl polysiloxane	Iodophors, sodium hypochlorite, chlorine dioxide, dual or synergized quaternary ammoniums
Reversible hydrocolloid	Iodophors, sodium hypochlorite
Compound	Iodophors, sodium hypochlorite

TABLE 37-2 Processing Methods for Impression Trays

Impression Trays	Processing Methods
Aluminum	Heat sterilize via autoclave, chemical vapor, dry heat, or ethylene oxide sterilization.
Chrome-plated	Heat sterilize via autoclave, chemical vapor, dry heat, or ethylene oxide sterilization.
Custom acrylic resin	Discard after intraoral use on patient, or disinfect with tuberculocidal hospital disinfectant for reuse for the same patient's next visit.
Plastic	Discard after use.

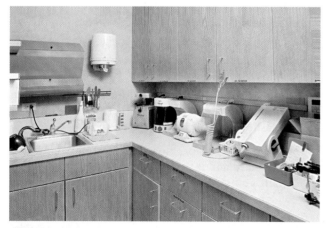

FIGURE 37.1
Dental office laboratory.

tant must label the custom impression tray if it will be needed in the future for a patient.

Once the disinfecting process is complete, the impression should then be rinsed and handled in an **aseptic** manner, avoiding any contamination by disease-producing microorganisms. Prostheses, occlusal registrations, and nonsterilizable equipment must be cleaned with soap and water and disinfected with a hospital-level disinfectant if they become contaminated. Again, care must be taken not to exceed manufacturer's recommendations for disinfectant time. Metal components may corrode if exposed to chemicals in excess of the recommended contact time. Chemical burns can also occur to human skin in sensitive persons if items are not rinsed before handling.

Articulators, case pans, and other equipment that have no contact with patients still require cleaning and disinfecting. Some equipment requires rinsing, drying, and lubricating. Prevention of contamination is better than having to use chemical agents on delicate equipment components. Any item that can withstand heat sterilization should be sterilized before reuse. Antimicrobial impression materials should be used if possible to reduce the amount of bioburden, or infectious agents, in the impression.

Why is it so important for laboratory safety and infection control procedures to be followed?

Dental Laboratory Equipment

Several pieces of equipment are utilized during the process of fabricating restorations, mouth guards, and bleach trays for patients. Some of these machines produce a bright light and very high heat and others rotate at a high rate of speed. The dental assistant should never operate or use any type of equipment without first reading the manufacturer's instructions on use, safety precautions, and maintenance.

Equipment Requiring Heat Sources

Alcohol torches, butane torches, and Bunsen burners are used for smoothing wax surfaces, setting teeth, and heating wax-carving instruments. They are also used for a variety of tasks that require an accurate and controlled pointed flame. Alcohol torches draw fuel through a wick from a reservoir near the top of the torch. It is important to periodically trim all irregular burned areas of the alcohol torch wick and to check the nozzle tip of alcohol and butane torches to ensure that they are free from obstructions. No torch should ever be left unattended when lit. Never attempt to fill the fuel reservoir on the torches with the flame lit.

A Bunsen burner requires a balanced air and gas mixture to produce a clean blue flame. It is attached to a gas valve by a rubber hose. The hose and connection should be inspected daily for loose connections and defects. The hose must be replaced when it shows signs of wear. Never leave an unattended burner lit. Avoid reaching over a lit burner. Ensure the gas valve is shut off completely when leaving the burner.

Vacuum Former

The vacuum former (Figure 37.2) is used for rapid fabrication of custom trays, mouth guards, splints for temporary crowns, night guards for bruxism, and bleaching trays. This machine softens a sheet of plastic with heat and then pulls it down onto the cast with suction. The heating element is housed inside a metal assembly at the top portion of the unit. Caution must be exercised when the machine is on because this area becomes very hot during use.

The sheet of plastic is placed and secured between a metal frame and a rubber gasket and then raised up to the heating element. A trimmed model is placed on the platform and the heat turned on. The heated plastic sheet hangs down over the model approximately 1 to 1.5 inches. The assistant grabs the handles of the frame and pulls the frame down onto the model and immediately turns on the suction to draw the hot plastic onto the model. The vacuum former gasket should be checked for cracks and the electric cord inspected before use. The unit should be unplugged after each use.

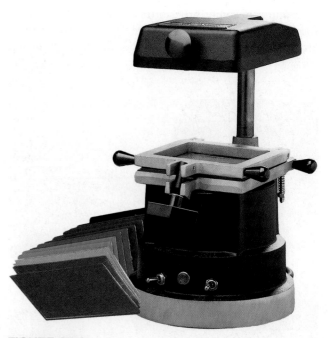

FIGURE 37.2
Vacuum former.
Courtesy Keystone Industries

Articulators and Facebows

The **articulator** (Figure 37.3) is a device designed to reproduce movements of a patient's mandibular arch in proper **centric occlusion** to the maxillary arch. In centric occlusion the cusps of the mandibular and maxillary posterior teeth contact each other as the patient's mouth closes. In ideal centric occlusion the mesial lingual cusps of the maxillary first molar occlude in the central fossa of the mandibular molars. Dental casts made from the patient's impressions are mounted onto the articulator with lab plaster. This allows the dentist and the dental technician to re-create the normal movements of the patient's jaw during the fabrication of a dental prosthesis so it will function properly.

Several types of articulators are available depending on the needs of the dentist, the dental technician, and the type of prosthesis being constructed. Some articulators are capable of simulating movements of the mandible and shape of the patient's condyle and include adjustable elements for horizontal rotation of the patient's jaw. An articulator may have a **facebow,** which is used to record the relationship of the maxillary arch to the horizontal axis rotation of the mandible.

The facebow requires three points of reference, which vary with the type of facebow used. Frequently, an ear-piece facebow is used for the two points of orientation. The facebow rests on the patient's face and the occlusal relationship is recorded by inserting wax, vinyl polysiloxane, or another material into the oral cavity. This records the patient's accurate horizontal bite relationship.

Dental Lathe

A **lathe** is a rotary machine used during grinding, finishing, and polishing procedures. The dental assistant should ensure that all burs and accessories are securely attached before turning on the lathe. The dental lathe has

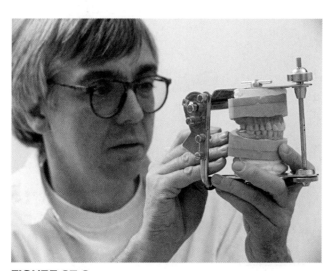

FIGURE 37.3
Articulator.

extensions at both ends. An adapter or chuck is used to secure a wide variety of rotary instruments onto either extension.

Instruments that can be attached to the lathe include acrylic burs, arbor bands, dental stones, and ragwheels. Arbor bands are circular sandpaper bands that are placed on rubber wheels to hold them in place. They are used to remove unwanted material during fabrication of dental prostheses. Ragwheels are made of cloth and are used to polish or buff dental prosthetic appliances so that they are smooth; some are made of leather and used to polish metals. Wet pumice and other polishing agents are used at the lathe with the rotating ragwheel. The ragwheel should remain wet while being used, otherwise it could become abrasive and scratch the item. A splatter guard prevents material from spraying the room, and a pan is used under the wheel to collect excess pumice material.

Flour of pumice is a very mild abrasive, such as that used in toothpaste, which can be mixed with water or disinfectant solutions to form a slurry paste to be used in conjunction with a dental lathe to polish dental appliances. Pumice is also available in a coarse grit when a stronger force is necessary such as on metal when prostheses are being made.

All brushes, ragwheels, and other laboratory tools should be sterilized between patients to prevent cross-contamination. If there is any question of possible contamination of an item, it should be treated as contaminated and cleaned and disinfected per manufacturer's instructions.

The pumice solution used at the polishing lathe should be dispensed following the unit dose concept. The **unit dose concept** prevents contamination of bulk supplies. The unit dose concept for pumice means that only enough pumice material should be dispensed and utilized for one patient's prosthesis. The pumice would then be discarded and the lathe and tray cleaned and disinfected.

When using the dental lathe it is important to wear protective glasses or goggles. Gloves and a mask should also be utilized when the dental assistant is working with the dental lathe. Never leave an unattended dental lathe running or attempt to stop the lathe by grasping the attachment with one's hands.

Mixing Bowls

Dental lab mixing bowls are made of flexible rubber or plastic material. They are used to mix alginate impression and gypsum materials. They come in small, medium, large, and extra large sizes depending on the size needed for the procedure. A spatula is used to blend the powdered alginate or gypsum and water together in the bowl. Mixing bowls should be disinfected by spraying with disinfectant and then wiping them dry for storage.

Disposable bowl liners and wooden spatulas may also be used. The liners fit into the flexible rubber bowls and are intended for a single use only. The wooden spatulas are also used once and then discarded. The bowl liners and disposable wooden spatulas maintain infection control issues and prevent cross-contamination between patients.

Vibrator

The vibrator (Figure 37.4) is used to move dental plaster or stone gypsum products when pouring a cast model. The impression is placed on the flat, top working surface of the vibrator as the gypsum material is poured into it in small increments. The vibrator increases the density of the mix by eliminating air bubbles from the mix prior to pouring and then ensuring that bubbles are removed as the model is poured. A control knob is used to adjust the intensity of the vibration from a gentle vibration to a vigorous pulsation.

To keep the vibrator clean, the rubber platform should be kept covered with a plastic cover and damp paper towels. The vibrator should be cleaned after each use so any stray gypsum materials are not allowed to harden on the unit. The vibrator's power cord and plug should be checked for defects before each use. The dental assistant must ensure that hair is pulled back from the face because this could be a serious safety hazard. If hair gets caught in any rotary dental equipment, the individual could be hurt.

Model Trimmer

A **model trimmer** (Figure 37.5) is used to trim and contour gypsum cast models. A model trimmer is an electrically operated machine that has a round abrasive wheel, a short working table, and a water-dispensing mechanism. The wheel rotates while water flows onto it, keeping it clean. Plaster and stone cannot be allowed to dry on the wheel surface because a dirty surface will diminish the trimmer's grinding efficiency.

Turn on the water before starting the model trimmer. When finished with the model trimmer, allow the water

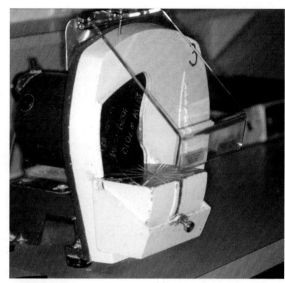

FIGURE 37.5
Model trimmer.

to run for one full minute to flush out particles from the trimmer drain and to prevent clogging of gypsum material in the plumbing lines. Light pressure should be used to press the cast model against the trimming wheel and to ensure that the water spray is sufficient to keep the wheel clean, but not too fast to splash the entire area.

The model trimmer unit should be periodically checked for leaks and cleaned frequently depending on the amount of usage. The power cord should be inspected for damage. Call a service technician if the unit does not operate correctly. When operating the model trimmer, the dental assistant must be sure to keep fingers away from the wheel and to wear safety glasses or goggles.

Dental Laboratory Instruments

Several instruments are commonly used in the dental laboratory, sometimes by the dentist and dental assistant during and between patient appointments. Lab spatulas have narrow or broad flexible blades. Broad blade spatulas are best for mixing alginate impression material because they allow the alginate to be pressed against the sides of the bowl, eliminating air bubbles and creating a creamy homogenous mixture. Lab knives are used to trim

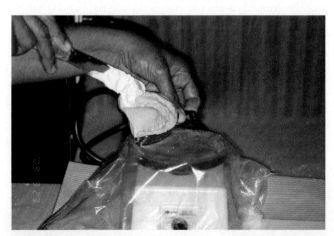

FIGURE 37.4
Vibrator.

Professionalism

Long hair must be tied back at all times when working in the dental laboratory. Hair that hangs down may not only become contaminated with aerosols containing patient's saliva, it is also a safety hazard if caught on the model trimming wheel. Long hair is not only an issue for laboratory procedures but for all dental procedures.

gypsum, dental compound, wax, custom trays, and other materials. The handles of spatulas and knives are usually made of wood or plastic. The blades must be kept dry to prevent rust. Wax spatulas are metal and designed to be used when manipulating hot wax during prosthodontic procedures. These instruments must be disinfected or sterilized and stored properly after each use.

What personal protective equipment should be worn by the dental assistant when operating the trimmer?

Diagnostic Cast Models

Dental cast models duplicate a patient's teeth and mouth structures for diagnostic purposes and are used as models for further fabricating of dental prostheses (Figure 37.6). They may also be used as an education tool by the dentist to explain characteristics to a patient regarding the patient's specific dental needs. Diagnostic casts can also show how a restoration will look when a treatment is complete. From the initial casts, dental prostheses are made that will fit the patient's jaw structure and resemble the other teeth. Cast models are made from quality dental impressions of the patient's teeth and oral structures. (See Chapter 36 for more information on dental impressions.)

Gypsum Materials

Gypsum products are used in dentistry to create diagnostic cast models of a patient's maxillary or mandibular arch. The most common gypsum products are plaster, stone, and die stone. Gypsum products are composed primarily of calcium sulfate dihydrate. A dihydrate is a substance consisting of two parts water to one part calcium sulfate. In the manufacturing process, gypsum is con-

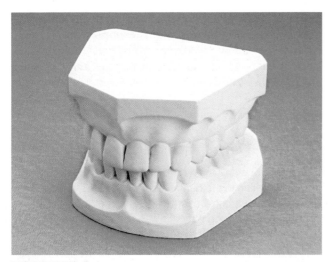

FIGURE 37.6
Dental model.

verted to plaster of Paris and artificial stone by a process called calcination, when the gypsum is heated. The heating process converts calcium sulfate dihydrate into calcium sulfate hemihydrate by removing water molecules. Hemihydrate is one-half part water and one part calcium sulfate.

Gypsum products are supplied in powder form. When mixed with water in the correct proportions a paste forms that hardens. Table 37-3 gives some general guidelines for the water-to-powder ratio, but remember that the ratio specified by the manufacturer should be followed for an optimum quality dental cast model. Before the material sets, it is soft and pliable and can be formed into a desired shape. During the setting process, gypsum gives off heat. This is called an exothermic reaction. Plaster powder particles are rough, irregular, and porous. Stone particles are fairly smooth, more regular in size, and dense. When plaster or stone is mixed with water, a hard substance is formed. During the setting period, a chemical reaction takes place in which the crystals of gypsum intermesh and become entangled with one another, giving the set material its strength and firmness.

The gypsum cast should be separated from the impression approximately 45 to 60 minutes after pouring. Prolonged contact between the alginate and the gypsum should be avoided. If not, a soft, chalky surface may be produced on the cast, which is undesirable. The model should not be separated from the alginate impression

TABLE 37-3 Recommended Water-to-Powder Ratio for Gypsum Products

100 Grams of Gypsum Product	Amount of Water
Dental plaster	45–50 mL
Dental stone	30–32 mL
Die (high-strength) stone	20–24 mL

until it is completely set. The dental assistant must wait until the model has passed its glossy stage and until the exothermic reaction is complete. If the cast is separated too soon, the teeth may break off and the patient will need to return to the office for another impression to be taken.

Plaster

Plaster of Paris is used for pouring cast models for preliminary study, for diagnostic reasons, to attach casts onto articulators, and for general use in the dental lab when strength is not important. Because of the porous and irregular particles, plaster requires more water to be added to the mix than when mixing stone. This creates a weaker cast. The initial setting time for most dental plaster is from 5 to 15 minutes and it is completely set within approximately 45 minutes. Removal of a cast from the mold too soon can result in fractures to the cast.

Stone

Dental stone is available in a yellow or buff color, requires less water to be added to the powder than when preparing plaster when mixing, and sets more slowly than plaster. When set, stone is harder, denser, and has a higher crushing strength than plaster. The harder stone casts provide excellent master casts for fabrication of dentures, bleach trays, athletic mouth guards, and temporary crown splints. Stone is more resistant to scratching and damage than plaster models.

Manufacturer's directions state to place the required water into a rubber bowl. The stone powder is then added slowly. All of the powder should be incorporated with the water before spatulating. Mixing of all gypsum should be thorough without whipping air into the mixture. Whipping can trap air bubbles that will weaken the cast and create defects in the model. Spatulation should be completed in 30 to 60 seconds. The bowl should be placed on a vibrator during mixing to cause air bubbles to rise to the surface. The initial setting time for artificial stone is usually 8 to 15 minutes and the final setting time is approximately 45 minutes. Stone models should be soaked in water before being trimmed to facilitate easier trimming and less wear and tear on the model trimmer wheel.

Die Stone

Die stone is the strongest gypsum product. It is used to create working casts for fixed prostheses and partial dentures. Die stone is most often poured by the dental laboratory technician from impressions made during the dental appointment, but some dentists may want to pour the model themselves. The die stone mix must not be too thick or too thin so that it flows into the dentition easily and yet is thick enough to maintain its strength.

What is the difference between dental plaster, dental stone, and die stone?

Pouring Dental Models

The dental assistant pours plaster and stone models in the dental office. An accurate cast can only be produced from a quality dental impression where correct preparation of materials has occurred. A minor mistake could cause a distorted cast. The impression would then need to be remade.

Dental impressions should be poured as soon as possible. They should be rinsed to remove saliva and any debris on the surface and sprayed with a disinfecting solution. An accurate water-to-powder ratio is necessary to preserve the properties of any gypsum product. As always, it is important to follow the manufacturer's directions to ensure correct usage of the product.

- Always use a clean, dry mixing bowl and spatula. The best time to clean a bowl and spatula is immediately after using them before the material has a chance to harden.
- Measure the volume of water and weigh the powder.
- Always add powder to water and not water to powder.

- Spatulate thoroughly by hand, incorporating all of the powder evenly throughout the mix until creamy. Avoid whipping the mix to avoid excess air bubbles.
- Vacuum mixing with a power mixer-investor helps to eliminate incorporation of air into the mix.
- Hold the bowl against a vibrator for a few minutes to cause trapped air to rise to the surface.
- Never add water to a mix that is too thick. This interferes with the setting properties. Discard the mix and start over.

The primary objective when pouring a dental cast is to capture all of the surface detail of the impression and to do so without introducing air bubbles. This is done by using a vibrator to make a thick gypsum mix that flows into all crevices of the impression.

What are the different methods by which a dental model may be poured?

A cast model has two parts: the **anatomic portion,** which includes the teeth and oral structures, and the base or art portion, on which the anatomic portion of the model sits (Figure 37.7). The anatomic part of a model should make up two-thirds of the model, whereas the art portion makes up one-third.

Factors that affect the setting time of gypsum products are water temperature, spatulation, and water-to-powder ratio. The cooler the water used, the longer the

material will take to set. The time and speed of spatulation affect the setting time and strength of gypsum. Rapid spatulation accelerates the setting time. When a high proportion of water is used, setting time is delayed and crushing strength is lowered, creating a weak model that is unusable for laboratory procedures. There are several ways to pour a cast, including the two-step method, the boxed method, and the inverted method.

- *Two-step pour method:* The two-step method requires the gypsum material to be poured into the impression first. A second mix is then used to create the base portion. The anatomic part is allowed to set and then the base portion is created separately using a spatula to form a flat patty. The anatomic portion is set on top of the base until the two portions harden together.
- *Boxed pour method:* The boxed pour method is similar to the two-step pour except boxing wax or a model base former is used to create the border for the base of the model. Boxing wax is placed around impressions after the cast is poured and used to make the base portion of the model by limiting the flow of the gypsum material.
- *Inverted pour method:* The inverted pour method is the most commonly used way to pour cast models. Both the anatomic portion and the base of the model are completed with one mix. The impression is poured first, then the rest of the gypsum material is used to create the base onto which the art portion is inverted and placed until the material is set (Procedure 37-1).

What might happen if a model is left in the impression to dry overnight?

Trimming Dental Models

Models should present a clean and neat appearance. After the setting period the models are separated from the impression. Do not let the alginate impression material become overdry before separating the cast. If this occurs, the cast might experience some surface damage or it might be inaccurate.

Using a lab knife the dental assistant cleans off the stone or plaster from the outside of the tray and begins to gently pry the tray from the cast. The dental assistant must be careful not to damage the cast during this process. Placing the knife between the tray and cast around all sides before separating them should loosen the tray without destroying the cast.

A stone model should be soaked in water for at least 30 minutes before trimming to help with the trimming process and put less wear on the model trimmer. Plaster models should not be soaked in water because plaster is a much less dense and more porous material than the stone.

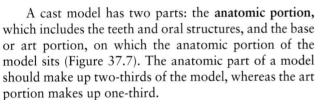

Maxillary model

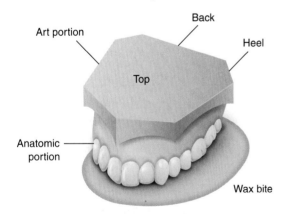

Mandibular model

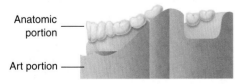

FIGURE 37.7
Anatomic and art portion of a dental cast model.

Procedure 37-1 Pouring Dental Models Using the Inverted Pour Method

Equipment and Supplies

- Maxillary or mandibular alginate impression
- Flexible rubber mixing bowl
- Lab spatula
- Tile or glass slab
- Plaster
- Water
- Vibrator

Procedure Steps

1. Measure room temperature water and weigh the powder. Add water to a clean, dry, rubber bowl. Add powder to the water and use a clean wide lab spatula to gently but quickly incorporate all the powder evenly into the mix until it is uniform and creamy. Avoid whipping the mix because whipping could incorporate air bubbles into the model, which is undesirable.

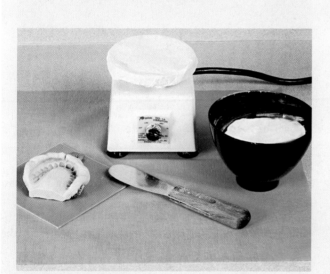

Preparing to pour a model.

2. Turn the vibrator on. Vibrate the mixing bowl for 30 seconds to one minute to bring any air pockets to the surface.

3. Hold the impression tray by the handle so that it rests on the vibrator. Place a small amount of plaster onto the impression at one end of the arch and let it quickly flow to the other side of the arch. Place another small amount of mixed plaster into the impression, ensuring that each tooth depression is filled in as gravity is used to cause the material to move around the impression. Touch the impression to the vibrator each time additional plaster is added.

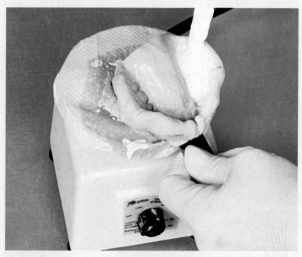

Begin pouring in small increments at the posterior of the impression.

4. After filling all teeth and covering critical surfaces of the impression, progressively larger amounts of the mix should be added. The intensity of the vibrator should be enough to cause the material to flow across the surface of the impression but not so intense that it creates bubbles.

5. Continue filling the impression to a level slightly above the height of the impression walls. Do not overfill. The plaster should not flow over the outside of the tray because it will interfere with separating the model from the tray.

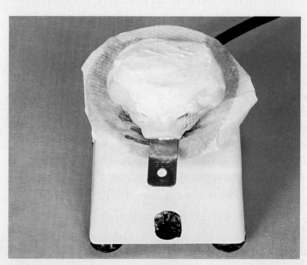

Fill the impression, but do not overfill it.

continued on next page

Procedure 37-1 *continued from previous page*

6. Set the impression down and turn off the vibrator. Using the spatula, place all of the remaining plaster from the bowl onto the tile or glass slab. If the plaster is thin, a small amount of powder may be mixed into the base material to make it stronger. Shape the base portion, utilizing the spatula to flatten it into an even patty with flat sides and just a larger width than the impression.

7. Invert the impression with the anatomic portion of plaster and place it onto the plaster patty. Bring up the posterior portion of the base material to meet the anatomic portion and smooth out the side and front of the base. Do not bring the sides of the base up to the tray because that could cause the tray to become embedded and locked into the base. For a mandibular cast use a narrow spatula to smooth and contour the tongue area of the base to ensure that it is flat while the plaster is still soft.

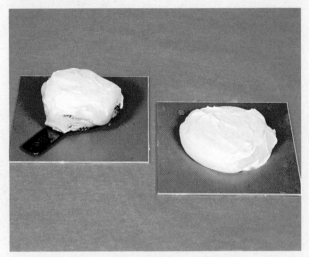

The anatomic portion ready to set with the art portion.

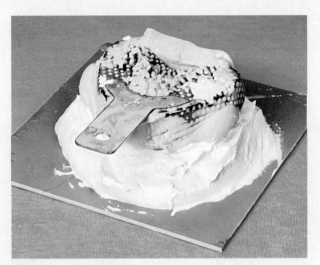

Smooth the sides of the base, but do not cover the tray.

A pencil should be used to mark trimming landmarks at the posterior, canine eminence, and between the central incisors. Trim the maxillary model first and then occlude the mandibular model with the maxillary model. Trim the mandibular model using the maxillary model's cuts as a guide. When trimming the base of both models, the dental assistant needs to examine each model to determine if there is any unevenness. The model should be placed on the model trimmer working table to assess whether it is parallel. If the impression tray was not seated evenly onto the arch, or the gypsum mix was too thin, the model will appear uneven or crooked. The base must then be trimmed or the model will not be cut evenly and important oral anatomy may be cut away. Always use eye protection when using the model trimmer (Procedure 37-2).

Ideal models have these characteristics:

- They clearly define three maxillary and three mandibular frenula.
- They should stand together on all sides without separating.
- They should have a visible tuberosity and retromolar pads.

- They should have a one-half inch base, clear and clean vestibule, and level teeth.
- They should present well with clean lines, without bubbles, and with all teeth visible when viewed from the facial.

Custom Impression Trays

A custom tray provides the dentist with an impression material carrier that allows for a more accurate impression than could be made from a stock tray. Custom trays are used to make the impressions needed to fabricate complete and partial dentures and long span bridges. Custom trays are fabricated from cast models to exclusively fit an individual patient (Figure 37.8).

The custom tray should be both strong and adjustable. It must withstand dimensional changes that can occur during the setting of impression material and hand pressure from the dental clinician while the impression sets. It needs to be adjustable in order to achieve a suitable and comfortable fit in the patient's oral cavity.

Procedure 37-2 Trimming Diagnostic Cast Models

Equipment and Supplies

- Cast stone or plaster models
- Pencil
- Laboratory knife
- Bowl of water
- Eye protection
- Model trimmer

Procedure Steps

1. After the heat from the setting process dissipates completely (approximately 45 minutes), trim any excess gypsum material from the outside of the tray with a lab knife and carefully separate the cast from the impression. Do not force the tray, or teeth may be broken during the process. The knife should be placed between the gypsum material and the tray to gently pry it loose all the way around the tray before separating the tray from the model.

2. Soak stone casts in room temperature water for at least 30 minutes before trimming.

3. Mark the maxillary cast with trimming marks between the central incisors, at the center of the cuspids, and posterior of the tuberosities. The mandibular cast will be trimmed to the shape of the maxillary cast.

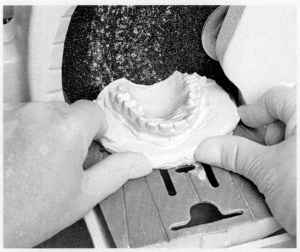

Trim posterior of the maxillary model.

5. Set the maxillary model on the counter to determine how even the base is and then place the model on the trimmer with the base of the model against the blade and put pressure where needed to even the base on the maxillary model. Make sure that when the anatomic portion of the model is placed on the table or counter the art portion is parallel with the countertop. (See top left image from page 590).

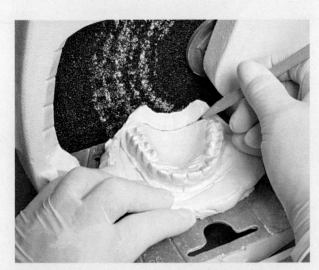

Mark the maxillary model with a pencil posterior of the tuberosities.

4. Put on eye protection and turn on the water to the model trimmer. Adjust water as needed to keep the wheel wet and turn on the model trimmer motor. Begin trimming the maxillary cast by placing the model onto the trimmer table and cut just enough on the posterior to create a flat surface. Cut to approximately 1/4 inch behind the maxillary tuberosities.

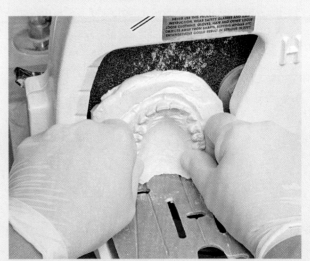

Trim the model base.

6. Cut the sides of the maxillary model using the cuspid as a guide so that the cut is parallel to the alveolar ridge, flared at the molar areas, and approximately one-quarter inch wide.

7. Turn the model using the lateral incisors and the line between the central incisors as a guide and trim until there is a point at the canine eminence. Do the same on

continued on next page

Procedure 37-2 *continued from previous page*

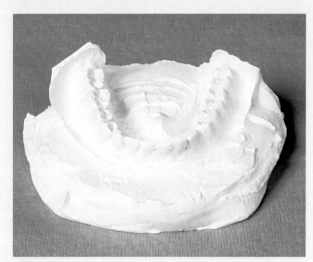

Examine how parallel the model is to the counter.

the next front cut, watching as you create a point between the central incisors and a point at the cuspid.

8. Trim the posterior of the mandibular model to at least one-quarter inch beyond the retromolar pads, then trim to even the base. Whichever model has the longest arch, the maxillary or mandibular, will be the guide for making the posterior cut even. Do not cut too close or the maxillary and mandibular landmarks will be ruined.

9. Put the maxillary and mandibular models together in proper occlusion. A bite registration may be necessary to provide an accurate occlusal relationship.

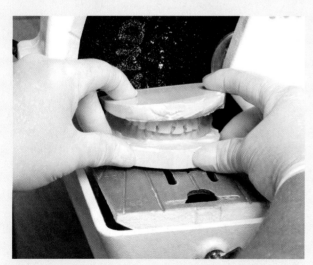

Place the models together to cut the posterior.

10. Place both models together and, using the maxillary cuts as a guide, trim the two sides and two front cuts of the mandibular model.

11. Separate the models and round the anterior portion of the mandibular model, keeping the canine eminence points created by the maxillary model guide.

12. Put the two models together again in proper occlusion and trim the heel on each side of the model to approximately one-half inch at an angle, ensuring that the maxillary tuberosities and mandibular retromolar areas are unharmed. (*Hint:* If the first side cuts are kept wide enough, these cuts will not damage the posterior arch landmarks.)

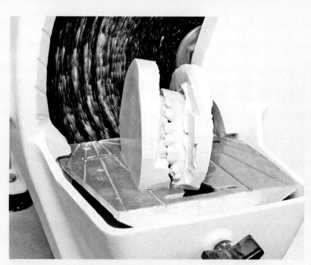

Models should balance together.

13. With the models together ensure that the posterior cuts are still even. Rinse both models well making sure that any debris from trimming is removed from the models or it will dry and create an inaccurate surface. Use a soft toothbrush and a moderate stream of water to gently remove any filing debris, but do not scrub the model because it may destroy the model and create holes—especially on plaster models.

14. Deposits from saliva bubbles should be broken off the surface of the models with a small instrument. Be extremely careful not to cause damage to the models. Rinse the models well again, dry, and label each model with the patient's name and date. Run water through the model trimmer to clean the pipe, and wipe down the outside of the trimmer.

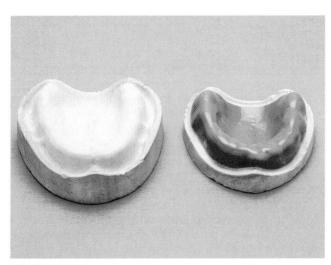

FIGURE 37.8
Maxillary custom tray.

The dentist considers the following key features when designing custom trays:

- The material from which the tray will be made
- The desired extension of the tray into peripheral and posterior areas
- The thickness of any spacer to be placed on the cast
- The location of any tissue
- The position and form of a handle if used

Custom tray design is based on the purpose of the tray and specifications needed by the dentist. The spacer thickness is determined by the type of material used to make the impression. The impression material used must have an optimal, even thickness to help improve dimensional accuracy while allowing ease of placement in the mouth. Wax or tin foil may be used and adapted to the model before custom tray construction in order to add space for the impression material. Perforations may be placed in the tray to allow for release of pressure during seating of the impression material and tray.

Tissue stops may be placed when constructing the tray to allow it to be located in the mouth while maintaining the desired spacing for the impression material. They are not essential in all cases. Tissue stops are valuable in creating fixed prosthodontics when using fairly fluid impression materials. They promote an accurate prosthetic–tissue relationship. The stops are made to hold the tray off the cast model by a distance equal to the thickness of the spacer. When the spacer is removed and the tray is placed in the patient's mouth, the stops hold the inner surface of the tray out of contact with the patient's tissue. The subsequent space between the tray and tissue is then later filled with impression material.

The tray must extend past the maxillary tuberosities on the upper arch and cover the retromolar pads on the lower arch. The lingual extension on the mandibular custom tray should cover the mylohyoid ridge at the floor of the mouth. See Chapter 5 for more information on the anatomy of the alveolar ridges on the maxillary and mandibular arches.

Tray handles are helpful when loading, placing, and orienting the custom tray but could cause distortion of the lip if not placed properly. The tray handle must be placed on the top of the tray arch at the midline to avoid distortion from the lip. The dentist determines whether a tray handle will be used. Problems with custom trays include the following:

- Border extensions too long or too short
- Tray too flexible due to insufficient thickness
- Tray cracked or damaged
- Improper handle position that interferes with border molding or insertion into the mouth
- Sharp or rough edges that may irritate the patient

Visible Light Cured Custom Trays

Light cured custom trays allow a longer time for manipulation of the material into the desired shape. Once molded into the correct form on the cast model, the tray is placed into the light curing unit (Figure 37.9) and hardened through a polymerization process. Polymerization is the setting process of uniting two or more monomers to form a polymer. It is a chemical process that causes two materials to harden.

Light cured custom trays are becoming more popular with dentists and labs because the material does not stick to fingers or models, reduces time, and eliminates odors and fumes caused by making self-cured methyl methacrylate custom trays. Visible light cure (VLC) resins are available in sheet, rope, and gel form. These are packaged in opaque containers so they are not exposed to light, which cause them to set (Procedure 37-3).

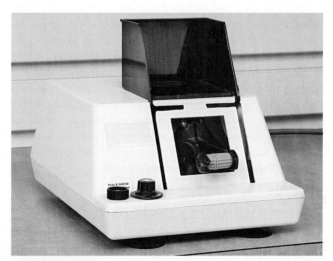

FIGURE 37.9
Light curing unit.

Procedure 37-3 Curing a VLC Impression Tray

Equipment and Supplies

- Cast stone model
- Pencil
- Baseplate wax
- Laboratory knife
- Petroleum jelly
- Opaque container of visible light cure resin
- Paper cup and plastic measuring vial
- Bowl of water
- Crown and bridge scissors

Procedure Steps

1. Outline the casts for the custom edentulous tray. Warm a piece of pink baseplate wax and apply it over the tissue-bearing areas of the cast. Trim wax layer to the tray outline. Place additional wax in any area that appears to have an undercut, which could get filled in with custom tray material and not allow it to release.

2. For stops, remove a small amount of wax from the residual ridge area at the midline and on each molar area with a blunt instrument. These will become tissue stops.

3. Coat the wax with a layer model release agent or petroleum jelly.

4. Remove a sheet of visible light cure (VLC) material from its protective pouch. Pull off a small piece and press into each of the holes in the wax spacers to serve as tissue stops. Lay the rest of the VLC material over the tissue surface of the cast. Form into a two-inch wafer for a maxillary tray and mold into a U-shape for a mandibular tray.

5. Give the material a moment to slump, or droop, onto the impression surface of the cast.

6. With wet or petroleum jelly–coated fingers, gently press material into place with no voids, onto the palate, the periphery rolls, and/or the lingual areas. Be sure the retromolar areas distal of the mandibular ridge and the maxillary tuberosity are completely covered.

7. Using a sharp instrument and/or scissors, trim excess material up to the custom tray outline. The material may be cut lightly beyond the outline and trimmed back after curing. Never trim the custom tray short of the outline on the cast.

8. Fabricate handles. Be careful because they may slump. Avoid placing tray handle material where it might cause distortion of the frenum and lip.

9. Put the cast with tray material into the visible light cure unit and process for two minutes.

10. Remove the cast and tray from the unit. Separate the cast and custom tray. Carefully remove the wax from inside the custom tray.

11. Return the tray to the curing unit and process for an additional six minutes.

12. Adjust and finish the borders of the tray to the outline drawn on the cast. Scrub tray with soap and water.

Acrylic Custom Trays

Acrylic custom trays are fabricated on the cast model using monomer and polymer materials called methyl methacrylate (Procedure 37-4). The powder is added to the liquid and mixed together until it reaches a doughy stage. While still in the doughy stage, the material is formed into the desired shape and then allowed to harden. An acrylic custom tray is a dimensionally stable material that is available in regular set, which is ready in five minutes, or extra-fast set, which is ready in three minutes. Acrylic custom tray materials must be used with proper ventilation due to the chemical fumes released by these materials.

Thermoplastic Custom Trays

Thermoplastic materials vary. Thermoplastic beads are put into very hot water, allowed to melt, manipulated while in a soft plastic stage, formed onto the cast model, and allowed to set. Other thermoplastic technology provides custom tray material for which the tray can be created in the patient's mouth or on a model within thirty seconds. The tray base is softened under hot water until pliable and then molded to the patient or on a model to form a custom tray. The tray is then removed and allowed to cool. Thermoplastic trays may be trimmed with slow-speed carbide burs or heated with a butane torch until pliable.

Why is light-cured custom tray material becoming the most popular material used for custom trays?

Dental Waxes

Many different waxes are used in dentistry. Waxes are supplied in various types, each intended for a specific purpose and designed to function to produce the best

Procedure 37-4 Constructing an Acrylic Custom Tray

Equipment and Supplies

- Cast stone model
- Pencil
- Baseplate wax
- Laboratory knife
- Petroleum jelly
- Bowl of water
- Auto-polymerization acrylic tray and baseplate material powder and liquid
- Paper cup, plastic measuring vial
- Slow speed handpiece with acrylic bur

Procedure Steps

1. For spacer, adapt one thickness of baseplate wax to the model. For stops remove small amount of wax from ridge area with a blunt instrument.

2. Soak model in room temperature water.

3. Fluff powder. Add one full measurement of powder to one vial of liquid in paper mixing cup. Mix with wood tongue depressor for one minute.

4. When mixture becomes stringy, remove and incorporate cold water. This will reduce exothermic heat when curing and prevent sticking.

5. With wet or petroleum jelly–coated fingers, knead for 30 seconds and then form into a 2 inch disc for a maxillary tray. For a mandibular tray, form into a U-shape. Save a small piece of the mix for a handle.

6. Place wafer on palatal area, overlapping the ridge, and gently push over the ridge to the periphery. Push excess toward posterior until proper and even thickness is formed. Trim excess with a knife.

7. Use the saved piece of material to form a handle and press into position with a drop of acrylic liquid. The handle, if used, should be positioned in the midline of the tray at an angle to avoid interfering with the upper lip or frenula.

8. If retention holes are desired, use a blunt instrument to perforate before the material sets.

9. Allow to cure for three minutes. To accelerate cure, place in hot water. To prevent wax spacer from melting, place in cool water.

10. An optional technique is to place a piece of foil on the model between the wax and the acrylic material. This prevents the wax from melting. If making stops, the dental assistant must remember to match cuts in the foil to the cuts in the wax spacer.

11. Trim with acrylic bur. Polish or flame to smooth edges if desired. Use acrylic bur to remove material at frenum landmarks.

---

possible results. The most commonly used waxes in dentistry include the following:

- *Baseplate wax:* Baseplate wax is used to create a spacer over the cast before a custom tray is made (Figure 37.10). This wax may be used to block out undercuts on cast models or for bite registration and to simulate the vertical dimension created by the teeth during denture and partial denture fabrication. Baseplate wax is pink and is available in sheets or U-shaped blocks.

- Inlay wax is used to prepare patterns. These patterns are reproduced in gold or other material in the fabrication of inlays, crowns, and fixed and removable partial dentures. Inlay wax is sometimes called casting wax (Figure 37.10).

- *Bite registration wax:* Bite registration wax has metal incorporated into the wax. The metal is copper or aluminum. Bite registration wax comes in U-shaped wafers. It is used to record the occlusal relationship between a patient's opposing arches and for the proper articulation of the maxillary and mandibular models.

- *Indicator wax:* Indicator wax is usually green in color and coated with a water-soluble adhesive on one side. It is used for registering occlusal contacts on teeth. The dentist may use it to evaluate high spots on restorations.

- *Sticky wax:* Sticky wax is made of beeswax, paraffin, and resin. It comes in orange and darker shades of blue, red, and violet. The resin gives the wax its adhesiveness and hardness. Sticky wax is useful in holding broken parts of a denture together during repair.

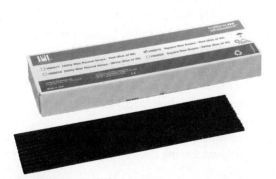

FIGURE 37.10
Baseplate and inlay wax.
Courtesy Coltene Whaledent

- *Utility wax:* Utility wax is a red or colorless wax that comes in rope form (Figure 37.11). It is extremely pliable and tacky at room temperature. It can be used on the periphery of impression trays to extend the tray or to make it a more comfortable fit for the patient.
- *Boxing wax:* Boxing wax may be used to provide a boundary for poured gypsum materials to make the shape for the model base (Figure 37.11). It comes in long strips 1.5 inches wide. Boxing the model base provides a barrier for holding the gypsum material in place as it sets and will reduce the time needed to trim a model.

What do you think might be the difference between dental wax and dental compound?

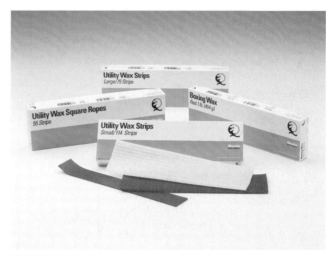

FIGURE 37.11
Utility wax and boxing wax.
Courtesy Quala, a registered trademark of American Dental Cooperative (ADC)

Compound

Dental compound is a thermodynamic material. It can be softened by warming and hardened by cooling. It is available in stick or wafer forms. Compound materials are used to customize and extend the periphery on a custom tray or may be used as a tray material for full dentures. Different colors of compound display slightly different thermodynamic behavior; they soften and harden at different temperatures. Red compound tends to soften at lower temperatures, but is not as accurate as gray stick compound, which softens at a slightly higher temperature but provides for greater detail for the purpose of border molding.

● SUMMARY

Many dental restorations are constructed outside of the patient's mouth in a dental laboratory. Specific supplies and equipment are necessary for these processes. Custom trays are prepared by the dental assistant for a patient's impressions. A dental impression is made of the patient's dental arches, which is the negative into which gypsum materials will be poured until it sets. Plaster and stone are the gypsum materials used in the dental lab by the dental assistant to create the positive cast model replicating the patient's oral cavity. The dental assistant then trims the cast models for an attractive and accurate reproduction of the patient's oral cavity. Casts are used in the dental office for preliminary study models or to fabricate custom trays, mouth guards, bleach trays, or splints for temporary restorations. An occlusal registration is taken for an accurate fit in the patient's mouth.

● KEY TERMS

- **Anatomic portion:** The portion of a model that includes the teeth and oral structures. p. 586
- **Articulator:** A device used to reproduce the patient's jaw movements. p. 582
- **Aseptic:** Free from contamination by disease-producing microorganisms. p. 581
- **Centric occlusion:** The position of the mandible when the teeth are biting fully together. p. 582
- **Facebow:** Part of an articulator that is used to record the relationship of the maxillary arch to the horizontal axis rotation of the mandible. p. 582

- **Gypsum:** Materials used to create diagnostic cast models of a patient's maxillary or mandibular arch. p. 584
- **Lathe:** A rotary machine used during grinding, finishing, and polishing procedures. p. 582
- **Model trimmer:** A machine used to grind and contour gypsum cast models. p. 583
- **Prostheses:** Artificial replacements for teeth and other oral structures. p. 579
- **Unit dose concept:** Prevents contamination of bulk supplies by dispensing only enough to complete the procedure. p. 582

CHECK YOUR UNDERSTANDING

1. Who is protected when proper procedures are followed in the dental lab?
   a. dental assistant
   b. dentist
   c. patient
   d. dental lab technician
   e. all of the above

2. The process of dispensing only enough material to complete a procedure is called what?
   a. preventing contamination of bulk supplies
   b. unit dose concept
   c. both of the above
   d. none of the above

3. What is the device called that is designed to reproduce movements of the mandibular arch in proper occlusal relationship to the maxillary arch?
   a. vibrator
   b. lathe
   c. articulator
   d. compound

4. What must the dental assistant do before starting the model trimmer?
   a. Put on safety glasses or goggles.
   b. Pull hair back and up off the collar.
   c. Turn on the water.
   d. All of the above.

5. What is the primary objective when pouring a dental cast?
   a. to capture all surface detail
   b. to vibrate air bubbles out of the gypsum material
   c. to create an accurate model of the patient's dental arches
   d. all of the above

6. Which of the following is a method for pouring gypsum models?
   a. two-step pour method
   b. boxed pour method
   c. inverted pour method
   d. all of the above

7. Which type of model should be trimmed first?
   a. maxillary
   b. mandibular
   c. it does not matter
   d. both models are trimmed together

8. What will get cut off if the cast models are trimmed too closely on the posterior?
   a. tuberosities
   b. retromolar areas
   c. mylohyoid ridge
   d. both a and b

9. How are VLC custom tray materials packaged?
   a. so they are not exposed to light
   b. in opaque containers
   c. both of the above
   d. none of the above

10. What is sometimes placed between layers of wax in bite registration material?
    a. aluminum
    b. copper
    c. compound
    d. both a and b

INTERNET ACTIVITY

- Go to http://trubyte.dentsply.com/pro/lab_step_1.shtml for great visuals and explanations of denture impressions for edentulous patients, including information about tissue stops and custom tray preparation.

WEB REFERENCES

- The Articulator www3.musc.edu/occlusion/handouts/10thearticulator.html
- British Dental Journal: The design and use of special trays in prosthodontics: guidelines to improve clinical effectiveness www.nature.com/bdj/journal/v187/n8/full/4800295a.html
- Heraeus-Kulzer www.heraeus-kulzer-us.com
- Organization for Safety and Asepsis Procedures www.osap.org
- Scrimpshire Dental Studio: Pouring Gypsum Models www.scrimpshire.com/docpage.cfm?doc_id=174
- Treatment Center Policies and Procedures: Infection Control dentalschool.bu.edu/treatment-policies/infection.html

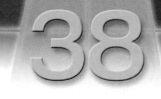

38
General Dentistry

Chapter Outline

- Cavity Preparation
- Restorations
  —Class I Restorations
  —Class II Restorations
  —Class III and IV Restorations
  —Class V and VI Restorations
- Veneers and Bonding
- Tooth Whitening

Learning Objectives

After reading this chapter, the student should be able to:

- Discuss the two areas of operative dentistry and the indications for both.
- Describe the two phases of cavity preparation.
- Identify and describe the standardized classifications of cavity preparations and restorations.
- Describe the assistant's role in cavity preparation and restoration procedures.
- Define a chairside veneer and describe the chairside veneer procedure.
- Discuss the differences in preparation and placement of amalgam and composite resin.
- Identify the clinical candidates for placement of direct bonding.
- Describe the procedures available for whitening teeth.

Preparing for Certification Exams

- Identify the different classes of preparations and restorations.
- Prepare for and assist with the various classes of restorations.
- Prepare for and assist with the placement of veneers.
- Describe the process of preparation and placement of amalgam and composite resin.
- Prepare and set up for whitening of teeth.

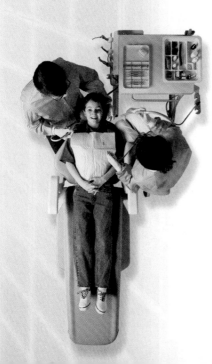

Key Terms

Aesthetic dentistry	Outline form
Axial wall	Pulpal wall
Bonding	Restoration
Cavity wall	Restorative dentistry
Diastema	Retention form
Line angle	Veneer
Operative dentistry	Whitening

In Illinois during the late 1880s, G. V. Black, "the grand old man of dentistry," related the clinical practice of dentistry to a scientific-based discipline. He created the foundation for dental education and provided the basis for cavity preparation and **restoration**. Because of Black and others, dentistry is recognized as an important member of the health care community.

Although the original practice of dentistry has branched into several specialties, operative dentistry continues to be the most active area of most dental practices. **Operative dentistry**, also known as general dentistry, is the art and science of diagnosis and treatment of defective teeth. The dental assistant must be well informed about the processes and procedures involved in operative dentistry because these are most commonly done in the general dental office.

Operative dentistry is divided into two areas, restorative dentistry and aesthetic dentistry. **Restorative dentistry** is intended to restore natural form and function to defective teeth by means of a direct or indirect restoration. The dental materials are most often dental amalgam, composite resin, or intermediate material. The indications for restorative dentistry include:

• Caries

• Restoration replacement or repair

Dental Assistant PROFESSIONAL TIP

The dental assistant is expected to know how to prepare a patient and assist the dentist in performing a restoration. Occasionally, the dentist has to change the treatment plan once the preparation has begun. Be aware of the change that is occurring and be prepared to pass different instruments or materials should the dentist call for them. For example, a Class I cavity is being prepared and the dentist finds decay on the mesial of the tooth. Now, the dental assistant will need a matrix system, which was not expected. The dental assistant may consider keeping such instruments close at hand.

• Fractured teeth

• Abrasion or erosion of tooth structure

Aesthetic dentistry is the area of operative dentistry meant to restore or emulate natural beauty. It is the means for improving the appearance of teeth with direct or indirect restorations or use of whitening procedures. The indications for aesthetic dentistry include:

• Malformed teeth

• Discolored teeth

• Fractured or traumatized teeth

• Misaligned or poorly spaced teeth

Cavity Preparation

To properly prepare and restore a tooth to its proper form and function, as well as to regain its aesthetic look, the dentist must know the anatomy of the tooth, especially the thickness of the enamel and the location and size of the pulp. Cavity preparation is the process of conservatively removing a defective or decayed tooth structure or failed dental restoration while leaving the maximum amount possible of healthy tooth structure to support a restoration. The objectives of cavity preparation are to:

• to remove all defects in the tooth
• to protect the pulp
• to conservatively locate the margins of the restoration
• to form the preparation so the restoration and tooth will function with the forces of chewing without fracture
• to allow for aesthetics

The dental assistant must understand the terminology and process of cavity preparation to be able to aid the dentist by delivering dental instruments and materials in the proper order and in a timely manner. Table 38-1 defines the terminology used when describing the anatomy of a cavity preparation; see also Figure 38.1.

The process of cavity preparation is divided into two stages, the initial preparation and the final preparation. In the initial stage of a cavity preparation, the **outline form** is created by extending the preparation in all directions until sound enamel supported by healthy dentin is reached and to obtain a sound pulpal floor. This also creates the **retention form,** which mechanically locks in the restorative material and prevents the material from being dislodged (Figure 38.2).

TABLE 38-1 Terminology Used to Describe the Anatomy of a Cavity Preparation

Cavity wall	All internal tooth surfaces of a cavity preparation.
Internal wall	Any cavity wall that does not extend to the external tooth surface.
External wall	Any cavity wall that does extend to the external tooth surface. *Example:* lingual wall, mesial wall, gingival wall.
Axial wall	Internal cavity wall that runs parallel to the long axis of the tooth.
Pulpal wall	Internal cavity wall that runs perpendicular to the long axis of the tooth; also known as the pulpal floor.
Gingival wall	The external wall/pulpal wall closest to the gingivae.
Line angle	The angle formed at the junction of two walls. The line angle is named by combining the names of the two walls. *Example:* the line angle formed by the mesial wall and the buccal wall is known as the mesiobuccal line angle.
Cavosurface margin	The junction of the wall of the cavity preparation and the external surface of the tooth.
Convenience form	Changes necessary to the basic outline form of a cavity preparation to allow for proper instrumentation.
Retention form	The shape of the cavity preparation that prevents displacement of the restorative material.

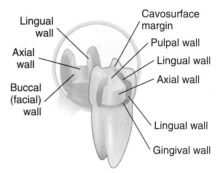

FIGURE 38.1
Anatomy of a cavity preparation.

(Figure 38.3), and placement of bases, liners, or other pulpal protective materials.

It is important to note that there are some differences in cavity preparation design depending on the restorative material to be placed. For example, a composite resin restoration does not require extensive retention grooves and notches because of the chemical bonding process that it uses, whereas an amalgam restoration relies more on mechanical retention.

What is the role of the dental assistant when it comes to restorations?

Restorations

G. V. Black created a classification system for cavities according to anatomic location, as well as by the type of treatment necessary. He labeled the classes as Class I through Class V. Since Black's initial description of the classes of cavity preparation, a sixth class has been added that is known as Class VI. The dental assistant must be able to identify the class of restoration the dentist will be preparing as well as the type of dental restorative material to be placed. This information tells the dental assistant

After the initial retention form has been created, the final phase of the cavity preparation can begin. This includes removal of remaining caries or old restorative material, placement of retention grooves and notches to help prevent the restorative material from dislodging

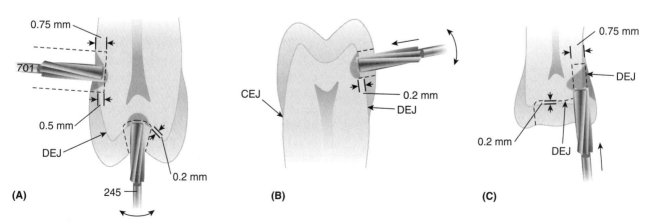

FIGURE 38.2
Creation of retention form in a cavity preparation.
DEJ (dental-enamel junction)
CEJ (cement-enamel junction)

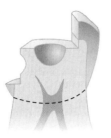

FIGURE 38.3
Retention grooves and notches are placed at the final phase of cavity preparation to help retain the dental material.

how to prepare for the patient's treatment. The dental assistant has these responsibilities:

1. Inform the patient of the procedure to be performed and answer any questions the patient may have. All dental offices should provide a written consent to be signed by the patient. This consent should inform the patient of all the pros and cons of the procedure to be performed at that appointment. (The dentist may prefer to provide this information.)
2. Be familiar with the procedure, materials, and instruments.
3. Prepare the instruments and materials to be used for the procedure.
4. Anticipate the dentist's next step.
5. Provide moisture control and good visualization for the dentist. This is best achieved with high-velocity suction and the air/water syringe.
6. Transfer dental hand instruments to the dentist.
7. Mix and transfer dental materials.
8. Always practice infection control.
9. Help to comfort the patient at all times.

In addition to these duties, if the state and the dentist allow expanded duties, the dental assistant will perform the expanded duties dental assistant (EDDA) or expanded functions dental assistant (EFDA) functions as necessary.

All nine steps are necessary whether the preparation is small or multisurface. Other steps may be added per the requirements of larger or more difficult restorations. In general, operative dentistry follows a consistent protocol, as outlined in Table 38-2.

Class I Restorations

The carious lesions requiring Class I restorations are typically found in the pits and fissures of the posterior teeth due to the patient's inability to clean these areas well. Class I cavities and restorations are usually small and found on a single surface of the tooth, but a single tooth may have numerous Class I cavities or restorations. Areas susceptible to Class I caries include (Figure 38.4):

A. Occlusal pits and fissures of the posterior teeth
B. Buccal pits and fissures of the posterior teeth
C. Lingual pits and fissures of the maxillary molars
D. Lingual pits of the maxillary incisors

TABLE 38-2 Consistent Protocol for a Restorative Procedure

1. Evaluate the tooth to be restored.
2. Deliver topical and local anesthetic if desired by the patient and recommended by the doctor.
3. Discuss with the patient the material to be placed.
4. Place moisture control items, cotton rolls, or dental dam.
5. Prepare the tooth for the restoration.
6. Apply the dental materials.
7. Carve or finish the restoration.
8. Check the occlusion and adjust as necessary.
9. Polish the restoration.
10. Provide verbal and written postoperative instructions.

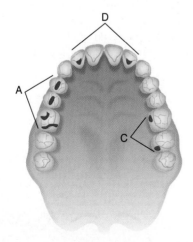
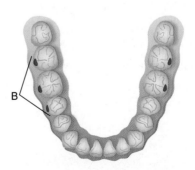

FIGURE 38.4
The various locations of Class I caries and restorations.

Class I cavity preparation and restoration may be the most common procedure in the general dental office. The procedure is rather simple. (See Procedure 38-1.) The dentist follows the pits and fissures identified as carious with a rotary hand instrument or dental drill handpiece. The bur of the instrument cuts into the enamel and dentin to remove the caries and creates an outline form that is smooth and without sharp angles (Figure 38.5). Then, as with removal of all caries, the dentist uses a caries indictor dye on the preparation. This dye marks remaining caries, allowing the dentist to move to the final phase of cavity preparation by removing the stained, carious tooth structure.

Class I cavities can receive either amalgam or composite resin. In modern aesthetic dentistry, most dentists place composite resin. Amalgam has fallen out of favor with patients due to the presence of mercury and its dark appearance. Occlusion must always be considered when placing a Class I restoration on the occlusal surface. After placement of the restoration, the dentist places a piece of articulating paper between the patient's maxillary and mandibular teeth. The patient bites and grinds on the paper to show how the teeth occlude on the restoration. The dentist adjusts the occlusion or bite as necessary and completes the procedure by polishing or burnishing the restoration.

Class II Restorations

Class II cavity preparations and restorations are an extension of the Class I into the proximal surfaces of the posterior teeth. Areas susceptible to Class II caries include:

1. Two-surface restoration of a posterior tooth
2. Three-surface restoration of a posterior tooth
3. Multisurface restoration of a posterior tooth

These preparations and restorations are named for the surfaces they include. For example, consider the case in which a premolar is found to have caries on the distal surface. The preparation and restoration must include the occlusal surface because access to the distal caries is through the occlusal and then into the distal proximal area. Therefore, the preparation and restoration is a disto-occlusal (DO). The Class II preparation may also include other surfaces as well, such as the mesial surface of the previous tooth, making the restoration a mesio-occlusodistal (MOD).

Class II preparations are somewhat more difficult than Class I preparations (Figure 38.6) (Procedure 38-2). Access to the proximal surfaces is obtained by preparing the occlusal surface for a Class I preparation first, then extending the preparation into the proximal area and dropping to create a box with a gingival wall and removing the proximal wall. The dentist must be careful to avoid damaging the adjacent proximal wall of the neighboring tooth.

The restorative material of choice is dependent on the size of the cavity to be restored. Many dentists place amalgam, but aesthetic dentistry and improvements in the composite resin and bonding materials have led other dentists to choose tooth-colored composite resins even for large Class II restorations. Due to the missing proximal wall or walls, the dentist must use a matrix system to create the proper shape and hold the material in place until the material is cured or set. (See Chapter 39 for a discussion of matrix systems.)

FIGURE 38.5
Typical Class I cavity preparation of a premolar.

FIGURE 38.6
Typical Class II cavity preparation of a premolar.

Procedure 38-1 Assisting with a Class I Restoration

Equipment and Supplies

- Restorative tray for appropriate dental material to be used including basic setup, hand cutting instruments, amalgam carrier, condensers, burnishers, carvers, plastic instrument, and articulating paper holder
- Local anesthetic setup (Some patients do not require anesthetic.)
- Dental dam setup (Some dentists do not use the dental dam.)
- High-volume evacuator (HVE) and saliva ejector
- High-speed and low-speed rotary handpieces
- Burs, often in a block (Each dentist has preferences.)
- Cotton products (pellets, rolls, 2 × 2 gauze squares, dry angles)
- Dental liner, base, bonding agent, and caries indicator dye
- Permanent restorative material of choice
- Articulating paper
- Polishing items
- Dental floss

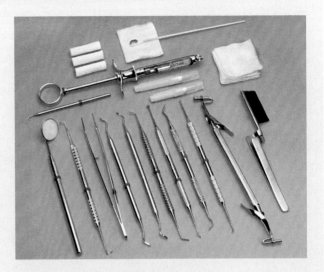

Assistant tray setup for a Class I restoration.

Procedure Steps

Assisting for a Class I Composite Restoration	Assisting for a Class I Amalgam Restoration
1. Deliver mouth mirror and explorer to dentist. (Dentist must examine tooth to be restored.)	1. Deliver mouth mirror and explorer to dentist. (Dentist must examine tooth to be restored.)
2. Assist dentist in the delivery of anesthetic, topical and local.	2. Assist dentist in the delivery of anesthetic, topical and local.
3. Place isolation items, cotton rolls, or dental dam (state permitting).	3. Place isolation items, cotton rolls, or dental dam (state permitting).
4. Deliver mouth mirror to dentist and inform dentist of the type of bur on the handpiece.	4. Deliver mouth mirror to dentist and inform dentist of the type of bur on the handpiece.
5. Adjust the light, retract the patient's cheek or tongue, and use the HVE and air/water syringe to keep the working area clear for the dentist.	5. Adjust the light, retract the patient's cheek or tongue, and use the HVE and air/water syringe to keep the working area clear for the dentist.
6. Transfer the necessary instruments to the dentist during the preparation as needed.	6. Transfer the necessary instruments to the dentist during the preparation as needed.

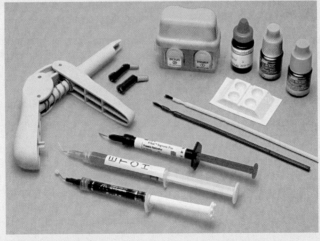

Dental materials setup.

continued on next page

Procedure 38-1 *continued from previous page*

Assisting for a Class I Composite Restoration	Assisting for a Class I Amalgam Restoration
7. Rinse and dry prepared tooth for the dentist to evaluate.	7. Rinse and dry prepared tooth for the dentist to evaluate.
8. Deliver caries indicator dye to the preparation, wait, rinse, and dry. (Repeat until tooth is clear of caries.)	8. Deliver caries indicator dye to the preparation, wait, rinse, and dry. (Repeat until tooth is clear of caries.)
9. If the preparation requires a base or liner, mix and deliver to the dentist.	9. If the preparation requires a base or liner, mix and deliver to the dentist.

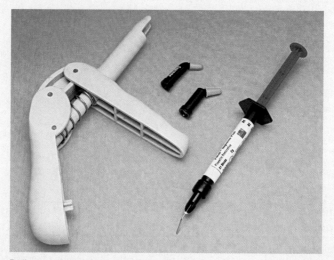

Delivery systems for composite resin.

10. Deliver etch and rinse. Then deliver bond and light cure.	10. Activate amalgam capsule and triturate.
11. Place an appropriate amount of composite resin on a paper pad and protect from light.	11. Fill the smaller end of the amalgam carrier and transfer to the dentist. The dentist may want both ends of the carrier filled. Alternate the condenser with the carrier. Continue to supply the dentist with more amalgam until the preparation is slightly overfilled.
12. Deliver the composite to the dentist with the composite placement instrument of the dentist's choice. The dentist will add material in increments, each followed by use of the curing light.	12. Exchange the condenser for the burnisher so the dentist can burnish the excess mercury to the tooth surface.
13. The dentist will use a high-speed handpiece with finishing burs to carve the restoration.	13. Deliver the carving instruments of dentist's choice until the restoration is complete.
14. The dental assistant will continue to use the HVE to remove particles and for retraction during the continued occlusal adjustments and finishing of the composite.	14. The dental assistant will continue to use the HVE to remove particles and for retraction during the continued carving and burnishing.
15. The assistant must still use the HVE to remove any pieces of composite as well as continue to retract the cheek, lip, or tongue.	15. The assistant must still use the HVE to remove any pieces of amalgam as well as continue to retract the cheek, lip, or tongue.
16. Remove all cotton and the dental dam. Rinse and dry the area.	16. Remove all cotton and the dental dam. Rinse and dry the area.
17. Place articulating paper between the maxillary and mandibular teeth to check the occlusion. The dentist will continue to adjust the occlusion until the bite is correct. Heavy colored marks will appear on the restoration in areas needing adjustment.	17. Place articulating paper between the maxillary and mandibular teeth to check the occlusion. The patient should bite down carefully and gently so as to not fracture the new restoration. The dentist will continue to adjust the occlusion until the bite is correct. Heavy colored marks will appear on the restoration in areas needing adjustment.

continued on next page

Procedure 38-1 *continued from previous page*

Assisting for a Class I Composite Restoration	Assisting for a Class I Amalgam Restoration
18. Inform the patient the composite material is cured and chewing is possible immediately.	18. Inform the patient not to chew on that side of his mouth. The amalgam will continue to harden for several hours after placement.
19. If the patient received anesthetic, inform her to avoid chewing until the anesthetic is gone so as to avoid biting her cheeks or tongue.	19. If the patient received anesthetic, inform him to avoid chewing until the anesthetic is gone so as to avoid biting his cheeks or tongue.
20. Inform the patient to call the office if she finds her occlusion is incorrect. She will need to return to the office for an occlusal adjustment.	20. Inform the patient to call the office if he finds his occlusion is incorrect. He will need to return to the office for an occlusal adjustment.

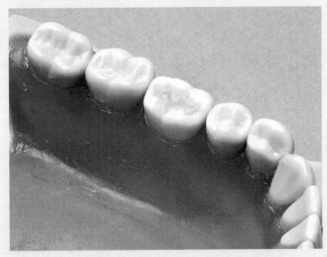

Composite restoration.

What should the dental assistant do if the new restoration breaks during the final carving and polishing?

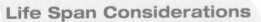

Life Span Considerations

Amalgam has proven to last numerous decades when placed in an appropriate environment. The patient must have excellent oral hygiene to prevent recurrent decay around the amalgam restoration. Composite resin dental material is relatively new compared to amalgam. Composite has greatly improved over time. The longevity of the new generations of composite is speculated to be longer than that of amalgam when placed in an ideal environment with excellent oral hygiene. The speculation is due to the fact that composites are improving with each new generation and research has only four decades of history. Research and development continues to provide the best materials to restore teeth to their proper form and function.

Class III and IV Restorations

Class III and IV preparations and restorations occur on the anterior teeth. Class III involves the proximal surfaces, whereas Class IV involves not only the proximal surface but the incisal edge as well. Class III preparations and restorations often require access to the caries through the facial or, more often, the lingual surface of the tooth (Figure 38.7).

As with Class II restorations, Class III restorations are named by the two surfaces included in the restoration. For example, caries on the mesial of tooth #8 will require access from the lingual and is known as a mesiolingual

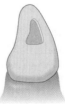

FIGURE 38.7
Typical Class III preparation of an anterior tooth.

Procedure 38-2 Assisting with a Class II Restoration

Supplies and Equipment

- Restorative tray for appropriate dental material to be used including basic setup, hand cutting instruments, amalgam carrier, condensers, burnishers, carvers, plastic instrument, and articulating paper holder
- Local anesthetic setup (Some patients do not require anesthetic.)
- Dental dam setup (Some doctors do not use the dental dam.)
- High-volume evacuator (HVE) and saliva ejector
- High-speed and low-speed rotary handpieces
- Burs, often in a block (Each dentist has preferences.)
- Cotton products (pellets, rolls, 2 × 2 gauze squares, dry angles)
- Matrix system setup
- Dental liner, base, bonding agent, and caries indicator dye
- Permanent restorative material of choice
- Articulating paper
- Polishing items
- Dental floss

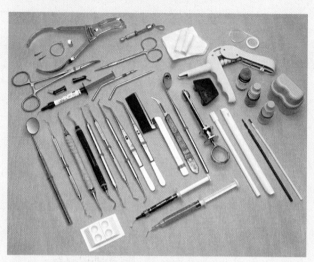

Assistant tray setup for composite restoration.

Procedure Steps

Assisting for a Class II Composite Restoration	Assisting for a Class II Amalgam Restoration
1. Deliver mouth mirror and explorer to dentist. (Dentist must examine tooth to be restored.)	1. Deliver mouth mirror and explorer to dentist. (Dentist must examine tooth to be restored.)
2. Assist dentist in the delivery of anesthetic, topical and local.	2. Assist dentist in the delivery of anesthetic, topical and local.
3. Place isolation items, cotton rolls, dry angle, or dental dam (state permitting).	3. Place isolation items, cotton rolls, dry angle, or dental dam (state permitting).
4. Deliver mouth mirror to dentist and inform dentist of the type of bur on the handpiece.	4. Deliver mouth mirror to dentist and inform dentist of the type of bur on the handpiece.
5. Adjust the light, retract the patient's cheek or tongue, and use the HVE and air/water syringe to keep the working area clear for the dentist.	5. Adjust the light, retract the patient's cheek or tongue, and use the HVE and air/water syringe to keep the working area clear for the dentist.
6. Transfer the necessary instruments to the dentist during the preparation as needed.	6. Transfer the necessary instruments to the dentist during the preparation as needed.
7. Rinse and dry prepared tooth for the dentist to evaluate.	7. Rinse and dry prepared tooth for the dentist to evaluate.
8. Deliver caries indicator dye to the preparation, wait, rinse, and dry. (Repeat until tooth is clear of caries.)	8. Deliver caries indicator dye to the preparation, wait, rinse, and dry. (Repeat until tooth is clear of caries.)
9. Deliver to the dentist the matrix system of the dentist's choice. If state regulations permit, the dental assistant may place the matrix system.	9. Deliver to the dentist the matrix system of the dentist's choice. If state regulations permit, the dental assistant may place the matrix system.
10. If the preparation requires a base or liner, mix and deliver to the dentist.	10. If the preparation requires a base or liner, mix and deliver to the dentist.
11. Deliver etch and rinse. Then deliver bond and light cure.	11. Activate amalgam capsule and triturate.

continued on next page

Procedure 38-2 *continued from previous page*

Assisting for a Class II Composite Restoration	Assisting for a Class II Amalgam Restoration
12. Place an appropriate amount of composite resin on a paper pad and protect from light.	12. Fill the smaller end of the amalgam carrier and transfer to the dentist. The dentist may want both ends of the carrier filled. Alternate the condenser with the carrier. Continue to supply the dentist with more amalgam until the preparation is slightly overfilled.
13. Deliver the composite to the dentist with the composite placement instrument of the dentist's choice. The dentist will add material in increments, each followed by use of the curing light.	13. Exchange the condenser for the burnisher so the dentist can burnish the excess mercury to the tooth surface.

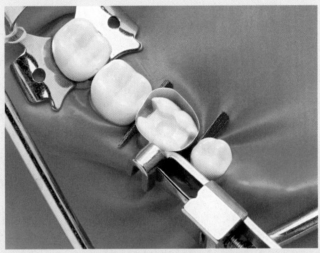

Condensing of composite resin into a Class II cavity.

14. The dentist will use a high-speed handpiece with finishing burs to carve the restoration.	14. Deliver the carving instruments of dentist's choice until the restoration is complete.

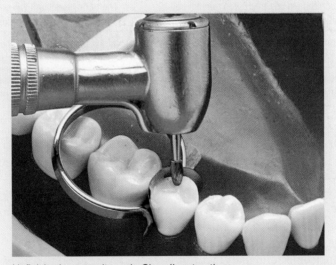

Unfinished composite resin Class II restoration.

15. The assistant must still use the HVE to remove any pieces of composite as well as continue to retract the cheek, lip, or tongue.	15. The assistant must still use the HVE to remove any pieces of amalgam as well as continue to retract the cheek, lip, or tongue.

continued on next page

Procedure 38-2 *continued from previous page*

Assisting for a Class II Composite Restoration	Assisting for a Class II Amalgam Restoration
16. Remove all cotton and the dental dam. Rinse and dry the area.	16. Remove all cotton and the dental dam. Rinse and dry the area.
17. Place articulating paper between the maxillary and mandibular teeth to check the occlusion. The patient should bite down carefully and gently so as to not fracture the new restoration, especially when the marginal ridge is too high. The dentist will continue to adjust the occlusion until the bite is correct. Heavy colored marks will appear on the restoration in areas needing adjustment.	17. Place articulating paper between the maxillary and mandibular teeth to check the occlusion. The patient should bite down carefully and gently so as to not fracture the new restoration. The dentist will continue to adjust the occlusion until the bite is correct. Heavy colored marks will appear on the restoration in areas needing adjustment.

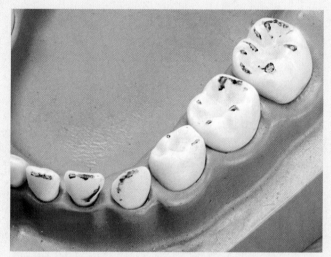

Marks created by use of articulating paper to mark areas for occlusal adjustment.

18. The dental assistant will continue to use the HVE to remove particles and for retraction during the continued carving.	18. The dental assistant will continue to use the HVE to remove particles and for retraction during the continued carving.
19. Inform the patient the composite material is cured and chewing is possible immediately.	19. Inform the patient not to chew on that side of his mouth. The amalgam will continue to harden for several hours after placement.
20. If the patient received anesthetic, inform her to avoid chewing until the anesthetic is gone so as to avoid biting her cheeks or tongue.	20. If the patient received anesthetic, inform him to avoid chewing until the anesthetic is gone so as to avoid biting his cheeks or tongue.
21. Inform the patient to call the office if she finds her occlusion is incorrect. She will need to return to the office for an occlusal adjustment.	21. Inform the patient to call the office if he finds his occlusion is incorrect. He will need to return to the office for an occlusal adjustment.

(ML) restoration of tooth #8. If the same caries involved the incisal edge of tooth #8, the Class IV restoration would be an incisomesiolingual (IML). It is more common to find a Class IV restoration involving both facial or labial and lingual surfaces wrapping over the missing incisal edge plus a proximal surface, making a four-surface restoration (Figure 38.8). Once again, the dentist must be careful not to damage the adjacent proximal surface of the neighboring tooth. A preparation

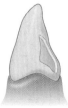

FIGURE 38.8
Typical Class IV preparation of an anterior tooth.

from the lingual helps to minimize the need to restore the aesthetic facial surface. Occasionally, it is impossible to avoid removing and repairing the facial surface of the anterior teeth.

The dentist will use composite resin to repair the aesthetic zone (Figure 38.9. Shade selection is very important when restoring the anterior teeth; also see Chapter 33 on dental materials). The dentist carefully manipulates the composite resin so that its form emulates that of the natural tooth. The matrix system used is known as mylar, a very thin plastic tape-like strip placed between the teeth and secured with a wedge (Figure 38.10). This clear matrix allows the curing light to penetrate through the matrix and into the composite resin for curing. Once cured, the restoration is finished and polished. There are numerous composite finishing systems. Typically, dentists have a preference for a particular finishing system.

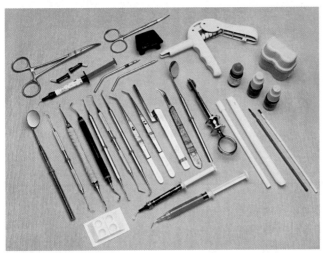

FIGURE 38.9
Composite resin tray setup.

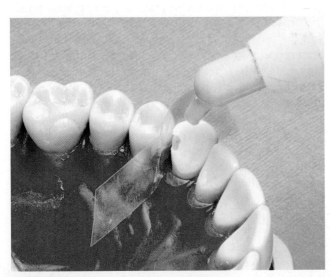

FIGURE 38.10
Placement of composite resin Class III restoration.

Class V and VI Restorations

Class V preparations and restorations are found on the gingival third of the facial or lingual surfaces of all teeth (Figure 38.11). These are one-surface cavities named for that same surface. For example, a Class V cavity on the buccal of #20 is called a buccal class V cavity, preparation, or restoration of tooth #20. Class V cavities may extend below the free gingival margin and disappear underneath the tissue. This gingival tissue will need to be retracted to access the caries, obtain visibility, and control moisture and hemorrhage. The dentist will have a protocol for this clinical situation such as a retraction cord or dental dam.

Class VI preparations and restorations are found on the incisal edge of anterior teeth or the occlusal cusp height of posterior teeth (Figure 38.12). This is also a one-surface preparation and restoration that is named for the surface affected. All dentists will use a composite resin material to restore incisal edges of the anterior teeth, but some dentists will use amalgam to restore the cusp tips of posterior teeth. The dental assistant uses the same setup for Class V and VI restorations as for the Class I restorations. See Procedure 38-1 to review these steps. (For more information on various matrix systems used in Class VI preparations, see Chapter 39.)

Veneers and Bonding

A **veneer** is a thin layer of tooth-colored composite resin or laboratory-created porcelain applied to the facial surface of a tooth. Placement of a chairside veneer is more commonly known as **bonding** or placing a *direct veneer,*

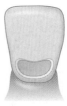

FIGURE 38.11
Class V cavity preparation.

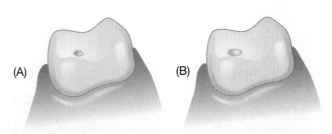

(A)　　　　　(B)

FIGURE 38.12
Class VI cavity preparation: (a) showing exposed dentin on mesiofacial cusp and (b) preparation of Class VI cavity.

Preparing for Externship

Discuss with your new dentist the materials and instruments she or he prefers for each of the classes of restorations. Be prepared before the first patient. Each dentist practices differently depending on the individual's education and continued education. Offices with multiple dentists will be more challenging to the dental assistant because each dentist has her or his own philosophy concerning preparations and dental materials. Again, always ask if you do not know what the dentist needs for each procedure.

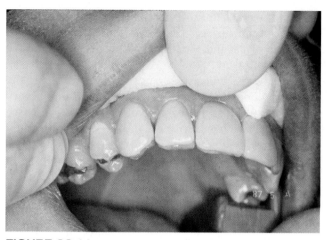

FIGURE 38.14
Teeth after bonding material has been placed.
Image courtesy Instructional Materials for the Dental Team, Lex., KY

as discussed in Chapter 33. For the purpose of this section, the procedure for assisting with chairside bonding is the priority. (See Procedure 38-3.) See Chapter 40 for further information on laboratory-created porcelain veneers. The chairside veneer is primarily an aesthetic procedure (Figures 38.13 and 38.14). Patients often request bonding, and dentists recommend bonding to:

- repair a tooth
- hide a defect on a tooth
- change the color of a tooth
- give the optical illusion of having straighter teeth
- close a space or **diastema**

Occasionally, the dentist prepares the tooth or teeth to allow removal of an imperfection or to allow for the necessary thickness of the composite material. It is important for the dental assistant to maintain a dry working field while the dentist is working. Bonding must be placed in a dry environment to obtain proper bonding of the composite resin to the tooth surface.

When placing bonding, the dentist uses various shades or colors of composite. It is helpful for the dental

assistant to manage the numerous shades the dentist has selected. Placement of bonding is a true skill. The dentist must sculpt the composite resin to emulate natural tooth color and form.

Tooth Whitening

Tooth **whitening** is the process of brightening stained, discolored teeth with in-office or at-home systems. Whitening is a simple means to rejuvenate a smile. The primary reasons to whiten teeth include:

- to reduce extrinsic stains, that is, stains from foods and liquids such as mustard, tea, and coffee
- to reduce the yellowing caused by the aging of teeth
- to reduce intrinsic stains such as those that result from the use of tetracycline and/or too much fluoride

Each and every patient will have a different response to whitening. The procedure is not guaranteed or permanent. The informed consent that the patient signs before the procedure should state this. The length of treatment and the longevity of the result are also variable. It has been reported that some severe intrinsic staining can be removed with lengthy use of at-home professional whitening products, but most patients need the one-time in-office procedure or a short two- to three-week use of an at-home professional product to obtain their goal. Most patients will need touch-up to the whitening depending on their eating, drinking, and other oral habits. (For more information on dental stains and polishing, see Chapter 48.)

In-office tooth whitening can typically be accomplished in just one hour. This procedure is ideal for the patient who desires a whiter smile in a very short period of time. For example, an important event like a wedding or reunion will cause a patient to want a whiter smile quickly. Patients must be informed, however, that the final shade cannot be determined prior to the procedure.

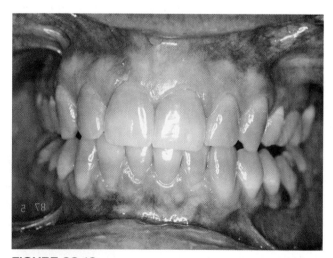

FIGURE 38.13
Discolored teeth before bonding.
Image courtesy Instructional Materials for the Dental Team, Lex., KY

Procedure 38-3 Assisting with a Chairside Veneer

Equipment and Supplies

- Restorative tray for appropriate dental material to be used including basic setup, hand cutting instruments, condensers, carvers, plastic instrument, articulating paper holder, patient safety glasses
- Local anesthetic setup (Some patients do not require anesthetic.)
- Dental dam setup (Some doctors do not use the dental dam.)
- High-volume evacuator (HVE) and saliva ejector
- High-speed and low-speed rotary handpieces
- Curing light and protective shield
- Burs, often in a block (Each dentist has preferences.)
- Cotton products (pellets, rolls, 2 × 2 gauze squares)
- Delivery brushes and mixing wells
- Mylar matrix system
- Composite resin shade guide
- Dental liner, base, etch, bonding agent, and caries indicator dye
- Permanent restorative (composite resin and delivery gun)
- Dental floss
- Articulating paper
- Finishing carbide burs
- Polishing items including abrasive strips, discs, cups, and polishing paste

Procedure Steps

1. Shade selection. The dentist may choose several shades to emulate the various areas of natural teeth.

2. Assist in the delivery of topical and local anesthetic if necessary.

3. Place moisture control items such as cotton rolls and dental dam (state permitting).

4. Deliver mouth mirror to dentist and inform dentist of the type of bur on the handpiece.

5. Adjust the light, retract the patient's lip, and use the HVE and air/water syringe to keep the working area clear for the dentist.

6. Transfer the necessary instruments to the dentist during the preparation as needed.

7. Rinse and dry prepared tooth for the dentist to evaluate.

8. Place mylar matrix system.

9. When placing composite resin, deliver etch and rinse. Then deliver bond and light cure.

10. Place an appropriate amount of composite resin on a paper pad and protect from light. Numerous shades may be used. Manage the materials carefully so as to give the dentist the correct shade at the correct moment.

11. Pass the dentist the instrument of choice for composite material. The plastic instrument is the most often utilized.

12. Have bonding agent available. The dentist may use a bonding agent to help manipulate the material.

13. Due to the thin layer, the composite may or may not be cured in layers. The dentist will give direction as to when to light cure.

14. The dentist will use a high-speed handpiece with finishing burs to carve the restoration.

15. The low-speed handpiece is used with a mandrel or attachment to place the final polish.

16. The assistant must still use the HVE to remove any pieces of composite as well as continue to retract the lip.

17. Remove all cotton and the dental dam. Rinse and dry the area.

18. Provide a large mirror for the patient to approve the restoration.

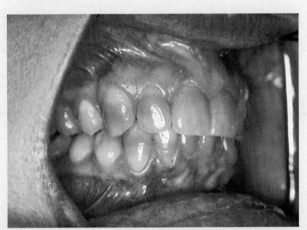

(A)

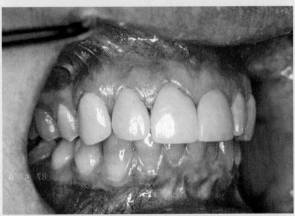

(B)

(a) Before placement of veneers and (b) after placement of veneers.
Images courtesy Instructional Materials for the Dental Team, Lex., KY

continued on next page

Procedure 38-3 *continued from previous page*

19. If the patient received anesthetic, inform her to avoid chewing until the anesthetic is gone so as to avoid biting her lips.

20. Provide the patient with oral hygiene instructions and advise her of the need to keep regular dental visits to help maintain the new veneers.

21. Inform the patient that composite resin will stain over time with the foods and liquids she eats and drinks.

22. Chairside veneers have limited longevity. They may chip and wear over time. Inform the patient to never bite into hard items such as ice or hard candy—such actions can fracture the bonding.

Steps for the in-office procedure are as follows:

• The gingivae are isolated by means of a dental dam, and/or a light-reflective resin barrier is used that is applied to the junction of the tooth with the gingivae to prevent the whitening material from touching the tissue.

• A very high-concentration whitening agent is applied to the facial surface of the teeth.

• A high-intensity light or laser is used to amplify the ability of the whitening agent.

Some controversy surrounds the use of high-intensity lights and lasers. The dental assistant needs to know the dentist's policy concerning the use of high-concentration whitening materials with high-intensity lights and lasers. It is also helpful to read the latest dental journals concerning these materials and procedures.

At-home whitening procedures are very common and may be professional or store bought. The at-home professional materials and procedures have been tested and proven to be efficient with great results. Once again, each patient will have an individual result. This procedure usually takes 10 to 14 days of use to achieve the desired result.

Legal and Ethical Issues

Each and every procedure should require the patient to sign a consent form for treatment. The patient must be fully informed of the procedure and the dental material to be used. Legal issues arise when the patient is not informed of all pros and cons, especially concerning the materials placed in the patient's mouth. It is the patient's right to be informed. The dental assistant often gives the patient the consent form while waiting for the dentist to enter the operatory. The patient will ask the assistant questions concerning the treatment. Be prepared to answer the patient's questions. If you do not know the answer, wait for the dentist. The signed consent for treatment form is to be kept with the patient's legal dental record.

Steps to using at-home professional whitening materials are:

• A custom tray is made from a model of the patient's teeth.

• The patient is provided with tubes of peroxide-based gel for application into the custom-fitted tray.

• The patient is instructed to wear the trays with the gel for a period of time based on the manufacturer's suggested use. Some gels require the tray to be worn for 30 minutes, whereas other gels are meant to be in place overnight.

Patients must be informed that they may experience some sensitivity with the use of any whitening product. As part of the verbal instructions and consent process, patients must be told to stop use of the whitening product immediately if they experience sensitivity. The use of a desensitizing toothpaste or a rinse containing fluoride will improve the condition. Once the sensitivity problem has improved, patients may continue use of the whitening product. If the sensitivity is severe, patients should be told to call the dental office.

Patients should also be informed that it is possible to overwhiten the teeth. This causes transparency of the enamel, giving the teeth a gray or blue appearance. The transparency is most often due to prolonged use of at-home whitening trays where the patient is in control of their use. Therefore, the patient must be aware of the proper use of the products.

The preparatory appointment for at-home whitening can be with the dental assistant, but the dentist must first examine the patient to confirm the patient is a good candidate for a whitening procedure. Prior to performing any duties, dental assistants must be clear on what duties are allowed by the state in which they practice. Typical duties performed during the preparatory appointment include the following:

1. The assistant informs the patient of the pros and cons of the procedure and provides the patient with the consent form.

2. An initial shade is taken in natural light and noted in the patient chart (Figure 38.15).

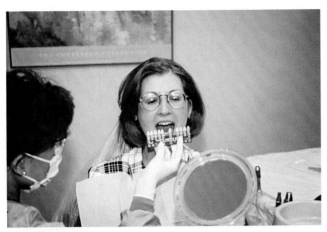

FIGURE 38.15
Dental assistant matching the patient's teeth to the shade guide to record initial shade of the teeth prior to whitening.
Image courtesy Instructional Materials for the Dental Team, Lex., KY

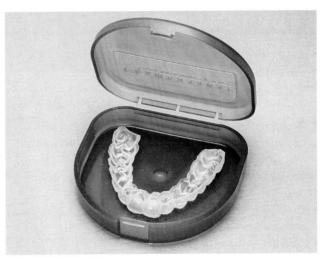

FIGURE 38.16
Custom whitening tray.

3. The assistant takes the impression for the tray models, usually with alginate impression material.

4. The patient is scheduled to pick up the whitening materials at a later date.

5. In the laboratory, the dental assistant pours stone into the models.

6. Once set, the models are trimmed and blockout material is placed on the facial surface of teeth to be whitened. This blockout material provides a well in the final tray so that the gel sits against the facial surface of each tooth.

7. With the use of the vacuum former, the tray material is pulled over the model and then trimmed to form the final whitening tray (Figure 38.16).

The appointment during which the patient picks up the whitening materials can also be with the dental assistant:

1. The patient tries the trays in his or her mouth to check for rough or sharp areas.

2. The dental assistant verbally goes over the at-home instructions.

3. The dental assistant shows the patient how much gel to place in each well of the tray.

4. The patient is scheduled to return for a shade check in approximately five to seven days to see if progress is being made.

5. During the return appointment, compare the initial shade taken on the day of the impressions with the new shade and show the patient the progress in the mirror.

Numerous over-the-counter materials for whitening teeth are available. These products are not as effective in achieving the change in shade as professional products administered and monitored by dentists. These products come in various forms including strips, brush-on whitening, and trays with preloaded gel. Most of these products have some benefit for patients and may be useful in certain situations.

SUMMARY

The most common procedures in the general dental office are the standardized Class I through VI restorations. It is important for the dental assistant to be able to recognize the procedure, prepare the operatory and patient for the procedure, and assist the dentist. The dentist relies on the dental assistant for support during these procedures.

Amalgam or composite resin is used in Class I, II, and V restorations, but aesthetics are kept in mind with the anterior teeth. Therefore, Class III, IV, and VI restorations require the use of composite resin to match the natural tooth structure.

Chairside veneers have become increasingly popular to change the shade, shape, or alignment of teeth. Bonding agents and composite resin are used to create a more aesthetic smile. In the last 20 years, the public has desired whiter teeth. Today, several methods are available for obtaining a whiter smile. In-office and at-home professional products are recommended by dental professionals to achieve the best result, although store-bought products are also available.

The changes seen in dentistry since G. V. Black developed the initial classification system for cavity preparations and restorations have been tremendous and will continue at a greater rate in the future.

KEY TERMS

- **Aesthetic dentistry:** Operative dentistry to emulate natural beauty; cosmetic dentistry.   p. 597
- **Axial wall:** Internal surface of a cavity preparation positioned parallel to the long axis of the tooth.   p. 598
- **Bonding:** Tooth-colored resin composite that is bonded, sculpted, hardened, and polished to tooth surfaces; usually used for aesthetic purposes.   p. 607
- **Cavity wall:** One of several walls of a cavity preparation.   p. 598
- **Diastema:** Space between two teeth; place where adjacent surfaces do not touch.   p. 608
- **Line angle:** Junction of two surfaces in a cavity preparation; cavity line angle.   p. 598
- **Operative dentistry:** Common term for restorative or aesthetic dentistry that restores decayed or defective teeth to proper form and function.   p. 597
- **Outline form:** The shape of the area of a cavity preparation.   p. 597
- **Pulpal wall:** The internal surface of a cavity preparation positioned perpendicular to the pulp of the tooth; the floor of the preparation.   p. 598
- **Restoration:** Measures taken to return a defective tooth to proper form and function with the use of a dental material.   p. 597
- **Restorative dentistry:** Area of dentistry that restores decayed or defective teeth to proper form and function; an area of operative dentistry.   p. 597
- **Retention form:** The shape of a cavity preparation; designed to prevent displacement of the dental material.   p. 597
- **Veneer:** Ultrathin layer of composite resin or porcelain bonded to the facial surface of teeth.   p. 607
- **Whitening:** Process of brightening stained, discolored teeth with in-office or at-home systems.   p. 608

CHECK YOUR UNDERSTANDING

1. Retentive notches and grooves are placed during which phase of cavity preparation?
   a. initial phase
   b. final phase
   c. notches and grooves are not required in cavity preparation
   d. both a and b

2. It is the responsibility of the dental assistant to
   a. be familiar with the procedure, materials, and instruments.
   b. prepare the instruments and materials to be used for the procedure.
   c. transfer dental hand instruments to the dentist.
   d. help to comfort the patient at all times.
   e. all of the above.

3. Class I cavities and restorations are found in all of the following locations except
   a. occlusal pits and fissures of the posterior molars.
   b. lingual pits of the maxillary incisors.
   c. buccal pits of the mandibular molars.
   d. between the anterior teeth.

4. Class V cavities and restorations are found
   a. on the incisal edges.
   b. on the occlusal cusp tips of molars.
   c. in the interproximal areas of anterior teeth.
   d. at the gingival third on the buccal and lingual surfaces of any teeth.

5. Chairside veneers give the same result as placing composite resin as bonding on the facial surface of teeth. What materials are needed to place chairside veneers or bonding?
   a. composite in numerous shades
   b. polishing system
   c. bonding system
   d. curing light
   e. all of the above

6. Bonding is used to
   a. improve the color of teeth.
   b. change the shape of teeth.
   c. close spaces between teeth.
   d. better align teeth.
   e. all of the above.

7. The patient can expect all of the following from bonding except
   a. limited longevity.
   b. staining potential.
   c. risk of chipping and fracture.
   d. poor cosmetic results.

8. Placement of Class III and IV restorations requires all of the following except
   a. Tofflemire matrix.
   b. composite resin.
   c. bonding agent.
   d. shade guide.
   e. polishing kit.

CHECK YOUR UNDERSTANDING (continued)

9. Professional whitening is used to remove all of the following types of stains except
   a. extrinsic stains from coffee, tea, and spaghetti sauce.
   b. staining of composite veneers.
   c. intrinsic stains from antibiotics.
   d. yellowing due to age.

10. Over-the-counter whitening products are
   a. ineffective.
   b. useful in certain situations.
   c. available in tray delivery systems only.
   d. damaging to tooth structure.

● INTERNET ACTIVITY

- Visit www.ada.org and find the video titled "Whiter Teeth (full-length)." Click and download the video. The dentist featured in the video is Dr. Jeff Morley, a cofounder of the American Academy of Cosmetic Dentistry.

● WEB REFERENCES

- About Cosmetic Dentistry   www.aboutcosmeticdentistry.com
- Academy of General Dentistry www.agd.org
- American Academy of Cosmetic Dentistry www.aacd.org
- American Dental Association www.ada.org
- Pierre Fauchard Academy www.fauchard.org

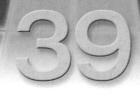

Matrix Systems
for Restorative Dentistry

Chapter Outline

- Posterior Matrix Systems
  - —Tofflemire Retainer
  - —Matrix Bands
  - —Wedges
- Anterior Matrix Systems
- Alternative Matrix Systems
  - —Automatrix System
  - —Sectional Matrices
  - —Anterior and Cervical Matrix Bands
  - —Other Matrix Systems for Primary Teeth

Learning Objectives

After reading this chapter, the student should be able to:

- Explain the application for a matrix system and discuss the universal matrix system.
- Identify the components of a Tofflemire retainer.
- Discuss the purpose of matrix bands and wedges.
- Describe the matrix systems available for anterior restorations.
- Compare the matrix systems for anterior teeth versus posterior teeth.
- Identify alternative matrix systems.
- Discuss the process for using an automatrix system.
- Discuss the process for using a sectional matrix.
- Identify the matrix systems utilized for pediatric patients.

Preparing for Certification Exams

- Assemble the retainer and matrix band.
- Identify the components of the Tofflemire retainer.
- Identify the various matrix systems.
- Place and remove the various matrix systems.

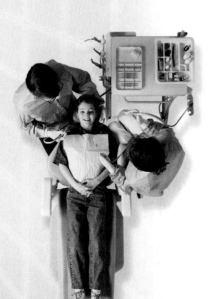

Key Terms

Automatrix

Celluloid strip

Matrix band

Matrix system

Mylar

Sectional matrix

Tofflemire retainer

Universal retainer

Wedge

Once a tooth has been prepared into a Class II, III, or IV cavity preparation (which means at least one of the interproximal walls is missing), a device must be placed to hold the material to the tooth in order to restore the tooth. Otherwise, the restorative material could not be controlled to re-create the natural form of the tooth. The device used to help the dentist to restore the proper form is known as a **matrix system.**

The matrix system's primary function is to restore anatomic contours and contact to the proximal tooth. Other capabilities that must be present in a matrix system are the ability to prevent impingement of restorative material on the gingival tissue and to create a smooth external surface.

Numerous matrix systems are available on the market. The qualities of these systems include rigidity for support of the restorative material and ease of application and removal.

In several states, the placement and removal of any matrix system is a procedure that can be performed by the dental assistant.

Posterior Matrix Systems

For the restoration of Class II posterior cavities, the most commonly used matrix system in the United States is the Tofflemire retainer and matrix band. Similar retainers are used throughout the world. As part of the tray setup for a Class II restoration, the dental assistant should have the matrix system assembled prior to beginning the procedure.

Dental Assistant PROFESSIONAL TIP

The setup and use of a Tofflemire system can be difficult and frustrating. Practice placing the matrix in the retainer often for different areas of the mouth. Do not show your frustration to the patient. If you need help, seek someone in the office to assist you. It is appropriate to place the matrix in the retainer as part of the setup tray prior to seating the patient.

Patient Education

After the use of a matrix to support a Class II restoration during placement, the amalgam will remain somewhat soft for several hours. The dental assistant must inform the patient to be very careful when eating for approximately 24 hours so as not to fracture the new amalgam restoration. The patient should avoid any hard or crunchy foods for 24 hours. If a composite resin is placed as a Class II restoration, the filling is very hard once light cured. The patient should call the dental office if the occlusion is too tall or high and make an appointment for an occlusal adjustment.

Tofflemire Retainer

The **Tofflemire retainer** or **universal retainer** is the mechanism used to hold the matrix band in position. The three styles of Tofflemire retainers are each used for specific circumstances. The universal retainer is usually positioned on the buccal side of the tooth, although it is possible to place the retainer on the lingual surface in special circumstances (Figure 39.1a). Should the Class II preparation

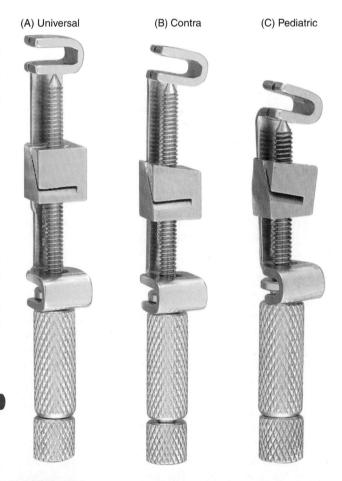

(A) Universal   (B) Contra   (C) Pediatric

FIGURE 39.1
Examples of Tofflemire retainers: (a) universal retainer, (b) contra-angle retainer, and (c) pediatric retainer.
Courtesy Miltex Inc.

TABLE 39-1 Anatomy of the Tofflemire Retainer

Outer knob	Locks the matrix band into place by tightening the spindle within the locking vise. • Hold the retainer with the U guides up. • *To tighten the band* into the retainer, turn the short knob away from you. • *To loosen the band* or locking vise, turn the short knob toward you. If the spindle comes out of the locking vise, simply place the tip of the spindle toward the access hole of the locking device and turn the short knob away from you.
Inner knob	Increases or decreases the size of the loop. When placing the band around the tooth, the smaller circumference of the band is in contact with the gingiva, and the long knob is tightened to decrease the size of the loop so that it is snug around the tooth.
Locking vise	A sliding body that holds the band and contacts the spindle to the band firmly. Contains a diagonal slot for the ends of the band. The diagonal slot faces the gingiva when placed on the tooth.
Spindle	Screw that fits into the locking vise to be tightened to hold the band firmly. When placing the band into the diagonal slot, the spindle must not be in the slot.
Head with three U-shaped guides	Positions the band for best access in placement of the matrix system on the tooth and access to the preparation.

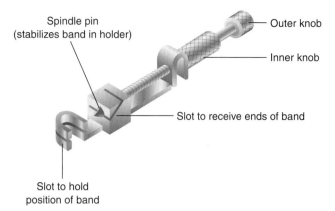

FIGURE 39.2
Anatomy of a Tofflemire retainer.

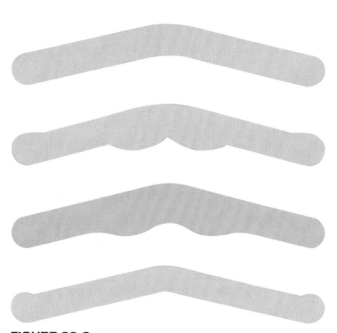

FIGURE 39.3
Common shapes of Tofflemire matrix bands.
Courtesy Miltex Inc.

require the loss of the buccal surface, the contra-angle retainer is designed to accommodate the lingual positioning (Figure 39.1b). A pediatric size retainer is available for small patients (Figure 39.1c). Table 39-1 and Figure 39.2 detail the anatomy of a Tofflemire retainer.

Matrix Bands

The **matrix band** is a strip or band placed so as to serve as a retaining outer wall that supports the restorative material to re-create proper form and function for the tooth. The bands used with the Tofflemire retainers are usually made of stainless steel, but titanium bands are also available. Other bands are celluloid or transparent plastic used for other types of restorations and materials. The stainless steel matrix bands most commonly used are the universal, extension, and pediatric bands (Figure 39.3).

The thickness of the universal matrix band is quite important. They may be as thin as 0.038 mm or much thicker for more rigidity. The universal band is utilized for a Class II preparation of minimum dimensions. The extension band is needed for Class II preparations where the gingival wall extends extremely apical. In this case,

the universal band does not have enough height to clear the occlusal table. The wings of the extension band provide the extra height required for proper form.

To assemble the retainer and matrix band, the operator must know which tooth and surfaces are to be restored (Procedure 39-1). When the band is curved to create a loop, there will be two edges, the occlusal edge and the gingival edge (Figure 39.4):

• The gingival edge forms a smaller loop than the occlusal edge. The gingival loop is the edge that comes in contact with the gingiva and prevents the restorative material from impinging on the gingiva and into the embrasure space. The embrasure space is the triangular space created by the gingiva and the two walls of proximal teeth apical to the contact of these two teeth.

• The occlusal edge forms the larger loop and is the edge toward the occlusal surface of the tooth.

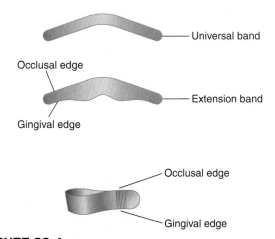

Universal band

Occlusal edge

Extension band

Gingival edge

Occlusal edge

Gingival edge

FIGURE 39.4
Matrix band formed into a loop.

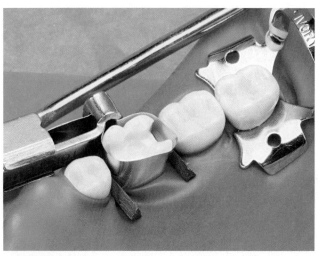

FIGURE 39.5
Wedge positioned from the lingual.

Prior to placement into the retainer, the band must be contoured to thin the band in the area of the interproximal contact. This will allow for an appropriate contact—one that is not too loose or too long. To contour the band, use a burnisher or the handle end of a mouth mirror and rub the inner surface of the band until the band begins to curl.

There are many choices for matrix systems. How do you decide what thickness of matrix band to use?

Wedges

When the matrix band is placed around the tooth, it alone does not provide the proper anatomic shape. A **wedge** is needed to provide the correct contour at the gingival edge. The wedge is usually triangular or anatomic in shape. This shape allows the wedge to fill the embrasure space and places pressure on the matrix to provide the proper contour for restoring Class II preparations. Cotton pliers are used to hold the wedge while it is being inserted into the embrasure space from the lingual or buccal aspect with light to moderate pressure (Figure 39.5).

Wedges come in numerous sizes and select shapes. The most common wedges are made of wood or plastic. There are even clear plastic wedges to aid in the placement of composite resin (Figure 39.6). Some considerations are important when selecting a wedge:

• It must be wide enough to place pressure on the apical and gingival walls of the Class II preparation.

• It must be slightly wider than the embrasure space to place enough pressure on the teeth so as to cause a slight separation of the teeth.

If the incorrect wedge is chosen, the proper contact and contour will not be achieved (Figure 39.7). When the wedge is too small, the band may not contact the wall of

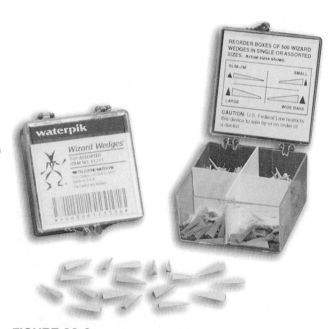

FIGURE 39.6
Numerous styles of wedges.
Courtesy Waterpik, Inc.

the tooth, creating a space for the material to flow between the tooth and the band beyond the gingival wall, hence impinging into the embrasure space and causing an overhang of the restoration. If the wedge is too large, it may create an indent in the matrix band and into the preparation box, causing cupping. Both situations result in an improper form for the restoration.

In many states, dental assistants and/or expanded duty dental assistants may legally place and remove the matrix system (see Procedure 39-2).

How do you secure a matrix for a Class II restoration when there is no adjacent tooth to the proximal box of the preparation?

Procedure 39-1 Preparing the Tofflemire Matrix System

Equipment and Supplies

- Basic setup: mouth mirror, explorer, cotton pliers, hemostat
- Tofflemire retainer
- Tofflemire matrix band
- Burnisher
- Paper pad
- Assortment of wedges

Procedure Steps

1. Examine the preparation with a mirror and note the location in the mouth and the depth of the proximal box.

2. Choose the type of matrix band to be used, for example, universal or extension. Consider the size of the tooth.

3. Burnish the middle of the band on a paper pad until the ends begin to curl to create a thinner area for proper contact. The spindle is released from the locking vise by turning the short knob toward yourself.

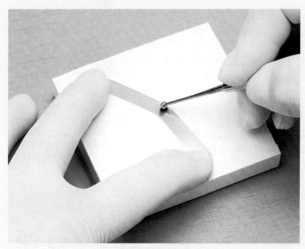

Contour the band until it begins to curl.

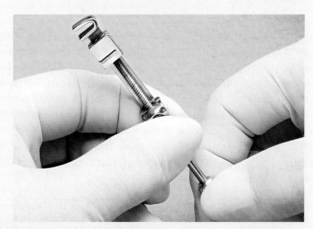

The spindle is released from the locking vise by turning the short knob toward yourself.

4. Hold the retainer so the diagonal slot and the U-guides are up. Turn the short knob away from you so the spindle is not visible in the diagonal slot.

5. Turn the long knob so the U-guides are close to the locking vise.

6. Make a loop with the band to form the occlusal and gingival edges. The occlusal edge is the larger of the two edges.

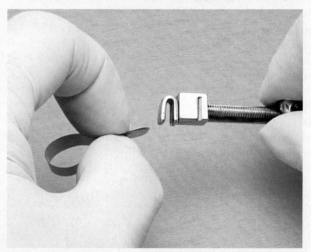

Fold band to form a loop and then place in the retainer, occlusal edge first.

7. With the diagonal slot of the retainer facing up, place the joined ends of the band into the diagonal slot of the locking vise, occlusal edge first.

8. Place the band into the proper guide slots. The location of the tooth to be restored determines which way to place the band into the guide slots, for example, maxillary, mandibular, right, or left.

9. Tighten the short knob to screw the spindle into the locking vise in order to hold the band in the retainer.

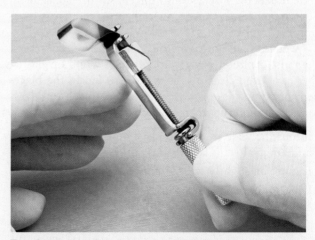

Turn the short knob to tighten the spindle into the locking vise.

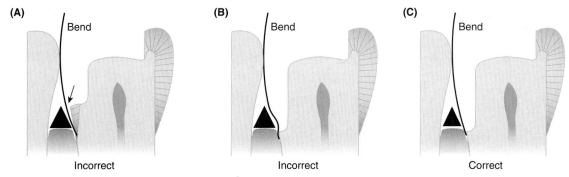

(A) Bend   Incorrect

(B) Bend   Incorrect

(C) Bend   Correct

FIGURE 39.7

Proper and improper placement of wedges: (a) A wedge too small for the embrasure space fails to place proper pressure against the band, allowing space for material to flow causing an overhang. (b) A wedge too large indents the band, creating a cupping effect. (c) The correct size wedge places proper pressure against the band and adjacent tooth.

Dental Assistant: Professional Tip

The practice of using Tofflemire retainers may last for a dentist's entire career, but dentistry is always evolving. New methods and materials are being developed at a rate of one every 18 months. In other words, some materials and instruments are obsolete within a year and a half. Most dentists cannot afford, or do not choose, to change their materials, instruments, or techniques that frequently. It is important, however, for the dentist and the dental assistant to be aware of the new technology, materials, and techniques. Reading industry journals and attending continuing education courses will help them accomplish this.

Anterior Matrix Systems

For the restoration of Class III or IV preparations or the repair of a fractured anterior tooth, a clear **Mylar** or **celluloid strip** matrix is utilized (Procedure 39-3). The matrix aids in placing, confining, and contouring the composite and also isolates the preparation and prevents the use of excess material.

Composite resin is the restorative material used for repairing anterior teeth. The material requires the use of a curing light. Therefore, the ideal matrix is clear to allow for light to penetrate into the material. A metal matrix is available but not often used. A metal matrix may actually scratch the composite resin. A retainer is not necessary to restore the anterior preparation.

To provide proper contour to the restoration, the polyester strip is shaped using the handle of the mouth mirror or cotton pliers. The strip is pulled several times along the metal instrument to create the proper contour. The strip is placed in the interproximal space and wedged from the facial or lingual to form a seal against the tooth to be restored. This also protects the adjacent tooth from the materials to be used.

Proper placement and isolation are very important due to the sensitivity of the composite materials and bond-

ing agents to moisture. If the preparation is near the gingiva, the tissue and the fluid in the sulcus are often a problem when managing the isolation of the area to be restored. Occasionally, a dry retraction cord placed into the sulcus prior to placement of the Mylar matrix and wedge will retract the tissue and control the sulcular fluids.

After the restoration has been cured, remove the wedge, matrix, and cord. Discard these items with other disposables. Use dental floss to check for proper contact with the adjacent tooth before polishing and finishing of the restoration.

Alternative Matrix Systems

Dental materials, techniques, and instruments are undergoing constant development. New matrix systems are created routinely. The dental assistant should be aware of new systems and be willing to help the doctor try new systems. Improvements in matrix systems can make placement of restorations much easier and more comfortable for the patient.

Automatrix System

One of the popular alternatives to the Tofflemire retainer is the **automatrix**. The advantage to the automatrix is the lack of a retainer. The automatrix is a band that is preformed into a loop with a small coil on its side. This coil is the auto-lock loop, which replaces the retainer. A tightening wrench is used to tighten the band around the tooth by placing the end of the wrench into the coil and turning it clockwise. To create good contact with the adjacent tooth, a shaping instrument or burnisher may be used to thin the matrix against the proximal tooth. The wedge can then be placed and the preparation filled with the material of choice.

Once the restoration has been placed, the wrench is used to loosen the band by turning it counterclockwise. The explorer is then placed in the lock-release hole to help remove the band from the tooth. When the band is loose, it can be cut away from the tooth. The restoration

Procedure 39-2 Placing and Removing Retainer, Matrix Band, and Wedge for a Class II Restoration by an Expanded Duties Dental Assistant

In many states, dental assistants and/or expanded duties dental assistants may legally place and remove the matrix system.

Equipment and Supplies

- Basic setup: mouth mirror, explorer, cotton pliers, hemostat
- Tofflemire retainer with matrix in place
- Burnisher
- Wedge
- Cotton rolls
- Floss

Procedure Steps for Preparation of the Matrix Band

1. The band often gets folded upon placement into the retainer. If this should occur, use the handle of a mouth mirror to open the loop.

2. Survey the size of the tooth and adjust the band accordingly by turning the long knob.

Procedure Steps for Placement of the Retainer and Matrix Band

1. Place the retainer along the buccal side of the tooth to be restored and lightly slide the band around the tooth with a rocking motion to get past the other proximal contact (if only one contact was removed in preparation). Leave a 1.0- to 1.5-mm lip along the occlusal surface.

2. Hold the band in place with one finger on the occlusal surface and tighten the band around the tooth by turning the long knob.

3. Check the contour of the band to the tooth with the explorer. The band can catch on the proximal box, creating a poor margin in the box.

4. Use the ball burnisher to adapt the band to the proximal tooth for a tight contact.

Procedure Steps for Placement of the Wedge

1. Select the proper wedge. The size of the embrasure will determine the size of the wedge.

2. Use the cotton pliers to hold the wedge with the flat edge toward the gingival. With moderate pressure, place the wedge from the lingual into the embrasure space. If both mesial and distal contacts need to be restored, then two wedges are needed.

3. Check the gingival floor in the proximal box to ensure that the band is tight against the tooth to seal the band to the wall of the tooth.

Procedure Steps for Removal of the Retainer, Matrix Band, and Wedge

1. Once the tooth has been filled and initially carved, loosen the retainer from the band by turning the short knob.

2. Place a finger over the occlusal surface and matrix band. Remove the retainer from the mouth by gently lifting it toward the occlusal surface, leaving the matrix band around the tooth.

3. With the cotton pliers, remove the wedge.

4. Remember that the amalgam is still soft. Very carefully remove the band by using a light seesaw motion to prevent the restoration from fracturing.

5. Final carving of the restoration is performed.

6. After the initial set of the restorative material, use floss to check the contact with the proximal tooth.

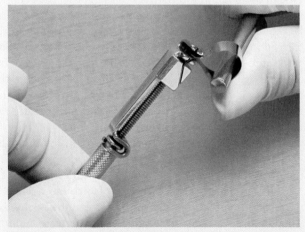

Opening of the matrix band after placement into the retainer.

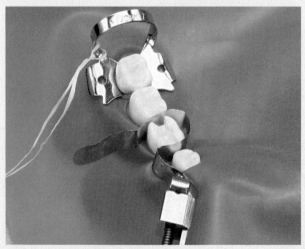

Removal of the retainer.

Procedure 39-3 Placing a Clear Polyester Matrix for Class III and IV Restorations

Equipment and Supplies

- Basic setup: mouth mirror, explorer, cotton pliers
- Clear matrix strip
- Wedges
- Cotton rolls
- Floss

Procedure Steps

1. Examine the tooth and preparation to be restored.

2. Contour the matrix band as necessary for the curvature of the tooth.

3. Place the matrix band interproximally, ensuring that the band extends beyond the gingival wall of the preparation.

4. Place the wedge into the embrasure using the cotton pliers.

5. After curing the composite, the wedge and matrix are removed and discarded.

6. Use floss to check for appropriate contact with the adjacent tooth.

7. The composite is then finished and polished.

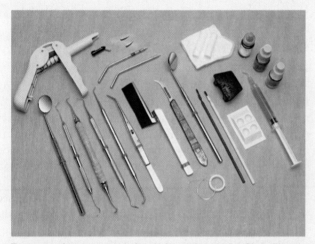

Tray setup for placement of a clear matrix strip for Class III and IV restorations.

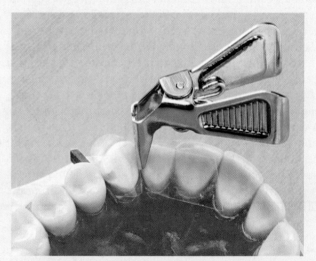

Completed placement of the clear matrix.

can be finished at that time. The automatrix is supplied to the dental office in a kit that includes the tightening wrench and numerous sizes of matrices. The matrices are available in metal and plastic.

Sectional Matrices

The **sectional matrix** is made of plastic or metal. This matrix system is usually supplied as a kit including numerous sizes of matrices, tension rings, and forceps for placement of the tension ring (Figure 39.8). The use of the tension ring provides for a tight contact to the proximal tooth. Again, to help create a good contact with the proximal tooth, the metal matrix can be thinned or burnished in the area that will contact the proximal tooth.

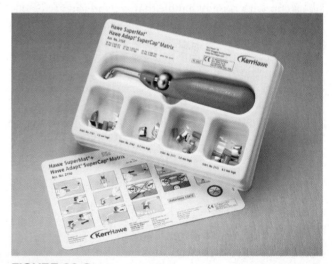

FIGURE 39.8
Sectional matrix kit.

The sectional matrix placement procedure begins with the placement of the matrix into the interproximal space followed by a wedge to secure the matrix to the tooth. The forceps are then used to place the tension ring with the prongs toward the gingiva. The tension ring causes the matrix to flex to create the contact. Burnish the matrix against the proximal tooth one more time to ensure good contact. Be careful to not bump or touch the tension ring while placing the restoration or when assisting the dentist in placing the restoration. The tension ring, if not completely secure, can dislodge and spring away from the teeth. This can startle the operator and the patient and may cause soft tissue damage. It is appropriate to tie a piece of floss to the tension ring in order to retrieve it from the patient's mouth should it dislodge. Once the tension ring is secure, the restoration can then be placed and cured.

The advantage to the sectional matrix in placement of composite resin is the ability to more easily access the restoration with the curing light. After the restoration is placed, the forceps are used to remove the tension ring. Cotton pliers are used to remove the wedge and sectional matrix. Sometimes the mosquito hemostat allows for a better grip on the small, tight sectional matrix. Inform the patient that there will be some pressure when removing the sectional matrix. The dental assistant should use a gentle rocking motion to dislodge the sectional matrix and avoid a sudden forceful tug. The edge of the metal sectional matrix is very sharp and will easily cut soft tissue. The sectional matrix is a single-use item and should be discarded with any other disposables used during the procedure.

Anterior and Cervical Matrix Bands

Another matrix system available to create the proper contour, especially for a Class V preparation, is known as a cervical matrix band. The matrix actually looks more like a cup with a small handle than a band (Figure 39.9). This system is also supplied in a kit with numerous sizes of bands to match the curvature of the gingival one-third of different teeth. Recall that the gingival area of the tooth is the portion of the tooth adjacent to the gingiva and sometimes referred to as the cervical area or the neck of the tooth.

The kit provides a handling instrument to hold the matrix to the tooth. The matrix is clear so composite resin

Professionalism

Occasionally, after removing the matrix of a Class II restoration, the contact is inadequate. If this should happen, remain calm and simply explain to the patient the importance of good contact with the proximal tooth. Prepare for the dentist to remove the new filling and place another restoration utilizing the same matrix or a new matrix per the dentist's request.

can be cured through it (Figure 39.10). These matrices can be used to restore other anterior preparations because they can provide a natural contour.

What type of matrix system would you choose for a young patient with a partially erupted adult tooth requiring a Class II restoration?

Other Matrix Systems for Primary Teeth

The use of a Tofflemire or universal retainer and matrix is difficult with a pediatric patient because of the size of a child's mouth and the size and shape of the primary teeth. Although a pediatric matrix band and retainer are available, other systems may be used. The most common types of matrix systems include the T-band and the spot-welded band.

The T-band is a narrow copper band literally shaped like the letter "T." This band is prepared by folding the wings into a U. Next, the opposite end of the band is placed into the U and the wings are closed (Figure 39.11). The free end may be pulled to adjust the size of the band. The band is placed on the tooth with the free end toward the buccal for access and adjustments. The band is tightened by pulling the free end of the loop and then secured by squeezing the wings. A very small wedge also will help secure the copper band.

A spot-welded band requires a small welding machine. A strip of stainless steel matrix is measured to one inch. The band is formed around the prepared tooth

FIGURE 39.9
Example of a cervical matrix.

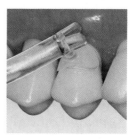

FIGURE 39.10
Cure-Thru clear cervical matrix.
Courtesy Premier Products

and held together with cotton pliers. The band is removed from the mouth and then welded together with the welding machine in three locations. Now, the matrix is ready for use in restoring a Class II primary preparation. Both the copper band matrix and the spot-welded matrix may be formed and placed by the dental assistant in many states.

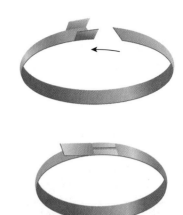

FIGURE 39.11
Preparation of a T-band.

Preparing for Externship

Be aware of and prepared to use numerous types of retainers and matrices. Review the systems preferred by the dentist before assisting him or her. Each dentist practices differently and with different materials. The dental supply company will send samples of new materials including matrix systems. Read the instructions and be prepared for changing systems and materials.

SUMMARY

The dental matrix is vitally important in creating proper anatomic contours, proximal contacts, and smooth external surfaces for all Class II, III, IV, and V restorations. The type of matrix system chosen for each type of restoration is dependent on the tooth to be restored, the size and shape of the restoration, the type of material to be used, and access to the preparation. Most posterior teeth requiring a matrix are properly restored using a Tofflemire or universal retainer and matrix. The matrices available for use with the Tofflemire retainer are supplied in numerous sizes, shapes, and thicknesses.

The automatrix and sectional matrix systems are alternatives to the Tofflemire system for restoring Class II preparations. Neither system requires a retainer. The automatrix system uses a tightening wrench to secure and loosen the preformed band. The sectional matrix system uses small kidney bean–shaped matrices and a tension ring to create the proper form and isolation. All three of these systems are available in metal and plastic.

Anterior teeth require a different type of matrix system. Class III and IV preparations as well as fractured anterior teeth require a Mylar or celluloid matrix. The Mylar matrix is a clear polyester material, which forms well to the contours of the teeth and allows for ease in placing and curing composite materials. Pediatric patients require matrices that are smaller and able to contour to their smaller teeth and mouths. The Tofflemire system has retainers and matrix bands suited to the pediatric patient, but other systems are available such as the copper T-band and the spot-welded band. All of these systems require a wooden or plastic wedge to help isolate the tooth preparation and contour the restorative material to the proper form. Depending on the laws of a state, the dental assistant can place and remove the matrix system.

Cultural Considerations

In other areas of the world, different types of retainers and matrices are used. For example, the Siqveland retainer is commonly used. It is somewhat similar to the Tofflemire retainer. It is also common for dentists in other areas of the world to reuse the matrix after it has been thoroughly scrubbed and sterilized. This is not often done in the United States. Dentists licensed in the United States dispose of the matrix after one use.

KEY TERMS

- **Automatrix:** Matrix system used to create a temporary wall to support the tooth restoration without using a retainer. p. 619
- **Celluloid strip:** Transparent polyester strip used to create a temporary wall to support the tooth restoration of an anterior tooth; often known as a Mylar strip. p. 619
- **Matrix band:** Strip or band placed so as to serve as a retaining outer wall that supports the tooth restoration to re-create proper form and function. p. 616
- **Matrix system:** The device used to help the dentist restore anatomic contours and proximal contact to the proximal tooth. p. 615

KEY TERMS (continued)

- **Mylar:** A trademarked, thin polyester film. p. 619
- **Sectional matrix:** Small kidney bean–shaped matrix that is held in place by a spring-loaded ring to create natural contacts and profile. The Palodent sectional matrix system is an example. p. 621
- **Tofflemire retainer:** Mechanism that holds the matrix band in position; also known as a universal retainer. p. 615

- **Universal retainer:** Mechanism that holds the matrix band in position; also known as a Tofflemire retainer. p. 615
- **Wedge:** Wood or plastic, usually triangular or anatomic apparatus placed in the embrasure space to secure the matrix to the tooth and provide the proper contour for restoring a Class II cavity. p. 617

CHECK YOUR UNDERSTANDING

1. All of the following are components of the Tofflemire retainer except the
   a. outer knob.
   b. inner knob.
   c. U bolt.
   d. locking vise.

2. Required qualities of a matrix system include
   a. rigidity.
   b. ability to create proper anatomic contours.
   c. ability to restore proper proximal contact.
   d. ability to prevent impingement of restorative material on the gingival tissue.
   e. all of the above.

3. The occlusal edge of the matrix band when formed into a loop is placed into which slot first?
   a. diagonal slot
   b. outer guide slot
   c. straight slot
   d. inner guide slot

4. The qualities of a wedge include all of the following except that
   a. it is wide enough to place pressure on the apical wall to hold the band in place.
   b. it is slightly wider than the embrasure space.
   c. it is made of wood or plastic.
   d. it is so snug against the tooth as to create a dimple in the proximal box preparation.

5. All of the following are appropriate matrices for restoring a primary tooth except
   a. extension bands.
   b. sectional matrix.
   c. T-band.
   d. both a and c.
   e. a, b, and c.

6. Anterior teeth may be restored utilizing which of the following matrices?
   a. Tofflemire matrix
   b. sectional matrix
   c. Mylar strip
   d. cervical band
   e. both c and d

7. Sectional matrix systems are primarily used to restore
   a. Class II restorations with composite resin.
   b. Class II restorations with amalgam.
   c. Class III restorations with composite resin.
   d. Class III restorations with amalgam.

8. The purpose of a matrix system is
   a. to provide support to the proximal wall to fill a Class II preparation.
   b. to create contact with the proximal tooth.
   c. to contour the restoration to a natural form.
   d. all of the above.

9. The primary problem created by a poorly fitting wedge is
   a. cupping.
   b. voids.
   c. overhang.
   d. both a and b.
   e. both a and c.

10. In several states, the dental assistant may legally
    a. prepare a tooth with a high-speed handpiece.
    b. place and remove matrix systems.
    c. place and remove wedges.
    d. isolate teeth to be restored.
    e. b, c, and d.

INTERNET ACTIVITY

- Go to www.columbia.edu/itc/hs/dental/operative/ matrixband.html. There you will find a video to download and play that demonstrates the parts of the Tofflemire retainer as well as other useful videos related to general dentistry.

WEB REFERENCES

- Free-Ed.net www.free-ed.net
- Kerr Sybron Dental Specialties www.kerrhawe.com
- Rihani International, Inc. www.rihani.com

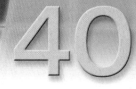

Fixed Prosthodontics

Learning Objectives

After reading this chapter, the student should be able to:

- Define fixed prosthodontics.
- Discuss the type of restorations involved in fixed prosthodontics.
- Discuss inlays and onlays and when they are used.
- Explain the reasons to place a veneer.
- Explain the types of crowns.
- Discuss the indications and contraindications for a fixed prosthesis.
- Explain the procedural steps for crown and bridge preparations.
- Discuss the importance of tissue management.
- Discuss the advantages of the current generation of milled ceramics.
- Explain patient care instructions for fixed prosthodontics.
- Describe the role of the laboratory technician.

Preparing for Certification Exams

- Differentiate between direct and indirect restorations.
- Perform and assist in the preparation of a fixed prosthesis.
- Perform and assist in the placement of gingival retraction.
- Prepare, mix, and deliver materials required for cementation of a fixed prosthesis.
- Describe the process for preparation and placement of a full crown.

Key Terms

Abutment

Cast post

Core buildup

Crown

Die

Fixed partial denture

Implant

Inlay

Maryland bridge

Milled restoration

Onlay

Pontic

Porcelain-fused-to-metal crown (PFM)

Prosthesis

Prosthodontist

Veneer

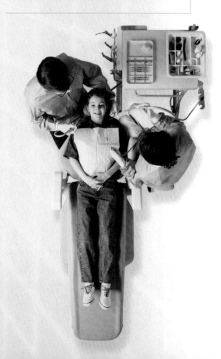

The act of chewing is the beginning of digestion. If teeth are missing, the digestive system has trouble functioning properly, which can cause numerous gastrointestinal problems. Every day teeth are lost due to neglect, trauma, periodontal disease, or systemic disease. Therefore, it is advantageous for a patient to replace a missing tooth or teeth not only for appearance but also for good health and nutrition.

A dental **prosthesis** is required to replace fractured or missing teeth. For the purposes of this chapter, the fixed prosthesis is the primary topic. A fixed prosthesis is cemented in place utilizing existing teeth or implants and is not removable like a traditional denture. It may restore a single decayed or fractured tooth or replace numerous missing teeth.

General dentists can treat most dental problems that require a fixed prosthesis, but on occasion, a patient may present with severe dental problems that are best served by a prosthodontist. A **prosthodontist** is a general dentist who has completed an additional three-year program in clinical practice and research in the dental specialty of prosthodontics. Prosthodontics is the dental specialty pertaining to the restoration and replacement of teeth.

This chapter discusses many procedures that the dental assistant may perform in some states but not in others. As with any dental practice, the dental assistant must know the regulations for the state in which he or she is working. The dental assistant for a fixed prosthetic procedure must be prepared to assist the dentist during technically difficult and lengthy procedures and perform the duties allowed by the state with great skill and professionalism.

Dental Assistant PROFESSIONAL TIP

Have confidence in front of the patient. When the dentist asks you to perform a task that takes place in the patient's mouth, approach the situation every time as if you had performed the task many times. Do not give the patient an opportunity to distrust you and your skills. If you are uncomfortable, request to see the dentist away from the operatory and patient and explain the problem. Even though this is a new experience for you, you have to perform the procedures at some point and become comfortable and confident. Experience is the key to excellence.

Treatment Planning

When a patient presents to the dental office, a complete dental and medical history must be collected including a list of current medications, a full mouth series of radiographs and photographs, a thorough intraoral and extraoral examination, and diagnostic models. The dental assistant in most states can collect much of this information, but the dentist must perform the examination.

Once all of the information has been collected, the dentist can develop a plan to restore the patient's mouth to natural form and function. The dentist will often provide the patient with more than one treatment option based on the patient's needs and desires. For example, a missing tooth may be replaced with an implant or a bridge. The patient has the right to know the pros and cons of each restorative option before committing to a treatment plan. Some treatment plans are very complex and can take months or years to complete.

A fixed prosthesis is indicated only when:

- One or two teeth are missing in the same quadrant
- Supportive tissues, bone, and gingiva are healthy
- Good adjacent teeth are available for abutments
- Patient has good general health

Legal and Ethical Issues

It is all patients' right to have all treatment options available in order to choose the best treatment plan for themselves. Even though the dentist may not provide certain treatment options, patients must be given those options and a referral if they choose to seek that treatment. For example, many dentists do not restore dental implants. They must still give the patient the option of restoring a missing tooth with a dental implant. It is considered malpractice if a dentist withholds various treatment options and then benefits from performing an alternative treatment that the dentist offers, such as providing a bridge to replace a missing tooth.

- Patient has a desire to have treatment
- Patient maintains good oral hygiene.

    Contraindications to fixed prosthetics include:

- Supportive tissues, bone, and gingivae are diseased
- Lack of good abutment teeth
- Patient has poor general health
- Patient is unable and/or unwilling to perform good oral hygiene practices
- Patient faces economic barriers

Indirect Restorations

Indirect restorations are fillings, crowns, bridges, and veneers created outside of the mouth by a laboratory technician and permanently cemented in the patient's mouth by the dentist. The prostheses are delivered to the office ready for placement. Some restorations are cast in metal, whereas **milled restorations** are made of ceramic. The teeth that anchor the restoration must be prepared to receive the cast or milled prosthetic. Once the restoration is seated or placed onto the tooth or teeth, the dentist makes minor adjustments to the occlusion or contacts.

Inlays and Onlays

Inlays and onlays are fixed prostheses that are placed into a prepared cavity. An **inlay** is a Class II restoration created in cast metal or milled ceramic. Class II preparation and restoration involve two surfaces, three surfaces, or multiple surfaces of a posterior tooth but not involve the cusps of the occlusal surfaces. (See Chapter 38 for more information.) An **onlay** is also a Class II restoration that is placed into a prepared cavity, but it covers the occlusal surface of one or more cusps.

    Gold has been the traditional material of choice for inlay and onlay restorations due to desirable characteristics such as malleability, biocompatibility, and tarnish resistance. Gold, though, is not the strongest material

Life Span Considerations

It is paramount for patients to be given instructions about the care and longevity of fixed prostheses. Many patients express the misunderstanding that full coverage of a tooth by a crown means that the tooth can never decay. This statement is false. Decay can occur at the margin of a restoration or root surface of any tooth with a general filling or fixed prosthesis. Patients should be given verbal and written instructions for oral hygiene including brushing, flossing, and using floss threaders and other hygiene products recommended by the dentist or hygienist. Restorations will last many years if placed properly and taken care of through excellent patient home care.

available. Recent technology has introduced milled ceramic, which is the strongest material available for inlays and onlays. Ceramic is bonded to the tooth structure to provide durability and strength. Other qualities of milled ceramics include resistance to temperature change and good aesthetics. On occasion, composite resin is used for inlays. A lab technician or the dentist in the office laboratory makes the restoration.

Patients may ask the dental assistant what material they should choose for their restoration. What factors would you consider when discussing the best materials for a fixed prosthesis?

Veneers

A **veneer** is an ultrathin layer of composite resin or porcelain bonded to the facial surface of teeth. The two types of veneers are direct and indirect veneers. Composite resin veneers, placed through the process of bonding, are direct veneers and were discussed in Chapter 38. They are considered direct veneers because they are created directly in the patient's mouth. Porcelain veneers are indirect veneers because the laboratory technician fabricates them after the dentist has prepared the teeth.

    Patients desire porcelain veneers for a number of reasons (Figure 40.1) such as to:

- repair a traumatic injury to a tooth or teeth.
- hide a defect in the enamel such as hypocalcification or fluorosis.
- change the color of the teeth.
- give the optical illusion of straighter teeth.
- close spaces or diastemas.

    The shade or color of the veneer or veneers is extremely important. Just about one of the most difficult things a dentist must do is match the shade of a single veneer to the natural tooth structure of the surrounding teeth. With modern technology and the cooperation of a good laboratory technician, the technician will meet with the patient in the lab or the dental office to look at the patient's natural tooth shade. Many companies specializing in color have developed technology that allows the lab technician or the dentist to digitally measure the shade of the surrounding teeth to ensure that each dental prosthesis matches not just the tooth being replaced, but the teeth surrounding it (Figure 40.2).

    Traditionally, the dentist or the dental assistant has a series of shade guides that are used to match the shade of the surrounding teeth and often will draw a map on a piece of paper to map the colors. It is also important to communicate to the lab technician the shade of the prepared tooth, often known as the stump shade. If the prepared tooth or stump is very dark, this information

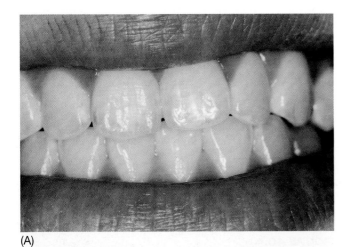

(A)

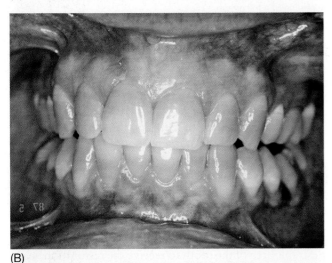

(B)

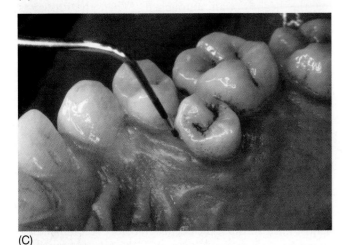

(C)

FIGURE 40.1
Reasons patients want veneers: (a) fluorosis, (b) tetracycline stain, and (c) crowding of teeth.
Images (b & c) courtesy of Instructional Materials for the Dental Team, Lex., KY

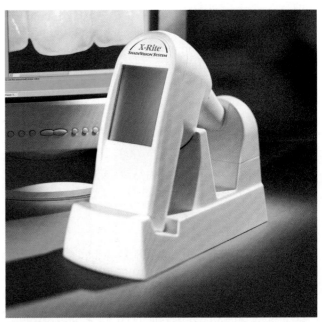

FIGURE 40.2
Example of a digital system used to map the shade of natural tooth structure.
Courtesy X-Rite Incorporated

The preparation by the dentist of the teeth to be veneered is conservative. In other words, the dentist tries to maintain as much enamel as possible because the cements used to adhere the veneer to the tooth bond better to enamel than dentin. Diamond burs and discs are most often used to reduce the tooth structure. Enough tooth structure has to be removed to allow for the thickness of the porcelain. The patient should be informed that the prosthesis will feel slightly thicker than the natural tooth structure.

Once the tooth has been reduced, the gingiva has to be retracted with retraction cords to create a dry field for the impression. The dental assistant can place the retraction cords in some states. Check the state regulations for duties that may be performed by the dental assistant. This skill takes practice so as to not damage the gingiva and periodontal attachment.

After the retraction cord has been left in the sulcus for approximately five minutes, the cords are removed and the impression is taken. The dentist or the expanded duties dental assistant makes and temporarily cements the temporary veneers. Again, in some states the dental assistant without expanded duty skills may also make and place temporary veneers. Occasionally, the preparation is so minimal that the teeth do not require temporaries.

At the patient's cementation appointment, the temporaries are removed and the veneers are tried on the prepared tooth structure. The patient should approve the shade and shape before permanent cementation takes place. If colored cement is required, the try-in paste or test color of the cement should be utilized. The veneers

allows the lab technician to mask the dark natural shade. The shade of the luting agent or cement is equally important. Most cement kits have numerous shades. Now with the use of a digital shade meter, the shade of the veneer does not need to be altered by colored cement; instead, a transparent cement gives the best results.

are then bonded to the tooth structure using a conventional bonding technique using etch, bond, and the veneer cement. After light curing, the excess cement is removed and final adjustments are made to the occlusion followed by a final polish of the adjusted area (Figure 40.3).

The dentist and the dental assistant are seating six veneers. Unfortunately, the last two veneers will not seat to the margins. Why might the veneers not seat properly? **?**

Crowns

A **crown** is a restoration that covers or replaces a major part of or the entire clinical crown of a tooth. A full crown covers the entire anatomical crown of a single tooth, usually to the free gingival margin (Figure 40.4). When the dentist diagnoses the need for a full crown on

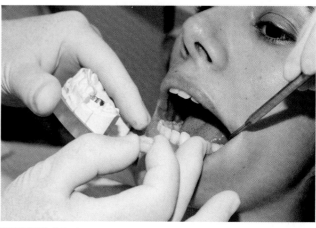

FIGURE 40.4
Example of a full crown.

a single tooth, the tooth has lost approximately 50% or more of its natural tooth structure to a failing restoration with recurrent decay or fractures of a cusp and cannot be reconstructed with a more conservative restoration.

In addition to the need for a crown, the tooth may require more retention to maintain the crown by placing a core buildup with pins or a post and core. A full crown is made of gold, semiprecious metal, porcelain-fused-to-metal, porcelain-fused-to-gold, or all ceramic.

Sometimes a single tooth exhibits a healthy buccal or lingual wall and the dentist elects to be conservative and preserve the natural tooth structure. This is known as a three-quarter crown. The preparation readies the less desirable area of the tooth to receive the restoration, leaving the healthy wall untouched. When the crown is seated, the healthy enamel is visible and the prepared area is now protected by the restoration.

Today, patients want aesthetics as well as strength from their dental prosthetics. The **porcelain-fused-to-metal crown (PFM)** achieves both for the posterior teeth. It is a full crown, first cast in metal and then covered with aesthetically pleasing porcelain to match the adjacent teeth. One of the only disadvantages is the difficulty the lab technician has in masking the dark color of the metal shell. Therefore, a PFM is not the best choice of crowns for the aesthetic, or smile, zone.

To achieve the best shade in the aesthetic zone, an all-ceramic crown is the right choice for most patients. The dentist must consider the occlusion before recommending all-ceramic restorations due to the risk of shearing or fracturing off some of the porcelain. Zirconia is the ceramic material with the greatest strength and is milled to perform like the casting performs for the PFM. The porcelain is then stacked on the milled shell to imitate the natural tooth structure. The advantage of the all-ceramic crown is that the shell is milled from ceramic that matches the stump shade of the natural tooth or a white shade to mask the dark color of the natural prepared tooth structure. This provides the patient with a much more natural looking prosthesis than a PFM (Figure 40.5).

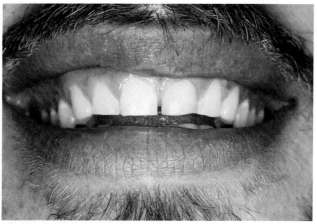

(A)

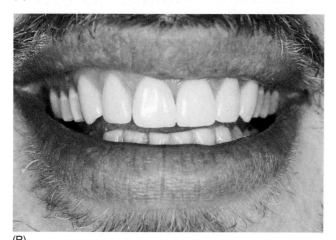
(B)

FIGURE 40.3
(a) A patient with worn anterior dentition and (b) same patient with final restorations.
McIntyre F. Restoring esthetics and anterior guidelines in worn anterior teeth. JADA 2000; 131(9):1279–1283. Copyright © 2000 American Dental Association. All rights reserved. Reprinted with permission.

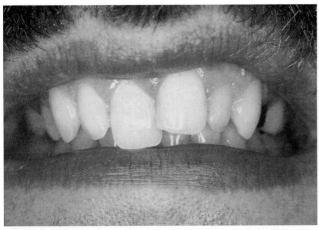

(A)

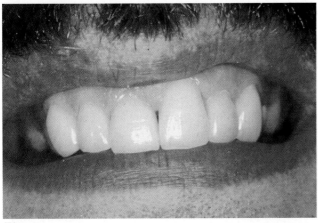

(B)

FIGURE 40.5
(a) A 40-year-old patient who requested nonorthodontic treatment for his imbricated upper anterior teeth. (b) Same patient after dentin-bonded all-ceramic crowns were placed at teeth #6 through #11. Gingival contouring or crown lengthening was suggested to the patient so the gingival level at teeth #8 and #9 would be similar. The patient declined this treatment.
Trevor Burke F.J., Qualtrough AJE, Hale RW Dentin-bonded all-ceramic crowns: current status. JADA 1998; 129(4): 455–460. Copyright © 1998 American Dental Association. All rights reserved. Reprinted with permission.

Fixed Partial Denture or Bridge

A **fixed partial denture,** also known as a fixed bridge, is a prosthetic replacement of one or more missing teeth cemented or attached to the abutment teeth or implant abutments adjacent to the space. The **abutments** are the natural teeth or implants used to support or anchor the fixed dental prosthesis. A fixed bridge consists of units, each pertaining to a tooth. For example, if a patient is missing a single tooth and the teeth on either side are going to be prepared for the bridge, the bridge is a three-unit prosthesis. The components of a bridge are the abutments and the **pontic,** which is the artificial tooth that replaces the missing tooth.

Depending on the design of the bridge, there can be more than two abutments. The dentist determines the design prior to preparation of the abutments. The num-

ber of teeth missing determines the number of pontics. It is not recommended to have too many pontics in a row. This will cause the structure of the bridge to be compromised and will place too much stress on the abutments. A nice alternative to a long bridge is an implant-supported bridge.

Most bridges are made of gold or porcelain-fused-to-metal. Technology is greatly improving the all-ceramic prosthetics, but the technology for using all-ceramic fixed bridges in the posterior of the mouth is still being developed. On the other hand, in the aesthetic zone, an all-ceramic bridge is possible because less chewing force is exerted on the anterior teeth. An excellent option for a missing anterior tooth is the **Maryland bridge** or resin-bonded bridge (Figure 40.6). This prosthesis is a type of fixed partial denture that does not require crowns, but instead has wings that are bonded to the lingual surfaces of adjacent natural teeth.

Traditionally, the Maryland bridge is fabricated like a PFM with a metal substructure and wings. The disadvantage to the metal wings is the transparency of the enamel of the abutments. The metal tends to show through the interproximal areas, creating a darkened area between the pontic and the abutments. Today, the darkness is not acceptable to patients; therefore, the all-ceramic restoration is the better choice.

The Maryland bridge is a great prosthesis for replacing a single anterior tooth without much preparation of the abutments. The lingual aspect of the abutments must be slightly prepared in the enamel to support the pontic. At cementation, the wings are bonded to the prepared

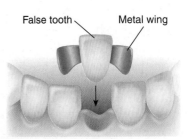

False tooth   Metal wing

FIGURE 40.6
The Maryland bridge technique.

lingual areas of the abutments. The excess cement is removed and the area checked for occlusion and then polished. The dental assistant should inform patients who have had a Maryland bridge placed to be aware and very careful of the types of foods they bite into and to never use their teeth as tools for fear of loosening or fracturing the Maryland bridge.

Implants

An **implant** is a screw-like device specially designed to be placed surgically within the mandibular or maxillary bone as a means of providing support for a dental prosthesis. When a tooth is lost, the patient has the option of having an implant placed rather than a bridge—providing the patient has sufficient bone. The advantage to placing the implant is that there is no need to cut on adjacent teeth for abutments. When given the choice, many people will elect to have an implant and save healthy tooth structure. If several teeth are missing in one quadrant, an implant bridge is a treatment plan option. In this case, two implants are placed, leaving room between them for a pontic. An implant-supported bridge is fabricated and cemented into place. For more information on implants, see Chapter 43.

A patient has been given treatment options for replacing an extracted tooth. The options are to place an implant or prepare for a bridge. The patient asks the opinion of the dental assistant. How will you respond to this patient?

Overview of a Crown Procedure

After diagnosis, the preparation and placement of a crown prosthesis takes two appointments unless the prosthesis is milled within the dental office. (Milled restorations are covered later in the chapter.) The first appointment involves shade selection, preparation of tooth structure, impression, and cementation of the provisional crown. The second appointment is typically a shorter appointment involving removal of the provisional crown, try-in, cementation of the final restoration, and adjustment of the occlusion as necessary.

Shade Selection

Today, most patients want an aesthetically pleasing prosthesis even on the posterior teeth. Therefore, a porcelain restoration is the option of choice and a shade must be selected. As with veneers, a shade may be chosen by the dentist, the lab technician, or the dental assistant (Figure 40.7). If the restoration is in the aesthetic zone, the dentist and patient may elect to have the lab technician digitally map the shades of the adjacent teeth to develop the

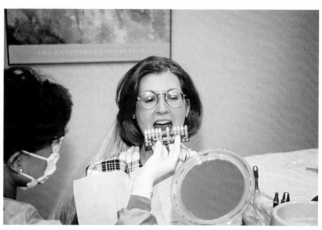

FIGURE 40.7
Choosing the shade before preparation.
Image courtesy Instructional Materials for the Dental Team, Lex., KY

shades of the restoration. Otherwise, the dentist or dental assistant will use the standard shade guides to closely map the adjacent teeth. A helpful hint is to take photos of the shade tabs next to the natural teeth and send these photos with the impression to the lab technician.

Preparation

The dentist begins the preparation of the tooth by reducing the occlusal surface and the vertical walls of the tooth to allow for the appropriate thickness of metal and/or porcelain and without compromising the pulp and strength of the remaining tooth structure. The preparation must also allow for *draw,* or the ability for the restoration to be fully placed and removed before cementation. Occlusal forces are also a consideration in the preparation design.

The dentist then creates a gingival margin in one of many shapes, depending on the material to be used for the restoration. The margin allows for the restoration to blend into the tooth with a smooth junction. The shape of the margin is created by the shape of the bur the dentist uses. For example, a chamfer bur has a rounded cutting end, which creates a rounded margin for a metal casting. The dentist is trained to know what bur and angle are necessary for each type of restoration. The dental assistant should know which burs the dentist prefers for each restorative procedure in order to have the operatory prepared for the procedure.

Retention for Crowns

Often, the anatomical crown of a tooth requiring a restorative crown has been damaged extensively or has undergone endodontic therapy. To achieve good retention and support of the restorative crown, the damaged or fractured area of the tooth must be rebuilt with a separate restoration. A **core buildup** is the restorative material that re-creates the lost tooth structure of the anatomical crown of a vital tooth. Some dentists use amalgam as a core material, but amalgam requires a hardening time and therefore the patient often has to return to the office at a later date for the actual preparation of the crown. More commonly, the dentist will remove any old amalgam, other restoration, and decay, and build up the lost tooth structure with self-curing or light-curing composite resin material. Reinforced glass ionomer cement may be used. If entire cusps are lost, it is necessary to add retention to the buildup.

Prior to placement of the buildup material, retention pins are placed into solid tooth structure by drilling pinholes followed by placement of the pins. The pins are carefully placed so as to avoid the pulp chamber. The buildup material surrounds the pins, helping to secure the material to the tooth.

An endodontically treated tooth often requires a post and core to restore the anatomical crown prior to crown preparation. A post can be cast or prefabricated. A **cast post** is a metal post created by a laboratory to be placed into an endodontically treated tooth to improve retention of a cast restoration. In order for the laboratory to create the post, post room is made by removing some of the gutta percha or other endodontic filling material in the endodontic canal to allow room for the post. An impression post made of plastic is placed into the canal while impression material is flowed into the same space. The resulting impression is sent to the lab for casting and finishing. The top of the cast post is also the core.

The patient returns to the office for cementation of the cast post and core, final preparation of the tooth, and impression for the crown. Prefabricated posts come in numerous sizes in a kit with post room drills (Figure 40.8). The dentist makes post room into the endodontic canal and uses the corresponding metal, ceramic, or fiber post to gain retention. The dental assistant mixes the cement for permanent placement of the post by the dentist. The post is cemented into the endodontic space, and a light-cured composite resin or amalgam is used to make

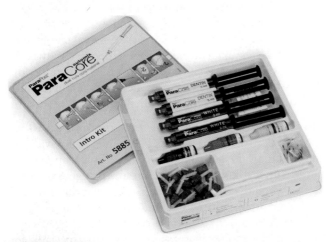

FIGURE 40.8
Post and core kit.
Courtesy Coltene Whaledent

the core. The dentist can then prepare the tooth for the crown. While the dentist prepares the canal or the tooth, the dental assistant must maintain a clear field for the dentist to work by retracting and suctioning the saliva.

Tissue Management

The final impression must show the entire gingival margin with clarity in order for the laboratory technician to make an accurate crown. Inevitably, the tissue is cut upon preparation of the tooth for the crown. Healthy tissue does not bleed very much, but unhealthy tissue or tissue that has had to adapt to a rough margin due to a poor restoration or fracture bleeds readily. Bleeding tissue does not allow for good flow of impression material around the gingival margin. Other fluid in the sulcus also creates a problem for the impression material. (See Chapter 36 concerning properties of impression materials.) Control of the gingiva, blood, and other fluids surrounding the preparation is called tissue management. The most common method of tissue management is the use of a gingival retraction cord. Not only does the cord control the fluids, it literally pushes the tissue away from the tooth, widening the gingival sulcus and exposing the prepared gingival margin.

Types of Retraction

There are three types of gingival retraction: chemical, mechanical, and surgical. The most common form of gingival retraction is chemical retraction with the use of a retraction cord containing chemicals that cause the tissue to shrink away from the tooth and/or to coagulate the blood and remove other sulcular fluids. Both mechanical and chemical retraction provide only temporary widening of the sulcus.

Retraction Cords Retraction cords vary in size and texture. They are available in untwisted, twisted, and braided. Untwisted cord must be manually twisted prior to use. As for thickness, the dentist will decide which size cords are necessary for the procedure. Cord size is determined by the condition of the tissue and the margins of the preparation (Figure 40.9).

Once the dentist decides which size of cord to use, the dental assistant cuts the cords to length. A good way for the dental assistant to determine the length of the cords is to wrap the cord around the little finger and cut the cord to this length. The circumference of the little finger is about the same circumference as an adult molar.

Cords are either nonimpregnated or impregnated. Nonimpregnated cords do not have chemicals in the cord. Impregnated cords contain astringent-vasoconstrictor agents to control bleeding and shrink the tissue. The chemicals most often used are epinephrine, ferric sulfate, and aluminum chloride. Epinephrine is a vasoconstrictor, so epinephrine cords are not to be used with cardiovascular patients. Epinephrine can increase blood pressure and create arrhythmias or an irregular heartbeat, placing the patient in cardiac danger. The patient's health history should be reviewed before use of any impregnated cord.

Ferric sulfate and aluminum chloride are available in a liquid or gel form. These chemicals are hemostatic or act to arrest bleeding (Figure 40.10). They are dispensed into a dappen dish where the nonimpregnated cords are soaked before placement, or a cotton pellet is soaked and then placed on the area that is hemorrhaging. Another means of delivering a hemostatic agent is by an infuser syringe, by which the agent is preloaded by the supplier into a syringe and easily injected into the sulcus.

The retraction cord is placed in the sulcus with the use of a cord-packing instrument (Procedure 40-1). This instrument has a blunt rounded end that is sometimes serrated. Some dentists and dental assistants prefer a plastic instrument due to the thin working end. The cord is gently pushed into the sulcus without damaging the

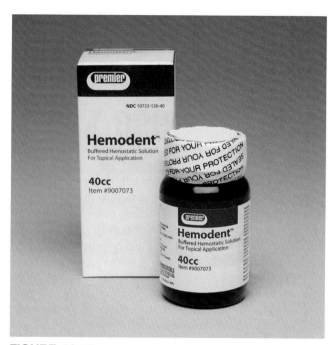

FIGURE 40.10
Various types of hemostatic agents.
Courtesy Premier Products

periodontal tissues. The sulcus is in the shape of a "V" with the narrowest part at the periodontal attachment. The best retraction is usually achieved by placing two cords, a smaller one placed first toward the periodontal attachment and then a larger cord placed at the opening of the sulcus.

Some states may or may not allow the dental assistant to place retraction cords. Other states may allow the dental assistant to place only cords that do not have hemostatic agents, which are considered a medication and must be administered only by a dentist. Always check the regulations for the state in which you work.

Mechanical Retraction   Mechanical retraction is occasionally necessary when other methods fail. The dentist uses mechanical retraction to force the tissue away from the tooth with the use of a temporary crown. The temporary crown extends beyond the gingival margin into the sulcus. The patient wears this temporary crown for several days and then returns to the office for the impression. Unfortunately, this type of retraction requires an extra appointment for the patient.

Surgical Retraction   Surgical retraction is used to remove hypertrophied or excess tissue interfering with the gingival margin. This tissue is removed with an electrosurge, surgical knife, or laser. An electrosurge is a device with a wand that holds a wire tip. A current runs through the wand to the tip to cut and cauterize the tissue. It effectively removes tissue and controls bleeding. Dental lasers are becoming increasingly popular, especially for tissue management. They perform in a manner similar to that of the electrosurge.

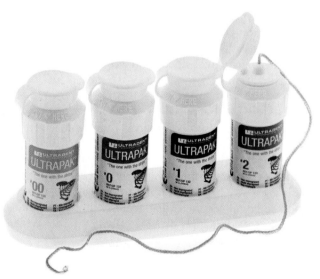

FIGURE 40.9
Examples of the different sizes of retraction cords available.
Courtesy Ultradent Products, Inc.

Procedure 40-1 Placing and Removing a Gingival Retraction Cord

Equipment and Supplies

- Mouth mirror
- Explorer
- Cotton pliers
- Cord-packing instrument
- Gingival cords of dentist's preference
- Scissors
- Hemostatic agent
- Dappen dish
- Cotton rolls

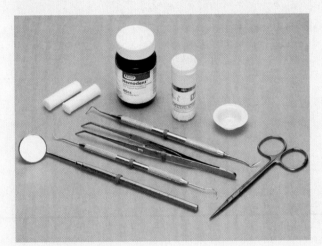

Retraction tray setup.

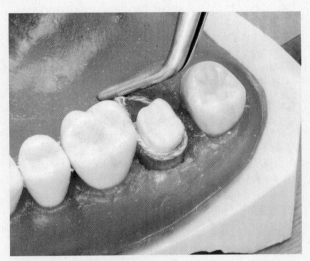

Retraction cord placement.

7. With the cord-packing instrument, gently pack the cord with light pressure into the sulcus. (*Hint:* Try to lightly push back toward the portion of the cord last inserted into the sulcus. Pushing forward stretches and drags the cord around the tooth.)

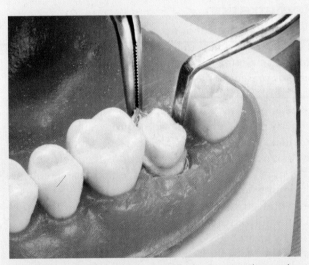

Use of the cord-packing instrument to place a retraction cord.

Procedure Steps

1. Gently rinse and dry the preparation; this allows for better visibility of the margins.

2. Isolate the quadrant with cotton rolls.

3. Cut an appropriate length of cord—longer for molars and shorter for anterior teeth. (*Hint:* Use the circumference of your little finger to gauge the length of cord for a molar.)

4. Place the cord or cotton pellets into the hemostatic solution if there is hemorrhaging of the tissue.

5. If using a hemostatic agent, inform the patient that the chemicals will taste bad.

6. Using the cotton pliers, make a loop with the cord and gently lay it around the prepared tooth at the margin or opening of the sulcus with the ends of the loop on the buccal side of the preparation. This placement allows for easy removal of the cords.

8. Once the cord is fully placed, the ends of the loop should be end to end. If the cord is too long, it can be cut with scissors. If it is too short, a new cord should be placed. Placing a small piece is not appropriate because it often gets left in the sulcus, creating a periodontal problem.

9. Depending on the dentist's preference, two cords of differing sizes may be used. Place the smaller of the cords first followed by the larger cord.

continued on next page

Procedure 40-1 *continued from previous page*

10. The cords should be left in the sulcus for approximately five minutes but not longer than seven minutes. (*Hint:* Set a timer.) Instruct the patient to remain still so as to keep the area dry and the hemostatic agent off the tongue. (*Hint:* Time is dependent on the type of hemostatic agent. Read the manufacturer's information on the agent.)

11. When time is up, the operator removes the cotton and the second cord while the assistant fills the impression tray. The operator removes the cord with the cotton pliers by grasping the end of the cord on the buccal side of the preparation. The cord is not removed until the impression is ready to be taken. The operator must keep the sulcus and preparation dry before the placement of the impression.

12. After the impression, the first cord must be removed. Do not forget about the cord—a severe periodontal problem can develop in a short amount of time if a cord is not removed.

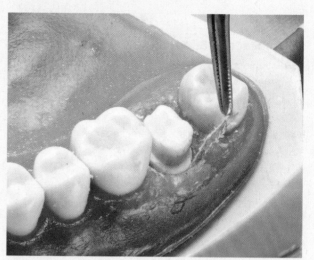

Use of cotton pliers to remove a retraction cord.

Final Impression and Bite Registration

The taking of the final or master impression is a vital step in the process of creating an indirect restoration. The preparation must be accurate. If any deformation or defect is present in the final impression, the final restoration fabricated at the laboratory will be faulty, resulting in the failure of the restoration to fit the prepared tooth properly. This is the point where proper gingival retraction makes the difference. The general reason for impression failure is the lack of proper tissue management. The laboratory cannot guess where the margins should be. The impression must be an accurate form of the prepared tooth and surrounding teeth in order for the laboratory technician to create a properly fitting restoration.

The dentist chooses the impression material to be used. Depending on state regulations, the dental assistant may be able to take the final impression. The procedure for mixing and delivering the impression material usually requires two people. A bite registration is necessary for the laboratory to articulate or fit together the models of the prepared and adjacent teeth with the opposing arch. The bite registration is a form of impression material placed in between the maxillary and mandibular arch. The dental assistant instructs the patient to close his or her mouth into a natural bite position and allow the material to set. See Chapter 36 for a discussion of the mixing and delivery of impression and bite registration materials.

Preparing for Externship

Get a defined job description from the dentist or office manager. Know exactly what your job entails. For example, some offices do their own general cleaning instead of hiring a janitorial team. Know if you are expected to perform such jobs. Be aware of the priorities. Patients always come first. All other duties fall second to whatever a patient requires or what the dentist needs to treat a patient.

Provisional Coverage

Provisional or temporary coverage of a prepared tooth is placed after the final impression has been created. The purpose of a provisional restoration is to:

- maintain function and aesthetics
- protect the prepared margins
- control the surrounding gingiva
- prevent shifting of the prepared and surrounding teeth
- reduce sensitivity of the prepared tooth

The patient must wear the provisional restoration until the final restoration is placed. It is temporarily cemented in place for ease of removal when necessary.

The patient must be informed that should the provisional restoration come off the prepared tooth prior to the final cementation appointment, the patient will need to return to the dental office to have it recemented. The duration for wearing the provisional is dependent on the time the laboratory technician requires to make the final restoration. In fixed prosthodontics, many cases are complex and require extended time for developing the final restorations. In such cases, the patient wears the provisional for a longer period of time. The expanded duties dental assistant can fabricate provisional restorations. Check your state regulations. Chapter 41 is dedicated to the types and uses of provisional coverage.

Cementation Appointment

The initial step at the cementation appointment is the removal of the provisional restoration. The dental assistant removes the provisional with a large spoon excavator, scaler, or hemostat. The instrument chosen should be able to grasp the provisional so that the provisional does not fall into the back of the patient's mouth upon removal. Once removed, the provisional should be kept in case a problem occurs with the final restoration.

The assistant can place the final restoration for the dentist to approve. Check the applicable state regulations to ensure that the dental assistant may place the crown at the try-in stage. Once the dentist approves the marginal fit, contacts, and occlusion, the dentist seats the restoration with permanent cement. The dental assistant mixes and delivers the cement to the restoration and delivers the restoration to the dentist for placement on the prepared tooth. Once the restoration is placed with permanent cement, it is very difficult to remove. Great care is taken to ensure that the restoration seats properly onto the prepared tooth. Should the restoration not seat properly, the margins would be open, creating a space for bacteria and eventual decay to occur. The occlusion would also be too tall, preventing the opposing teeth from properly closing.

The dentist decides which cement or luting agent is to be used. The dental assistant must be familiar with the manufacturer's recommendations for mixing and placement of the cement into the internal surface of the restoration. Most restorations require only a thin layer of cement due to the very thin space allowed for the cement between the prepared tooth and the restoration. Excess cement will flow out around the margins and must be removed to avoid periodontal irritation. In some states, the dental assistant can perform this step. See Chapter 35 for more details concerning dental cements.

Overview of a Bridge Procedure

The setup and preparation of a fixed bridge is nearly the same as for a fixed single crown (see Procedure 40-2). The only difference involves a possible third appointment. The first appointment is the preparation and provisional appointment, followed by a framework try-in appointment, and finally the cementation appointment.

Preparation

The only difference in the preparation of a fixed single crown and a bridge is the number of teeth prepared. Because more teeth are involved, the appointment time is longer. The abutment teeth are prepared for full crowns or onlays. After the preparations, the procedure continues with tissue management, impressions, and provisional coverage. All of these procedural steps are the same as with a single crown. The impressions, bite registration, and laboratory prescription are all sent to the laboratory for fabrication.

Framework Try-In

Prior to the second appointment, the dental assistant ensures that the laboratory has returned the impression, model of the prepared teeth, and the metal framework to the dental office. Items being delivered to or returned from the dental laboratory are referred to as a *laboratory case* or just a *case*.

When the patient arrives, the dental assistant can remove the provisional and remaining cement. The framework is placed on the prepared teeth. The dentist checks the fit and marginal integrity. If the framework does not fit properly, the dentist may cut or section the framework to get individual abutments to fit and cure them together to the proper fit or a new impression is taken. Regardless of which technique the dentist chooses, the laboratory will make a new framework and the try-in appointment is repeated. If the framework fits, an impression is taken with the framework left in place. When the impression is removed, the framework will be left in the impression. This is known as a pick-up impression and allows the laboratory to know the shape and positioning of the soft tissue. The soft tissue is important because the pontic must appear as if it is emerging from the tissue like a natural tooth yet be accessible for the patient to clean underneath it. The provisional is again cemented with temporary cement and the patient is scheduled for the final cementation.

Why might the metal framework for a fixed partial denture or bridge not fit properly?

Cementation Appointment

Prior to the patient's cementation appointment, it is important for the dental assistant to ensure that the prosthesis has arrived in the dental office. Sometimes the patient's prepared teeth are very sensitive. If this is an issue, then local anesthetic may need to be required. The provisional is removed and the preparations cleaned and dried. The final prosthesis is placed on the prepared teeth. The dentist checks the margins, contacts, and occlusion and makes adjustments as needed. The patient should approve the final shade before cementation. Finally, the prosthesis is cemented with permanent cement (See Procedure 40-3).

Procedure 40-2 Assisting with a Crown or Bridge Restoration

Equipment and Supplies

- Restorative kit including:
  - Mouth mirror
  - Explorer
  - Cotton pliers
  - Air/water syringe
  - Spoon excavator
  - Scissors
  - Hemostat
  - Spatula
  - Other instruments required by the dentist
- Local anesthetic setup
- Gingival retraction setup
- Provisional coverage setup
- Impression and bite registration setup including the impression trays
- High-speed and contra-angle handpieces and burs
- Shade guide
- High-volume evacuator (HVE) and saliva ejector
- Cotton products (pellets, rolls, 2 × 2 gauze squares, dry angles)
- Articulating paper and holder
- Dental floss

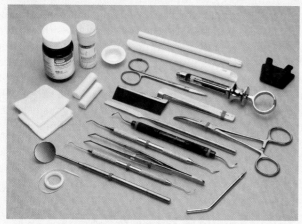

Tray setup for crown and bridge preparation.

Procedure Steps Prior to Preparation of the Tooth

1. Assist in administration of local anesthetic.

2. If an alginate impression is needed for use in making the provisional or for the opposer (the opposite arch from which the restorative work is to be completed), take it at this time.

3. If a stent for making of the provisional is needed, take it at this time. A stent is a small impression of the tooth prior to preparation that is usually made with an alginate impres-

sion, bite registration, or a small thermoplastic disc. It is used to make the temporary crown after preparation.

4. If the final impression requires a two-stage silicone impression, take the first stage impression at this time.

5. If the final restoration is tooth colored, take the shade at this time.

Procedure Steps for Preparation of the Tooth

1. Maintain a clear operating field with use of the HVE to retract the lips and tongue and to remove water and debris.

2. The dentist uses diamond burs to quickly cut away decayed or fractured portions of the tooth. Other shaped burs define the appropriate shape of the preparation.

3. The dentist or dental assistant places the gingival retraction cords.

4. Ready the final impression materials.

5. Rinse and dry the preparation.

6. Transfer the cotton pliers to the dentist for cord removal.

7. Assist the dentist or other assistant in placement of the light-body impression materials.

8. Fill the impression tray with heavy-body impression material.

9. Receive the light-body delivery system (usually a syringe or impression gun) from the dentist while delivering to the dentist the impression tray in correct alignment for the dentist to grasp and insert directly onto the prepared area in the patient's mouth.

10. Watch the clock for the appropriate setting time according to the recommendations of the impression material's manufacturer.

11. The dentist or the dental assistant can remove the impression tray. Check the state regulations.

12. Rinse the patient's mouth. Many impression materials have a poor taste.

13. Take the bite registration.

14. Remove any remaining gingival retraction cords.

15. Fabricate the provisional restoration and cement with temporary cement.

16. Give the patient provisional restoration care instructions.

17. Schedule the patient for the permanent cementation appointment.

18. After the dentist writes the laboratory prescription, prepare the case for delivery to the laboratory technician.

Procedure 40-3 Assisting in the Cementation of a Fixed Prosthesis

Equipment and Supplies

- Restorative kit including:
  - Mouth mirror
  - Explorer
  - Cotton pliers
  - Air/water syringe
  - Spoon excavator
  - Scissors
  - Hemostat
  - Spatula
  - Other instruments required by the dentist
- Cast or milled restoration delivered from the laboratory
- Bonding setup and/or cementation setup (per dentist's preference)
- High-speed and low-speed rotary handpieces
- High-volume evacuator (HVE) and saliva ejector
- Articulating paper and holder
- Cotton products (pellets, rolls, 2 × 2 gauze squares, dry angles)
- Scaler to remove excess cement
- Burs and porcelain or gold polishers
- Dental floss

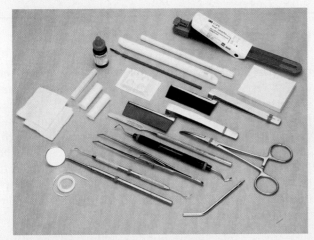

Tray setup for cementation of a fixed prosthesis.

Procedure Steps

1. Place restoration onto the model returned from the dental laboratory for inspection by the dentist. If the crown is not returned from the lab as "disinfected," the dental assistant must disinfect it prior to the dentist placing it in the patient's mouth.

2. Transfer the restoration to the dentist for placement onto the prepared tooth.

3. Transfer the mouth mirror and explorer to the dentist.

4. Hold the restoration in place with cotton pliers for the dentist to check the contacts of the restoration with the adjacent tooth.

5. Place cotton rolls to help keep the preparation dry.

6. When the dentist signals, mix the cement and quickly apply the cement in a thin layer to the internal surface of the restoration.

7. Transfer the restoration to the dentist for placement.

8. The dentist places the restoration with firm finger pressure. The patient then bites on a cotton roll or wooden stick to seat the restoration completely.

9. Once the cement reaches its initial set after three to five minutes, the excess may be removed. Use a controlled fulcrum to maintain stability when removing the excess cement.

10. Use the tip of the explorer or scaler to slightly extend into the sulcus to lift up on the excess cement. Use lateral pressure against the restoration. This procedure often requires the removal of cement subgingivally. Many states do not allow the dental assistant to use any instrument subgingivally. Check state regulations for allowed dental assistant duties.

11. To remove the excess cement in the embrasure space, tie a knot in a piece of dental floss and carefully pull the knot through the embrasure space to dislodge the cement.

12. After the cement is removed, the dentist checks the occlusion, adjusts if necessary, and polishes the restoration with the contra-angle and slow-speed polishers.

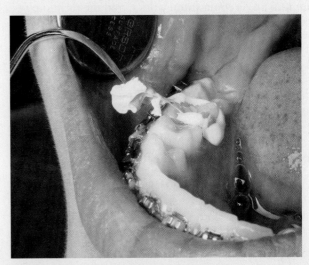

Excess cement around the permanent restoration.

Machined Restorations

Today, all-ceramic restorations are the most aesthetic dental restorations available. Zirconia and alumina milled frameworks finally give the dentist and patient a life-like restoration. The days of relying on porcelain to mask the dark metal framework of a PFM are gone. All-ceramic restorations are best utilized in the aesthetic zone, but recently dentists have begun to use them on some posterior teeth. They are not recommended for restoring second or third molars at this time. There are some limitations to the use of all-ceramic restorations, however. For example, excessive forces due to clenching or grinding may result in fracture of an all-ceramic restoration. Patients that clench or grind their teeth must agree to wear a night guard if they desire to have all-ceramic restorations. The night guard helps prevent excessive forces on the restorations protecting against failure or fracture of the ceramic.

Ceramic restoration systems work by scanning the model of the prepared tooth and storing this information. The machine then cuts or mills a block of Zirconia or alumina ceramic in the shape of the tooth to fit the model it just scanned. This creates the framework or substructure of the restoration. This technology is known as CAD/CAM or computer-aided design/computer-assisted manufacturing. It is used in many ceramic applications in numerous industries.

Once the milling is complete, the laboratory technician stacks or builds the aesthetic porcelain on the exterior of the ceramic framework to create a life-like restoration. The restoration is then fired in a kiln and polished. It is now ready for placement into the patient's mouth. Since 1995, the CEREC milling system has been available to dentists to mill the all-ceramic restorations in the office during the preparation appointment. This allows the patient to have the restoration permanently cemented the same day as the preparation. There are now numerous systems that mill alumina or Zirconia frameworks, and the technology is ever changing for the better.

Patient Instructions

Many patients believe that they cannot get decay or infection once a fixed prosthesis has been placed. It is very important for the patient to receive verbal and written instructions for home care of the patient's new restorations. Instructions include the following:

- Good home care is necessary for the longevity of the fixed prosthesis.
- Brush and floss with good technique at least twice daily. (Other products such as interproximal brushes may also be demonstrated to the patient.)

- In the case of a bridge, use floss threaders to clean under the pontic or artificial tooth and the sides of the abutments associated with the pontic.
- Superfloss can also be used to clean underneath the bridge. Superfloss is a piece of floss that has a stiff end for threading underneath the bridge, regular floss in the middle, and an end section that is similar to yarn to lift any plaque from the prosthesis or tooth structure. The yarn-like section provides a texture to better grab and remove the plaque from the prosthesis.
- Continue to have regular visits with the hygienist to help maintain overall oral health.

Role of the Laboratory Technician

The roles of the dental laboratory and the laboratory technician are vital. Fixed prostheses cannot be created without their assistance. The laboratory technician is trained at a two- or four-year school and receives a certificate or degree in dental technology.

The technician receives the impression, bite registration, and prescription. The impression is poured into models. The models are trimmed and dies cut. A **die** is a precise replica of a prepared tooth created from an impression used by the dental laboratory technician to make the cast or milled restoration. See Chapter 37 for a more complete description of laboratory procedures. For fixed prosthodontics, the dental laboratory technician fabricates the restoration according to the laboratory prescription completed by the dentist.

Laboratory Prescription

The laboratory prescription gives the dental laboratory technician all of the information needed to fabricate the desired restoration. Many laboratories provide the prescription forms they want the dentist to complete. Other prescription forms are bought through the local dental associations. All laboratory prescriptions are duplicated. The dentist and the laboratory must keep a copy of the prescription for at least two years or as required by state law. Dentists are advised to keep a copy of the prescription in the patient's chart. The prescription should contain the following information:

- Dentist's name, license number, address of the office, phone number, and signature
- Patient's name or identification number
- Type of prosthesis to be fabricated
- Type of materials to be used in fabrication
- Exact shade of restoration and any anatomic characterization
- Preparation date and date the case is expected to be back to the dental office

SUMMARY

Fixed prosthodontics is the art and science of restoring defective or damaged teeth and/or replacing missing teeth. Other than general dentistry, fixed prosthodontics procedures are the most common type of procedure in the general dental office. Many cases are complex, however, and require the expertise of a prosthodontist.

Fixed restorations are indirect and usually require two appointments and a provisional restoration. Depending on the dentist and state regulations, the dentist may rely on the dental assistant to perform some of the procedural steps such as packing the cords, mixing and sometimes

taking impressions and bite registrations, making the provisional restoration, and choosing the shade. Inlays, onlays, veneers, crowns, and bridges all require four-handed dentistry in the operatory and a laboratory technician to fabricate the final restoration. Many steps must be accurate to develop the best restoration for the patient. It is the patient's responsibility to maintain the restoration with excellent home care. The placement of porcelain veneers have become one of the most popular cosmetic procedures in the United States.

KEY TERMS

- **Abutment:** A natural tooth or implant used to support or anchor a fixed or removable dental prosthesis. p. 631
- **Cast post:** Metal post created by a laboratory to be placed into an endodontically treated tooth to improve retention of a cast restoration. p. 633
- **Core buildup:** The restorative material that re-creates the lost tooth structure of the anatomical crown (also known as just a *buildup*); part of the cast post that extends into the anatomical crown. p. 632
- **Crown:** A restoration covering or replacing a major part of or the entire clinical crown of a tooth. p. 630
- **Die:** A precise replica of a prepared tooth created from an impression used by the dental laboratory to make the cast or milled restoration. p. 640
- **Fixed partial denture:** A prosthetic replacement of one or more missing teeth cemented or attached to abutment teeth or implant abutments adjacent to the space. p. 631
- **Implant:** A titanium, screw-like device specially designed to be placed surgically within the mandibular or maxillary bone as a means of providing for a dental prosthesis. p. 632
- **Inlay:** A cast or milled restoration designed to fill a Class II cavity preparation. p. 628

- **Maryland bridge:** A type of fixed partial denture that does not require crowns, but may require a minimally invasive preparation to the lingual aspect of the adjacent teeth; also known as a resin-bonded bridge. The wings of the prosthesis are bonded to the lingual surfaces of adjacent natural teeth. p. 631
- **Milled restoration:** A precision-cut piece of ceramic that fits a die for a crown, inlay, or onlay. p. 628
- **Onlay:** A cast or milled restoration designed to cover the occlusal surface of at least one cusp of a posterior tooth. p. 628
- **Pontic:** An artificial tooth on a fixed partial denture or bridge. p. 631
- **Porcelain-fused-to-metal crown (PFM):** An indirect restoration in which porcelain is fused to the external surfaces of a casting to imitate the appearance of natural tooth structure; usually provides full coverage. p. 630
- **Prosthesis:** A replacement for a missing tooth. p. 627
- **Prosthodontist:** A dental specialist whose practice is limited to the restoration of the natural teeth and/or the replacement of missing teeth with artificial substitutes. p. 627
- **Veneer:** Ultrathin layer of composite resin or porcelain bonded to the facial surface of teeth. p. 628

CHECK YOUR UNDERSTANDING

1. Fixed prosthodontics is defined as
   a. the area of dentistry focused of the placement of direct restorations.
   b. the area of dentistry focused on root canal therapy.
   c. the area of dentistry focused on the replacement of fractured or missing teeth.
   d. the area of dentistry focused on the removal of teeth.

2. Which of the following are required for an indirect restoration?
   a. two appointments
   b. a provisional restoration
   c. a laboratory technician
   d. permanent cementation
   e. all of the above

CHECK YOUR UNDERSTANDING (continued)

3. A crown differs from an onlay in that a crown
   a. covers the occlusal surface.
   b. has margins extending to the gingiva at some point on the preparation.
   c. can be made of gold or ceramic.
   d. preserves healthy portion of the tooth.

4. An abutment is
   a. the artificial tooth between two prepared teeth.
   b. sometimes an implant.
   c. the supporting tooth of a bridge.
   d. both a and c.
   e. both b and c.

5. The expanded duties dental assistant can perform all of the following steps in a fixed prosthesis procedure except
   a. taking the bite registration.
   b. developing the treatment plan.
   c. making the provisional restoration.
   d. packing the gingival retraction cords.

6. The purpose of a hemostatic agent is
   a. to shrink the gingival tissue and control bleeding and sulcular fluids.
   b. to help the margin have a smooth surface.
   c. to physically push the tissue away from the prepared tooth.
   d. to provide the operator with a better view of the prepared margins.
   e. both a and d.

7. Why is it important to provide the laboratory technician with an accurate impression?
   a. to allow the technician to know the exact location of the prepared margins

   b. to have the most accurate restoration for placement on the prepared tooth
   c. to avoid gaps or spaces at the margin of the tooth with the restoration
   d. all of the above

8. How does a bridge preparation and appointment differ from a crown preparation?
   a. The bridge appointment is longer.
   b. A bridge requires only a single preparation.
   c. A bridge often requires three appointments.
   d. a, b, and c.
   e. Both a and c.

9. The laboratory prescription should contain all of the following except
   a. the patient's address and phone number.
   b. the type and shade of the restoration to be fabricated.
   c. the dentist's signature.
   d. the type of material to be used for the restoration.

10. Milled ceramics
    a. are aesthetically superior to other restorations.
    b. can be made in the office with the proper equipment.
    c. are made of alumina or Zirconia.
    d. can be placed on anterior and some posterior teeth.
    e. all of the above.

INTERNET ACTIVITY

• Visit www.ivoclar.com. Click on the Products tab. On the left side of the screen there is a Video tab. Click and view several of the video clips. The video titled "Variolink II and IPS" shows the removal of temporary crowns, retraction cord placement, and cementation of crowns. These videos are created and sponsored by Ivoclar and feature their products.

WEB REFERENCES

• Academy of Prosthodontics www.academyprosthodontics.org
• American Academy of Fixed Prosthodontics www.fixedprosthodontics.org
• American College of Prosthodontics www.prosthodontics.org
• American Dental Association www.ada.org
• Dental Compare: The Buyers Guide for Dental Professionals www.dentalcompare.com
• Dental-Videos.com www.dental-videos.com
• Ivoclar Vivadent www.ivoclar.com

41

Provisional Coverage

Learning Objectives

After reading this chapter, the student should be able to:

- State the importance of provisional restorations.
- Explain the criteria for the use of provisional restorations.
- Describe techniques for fabricating provisional restorations.
- List the different types of provisional materials.
- Demonstrate fabricating a custom provisional crown or bridge.
- Demonstrate fabricating a provisional aluminum crown.
- Demonstrate giving home care instructions to a patient following delivery of a provisional restoration.

Preparing for Certification Exams

- Fabricate and place temporary crowns where allowed by state regulations.

Key Terms

Aesthetics	Margin
Contour	Polymerization
Dual-curing process	Provisional
Embrasure	Self-curing process
Exothermic reaction	Stent
Fabricated	

Chapter Outline

- Criteria for Provisional Fabrication
  - —Mechanical Criteria
  - —Biological Criteria
  - —Aesthetic Criteria

- Types of Provisional Coverage
  - —Direct Technique
  - —Indirect Technique
  - —Custom Provisional Coverage
  - —Preformed Polycarbonate Provisional Crowns
  - —Celluloid Provisional Crowns
  - —Aluminum Provisional Crowns

- Provisional Restoration Materials
  - —Methacrylate
  - —Bis-Acryl Composites
  - —Bis-GMA Composites

- Home Care Instructions

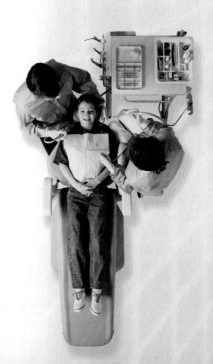

Provisional restorations

are fabricated to protect the prepared tooth/teeth structure during the period between the tooth preparation and seating of the final restoration. The provisional restoration is referred to as a temporary prosthesis or an interim restoration. The term **provisional** may refer to a temporary crown, inlay, onlay, or bridge that is designed to protect the prepared tooth or teeth while the permanent prosthesis is being **fabricated,** or constructed, by the dental laboratory technician.

The temporary restoration is created to cover the entire tooth with a natural appearance. Proper occlusal/incisal anatomy with sealed margins and proximal contacts between the teeth is important for a successful temporary restoration. Several techniques and materials are available to the dental clinician for this purpose. The dentist, the dental assistant under supervision of the dentist, or the dental lab technician will construct the provisional.

Although it is temporary, a provisional restoration fulfills many requirements for both the patient and the dentist and complements the quality of dentistry provided by the facility. The provisional restoration should:

- protect the prepared teeth.
- allow for healing of the soft tissues.
- maintain proper relationship of the contacts between the teeth.

- provide interim function for the patient.
- provide for aesthetics and phonetics.

Provisional restorations are most often required for a two-week period, but may be needed for longer depending on the needs of the patient and the patient's treatment plan (Figure 41.1). The patient may need to wear the provisional for six months or longer while the bone and gingival tissues heal around an implant. These types of provisionals must be strong enough to provide long-term service.

After the provisional restoration has been properly trimmed and adjusted, it is cemented with temporary cement. Preformed provisional restorations are only available and useful for single temporary crowns and are lined with acrylic resin to achieve a proper fit. Multiunit bridge preparations require custom-made provisional restorations. Various acrylic resin materials for fabricating provisionals are available, some of which have been utilized for many years. Newer products have improved the delivery of provisional resins in addition to their quality.

Dental Assistant PROFESSIONAL TIP

Fabricating quality provisional restorations takes experience and skill. Skills can be learned through concentrated practice and attention to detail. The dental assistant must understand the proper contours of teeth and how they contact each other. The embrasure spaces are extremely important to contour and smooth accurately.

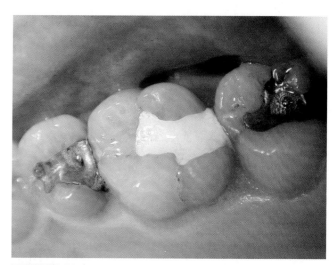

FIGURE 41.1
A provisional restoration.
Image courtesy Instructional Materials for the Dental Team, Lex., KY

Criteria for Provisional Fabrication

Provisional restorations should protect the teeth against invasive microorganisms, food, and saliva. In addition, for anterior teeth, the appearance of temporary restorations is important. The provisional restorations should also prevent conduction of hot and cold temperatures for the patient's comfort. Maintaining accurate proximal contacts between the teeth and the proper occlusal relationship between the maxillary and mandibular arches prevents drifting of the dentition. If the temporary restoration does not fit properly in these areas, the permanent restoration may not adapt into the space correctly and will need to be adjusted prior to cementing.

Temporary restorations require good adaptation to the tooth at the margin (Figure 41.2). The **contour** is the overall shape of the provisional, which must approximate the original natural tooth form. The **embrasure** spaces of the provisional must be properly created and formed to the accurate outline of the tooth. Embrasures are the V-shaped spaces formed by the contour and position of adjacent teeth. It is essential that the interproximal embrasure spaces between the teeth be designed accurately on the provisional restoration. They must be shaped and rounded smooth and flush with the marginal edge of the restorative preparation.

Proper contouring of provisionals can assist in the patient's maintenance of periodontal health by allowing access to the soft tissues during oral home care. Provisional restorations must satisfy mechanical, biological, and aesthetic factors, all of which relate to each other. A properly constructed temporary will have the following characteristics:

- It will be smooth and polished so it does not irritate the tongue, lips, cheeks, or gingival tissues.
- It will provide the appropriate occlusal form and relationship to any opposing teeth.
- It will provide appropriate proximal contact relationships with unprepared adjacent teeth to prevent drifting.
- It will provide acceptable aesthetics if placed in the anterior area of the mouth.

Mechanical Criteria

A provisional restoration must function during the length of time the patient wears it. A large amount of stress is placed on provisional crowns and bridges during chewing, and the provisional crown or bridge should be strong enough to withstand that stress. The strength of the material selected by the dentist and the design of the provisional influences the durability of the interim restoration. This is less of a concern with single-unit teeth than with multiple-unit bridges.

Fixed provisional bridges function as a beam to extend over the area where the teeth are missing. The greater the length of the bridge span, the higher the chance exists for the restoration to flex. This creates high stress at the connections where the teeth on either side of

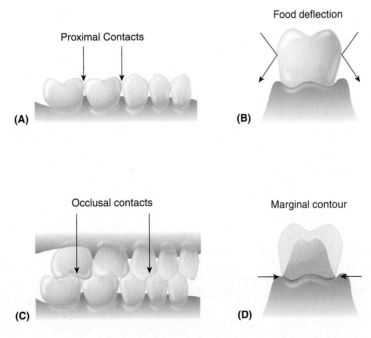

FIGURE 41.2
Features of a sound temporary restoration: (a) Correct proximal contacts, (b) proper tooth contours, (c) proper occlusal contacts, and (d) correct fit at the preparation margins.

the missing tooth or teeth must support the provisional bridge. Therefore, to reduce the potential for fracturing, the abutment connectors of the temporary bridge should be larger than those on the final restoration.

Reinforcement of a provisional bridge should also be considered when oral habits such as clenching or grinding are present. When a patient must wear the provisional for a prolonged period of time, the crown or bridge may need to be removed and reseated more than once. If it is strong enough it will not fracture upon removal.

What could happen to a provisional bridge if it is not strong enough? What oral habits might cause this problem to occur? **?**

Biological Criteria

Proper contours of the provisional and adaptation at the margin help the patient maintain the periodontal health of the tooth-supporting structures. A provisional restoration needs to seal and insulate the prepared tooth from injury and recurring decay. The temporary crown or bridge should fit well at the margin where the restoration meets the tooth structure to prevent saliva from leaking onto the recently cut dentinal tubules. (See Chapter 8 for more information on dentinal tubules.) This also prevents sensitivity to hot and cold temperatures for the patient during the interim time before the permanent restoration is cemented in the mouth.

To prevent sensitivity, the temporary should extend to the margin of the tooth preparation but not beyond. It should fit the tooth snugly so food and plaque do not get caught under the margin area, which can cause gingival irritation and bleeding. If the provisional is to be worn for a long period of time, dental caries may occur and the permanent restoration will no longer fit the tooth properly.

All provisional materials produce some heat during their setting time. This exothermic setting temperature may have an adverse effect on the tooth pulp while the temporary crown or bridge is being made. The dental assistant must be aware of this and ensure that the provisional is not allowed to sit on the tooth for too long. The newer dual-cured materials prevent this problem, although they are more expensive to use.

To allow the patient to keep the provisional restoration clean, the provisional must have a good fit at the margin, the proper contour, and a smooth surface. A temporary that extends beyond the margin into the gingival tissues will become an irritant to the tissue and cause plaque buildup and inflammation. The longer the provisional restoration must be worn by the patient, the more any deficiencies in its fit and contour will adversely influence the health of gingival tissues. If the restoration's margins are inadequate or rough, the gingiva will be affected. Any inflammation will cause bleeding, possible

gingival recession, and may affect the fit of the final restoration and the patient's periodontal health.

The provisional restoration also needs to be able to maintain the teeth in a stable position. A stable provisional is less likely to allow teeth to shift during the interim period before the final restoration is seated. Any movement, even minor, will require adjustments or even a possible remake of the final restoration. Adequate maxillary and mandibular occlusal relationships, as well as proximal contacts, will prevent drifting and extrusion of teeth that can affect the fit of the final restoration. Proper contouring and adequate adaptation of the provisional to the margin should maintain teeth in their accurate position. Correct shaping of the temporary crown or bridge will maintain the relationships between the teeth, prevent food impaction into the soft tissues, and allow the patient to clean the area well during home oral hygiene procedures.

What might happen if the margin of the temporary crown or bridge does not fit well? How can these problems be prevented? **?**

Aesthetic Criteria

Aesthetics, sometimes spelled *esthetics*, refers to how the provisional restoration looks in the mouth. This is especially important in the anterior of the mouth. How well the provisional matches the color, contour, and shape of the other teeth is important to the patient. Selection of which provisional material to use determines how well the teeth will match. Provisional materials are available in various tooth shades that can be selected by the dental assistant. Some temporary resin materials may absorb stains from coffee, tea, or other dark beverages, especially if the restoration is not well polished.

Types of Provisional Coverage

Numerous techniques and materials can be used to achieve a successful temporary restoration. Regardless of the material used to construct a provisional, the most

Patient Education

Educating patients on how to care for their provisional restoration is extremely important. The dental assistant has an obligation to take the time to make sure instructions are clear and well understood. The patient must comprehend that if the provisional falls out during the interim period while the permanent restoration is being made by the dental laboratory, the permanent restoration may not fit. The patient must also realize that the gingiva can quickly become inflamed if plaque is allowed to remain. Results of the final restoration will not be the quality that the patient or the dentist desires if the foundation is not solid. This is especially true if the provisional is placed on implants. The foundation must be kept clean for a long period of time for the bone to be healthy and strong.

common method used to record the shape and size of a tooth before it is prepared and impressions made is through the use of a stent matrix or template. A **stent** is any material used to make a mold of the original contour of a tooth or teeth. The stent provides a preliminary shape for the provisional and simplifies custom fabrication of the temporary crown or bridge (Figure 41.3).

Stents can be created by using various methods and several different choices of materials. A stent is often utilized when a fixed bridge is needed by the patient, especially when implants are involved. The technique used most often is to make the stent and provisional during the patient's appointment. Methods used to create a stent matrix involve the use of:

- a vacuum-formed custom tray.
- an alginate impression.
- a polyvinylsiloxane impression.
- a thermoplastic disc.

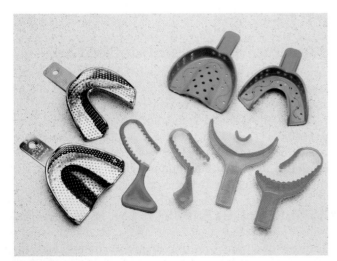

FIGURE 41.3
Provisional stents.

There are also several types of preformed provisional restorations that can be utilized as stents for fabricating a provisional crown. A preformed provisional single-unit crown can be made from polymer, polycarbonate, celluloid, copper, or aluminum material.

Following tooth preparation by the dentist, the provisional material is mixed and placed into the stent. A lubricant may be placed into the stent first to ensure that the temporary material does not adhere to the tooth or model. It is then seated over the prepared teeth or model. After the material enters a rubbery stage, it can be removed from the stent and is easily trimmed with scissors or a scalpel blade. Due to the malleability of the temporary material at this phase, the dental assistant must be careful not to distort the provisional.

The provisional is then reseated onto the tooth or model preparation and the material allowed to completely harden, after which further adjustments are made to achieve a proper fit. When completed, the provisional material will fill in the space between the tooth preparation and the original shape of the tooth, which will satisfy aesthetics and provide for tooth function and stabilization of the arch.

Direct Technique

Most dentists use a direct technique to fabricate provisional restorations. With this method the provisional restoration is made directly on the patient's tooth. The advantages of the direct technique include time efficiency and the low cost of traditional provisional materials. An additional advantage of the newer dual-cured resin materials is the shorter time of temperature rise during polymerization. Self-cured materials cause a significantly higher temperature rise during polymerization than dual-cured materials. **Polymerization** is the chemical setting process of resin materials. The disadvantage of the direct technique is the high temperatures created as both the self-curing and dual-curing resins harden. When using this method, the dental assistant must be very aware of the heat released by the chemical setting reaction of acrylic resins. As acrylics set, the high temperatures given off might harm surrounding oral tissues and the dental

Professionalism

Excellent dental assisting skills are perfected through experience and persistence. The dental assistant who can construct quality provisionals will quickly become valuable to the dentist and advance in his or her career. Continuing education courses are frequently offered to expand the skills and knowledge of the dental team. The dental assistant should attend seminars as often as possible to learn techniques and understand how to work with the newest resin materials.

pulp of the tooth. The chemical reaction that produces heat during the setting of acrylic resins is called an **exothermic reaction**. Air or water can be used to cool the tooth during the setting time. This helps prevent too high a temperature for the patient. Removing the temporary crown from the prepared tooth before the acrylic resin material completes curing also prevents the tooth from becoming too warm; however, the material must be set hard enough to avoid distortion to the temporary crown.

Indirect Technique

The indirect technique of creating provisional restorations is more time consuming than the direct technique. The indirect method requires that impressions for study models be taken before the patient's crown or bridge preparation appointment. The dental laboratory technician, the dentist, or the dental assistant fabricates the temporary crown on the model rather than in the patient's mouth so it is ready when the patient returns for the preparation appointment. The tooth or teeth to be prepared must be cut on the model by the dentist. The dental lab technician may prefer this method particularly with complex cases. The lab technician may use wax to design aesthetic anterior restorations and provisional restorations.

This preliminary procedure of fabricating a temporary restoration assists the dental laboratory technician prior to fabricating the permanent restoration. The dental assistant will create a gypsum model from the impressions and fabricate the stent matrix from the cast model to create an accurate replica of the patient's tooth or teeth before they are prepared for the crown or bridge.

Advantages of the indirect technique include less chair time for the patient, a preliminary design of the tooth/teeth preparation as well as the permanent restoration, and better control of heat released during polymerization. The disadvantages of this method are the time required to complete the provisional and the additional expense due to time spent by the dentist and/or the dental laboratory technician.

What must be created or made before a provisional restoration can be fabricated? What is released during the chemical setting process of acrylic materials? What is the advantage of the newer dual-cured resin materials?

Custom Provisional Coverage

To fabricate a custom provisional, the material is mixed and placed in an impression or stent, which is then seated over the patient's prepared tooth or teeth for the direct method, or on the model for the indirect method (Procedure 41-1). After approximately two to three minutes, depending on the material used, it will enter a rubbery stage. At this point the provisional can be removed from the stent and the excess material promptly trimmed with scissors or a scalpel blade. Excess material that must be removed and does not belong to the proper shape of the provisional is called *flash*.

The provisional is then reseated onto the preparation or preparations while still malleable (i.e., while it is still able to be formed). If the material used is one that undergoes an exothermic reaction, the temporary must be kept cool with a water spray during the polymerization stage so the tooth does not get too hot. If the provisional material is dual cured, the restoration is partially light cured with a standard handheld light curing unit until it becomes firm. It is then removed and the final curing process is complete in 20 to 60 seconds, depending on the manufacturer's directions for the particular material. The provisional is then trimmed to its final shape with acrylic burs, discs, or other rotary instruments. During the rubbery stage the dental assistant must be very careful not to distort the provisional or it will need to be remade.

Preformed Polycarbonate Provisional Crowns

Preformed polycarbonate provisional crowns are available for both anterior and bicuspid posterior teeth. They are available in a variety of shapes and sizes. Polycarbonate crowns are lined with a provisional material and trimmed to fit the tooth preparation. The crown matrix remains part of the restoration. Preformed provisional restorations are useful for single-unit temporary crowns only.

Celluloid Provisional Crowns

Celluloid crown form provisionals are available only for premolars and anterior teeth. They are clear shells and must be cut to fit the tooth shape and height. Celluloid crown forms are then lined with the provisional resin material, after which the celluloid matrix is removed from the form prior to temporary cementation.

Aluminum Provisional Crowns

Aluminum shell crowns are available only for posterior teeth where aesthetics is not a concern. They are available in a variety of sizes and organized in the box according to right and left sides in addition to maxillary and mandibular shapes (Figure 41.4). A measurement device is included in the kit to help with selecting the proper size of aluminum crown. Aluminum shells are marked on the inside with a number referring to their size.

Aluminum crowns may be lined with acrylic resin material to create a better fit, to help insulate the prepared tooth from heat and cold, and to provide a stronger provisional restoration. To create an ideal aluminum provisional, the aluminum shell can be removed from the acrylic provisional. If the shell is not removed,

Procedure 41-1 Fabricating and Placing a Custom Provisional Bridge

Dental assistants should be sure to check with their state practice laws to determine what tasks they are allowed to perform versus the tasks that are to be accomplished by the dentist.

Equipment and Supplies

- Basic setup: mirror, explorer, cotton pliers
- Cement spatula, mixing pad, temporary cement
- Saliva ejector, high-volume evacuator tip (HVE), air/water syringe tip
- Crown and bridge scissors
- Bis-acryl automix cartridge and delivery system
- Slow-speed motor
- Assortment of acrylic burs, discs, and mandrels
- High-speed handpiece with diamond burs
- Articulating paper
- Floss

Procedure Steps

1. Prior to preparation for the bridge, while the anesthetic is taking effect, take a quadrant impression with alginate impression material. Cut out the pontic area with a scalpel blade. Remove any interdental gingival areas to provide bulk for the temporary restoration and so the impression will seat correctly later. Wrap the impression in a wet paper towel to keep moist so it does not distort when drying out.

2. Inform the patient that you are going to make a temporary bridge, which will allow the teeth to function normally while the permanent bridge is being fabricated by the dental laboratory. Select a tooth shade if appropriate.

3. Clean and dry the teeth. Fill the impression with the bis-acryl provisional material, placing extra material into the pontic area. To prevent air bubbles, dispense provisional material onto the occlusal (or incisal) surfaces and then bring the tip of the material gingivally, slightly overbuilding it.

4. Insert the impression back into the mouth over the prepared teeth. Hold firmly in place for approximately two to three minutes. Check that the material is still in its rubbery stage with an instrument. If left to set too rigid, removal may be difficult.

5. Remove the provisional bridge together with the impression from the prepared teeth. While still rubbery, excess material may be cut with crown and bridge scissors. Allow five additional minutes for the material to set. Evaluate the provisional bridge for fit, voids, and thin areas.

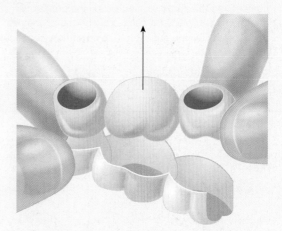
Remove the acrylic resin bridge from the formed stent matrix.

6. Mark the margins and proximal contact with a pencil to ensure these areas do not get trimmed away. Trim the margin areas to shape with slow-speed acrylic burs. Trim the embrasure areas with discs on a mandrel while using a fulcrum and eye protection.

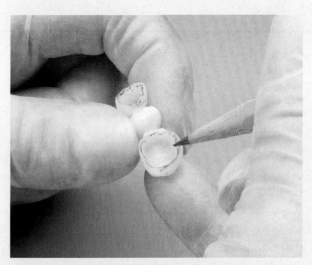
Mark the interproximal contacts with a pencil.

7. Place the bridge onto the prepared teeth and ask the patient to carefully close the teeth together while you hold articulating paper between the maxilla and mandible. Note high spots and adjust the occlusion with slow-speed round burs. Polish with a wet ragwheel and pumice. Rinse and dry the abutment teeth well.

8. Rinse the patient's tooth to clean it and dry it well. Place cotton rolls on the buccal and lingual areas and instruct the patient to hold her mouth open while you mix the cement.

continued on next page

Procedure 41-1 *continued from previous page*

9. Mix the temporary cement or place automix temporary cement into the abutment teeth. Line the provisional abutments and place the temporary bridge on the prepared teeth. Tell the patient to bite down firmly on a cotton roll.

10. Allow the temporary cement to set. Remove excess cement from around the margin.

11. Floss the gingival sulcus to remove cement from under the gingiva. Pull the floss out through the side so the temporary bridge will not be loosened. Use a bridge threader to floss under the pontic. Rinse the area well.

12. Give the patient a mirror and show her how to clean under the pontic and abutment areas. Provide postoperative instructions.

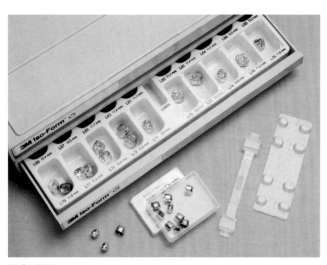

FIGURE 41.4
Selection of aluminum crowns.

the metal will react with acidic beverages or food and produce an unpleasant taste for the patient.

The dental assistant will try the shell on the prepared tooth and trim it to fit, adjust any proximal contacts, and then smooth any sharp areas with a green stone, a sandpaper disc, or contouring pliers (Procedure 41-2).

What could happen if the aluminum crown form is left on as part of the provisional restoration? What are some foods and drinks that should be avoided when wearing a provisional aluminum crown? **?**

Provisional Restoration Materials

Numerous materials are available for use in constructing provisional restorations. Advances in technology continue to lead to improvements in the strength, shade choices, setting characteristics, and clinical techniques used for provisional materials. All provisional restorative materials have their advantages and disadvantages as well as desirable and undesirable properties. The success-

ful outcome of a temporary crown or bridge depends on which method is utilized for its fabrication.

Methacrylate

Methacrylates have been used successfully for many years. The methacrylate group is acrylic or plastic, most often mixed as a powder/liquid system, and include methyl-methacrylate, ethyl-methacrylate, and vinylethyl-methacrylate.

Advantages to methacrylates are that they are fracture resistant and can be easily polished. Disadvantages include the higher capacity for shrinkage, the heat generated during polymerization, and less aesthetic appeal when compared to the newer provisional materials. Another disadvantage is the unpleasant odor that the material produces.

Methyl-methacrylate, ethyl-methacrylate, and vinylethyl-methacrylate materials set through a **self-curing process**, which causes the materials to harden when the monomer and polymer chemicals are mixed. The methylethyl-methacrylate materials are supplied in a powder/liquid system (Figure 41.5). They are mixed as a base and catalyst

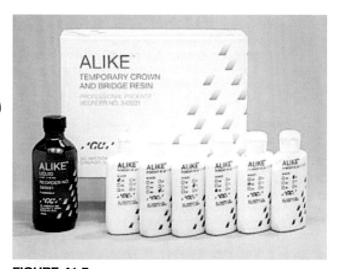

FIGURE 41.5
Methyl-methacrylate acrylic resin powder and liquid.
Courtesy GC America, Inc.

Procedure 41-2 Fabricating and Placing an Aluminum Shell Provisional Restoration

Dental assistants should be sure to check with their state practice laws to determine what tasks they are allowed to perform versus the tasks that are to be accomplished by the dentist.

Equipment and Supplies

- Basic setup: mirror, explorer, cotton pliers
- Cement spatula, mixing pad, temporary cement
- Saliva ejector, high-volume evacuator tip (HVE), air/water syringe tip
- Assortment of aluminum shells
- Crown and bridge scissors
- Contouring pliers
- Hemostats
- Dappen dish
- Methyl-methacrylate acrylic powder and liquid
- Slow-speed handpiece
- Assortment of acrylic burs, green stones, and discs
- Articulating paper
- Floss

Procedure Steps

1. Inform the patient that you are going to make a temporary crown, which will allow the tooth to function normally while the permanent crown is being fabricated by the dental laboratory.

2. Use the measurement device included in the aluminum shell kit to measure the mesiodistal distance of the tooth needing the temporary. If a shell is selected that is slightly larger or smaller than necessary, it is soft enough to be shaped to the proper proportions with the contouring pliers.

3. Use cotton pliers to remove aluminum crowns from the box so as not to cross-contaminate the container. Try the shell on the prepared tooth. If the shell is too large, the proximal contact areas can be adjusted with the green stone. If the shell is too small, place the aluminum crown on the stretching block provided with the temporary crown kit, and stretch the margins slightly. Contouring pliers may also be used to stretch the aluminum crown to size. Disinfect any crown that has been tried on.

4. Aluminum shells must be trimmed from the marginal areas on the mesial and distal sides in order to seat completely on the tooth preparation. Using crown and bridge scissors, cut small slivered shapes from these areas. Trim the mesial and distal margins of the shell until the occlusal height of the crown is correct. Be sure to follow the contour of the gingival tissue.

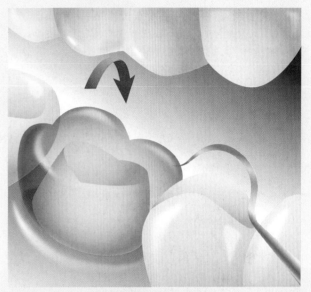

Aluminum crown being fitted for height.

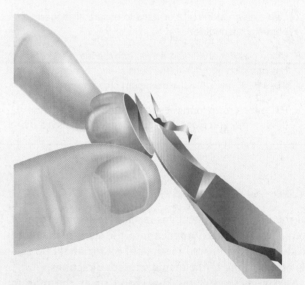

Aluminum crown being cut at the mesial and distal interproximal areas.

5. Try the shell back on the prepared tooth. It should extend to or slightly past the finish line of the preparation. Trim away any areas on the aluminum crown that impede on the gingival tissues enough to cause them to blanch.

6. Using the contouring pliers, smooth the aluminum crown and contour it so that it is wider at the proximal contact and more narrow at the gingiva. Pulling the pliers side to side will also smooth rough edges.

continued on next page

Procedure 41-2 *continued from previous page*

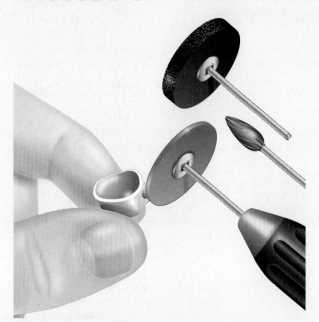

Smooth the jagged edges of the provisional.

7. Use a green stone and/or discs to ensure all jagged edges are smoothed.

8. Place powder and liquid acrylic into the large end of the dappen dish and mix to the consistency of honey. Place the acrylic resin into the aluminum crown form.

9. Place the crown form with acrylic onto the tooth and press firmly into place. When the excess resin feels rub-bery, remove the crown matrix carefully. For the next two to three minutes, continue placing the aluminum crown on and off the tooth. If it remains on the tooth, the acrylic resin will become too hot for the tooth pulp to tolerate. If left off the tooth for too long, the acrylic will shrink and it will no longer fit on the tooth.

10. When the acrylic is hardened, remove the aluminum shell by cutting with crown and bridge scissors and bending with the hemostats until it is completely removed. Try it on the tooth and have the patient close together on the articulating paper. Adjust the occlusion with the acrylic bur or green stone.

11. Using a lathe, a wet ragwheel, and pumice, polish the temporary crown until it is smooth. Rinse it well.

12. Rinse the patient's tooth to clean it and dry it well. Place cotton rolls on the buccal and lingual areas and instruct the patient to hold his mouth open while you mix the cement.

13. Mix the temporary cement. Fill the provisional crown and place it on the prepared tooth. Tell the patient to bite down firmly on a cotton roll.

14. Allow the temporary cement to set. Remove excess cement from around the margin. Floss the gingival sulcus to remove cement from under the gingiva. Pull the floss out through the side. Rinse the area well.

15. Give the patient a mirror and show him how to clean the provisional with floss by pulling it out the sides of the crown. Give postoperative instructions.

---

until the proper consistency is reached to form a rope of material which is then applied into the stent matrix and placed onto the prepared tooth until set for about 60 seconds or according to the manufacturer's directions.

Methyl-methacrylates have good fit at the **margin** (the junction where the provisional meets the tooth structure), are easily polished, and durable. Some methyl-methacrylates polymerize through a dual-curing process. Disadvantages of this material are its high exothermic reaction, low resistance to abrasion, and high shrinkage during polymerization.

Ethyl-methacrylates polish well, demonstrate minimal exothermic reaction, have good resistance to staining, and have a low rate of shrinkage while setting. However, they are not as hard or durable as the methyl-methacrylate resins. Vinylethyl-methacrylate materials are easily polished, exhibit minimal exothermic reaction, are resistant to abrasion, have good resistance to stain-

ing, and are flexible. They have the disadvantages, however, of not being as aesthetically pleasing nor as resistant to fractures as other materials.

Bis-Acryl Composites

Bis-acryl composites (Figure 41.6) are also known as bis-acryl resins. They are more aesthetic than the methacrylates, but are also more brittle and may not be suitable for provisional bridges. They work well, however, for single-unit crowns. Advantages of bis-acryl composites are their good fit at the margin, low exothermic reaction, resistance to abrasion, low shrinkage upon setting, excellent ability to be polished, and their availability in self-cured or dual-cured versions. Disadvantages of bis-acryl resins are that they are less resistant to stain, more brittle, and more expensive than the methacrylate group; they come in a limited selection of shades; and they are not as easy to repair.

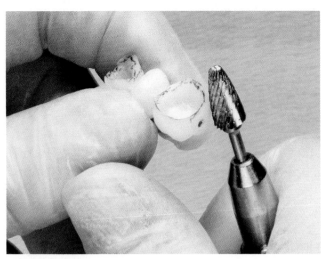

FIGURE 41.6
Bis-acrylic composite provisional.

Bis-GMA Composites

Bis-GMA resins have the fracture resistance of the methacrylates along with improved aesthetics, which allows for use in the anterior areas of the mouth where good aesthetics is essential. The resistance to fracture of this provisional material allows for its use when a longer-span bridge is necessary. Bis-GMA composite provisional restorative material also has a good marginal fit, good ability to be polished, and a very low exothermic reaction. It is resistant to abrasion, has a very low rate of shrinkage when setting, has good color selection and shade stability, is strong, and dual cured.

Bis-GMA composite resins are easily repaired by adding other composite resin materials. These materials are supplied as a cartridge system in which two syringes are placed side by side, one base and one catalyst. They are mixed together as the dental assistant squeezes the trigger on the handheld device and the materials are extruded through a mixing tip, which causes them to begin the setting process. These materials then go through a **dual-curing process** in which an application of

a visible light is necessary for the final set or curing of the material. The advantage of dual-cured resin materials is their lower temperature during polymerization compared to that of self-cured resins.

Which provisional restorative material has been used for many years? Which provisional material is more brittle and better suited for single crowns than multiple-unit bridges? Which provisional materials are dual cured?

Home Care Instructions

Explaining to patients how to care for a temporary crown, inlay, onlay, or bridge is extremely important to ensure the final restoration will fit properly when it comes from the dental laboratory. It is also essential for patients to understand how the provisional is cared for during the interim period. How the provisional is cared for determines the health of the surrounding tissues when the permanent crown or bridge is cemented in place.

The dental assistant has the important responsibility of explaining to the patient how to take care of the provisional restoration. The postoperative instructions to the patient should consist of these instructions:

- The restoration may be plastic or some other material and is only meant to serve the patient's needs and protect the tooth while the permanent crown or bridge is being made.

- Because the temporary restoration does not fit the mouth as perfectly as the permanent one will, the tooth (or teeth) may be sensitive to cold, hot, and sweets. It is important for the patient to come back to the office if the patient experiences extreme sensitivity.

- The temporary restoration cement requires about 45 minutes to set, so the patient should not chew anything during that period of time. If the gingiva is tender the patient should rinse with warm saltwater two to three times a day until the tooth feels normal.

- Certain foods will stick to the temporary crown, so the patient should not chew gum and should avoid sticky foods that might pull it loose during the interim period of time.

- Temporary restorations are not strong and could break or come off. If the restoration does loosen and come off, the patient must call the office immediately. The patient could go to the store and buy some Fixodent and place a small amount inside the provisional and place it back on the tooth until the patient can get in to see the dentist.

- The dental assistant must make sure the patient understands that the provisional cannot be left out of the

Cultural Considerations

Communication barriers exist even when people speak the same language and come from similar cultures. The dental assistant will occasionally need to explain dental procedures and especially home care instructions to patients who cannot understand what words are being spoken. A good dental assistant uses gestures and any visual aids feasible to explain to patients what is necessary to ensure the information is understood. The dental assistant should also emphasize the importance of completing the full treatment once started and ensure the patient understands that provisional crowns are temporary and not permanent.

mouth because the teeth will move and the final crown or bridge will not fit, and the tooth could be very uncomfortable and sensitive.

- The patient should know how to properly clean the provisional restoration. It should not be brushed or flossed too vigorously, but it is important to keep the area clean with a gentle touch.

- The provisional should be flossed daily but instead of pulling the floss up through the contacts of the teeth, it should be pulled out through the side so the area is cleaned but the restoration is not pulled loose.

- If the provisional is a multiunit bridge, the patient must be shown how to clean the interproximal areas around each abutment as well as how to clean underneath a bridge to keep the pontic area from building up plaque.

- The dental assistant should also explain to the patient how to clean the final restoration, how to use a bridge threader (Figure 41.7) for the provisional, and how to clean the permanent restoration.

- The patient may be instructed in the use of a Waterpik-type device to keep the provisional and permanent restoration clean.

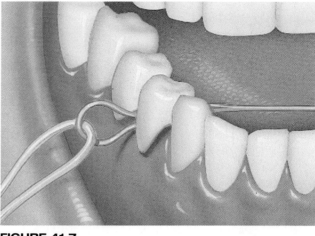

FIGURE 41.7
Bridge threader.

What are some of the postoperative instructions the dental assistant should explain to the patient? How should a bridge be cleaned?

Preparing for Externship

The dental assistant should prepare for externship by taking time to study the shape and form of teeth (morphology) and to gain experience with creating provisionals on models while still in the school environment. A dental assistant student should continue to practice fabricating provisional crowns and bridges on typodont models as often as possible before going to externship. During externship the dental assistant should watch and learn from the dentist or expanded functions dental assistant to see various techniques and materials utilized for provisional fabrication on behalf of patients.

SUMMARY

A provisional restoration must provide function, comfort, and aesthetic replacement for the prepared tooth structure while the permanent crown or bridge is being made at the dental laboratory. Fabrication of acceptable provisional restorations requires an assortment of clinical activities, material selection, and techniques. Several materials are successfully used to create temporary restorations. Provisional restorations must fit well at the margins and the proximal contacts and must provide an occlusal relationship between the maxillary and mandibular arches.

It is the responsibility of the dental assistant to show the patient how to properly care for the provisional while the permanent restoration is being fabricated by the dental laboratory. Ideally, temporaries should be similar to the final restoration by providing pleasing aesthetics to enhance the patient's self-image. A good provisional also gives the patient confidence in the skills of the dental team.

KEY TERMS

- **Aesthetics:** Refers to how the provisional restoration looks; also spelled esthetics.   p. 646
- **Contour:** The overall shape or form of the original tooth structure.   p. 645
- **Dual-curing process:** A process in which the material begins to harden through self-curing and then requires a final cure with a visible light unit.   p. 653

- **Embrasure:** The V-shaped space formed by the contour and position of adjacent teeth.   p. 645
- **Exothermic reaction:** A chemical reaction that produces heat during the setting of a material.   p. 648
- **Fabricated:** Made or constructed.   p. 644
- **Margin:** The junction where the provisional meets the tooth structure.   p. 652

KEY TERMS (continued)

- **Polymerization:** The chemical setting process of resin materials. p. 647
- **Provisional:** A temporary crown or bridge that is made to cover and protect the prepared tooth or teeth while the permanent prosthesis is being fabricated. p. 644
- **Self-curing process:** The hardening or setting process when two chemical materials are mixed. p. 650
- **Stent:** Any material used to make a mold of the original contour. p. 647

● CHECK YOUR UNDERSTANDING

1. Who will fabricate the provisional restoration?
   a. the dentist
   b. the dental assistant, where allowed by state policies
   c. the dental laboratory technician
   d. all of the above

2. To promote oral hygiene of the provisional restoration, the dental assistant must help the patient understand which of the following:
   a. where plaque is found
   b. how to floss the provisional
   c. how to brush the provisional
   d. how to remove plaque under the pontic of a bridge
   e. all of the above

3. A provisional restoration should
   a. have open contacts.
   b. have tight contacts.
   c. adapt to the margin.
   d. be longer than the margin.
   e. both b and c.

4. What is the chemical reaction called that gives off heat during the setting of dental materials?
   a. dual-cured
   b. exothermic
   c. stent
   d. fabrication

5. What is the mold of a tooth called before the tooth is prepared for the permanent restoration?
   a. dual-cured
   b. exothermic
   c. stent
   d. fabrication

6. What are the primary criteria categories for provisional restorations?
   a. self-cured, light-cured, and exothermic
   b. stent, mold, template, matrix
   c. mechanical, biological, aesthetic
   d. polymer, polycarbonate, celluloid, aluminum

7. Dual-cured resins
   a. set through self-curing only.
   b. set through light curing only.
   c. set through self-curing and light curing.
   d. do not require polishing.

8. If the provisional loosens or falls out and is not replaced, the teeth will
   a. shift.
   b. drift.
   c. extrude.
   d. move.
   e. all of the above.

9. Why should the dental assistant mark the contacts and margins of the provisional with a pencil?
   a. for aesthetic reasons
   b. so the provisional is strong
   c. to ensure the contacts are not lost
   d. for good adaptation to the margins
   e. both c and d

10. Correct shaping and contouring of the provisional will
    a. maintain the relationship between the teeth.
    b. prevent food impaction from the gingival tissues.
    c. allow the patient to clean the provisional properly.
    d. all of the above.

● INTERNET ACTIVITIES

- Go to www3.musc.edu/PRO-folder/Lectures/Lec.8.Preformed/preform.1.htm to learn how to construct preformed polycarbonate, celluloid, and aluminum provisionals.

- Visit http://advantagedentalinc.com/demonstration.html for directions on how to create custom temporary restorations using thermoplastic discs for the stent matrix.

● WEB REFERENCES

- Aurum Ceramic Product Collection www.aurumgroup.com/usa/default.htm
- In Vitro Comparison of Peak Polymerization Temperatures of 5 Provisional Restoration Resins www.cda-adc.ca/jcda/vol-67/issue-1/36.html
- 3M ESPE http://solutions.3m.com/wps/portal/3M/en_US/3M-ESPE/dental-professionals/

42

Removable Prosthodontics

Key Terms

Alveoplasty	Occlusal
Complete denture	Overdenture
Connectors	Partial denture
Denture base	Reline
Edentulous	Rests
Framework	

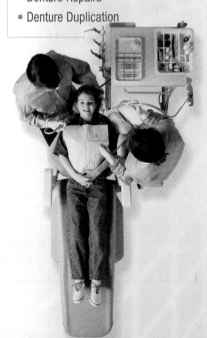

The main purposes of removable prosthetics are to replace and restore the function of the teeth, to stabilize the arch, and to improve the patient's overall health and aesthetics. Most patients would prefer to have a fixed prosthodontic, but for some cases this is not a choice of treatment. Considerations that indicate whether this type of treatment is possible include the patient's oral and overall health conditions and cost factors. The patient must have adequate bone structure to assist in the successful wearing of the prosthesis.

The difference between a fixed prosthesis and a removable one is that a removable prosthesis can be removed from the mouth for cleaning, repair, and examination. A fixed prosthodontic is a bridge that replaces one or more teeth; it is permanently cemented in place and cannot be removed for cleaning. The cleaning of a fixed prosthetic is done by correct toothbrushing and flossing and the use of a floss threader to clean underneath where the missing tooth has been replaced by a pontic.

A removable dental prosthesis is a fabricated substitution that is designed to replace missing oral structures and the teeth. The patient who is without teeth is referred to as being **edentulous**. There are three types of removable prostheses: the partial denture, the complete (full) denture, and the overdenture.

Dental Assistant PROFESSIONAL TIP

Remember that patients can be sensitive about wearing dentures. As a courtesy to patients, provide them with a tissue for privacy and mouthwash to freshen their mouths when patients are asked to remove their dentures. Be extremely careful cleaning and polishing the prosthesis. Hold the prosthesis securely in order to avoid dropping it. Before making adjustments, know the protocol of the office.

A **partial denture** is designed to replace one or more teeth in an arch. The partial denture is retained and supported by the underlying tissues and remaining teeth. The initial construction for the partial denture begins with a metal framework. The **framework** is designed to support the units and necessary components of the partial denture.

A **complete denture** replaces all of the teeth in a full arch, either the mandible or the maxilla. The complete denture is supported and retained by the underlying gingival tissues and bone, alveolar ridges, hard palate, and oral mucosa. The **denture base** is the initial component that holds the denture teeth.

The **overdenture** is designed to fit over retained roots, remaining teeth (most often cuspids), or an endosseous implant, which is surgically inserted into the alveolar process.

If the patient is a current denture wearer and is having difficulty wearing a lower denture, what would be some reasons for the difficulties? What additional treatment procedures could possibly help with these difficulties?

History of Removable Dental Prostheses

The use of complete sets of dentures has been found dating back to the 15th century. During this time, teeth were carved from bone or ivory and in some cases actual teeth from dead or living donors were used. These teeth rotted over time and the denture was uncomfortable for the patient to wear. The first porcelain denture was constructed in the 1700s. In the 1800s vulcanite was used to create dentures. In the late 19th century and early 20th century, metal such as gold was used as well. Later in the 20th century acrylic resin and other plastics became popular materials for fabricating dentures.

Modern technology has offered considerable advances in the quality and safety of the denture materials being used today. Today, lightweight materials including synthetic plastic resins and alloy metals allow for better support and fit, which allow for more comfort. With the ongoing perfecting of dental implants, dentures are now secured to the bone via an implant and the overdenture. Overall aesthetics continues to improve as well with better tooth shades and shapes to create a more natural look.

Factors Influencing the Choice of a Removable Prosthesis

Many factors must be considered prior to a patient receiving a removable prosthesis. The first step in any treatment is a thorough diagnosis. This is achieved through methods such as obtaining a complete health history and conducting an oral examination.

A complete health history consists of each question being answered by the patient to determine any past or present health conditions that could affect the outcome of the treatment plan. It is important that all questions on the health history be answered. The health history is considered a legal document in a court of law.

A common question that should be asked each time a patient is seen in the office for treatment is "Has there been a change in your health history or personal information since we saw you last?" If the answer is yes, have the patient include the change on the health history, date it, and have the patient initial it. Helpful records that should be requested from the patient and accompany the health history form include previous study models, radiographs, and photographs of the patient from the lateral and frontal view.

Consultation Appointment

After the patient has had her initial oral examination and the dentist has concluded that the patient is a good candidate for a removable prosthesis, the next appointment for the patient will be a consultation. The consultation is an appointment at which the dentist discusses the diagnosis and recommended treatment. The diagnostic aids gathered at the initial appointment are present for discussion and used as support for the diagnosis.

To prepare for the consultation appointment, the assistant should prepare the operatory or consulting room by mounting the radiographs on the light view box and placing the study models, patient facial photographs, and any other forms of visual aids where they are easily accessible to the dentist. The consultation appointment is held for the purposes of discussing the proposed treatment and financial arrangements and allowing the patient time to ask questions and discuss concerns.

What items are necessary for the assistant to have in the operatory during the consultation appointment?

Life Span Considerations

The treatment age for a person who needs a removable prosthodontic treatment can range from young to old. Determining factors include the patient's dental needs and socioeconomics. The patient who receives a dental prosthesis at a young age is more likely than an older patient to need implants for retention due to resorption of tissue and bone as the younger patient ages.

Removable Partial Denture

The partial denture is designed to replace missing teeth and to preserve the hard and soft tissues of the arches. In addition to replacing missing teeth, the design of the partial is intended to reestablish proper occlusion and evenly distribute the pressures on the abutment teeth (the natural teeth that provide support for the partial).

It is important for the abutment teeth to be without defect. If a defect or decay is present, the teeth or tooth must be completely restored prior to taking the impression for the construction of the partial to provide an accurate fit for the framework and the necessary strength needed to support a partial denture.

Considerations for Partial Denture Treatment

A number of factors need to be examined prior to a patient receiving a removable partial denture:

- Is there a tooth for a distal attachment? If there is no tooth for a distal attachment, then a partial is one choice to restore the function of the quadrant.
- Does the patient exhibit an interest in wearing a removable partial denture?
- Does the patient demonstrate ability and motivation to adjust to the wearing and maintaining of a removable partial denture?
- Can the patient physically and/or emotionally tolerate the wearing of dentures? Physical effects can include gagging.
- Is the patient willing and able to comply with the necessary oral hygiene regimen needed to ensure that the abutment teeth stay free of plaque?

Regular dental exams and teeth cleanings are encouraged to ensure that all remaining teeth and bone stay healthy. The dentist will discuss with the patient the patient's feelings about her overall oral health and her feelings with regard to the wearing of a removable or full prosthesis. In many instances wearing a removable prosthesis successfully takes commitment and persistence on the part of the patient.

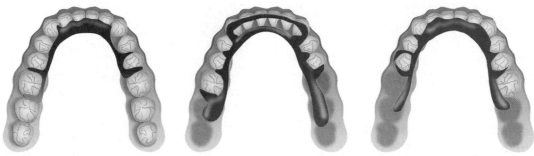

FIGURE 42.1
Mandibular processed partial denture with rests on the mesial surfaces of the first bicuspids.

If a patient who is mentally challenged needs to have extractions and is accompanied by his full-time caregiver, what home care instructions would be given and to whom and why?

Advantages of a Removable Partial Denture

For the patient with extreme financial difficulties, advanced periodontal disease, and a lack of ability to care for one's own natural teeth, a removable denture is often the only option for dental treatment. It is always best to attempt to keep all natural teeth when at all possible. The advantage of a removable prosthetic is that it replaces missing teeth and structure for function and aesthetics.

The partial denture can replace several teeth that are missing in a long span on both arches and in all quadrants. The partial denture is designed to provide support to any periodontally compromised teeth and can be worn by young or old patients. The young patient may require a removable temporary partial design to replace missing deciduous teeth. The prosthetic is called a flipper. It is designed to hold the spot for the permanent teeth to ensure correct eruption. The design of the partial denture is such that if additional natural teeth are lost, they can possibly be added to the existing partial; however, this cannot always be guaranteed. It depends on which teeth are the "rests." If the teeth that are lost are "rests" (see next section), the partial will have to be completely remade at additional cost to the patient.

Components of a Removable Partial Denture

The components of the removable partial denture include the rests, connectors, denture base, metal framework, retainers, and artificial teeth (Figures 42.1, 42.2, and 42.3). The **rests** are the part of the partial denture that contacts a tooth by resting on top of the occlusal surface of the prepared tooth to provide vertical and horizontal support. The rests are designed to control the position of the partial denture in relation to the teeth and supporting structures. Often

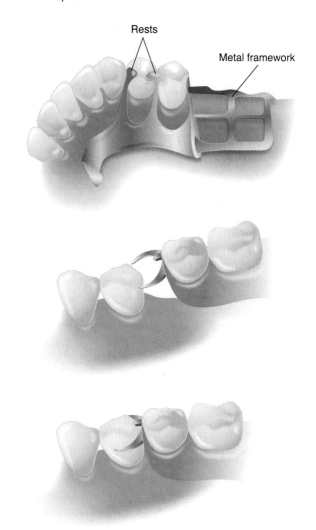

FIGURE 42.2
Mandibular unprocessed partial denture, displaying metal framework, connector, and rests.

the dentist will make a small preparation on the occlusal, incisal, or lingual surface on the tooth so the rest(s) can sit in the arch in correct occlusion. The preparation can be prepared using a round or egg-shaped carbide or diamond bur. This is most often done without anesthetic.

The **connectors** connect the different parts of the partial into one working unit. The connectors hold the working parts in the proper position and equally distribute the

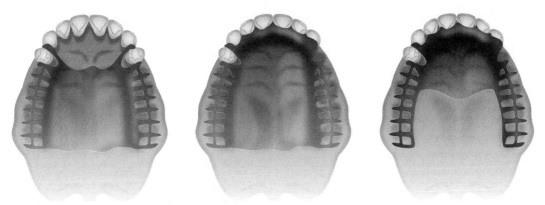

FIGURE 42.3
Maxillary unprocessed partial denture, displaying metal framework, rests, connector, and palatal strap.

stresses of mastication. The connector is divided into minor and major connectors. The major connector on the mandibular is often a bar or plate-type design, and it connects the left and right quadrants on the partial. The maxillary is often a bar, a strap, or a full palatal plate.

The stress breaker (hinge) may be built into the partial. It is not as common today to see the stress breaker due to current design changes, but you may see some on occasion. This is a metal device that relieves pressure on the abutment teeth during the mastication process.

The minor connectors are rests and clasps that provide both vertical and horizontal support to an abutment tooth and clasps that are connected to the major connector. These connectors protect against food impaction by filling the tooth and tissue junctions. The clasp(s) and rest(s) maintain the integrity of the arch by a mesial and distal bracing action.

The retainer is often referred to as a clasp. The retainer contacts the abutment teeth and prevents movement of the partial when chewing and swallowing. The design of the retainer is one of two types: one type encircles and adapts to the abutment tooth or teeth and the other, a bar type, extends from the gingival to the occlusal of the tooth.

The denture base is the part of the partial denture that is constructed to look like gingival tissue. It is often made of acrylic with fibers to enhance the natural appearance. The artificial teeth are held into the denture base. The artificial teeth are constructed of either acrylic or porcelain and are held into the denture base with either holes or pins in the underside of the teeth, or in the case of acrylic, they are actually bonded directly to the denture base. The teeth come in numerous sizes, shapes, and shades.

Removable Partial Denture Appointments and Procedure

Once the patient has had a thorough examination and either a prophylaxis or periodontal treatment performed, the procedure for the construction of the removable partial denture can begin. It is imperative that the oral structures, remaining teeth, gingival tissues, and alveolar bone be in a healthy state to ensure overall success of this procedure. The objective of the treatment is to replace the missing teeth.

To begin the procedure, the dentist makes adjustments to the occlusal surfaces of the remaining teeth to allow for clearance of the metal framework between the arches. The buccal and lingual surfaces are contoured to allow for the partial to be easily inserted and removed by the patient. If the teeth are unable to be contoured to achieve the desired angulations, then the abutment teeth need to be crowned to create the desired contour.

Once the adjustments are made and the contours are achieved, then the final impression and wax bite is taken. A desired tooth shade is selected. These are then all sent to a dental laboratory for initial processing. The final impression and wax bite is disinfected prior to being sent to the dental lab. In many cases the dental laboratory will send back to the dental office a wax try-in, which is the partial prepared in a wax form only for the purpose of "trying it in" to evaluate the overall fit and to establish the patient's correct bite. The wax bite is then secured to the metal framework for stabilization purposes (Procedure 42-1).

After the procedure, the patient should be educated on how to take care of his teeth so that loss of more teeth in the future can be minimized. If left undisturbed, plaque (biofilm) leads to periodontal disease, which will result in additional tooth loss. The dental team is responsible for offering the patient oral hygiene instructions so the patient is aware of where he is leaving plaque when he brushes and flosses his teeth. The patient is strongly encouraged to comply with the oral hygiene instructions. If the patient has to have additional natural teeth removed (extracted) in the future, adding the lost teeth onto the existing partial is a common dental practice.

Complete (Full) Dentures

When a patient presents with missing teeth, in order to replace the lost teeth, a complete denture is constructed to restore lost function and aesthetics for the dental

Procedure 42-1 Making a Final Impression for a Partial Denture

Equipment and Supplies Needed

- Basic setup and mouthwash
- Custom tray or stock tray, tray adhesive
- Periphery wax for border molding
- Tooth shade guide
- Bite registration material
- Dispensing gun, mixing tips, mixing pad, and spatula
- Lab prescription form

Procedure Steps

1. The dentist places the custom or stock tray in the patient's mouth to determine fit.

2. The dentist places periphery wax on the rim of the impression tray for contouring.

3. The dental assistant applies tray adhesive to the inside and borders of the impression tray and lets it completely dry.

4. The dental assistant mixes the impression material using either a two-part system or cartridge method and load the impression tray. (The dentist places the impression tray.)

5. The dentist removes the impression tray from the patient's mouth when the impression material has completely set.

6. The dentist takes the occlusal bite registration and select the tooth shade.

7. The dental assistant disinfects the impression and occlusal bite registration by spraying it with a disinfecting solution and placing it in a sealed container for the dental lab to pick up and process.

8. The dentist completes the lab prescription form informing the dental lab technician what is needed for the denture case. The prescription form must be signed by the dentist in order for the dental lab technician to process the denture case.

patient. The denture is supported by the alveolar bone and oral mucosa. The conditions of the alveolar bone due to hereditary defects or periodontal disease determine the support or lack of support for the denture.

Considerations and Indications for Complete (Full) Dentures

Complete dentures might be a necessary treatment for a number of reasons. For instance, if a dental patient were not motivated or able to maintain her existing teeth, such a patient would be a candidate for a full denture. Also, if a patient has advanced periodontal disease and accompanying bone loss, treatment with a full denture is the clear choice. Sometimes patients who have had full dentures must obtain a new set of dentures due to wear and dimensional changes.

Regardless of the reason for wearing a denture, the patient who is to receive complete dentures must have a positive attitude about wearing a denture. Dentures are not like natural teeth (dentition). They are artificial replacements (appliances) and the patient must learn to adapt to the dentures and learn to use them. The patient must be committed and persistent in his or her efforts at adjusting to the denture. As with anything new, there is an adjustment period.

The dental team is responsible for educating the patient about how to become a successful denture wearer.

Patient Education

Patient education is vital when a patient gets a dental prosthesis. The patient is transitioning from a natural function to a new learned function and may have expectations that are unachievable. Learning how to wear dentures takes commitment and persistence on the patients' part, so they will need encouragement and education by the dental team. Dissatisfaction with dentures can often be traced back to the lack of patient education. Be sure to communicate effectively with patients to minimize their frustration and dissatisfaction with their dentures.

Dental practices often have pamphlets and patient education videos for the new denture patient to view. The patient should be in overall good health and with healthy alveolar ridges (mandibular and maxillary bones) and oral mucosa (gingival tissues). If the denture does not fit the alveolar ridges properly, degeneration of the ridges can occur at a much faster rate. If the patient experiences weight loss, dentures will lose their proper fit and they will need to be relined to improve their fit. Impaired health may contribute to a lack of muscle coordination, which is needed to keep the dentures in place.

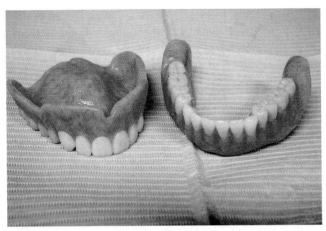

FIGURE 42.4
(Full) complete maxillary and mandibular denture.
Image courtesy Instructional Materials for the Dental Team, Lex., KY

Components of Complete Dentures

The two basic components of a complete denture are the base and the denture teeth (Figure 42.4). The base is made of acrylic and often has an embedded mesh screen for additional strength. The acrylic is impregnated with pigmentation and fibers to create a natural appearance. The different skin tones of people are often reflected in variations in the color of their gingivae—not all gingivae are pink. The base covers the alveolar ridges and gingival tissues. The artificial denture teeth are embedded in the denture base, as with a partial denture.

The denture teeth are constructed of acrylic resin (plastic) or porcelain. Porcelain teeth resist stain better than acrylic resin teeth, but are more brittle. In addition, porcelain teeth are noisy—they make a clacking noise when they occlude—and will cause faster resorption of the alveolar ridge. Acrylic resin teeth are easier to adjust and polish than porcelain teeth. The posterior denture teeth are either nonanatomic or anatomic. Nonanatomic posterior teeth do not have detailed anatomy on the occlusal surface. They are designed to provide additional strength for patients who have poor alveolar ridges to retain dentures. In contrast, anatomic teeth resemble natural teeth in that they have detailed anatomy on the **occlusal** surface.

Cultural Considerations

Certain cultures request specific characterizations to be made to prostheses, such as a gold tooth or teeth. Many dental laboratories can accommodate most special requests for characterizations. It is the responsibility of dental team members to listen to patients and respond to any specific requests that may be made.

Immediate Dentures

The patient who has been diagnosed as needing a complete (full) denture and who has existing natural teeth has two options for treatment. The patient could have all of his remaining teeth extracted at one appointment and have an **alveoplasty**, in which his alveolar ridges are shaped and contoured. If it weren't for immediate dentures, this patient would be without dentures for four to six months in order to allow for healing. Instead, immediate dentures would be used as a prosthesis, serving as a protective covering for the surgical area. The disadvantage of this treatment is that the patient has a restricted diet and poor aesthetics for that time frame.

The second treatment approach would be to extract only the posterior teeth and allow for complete healing (four to six months). The denture is constructed while healing takes place. Once the healing occurs, the patient returns, his anterior teeth are extracted, and the denture is inserted. An advantage of this second treatment approach is that patients do not have all of their teeth removed and their diet is not as restricted. Also with this second treatment option it is easier for the dental lab to re-create natural aesthetics and the denture serves as a compress or bandage to protect the healing tissues.

The second treatment approach is the one most frequently chosen by patients. A disadvantage of the immediate denture is that there is no opportunity for a try-in to evaluate the fit of the denture prior to delivery. This creates the need for the patient to have the denture relined in four to six months once final healing has been achieved (Figure 42.5). Due to this relining issue, the cost of the second treatment approach is higher than the first approach.

Overdentures

Overdentures are a full denture. This denture must be supported by the bony ridge, oral mucosa, and two or more remaining teeth or implants. When patients wear dentures over long periods of time, they experience a loss of alveolar bone and tissue due to the pressures placed on the oral mucosa and alveolar bone. The arch most susceptible to this occurrence is the mandible. The shape of the mandible is like a horseshoe. It is thinner than the maxilla and because the mandible takes the majority of the force from the bite, the alveolar bone dissolves over time. This process causes the lower denture to lose its proper fit over time.

As a rule, the upper denture is much easier for the patient to adapt to than the lower denture, mostly due to stability and adherence issues. A maxillary denture that fits well is held in place through suction being created by the extension or border areas of the denture base; this is not achieved with the mandibular denture. Once the lower denture loses its original fit to the bone and tissues,

(A)

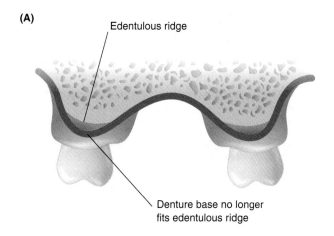

Edentulous ridge

Denture base no longer
fits edentulous ridge

(B)

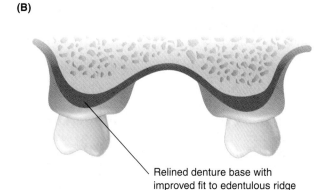

Relined denture base with
improved fit to edentulous ridge

FIGURE 42.5
(a) Ill-fitting maxillary denture and (b) improved fit with denture reline.

the denture tends to float on the alveolar bone. This causes the patient irritation to the tissues and stress in the wearing of the denture.

An overdenture is designed with either a snap or magnet capability to fit over the retaining device. It is imperative that the patient be diligent with proper oral hygiene and have regular dental hygiene visits for dental checkups. Dental visits and proper home care ensures the success of the dental implant and overdenture.

Home Care Instructions for Denture Wearers

The patient must be given certain specific instructions regarding denture wearing and how to care for the new prosthetic. The prosthetic appliance is constructed of acrylic, which is subject to dimensional changes due to drying out and improper handling; therefore, proper care of the prosthetic is very important.

The following instructions should be given both verbally and in writing to denture wearers:

1. Keep dentures in liquid when not being worn to prevent dimensional changes.
2. Remove the denture(s) or partial(s) and rinse the mouth daily.

3. Brush the outside and inside of the denture with a denture brush. Dentures will stain and build up calculus just like natural dentition. Be very careful not to drop the denture or partial while brushing. Brushing should be done over the sink with some water in it.
4. Use nonabrasive toothpaste to clean the denture and an over-the-counter commercial denture cleaner for overnight soaking.
5. Rinse the denture thoroughly after removing from the soaking solution before inserting it back into the mouth.
6. Leave the prosthetic out of the mouth overnight to allow oral tissues to breathe and to relieve the pressure applied by the prosthetic.

Denture Relining

Over time, a removable dental prosthesis will lose its original fit to the tissue and bone due to anatomic changes on the upper and lower ridges. This occurs from the pressures of the patient's denture on the alveolar bone (ridges) causing the tissue and bone to shrink. The **reline** process adds a new layer of hard acrylic to the internal portion of the denture, which restores the overall fit of the dentures.

Often oral tissues become inflamed if the patient uses an ill-fitting denture. In such cases, a tissue conditioning treatment must be performed. Tissue conditioning is a procedure done in the dental office. This procedure uses a soft and soothing acrylic material that provides a cushion to the ridges to allow for healing prior to the permanent reline, which is done by a dental lab technician. The patient is instructed to wear the dentures with the tissue conditioner in place for a few weeks prior to the permanent lab reline.

Denture Repairs

At times, a denture or partial denture will need to be repaired. Replacing a lost tooth from a denture is a common repair and can be done in the dental office; a more complex repair may need to be sent out to the dental lab. Commercial over-the-counter denture repair kits are available; however, they are not recommended by the dental community. If the fit of a denture is altered, it could cause discomfort and damage to the alveolar bone and tissue. A professional repair performed by a dentist can in most cases be done the same day with little inconvenience to the patient.

Professionalism

Be a good listener to prosthodontic patients. Empathize with their concerns and offer positive feedback and encouragement. Provide patient education to minimize a patient's anxieties.

Extensive denture damage may need to be repaired by a laboratory technician. When the patient leaves the denture to be repaired either on site or by an off-site technician, the denture is disinfected prior to being handled during the repair process. When a denture or partial is repeatedly repaired, the integrity of the denture is often reduced. In such cases, the dentist may want to recommend that the patient have a new denture constructed to restore its initial integrity and fit, which will help protect the ridge and tissue.

Denture Duplication

A duplicate denture is often constructed for patients as a courtesy and is something that can come in handy for patients if they ever have to be without their original denture. Denture wearers will often have to leave their dentures with the dentist for difficult repairs and for reline procedures. The duplicate denture will allow denture wearers to resume normal daily functions without the embarrassment of not having their teeth.

SUMMARY

A removable prosthesis is not the most desirable of dental treatments, but it does serve a purpose. It is important for missing teeth to be replaced because teeth are designed to occlude one another and to have lateral contact. When teeth are lost, a removable prosthesis can prevent the other teeth in the arch from either extruding or drifting due to lost support.

Advancements in dentistry with dental implants have greatly benefited patients who wear full dentures. The implant placed with an overdenture has improved the overall fit on the lower arch and provides patients with better mastication and confidence when wearing and using the prosthesis. A very important part of the success of the implant and overdenture is good oral hygiene and proper plaque removal every 24 hours. Proper oral hygiene greatly assists the patient in keeping the implants healthy.

A primary role of the assistant with regard to the patient wearing any removable prosthesis is patient education in the area of oral hygiene and proper care of the denture or partial denture. The dental assistant can be very helpful in the denture adjustment procedure by talking with the patient and informing the dentist about the patient and any concerns. Some states allow the dental assistant to perform minor adjustments and to clean and polish the denture under the direct supervision of the dentist. Always refer to the appropriate state's dental practice act to determine the laws and rules that govern allowable procedures.

Preparing for Externship

Knowledge of prosthodontic procedures and how to care for patients with removable prosthodontics is an important responsibility of a dental assistant. Be sure to review procedures and ask questions prior to procedures being performed. Practice providing patient instructions about denture wearing by role-playing this activity with friends or family members.

KEY TERMS

- **Alveoplasty:** Surgical procedure performed to shape and contour alveolar ridges.   p. 663
- **Complete denture:** Dental prosthesis that replaces all missing teeth in a full arch or arches.   p. 658
- **Connectors:** Elements of a partial denture that unite the working parts into one unit.   p. 660
- **Denture base:** Referred to as the saddle, it holds the denture teeth and acrylic that covers the alveolar ridges.   p. 658
- **Edentulous:** Without teeth.   p. 658
- **Framework:** Metal skeleton of a removable partial to which remaining units are attached.   p. 658
- **Occlusal:** Chewing surface of the posterior (back) teeth located on the molars and bicuspids.   p. 663
- **Overdenture:** Denture base that rests on the endodontically retained prepared teeth or on an implant instead of the tissue and bone.   p. 658
- **Partial denture:** Dental prosthesis that replaces one or more missing teeth in an arch or arches where at least one natural tooth remains.   p. 658
- **Reline:** Process to improve the internal fit of the dental prosthesis (full, partial, or overdenture) by resurfacing the tissue side of the prosthesis.   p. 664
- **Rests:** Element of a removable partial denture that makes contact with a tooth to provide vertical and horizontal support.   p. 660

CHECK YOUR UNDERSTANDING

1. The primary function of a removable prosthetic is to
   a. replace and restore the function and aesthetics of the teeth.
   b. provide the patient with a protective hard covering to protect tender gum tissue.
   c. give the patient the option to wear teeth or not.
   d. restore decayed teeth.

2. What are the types of removable prosthetics?
   a. partial denture
   b. full (complete) denture
   c. overdenture
   d. all of the above

3. Why are dentures not needed as often today as they used to be?
   a. earlier diagnosis and treatment for periodontal disease
   b. patient education in oral hygiene with monitoring
   c. HIPAA regulations
   d. both a and b

4. What are some indications for partial denture treatment?
   a. family history of oral cancer
   b. poor bone support for remaining teeth
   c. patient not able to comply with necessary oral hygiene care due to mental or physical illness
   d. both b and c

5. What treatment choices are available if no tooth is present for a distal attachment for fixed prosthodontics?
   a. extract remaining teeth and place a full (complete) denture
   b. dental implant

   c. partial denture
   d. both b and c

6. What tools are available for patient education about wearing dentures?
   a. plaque (biofilm) disclosing liquid
   b. in-office patient education videos
   c. educational pamphlets
   d. all of the above

7. The overdenture is designed to fit into or onto what device(s), which adds support to the denture?
   a. posterior ridge of acrylic
   b. endodontically treated retained root tips
   c. dental implants
   d. both b and c

8. What is a cause for additional tooth loss when wearing a partial denture?
   a. faulty design of the prosthesis
   b. lack of oral hygiene
   c. untreated periodontal disease
   d. all of the above

9. The patient's ability to wear dentures relies on which of the following important aspects?
   a. size of the tongue
   b. size of the jaw
   c. commitment and persistence
   d. family history

10. The metal skeleton of a removable partial to which remaining units are attached is called the
    a. framework.
    b. template.
    c. flange.
    d. retainer.

INTERNET ACTIVITY

- Go to www.dentures.com and find the "what to expect video" by clicking the Considering Dentures box and then What to Expect Video.

WEB REFERENCES

- Dental-Professional.com   www.dental-professional.com/News_Articles.aspx?NewsID=News035
- Everything You Need to Know About Dentures   www.denturehelp.com/Pages/home.html
- MyDentureCare.com   www.mydenturecare.com/products.aspx

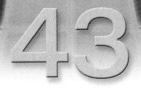

43

Dental Implants

Learning Objectives

After reading this chapter, the student should be able to:

- Describe the process of correct patient selection to receive dental implants.
- Describe the indications and contraindications for dental implants.
- Identify all types of dental implants and their appropriate function.
- Explain the surgical technique used in dental implantation.
- Understand dental implant maintenance.
- List the duties that are required to assist in a dental implant surgery.

Preparing for Certification Exams

- Receive and prepare patients for treatment, including seating, positioning chair, and placing napkin.
- Prepare surgical armamentarium.
- Identify intraoral anatomy.
- Apply topical anesthetic to the injection site.
- Transfer dental instruments.
- Maintain field of operation during dental procedure through the use of retraction, suction, irrigation, drying, placing, removing cotton rolls, and so forth.
- Demonstrate understanding of the OSHA Bloodborne Pathogens standard.
- Perform sterilization and disinfection procedures.
- Provide patient preventive education and oral hygiene instruction.
- Monitor and respond to postsurgical bleeding.

Key Terms

Alveolar bone	Osseointegration
Dental team	Osteonecrosis
Endosteal implant	Stent
Implant	Subperiosteal implant
Mini implant	Titanium
Mucoperiosteum	Transosteal implant

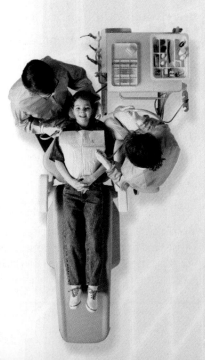

Dental implants are used to replace missing or extracted teeth.

In a dental implant, **titanium** posts are placed directly into the **alveolar bone** (Figure 43.1). Dental implants represent a great advancement in modern dental care. Implants hold the artificial teeth (abutments) in place in a manner similar to that of the natural root system.

The "traditional" implant process involves several steps and may take from three to nine months for completion, at which time the implant has achieved full **osseointegration** (i.e., the healthy bone has fused to the metallic implant). If necessary, to generate substantial bone for placement of an implant, the dentist may want to consider using allografts. This involves the use of either bone harvested from the patients themselves or manufactured products for bone and tissue regeneration. Some examples of manufactured products include Biomend and Biomend Extend.

Dental specialists may or may not be involved in every implant case; however, if necessary, they can be called on for their expertise. Having entered the dental mainstream, implants are increasingly thought of as the standard of care for tooth replacement. Long-term success is determined by many factors including, but not limited to, proper case/patient selection, the implant type and placement, the clinical expertise of the **dental team,** and routine maintenance of the implant as well as the surgical area

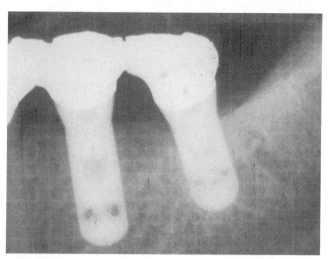

FIGURE 43.1
Radiograph of a dental implant.

during healing. The average long-term success rate of single-tooth implants is approximately 90% for patients who maintain and care for them properly.

The Dental Implant Patient

Patient selection for a successful implant result is dependent on many factors. A thorough medical history and evaluation must be accomplished and are vitally important to the success of the implant. For instance, systemic diseases that suppress the immune system can delay the healing process and therefore affect the potential success of the implant. Examples of these diseases include AIDS/HIV, diabetes, and cancer (for which chemotherapy has been used as a treatment). Patients who have a systemic disease or who take medications for such diseases must be identified prior to any dental treatment.

Recently, a category of drugs called bisphosphonates, used in the treatment of **osteonecrosis**, metastatic cancer of the bone, and Paget's disease, has been identified as adversely affecting the ability of bone to heal after surgery. Evidence suggests that bisphosphonates are linked to osteonecrosis that occurs after various types of dental surgery such as implants and extractions. Osteonecrosis of the maxilla and mandible is associated with decreased blood flow to bone that has been exposed during surgery (Figure 43.2). This results in a lack of healing in the surgical area.

Dental assistants must ask potential implant patients about the possible use of bisphosphonates when gathering their medical history. Another important piece of information that should be gathered in the medical history includes finding out whether the patient is allergic to any materials used during the implant procedure such as latex, eugenol, iodine, certain metals, and medications.

Dental Assistant PROFESSIONAL TIP

Remember that dental implants represent a huge investment in time, money, and commitment. Always be sensitive to your patient's questions and insecurities, and respond with truthfulness, empathy, and encouragement. Remember that there are no dumb questions.

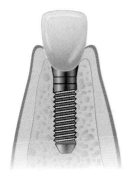

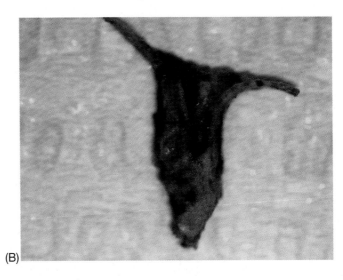

FIGURE 43.2
(a) Natural tooth with implant and (b) necrotic interproximal bone removed during debridement.

Nase JB, Suzuki JB. Osteonecrosis of the jaw and oral bisphosphonate treatment. JADA 2006;137(8): 1115–1119. Copyright © 2006 American Dental Association. All rights reserved. Reprinted with permission.

Legal and Ethical Issues

Informed consent is of particular concern legally for both the dentist and patient. Implants represent such a large investment in time and money that both parties must mutually understand all of the risks and consequences involved in detail. Informed consent must be in writing and detail the different treatment options available (including no treatment), the costs of all procedures, the sequence and course of treatment, the possible risks of failure and retreatment, and the commitment of post-placement maintenance.

Suppose that during the medical history review you notice that the implant candidate uses a drug such as Aredia or Zometa (both examples of bisphosphonates). Why is it important to bring this to the attention of the doctor?

Emotional and Psychological Profile

Another factor in patient selection is the emotional and psychological profile of the patient. It is important for the dental team to identify the patient's ability to cope with the upcoming surgical procedure and maintenance plan. The patient's overall outlook and realistic expectations of the risks involved are important considerations, because the implant process is very complex and can be very stressful at times. The patient's ability to understand and cope with these stressful times is indicative of overall patient satisfaction and ultimately the final success of the implant.

Examination of Teeth and Surrounding Oral Structures

Another important issue for consideration that may help determine successful patient selection for an implant comes directly from the clinical examination. The presence or absence of periodontal disease must be screened for and evaluated when selecting potential implant candidates. The level, density, height, and width of alveolar bone present must be carefully analyzed because these factors directly affect the ability to place and retain the implant. In addition, the condition of all oral tissues is an area of concern and should be analyzed in relation to the potential success of the implant.

The final, but very important consideration is the patient's ability and willingness to keep the oral environment clean and disease free. This consideration should be noted and reinforced in the overall analysis. This assessment of oral hygiene may be determined by a dental assistant using disclosing agents to determine plaque levels or may be done by a licensed provider (dentist or dental hygienist) who will use other techniques that dental assistants are not allowed to do as dictated by state rules and regulations.

Radiographic Evaluation

The radiographic evaluation is crucial in determining whether a patient is a potential candidate for implant placement. Although most often extraoral radiographs are exposed to determine implant possibilities, a combination of intraoral and extraoral radiographs may be ordered by the dentist. A computed tomographic (CT) imaging scan may also be requested depending on which type of implant is to be used. The CT scan can provide yet another key component in the evaluation process.

Fabrication of Dental Casts and Surgical Stents

Diagnostic dental casts (study models) serve as a physical three-dimensional model that can provide valuable information for the implant process. Occlusion, tooth shape, and tooth position are all important factors in the evaluation process and are assessed by using dental casts. In addition, the dental casts can be used to fabricate (indirectly) the surgical **stent** that is used to aid the dentist in positioning the implant in its exact and final position.

Educating Patients About Implants

On completion of the evaluation process and the successful determination that a patient is an appropriate candidate for an implant or implants, the next step is to fully educate the patient about what to expect and what is involved during various phases of the implant process. It is the role of the implant team to stress that the patient maintain a positive attitude with a thorough understanding of the procedure. The patient must be educated as to the long-term commitment required for proper care of the implant during all phases of treatment, especially home care and recall visits.

The patient must also understand the risks associated with implant placement and be willing to accept these risks. The patient should be informed that a potential risk may include re-treatment or failure if osseointegration fails to occur. It is imperative that patient education be viewed as one of the most important keys to successful implant treatment, and it is the job of the implant team to provide all of the tools necessary to accomplish this feat.

How is each member of the implant team responsible for or involved in the success of a patient's implant? **?**

Indications for Implants

The role of an implant and its indications are varied. When a patient has insufficient bone to adequately retain a full upper or lower denture or when the patient's teeth are not adequate to support removable prostheses, implants may be utilized. Implants may also be used to improve a patient's aesthetics, thus improving the patient's psychological attitude about his or her appearance and the function of his or her dentition.

Contraindications for Implants

There are contraindications to a patient receiving dental implants. Implants require an adequate amount of space and bone to be successful in the long term. If adjacent teeth are spaced closely together, then an implant may not be successful. Bone support with insufficient density

can lead to poor osseointegration and may ultimately compromise the success of the implant.

As previously discussed, certain medical conditions may also adversely affect the healing phase and ultimately the success of the implant. Patients who habitually grind their teeth (bruxism) or have other contradictory oral habits may be poor implant candidates. Patients with unusual anatomic structures may also present treatment challenges. Also, patients who are unwilling or unable to follow the meticulous postimplant placement maintenance and care, such as meticulous daily home care and follow-up recall visits with the dentist and hygienist, may represent a group not best suited for the implant process.

Types of Implants

Implants can be divided into four basic types: subperiosteal implants, endosteal implants, transosteal implants, and mini implants. A **subperiosteal implant** is most often used for patients who have insufficient bone to support and secure full maxillary or mandibular dentures. This situation is most often encountered with patients who have suffered severe resorption of the mandible. Severe resorption of the mandible can be defined as bone (tissue) that has been reabsorbed by the body due to either infection or irritation to the point of not being sufficient in amount to maintain/retain an implant.

Subperiosteal implants are typically made of titanium and are placed to rest on the superior border of the mandibular ridge, with posts or bars rising above the **mucoperiosteum** (gingival level) (Figures 43.3 and 43.4). This type of implant can be placed using either a single-step surgical technique or a two-stage surgical treatment sequence. Single-step surgeries are performed when both the implant and the hex (tooth portion) are placed at the same appointment. Two-stage surgeries entail placement of the implant at one appointment with a two- to six-month healing phase for osseointegration before the second surgery for placement of the hex.

An **endosteal implant** is surgically placed in the bone and can be used to replace a single tooth or multiple teeth. They are also often used for patients who are

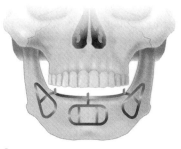

FIGURE 43.3
Example of subperiosteal implant.

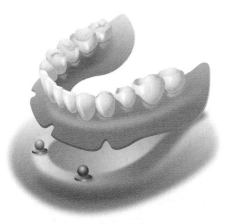
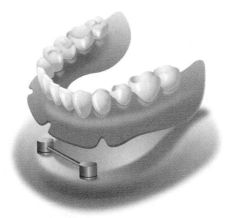

FIGURE 43.4
Example of two different types of implant stabilization for dentures.

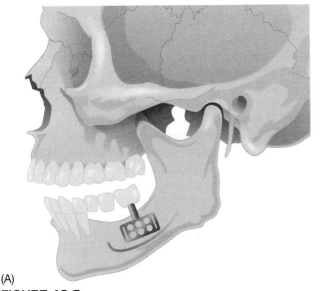
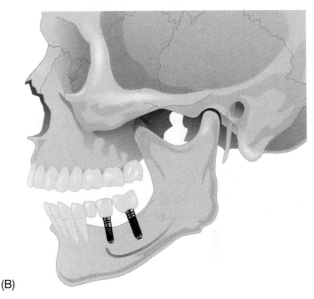

(A)   (B)

FIGURE 43.5
Examples of two different types of endosteal implants: (a) blade implant and (b) screw implant.

totally edentulous (Figure 43.5). Bone structure must be sufficient and allow at least two millimeters between the implant and the mandibular nerve canal when replacing mandibular teeth. There are four types of endosteal implants: blade, screw, cylinder, and transitional. The endosteal implant requires a two-stage surgical treatment sequence. (See Chapter 40 for more information on the relationship between prosthetics and the completed implant process.)

Transosteal implants are used for patients with the most severe resorption of the mandibular ridge and are usually the last resort for this type of situation (Figure 43.6). The transosteal staple is the most common type of transosteal implant used. Transosteal implants are inserted through the inferior border of the mandible and positioned into the edentulous area starting from the inferior border.

Mini implants have been designed specifically for denture instability (Figure 43.7). This type of implant

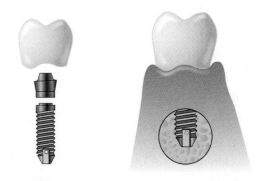

FIGURE 43.6
Transosteal implant.

uses a minimally invasive, microsurgical, single-step technique. With this technique the implants are screwed directly into the bone with no waiting period for osseointegration to occur. These implants can be loaded with the weight of the denture immediately after insertion.

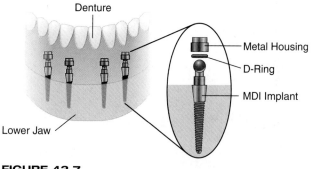

FIGURE 43.7
Mini implant.

Life Span Considerations

The treatment age for patients who are interested in the process of implantation can vary greatly. However, very young patients with incomplete bone formation and elderly patients with advanced bone resorption may not be appropriate candidates.

Preparation for Implantation

After choosing the appropriate implant for inpatient treatment, preparation for the surgical phase of the process can begin. Informed consent must be obtained and reviewed prior to surgery. Informed consent is used to protect the dental team from liability and to educate the patient of the risks, possible complications, and treatment options (which include doing nothing).

The informed consent form should be in writing and should fully and explicitly explain the sequence of treatment and provide a detailed approximate time frame. The dental assistant's role in obtaining informed consent is multifaceted. The dental assistant may explain the procedure (using the written form) to the patient, act as a witness to the patient's signature by signing the form after the patient has signed, and/or serve as interpreter if the patient does not speak English.

As a part of the dental implant team, what is your role as a clinical dental assistant in implant surgery? **?**

Preparation for Surgery

It is the responsibility of the dental assistant to prepare the operatory, instruments, materials, and supplies (armamentarium) for both the first and, if necessary, the second surgery. The following items may be required for surgery (note, however, that surgical setups vary according to the dentist's preferences):

- IV sedation and local anesthetic setup
- Rongeurs
- Mouth mirrors

- Surgical curette
- Surgical evacuation tip
- Tissue forceps and scissors
- Tongue and cheek retractors
- Sterile gauze and cotton pellets
- Hemostat
- Low-speed surgical handpiece
- Bite block
- Sterile template (surgical stent)
- Oral rinse
- Sterile surgical handpiece
- Betadine
- Scalpel and blades
- Periosteal elevator
- Implant instrument kit
- Sterile implant kit(s)

In addition to being responsible for the tray setups for implant surgery, the dental assistant may assist the doctor with intravenous sedation if utilized. (The dental assistant should check the applicable state practice laws to determine what duties are allowed.) The dental assistant assists the doctor with the transfer of instruments, stent placement, handpiece usage, and other specific implant equipment or materials as required during the procedure.

Throughout the procedure the dental assistant must adhere to infection control protocols for the safety of both the patient and the other dental team members. After the surgery has been completed the dental assistant reviews the postoperative instructions with the patient and/or patient escort before patient dismissal.

After the patient has left the operatory, the dental assistant is responsible for cleaning up, disinfecting the treatment room, and processing and sterilizing the instruments. Infection control protocols and OSHA's Bloodborne Pathogens guidelines must be followed. (See Chapter 12 for more information related to infection control.) Some implant surgeries may require the use of an additional assistant. This individual is commonly known as a "floater."

How does the single-stage surgical implant technique and the two-stage technique vary? How are these techniques similar? **?**

Dental Implant Maintenance

The maintenance and home care of dental implants are important components in maintaining the integrity of the implant. Home care for implants requires meticulous oral hygiene. Maintaining and adhering to a daily routine are essential to the long-term success of a dental implant.

All brushes and instruments used in the care of implants must be made of plastic with no metal components. Metal can scratch and damage the titanium surface

Preparing for Externship

The dental assistant should review with the general dentist the roles of all members of the dental team involved with patient implant treatments. This will aid in communicating to the patient the role that the various members of the dental team have in working together to ensure the success of the implant procedure. Communicating this information can help the patient feel more confident in the overall outcome of the treatment.

Cultural Considerations

Because dental implants represent the cutting edge in high-tech dentistry, one obstacle that may be encountered when working with patients from different cultural backgrounds is communication. The language barrier that results may hinder the dental team in the education process when explaining the intricate aspects involved with the implantation process. Subjects such as surgical techniques, osseointegration, and the restoration process may require visual aids and other innovative communication techniques to successfully educate the patient.

of the implant. Toothbrushes and adjunct cleaning tools should always be angled toward the occlusal surface to avoid tissue irritation and/or damage (Figure 43.8). Plaque builds up on implants just as on natural teeth and dental prostheses and, therefore, must be removed daily—ideally after every meal using a soft toothbrush and flossing with dental tape or ribbon.

Patients may also wish to use an antimicrobial mouth rinse such as 0.12% chlorhexidine gluconate, which can be applied directly to a toothbrush or floss before use. The use of a rinse can also be helpful during the initial healing phase when mechanical removal of plaque is not indicated. Oral irrigators that direct water spray to remove food debris and plaque from around the

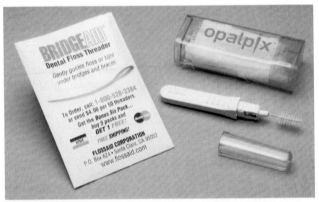

FIGURE 43.8
Home oral health care adjuncts for use with dental implants.

implant can be used, but the patient should be cautioned to direct a gentle spray horizontally and not vertically into the gingival sulcus to avoid tissue damage.

Routine recall visits to the dentist and hygienist are also a vital step toward maintaining a healthy dental implant for maximum longevity. The dental professional can reach areas that the patient cannot reach, and can use specialized plastic graphite, Teflon, or nylon instruments to remove any calculus that may build up over time.

The Future of Implants

Future trends in implantology are limitless. Currently, the focus is on single-tooth implants placed in one surgical appointment. The advantages of this technique include reduced chair time, elimination of a second surgical procedure, the ability to use an immediate denture, and preservation of crestal bone.

Perhaps most importantly, implants provide improved psychological benefits to the patient as he or she receives an aesthetic restoration on the day of implant surgery. Choosing an implant system that has the ability to provide maximum desired results for the patient is the ultimate goal. Implants may now be started and completed in just a few hours depending on the patient needs and the office. Technology used for dental implants is constantly being researched and improved.

SUMMARY

The use of dental implants is becoming increasingly more common and desirable for patients and providers alike. Successful implant placement is determined by many factors including adequate bone levels, patient health, desire to maintain implants, and the expertise of the dental team. Knowledge of a patient's medical and dental health history is an absolute requirement for patient selection. A clinical dental examination and radiographic examination are performed to determine the ultimate compatibility of the implant and the patient. Professional home care instructions and follow-up care are the true keys to suc-

cess of a patient's implant and are often the responsibility of the dental assistant.

Professionalism

The ability to empathize with patient concerns and to provide encouragement as well as positive feedback in a professional manner helps the dental assistant achieve the final goal of patient satisfaction.

KEY TERMS

- **Alveolar bone:** The bone that supports the teeth of both the mandible and maxilla.   p. 668

- **Dental team:** Team consisting of various dental specialists such as periodontists, prosthodontists, and oral maxillofacial surgeons; also includes general dentists, dental hygienists, and dental assistants.   p. 668

- **Endosteal implant:** Implant that is surgically placed in the bone. Four types are available: blade, cylinder, screw, and transitional (provisional).   p. 670

- **Implant:** A surgically positioned metallic framework or screw placed directly in or on the mandibular or maxillary ridges.   p. 668

- **Mini implant:** A threaded implant placed using minimally invasive microsurgery for long-term denture stabilization.   p. 671

- **Mucoperiosteum:** Membrane that is formed by the combination of the mucosal and periosteal surfaces.   p. 670

- **Osseointegration:** A biological bonding process that fuses healthy bone to a metallic implant, usually titanium.   p. 668

- **Osteonecrosis:** Bone death resulting from poor blood supply to an area of bone.   p. 668

- **Stent:** A sterile, clear acrylic template positioned over the alveolar ridge that enables the location of the exact position of a dental implant.   p. 670

- **Subperiosteal implant:** Implant that is placed on top of alveolar bone with abutment posts or bars rising above the mucoperiosteum; used primarily when the alveolar bone has atrophied (wasted away), usually as a result of a failed or poorly fitting denture.   p. 670

- **Titanium:** Type of metal that is most compatible with human tissues and bone.   p. 668

- **Transosteal implant:** Implant that is inserted through the mandible from the inferior border.   p. 671

CHECK YOUR UNDERSTANDING

1. What category of medication is responsible for postoperative osteonecrosis?
   a. narcotics
   b. nonsteroidal anti-inflammatory drugs (NSAIDs)
   c. bisphosphonates
   d. antibiotics

2. Contraindications for dental implants include
   a. loose dentures.
   b. high palatal vault.
   c. congenitally missing teeth.
   d. none of the above.

3. Which of the following is not a type of dental implant?
   a. circumoral
   b. transosteal
   c. blade
   d. subperiosteal

4. What is the long-term success rate of single-tooth implants?
   a. 50% to 60%
   b. 75%
   c. 80% to 90%
   d. approximately 90%

5. Tools used in the evaluation process for dental implants include which of the following?
   a. x-rays
   b. blood calcium levels
   c. diagnostic casts
   d. both a and c

6. Most implants are made of
   a. stainless steel.
   b. gold.
   c. titanium.
   d. palladium.

7. Diseases that may suppress the immune system and delay the healing of implants include which of the following?
   a. diabetes
   b. AIDS
   c. cancer
   d. all of the above

8. Members of the implant team may include which of the following?
   a. prosthodontist
   b. endodontist
   c. periodontist
   d. both a and c

9. Dental implant maintenance does not include which of the following?
   a. office recall visits
   b. daily flossing
   c. taking implant out daily and soaking overnight
   d. use of plastic hygiene aids

10. Indications for dental implants include which of the following?
    a. stabilization of loose dentures
    b. support of partial dentures
    c. replacement of congenitally missing teeth
    d. all of the above

INTERNET ACTIVITY

- Go to http://ocw.tufts.edu/Content/10/readings/ 244658 and research the current success rate of implants in general.

WEB REFERENCES

- American Academy of Periodontology   www.perio.org/consumer/zm.htm
- The Humboldt-Del Norte Dental Society   www.hdnds.org/icase.htm
- University of Virginia   www.healthsystem.virginia.edu/uvahealth/adult_oralhlth/implants.cfm
- World Center for Implantology   www.enexus.com/dental-implant/doctor.htm

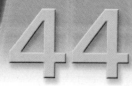

Endodontic Procedures

Learning Objectives

After reading this chapter, the student should be able to:

- Identify the causes of pulpal damage.

- List the different symptoms of pulpal damage.

- Describe the various tests used for endodontic diagnosis.

- Explain the steps for endodontic procedures.

- Describe endodontic instruments, accessory instruments, and medicaments necessary for endodontic treatment.

- Demonstrate assisting during endodontic extirpation and obturation procedures.

- Describe three surgical endodontic procedures and state their purpose.

Preparing for Certification Exams

- Prepare procedural trays/armamentaria setups.

- Place and remove dental dam.

- Expose and process dental radiographs.

- Using the concepts of four-handed dentistry, assist with basic intraoral endodontic procedures.

- Maintain field of operation during dental procedures through the use of retraction, suction, irrigation, drying, placing and removing cotton rolls, and so forth.

- Transfer dental instruments, mix dental materials, and place temporary fillings.

- Demonstrate understanding of the OSHA Hazard Communication standard.

- Provide preoperative and postoperative instructions.

- Perform sterilization and disinfection procedures.

- Monitor and respond to postsurgical bleeding.

Key Terms

Apicoectomy	Obturate
Debridement	Percussion
Endodontics	Periapical abscess
Extirpation	Pulpitis
Irreversible pulpitis	Reversible pulpitis
Necrotic pulp	

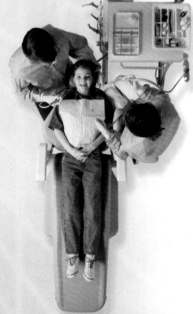

Endo is the Greek word for "inside" and *odont* is the Greek word for "tooth"; therefore, endodontic treatment involves treating the inside of the tooth. **Endodontics** is the specialty involving the treatment of the tooth pulp and periapical tissues. The pulp extends from the crown of the tooth to the tip of the root, which is called the apex. Periapical tissues, also called periradicular tissues, are those tissues around the apex of the tooth. This is where the pulp connects with tissues surrounding the tooth, such as blood and nerve vessels, periodontal ligaments, and alveolar bone. The tooth pulp contains nerve vessels, blood vessels, connective tissue, fibroblasts, macrophages, and lymphocytes.

Pulpal tissues nourish the tooth during its growth and development. When the pulp becomes infected, the infection must be removed or it will spread to the bone that surrounds the tooth. This can cause severe pain and if left untreated may even become life threatening. The infection will cause the bone to resorb. Resorption is destruction of the bone, which causes the tooth to loosen over a period of time. When resorption occurs the patient may lose one or more teeth in the area. The infection must be removed either through root canal (endodontic) therapy or by an extraction. The goal of endodontics is to retain the natural tooth in the arch.

All general dentists are capable of treating the tooth with endodontic therapy, or the patient may be referred to an endodontist, which is a dentist who specializes in root canal treatment. To become an endodontic specialist, a dentist completes dental school and attends advanced training in endodontics for an additional two years. General dentists refer difficult-to-treat

---

Dental Assistant   PROFESSIONAL TIP

Patients should be educated to realize that when tooth pulp becomes infected, the infection must be removed or it will spread to the bone that surrounds the tooth, which will cause the tooth to loosen over a period of time. The dental assistant can explain how the infection must be removed either through root canal therapy or by extracting the tooth. Patients should understand that the goal of endodontics is to retain the natural tooth in the arch. If the natural tooth in the arch is not retained, then a bridge may be required later.

---

cases to an endodontic specialist. Endodontic therapy can be performed only if the root canals are accessible and are able to be adequately cleaned of debris and thoroughly sealed.

Causes of Pulpal Damage

The pulp can be injured in several ways. The most common causes of pulpal nerve damage are severe tooth decay and either acute or chronic trauma. Pulpal irritation may occur through microbial, mechanical, or chemical irritation. Microbial irritation is most often brought on by destructive tooth decay reaching the inside portion of the tooth and allowing harmful bacteria to enter the pulp. The pulp is affected before actual invasion by bacteria when bacterial by-products pass through the dentinal tubules into the pulp chamber. Carious lesions (caries) contain numerous species of bacteria. As decay progresses toward the pulp, the intensity of the microbial irritation increases. The result of microscopic organisms entering the pulp chamber is inflammation and infection.

Mechanical irritants to pulpal tissues include trauma to the tooth from a blow, deep restorations, biting on a hard object, or excessive movement of the tooth, which may disrupt the blood and nerve supply. A blow to a tooth may occur from an accident, a fall, or an athletic sports injury. A tooth may be forcibly knocked out of its socket, disrupting the blood and nerve supply to the tooth. A tooth can become cracked or broken from biting on something such as a bone while eating. It can also break or chip from a traumatic accident. Deep restorations may disturb the tooth pulp even when medications are placed between the restoration and the tooth pulp.

Heat generated during the cutting of a tooth with deep caries may damage the pulp beyond its ability to repair itself. During restorative treatment, the dentist and dental assistant play major roles in keeping both the tooth and the high-speed handpiece cooled with water during preparations. When the bur rotates at a high rate of speed, heat is generated through the friction of the bur cutting tooth enamel and dentin. Water running through the high-speed handpiece cools the bur. The dental assistant also keeps the tooth clean and cool with the air/water syringe. The high-volume evacuator suctions excess water out of the oral cavity.

Deep temporary or permanent restorations placed near the pulp may cause chemical irritation from the restorative materials. Damage to pulpal tissues (Figure 44.1) results from:

- Aggressive tooth decay reaching the pulp chamber
- Trauma to the tooth due to a physical blow that separates the tooth from the nerve supply, either recently or in the past
- Trauma to the tooth due to a complete or incomplete fracture
- Mechanical and thermal irritation from tooth preparation
- Chemical irritation when restorative materials are placed too close to the pulp

Symptoms of Pulpal Damage

The most common symptom of pulpal damage is pain. Each individual patient will experience symptoms differently. Symptoms of pulpal damage may include:

- Oversensitivity of the tooth to hot or cold food and beverages
- Pain or discomfort from the tooth when chewing or biting
- Facial swelling due to a periapical abscess
- Aching of the tooth without a definable reason, possibly keeping the patient awake at night

Note, however, that sometimes there are no obvious symptoms.

The patient may develop an acute toothache with sharp and throbbing pain that is usually worse when lying down (a result of the infection settling in one area

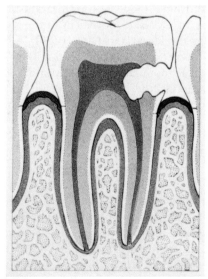

FIGURE 44.1
A tooth with extensive pulpal damage.
© Dorling-Kindersley

of the head). The patient may or may not be aware of having decay in that tooth or may remember experiencing trauma to the affected tooth. Inflammation of the pulpal tissue may be acute and severe and may keep the patient awake at night, or the pulpal inflammation may be chronic with mild to dull pain. **Pulpitis** is inflammation of the tooth pulp that may be reversible or irreversible—or the pulp may already be dead. A **periapical abscess** is an infection from within the tooth that spreads out through the tooth's apex and into the surrounding bone.

Reversible Pulpitis

A vital pulp is alive and will have a reaction to cold temperatures and other tests performed by the dentist. When restoring a tooth with deep caries, the dentist will often remove the caries and place a medicated sedative temporary filling to soothe, the inflamed pulp, to prevent further irritation, and to allow the symptoms to subside.

Deep decay produces an inflammatory response in the pulp tissue from the abundance and replication of the bacteria present. Inflammation is the body's response to infection and provides increased blood flow to the area so that phagocytes (cells that ingest microorganisms) within the white blood cells can consume and destroy the foreign organisms. Pus is produced from this process as the immune system disposes of harmful toxins. Removal of deep caries near the pulp may cause pulpal irritation. Placement of a sedative filling with calcium hydroxide gives the tooth a chance to produce reparative dentin and heal itself. If the tooth is able to respond to the treatment and the patient's symptoms subside this is called **reversible pulpitis.**

Irreversible Pulpitis

When inflamed tooth pulp is unable to respond to treatment and the patient's symptoms of pain continue, this is called **irreversible pulpitis.** There may not even be any visual changes on a periapical radiograph. When a tooth is diagnosed with irreversible pulpitis, endodontic treatment is indicated as long as the tooth is restorable and there are no signs of a root fracture. The only alternative to root canal therapy is extraction of the tooth.

Pulpal Necrosis

Necrotic pulp is nonvital pulp that is infected and dead (Figure 44.2). Necrotic pulp has been deprived of its blood and nerve supply and is no longer composed of living tissue. A nonvital tooth will not respond to heat, cold, or electrical stimulation. Nonvital pulp may range from being asymptomatic to being very sensitive. For instance, some patients may not realize they have an infection, whereas others may experience severe discomfort. A periapical lesion will appear on a radiograph if the bacterial infection extends into the bone surrounding the apex of the tooth. As a patient's condition progresses from pulpitis to pulpal necrosis, the patient may experience excruciating pain caused by fluid and gaseous pressure within the confined space inside of the tooth. The tooth must either be extracted or be treated endodontically.

Periapical Abscess

A periapical abscess usually results from an infection of pulpal tissue, causing the pulp to die (Figure 44.3). This type of infection causes fluids and by-products to build up within the walls of the pulp chamber and root canal(s). The periapical abscess is formed when these materials escape through the apical foramen of the tooth. An area of pus and fluid accumulation forms in the bone surrounding the apex of the tooth. As the pressure builds up, a channel can form through a path of least resistance in alveolar bone or the soft tissue. This channel is called a fistulous tract or fistula. When the pus reaches soft tissue, facial swelling can occur.

If the infection is not treated, the patient may have an elevated temperature, a general feeling of malaise, throbbing pain in the affected area, and possibly swollen lymph nodes. If the inflammation spreads out into the connective tissues of the face, it becomes cellulitis. Cellulitis is a serious bacterial infection that may become life

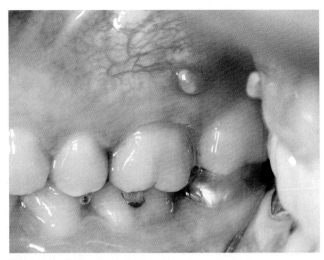

FIGURE 44.3
Periapical abscess draining to gingiva.
Image courtesy Instructional Materials for the Dental Team, Lex., KY

threatening. It appears as a swollen, red area of the skin that feels hot and tender and may spread rapidly. The dentist will incise and drain the abscess and prescribe antibiotics as needed.

Incision and Drainage

An acute periapical abscess may require incision and drainage (I&D) to eliminate the area of infection. This treatment is indicated when swelling and infections are localized in the alveolar bone with a clearly defined area on the mucosa. The I&D procedure is generally spread over several visits to ensure the infected pulp and associated bacteria have been adequately drained.

The I&D procedure involves the dentist incising, or lancing, the area and expressing the exudate (pus). Note that local anesthesia may not be as effective during an I&D procedure due to the severe infection present. During the procedure, the dental assistant needs to keep the high-volume evacuator or a 2 × 2 gauze square close to the incision site to absorb the exudate. If indicated, a drain will be placed to provide short-term drainage and to prevent the opening from closing prematurely until infection drains from the area. The dentist may prescribe antibiotics for the patient. Once the infection is controlled and the swelling and tenderness subside, the dentist will treat the tooth endodontically.

What are some causes of damage to the pulp that may cause a tooth to require endodontic treatment?

Endodontic Diagnosis

When diagnosing an endodontic condition, it is important for the dentist to diagnose the correct tooth and to

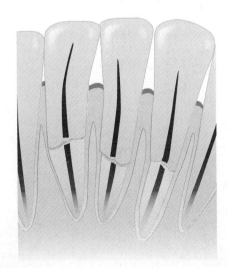

FIGURE 44.2
Fractured incisors leading to necrotic pulp.

determine what damage has already occurred. The patient's dental history is a valuable aid to the dentist because it may provide important information regarding previous injuries to the teeth.

Frequently, patients are unable to point to a specific tooth, and the dentist must determine which tooth is causing discomfort to the patient. The dentist begins with a clinical examination of the oral cavity. This allows a visual inspection of the patient's mouth, which may provide clues to the nature of the patient's problem. The dentist examines the area for discoloration of the teeth, broken crowns, caries, swelling, or abnormally soft tissue. Swelling is a sign of a severe periapical abscess. Many tests are available to the dentist to use as tools to diagnose the need for endodontic treatment. Among these tests are radiographs, percussion, palpation, and mobility tests, periodontal probing, cold and heat tests, electric pulp tester, and transillumination and anesthetic tests.

Radiographs

Radiographs are the most valuable diagnostic tool used in dentistry. The dental clinician uses radiographs to evaluate structures that cannot be seen by clinical examination. Darkening of the tooth or radiolucency at the apex of a tooth is an indication of periapical pathology (disease) and the potential need for endodontic treatment. Excessive bone loss in this area occurs in response to infected or dying pulp and appears as a dark radiolucent area surrounding the apex of the root. This radiolucency indicates a loss of bone. Radiographs also reveal possible causes of injury to the pulp before bone resorption occurs. Deep caries, fractures, and previous pulpal exposures are examples of pulpal injuries that can be detected on a radiograph.

An accurate radiograph can reveal root length, curvature of the root, and abnormal calcification of pulpal areas (Figure 44.4). This information is helpful when determining if the tooth can be treated successfully with endodontic therapy. A radiograph that is properly exposed and processed becomes the permanent record of

Preparing for Externship

Radiographs are the most valuable diagnostic tool used in dentistry. Elongation and foreshortening of a radiograph makes it difficult for the dentist to estimate the working length of a root canal. The dental assistant should spend time studying proper paralleling and bisecting angle x-ray techniques and practice taking films that do not create elongation and foreshortening errors.

the patient's condition and can be used as a baseline for future reference. The dentist will compare initial radiographs with postoperative radiographs to determine if treatment was successful. Conventional or digital radiographs are exposed throughout the endodontic procedure to establish the length of the tooth roots, to provide a working length for endodontic instruments, to confirm that the root canal filling material is located properly one to two millimeters from the tooth apex, and to obtain a final film as a record of the finished endodontic procedure. Radiographs are needed to process dental insurance claims or to get preauthorization on certain procedures such as crown and bridge treatments.

Percussion

A **percussion** test is the gentle tapping on the crown of the tooth to determine if the infection and inflammation have reached the periodontal tissues at the apex of the tooth (Figure 44.5). The back end of a mirror handle or any blunt instrument can be used to tap lightly on the tooth. The inflamed area is stimulated if a periapical infection exists and the patient will feel discomfort, which helps the clinician establish which tooth is involved and how severe the infection is. Teeth on each side of the affected tooth should also be tapped in order to compare the patient's reaction.

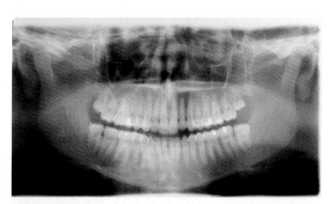

FIGURE 44.4
A radiograph of a periapical abscess.

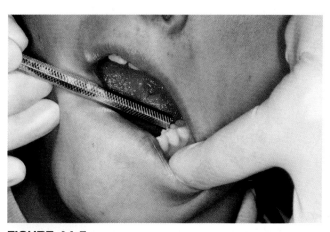

FIGURE 44.5
Percussion test.
Image courtesy Instructional Materials for the Dental Team, Lex., KY

Palpation

In a palpation test, a finger or fingers are used to apply light pressure to areas of the mouth. This is done to detect swelling, pain, or abnormally firm tissues. The dentist gently presses his or her fingers against the soft tissues that cover the bone and apices of the teeth and compares the way they feel with other areas of the mouth (Figure 44.6). (*Apices* is the plural of *apex* and means more than one root tip.)

Mobility

A mobility test is done to establish abnormal movement of a tooth in comparison with other teeth. The dentist places the tooth between the handles of two instruments and applies pressure to both sides to assess tooth movement (Figure 44.7). Mobility of a tooth indicates permanent loss of the tooth's supporting bone structure. Bone loss occurs after a long period of infection and will be evident if an infection has been present for some time. The dentist may want to use a periodontal probe to examine the bone level and decide if prognosis for endodontic treatment is good or if the bone level is beyond the level that is needed to restore the tooth. A periodontal probe can only give an indication of bone loss during a soft tissue examination. A true diagnosis of bone loss is only done through a radiographic examination.

Cold Test

A cold test is done by placing something cold on the tooth. This can be done with a small piece of ice or ethyl chloride sprayed on a cotton-tipped applicator and applied to the crown of the tooth. The tooth should first be dried. The ice may be held with a 2 × 2 gauze square or the cold cotton-tipped applicator held onto the gingival third of a tooth crown (Figure 44.8). If the pulp is inflamed, the patient will experience a lingering sensation to cold.

Heat Test

Infected teeth react quickly to heat. Most often a heat test is done by isolating the tooth with cotton rolls and drying it, then melting a gutta percha point (discussed later in this chapter) and immediately applying it to the suspect tooth (Figure 44.9). If the patient reacts with a painful response that lingers for a few seconds after the heat is removed, pulpitis is most likely present. If the patient experiences intense pain, the pulp is irreversible, and an endodontic procedure will be necessary to save the tooth by removing the infected pulpal tissue. If the patient does not experience any discomfort, the pulp is necrotic, meaning already dead. Both irreversible pulpitis and necrotic pulp require endodontic treatment for the tooth to remain in the mouth and not cause loss of bone over time.

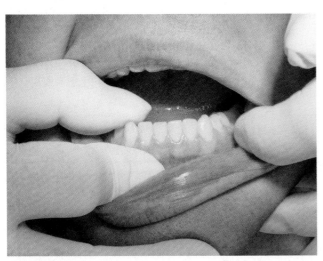

FIGURE 44.6
Palpation test.

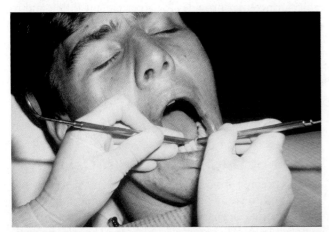

FIGURE 44.7
Test of mobility.
Image courtesy Instructional Materials for the Dental Team, Lex., KY

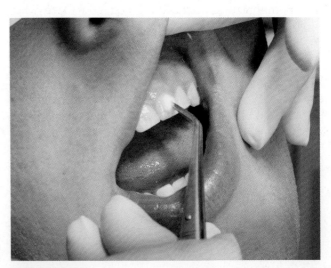

FIGURE 44.8
Ethyl chloride frost.

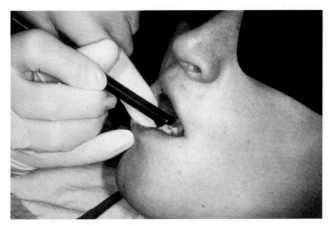

FIGURE 44.9
Heat test.
Image courtesy Instructional Materials for the Dental Team, Lex., KY

Electric Pulp Tester

An electric pulp tester sends a small electric current through the tooth to detect the vitality of the tooth (Figure 44.10). Tooth vitality tells the clinician the condition of the pulp and whether it is alive and vital, dying, or already dead and necrotic.

To conduct the test, the tooth is first dried. Toothpaste is used as a medium to conduct the electric current. The pulp tester is turned on and set for manual or automatic mode. A digital readout informs the clinician of the electric pulses being delivered to the patient's tooth. The tip of the pulp tester is never placed on a restoration but on sound enamel tooth structure on the crown of a tooth. Electric pulp testers work gradually enough that the patient feels the stimulus to the tooth long before it becomes painful. The patient usually describes a warm feeling.

If the tooth is vital, it responds quickly to the applied voltage. If the tooth is dying, it does not respond until a higher voltage is applied. If the tooth is necrotic, it will probably not respond to an electric current. Newer pulp testers automatically reduce the voltage to zero when

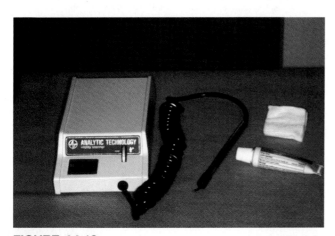

FIGURE 44.10
Pulp vitality tester.

delivery of the programmed dose is achieved rather than the clinician needing to reset the voltage as with a manual pulp testing unit. Testing of the pulp must be used along with other tests to allow for a proper diagnosis.

Transillumination

If the dentist suspects the tooth may be fractured, he or she may use a fiber-optic light to diagnose a fractured crown. The fiber-optic light provides an intense concentrated light that may be passed through the tooth. This is done most effectively on anterior teeth because of their structure and location in the arch. The light transmits through the enamel and dentin, permitting detection of a fractured crown or even a carious lesion.

Anesthetic Test

If the patient is having difficulty deciding which tooth has been causing the discomfort and the other diagnostic tests just discussed have been unable to positively determine exactly which tooth is involved, the dentist will use his or her educated judgment derived from the tests and administer local anesthetic for the tooth most likely infected. If the patient's discomfort is relieved by the anesthesia, then the accurate tooth has been identified. However, profound anesthesia is not always achieved due to persistent infection in the area.

What tests are used to analyze the need for a tooth to have endodontic treatment?

Endodontic Procedures

Endodontic treatment begins with the initial access into the pulp chamber. This often involves removal of tooth decay. Once the affected pulp chamber is exposed, the infection and infected pulp are removed. The areas surrounding the pulp chambers and pulp canals are carefully cleaned, enlarged, and shaped to provide a clean bondable surface that provides for a permanent filling and to prohibit any further infection from occurring. In the case of reversible pulpitis, medications are placed that may help calm the tooth and prevent the need for endodontic treatment. Indirect and direct pulp capping may soothe irritation of pulpal tissues. Root canal therapy may take one or more appointments based on the number of canals and the degree of infection.

Indirect and Direct Pulp Capping

In an attempt to protect the pulp against additional injury and to stimulate pulpal regeneration, a protective biocompatible agent or medicated liner is applied over an exposed or nearly exposed vital pulp. This treatment is referred to as pulp capping. When the pulp is exposed during tooth preparation or through traumatic injury,

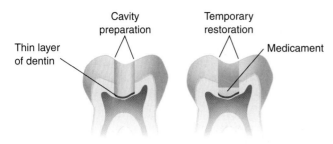

FIGURE 44.11
Direct and indirect pulp capping.

placing a pulp cap directly over the exposed pulp is called direct pulp capping. If deep caries are present and danger of exposing the pulp exists, placing a pulp cap over a layer of remaining dentin is referred to as indirect pulp capping (Figure 44.11).

The objectives of direct and indirect pulp capping are to seal the pulp against bacterial leakage, encourage the pulp to wall off the exposure site by initiating repair of the dentin, and maintain the vitality of the underlying pulp tissue regions. If pulp capping is not effective, the pulp will need to be treated endodontically.

Pulpotomy

A pulpotomy is the removal of the entire coronal pulp in the pulp chamber, leaving only the vital pulp within the roots (Figure 44.12). The pulp is then retained in the root canals and treated with medication to preserve its vitality and function. Root canal therapy is completed at a later date if indicated. Complete **extirpation** (removal of infected pulp tissue) is almost impossible in primary teeth

because the apices of primary teeth are not fully closed and there may be resorption of root structure due to permanent succedaneous teeth.

Indications for a pulpotomy are caries in exposed primary teeth when retention of the tooth in the arch is more advantageous than extracting the tooth. A pulpotomy procedure may be performed on a young permanent tooth to maximize the opportunity for the root apex to develop and close (apexogenesis). A pulpotomy is also indicated when inflammation is confined to the coronal portion of the pulp. A pulpotomy is contraindicated when there is a fistula or an abscess, when the tooth crown is nonrestorable, or when there is profuse hemorrhage, extreme tenderness to percussion, mobility of the tooth, necrotic pulp, or the presence of pulp stones.

Pulpectomy

The most common endodontic procedure is a pulpectomy, which is the removal of the entire pulp from the pulp chamber and from the root canals of a nonvital tooth. A pulpectomy is the treatment of choice for primary teeth in order to keep the tooth and hold the space for the erupting permanent tooth, but a pulpectomy may also be performed on permanent teeth. Primary teeth have an increased number of accessory canals, making complete extirpation of the pulp and debridement of the canal more difficult. The necrotic pulpal tissue in the root canals is removed, cleaned, and filled with cement.

Indications for a pulpectomy are a cooperative patient, teeth with poor chance of vital pulp treatment, its strategic importance for space maintenance, absence of surrounding bone loss from infection, and expectation of the ability to restore the tooth in the future.

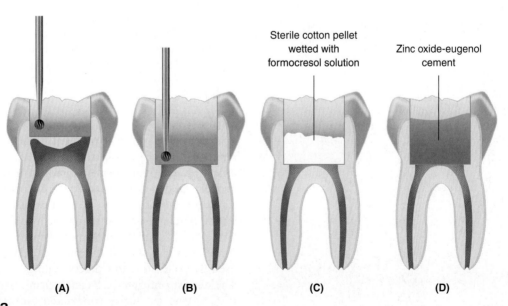

| (A) | (B) | (C) | (D) |

FIGURE 44.12
Pulpotomy procedure: (a) prepare tooth, (b) remove pulp, (c) place dry or medicated cotton pellet, and (d) place zinc oxide-eugenol temporary restoration.

What is the difference between a pulpectomy and a pulpotomy? Explain why these procedures are done rather than a complete endodontic procedure.

Access Opening

During a pulpectomy, after anesthetic is administered and the dental dam is placed, the dentist cuts through the enamel and dentin with a high-speed handpiece bur. The dentist then uses a slow-speed handpiece round bur and possibly a spoon excavator to remove all decayed tooth structure. The tooth opening is then deepened and widened to allow the dentist straight access into the pulp chamber or chambers.

The dentist must achieve good visibility and direct access for endodontic instruments to enter the pulp canals. The dentist will determine the precise location of each root canal with an endodontic explorer. The dentist then uses an endodontic broach to remove the infected pulpal tissue. A radiograph is exposed at this time to determine the exact length of the root canal or canals being treated. A file or files are placed down into each canal of the tooth before the x-ray is taken. These files are then measured in millimeters to obtain an accurate working length for filing and filling of the canal(s) (Figure 44.13). When the dental assistant takes a radiograph of the patient's tooth with the files in place, he or she must be sure to tell the patient not to close her mouth because the files are protruding from the tooth.

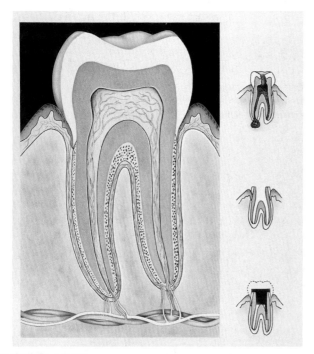

FIGURE 44.13
Root canal procedure involving the removal of pulp and filing of the root canal.

Cultural Considerations

The dental assistant has the important role of explaining to patients why a tooth should be saved through endodontic therapy rather than lost due to an extraction. When faced with a language barrier, the dental team can help the patient understand endodontic therapy through the use of visual aids such as videos, pamphlets, or drawings. Although some cultures have varying views regarding the loss of teeth, the dental team should still explain how endodontic treatment may save a tooth as well as the supporting bone structure.

Shaping and Cleaning

Each root canal must be prepared and shaped to create a continuous opening that tapers toward the apex of the tooth. The dentist uses specialized instruments after reading the radiograph. These instruments are used in a step-up process to shape the inside area of the canal. Removing debris, including necrotic nerve tissue, from the root canal within a tooth is called **debridement**. This step-up process cleans and removes debris from the canal walls during the widening of each canal through graduated file sizes. The dentist begins with a smaller file or reamer and uses the next larger size to increase each canal's width. Tapered files are used either by hand or with a rotary instrument in a slow-speed handpiece. The dentist files the canal to within two to three millimeters inside of the tooth apex. Files are used to manually clean the sides of the canal walls.

The dentist also uses cleaning agents to help thoroughly clean the inside of the tooth. Chemical agents used to irrigate the root canals are often bactericidal. They lubricate the canals and dissolve tissue and debris. After cleaning agents are used, they must be rinsed out of the tooth with water or saline solutions. Absorbent paper points are used to absorb all moisture from within the root canals and completely dry them out following debridement and irrigation.

Obturation

It is important to get a good seal at the apex of the root and to completely fill the root canals without voids. Periapical disease will most often result if the apex is not properly sealed at the root tip. The most common material used to **obturate**, or fill, root canals is gutta percha. Gutta percha is a thermoplastic rubber-like material. Gutta percha points are tapered so they ideally fit the canal after it is shaped. Endodontic sealing cements are used to hold the gutta percha filling material in place. The dentist obturates the canals using lateral condensation, warm, vertically compacted gutta percha, Thermafil, or injection techniques. The dentist uses a master gutta percha point that is the width and length of the last file used in each canal. The dental assistant takes a radiograph of the master gutta percha point to ensure it reaches within less than one millimeter of the apex before the cement is mixed.

It is important for the proper size cone/point to be used to ensure a good seal at the apex of the tooth. The dental assistant mixes the endodontic sealer, and the dentist or dental assistant places it on the master cone. The dentist inserts the gutta percha into the canal. Accessory gutta percha points are placed in the canal to fill up the canals. Specialized instruments are used by the dentist to laterally condense each accessory gutta percha point in the canal. When each canal is filled, an instrument is heated and used to condense the gutta percha in the pulp canal to ensure that it is filled. A radiograph is taken to ensure that a complete fill and good seal has been achieved.

Final Restoration

After the root canal has been completely filled, temporary restorative materials can be used to fill the tooth and seal it from moisture contamination. The dentist can either continue to prepare the tooth for a permanent restoration or refer the patient to another dentist for the permanent restoration procedure. An endodontist will refer the patient back to the general dentist for a post and core procedure and a crown preparation (Figure 44.14).

The final restoration required for a tooth depends on the amount of tooth structure remaining after the caries is removed. To eliminate future problems with the tooth, an immediate permanent restoration should be placed whenever possible. Temporary restorations do not effectively prevent contamination for extended time periods. The dental assistant can help the dentist ensure that the patient understands when a restoration is temporary and the importance of replacing it as soon as possible with a permanent filling. A permanent filling must be done in order to protect the tooth against fracture and recurrent decay.

Patient Education

Preventing contamination of the filled root canal between completion of endodontic treatment and the final restoration of the tooth should be a primary concern for the patient. To eliminate future problems with the tooth, an immediate restoration should be placed whenever possible. Temporary restorations do not effectively prevent contamination for extended time periods.

The dental assistant can help the dentist ensure that the patient understands when a restoration is temporary and that it must be permanently replaced as soon as possible to protect the tooth against a future fracture. Patients should be educated by the dental team to understand that they must accept some of the responsibility in following through with recommended treatment and to protect the investment in time and money that has been put into saving the tooth.

Post and Core Buildup

Following endodontic treatment the tooth still needs to be restored to proper form and function. Endodontically treated teeth are usually already broken down and will become brittle with time because they no longer have a moisture supply via blood and nerve vessels; therefore, a post and core are needed to build up the tooth (Figure 44.15). All endodontically treated teeth will require a crown as a final restoration to prevent future problems.

Post Placement of a post within a tooth is performed on endodontically treated teeth. The post will be placed within one or two root canals. The purpose of a post is to retain a core that is needed because of extensive loss of tooth crown structure. The post serves to supply extra support for a core when sufficient tooth structure does not exist.

There are two main categories of posts: custom fabricated and prefabricated. Custom-fabricated cast gold post and core techniques have been used for many years

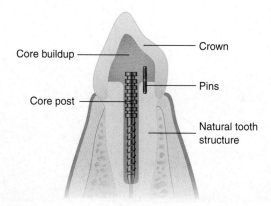

FIGURE 44.14
Endontically treated tooth with a core post, a core buildup, and a retention pin.

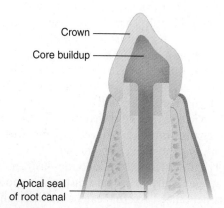

FIGURE 44.15
Nonvital tooth with a post and core buildup.

to provide a foundation to support the final crown restoration following endodontic treatment. Cast post and core procedures require two visits and fabrication in a dental laboratory. There are many types of commercially available prefabricated posts with various shapes, designs, and materials. Common prefabricated posts are made of stainless steel, titanium, gold-plated brass, ceramic, and fiber-reinforced polymers. Prefabricated posts are placed within the tooth after some gutta percha material has been removed from one or more canals with a Peeso reamer (explained later in this chapter). The post is then held in place with permanent cement and a core filling material.

Core Buildup   A core buildup is required when there is extensive loss of natural tooth structure. Placement of pins for additional retention is also evaluated by the dentist. The optimal buildup material will have adequate strength, be biocompatible, exhibit a high level of resistance to bacterial leakage, and be insoluble and dimensionally stable in the presence of oral fluids.

The most common core buildup materials are gold, amalgam, and composite. The goal of the core buildup is to establish the greatest stability and longevity of the restoration. This requires building a highly retentive stable structure around a post following endodontic treatment of a tooth. A crown is usually needed as the final restoration to effectively strengthen the tooth.

Why is it important to place a crown on a tooth following endodontic treatment? What is the purpose of a post and a core?

Instruments and Accessories

Endodontic instruments and accessories are often prepared in sterile packs or kits. A standardized setup can be used during each phase of treatment and supplemented with other items needed to complete the treatment. Before a canal can be filled, it must be completely cleaned. A patient suffering from an acute periapical abscess may experience severe discomfort. This pain is due to inflammation in the pulp canal and/or periapical tissues. When the pulp chamber is opened and the pressure released, the discomfort is relieved.

Once the pulp chamber is opened, broaches can be used to remove pulp tissue from the canal. The canal is then irrigated and debrided with reamers and files. The pulp canals are then dried and cotton pellets with medication are placed in the pulp chamber. The dentist places a temporary restoration to seal off moisture to the inside of the tooth until the next appointment.

Small hand-operated endodontic instruments and supplies are generally placed on a disposable sponge or in a compartmentalized box that can be sterilized and maintained in an orderly fashion. Several accessory items such as instruments, filling materials, medications, irrigating solutions, and cements must be readily available for use during endodontic procedures.

Dental Dam

A dental rubber dam (Figure 44.16) is essential during all endodontic procedures to keep the tooth isolated and to maintain a sterile field. This prevents contamination of the root canals by saliva, prevents small endodontic instruments from going down the patient's throat, and keeps infected tissues, debris, medicaments, and irrigating solutions from entering the patient's mouth. The dental dam improves visibility for the dentist, therefore improving the efficiency of the procedure.

Endodontic Explorer

The endodontic explorer (Figure 44.17) is most often a double-ended instrument that has long, tapered, and flexible pointed tips that create greater tactile feel for the dentist to detect root canal openings within a tooth. These instruments are angled from their shank in order to provide access to the pulp canal inside the tooth. They are used to locate canal openings and explore the pulp chambers and canals.

Endodontic Spoon Excavator

Endodontic spoon excavators (Figure 44.18) are long, double-ended excavators designed specifically for endodontic treatment. These instruments are similar in shape to a regular spoon excavator but have a longer shank. They allow for detection of caries or coronal pulp tissue or for removal of cotton pellets that may be deep inside the crown of the tooth.

Broaches

A root canal broach is used to remove the infected pulp tissue from within a tooth's pulp canal. Broaches are thin, flexible, tapered, and pointed, with a series of sharply

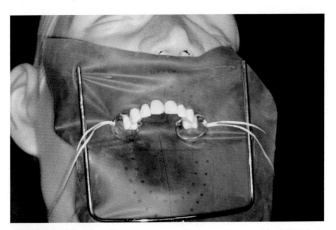

FIGURE 44.16
Rubber dam prevents debris from going down patient's throat.
Image courtesy Instructional Materials for the Dental Team, Lex., KY

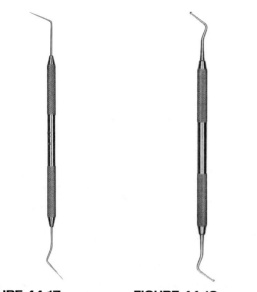

FIGURE 44.17
An endodontic explorer.
Courtesy Hu-Friedy

FIGURE 44.18
An endodontic spoon excavator.
Courtesy Hu-Friedy

pointed barbed projections that curve backward. The broach is introduced slowly into the root canal by the dentist until gentle contact is made with the canal walls. The dentist rotates the broach in a manner designed to entangle the pulpal tissue in the protruding barbs. The broach is then withdrawn directly from the canal. If successful the entire pulp is removed. These instruments are fragile and used with care to avoid breakage. Broaches are disposed of in a biohazard sharps container after one use. They come in several sizes similar to the sizes of reamers and files.

Reamers

Root canal reamers (Figure 44.19) are used to enlarge the pulp canal after broaches have been used. Reamers may be used with a reaming action (rotary cutting) or a filing action (scraping or pulling stroke). Reamers are tapered and pointed with spiral cutting edges. The cutting edges of reamers are farther apart than those found on endodontic files.

Reamers are available in many sizes beginning with size 10 and continuing in intervals of 5 up to size 60 or intervals of 10 through size 140. The dentist may use several reamers during one procedure, usually beginning with a relatively small size. The dental assistant prepares the next larger size each time the canal has been reamed to the desired diameter. This is called a step-up process.

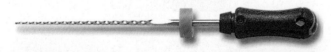

FIGURE 44.19
An endodontic hand reamer.
Courtesy DENTSPLY/Maillefer

Files

Root canal files are used after broaches and reamers (Figure 44.20). Root canal files look like reamers; however, the file threads and cutting edges are much finer and closer together. Files come in different styles: K-type, H-type (Hedstrom), and S-type, which are different in terms of their physical properties such as flexibility, resistance to fracturing during rotation, and method of manufacture.

Standard numerical size designations and color coding are the same for all root canal files. Sizes begin with size 8 and continue through size 140. Files also come in different lengths including 21, 25, and 27 mm. Files are available in carbon steel, stainless steel, or a nickel-titanium alloy. The newer titanium files have the advantage of greater strength and more flexibility, allowing them to have a longer working life.

Files and reamers are sterilized between use with dry heat, an autoclave, or a bead sterilizer. They are disposed of in a biohazard sharps container when damaged or no longer of use.

The K-type files (see Figure 44.20) are made of carbon steel and are tapered and pointed with tight spiral cutting edges arranged so that the cutting occurs with a rotating stroke. When the dentist pulls the instrument out of the tooth, the cutting edges scrape against the walls, removing necrotic tissue.

Hedstrom files (see Figure 44.20) are manufactured through a different process than K-type files. They are shaped like a series of cones that become larger from the tip toward the handle. The sharp blades of these files cut aggressively and are used in a push–pull motion and not rotated as the K-type files.

S-type files are made of stainless steel as opposed to carbon steel. Stainless steel bends more easily, is not as brittle, is less likely to break compared with carbon steel, and can be autoclaved without becoming dull. They have an S-fluted design. Hand and rotary files are also available in nickel titanium. Files are often stored in an endodontic file organizer, as shown in Figure 44.21.

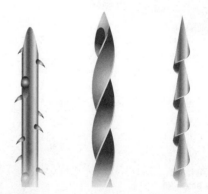

FIGURE 44.20
From left to right, a barbed broach, a K-type file, and a Hedstrom.

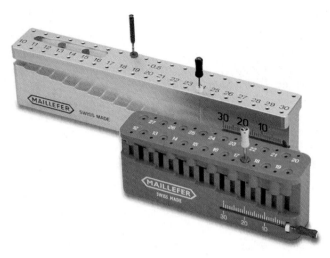

FIGURE 44.21
The EndoMbloc endodontic file organizer with a file being measured to length.
Courtesy DENTSPLY/Maillefer

Endodontic Stops

Endodontic stops (Figure 44.22) are small round pieces of rubber, plastic, or silicone. They are placed on the reamers, files, or even broaches to mark the measurement of the root canal. This prevents injury or perforation of the apex and periapical tissues of the tooth by preventing an instrument from extending out through the tooth root.

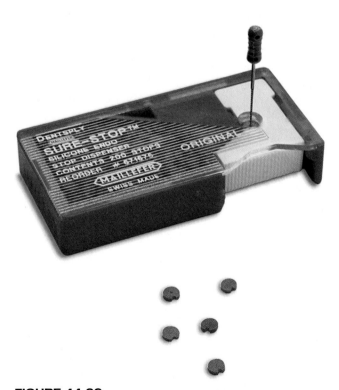

FIGURE 44.22
Endodontic stops kit.
Courtesy DENTSPLY/Maillefer

Endodontic Measuring Gauges

Precise measurements of the length of a root canal are vital to the success of endodontic therapy. The dentist or dental assistant uses a measuring gauge (Figure 44.23) to determine the working length of broaches, files, and reamers. There are many designs for endodontic rulers. All endodontic rulers measure files, reamers, and broaches in millimeter increments in various designs.

Why is the use of a dental dam so important for endodontic procedures?

Bead Sterilizer

The bead sterilizer can be used chairside during the root canal procedure to sterilize files and reamers between uses in different canals. Bead sterilizers use glass beads and generally heat up to around 425°F so only 15 seconds is required to sterilize a file. The dental assistant should ensure that any debris is removed from reamers and files before they are placed in the bead sterilizer. Other methods for sterilizing files and reamers include using a steam autoclave or dry heat.

Paper Points

Absorbent paper points (Figure 44.24) are used to completely dry out the root canals following debridement and irrigation. Paper points are highly absorbent, rolled, sterile paper cones that are tapered to fit into the root canal. They are available in assorted sizes from extra fine to coarse.

Lentulo Spiral

The lentulo spiral (Figure 44.25) is designed to transport endodontic sealer, cement, or medicaments into the finished root canal before placement of the master gutta percha point. It is used on a slow-speed handpiece with a latch-type contra-angle. It is flexible and tapered in design.

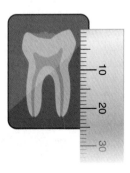

FIGURE 44.23
Endodontic millimeter ruler.

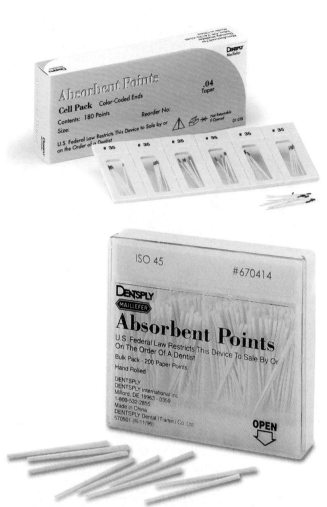

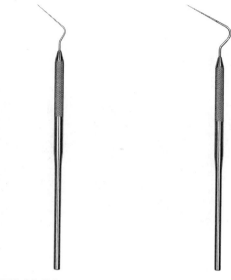

FIGURE 44.26
An endodontic spreader (left) and condenser (right).
Courtesy Hu-Friedy

FIGURE 44.24
Absorbent paper points.
Courtesy DENTSPLY/Maillefer

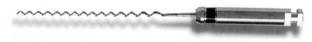

FIGURE 44.25
A lentulo spiral.
Courtesy DENTSPLY/Maillefer

Endodontic Spreader

The endodontic spreader (Figure 44.26) has an angled working end that is long and tapered to a point. This instrument is single ended and designed to condense root canal filling materials horizontally against the walls of the prepared root canal and to create a space for another gutta percha point. This process is called vertical and lateral condensation.

Endodontic Condenser

Endodontic condensers (see Figure 44.26) have an angled working end that is long and tapered but with a flat tip. It is used to condense root canal filling materials verti-

cally into the root canals. Some endodontic condensers have millimeter serrations to help the dentist evaluate the penetration depth of the instrument. The endodontic condenser, also called an endodontic plugger, can be heated to high temperatures for quick removal of excess gutta percha. An instrument called a Glick #1 is a double-ended instrument with an endodontic condenser on one end and a Woodson blade on the other. The dentist condenses or packs the gutta percha material in the pulp chamber using the condenser/plugger or the Glick #1 following the endodontic seal procedure and uses the other blade end to place temporary cement over the area.

Gates Glidden Burs

Gates Glidden burs (Figure 44.27) are football shaped and have pointed noncutting tips that create funnel-shaped openings into the root canals to permit straight access for reamers and files. They are used in a slow-speed contra-angle to enlarge the root canal. The number of bands at the base of the bur indicates its size. Gates Glidden burs are numbered 1 through 6 where the larger number indicates a larger bur width.

Peeso Reamers

Peeso reamers (Figure 44.28) resemble a Gates Glidden bur but have a straight fissure shape and end cutting capabilities. They are used carefully in a slow-speed contra-angle to remove some of the gutta percha filling material in preparation for a post. The dentist carefully follows the root canal so as not to perforate the canal. Peeso reamers have long shanks. Several sizes and kits are available for use.

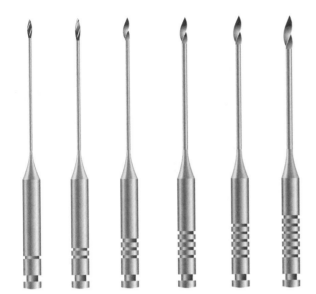

FIGURE 44.27
Gates Glidden burs with elliptical cutting edge tips.

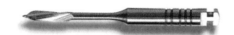

FIGURE 44.28
Peeso reamer with long parallel blades.
Courtesy DENTSPLY/Maillefer

Apex Finder

The apex finder (Figure 44.29) is an electronic measuring device for assessing the exact length of the root canal. It works by measuring gradients in electrical resistance when a file passes from dentin to apical tissue. Apex finders are especially useful when the root is curved.

Endodontic Handpiece

Endodontic handpieces are specifically designed as an alternative to handheld instruments. They help reduce the time needed for root canal preparation and prevent hand fatigue for the dentist. These handpieces remove tooth structure rapidly, require a light touch, and have a low torque so that the rotation rate is slower than that of conventional high-speed handpieces. Endodontic handpieces are more effective for canals that are not curved due to the possibility of perforating the side of the tooth root. They are available as air-driven or electric handpieces, and some endodontic handpieces have built-in apex locators.

What are the differences between the shanks on the Gates Glidden burs and the Peeso reamers? Why would these types of burs only be used in slow-speed handpieces? **?**

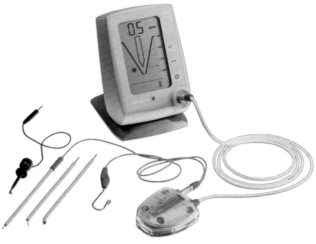

FIGURE 44.29
An apex finder.
Courtesy Sybron Dental Specialties

Medicaments and Materials in Endodontics

The persistence of bacteria in the root canal system may lead to the failure of endodontic treatment. Many medications such as phenol, iodine, formocresol, and antibiotics may be used for disinfection of the root canal. Camphorated parachlorophenol is used as an intracanal medicament often due to its antimicrobial effect within the root canals of endodontically treated teeth. RC Prep, or Root Canal Prep, may be used in conjunction with sodium hypochlorite to create fine oxygen bubbles. This bubbling action helps to lift out pulp debris and shavings from within the canal. It also bleaches, cleans, and disinfects the canal walls.

Irrigating Solutions

The most common solutions used to clean away the debris from the root canals created by endodontic files are sodium hypochlorite and hydrogen peroxide. Sodium hypochlorite is common household bleach. Both sodium hypochlorite and hydrogen peroxide mixed with water provide effective antimicrobial solutions. Saline and distilled water solutions are also frequently used to rinse out root canals during endodontics.

Endodontic Sealer

Endodontic sealer cement (Figure 44.30) is used with gutta percha obturation material. The sealer fills discrepancies between the root filling and the canal wall. It also acts as a lubricant to help seat the gutta percha cones and fills in any accessory canals. Root canal sealers and cements are available as zinc oxide-eugenol, calcium hydroxide, and glass ionomer materials in paste or capsule dispensing systems. The sealer is mixed and placed into the canal using paper points, files, directly with gutta percha, or with a lentulo spiral and slow-speed handpiece.

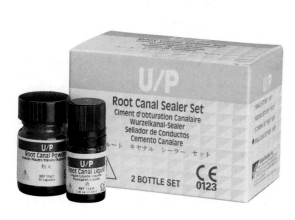

FIGURE 44.30
Root canal sealer.
Courtesy Sultan Healthcare

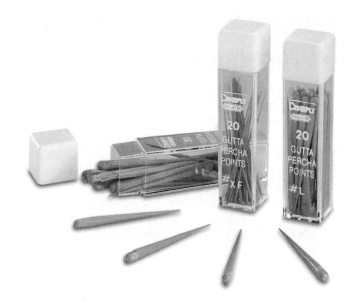

Gutta Percha

Gutta percha is a pink-colored type of plastic that has been the choice for root canal filling materials for many years. It softens when heated and is easily molded. When cooled it maintains its shape well. After the dentist uses instrumenting techniques to clean and debride the canal(s), the canal is dried and a master gutta percha point (Figure 44.31) is placed into the prepared tooth. The dentist first places a master gutta percha point that coincides with the endodontic file size used last, and then the dental assistant passes accessory gutta percha to the dentist until the tooth canals are completely filled.

Gutta percha points are made to the specifications of the American Association of Endodontics. The sizes vary from extra fine, fine, and medium to large. They also come in sizes corresponding to reamer and file sizes.

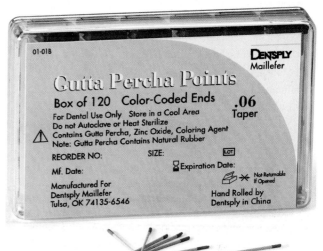

FIGURE 44.31
Gutta percha points.
Courtesy DENTSPLY/Maillefer

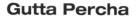

What are the most common solutions used by the dentist to irrigate the canal(s) during endodontic treatment?

Overview of Endodontic Treatment

To begin endodontic treatment, the dentist must first gain access to the root canal within a tooth with a high-speed handpiece and friction grip bur. A proper preparation helps identify accessory (extra) canals and gives a clear, unobstructed view to all canal openings. Next the coronal pulp is removed by using a round bur in a slow-speed handpiece or an endodontic spoon excavator.

The openings of the root canal(s) are located and enlarged if necessary with Gates Glidden burs. The pulpal tissue is then extirpated (removed) with a broach, after which the canal is debrided using reamers and/or files. After irrigating the canal, it is dried with paper points. The canals are then obturated (filled) with gutta percha, and the crown of the tooth is restored.

The endodontic procedure can be completed in one visit or over the course of several visits depending on the severity of the infection and the preference of the dentist (Procedure 44.1).

Life Span Considerations

The dentist may perform a pulpectomy or a pulpotomy on a primary tooth in order to keep the tooth so that it can hold space for the erupting permanent tooth. This will maintain the tooth free of infection until the permanent tooth erupts.

Procedure 44-1 Assisting with an Endodontic Procedure

Equipment and Supplies Needed

- Basic setup: mirror, explorer, locking cotton pliers
- Anesthetic setup
- Rubber dam setup
- Saliva ejector, high-volume evacuator (HVE) tip, air/water syringe tip
- Slow-speed handpiece and a #4 or #6 round bur
- Assortment of acrylic burs, discs, and mandrels
- High-speed handpiece and a #556 or #557 bur or burs preferred by the dentist
- Broaches, files, reamers
- Endodontic spoon excavator, spreader, condenser
- Woodson, articulating paper, floss
- Irrigating syringe, irrigating solution
- Bead sterilizer, butane torch, or other heat source
- Paper points, small cotton pellets
- Medication
- Temporary filling material
- Endodontic ruler and stops
- X-ray film, lead apron

Procedure Steps

1. The dental assistant passes the mirror and explorer to the dentist and then passes a 2 × 2 gauze to dry the muccobuccal fold and the topical anesthetic. The dental assistant passes the anesthetic syringe. When the dentist completes placing the anesthetic, the dental assistant rinses the area with the air/water syringe and aspirates excess water with the HVE tip.

2. The dental assistant or dentist places the rubber dam on the affected tooth. The dental assistant should inform the patient of the purpose of the dental dam and that if there are any concerns to let the dental team know.

3. The dentist creates an opening in the tooth with the high-speed handpiece and bur. The dental assistant should keep the rubber dam free of debris but be sure to stay out of the dentist's line of vision.

4. The dentist uses the slow-speed handpiece and round bur to remove caries and to access the pulp chamber. The dental assistant may quickly rinse the area to improve the dentist's field of view.

5. The dentist may want to use the endodontic spoon excavator to remove caries and the endodontic explorer to locate the pulp chamber and canal openings.

6. The dental assistant passes a barbed broach for the dentist to remove pulpal tissues from within the root canal. The dentist may want several broaches, especially if the tooth has more than one root.

7. The dental assistant passes a #10 or #15 reamer with stoppers to measure the length of each canal. The dental assistant exposes a radiograph so the dentist can measure the length of each canal with the file(s) or reamer(s) in place. The radiograph and working length of each canal are recorded in the patient's chart.

8. The dental assistant passes additional files in progression until the proper width and length of the canal are achieved. The size and length of the final file used are recorded in the patient's chart.

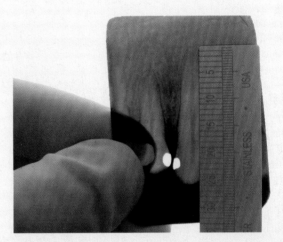

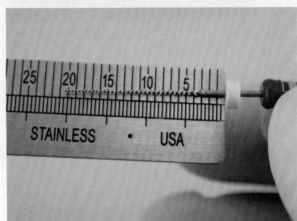

Measuring a file length with a radiograph.
Images courtesy Instructional Materials for the Dental Team, Lex., KY

9. The dental assistant passes the irrigating syringe with irrigating solution to the dentist. The dentist irrigates the canal(s). The dental assistant must keep the tip of the HVE very close to the tooth so the irrigating solution is efficiently aspirated and not allowed to splash the patient or the dental team.

continued on next page

Procedure 44-1 *continued from previous page*

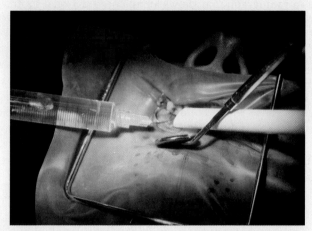

Irrigating a root canal.
Image courtesy Instructional Materials for the Dental Team, Lex., KY

10. The dental assistant passes paper points with locking cotton pliers and continues to pass paper points until the canal or canals are completely dry.

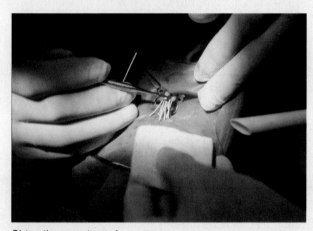

Obturating a root canal.
Image courtesy Instructional Materials for the Dental Team, Lex., KY

11. The dental assistant passes a small cotton pellet containing medication to the dentist who places it in the tooth. (At this point the dentist places a temporary filling material into the tooth or continues to obturate the canal and completes the root canal treatment. If a tooth is severely infected, the dentist may elect to have the patient return at a later date to complete the endodontic therapy.)

12. A master gutta percha point is selected that matches the width size of the last file used in each canal. The dental assistant exposes a radiograph to verify the proper length and seal.

13. The dental assistant mixes the endodontic sealer to a creamy consistency and passes it to the dentist, so he or she can coat the tip of the master gutta percha point. The dentist places the gutta percha with cement into the canal. (Some dentists will use a lentulo spiral to place the endodontic sealer deep into the canal before placing the gutta percha point.)

14. The dental assistant passes the endodontic spreader and additional accessory gutta percha points and continues to pass the spreader and an additional point until each canal is full.

15. The dental assistant passes the endodontic condenser and prepares the torch. The dental assistant holds some 2 × 2 gauze squares and holds the HVE tip close to the tooth.

16. The dentist heats the tip of the endodontic condenser and melts off the excess gutta percha material. It is important to adequately heat the instrument to avoid removal of the gutta percha filling from the canal. The dental assistant ensures that the HVE tip aspirates any smoke and receives the melted gutta percha from the dentist with a 2 × 2 gauze.

17. The dental assistant prepares the temporary filling material and passes the Woodson. The dentist places the filling. The dental assistant passes a lightly dampened cotton applicator to the dentist, who uses it to smooth the temporary restoration.

18. The dental assistant uses the HVE and air/water syringe to ensure that the rubber dam is rinsed free of debris. The rubber dam is removed and the dental assistant freshens the patient's mouth by rinsing and aspirating.

19. The dental assistant dries the tooth and passes the articulating paper to the dentist who will ask the patient to lightly tap the teeth together. If necessary, the dentist will adjust the occlusion with the Woodson, cotton applicator, or a round bur and slow-speed handpiece.

20. The dental assistant exposes a final radiograph and provides postoperative instructions to the patient.

Surgical Endodontics

The goal of surgical endodontics is to eliminate any source of apical infection emanating from the tooth root. It is important for all necrotic tissue to be eliminated so the alveolar bone can repair itself. Sometimes calcium deposits make it impossible for the dentist to reach the end of the root to seal it off. Surgery is also performed to treat a damaged root surface or a persistent infection in the surrounding bone.

Apicoectomy

Apico means "apex" and *ectomy* means "to cut off" or "surgically remove." An **apicoectomy**, therefore, is a surgical removal of the apical portion of the tooth. This is accomplished through a surgical opening in the overlying bone and gingival tissues. An apicoectomy is usually performed in conjunction with periapical curettage after the body fails to heal following endodontic therapy. Periapical curettage is the surgical removal of apically inflamed tissue. Some dentists place donor bone into the surgical site around the removed root to improve bone growth following dental surgery. Conditions that may indicate the need for an apicoectomy include:

- Persistent local infection following endodontic treatment
- Endodontic filling materials or medications extruded into the periapical tissues
- A broken instrument lodged in the canal, preventing complete obturation
- Obstruction caused by a calcified root canal or a pulp stone
- Extreme curvature of the canal, preventing access to the apex of the root

The apicoectomy is performed on a tooth where the root canal failed. This procedure is most often performed by an endodontist or oral surgeon and is an alternative to having the tooth extracted (Procedure 44-2). Figure 44.32 is a radiograph that shows an apicoectomy on a tooth.

Retrograde Filling

A retrograde filling is used to seal the apical end of a root canal by placing restoration material into the root apex. This is usually done in conjunction with an apicoectomy (Procedure 44-2). Following the surgical removal of the apex of the tooth, a small filling is placed to seal the root canal. Retrograde filling materials include EBA cement, IRM, zinc-free high-copper amalgam, and mineral trioxide aggregate (MTA).

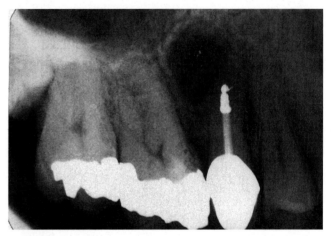

FIGURE 44.32
A radiograph showing an apicoectomy on a tooth.
Image courtesy Instructional Materials for the Dental Team, Lex., KY

Procedure 44-2 Assisting with an Apicoectomy and Retrograde Filling

Equipment and Supplies Needed

- Surgical setup: mirror, scalpel and blade handle, periosteal elevator, curette
- Retrograde filling instruments and material
- Surgical high-volume evacuator (HVE) tip, air/water syringe tip
- Slow-speed handpiece
- High-speed handpiece with surgical burs

Procedure Steps

1. The dentist makes a flap in the gingival tissue. The assistant may be asked to retract while the dentist creates a window in the bone at the apex of the root.

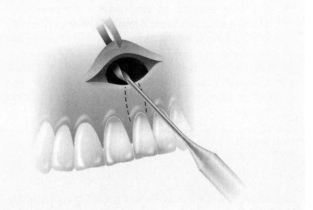

An incision and flap with bone removal during an apicoectomy.

continued on next page

Procedure 44-2 *continued from previous page*

2. When the root tip is exposed, the dentist uses the high-speed handpiece and surgical bur to cut and section the apex of the tooth and uses the surgical curette to remove all diseased alveolar bone tissue. The assistant should have several squares of 2 × 2 gauze available and continue to rinse the area and aspirate debris as necessary.

3. The dentist prepares the apex of the tooth with the high-speed bur or with other technology such as ultrasonics.

4. The assistant mixes and passes the retrograde filling material to the dentist, who places it into the opening in the apex of the tooth.

5. The area is cleaned and sutures placed.

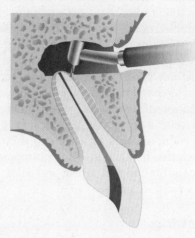

A high-speed handpiece and bur removes bone and exposes the apex.

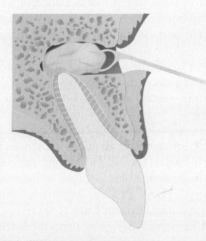

Removing infection at the apex: apical curettage.

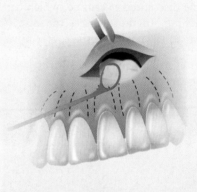

Gauze being used as necessary while rinsing the area and aspirating debris.

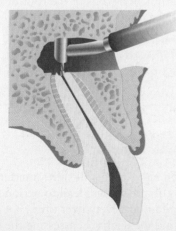

Preparing the root apex for a retrofilling.

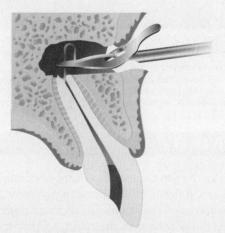

Placing a retrograde filling into the apex.

Root Amputation

Occasionally a multi-rooted tooth requiring endodontic treatment may have a root that is impossible to seal or is affected by periodontal disease. When the other roots of the tooth are treatable, rather than extracting the entire tooth, the untreatable root is amputated and removed (Figure 44.33). The opening to which the amputated root was attached is sealed with filling material similar to that used in an apicoectomy procedure. The retained section of the tooth is treated endodontically before amputation.

A root amputation procedure is especially indicated when the infected tooth is needed as an abutment support for a bridge. The endodontist or oral surgeon will use a treatment approach that helps control any postoperative swelling and discomfort for the patient including prescribing medication and ice packs.

Tooth Bleaching

Chemical agents may be used to remove discoloration from the crowns of nonvital teeth. Nonvital teeth may discolor because of pulpal hemorrhage into the dentinal tubules following traumatic injury of the tooth, or a nonvital tooth may become discolored over time, which can be treated with bleaching. In most cases, the discoloration poses no threat to the health of the tooth; how-

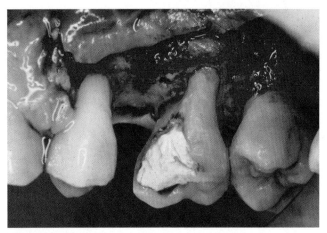

FIGURE 44.33
Surgical exposure of tooth #14. The mesiobuccal root has been removed and positive osseous contours established.
Hempton T, Leone C. A review of root resective therapy as a treatment option for maxillary molars. JADA 1997;128(4): 449–455. Copyright © 1997 American Dental Association. All rights reserved. Reprinted with permission.

ever, the appearance of the discolored tooth may be improved dramatically by bleaching the tooth from the inside following root canal treatment.

The technique for bleaching nonvital teeth involves the placement of a thick white paste composed of sodium perborate and Superoxol in the pulp chamber and placing a temporary restoration. The procedure will need to be repeated several times before a permanent restoration is placed in the tooth.

Lasers, Endodontic Microscopes, and Ultrasonics

Dental lasers are being used for certain procedures including endodontics and apicoectomies. Many laser procedures performed do not require anesthesia for patient comfort. The dentist uses the laser handpiece to create an opening for root canal therapy. After accessing the canal, the laser handpiece and a series of flexible fiber-optic tips clean and debride the root canal system. The laser handpiece incises gingival tissue and bone, removes the diseased root tip, and prepares an apex for a retrofilling during apicoectomy procedures.

The endodontic operating microscope makes visualization of the surgical area much easier for the endodontist. It allows enhanced magnification and illumination of the root surface, making it possible for the dentist to see fractures, missed and lateral canals, adjacent canals, perforations, and defects within a tooth. These surgical microscopes facilitate a more thorough debridement of infected tissue. Endodontic microscopes are also used to closely inspect retrofillings during apicoectomies. Miniature instruments have evolved to be used during microsurgery. They include explorers, mirrors, carriers, pluggers, and ultrasonic tips.

Ultrasonics has been used in dentistry for several years. The technology has evolved into an extremely accurate method of creating retrofilling preparations. The endodontic surgeon is able to prepare retrocavities that are parallel to the long axis of the root of the tooth while minimizing the removal of bone.

Why are dentists using dental laser technology along with microscopes for endodontic surgery?

● SUMMARY

When the nerve or pulp tissue of a primary or permanent tooth is infected, it needs to be treated to prevent a dental abscess and loss of the tooth. The ultimate objective of these procedures is to save the tooth, so that it will maintain the integrity and function of the dental arch. The only alternative to endodontic therapy is to extract the infected tooth. Unless the tooth is replaced, the

adjoining teeth on either side will shift, interfering with mastication. Loss of a tooth will lead to periodontal disease and loss of additional teeth over time.

Several tests aid the dentist in assessing the health of dental pulp. The most important assessment for the dentist is a radiograph. An accurate representation of the tooth is necessary for the dentist to be able to measure the proper length of each tooth root. Pulpal tissues within the tooth are removed with an endodontic broach and then the canals are cleaned, smoothed, and filed before filling with gutta percha.

The dental assistant must become familiar with the many instruments and accessory materials designed specifically for endodontic treatment. Surgical endodontic therapy may be required in cases of acute long-standing infection.

KEY TERMS

- **Apicoectomy:** The surgical removal of the apical portion of a tooth.   p. 695
- **Debridement:** Removal of debris, including necrotic nerve tissue, from a tooth root canal.   p. 684
- **Endodontics:** The specialty that involves the treatment of the tooth pulp and periapical tissues.   p. 677
- **Extirpation:** Removal of infected pulp tissue within a tooth.   p. 683
- **Irreversible pulpitis:** Condition in which inflamed tooth pulp is unable to respond to treatment and the patient's symptoms of pain continue.   p. 678

- **Necrotic pulp:** Nonvital pulp that is dead and gangrenous.   p. 679
- **Obturate:** To fill the root canals of a tooth.   p. 684
- **Percussion:** Gentle tapping on the crown of the tooth.   p. 680
- **Periapical abscess:** Infection from within the tooth that spreads out through the apex and into the surrounding bone.   p. 678
- **Pulpitis:** Inflammation of the tooth pulp.   p. 678
- **Reversible pulpitis:** Condition in which inflamed tooth pulp is able to respond to treatment.   p. 678

CHECK YOUR UNDERSTANDING

1. What are the causes of pulpal damage?
   a. microbial damage
   b. mechanical damage
   c. chemical irritation
   d. all of the above

2. What term describes the type of inflammation of a tooth pulp that is able to respond to treatment?
   a. reversible pulpitis
   b. irreversible pulpitis
   c. necrotic pulp
   d. none of the above

3. What term describes the type of inflammation of a tooth pulp that does not respond to treatment?
   a. reversible pulpitis
   b. irreversible pulpitis
   c. necrotic pulp
   d. periapical abscess

4. What is another name for nonvital pulp?
   a. reversible pulpitis
   b. irreversible pulpitis
   c. necrotic pulp
   d. periapical abscess

5. What is the most valuable tool a dentist uses to diagnose problems with a tooth?
   a. cold test
   b. heat test
   c. palpation
   d. radiograph

6. What is used to fill the root canal during an endodontic procedure?
   a. broaches
   b. files
   c. reamers
   d. gutta percha

7. During an endodontic treatment, which of the following is performed?
   a. post
   b. core buildup
   c. crown preparation
   d. all of the above

8. What is the purpose of a dental dam during an endodontic procedure?
   a. isolate the tooth
   b. maintain a sterile field
   c. prevent small instruments from falling in the patient's throat
   d. keep debris from going into the patient's throat
   e. all of the above

9. Which instrument is used to extirpate the tooth pulp during a root canal procedure?
   a. broach
   b. file
   c. reamer
   d. spreader

10. What procedure is performed when endodontic treatment fails to control an area of infection?
    a. retrograde filling
    b. periapical curettage
    c. apicoectomy
    d. all of the above

● INTERNET ACTIVITY

- Go to www.uic.edu then use the site's Google Search option to search for "depts/endo." On the search results page, choose UIC Department of Endodontics to view an apicoectomy performed with an endodontic microscope. Real Player is necessary to view this presentation.

● WEB REFERENCES

- Academy of General Dentistry   www.agd.org
- Advanced Endodontics of Houston   www.advanced-endodontics.com/surgical_therapy.html
- Advanced Endodontics of Westchester, PLLC   www.westchesterendo.com/doct_microsurgery.html
- Brazilian Dental Journal   www.forp.usp.br/bdj/t0182.html
- Dental Resources   http://dentalresource.org/topic58pulpotomypulpectomy.html
- The Endo Experience   www.endoexperience.com/emergencydiagnosis.htm
- Joseph S. Dovgan, DDS   www.endodovgan.com/Endoinfo_NSRET.htm
- The Journal of the American Dental Association   http://dental.case.edu/classnotes/year3/end/lectures/lecture1.pdf
- The Journal of the American Dental Association   http://jada.highwire.org/cgi/content/full/136/5/611
- University of Illinois at Chicago College of Dentistry Department of Endodontics   www.uic.edu/depts/endo/apico.html

45

Periodontal Procedures

Learning Objectives

After reading this chapter, the student should be able to:

- Define the terminology associated with periodontal procedures.
- Discuss the components of the periodontal examination.
- Describe the various instruments associated with periodontal procedures.
- Discuss the rationale for nonsurgical periodontal treatment.
- Explain the different surgical procedures for periodontal treatment.
- Discuss the advantages of using lasers.
- Describe safety features associated with the use of lasers.

Preparing for Certification Exams

- Place and remove periodontal dressings.
- Remove sutures.
- Monitor and respond to postsurgical bleeding.

Chapter Outline

- The Periodontal Practice
- The Periodontal Examination
  - Biofilm
  - Calculus
  - Gingival Appearance
  - Periodontal Probing Depths
  - Tooth Mobility
  - Suppuration
  - Furcation Involvement
  - Recession
  - Width of Attached Gingiva
  - Occlusion
  - Radiographic Evaluation
- Periodontal Instruments
  - Periodontal Probe
  - Naber's Probe
  - Explorers
  - Scalers
  - Curettes
  - Sonic and Ultrasonic Instruments
  - Scalpel
  - Periodontal Knives
  - Pocket Markers
  - Hemostats
  - Tissue Forceps
  - Needle Holders
  - Soft Tissue Rongeurs
  - Periodontal Scissors
  - Periosteal Elevators
- Nonsurgical Periodontal Treatment
- Surgical Periodontal Treatment
  - Procedures for Treatment of Mucogingival Defects
  - Procedures for Gaining Access
  - Procedures for Removing or Reshaping the Gingiva
  - Procedures for Treatment of Osseous Defects
  - Procedures for Regeneration of the Periodontium
  - Crown Lengthening Surgery
  - Periodontal Dressing Materials
- Lasers in Periodontics
  - Advantages of Laser Surgery
  - Laser Safety

Key Terms

Biofilm	Periodontal debridement
Calculus	Periodontal pocket
Exudate	Periodontal probe
Frenectomy	Periodontitis
Furcation involvement	Recession
Gingivectomy	Scaling
Gingivoplasty	

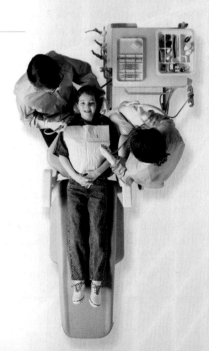

The dental assistant is often the individual who serves as a source of information for the patient. By understanding the various treatment options available for periodontal patients, the assistant can aid the patient in understanding the complexities that often go hand in hand with any type of treatment option. In addition, full knowledge of the instruments and materials needed for periodontal treatment is an extremely valuable asset of the dental assistant.

How might the members of the dental team vary in a periodontal practice versus a general dental practice?

The Periodontal Practice

The periodontal practice is a specialty practice that concentrates on the cause, diagnosis, treatment, and prevention of periodontal conditions and diseases. The periodontist is a dentist who has undergone an additional two years of residency upon successful completion of four years of dental school. The scope of practice for the periodontist does not include restorative procedures.

In addition to the periodontist, the periodontal practice typically has one or more registered dental hygienists. The number of hygienists depends on state regulations. The hygienist may perform initial therapy on patients in addition to treating patients who require periodontal maintenance. Additional education is not required for the dental hygienist to work in the periodontal practice. However, certain states do allow registered dental hygienists with appropriate certification to administer local anesthesia. This greatly assists in time management during nonsurgical periodontal procedures.

The dental assistant is an essential member of the team in the periodontal practice. The dental assistant

Dental Assistant PROFESSIONAL TIP

As a dental assistant, you may be required to review postoperative instructions with patients. Patients may be overwhelmed following surgical procedures, so in addition to oral instructions, the dental assistant should make sure that the patient is given written instructions as well. These instructions should include both professional and layman's terminology so that the patient can easily understand his role in promoting healing. Following verbalization of instructions, the dental assistant should have the patient repeat those instructions back to ensure understanding and promote compliance.

assists the periodontist during surgery and postoperative appointments, exposes and processes radiographs, and assists with numerous other procedures. (Refer to Chapter 2 for additional information on the duties and responsibilities of the dental assistant.) The role of the dental assistant can vary depending on the duties specified by state practice laws.

Support staff for a periodontal practice can include a receptionist, possibly a circulating dental assistant, a hygiene assistant, and an insurance and billing clerk. Additional personnel may be required depending on the volume of regularly treated patients.

Periodontal practices often depend on referrals from general dentists. In many cases, a general practice will treat patients with milder forms of periodontal disease or conditions; however, in the case of severe periodontal disease, the general dentist may refer the patient to a periodontist for more extensive treatment. The periodontal team and the dental team must establish a line of communication and form a partnership in order to co-manage these patients.

The Periodontal Examination

The periodontal examination is an essential component of the overall oral health assessment and is usually performed by either the dentist or the dental hygienist, depending on the practice. If the dental hygienist performs this procedure, the dentist will often reevaluate any aspect that seems beyond the normal limits. The examination should include an evaluation of the plaque biofilm, calculus deposits, gingival appearance, periodontal probing depths, bleeding, suppuration, tooth mobility, furcation involvement, gingival recession, occlusal analysis, and an interpretation of radiographic findings.

Legal and Ethical Issues

Unfortunately, periodontal disease can go undiagnosed for a significant period of time, especially if patients are not receiving the necessary treatment that they need in order to preserve their oral health. A patient may present at your office with complaints of misdiagnosis or treatment of periodontal disease. As a dental assistant, you may be faced with such comments as "Why wasn't I told this before now?" or "I should have been treated for this problem years ago." It is the dental assistant's responsibility to appease the patient without rendering any malicious or ill-intent comments about the previous treatment the patient received. You should be prepared with a well-versed statement that expresses your concern for the patient but does not provide any negative views for which you could potentially be held legally accountable.

TABLE 45-1 Descriptors Used in Assessing Gingival Appearance

	Healthy Gingiva	Changes in Gingiva
Color	Pink, light pink, pale pink	Red, bright red, bluish red
Consistency	Firm, resilient	Edematous, spongy, fibrotic
Contour/Shape	Fills embrasures, follows contour of the teeth, knife-edged, pyramidal	Blunted, recessed, punched out, swollen, rolled, cratered
Size	Fits snugly around the tooth	Enlarged

Biofilm

Biofilm is a community of numerous types of bacteria as well as other organisms that easily adhere to surfaces in the oral cavity. The presence of biofilm (formerly called dental plaque) indicates the potential for gingival problems. A patient's oral hygiene can be determined by assessing the presence of plaque. The presence of plaque is determined visually and with the use of an explorer.

Disclosing solution can also be very helpful in determining a patient's oral hygiene. Disclosing solution, which comes in tablets or liquid, colors or stains the plaque temporarily so an assessment of the patient's oral hygiene can be determined. If plaque is present, then further discussion with the patient regarding the importance of plaque removal is required. An evaluation of the patient's manual dexterity may provide insight into the patient's ability to do an adequate job of plaque removal.

Calculus

The presence of **calculus,** which is plaque that has had time to harden, should be documented as well as plaque. The amount of calculus and whether it is slight, moderate, or heavy should be noted, as well as whether the calculus is supragingival, subgingival, or both. The presence of calculus, determined by a visual inspection or with an explorer specifically designed to detect calculus, indicates that the patient's home care regimen is not adequate and that the patient may need instruction and guidance on developing a more appropriate home care regimen. In addition, this could indicate the need for more frequent recall visits.

Gingival Appearance

Even subtle changes in appearance of the gingivae can indicate that the patient may have some existing health issues. These changes may indicate the onset of the inflammatory process and be an indicator of further treatment. Changes in the color, consistency, contour, location, or position and shape of the gingivae should be noted. A description of both the marginal and papillary gingivae should be documented. Refer to Table 45-1 for a comparison of how gingiva looks when it is healthy versus when it is diseased.

Periodontal Probing Depths

It is crucial for the periodontal probing depths to be measured at regular intervals and recorded in the patient's chart. Either the dentist or the dental hygienist will perform this procedure at each visit. A normal sulcus has a probing depth of 3 mm or less. A pocket depth of greater than 3 mm is called a **periodontal pocket.** Six measurements are taken per tooth, one on each of the following locations: distobuccal, buccal, mesiobuccal, distolingual, lingual, and mesiolingual.

Probing depths are recorded to the next higher whole number if the reading falls between two full numbers; for example, a reading of 4.5 mm is recorded as 5 mm. At times, there will be a discrepancy between two clinicians when probing. In most clinics, a 1-mm probing depth difference is considered acceptable between operators. Any bleeding noted upon probing should be documented in the patient's chart. Bleeding is an indication of inflammation and should be monitored accordingly.

Tooth Mobility

Tooth mobility is the measurement of movement of a tooth in its socket (Table 45-2). The loss of bone support around a tooth can result in increased mobility as does trauma or occlusal forces. To assess horizontal mobility, the ends of two single-ended instruments are used to push on the tooth in a buccolingual direction or in the direction from the cheek toward the tongue. Vertical tooth mobility is determined by exerting pressure on the occlusal or incisal surface of the tooth. The scale increases as the degree of tooth mobility increases, which

TABLE 45-2 Mobility Rating

Classification	Description
Class I	Up to 1 mm of horizontal movement in a buccolingual direction
Class II	Greater than 1 mm of horizontal movement in a buccolingual direction
Class III	Greater than 1 mm of horizontal displacement plus vertical displacement since the tooth is depressible in the socket

could indicate that there has been trauma or an increase in loss of support.

Suppuration

Suppuration is also known as pus. Tissue fluid, dead cells, and polymorphonuclear leukocytes are all components of pus. Suppuration can be visible during probing or upon applying digital pressure at the base of the pocket surrounding the tooth. The presence of this slightly whitish to yellowish purulent **exudate** is a positive indicator of inflammation of the pocket.

Does bleeding when flossing indicate a problem with the gingivae?

Furcation Involvement

A furcation is the area of a multi-rooted tooth where the root divides. **Furcation involvement** is the result of periodontal infection that causes the loss of the interradicular bone between multirooted teeth. With the use of a furcation probe, such as the Naber's probe, detection and documentation of any issues related to furcation involvement is an important component of the periodontal examination.

There are four basic classifications of furcation involvement, with each being represented by a symbol. In a Class I furcation, the concavity or indentation above the furcation can be felt with the probe, but it cannot enter the furcation. With a Class II furcation, the probe can partially enter the furcation, but it is not able to pass completely through the furcation. In a Class III furcation, the probe on the mandibular molars can pass completely through the furcation, and on the maxillary molars, the probe can pass through the mesiobuccal or distobuccal roots and touch the palatal root. In a Class IV furcation, the involvement is the same as for Class III except the entrance to the furcation is clinically visible due to recession of the gingiva. Various symbols are used for classifying furcation involvement, as listed in Table 45-3.

Recession

Recession is the physical result of the apical migration of the epithelial attachment (Figure 45.1). Recession is measured using the periodontal probe from the cemen-

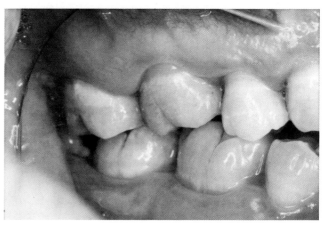

FIGURE 45.1
Gingival recession.

toenamel junction (CEJ) to the gingival margin. The CEJ is the junction where the crown and the root meet. Recession can be due to trauma such as brushing too vigorously, rapid tooth movement, extensive restorative treatment that may affect the gingivae, or **periodontitis**. As a result of recession, the papillae may be blunted or rounded.

Width of Attached Gingiva

The width of attached gingiva is an important characteristic to record as well. The attached gingiva prevents the free gingiva from being pulled away from the tooth. Areas with no attachment are subject to problems should a restoration in that area be necessary. The width of attached gingiva on the facial surface of the maxillary anteriors is 3.5 to 4.5 mm, and on the mandibular anteriors it is 3.3 to 3.9 mm. On the maxillary premolars the width is 1.9 mm, and 1.8 mm on the mandibular premolars. The width of attached gingiva is not measurable on the palatal aspect because the difference between the attached gingiva and palatal mucosa cannot be measured.

To measure the width of attached gingiva, measure from the gingival margin to the mucogingival junction. The mucogingival junction is the area that marks the connection between the attached gingiva and the alveolar

Life Span Considerations

Although most patients who are being treated for periodontal disease are adults, at times children will need some type of periodontal treatment. Children are frequently referred for a periodontal examination prior to undergoing orthodontic treatment. The dental assistant should be prepared to treat a wide age range of patients in a periodontal practice. Being able to closely identify with both the geriatric population as well as youngsters will help the dental assistant develop rapport with all types of patients.

TABLE 45-3	Charting Symbols for Furcation Classifications
Class I furcation involvement	⋀
Class II furcation involvement	Δ
Class III furcation involvement	▲
Class IV furcation involvement	◆

mucosa. The alveolar mucosa will appear darker than the gingiva due to the underlying blood vessels. Next, the probing depth in that area should be noted. By subtracting the probing depth from the total width of the gingiva, the width of attached gingiva is obtained.

Apical migration of the gingival margin past the CEJ is known as what? How would you inform the patient of what is going on in this case? **?**

Occlusion

The patient's occlusion should be thoroughly evaluated and recorded. Any excessive force or occlusal abnormality could potentially contribute to more serious problems. The condition of tongue thrusting can also cause problems to develop due to the constant pressure of the tongue during swallowing. This can lead to protrusion of the anterior teeth, particularly the maxillary anteriors.

Radiographic Evaluation

The use of radiographs can be very helpful in assessing the periodontium (Figure 45.2). When an individual has good oral health, the appearance on radiographs of the crest of the alveolar bone is about 1 to 1.5 mm apical to the CEJ. Although it is not necessary to use a periodontal probe to measure the actual distance, one should have an understanding of this measurement. This measurement means that the dental assistant should see that the alveolar bone is 1 to 1.5 mm down on the root surface in a healthy periodontium. The level of horizontal bone should be parallel to an imaginary line drawn from the CEJ on one tooth to the adjacent tooth. When a patient develops periodontal disease, there may be a loss of either horizontal or vertical bone or both.

Frequently, a full mouth series of radiographs is exposed for periodontal patients. In cases where bitewing radiographs are indicated, vertical bitewings are the radiograph of choice in contrast to the traditional horizontal ones.

When the tooth has horizontal mobility greater than 1 mm and can also be depressed in the socket, this is known as what class of mobility? What does this tell you about what is going on with the patient? **?**

Periodontal Instruments

A variety of instruments are utilized in the treatment of periodontal conditions. The majority of these instruments require that they maintain a sufficiently sharp cutting edge. It is essential for the dental hygienist or the

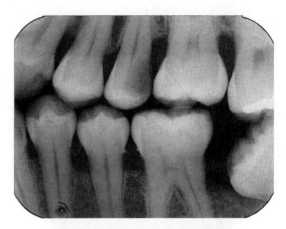
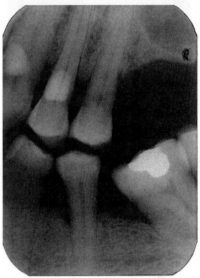

FIGURE 45.2
Radiographs can be helpful in assessing the periodontal status of a patient.

dental assistant to assess these instruments on a regular basis to ensure their sharpness. A dull instrument hinders the clinician in treatment. A sharp instrument, on the other hand, enables the clinician to be more thorough and efficient while reducing operator fatigue. A sharp instrument will also reduce the possibility of traumatizing the gingival tissues.

Currently, several methods are used to maintain instrument sharpness. The traditional sharpening stones and test sticks are still used, but have become less popular with the development of other devices such as the Sidekick by Hu-Friedy, which provides a sharp cutting edge with little effort on the part of the hygienist or assistant.

Periodontal Probe

The **periodontal probe** is a calibrated instrument used to diagnose the periodontal condition (Figure 45.3). The probe can be compared to a ruler. The instrument is marked off in millimeters at specific intervals depending on the manufacturer of the probe. These intervals allow

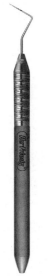

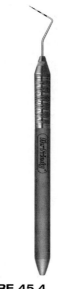

FIGURE 45.3
An example of one type of periodontal probe.
Courtesy Hu-Friedy

FIGURE 45.4
A color-coded probe used to measure a periodontal sulcus.
Courtesy Hu-Friedy

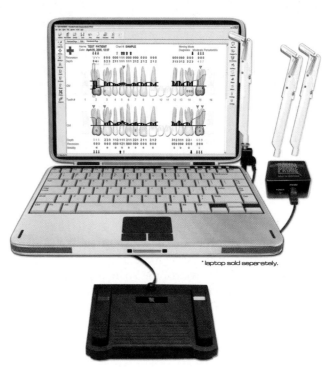

* laptop sold separately.

FIGURE 45.5
The Florida Probe is an example of one of the automated probing systems that are available.
Courtesy Florida Probe Corporation

for accurate measurement of the periodontal pocket. After the probe is inserted into the sulcus, a walking motion is used to gently move the probe around the tooth. The measurement is taken from the base of the pocket to the gingival margin. A total of six measurements are taken per tooth and recorded. When bleeding or exudate is present it is noted. The probe can also be used to measure the width of attached gingiva, recession, and any intraoral lesions. Periodontal probes can be flat, round, or oval and made of metal or plastic. They can also be color coded (Figure 45.4).

Advancements in modern technology have led to commercially available automated computerized probes (Figure 45.5). Automated probes allow the practitioner to perform the probing while the computer records the readings. These systems can be voice or foot controlled to reduce cross-contamination.

Naber's Probe

The Naber's probe (Figure 45.6) is a curved instrument that is calibrated similar to the periodontal probe. This instrument is used to locate not only the entrance to furcations, but also the degree of horizontal bone destruction.

Explorers

Explorers are usually thin, curved instruments that provide the maximum in tactile sensitivity (Figures 45.7 and 45.8). These instruments are typically classified as diagnostic, assessment, or evaluation instruments. They are used to detect calculus, faulty or defective margins on restorations, carious lesions, tooth irregularities, and furcations.

Scalers

Scalers are instruments that are used for **scaling**, which is the removal of supragingival and/or subgingival calculus. In some cases, scalers may be used subgingivally if the gingival margin is distended to allow access without traumatizing the tissue.

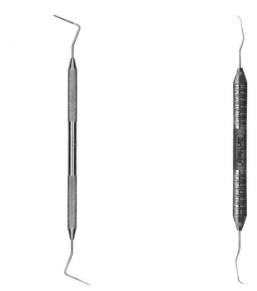

FIGURE 45.6
The Naber's probe is used to determine furcation involvement.

FIGURE 45.7
The ODU explorer is used to detect calculus, tooth irregularities, and faulty restorations. It is more easily adapted to deeper pockets than the pigtail explorer.
Courtesy Hu-Friedy

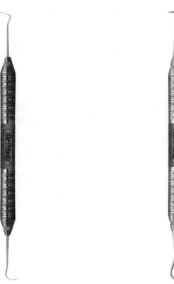

FIGURE 45.8
The pigtail explorer is used to detect calculus, tooth irregularities, and faulty restorations.
Courtesy Hu-Friedy

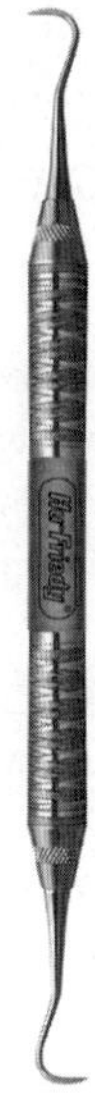

FIGURE 45.9
Sickle scaler H6/7.
Courtesy Hu-Friedy

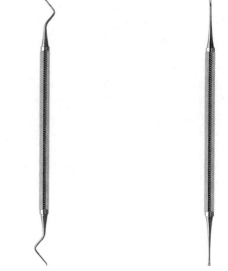

FIGURE 45.10
Hoe scaler.
Courtesy Hu-Friedy

FIGURE 45.11
Darby-Perry chisel scaler.
Courtesy Hu-Friedy

Sickle Scalers

Sickle scalers can be curved or straight (Figure 45.9). The cross section of a sickle scaler is triangular in shape. There are two cutting edges per end on the sickle. The face and the two lateral surfaces of the scaler meet to form a sharp tip. Because of this sharp tip, the sickle is not recommended for subgingival scaling. Both the curved and straight sickle scalers are available with an angulated or straight shank. Each type has advantages for allowing easier access to particular areas in the mouth for instrumentation.

Hoe Scalers

The hoe scaler (Figure 45.10) is used to remove large, tenacious deposits of supragingival calculus. The hoe has a single cutting edge that is beveled at a 45-degree angle to the end of the blade. The blade is turned at a 90-degree angle to the shank. A pull stroke is used with the hoe. It is most often used on posterior teeth on the buccal and lingual aspects.

Chisel Scalers

The chisel scaler (Figure 45.11) is a push instrument that has a single straight cutting edge with a continuous blade. Due to the design of the chisel, it is more easily adapted to the anterior region than other regions.

File Scalers

The file scaler (Figure 45.12) crushes and breaks down calculus prior to the use of curettes. The file can also be used to remove overhangs from restorations. The file is not recommended for use on root surfaces because its design does not allow for adequate adaptation to the curvature of roots. The file is considered a pull instrument with multiple cutting edges lined up in a series. The blades are at 90-degree angles to the shank. Because of its multiple cutting edges, its tactile sensitivity is decreased.

Curettes

The curette is an instrument that can be used to remove calculus, dental plaque, or biofilm. It is also used to smooth roughened root surfaces. The design of the curette allows for use subgingivally as well as supragingivally. Unlike the scaler, the cutting edges curve to meet at a rounded end called the toe. There are two basic types of curettes: the universal curette and area-specific curette.

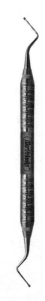

FIGURE 45.12
Hirschfeld file scaler.
Courtesy Hu-Friedy

Universal Curettes

The universal curette (Figure 45.13) can be adapted for use in any area of the mouth. There are two cutting edges per end, and the working ends are usually paired mirror images. The face of the universal curette is perpendicular, or at a 90-degree angle, to the lower shank.

Several types of universal curettes are available. Because of their design, they are good to use for specific amounts of calculus. For example, the thicker the shank, the better this instrument would be for heavy, tenacious calculus removal versus one that has a thin shank, which would be used for removal of less thick and less tenacious deposits of calculus.

Area-Specific Curettes

Area-specific curettes (Figure 45.14) are also known as Gracey curettes. Dr. Clayton H. Gracey created these instruments to allow for easier access to periodontal pockets. The face of the Gracey curette is at a 70-degree angle to the shank, and there is only one cutting edge per end. Each instrument is designed for adaptation to specific areas of the mouth. The original seven consist of the 1/2, 3/4, 5/6, 7/8, 9/10, 11/12, and 13/14. The original seven were first developed by Dr. Gracey. Modifications to these original instruments have been made to give the clinician additional instrument choices.

Extended Shank Gracey Curettes   In addition to the original area-specific curettes, Gracey curettes with extended shanks have been designed for access to pockets greater than 4 mm. These curettes have been modified to have a thinner working end—approximately 10% thinner—than the standard Gracey curette. They also have a lower shank that is 3 mm longer than the standard Gracey curette. These instruments may also be called the "after-five Graceys."

Miniature Gracey Curettes   Miniature Gracey curettes have been designed for easier access to root concavities, anterior roots, furcations, and narrow pockets greater than 4 mm. These instruments have a longer, lower shank and a thinner working end that is half the length of the standard Gracey curette.

Sonic and Ultrasonic Instruments

Sonic and ultrasonic instruments have become increasingly popular over the years. These instruments can remove hard, tenacious deposits of calculus much more quickly than traditional hand instruments. Both devices generate heat, thus they both use water as a cooling mechanism in addition to its use to flush out the pocket.

Sonic scalers attach directly to the high-speed handpiece and vibrate at between 3,000 and 8,000 cycles per second.

Sonic and ultrasonic instruments are used frequently in cases where the patient is sensitive or the patient does not have as much tenacious calculus. Ultrasonic scalers generate vibrations between 20,000 and 50,000 cycles per second. Ultrasonics can be either magnetostrictive or piezoelectric. The conventional tip motion for the magnetostrictive is elliptical, whereas the tip motion for the piezoelectric is linear in pattern. Several tip designs are available (Figure 45.15), such as the straight tip with internal flow water delivery, the beavertail tip for supragingival calculus removal, the thin periodontal tip, and the ball point tip which has an 0.8-mm ball-end for adaptation in the furcations.

Scalpel

The scalpel is used for removal of gingival tissue during periodontal surgery. The surgical scalpel is also known as

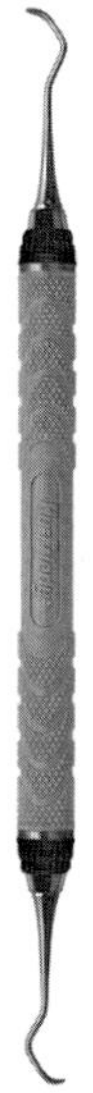

FIGURE 45.13
The Columbia 13/14 is one example of a universal curette.
Courtesy Hu-Friedy

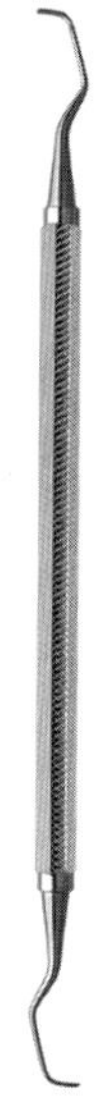

FIGURE 45.14
An area-specific curette.
Courtesy Hu-Friedy

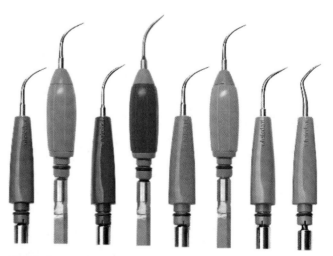

FIGURE 45.15
Ultrasonic inserts.
Courtesy Coltene Whaledent

the Bard-Parker scalpel. The scalpel has a metal handle that can be sterilized and a disposable blade. The blades are available in different sizes and shapes, as shown in Figure 45.16. Completely disposable scalpels can also be purchased. The safety scalpel is an innovative design that comes with a protective sheath that covers the blade, thus reducing the risk of injury from the blade.

Periodontal Knives

Periodontal knives are used to remove gingival tissue during surgery. They are often called gingivectomy knives. There are two commonly used types of knives: Orban and Kirkland knives. Orban knives are interdental knives. They are used for removal of gingival tissue in the interdental area. They are spear shaped and have cutting edges on both sides of the blades. Kirkland knives are the most commonly used knives in periodontal surgery (Figure 45.17). They are shaped like kidneys and are most often double ended.

Which instrument is used to determine if a furcation involvement is present?

Pocket Markers

Pocket markers (Figure 45.18) have pointed tips that are used to make small, minute perforations in the gingival tissue. Pocket markers are similar in appearance to regular cotton pliers.

Hemostats

Hemostats are forceps-style instruments with locking handles that are manipulated with only one hand. They

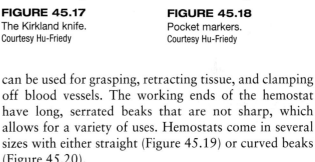

FIGURE 45.17
The Kirkland knife.
Courtesy Hu-Friedy

FIGURE 45.18
Pocket markers.
Courtesy Hu-Friedy

can be used for grasping, retracting tissue, and clamping off blood vessels. The working ends of the hemostat have long, serrated beaks that are not sharp, which allows for a variety of uses. Hemostats come in several sizes with either straight (Figure 45.19) or curved beaks (Figure 45.20).

Tissue Forceps

Tissue forceps (Figure 45.21) are designed like a hemostat. The beaks are curved at right angles to each other, and they are useful for holding tissue in place or for retracting tissue during surgery.

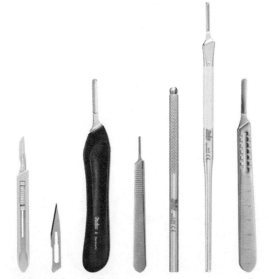

FIGURE 45.16
Various sizes and types of scalpels.
Courtesy Miltex, Inc.

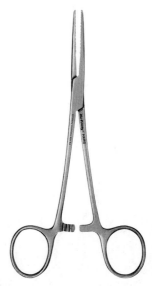

FIGURE 45.19
Straight hemostat.
Courtesy Hu-Friedy

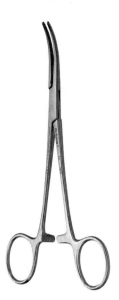

FIGURE 45.20
Curved hemostat.
Courtesy Hu-Friedy

Needle Holders

Needle holders are forceps with straight beaks. The beaks are shorter than those of the hemostat. The holders have several fine serrations with a groove down the center of each beak, which allows for ease of handling the suture needle. The needle holders come in various sizes and shapes (Figures 45.22 and 45.23).

Soft Tissue Rongeurs

Soft tissue rongeurs (Figure 45.24) are hinged-type pliers that can be used to shape the soft tissue and remove bony fragments. These instruments are also commonly referred to as nippers.

Periodontal Scissors

Periodontal scissors (Figures 45.25 and 45.26) are basically used to remove tissue tags or for cutting sutures. The blades are thin and long.

Periosteal Elevators

Periosteal elevators (Figures 45.27 and 45.28) are double ended with a round, bladed end and a long, tapered end. They are used to retract the soft tissue away from the bone during periodontal surgery.

Nonsurgical Periodontal Treatment

The goal of nonsurgical periodontal treatment (NSPT) is to return the gingival tissues to a healthy state that can be maintained by the clinician and the patient. To do so, systemic risk factors must be reduced, local risk factors for periodontal disease eliminated, and the bacterial load controlled.

To reduce the systematic factors associated with periodontal disease, the patient's medical history should be

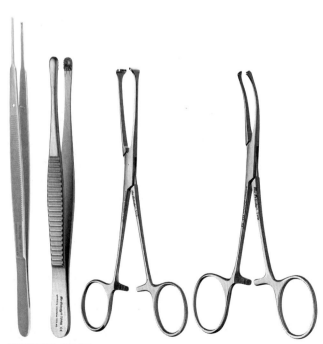

FIGURE 45.21
Several different sizes and types of tissue forceps.
Courtesy Hu-Friedy

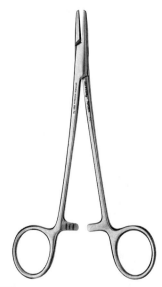

FIGURE 45.22
Grooved needle holder.
Courtesy Hu-Friedy

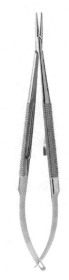

FIGURE 45.23
Micro straight needle holder.
Courtesy Hu-Friedy

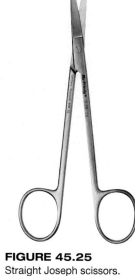

FIGURE 45.25
Straight Joseph scissors.
Courtesy Hu-Friedy

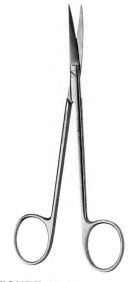

FIGURE 45.26
Curved Joseph scissors.
Courtesy Hu-Friedy

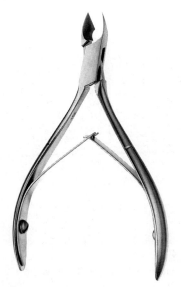

FIGURE 45.24
Soft tissue rongeurs or nippers.
Courtesy Hu-Friedy

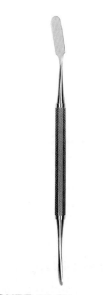

FIGURE 45.27
Prichard periosteal elevator.
Courtesy Hu-Friedy

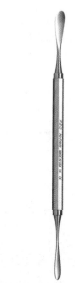

FIGURE 45.28
Benque periosteal elevator.
Courtesy Hu-Friedy

thoroughly evaluated. Any patient with a family history of diabetes should be referred to his or her family physician to determine if the patient has this condition. In addition, any patient who smokes should receive tobacco cessation counseling because smoking is a risk factor for periodontal disease. Other risk factors include any disease affecting the immune system and nutritional deficiencies.

Local risk factors can also include faulty or defective restorations. This can lead to retention of plaque over time, which then contributes to the damage of the periodontium. Any local risk factors should be eliminated accordingly.

The control of the bacterial load involves both the patient and the clinician. First, an appropriate oral health care regimen should be developed, and it should be

patient specific for each patient's condition and abilities. For instance, if the patient has limited dexterity, flossing may not be an option. The use of other interdental aids such as an electric toothbrush may be more beneficial to this particular patient. After developing an individual oral health care routine, the patient must receive professional treatment for the removal of calculus and bacterial by-products. If not thoroughly removed, the inflammatory process will continue.

Nonsurgical periodontal treatment is usually achieved through the use of both ultrasonic instrumentation and hand instrumentation. Multiple appointments may be necessary in which the clinician completes **periodontal debridement** by quadrants or sextants. A full-mouth debridement is classified as one that is completed in one or two appointments within a 24-hour time span. Following the procedure, a reevaluation appointment should be made after four weeks have passed to assess tissue response. Nonresponsive sites may show signs of inflammation and bleeding upon probing. These sites should be instrumented again using an ultrasonic instrument for plaque removal. After this additional instrumentation, these sites should be reassessed.

Upon completion of mechanical debridement and evaluation, additional therapy options may be warranted. Professional subgingival irrigation with an antimicrobial agent may be performed. However, studies have shown that this method has only a limited benefit, if any, over instrumentation alone. The use of a controlled-release, local delivery system for antibiotics or antimicrobials may also be recommended. Such systems place the agent in the periodontal pocket and gradually release it over several days. The agents used include:

- *Actisite*, a tetracycline hydrochloride fiber produced by Alza Pharmaceuticals.
- *PerioChip*, a chlorhexidine gluconate chip produced by Perio Products, Ltd.
- *Arestin*, a minocycline HCl powered microsphere produced by OraPharma, Inc.
- *Atridox*, a doxycycline hyclate gel produced by Atrix Laboratories.

Most of these products are biodegradable, with the exception of the Actisite fiber. Patients must return to the office after 10 days to have the Actisite fiber removed. Current research has shown only a small increase in attachment following the use of such products. (Refer to Chapter 14 on periodontal disease and attachment loss.)

Surgical Periodontal Treatment

As the periodontal condition worsens, the need for periodontal surgery increases. It is essential that all members of the dental team have a basic understanding of the indications for periodontal surgery, treatment options and the benefits of each type of treatment, and the risks involved with treating or not treating the condition. Depending on the type of treatment, risks of treatment may include additional sensitivity to cold due to increased root exposure, postoperative discomfort, swelling, and the appearance of longer teeth. If the option of no treatment is chosen, then the periodontal condition could worsen.

Procedures for Treatment of Mucogingival Defects

Treatment for mucogingival defects involves surgery that may increase the width of attached gingiva, eliminate frenum pulls, and cover exposed roots. This type of surgery is often referred to as periodontal plastic surgery.

Free Gingival Grafts

A free gingival graft is often performed in areas where there is insufficient or inadequate attached gingiva and/or recession (Figures 45.29 and 45.30). The donor tissue is taken from the hard palate and includes both surface epithelium and the underlying connective tissue. It is then sutured into the prepared receptor site. This procedure helps to thicken the attached gingiva. It is essential that the surgery site not be disturbed during the healing process.

Connective Tissue Grafts

Like a free gingival graft, a connective tissue graft also involves harvesting connective tissue from the palate, but a connective tissue graft usually results in a more natural color of the graft. The donor graft is placed under a small flap at the receptor site. As with free gingival grafts, it is essential that the surgery site not be disturbed during the healing process.

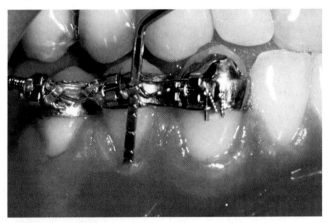

FIGURE 45.29
Chronic inflammation of the gingiva because there is not enough attached gingiva.
Image courtesy Instructional Materials for the Dental Team, Lex., KY

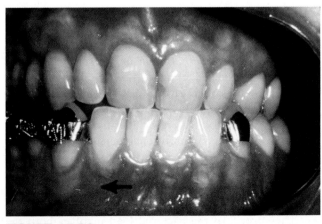

FIGURE 45.30
Area where gingiva has been attached.
Image courtesy Instructional Materials for the Dental Team, Lex., KY

Allografts

The use of allografts is becoming increasingly popular. An allograft is a graft that comes from a donated source. The graft material is processed and decellularized to extract any living cells. The manufacturers of allografts carefully screen all donors and are guided by government guidelines that scrutinize any type of transplant.

The advantage to this type of surgery is that a second surgery site is not required. The disadvantages include the fact that the graft does come from another human which could mean a greater chance of rejection, it is more costly, and it is more tedious for the periodontist to perform than the traditional connective tissue graft.

Frenectomy

A **frenectomy** is the surgical removal of the frenum including the attachment to the underlying bone. A triangular section is excised along with the frenum. A maxillary labial frenectomy is often indicated when the dentist feels that a diastema is too large interproximally between teeth #8 and #9 and the frenum is very close to the marginal gingiva. A lingual frenectomy is performed when the patient has a condition known as ankyloglossia (meaning "tongue tied") in which the lingual frenum is too close to the tip of the tongue. This can impede speech development and needs to be corrected.

Procedures for Gaining Access

Periodontal access surgery allows for access to the root for a more thorough debridement and to establish an environment for gingival tissue to reattach to the root surface. This type of surgery is also known as periodontal flap surgery or flap surgery. The access procedures used are the open-flap curettage, the modified Widman flap, and the excisional new attachment procedure. All three procedures are similar with only subtle differences in technique. However, it should be noted that the American Academy of Periodontology no longer recommends the use of the curettage procedure and instead emphasizes the use of the other two.

The modified Widman flap incorporates three incisions to separate the pocket lining from the tooth. The tissue is moved to allow access and then returned to its original position and sutured. The excisional new attachment procedure (ENAP) does not include elevating the flap past the mucogingival junction.

Procedures for Removing or Reshaping the Gingiva

This type of surgery is considered excisional because tissue is removed from the pocket. The two types of excisional periodontal surgeries include the gingivectomy and the gingivoplasty.

A **gingivectomy** is the surgical removal of gingival tissue. In the past, the gingivectomy was used as a treatment for patients with periodontitis. Today, the gingivectomy is limited to those cases in which gingival enlargement is present due to the use of certain medications, such as phenytoin, cyclosporine, and calcium channel blockers. The tissue is marked using pocket markers and then excised away to allow for easier access for the patient and to improve aesthetics. Note that as long as the patient continues on these medications, which often must be the case, there is the potential for the gingival tissue to become enlarged again. Often, patients may require an additional gingivectomy procedure at a later date.

A **gingivoplasty** is the surgical reshaping of the gingival tissue. This surgery is often performed to correct small craters or clefts and is usually only performed in localized areas. At times, the gingivoplasty may be performed following a gingivectomy.

Procedures for Treatment of Osseous Defects

Periodontal infection can result in changes in the architecture of the bone. Surgery may be required in an attempt to correct these changes. Surgery for the treatment of osseous defects includes ostectomy and osteoplasty. The ostectomy removes alveolar bone along with periodontal fibers that support the tooth. The osteoplasty removes only nonsupporting bone or bony ledges. As with other types of periodontal surgery, these two procedures are often performed in conjunction with one another. Once the flaps are elevated, chisels and burs are used to modify the bone to establish an alveolar form that provides a physiologic outline for the gingival tissue to follow. This new outline establishes the anatomic shape, which is free from bone ledges or craters. Hopefully, there is a minute loss of the bony attachment during surgery.

Procedures for Regeneration of the Periodontium

Periodontal regeneration surgery attempts to restore periodontal tissues that have been lost due to periodontal disease. By performing these surgical procedures, the periodontist attempts to stimulate the development of new alveolar bone, new cementum, and new periodontal ligament on the root. The two types of surgeries include bone grafting and guided tissue regeneration.

Periodontal bone grafting involves the placement of bone in an area in an attempt to encourage the body to rebuild alveolar bone. This type of surgery can be further categorized based on the source of the graft material.

The autograft is a surgical procedure in which bone is harvested from the body of the patient. The bone can be taken from the patient's jaw, tori, or the maxillary tuberosity. In addition, bone can be taken extraorally from such sites as the sternum or the iliac crest. Often, this type of bone is used in an attempt to ensure biocompatibility.

The allograft is one in which the bone comes from cadavers. Bone banks provide this type of bone. Cadaver bone is the most commonly used allograft material. The bone is freeze dried and demineralized with a solution of hydrochloric acid. This process helps reduce the risk of any type of transmission of disease.

A xenograft is a graft in which the graft material is taken from another species. Typically this bone comes from bovines (cows) or porcines (pigs). The bone is treated; however, a high risk remains that an antigenic reaction will occur with use of this material.

An alloplast is a synthetic bone material made from ceramics or hydroxyapatite mineral. Research suggests that this type of material serves better as a filler rather than for bone regeneration.

Guided tissue regeneration is still considered a relatively innovative concept in periodontal surgery. This technique suggests that improved and more effective healing occurs by allowing selected cells to grow and by excluding certain cells. Polylactic acid with citric acid ester membranes and polytetrafluoroethylene (Gore-Tex) membrane are examples of such barrier membranes. This type of surgery is indicated in areas of infrabony defects and furcations. *Infrabony* means that the junctional epithelium forming the base is located apical, or toward, the root apex, to the crest of the alveolar bone. With guided tissue regeneration, healing cells are encouraged to reproduce from the periodontal ligament and bone, not the epithelium. Note that the manufacturers of such barriers do not recommend the use of these barriers in patients who are smokers due to a less predictable response.

Crown Lengthening Surgery

Crown lengthening surgery or crown extension surgery is performed when a fixed prosthesis such as a crown, bridge or even a veneer needs to be placed (Figures 45.31, 45.32, and 45.33). Some of the gingiva and alveolar bone is removed from the neck of the tooth to make the crown longer. This may be indicated in cases where the crown

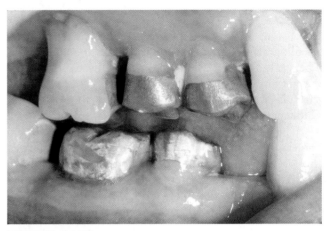

FIGURE 45.31
Before a crown lengthening procedure. The procedure must be done to provide enough tooth structure above the gum line to support a crown.
Image courtesy Instructional Materials for the Dental Team, Lex., KY

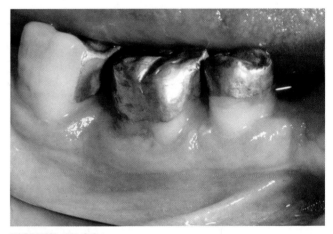

FIGURE 45.32
Picture of teeth following a crown lengthening surgery.
Image courtesy Instructional Materials for the Dental Team, Lex., KY

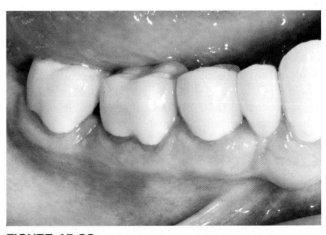

FIGURE 45.33
Mandibular quadrant with crown following crown placement.
Image courtesy Instructional Materials for the Dental Team, Lex., KY

has become fractured or damaged due to extensive caries. This type of surgery may be indicated in a healthy periodontium and involves the creation of an apically positioned flap with osseous surgery.

Periodontal Dressing Materials

A periodontal dressing serves as a protector for gingival and periodontal tissues following periodontal surgery. Several types of dressing materials are available. The most commonly used dressing materials include self-cured dressings or light-cured dressings. The self-cured dressing is one in which two materials come packaged separately in two tubes. The materials are then dispensed in a strip similar to toothpaste. The two strips are mixed together and applied to the site.

The advantage of the light-cured system is that it allows for more working time for the dental assistant. The dressing is applied only in the area needed in a small ribbon. The material is then lightly pressed into the embrasures to ensure that it is retained.

Prior to placement of either type of dressing, bleeding at the surgical site should be controlled. Postoperative instructions should be given to the patient both verbally and in writing. An emergency contact number should also be given prior to the departure of the patient.

Approximately one week postoperatively, the patient returns to the clinic for a follow-up appointment. At this time, if the periodontal dressing has not been dislodged and removed by the patient, the assistant may be required to remove the dressing. (Dental assistants should check their state dental practice laws to understand what procedures can be legally performed.) The dressing material, by this time, has hardened significantly and is easily dislodged using the end of a curette or spoon evacuator. Once slightly dislodged, cotton pliers can be used to capture the material and completely remove it from the patient's mouth.

Lasers in Periodontics

The use of lasers was first introduced in dentistry in the latter portion of the 20th century. Since that time, they have been increasingly used for a variety of purposes. Presently, the Food and Drug Administration has approved lasers for gingival curettage, diagnosis of pit and fissure caries, caries removal, soft tissue excision and incision, and cavity preps. In periodontal practices, lasers have been used for periodontal surgery, enhanced root instrumentation, removal of calculus, and to reduce subgingival bacteria.

Each type of laser differs in wavelength and waveform, and anyone planning on incorporating lasers into practice needs to have extensive training prior to use. The most frequently used lasers in periodontics are the Nd:YAG, diode, erbium, and carbon dioxide lasers.

Cultural Considerations

Patients often do not understand the rationale of investing money in the treatment of a disease that for the most part may be pain free. This is often the case for individuals who grew up in particular cultures or locations in which it was automatically assumed that losing one's teeth as an adult is a normal part of life. By explaining periodontal treatment to patients, the dental assistant can encourage patients to maintain their oral health and potentially save their teeth for the entirety of their adulthood.

Advantages of Laser Surgery

The most frequently touted benefits or advantages of laser surgery over traditional surgery include the following:

- The control of bleeding, or hemostasis, is extremely fast.
- Postoperative swelling, pain, and trauma to surrounding tissues are reduced compared to traditional surgery.
- The surgical field is dry.
- The possibility of bloodborne contamination is reduced.
- Various procedures can be completed in less time.

Note, however, that current literature does not support any claims of superior results following laser treatment. Because no science-based evidence or critical review of the literature has been provided, the American Academy of Periodontology at the time of this writing does not recommend laser treatment over the conventional periodontal therapy. Instead, laser treatment should be used as an adjunct to conventional periodontal therapy.

Laser Safety

Laser safety is of ultimate concern for both the patient and the entire dental staff. Appropriate training is strongly recommended for anyone operating this type of equipment. Note, too, that lasers differ based on the manufacturer, so it is essential that the staff be trained on a particular laser based on its manufacturer's recommendations.

The office should designate one individual to serve in the capacity of laser safety officer (LSO). A well-trained dental assistant can serve in the capacity of LSO. The LSO should be fully and completely trained in all laser systems used in the office. The LSO should also recommend the use of any personal protective equipment, ensure the posting of appropriate warning signs, follow maintenance and calibration procedures, supervise staff who work with the laser equipment, and document and report any incidents.

Some key elements must be considered as basic guidelines to follow when using lasers:

- Both the dental staff and the patient should wear safety glasses with side shields during the procedure.
- Surrounding tissues that are not to be treated should be protected with wet gauze packs.
- A high-volume evacuator should be used to draw off the plume as the tissue vaporizes.
- Matte-finished instruments, instead of glossy ones, should be used to ensure that the laser's light is not reflected.

Preparing for Externship

In preparing for your externship, you should be familiar with periodontal terminology and surgical procedures. In addition, you should be able to accurately identify all instruments used in periodontal procedures and know their uses. If needed, you can prepare 3 × 5 flash cards with terms, surgical procedures, and pictures of instruments so you can quiz yourself prior to your externship.

● SUMMARY

Periodontics is the dental specialty that deals with the prevention, diagnosis, and treatment of diseases and conditions of the structures that surround and support the tooth. The general dentist may initially treat patients with a periodontal condition if the condition is mild and maintainable. If the condition is advanced, the general dentist may refer the patient to a periodontist if the dentist feels that the patient needs additional measures or that

the patient can no longer be maintained appropriately in his or her clinic or office. By understanding the components of the periodontal evaluation, the numerous instruments utilized in periodontal treatment and diagnosis, the rationale for nonsurgical periodontal treatment, and the surgical options available to the patient, the dental assistant will be a valuable resource for the patient.

● KEY TERMS

- **Biofilm:** Consists of many types of bacteria and other organisms that form an organized colony that adheres to surfaces; previously called *dental plaque.* p. 701
- **Calculus:** Plaque that has hardened or calcified; commonly referred to as tartar. p. 701
- **Exudate:** A fluid-type substance that forms as a result of the inflammatory process; the fluid contains bacteria, leukocytes or white blood cells, dead cells, degenerated tissues, and tissue fluid. p. 702
- **Frenectomy:** Surgical removal of the frenum. p. 711
- **Furcation involvement:** Loss of interradicular bone between multirooted teeth as a result of periodontal infection. p. 702
- **Gingivectomy:** Surgical excision of the gingiva. p. 711
- **Gingivoplasty:** Surgical reshaping of the gingival tissue. p. 711
- **Periodontal debridement:** The removal of calculus, plaque, and its by-products from the coronal and root

surfaces and tissue wall and pocket to promote healing. p. 709
- **Periodontal pocket:** A sulcus that has deepened beyond three millimeters due to some type of pathology. p. 701
- **Periodontal probe:** An instrument that is demarcated at specific units of measurement and is used to determine the depth of the periodontal sulcus or pocket. p. 703
- **Periodontitis:** Inflammation of the periodontium. p. 702
- **Recession:** Apical migration of the gingival margin leading to exposure of the cementoenamel junction. p. 702
- **Scaling:** The removal of biofilm, calculus, and stains from the crowns and roots of teeth. p. 704

● CHECK YOUR UNDERSTANDING

1. A patient is preparing to undergo orthodontic treatment. The orthodontist has referred the patient to the periodontist first for an evaluation of tooth #22. There is 2 mm of recession, a 2-mm pocket depth on the facial aspect, and an inadequate amount of attached gingiva. The procedure of choice for this area will be
   a. crown lengthening surgery.
   b. flap curettage.
   c. gingivectomy.
   d. free gingival graft.
   e. pocket elimination surgery.

2. A patient fractured tooth #3 and the dentist wishes to do a crown. However, the remaining part of the crown is insufficient for a crown prep, so the patient was referred to a periodontist for treatment. The procedure that the dentist wants the periodontist to perform is most likely
   a. pocket reduction surgery.
   b. connective tissue graft.
   c. crown lengthening surgery.
   d. free gingival graft.
   e. pocket regeneration surgery.

3. A patient presents with severe periodontal disease, radiographic bone loss, and light to moderate subgingival calculus. The periodontist has already used an ultrasonic device and now needs additional instruments. The instrument of choice will be
   a. sickle scalers.
   b. file scalers.
   c. area-specific curettes.
   d. a periodontal probe.
   e. a Naber's probe.

4. The instrument of choice in assessing the presence of subgingival calculus, faulty restorations, and root irregularities is the
   a. tissue forceps.
   b. hemostat.
   c. explorers.
   d. soft tissue rongeurs.
   e. Naber's probe.

5. A patient has been taking the medication Dilantin which is known to cause gingival enlargement (overgrowth or hyperplasia). In order for the patient to do an adequate job with home care, the surgical procedure most likely to be recommended will be

   a. a gingivectomy.
   b. a frenectomy.
   c. a free gingival graft.
   d. a connective tissue graft.
   e. osseous surgery.

6. A patient is preparing for orthodontic treatment and is referred to a periodontist for an evaluation. There is a diastema present between teeth #8 and #9. It is also noted that the maxillary labial frenum is relatively low on the gingival margin. The treatment of choice will be
   a. a connective tissue graft.
   b. scaling.
   c. a frenectomy.
   d. a gingivoplasty.
   e. none of the above.

7. A patient presents with heavy supragingival and subgingival calculus. The first instrument to be used in the treatment aspect will most likely be
   a. ultrasonic instruments.
   b. sickle scalers.
   c. extended shank Gracey curettes.
   d. a hemostat.
   e. periodontal scissors.

8. An instrument that can be used throughout the mouth, both supragingivally and subgingivally, for calculus removal and debridement is
   a. a periosteal elevator.
   b. a universal curette.
   c. a sickle scaler.
   d. soft tissue rongeurs.
   e. needle holders.

9. The instrument of choice for measuring periodontal pockets, gingival recession, and the width of attached gingiva is the
   a. scalpel.
   b. explorer.
   c. universal curette.
   d. hemostat.
   e. periodontal probe.

10. When a patient loses the bone between the roots of multirooted teeth, this is called
    a. furcation involvement.
    b. mobility.
    c. gingivitis.
    d. gingivectomy.
    e. suppuration.

INTERNET ACTIVITY

- As a dental assistant, you should be prepared for questions involving periodontal surgery. With the Internet, patients are becoming more educated about oral health topics. To better prepare for any potential questions, go to www.perio.org and download, review, and utilize the information provided under "Periodontal Procedures."

WEB REFERENCES

- American Academy of Periodontology   www.perio.org
- American Dental Association   www.ada.org
- American Dental Hygienists' Association   www.adha.org
- British Dental Association   www.BDA-dentistry.org.uk
- Medline Plus   www.nlm.nih.gov/medlineplus/gumdisease.html

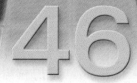

46

Oral Surgery Procedures

Learning Objectives

After reading this chapter, the student should be able to:

- Describe the specialty of oral and maxillofacial surgery.
- Explain certain medical conditions that may compromise a patient's well-being during surgery.
- Identify the various surgical instruments and tray setups and describe their functions.
- Demonstrate aseptic procedures followed in an oral surgery office.
- Explain various oral surgical procedures.
- Explain the function of sutures and demonstrate suture removal.
- Demonstrate the preparation and dismissal of the patient before and after surgical treatment including pre- and postoperative instructions.
- Describe possible postsurgical complications.

Preparing for Certification Exams

- Demonstrate tray setups for extractions and impactions.
- Demonstrate tray setups for incision and drainage.
- Demonstrate tray setups for oral examination.
- Demonstrate tray setups for suture placement and removal.
- Demonstrate tray setups for treatment of dry socket.
- Demonstrate assisting with extractions and impactions using four-handed dentistry.
- Demonstrate assisting with postoperative treatment and complications.
- Demonstrate assisting with suture placement and removal.
- Prepare, mix, and store postextraction dressings.
- Demonstrate providing patient with oral and written pre- and post-treatment instructions.

Key Terms

Alveolitis
Ankyloglossia
Crepitus
Diastema

Exodontia
Luxate
Malady
Malignant

Chapter Outline

- Indications for Oral and Maxillofacial Surgery
- The Oral Surgeon
- The Dental Surgical Assistant
  —Ethical and Legal Ramifications
- The Surgical Setting
- Specialized instruments and Accessories
  —Bone Files
  —Dressing Pliers
  —Elevators
  —Forceps
  —Hemostats and Needle Holders
  —Mouth Props and Mouth Gags
  —Operating Lights
  —Retractors
  —Rongeurs
  —Scalpels/Surgical Blades and Blade Removal Device
  —Scissors
  —Surgical Aspirators
  —Surgical Burs and Handpieces
  —Surgical Chisels and Mallet
  —Surgical Curettes
  —Surgical Preset Trays
  —Suture Needles and Materials
- Surgical Asepsis
  —Care and Sterilization of Surgical Instruments
  —Surgical Attire, Scrub, and Hand Washing
- Surgical Preparation
  —Medical and Dental History
  —Intraoral and Extraoral Examination
  —Vital Signs
  —Radiographs
  —Preoperative Instructions
  —Informed Consent
  —Patient Preparation
  —Pain Control in Oral Surgery

- Surgical Procedures
  —Alveolectomy and Alveoloplasty
  —Arthrotomy
  —Biopsy
  —Cleft Lip, Palate, and Tongue
  —Cyst Removal
  —Drainage of Facial Infections
  —Exodontia
  —Exostosis
  —Fractures
  —Frenectomy
  —Genioplasty
  —Gingivectomy and Gingivoplastomy
  —Implantology
  —Oral Pathology and Tumors
  —Periodontal Flap Surgery
  —Surgical Endodontics
  —Surgical Orthodontics
- Sutures
  —Types of Sutures
  —Instruments for Sutures
  —Suture Removal
  —Postoperative Instructions for Sutures
- Instructions for Patient Care
  —Preoperative Instructions
  —Postoperative Instructions
- Postsurgical Complications

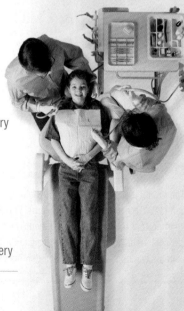

Oral and maxillofacial surgery is a specialty of dentistry that involves the diagnosis and treatment of diseases, injuries, and defects of the hard and soft tissues of the oral and maxillofacial region. The Egyptians are believed to have been the pioneers of oral surgery (1600 or 1700 BCE) followed by the Greeks. Hippocrates (460 BCE) described the treatment of jaw fractures and advised the removal of decayed teeth. Al-Zahrawi (936–1013 CE), or Albucasis, is famous for his 30-volume medical encyclopedia *Al-Tasrif li man ajaz an-il-talif* (English translation: "An aid to him who lacks the capacity to read big books"). He mentions the problem of non-aligned or deformed teeth and procedures to rectify these defects. He also discusses the procedure for preparing and setting artificial teeth made from animal bones. French surgeon Ambroise Paré (1510–1590) described the methods of transplanting and implanting teeth and also described obturators for cleft or perforated palates, extracted teeth, drained dental abscesses, and set jaw fractures.

In April 1947, the American Board of Oral Surgery was approved by the Council on Dental Education of the American Dental Association and authorized to proceed in the certification of specialists in oral surgery. Certified oral and maxillofacial surgery assistant (COMSA) is a Dental Assisting National Board recognized

title for dental assistants with specialized training in oral surgery.

Indications for Oral and Maxillofacial Surgery

Patients may need oral and/or maxillofacial surgery for various reasons:

- They have decayed or nonvital teeth that cannot be restored and need extraction.
- The removal of impacted teeth and fractured or retained root fragments is necessary.
- Certain pre-prosthesis procedures, such as removal or shaping of overgrown soft and hard tissues, or extraction to aid in orthodontic treatment are necessary.
- They have cysts and tumors (either part of the lesion or the entire lesion along with some normal tissues) that must be removed for microscopic studies.
- A surgical incision must be made to drain oral infections so that the infection does not spread to any of the vital organs via the bloodstream.
- They have snoring or sleep apnea issues that are addressed by adjusting the posterior palatine muscles.
- To stabilize fractured bones in the maxillofacial area, either by using intermaxillary fixation wiring or bone plating.
- A child born with a cleft lip and palate or someone who has experienced a trauma or accident resulting in facial deformity can benefit from surgery. Certain specialized reconstructive and cosmetic surgeries can be done to repair the deformity.
- Surgery is needed in the temporomandibular joint (TMJ) area to address continuous stress or trauma to the TMJ area. If left untreated this can result in crepitus. **Crepitus** is a medical term that describes the grating, crackling, or popping sounds and sensations experienced under the skin and joints.
- The presence of stone(s) in the salivary glands, or sialolithiasis, which can cause pain and infection, can be addressed through surgery.
- Missing teeth are needing to be replaced with the use of implants.

The Oral Surgeon

An oral surgeon is a specialist who treats the anatomic area of the mouth, jaws, face, and their associated structures. Oral surgeons, after receiving a four-year doctor of dental surgery (D.D.S.), doctor of dental medicine (D.M.D.), or bachelor's of dental surgery (B.D.S.) degree in dentistry, continue their education and complete an additional four to six years of specialty training. (*Note:* The D.D.S. and D.M.D. degrees are the same degree

Dental Assistant PROFESSIONAL TIP

The mouth is a doorway to overall health. Neglecting one's oral health can result in general health problems. The dental assistant often has an important relationship with patients and may be able to affect patients' behavior. If the dental assistant exhibits good oral hygiene, patients will be encouraged to model this behavior.

approved by the Commission on Dental Accreditation (CODA) in the United States, whereas the B.D.S. is equivalent to the D.D.S. and D.M.D. in Europe and many countries in the Eastern part of the world.)

Some residency programs integrate a medical education as well and confer an appropriate medical degree (M.D.). The American Board of Oral and Maxillofacial Surgeons (ABOMS) is the certifying board for the specialty of oral and maxillofacial surgery in the United States. This board conducts certification examinations for the certification of specialists in oral surgery. After completion of their main degrees, one- or two-year fellowships can be taken to expand the scope of practice to areas such as head and neck cancer, cosmetics, or craniomaxillofacial surgery.

The Dental Surgical Assistant

The dental surgical assistant performs many specialized tasks requiring both interpersonal and advanced technical skills: (1) pre- and postsurgical patient assessment and monitoring, (2) use of specialized surgical instruments, (3) assisting with surgical procedures, (4) performing surgical asepsis and scrub, (5) assisting with pain control techniques, and (6) delivery of pre- and postsurgical instructions.

Dental assistants who choose to become surgical assistants do so by completing a specialized surgical assistant academic program or by obtaining on-the-job training. Advanced credentials for being a surgical assistant can be obtained through any recognized agency, such as the Dental Assisting National Board (DANB). However, effective January 1, 2000, the COMSA examination was discontinued due to low participation. Current COMSAs can continue to renew their credentials annually. The American Association of Oral and Maxillofacial Surgeons (AAOMS) offers several advanced training and certification programs. The surgical assistant may also need certification in advanced life support and/or intravenous (IV) administration.

How can an oral surgery assistant eliminate any risk factors leading to a lawsuit in a surgical office?

Ethical and Legal Ramifications

As with any dental procedure, it is important to ensure that the members of the dental team are well trained and qualified to provide quality patient care. In the practice of maxillofacial surgery, there is much the dentist and the dental team members can do to reduce legal vulnerability. Sound office practice management procedures may contribute significantly to minimizing legal risks. Clear communication is another important tool in managing almost all kinds of risks. Therefore, before starting any surgical procedure, the oral surgeon must explain the entire procedure to the patient. This should be done orally and in writing. The surgeon should also ensure that all questions are answered to the level of the patient's understanding. This helps prevent a situation later in which the patient might ask "Why didn't you tell me this before?"

It is the responsibility of the surgical assistant to make sure that all consent forms are signed by the patient, in front of a witness, and countersigned by the oral surgeon with all current dates indicated. During or immediately after the procedure, all details related to the procedure should be documented. Medication given and the status of the patient before, during, and after the surgery should be noted. The surgical assistant must make sure that a family member or friend is available to take the patient home after the surgical procedure has been performed. Postsurgical instructions must be given to the patient, both orally and in writing. It is also beneficial to explain the postsurgical instructions to the family member or the escorting friend, because they can help the patient at home with follow-up on instructions. All questions the patient has should be answered prior to the patient leaving the office.

The Surgical Setting

Dental surgical procedures can be completed in a private dental office or in a hospital operating room. Most dental surgical procedures are performed in surgical suites found in oral surgeons' offices. These suites are similar to, but smaller in size than hospital operating rooms. Any outpatient dental surgical procedure can safely and efficiently be performed in an office setting as long as the necessary equipment, supplies, and trained staff are available.

By performing dental surgeries in the dental office, the high costs and the inconvenience of hospitalization can be avoided. When an oral surgical procedure is to be performed in a hospital setting, the maxillofacial surgeon and the surgical assistant must be preapproved by the hospital administration to use the hospital facilities. This approval is based on the individual's credentials to practice oral surgery procedures. Other specialists who may be part of the oral surgery team include a general surgeon, a cosmetic surgeon, an implantologist, and an oncologist.

Specialized Instruments and Accessories

Surgical instruments are designed to apply adequate pressure in specific areas to loosen, retract, and remove bone, soft tissues, or teeth. They are made from stainless steel and can be reused after sterilization or they are disposable. A surgical assistant must have thorough knowledge of all dental surgical instruments and their functions and must also know how to sterilize, organize, and transfer them. All dental surgical instruments are classified as critical instruments and must be thoroughly cleaned and sterilized after each use (unless they are the disposable type).

Bone Files

One type of specialized surgical equipment is a bone file (Figure 46.1). A bone file is usually a double-ended instrument with a rounded working end with serrations.

It is used in a back-and-forth motion to trim and smooth the bone after a tooth has been extracted.

Dressing Pliers

Dressing pliers (Figure 46.2) are tweezers of various sizes and designs with pointed beaks. The handle or working end of the instrument has serrations for good grip. Some dressing pliers have locks that prevent slippage of the gripped items.

Elevators

Elevators are surgical instruments used to raise a tooth from its socket. Various types of elevators can be used in dental surgery. The most commonly used elevators are straight elevators. A straight elevator has a handle, a straight shaft, and a rounded, scoop-shaped tip. The tip is used to create space between the bone and the root. It may have serrations to aid in the removal of root fragments, and a flat back to gain leverage. Straight elevators are available in small and large sizes. Periosteal elevators are one type (Figure 46.3). These are mainly used to lift full-thickness soft tissue flaps or loosen the periosteum tissue from bone. The tips require protection and need to be kept very sharp, otherwise shredding of the flap can occur. The most common types in use are the double-ended type. Other available types include the periosteotome, Fedi, and Ochsenbein chisels.

Exolever elevators are used to elevate or **luxate** the tooth from its natural socket (Figure 46.4). The tips of these instruments are designed to be used in a mesial or distal, and maxillary or mandibular area. The handles of exolever elevators can be either the grasp type or T-handled for extra leverage. Exolever elevators are commonly known as root tip elevators.

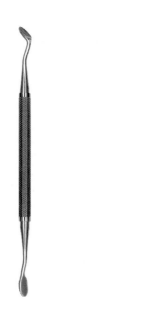

FIGURE 46.1
A bone file.
Courtesy Hu-Friedy

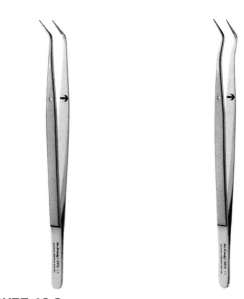

FIGURE 46.2
Dressing pliers: College dressing pliers and dressing pliers.
Courtesy Hu-Friedy

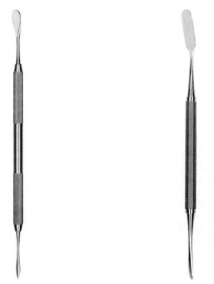

FIGURE 46.3
Periosteal elevators: Kramer-Nevis periosteal and Prichard periosteal.
Courtesy Hu-Friedy

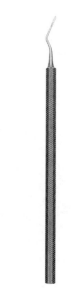

FIGURE 46.5
A root tip pick.
Courtesy Hu-Friedy

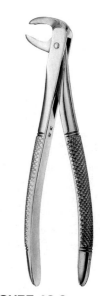

FIGURE 46.6
Dental forceps.
Courtesy Hu-Friedy

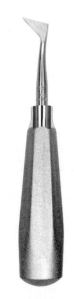

FIGURE 46.4
A Cryer elevator.
Courtesy Hu-Friedy

Apical elevators are used to loosen and elevate the broken parts of the roots. These elevators are designed with thinner handles and longer shanked tips than normal elevators. These are also known as root tip picks (Figure 46.5).

Forceps

Forceps (Figure 46.6) are another important instrument used during oral surgery. These instruments have a handle, a neck, and a nib or beak. The beaks of tooth-extracting forceps are designed to grasp the tooth with maximum contact on the facial-lingual surface of the root(s) just below the cervix. The inner surface of each of the two beaks is concave and the outer surface is convex.

Forceps types can be remembered by either the number indicated on the instrument or by identifying the forceps by shape. Most forceps are designed as right- or left-sided pairs and are numbered with an R (right) or L (left), such as 53R or 53L forceps. Universal forceps are designed to be used on both the left and right sides.

The shape of the forceps is designed to accommodate various teeth anatomy such as the maxillary or mandibular area, right or left, anterior or posterior. The curve of the shank of the forceps identifies its use for either upper or lower teeth. Both beaks of maxillary forceps are usually angled away from the curvature of the handles. These varying angles make it easier to reach various parts of the arch so that the tip of the beak can fit into the trifurcation of the maxillary molar tooth. Furcation is the area of the tooth where roots are dividing into two (bifurcation) or three (trifurcation). The beaks of mandibular forceps are usually at a very sharp angle or almost at a right angle to the shank, and in the same direction as the curvature of the handles. This makes it easier to reach different parts of the mandibular arch. The overall shape of the forceps, from the beak to the handle, can usually provide quick identification of the arch for which it is designed. The S-, I-, and Z-shaped forceps are used on the maxillary arch. Forceps that are C and L shaped are used on the mandibular arch.

The width of forceps is wide or narrow to fit the anterior or posterior teeth. For example, forceps #17 has a wider beak than #171. "Cow horn" forceps are one of the special kinds of forceps designed with pointed beaks to fit into the furcation of molar roots. Forceps are often selected based on the dentist's personal preference.

New dental forceps that are designed based on physics are now available. These forceps apply pressure to a cushioned side that rests around the tooth by removing the tooth from a patient's gingiva and bone. The forceps comes with first and second pivotally connected handles, including a user grasping portion. The end of the first handle ends in an arcuately (meaning "in the form of a bow") extending tooth extracting beak. The second handle of the forceps provides an opposing and offset support by exhibiting a support surface with an ergonomic configuration that is comparable to the patient's gingiva. The handles are subsequently rotated in an outward fashion away from the patient's gingiva to forcibly dislodge the tooth from the patient's gingiva and bone. This reduces the patient's anxiety during extraction by eliminating the extraction sound and also eliminating the need for an elevator prior to the extraction.

Hemostats and Needle Holders

Hemostats and needle holders (Figure 46.7) are used frequently in dental surgery. These instruments look much like scissors with locking joints and serrated beaks. Hemostats have long beaks in various straight or curved lengths. They can be used as a type of clamp or as a holding device to transfer other instruments. Needle holders have a beak that is rounded and blunt with serrated crisscrossed edges inside the beak to assist in holding a needle. There may be a longitudinal cut in the center of the serration for extra grip.

Mouth Props and Mouth Gags

Mouth props (Figure 46.8) are used for keeping the mouth open while a dental procedure is being performed. They are small, medium, or large pieces of hard rubber. Mouth props are also known as bite blocks. A safety feature while using small bite blocks would be to tie dental

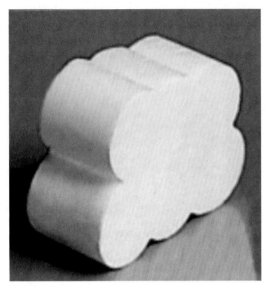

FIGURE 46.8
EZ-Prop mouth props.
Courtesy DENTSPLY/Rinn/MPL

floss to them to prevent them from slipping into the throat. Mouth props are available as a disposable item.

Another style of mouth prop, a mouth gag, is a scissors-like instrument with padded ends instead of blades (Figure 46.9). The padded ends are placed into the tooth occlusion while in a "bite," and later used to spread the jaws apart while the patient is asleep during surgery.

Operating Lights

Several types and sizes of operating lights are available (Figure 46.10). Dentists can choose whichever works best for them. It is the job of the dental assistant to adjust the light to keep the surgical field properly lighted throughout

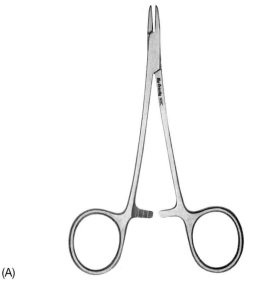

(A)

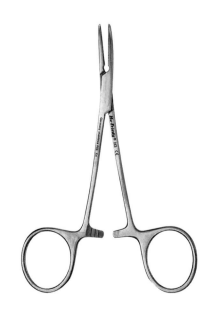

(B)

FIGURE 46.7
(a) Hemostat and (b) needle holder.
Courtesy Hu-Friedy

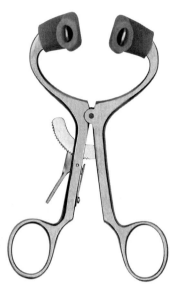

FIGURE 46.9
Mouth gag.
Courtesy Hu-Friedy

the procedure. Infection control barriers are placed on the light handles preoperatively while asepsis is being performed.

In addition to the standard operating light, the dental surgeon may use loupes with lights or separate headlights. A loupe is a type of magnification device or special pair of eyeglasses that is used to see things close up. The light-emitting diode (LED) dental loupe light provides an up to 18,000 lux (unit of illuminance) patch of bright homogenous light. The light is simply clipped to the front of the loupe bar (the bar between the two eyepieces that

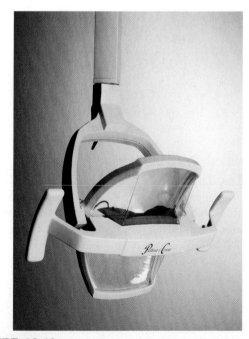

FIGURE 46.10
Operating light.

sit on the nose when wearing the loupes) and is powered by a small, rechargeable lithium battery that provides more than four hours of continuous use. Two batteries and a desk-top charging unit, which doubles as a holder for the batteries and loupes, are supplied as standard. In this way, one battery can be recharging while the other is in use. The LED is easy to fit and can be easily adjusted to work with most types of loupes and eyeglass frame combinations (where the loupes are fitted into prescription eyeglasses). An optional "universal clip" is also provided with the LED light that allows it to be fitted to other kinds of loupes, made by various manufacturers.

Retractors

Retractors are used for holding tissues away from the operating field. Three types of retractors are used in surgery. Tissue retractors are a hemostat-type device with notched tips to hold tissue, or claw-like blades with holding tips. Tissue retractors are used to retract and hold tissue during surgical procedures. The tongue retractor (Figure 46.11a) is an instrument with a long shaft and padded or serrated edges. This retractor is used to grasp and hold the tongue. Cheek retractors (Figure 46.11b) may be bent, wire-shaped or flat devices with curved handles that are used to scoop and hold cheek tissue. These retractors are made of metal or plastic.

Rongeurs

Rongeurs (Figure 46.12) are used for nipping uneven or unwanted bone pieces by contouring and shaping the bone after extraction as an aid to proper healing of the alveolar ridge. These instruments are similar to forceps but have a spring in the handle to provide a "nipping" action. Their beaks are either sharp cutting points (ends) or round-sided (blades), which are used to snip off bony edges and rough areas.

Scalpels/Surgical Blades and Blade Removal Device

Scalpels (Figure 46.13) are surgical knives with a disposable or reusable handle. Disposable scalpels are supplied in sterile sealed packages. Surgical blades come in various shapes and sizes and are used to make precise incisions into the soft tissues with the least damage to the tissue. The smaller the amount of tissue damage, the easier the healing process with minimal or no scarring. The size and shape of the blade can be selected based on the procedure performed. The most commonly used blades include blade #15 for most surgical procedures and blades #11 and #12, which are used to incise and drain lesions. The blades of scalpels are categorized as sharp instruments and, therefore, must be discarded into an approved sharps container. To avoid any potential injury while attaching or removing a blade, extra care must be

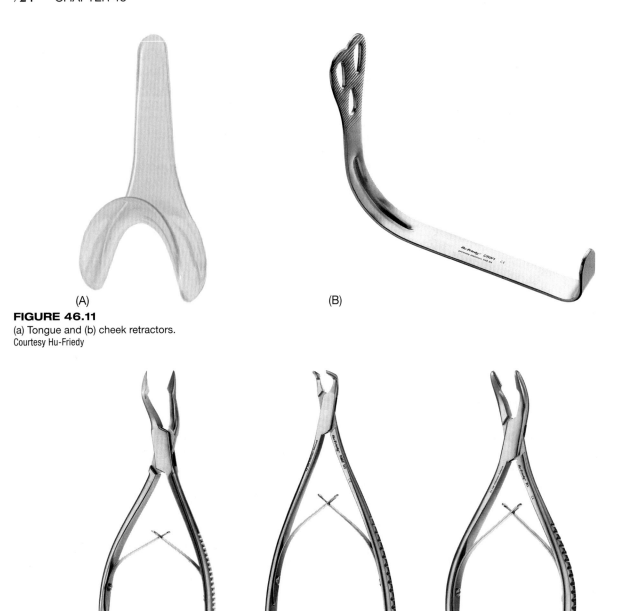

FIGURE 46.11
(a) Tongue and (b) cheek retractors.
Courtesy Hu-Friedy

(A)   (B)

FIGURE 46.12
Various types of rongeurs.
Courtesy Hu-Friedy

utilized, by using either retractable blades (Figure 46.14) or a mechanical blade removal device (Figure 46.15).

Scissors

Various specialized scissors are used in oral surgery. Tissue scissors (Figure 46.16) have a long handle with a serrated blade edge that is used to grasp and hold the tissue during cutting. Suture scissors (Figure 46.17) are smaller with one curved, half-moon blade that is inserted under the suture thread during cutting. Bandage scissors are used to cut materials and dressings during surgery (Figure 46.18). They usually have one long, blunted blade tip to insert under material.

Surgical Aspirators

Surgical aspirators are suction tips with long handles and narrow tip openings (Figure 46.19). The narrow tip is designed to hold and not to suction in any broken piece of tooth or bone during the surgical procedure. Surgical aspirators can be either disposable or made of metal. They are used to aspirate sockets, deeper throat areas, and surgical sites.

It is a good idea to keep several aspirators handy while surgery is being performed in case any aspirator gets blocked by a piece of tissue or bone that accidentally did get past the narrow tip. If this occurs, the blocked aspirator can be replaced with a new one.

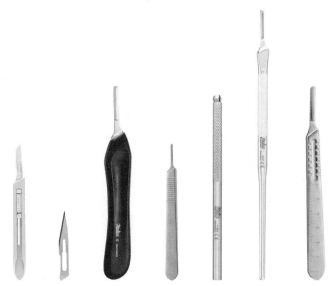

FIGURE 46.13
Various sizes and types of scalpels.
Courtesy Miltex, Inc.

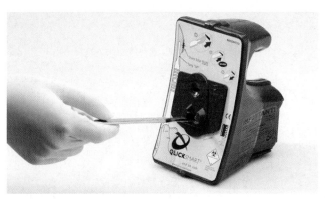

FIGURE 46.15
Blade removal device.
Courtesy www.quicksmart.com

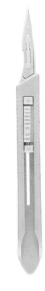

FIGURE 46.14
A retractable blade.
Courtesy Miltex, Inc.

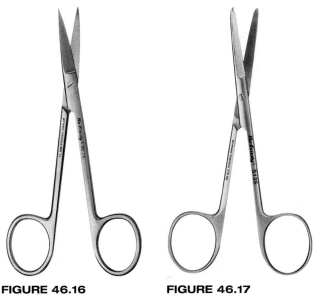

FIGURE 46.16
Tissue scissors.
Courtesy Hu-Friedy

FIGURE 46.17
Suture scissors.
Courtesy Hu-Friedy

To prevent the suction tip from becoming blocked, the dental assistant should have a cup of water available to flush away any tissue or bone piece in the suction tip.

Surgical Burs and Handpieces

Surgical burs (Figure 46.20) are similar to dental burs but they are larger in size and are used to remove bone, to expose root tips, or to divide teeth in preparation for sectioning and removal. They are used with a surgical handpiece (Figure 46.21). The handpieces are power devices that hold inserted rotary instruments in place. Handpieces are classified based on their revolutions per minute as slow speed, high speed, or ultra high speed. Surgical

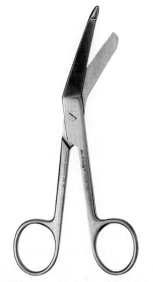

FIGURE 46.18
Bandage scissors.
Courtesy Hu-Friedy

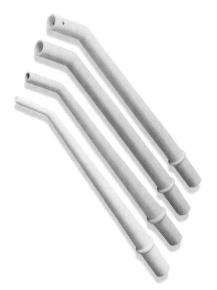

FIGURE 46.19
Various types of aspirating tips.
Courtesy Young Dental

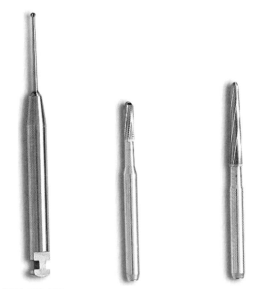

FIGURE 46.20
Various types of surgical burs.
Courtesy DENTSPLY/Maillefer

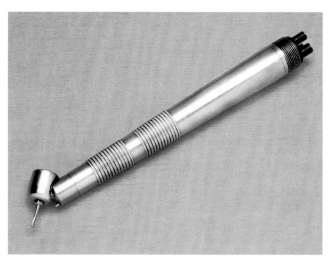

FIGURE 46.21
A surgical handpiece.

handpieces are slow speed because they are used for precise surgical work.

For decades, surgical handpieces with burs have been the standard cutting instrument for general dental work. It has been realized for some time, however, that these air turbine handpieces have significant disadvantages: their cutting efficiency and speed control are poor and they make it difficult to maintain asepsis. New technology has provided dentists with various options for cutting instruments including electric handpieces that are more efficient than air turbines. Cavity preparation is quicker, more precise, and less traumatic with modern electrical technology than is possible with air turbines.

Nitrogen-powered handpieces are another choice. These types of handpieces come in a system that provides one or more handpieces, each driven by pressurized nitrogen gas contained in a portable tank. A water reservoir is provided for medicated water to be applied to the tooth site. The system has two channels to which either a conventional dental handpiece or an abrasive handpiece can be attached. When two abrasive handpieces are attached, two different abrasive materials may be used by the system, one material for cleaning and one material for cutting or abrading.

Surgical Chisels and Mallet

Surgical chisels are longer, thicker, and heavier than regular tooth chisels. They are available in small, medium, and large blade-width tips. Surgical chisels are used with a mallet (Figure 46.22) to chip away bone and to apply enough force to section impacted molar teeth, which are then removed in sections. A surgical mallet is a hammer-shaped device used to apply pressure to chisels. It may have a plain metal face or removable nylon padded facing.

Surgical Curettes

Surgical curettes (Figure 46.23) are hand instruments with a spoon-shaped face that are inserted in the socket or surgical site to remove infectious material, lesions, and/or debris. A surgical curette is larger than a dental operative curette, but similar in shape. Curettes may be single or double ended.

Surgical Preset Trays

Hand instruments and other related accessories for a surgical procedure can be prepared, stored, and transported together as a preset tray (Figure 46.24), also known as a preset cassette. The sterile tray can be set up prior to the patient being seated or brought into the surgical operatory.

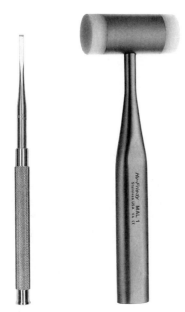

FIGURE 46.22
A surgical chisel and mallet.
Courtesy Hu-Friedy

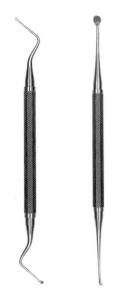

FIGURE 46.23
Surgical curettes.
Courtesy Hu-Friedy

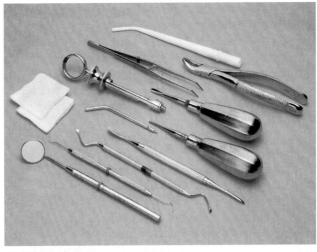

FIGURE 46.24
Tray set-up for surgical examination.

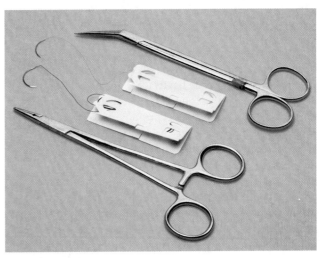

FIGURE 46.25
Surgical needles.

All items on the surgical tray are normally organized in order of use and are readily available for the procedure, making for a smooth and efficient working environment.

Suture Needles and Materials

Sutures are used to close a wound or incision. To suture a wound, suture thread, a suture needle (Figure 46.25), a needle holder, and suture scissors are required. The suture threads can be made of either resorbable or non-resorbable material. Resorbable suture material of gut or collagen substances does not require removal after the wound has healed. A nonresorbable material of silk or nylon requires removal in five to seven days, depending on the healing condition. The needle used for suturing is either straight or curved. Needles are available in various sizes with a rounded or cutting end. They are commonly sized 1/2 or 1/4.

Why are oral surgical instruments designed with certain specific shapes?

Surgical Asepsis

The surgical dentist and staff are classified under OSHA's infection control standard as Category I, which includes all tasks performed that involve exposure to blood, body fluids such as saliva, and body tissues. Surgical asepsis is the procedure done to reduce or eliminate contaminants, such as bacteria, viruses, fungi, and parasites, from entering the operative field to prevent infection.

The goal of surgical asepsis is to eliminate infection. Surgical asepsis eliminates the possibility of transmitting agents such as bacteria and viruses from one surface to another. It is essential to maintain surgical asepsis based on aseptic principles and rituals with an understanding as to how and why surgical asepsis is performed. Rituals or steps in surgical asepsis may actually enhance learning and efficiency in the operating room even though they may or may not directly affect nosocomial (originating or taking place in a hospital) infection rates. Infections are considered nosocomial if they first appear during 48 hours or more after hospital admission or within 30 days after discharge.

Cleanliness is the first step in asepsis. The modern concept of asepsis evolved in the 19th century when Ignaz Philipp Semmelweis first showed that if a doctor and/or midwife washed his or her hands prior to delivery, there was a reduction in women having puerperal fever. Semmelweis also witnessed that midwives who routinely washed their hands prior to delivery had a lower patient fatality rate than did the medical students who did not routinely wash their hands. Puerperal fever or childbed fever is a serious form of septicemia contracted by a woman during or shortly after childbirth or abortion. It is thought that it was spread due to unsanitary conditions, but it can be caused by the naturally occurring Group A streptococcus bacterium, among others.

Later, Joseph Lister introduced the use of carbolic acid as an antiseptic. Lister also promoted the idea of sterile surgery while working at the Glasgow Royal Infirmary. Lawson Tait, a Scottish surgeon, practiced asepsis, introducing principles and practices that have remained valid to this day. His emphasis on aseptic techniques reduced surgical mortality significantly. Antiseptics are used to reduce or kill germs and are applied to skin and wound surfaces. Disinfectants are chemicals applied to inert surfaces and are usually too harsh to be used on biological surfaces.

Currently, the technique used for asepsis includes a series of steps that complement each other. The surgical operatory room is laid out according to specific guidelines, subject to regulations concerning filtration and air flow. Filtration is the process of using a filter to mechanically separate a mixture of solids and fluids. This basically removes bacteria from the environment. The air flow is established in such a way that the surgical area is receiving fresh air while the contaminated air is expelled through an exhaust system.

The operatory should always be kept clean between surgical cases. All members of the surgical team are required to wash their hands and arms with a germicidal solution prior to any operative procedure. Operating surgeons and nurses perform a surgical scrub following guidelines written by the Centers for Disease Control and Prevention (CDC). These guidelines involve washing hands with and without a brush for a prescribed amount of time. Instruments that are not disposable are sterilized through autoclaving. Disposable instruments are used only once. Dressing material is sterile. Dirty and biologically contaminated materials such as saturated cotton rolls and dressing materials are subject to regulated disposal.

Care and Sterilization of Surgical Instruments

Critical instruments, which includes instruments that penetrate soft tissue and bone, must be sterilized. Critical instruments include needles, scalpels, and all other surgical instruments such as dental explorers, dental burs, and endodontic instruments. During the 19th century, Ernst von Bergmann, a German surgeon from Latvia who introduced heat sterilization of surgical instruments, introduced the autoclave. The autoclave is a device used for the sterilization of surgical instruments. Prior to instrument sterilization or disinfection, certain tasks must be carried out. For example, patient debris and body fluids must be removed from the instruments and surfaces using a disinfectant.

Utility gloves should be worn when cleaning instruments. Utility gloves are thick gloves used for "dish washing" or cleaning instruments and are not regulated by the Food and Drug Administration (FDA). Utility gloves should be cleaned and disinfected after use and discarded when they become cracked or punctured.

Instruments should be cleaned in an ultrasonic cleaner and prepackaged before processing through the sterilizer to protect them from contamination after sterilization. Only the wrapping material designed for the particular method of sterilization such as muslin, clear pouches, or paper should be used. Wrapping material should be either self-sealing, heat sealed, or double folded and sealed with the appropriate tape. The CDC recommends that an internal chemical indicator be used inside all bags or cassettes to ensure that the steam has penetrated the wrapping and sterilization has occurred.

Although no documented cases of disease transmission have been associated with dental handpieces, sterilization between patients with acceptable methods that ensure internal as well as external sterility is recommended. The inside lines of high-speed handpieces may become contaminated when patient fluids are retracted back through air/water openings. If the handpiece is not properly processed, the retracted fluids may enter the mouth of the next patient. For proper sterilization of handpieces, the manufacturer's instructions must be followed.

Note that the CDC 2003 guidelines for Infection Control in Dental Health Care Settings recommend that sterile water or saline water is used during surgical procedures.

Surgical Attire, Scrub, and Hand Washing

To maintain asepsis, appropriate clothing is required. Scrubs, which include a set of pants and top made of cotton materials, are worn under a sterile gown (Figure 46.26). Surgical caps are worn to confine the hair so that the surgical site does not get contaminated. Disposable covers are placed over shoes. Protective eye wear is worn to shield the eyes from spatters of contaminated materials and fluids. Face masks are used to protect the oral and

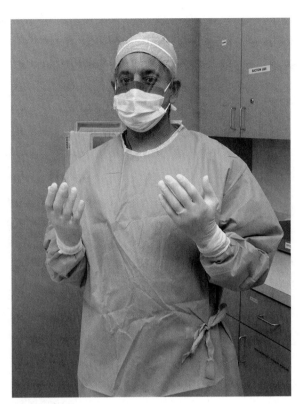

FIGURE 46.26
Surgical attire.

nasal mucosa from body fluid splatters. They should be changed when visibly soiled or wet.

The CDC 2003 guidelines for Infection Control in Dental Health Care Settings recommend that sterile gloves be worn during surgical procedures and during patient examinations and procedures. Latex gloves have proved effective in preventing transmission of many infectious diseases to health care workers, although note that some workers may have an allergic reaction or sensitivity to latex. According to the American College of Allergy, Asthma, & Immunology (ACAAI), it is estimated that 3%–17% of health care workers are latex sensitive. Therefore, nonlatex gloves, such as vinyl or nitrile, are commonly used in health care. Nitrile gloves are a commonly used nonlatex type of glove that is made from a synthetic polymer. These gloves do not contain any protein so they are less likely to cause irritation and allergic reactions. They provide a high degree of softness, sensitivity, feel, and flexibility. The nitrile material reacts to the body temperature and conforms to the shape of the hand, making them exceptionally snug.

Between patients, gloves must be removed and hands must be washed and regloved. Hands should be washed at the start of the day, before gloving, after removal of the gloves, after touching any contaminated surface, and at the end of the day (Figure 46.27). Hand washing with water

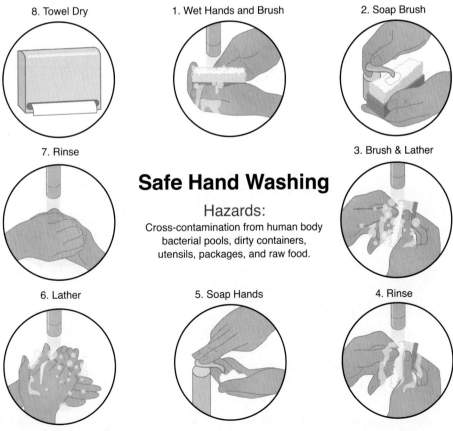

8. Towel Dry

1. Wet Hands and Brush

2. Soap Brush

7. Rinse

Safe Hand Washing

Hazards:
Cross-contamination from human body bacterial pools, dirty containers, utensils, packages, and raw food.

3. Brush & Lather

6. Lather

5. Soap Hands

4. Rinse

FIGURE 46.27
Safe hand washing techniques.

Procedure 46-1 Completing a Surgical Scrub

Supplies

- Antimicrobial soap
- Sterile surgical scrub brush
- Sterile disposable towels

Procedure Steps

1. Remove all jewelry from hands and arms.

2. Wet hands and forearms up to the elbow with warm water for 30 seconds.

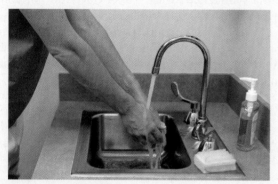

Wet hands and forearms.

3. Dispense about 5 mL of an antimicrobial soap into cupped hands and rub all over the wet area to make lather for 30 seconds.

4. Clean under fingernails with a nail stick or sterile scrub brush. (*Note:* Fingernails must be clipped.)

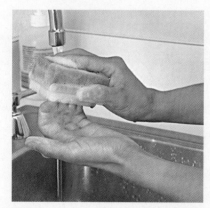

Nail scrubbing.

5. Rinse thoroughly for 30 seconds under tap water.

6. Repeat the procedure with soap but now without the scrub brush for another 30 seconds. (*Note:* Do not use a scrub brush on the skin because it is too stiff and may cause microscopic abrasions.)

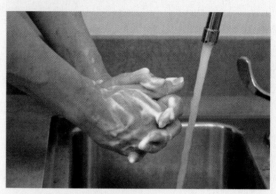

Lathering the soap over wet areas.

7. Finally rinse with warm water, beginning at the finger tips and moving the hands and forearms through the water and up so that the water drains off the forearms last. This is done to prevent hands from recontamination.

8. Close the tap either by pedal control or by the end of the elbow. Motion-sensitive taps are a good option. Do not touch anything with bare, cleaned hands. (*Note:* Once the hands have been washed, they must be kept above the navel level, because the area below the navel is considered unclean in a hospital surgical setting.)

9. Dry hands and forearms thoroughly with disposable sterile towels.

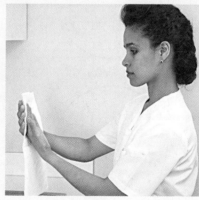

Drying arms.

10. Apply antimicrobial lotion. This is recommended before gloving because it protects the skin from drying and cracking.

11. Don sterile gloves (see Procedure 46-2).

Note: If no instructions are provided with the formulation of scrub soap, two 5-minute scrubs of hands and forearms followed by rinsing are performed.

Procedure 46-2 Donning Surgical Gloves

Supplies

- Pair of double-wrapped, sterile, appropriately sized surgical gloves
- Hand cream (if needed, prior to gloving)

Procedure Steps

1. Perform surgical scrub (see Procedure 46-1).

2. Select the appropriate glove size and inspect the package to make sure it is intact, dry, and sealed.

3. Check the expiration date on the package.

4. Place the sterile package on a clean, dry surface above waist height with the cuffed end of the gloves toward you. (*Note:* Consider anything held below the waist level contaminated.) Do not place a sterile glove package on a wet surface.

5. Open the sterile glove wrapper by touching the outside of the pack only. Do not touch the outside of the glove with your bare hands or the inside of the glove with a gloved hand.

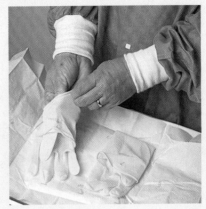
Donning glove on right hand.

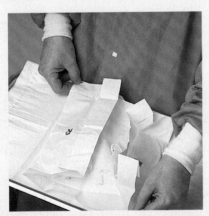
Surgical gloves on an open package.

6. Keep hands inside gown sleeves while grasping the cuff of the glove for the dominant hand.

7. Lay glove on forearm of the dominant (right) hand, with the palm of the glove facing down, glove fingers pointed toward elbow, and glove thumb positioned on thumb side of dominant hand (right hand).

8. Grasp the inside glove cuff with the right hand.

9. With the nondominant (left) hand, pull the dominant (right) hand glove cuff over the cuff of the gown by grasping the folded inside edge of the cuff, because the folded inside edge will be placed against the skin and thus will be contaminated. The outside portion of the glove must not be touched by an ungloved hand because it must remain sterile.

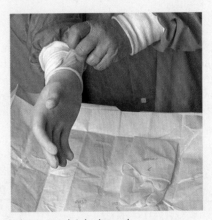
Right hand glove completely donned.

10. Pull the cuff onto the dominant hand using the thumb and fingers of the nondominant hand to avoid touching the rest of the glove.

11. Place second glove on the forearm of the nondominant (left) hand with the palm of the gloved dominant (right) hand with fingers pointed toward the elbow, and gloved thumb on thumb side of the nondominant (left) hand.

12. Grasp the inside glove cuff with the nondominant hand through the gown, being careful to keep fingers inside the gown.

13. Grasp the sleeve of the gown and the cuff of the glove and pull the glove onto the nondominant (left) hand, making sure that the thumb of the right gloved hand is not touching the cuff. Do not try to adjust the fit until you have donned both gloves.

14. Adjust the fingers in both gloves.

continued on next page

Procedure 46-2 *continued from previous page*

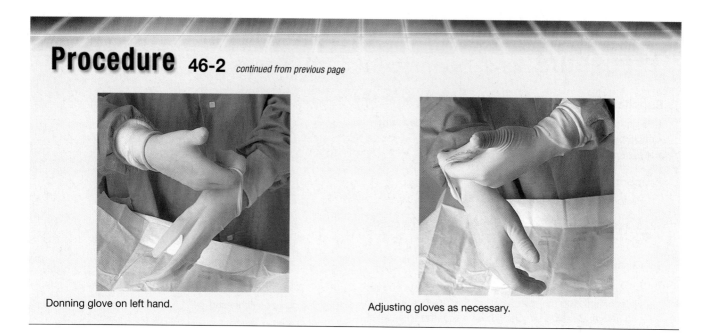

Donning glove on left hand.

Adjusting gloves as necessary.

and plain soap is adequate for patient examination and nonsurgical procedures. For surgical procedures, an antimicrobial hand scrub should be used (Procedure 46-1).

The surgical scrub is performed by all the members of the surgical team prior to donning sterile gloves and before performing a surgical procedure (Procedure 46-2).

Why is surgical asepsis necessary prior to performing a surgical procedure?

Surgical Preparation

Before a surgical procedure is performed, certain steps are taken to ensure the procedure is performed with minimal risk and maximum infection control. These steps include obtaining a complete and detailed medical and dental history from the patient. In some cases, written permission from the patient's primary care physician is required. Surgery can be delayed if certain medical conditions exist.

Medical and Dental History

Some patients have no abnormal physical signs at the time they present for a clinical examination, therefore obtaining an accurate diagnosis rests entirely on taking a complete history. Information first noted on the health history form includes the patient's name, age, sex, marital status, and occupation. The nature of the complaint and its duration should be recorded in the patient's own words. History of past illnesses, operations, and accidents should be included along with information on cardiovascular conditions and allergies. Family history should be included when relevant. It may be necessary to

talk to a relative or friend accompanying a patient when the patient does not provide clear answers. The site, severity, time, and mode of onset of the pain is recorded on the history form.

As a dental assistant, it is important to be knowledgeable about how a patient's past or current health history can affect her dental care. For instance, if a patient is on birth control pills, postsurgical pain may be more severe. It is also important to understand that if a patient is on birth control pills, certain antibiotics should not be prescribed because they may decrease the effectiveness of the pill. If a patient is pregnant, it is recommended that the woman wait to have any major nonurgent dental treatment performed until after the child is born. The first trimester is the most important and crucial stage of pregnancy because most of the baby's organs are formed during that stage. For this reason, when a procedure is necessary, it is best performed during the second trimester to minimize any potential risk. Dental work is also not recommended during the third trimester because the dental chair tends to be too uncomfortable for the mother. Patients in childbearing years should be educated on the importance of maintaining good oral hygiene. Women who are pregnant and have periodontal disease are at a higher risk of giving birth to low birth weight or preterm babies.

Patients with arthritis are given extra care because the disease limits their joint mobility, which can make dental procedures very painful. Many drugs used to treat asthma, such as adrenergic agonists, have side effects that involve the mouth and throat, which can cause dry mouth. Corticosteroids can cause dry mouth and also can make patients susceptible to fungal infections. Cromoly, another drug, can increase saliva production, while leaving a bad taste and burning sensation in the mouth.

Asthma patients should be advised to bring inhalers to each appointment to reduce any risk.

For patients with diabetes, dental procedures should be as short and as stress free as possible. It is recommended that these patients make their appointments in the morning because the blood glucose level is better controlled at this time of the day. Current blood sugar levels should be checked at every appointment. Any premedication prescribed by the dentist must be taken prior to a surgical procedure. If the patient's sugar is not under control, any nonemergency procedures must be postponed. The patient with diabetes should be informed that postsurgical healing can be delayed due to the diabetes.

Biophosphates are medications prescribed for patients with osteoporosis, the loss of bone strength and density, and also for those on chemotherapy. Popularly prescribed biophosphates include Avedia, Zometa, or Fosamax. One of the worst side effects of biophosphates is osteonecrosis of the jaw. Osteonecrosis is a condition that may result in permanent and painful destruction of the jaw bone and is therefore a serious concern for dentists. For patients who develop osteonecrosis, the loss of jaw bone can be aggravated by tooth extractions, oral surgery, deep scaling, and even dentures rubbing against the jaw.

Intraoral and Extraoral Examination

In surgical practice a preliminary general examination of the patient is performed prior to examining the problem area. Clinical examinations should be conducted methodically in order to ensure that no area goes unnoticed. This examination provides detailed information related to the patient's overall oral health. The surgical assistant can assist in performing the detailed intraoral and extraoral examination.

Vital Signs

Vital signs are often taken by the surgical dental assistant in order to assess the most basic body functions. Four vital signs are standard in most medical settings: temperature, pulse rate, blood pressure, and respiratory rate.

Body temperature can be checked by a thermometer. Previously, the average oral temperature for healthy adults had been considered to be 37.0°C (98.6°F), whereas normal ranges were between 36.1°C (97.0°F) and 37.8°C (100.0°F). Recent studies suggest that the average temperature for healthy adults is 36.8°C (98.2°F).

A patient's pulse rate can be checked by placing one's finger (index finger or third finger) on a major vein and counting the beats. These beats, or the movement felt under the vein, represent the rate at which blood is being pumped by the heart. The pulse can be recorded by counting the number of movements per minute. A normal pulse rate for a healthy adult, while resting, can range from 60 to 100 beats per minute (bpm). During sleep, this can drop to as low as 40 bpm; during strenuous exercise, it can rise as high as 200 to 220 bpm.

Blood pressure can be measured by using a sphygmomanometer. Typical values for blood pressure for a resting, healthy adult human are approximately 120 mm Hg systolic and 80 mm Hg diastolic (written as 120/80 mm Hg), with large individual variations. Normal systolic blood pressure can range from 110 to 140 mm Hg, whereas normal diastolic can range from 70 to 90 mm Hg.

The respiratory rate is the number of breaths a person takes per minute. This can be checked by a surgical assistant by listening to a patient's breathing sounds through a stethoscope. The stethoscope is placed on the patient's chest or back. Average respiratory rates vary based on age. For instance, newborns average 44 breaths per minute, infants 20 to 40 breaths per minute, preschool children 20 to 30 breaths per minute, older children 16 to 25 breaths per minute, and adults 12 to 20 breaths per minute.

The phrase "fifth vital sign" usually refers to pain, as perceived by the patient on a pain scale of 0 to 10, with 10 being the worst pain.

Vital sign information should be recorded on the patient history form. (For further information on vital signs see Chapter 23.)

Radiographs

Radiographs are sent to the oral surgeon from a general practice office and usually include chest x-rays. Head and neck radiographs can be taken when required. Most commonly used dental radiographs are periapical views for extractions, but extraoral radiographs such as panoramic, lateral skull, or cephalometric radiographs may also be required. (Refer to Chapters 31 and 32 for more details on radiographs.)

Preoperative Instructions

The oral cavity is a portal of entry as well as the site of disease for microbial infections that affect general health. It is very important for a patient to follow preoperative instructions prior to a scheduled appointment. Therefore, it is necessary to explain verbally and provide a written document for all preoperative instructions. These instructions may include taking certain prescribed medications, not eating food or drink for certain hours prior to the procedure, and not drinking alcohol.

Streptococcus viridans is a bacteria that can lodge on the heart valves, inflame the myocardium, and cause ulcerations on the inner walls of the artery. Due to the belief that patients with heart conditions were at a higher risk of acquiring this bacterium, the American Heart Association (AHA) had recommended that these patients take a dose of antibiotics prior to a dental treatment. In 2007, new guidelines were developed by the AHA due to various studies being done about the effectiveness of antibiotics prior to dental treatment. The AHA now recommends that patients only take antibiotics prior to dental procedures if the following conditions exist: artificial heart valves, a history of infective endocarditis and certain specific serious congenital heart conditions that have been present since birth, and a cardiac transplant that develops a problem in a heart valve. Patients with congenital heart disease are advised to check with their cardiologist for written clearance prior to having a surgical procedure performed.

Informed Consent

Informed consent is a legal condition which means that a person has given consent based on an understanding of the facts and implications of a procedure. An informed consent document identifies and explains details about the surgical procedure, including all risks involved in the treatment. Before starting a surgical procedure, a patient must sign an informed consent form. Informed consent for a patient under 17 years of age must be signed by a parent or a legal guardian.

Patient Preparation

Before taking the patient to the operatory, make sure that all preoperative instructions have been followed. The patient is given a clean gown to wear prior to the procedure. The facial area where surgery is to be performed is washed, shaved (if necessary; for instance, if a male patient has a beard), and the skin is wiped with a germicide.

Pain Control in Oral Surgery

Pain and the fear of pain in dentistry are controlled by using various pain control techniques. If a procedure is done in a dental office, then nitrous oxide/oxygen and local anesthesia are usually used to help control patient pain during the procedure. Before injection of local anesthetics by the dentist or expanded functions dental hygienist, the dental assistant applies topical anesthesia on the injection site for three to five minutes as indicated by the dentist. This is done to avoid the needlestick pain of the local anesthesia. A commonly used topical anesthetic agent is lidocaine and commonly used local anesthetic agents include lidocaine and mepivacaine. Local anesthetic agents can be combined with a vasoconstrictor medicine such as epinephrine. Epinephrine is added in various concentrations to increase the induction time of local anesthetic agents and also to constrict blood vessels at the surgery site to control blood loss. Epinephrine should not be used on patients with cardiac problems.

General anesthesia is typically used with procedures done in hospital settings. Sometimes, premedication with an analgesic and/or sedative is required prior to starting a procedure. The sedatives used are antianxiety agents such as Valium, Versed, and Demerol, intravenous sedation or inhalation sedation.

New methods for performing oral surgery and addressing pain issues continue to be developed. One new option for pain control in oral surgery is the WAND. The WAND is a computer-controlled local anesthesia system that injects anesthetic at a constant, slow rate with controlled pressure. The WAND does not look like a syringe and, therefore, may be less feared by a patient.

Advancements made in surgery, such as the surgical laser, have also helped to improve patient care. Surgical laser procedures can be done without bleeding and with decreased scarring and swelling, decreased postoperative pain, and more rapid healing than traditional surgical procedures.

What is an informed consent form and why is it important to have patients sign this form?

Surgical Procedures

Extractions are commonly performed in an oral surgeon's offices and include multiple extractions, impaction removal, alveoplasty, biopsy, and dental implant surgery. These and other surgical procedures are discussed next.

Alveolectomy and Alveoloplasty

An alveolectomy is usually performed to remove alveolar bone crests that may remain after tooth extraction. The smooth bone ridge that results prepares the patient for denture wear. An alveoloplasty is a surgical contouring and shaping of irregular bone remnants after a surgical procedure, such as multiple extractions. Commonly used surgical instruments for these two procedures include bone rongeurs and bone files. Surgical burs can be used in addition to the surgical handpiece.

Arthrotomy

An arthrotomy is the reconstruction and alignment of the mandible for TMJ disorders. The mandible may be altered to obtain one of three movements. A retrusive arthrotomy involves positioning of the condyle of the mandible in its most retrusive position. A protrusive arthrotomy involves positioning of the mandible forward to place it in a normal occlusion with the maxilla. A lateral arthrotomy involves positioning of the mandible to the side, which could be mesolateral (toward the center of the face), or distolateral (toward the outside of the face).

Biopsy

A tissue biopsy is another surgical procedure performed by an oral surgeon. There are three types of biopsies: An incision biopsy is done to remove a wedge-shaped section of affected tissue along with some normal adjacent tissue. An excision biopsy is done to remove the entire lesion of affected tissue with some underlying normal tissue. An exfoliative biopsy involves scraping a layer of cells from the surface of the lesion and spreading the cells on a glass slide for microscopic study. A brush biopsy is a type of exfoliative procedure (Figure 46.28).

A surgical assistant helps with tray setup and has a biopsy sample collection bottle ready. The bottle should have all of the required information on it and on the accompanying slip from the lab. Required information includes name, age, sex, date the specimen was collected, the site and size of the specimen, and the contact information for the doctor. A note can also be added as prescribed by the oral surgeon.

Cleft Lip, Palate, and Tongue

A cleft lip, palate, and tongue are congenital disorders. A cleft lip is formed due to failure of the median nasal process and one or both maxillary processes to fuse (Figure 46.29). A cleft palate is formed due to failure of the palatal parts of the maxillary and median nasal processes to fuse. A cleft or bi-fid tongue is the result of failure of the tongue muscles to fuse.

This failure of muscles to fuse can happen for hereditary reasons or because of physical or emotional trauma while the fetus is still in the womb. These clefts can result in malnutrition, difficulty breathing, a fear of choking, and emotional stress. An oral and maxillofacial surgeon along with a pediatrician and cosmetic surgeon can close these defects by making some incisions to loosen the muscles and then suturing them together to close the defect. Sometimes a bone graft can also be used to close these defects to construct a bony ridge.

After the surgical procedures are done the patient is provided with a removable or fixed prosthesis, which may include obturators. Following or in conjunction with all of these procedures, speech therapy is also provided by a speech/language pathologist to help the patient learn to control the oral muscles needed to produce understandable speech.

Cyst Removal

Cysts are fluid-filled or semisolid fluid-filled sacs (Figures 46.30 and 46.31). Some of the most common cysts found in the oral cavity are dentigerous, radicular, ranula, or mucocele. A dentigerous cyst is a sac of fluid containing

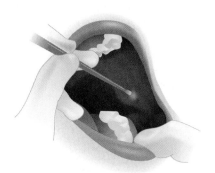

FIGURE 46.28
A dentist performing a brush biopsy.

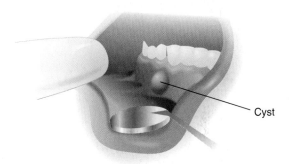

FIGURE 46.30
An oral cyst.

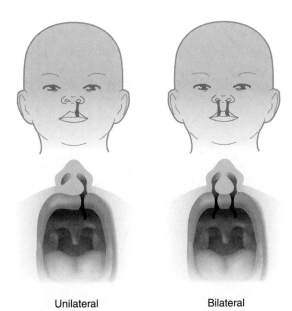

Unilateral   Bilateral

FIGURE 46.29
Appearance of unilateral and bilateral cleft lips and palates.

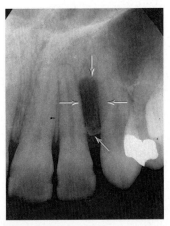

FIGURE 46.31
A radiograph of an oral cyst.

teeth. A radicular cyst is located alongside or at the apex of a tooth root. A ranula is a cystic tumor found on the underside of the tongue or in the sublingual or submaxillary ducts. Mucocele cysts form as a result of blockage of the opening of a minor salivary gland, resulting in a cystic sac underneath the oral mucosa. These cysts must be removed surgically because they can destroy bone as a result of the pressure they place on the bone. Small cysts can be removed in a dental surgical unit under local anesthesia by complete excision of the lesion, whereas larger cysts are excised under general anesthesia.

Drainage of Facial Infections

A facial infection drainage procedure is performed for a periodontal abscess or cellulitis. An incision is made into the affected area and an opening is obtained to remove and drain infected matter. In some cases, a small piece of rubber dam or iodoform gauze or even sterile glove material is inserted into the incision to maintain the opening for drainage. The surgical assistant assists during the procedure and with the postsurgical dressings.

Exodontia

Exodontia is removal or extraction of a tooth. The term *simple extraction* is usually used when a single tooth is extracted with the help of forceps and no surgical incision is performed. Surgical extraction involves removal of multiple teeth, malpositioned teeth, or impacted teeth. A multiple extraction involves the removal of two or more teeth during one procedure. When multiple teeth are extracted, the alveolar bone has to be removed and smoothed to prepare the ridges for denture or appliance wear. This reduction procedure is called an alveolectomy (see earlier section).

In a full mouth extraction, all teeth in the oral cavity are removed. Immediate dentures may be inserted over the sutured site at the time of surgery. A surgical template is used as a guide for the alveolectomy and resection of the area before placement of the immediate denture.

Impaction simply means a hindrance to eruption. There are various types of impaction (Figure 46.32). A soft tissue impaction occurs when the tooth is covered with tissues of the periodontium. Consequently, an incision is required to expose the tooth for extraction. A bone-and-tissue-impacted tooth is covered with tissue and bone. Bone-impacted teeth are typed and named for the tilt angle of the impaction. Horizontal impaction occurs when the tooth is horizontally tilted, for instance, leaning parallel to the floor at various angles where the crown may be perpendicular to an adjacent tooth crown. In vertical impaction, the tooth is in an upright position but in proximity to, or under, the crown of a nearby tooth. In distoangular impaction, the crown of the tooth is slanted toward the distal surface and covered by tissue

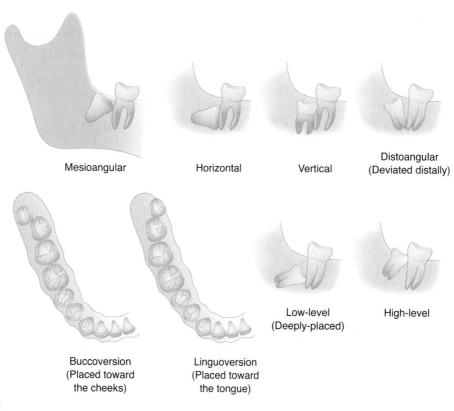

FIGURE 46.32
Types of impaction.

and/or bone, whereas in mesioangular impaction, the crown of the tooth is mesially tilted and covered by tissue and/or bone. In transverse impaction, the tooth is situated sideways to the adjacent teeth and occlusal plane and is covered by tissue and/or bone.

Exostosis

Exostosis is bony overgrowth. This overgrowth can be surgically removed and smoothed in preparation for dentures. A torus is an excessive bone growth. If a torus is on the lingual side of the mandible, it is termed *torus mandibularis*. If it is in the roof of the mouth, it is termed *torus palatinus*. Sometimes these tori can be used as a retention aid in constructing prostheses, but if they are big and irregular then they will require excision through a surgical procedure (Figure 46.33).

Fractures

A closed fracture reduction involves repair with intermaxillary fixation (IMF), tooth wiring, or ligation methods in which the teeth are "wired together" in proper alignment awaiting bone healing. In an open fracture reduction, a more complicated procedure involving an osteotomy and rigid fixation is performed where bone plate, mesh, pins, grafts, and other fixation devices can be used. Open reduction requires not only alignment by fixation of the teeth but also repositioning and correction of fractures after surgical access through the periosteum. Figure 46.34 shows a fractured tooth.

Surgical assistants can help with assisting and also with tightening and cutting the wires used in closed fracture reductions. They can also help with inserting and removing nasal food tubing and care of oral hygiene.

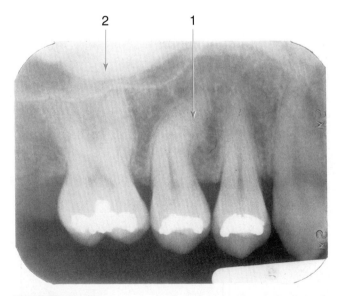

FIGURE 46.33
Torus palatinus. Note the overgrowth of bone on the midline of the palate.

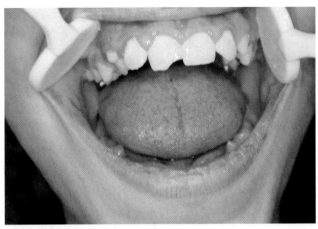

FIGURE 46.34
Fractured tooth.
Image courtesy Instructional Materials for the Dental Team, Lex., KY

Why might a closed fracture reduction be needed?

Frenectomy

A frenectomy is performed on the maxillary labial frenum to correct a **diastema**, or on the mandibular lingual frenum to correct **ankyloglossia** (Figure 46.35). A frenectomy can also be performed to reposition the frenum for orthodontic purposes to close the diastema between the central incisors.

Genioplasty

A genioplasty is plastic surgery of the chin or cheek, involving contouring or shaping of the bone for restorative or cosmetic purposes. Chin size is classified in six ways. Macrogenia is a large or excessive chin. Microgenia is an undersized chin.

A deficient chin occurs when there is excessive bone in one direction and deficient bone in another, classified

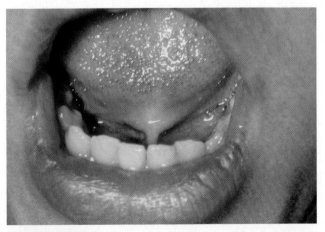

FIGURE 46.35
Ankyloglossia.

as lateral excessive. An asymmetrical chin occurs when there is a lack of balance of size and shape on opposite sides, and sometimes an excess of soft tissue will present a chin that looks abnormal in size and results in pseudo-macrogenia. "Witch's chin" is simply soft tissue ptosis.

Gingivectomy and Gingivoplastomy

A gingivectomy is a surgical excision of unattached gingival tissue, whereas a gingivoplasty or gingivoplastomy is surgical recontouring of gingival tissues (Figure 46.36). This is done sometimes to reduce gingival hyperplasia, which may have resulted from gingivitis due to pathology or medication. A surgical dental assistant helps with postoperative gingival dressing application and removal. (Chapter 45 discusses gingivectomies in more detail.)

Implantology

An oral surgeon along with the dental surgical team can independently perform implant procedures or can assist a general dentist or an implantologist. Dental implants are discussed in detail in Chapter 43. The procedure requires incision of the oral mucosa and preparing of the alveolar or jaw bone, and it can take up to nine months to complete.

Oral Pathology and Tumors

Oral pathology is a **malady** and basically refers to lesions present in the intra- and extraoral regions of the mouth. The term *tumor* merely means "swelling," but it is commonly interpreted to mean "cancer." Cancerous tumors are **malignant** (Figure 46.37). By contrast, benign tumors are not considered life threatening or deadly.

Leukoplakia is the formation of white patches on the mucous membrane of the oral cavity that cannot be scraped off and can be premalignant. A fibroma is a benign, fibrous, encapsulated tumor of connective tissue. A papilloma is a benign epithelial tumor of the skin or mucous membrane. A hemangioma is a benign tumor of dilated blood vessels. A granuloma is a granular tumor

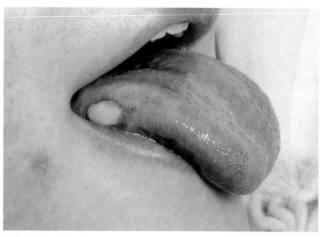

FIGURE 46.37
Malignant tumor on the tongue.

that usually occurs along with other diseases. A melanoma is a malignant, pigmented mole or tumor. A basal or squamous cell carcinoma is a malignant growth of epithelial cells. All of these maladies require close observation, and a biopsy may be indicated to confirm the diagnosis.

Complete excision is performed for most oral pathologies, along with the removal of some normal tissues to avoid later growth and spread of the disease. Most of these excision procedures are performed under general anesthesia in a hospital setting.

Periodontal Flap Surgery

Periodontal flap surgery is a procedure in which tissues are sectioned and removed. This may be necessary because of extensive singular pocket involvement or when, during tooth eruption, tissue flap coverage of erupting teeth, particularly third molars, obstructs or impacts food around the crown, causing gingival irritation and an infection termed pericoronitis.

Surgical Endodontics

An apicoectomy (Figure 46.38) usually requires opening of the periodontium, including some alveolar bone, and

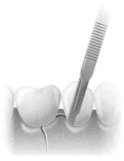

FIGURE 46.36
Incising the gum margin.

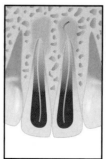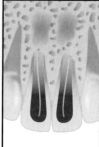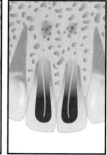

FIGURE 46.38
Apicoectomy of anterior teeth.

exposure with removal of the root apex. (See Chapter 44 for more about apicoectomies.) Many times this surgery is followed by a retrofill root canal treatment.

The surgical assistant must take care that the fractured part of the root apex is not sucked in by the aspirator because it must be kept to prove that all parts of the fractured tooth were removed. This is necessary in case any legal questions arise about the procedure. All details must be documented. It is recommended that a photo of the extracted broken pieces be taken and saved in the patient's record.

Surgical Orthodontics

Orthognathic surgery is surgical manipulation of the facial skeleton to restore facial aesthetics and proper function to patients with congenital, developmental, or trauma-affected conditions. An oral surgeon can perform these procedures along with an orthodontist and a cosmetic surgeon.

Sutures

Sutures are stitches used to hold together skin, internal organs, blood vessels, and all other tissues of the human body after they have been severed by injury or surgery. Sutures are basically used to repair tissues, facilitate healing, and keep the wound closed to prevent potential infection. Sutures must be strong, nontoxic, hypoallergenic, and flexible. They must lack the "wick effect," which simply means that sutures must not allow fluids from outside of the body to penetrate them—such penetration could easily cause infection.

Types of Sutures

The two basic types of sutures are absorbable and nonabsorbable. Nonabsorbable sutures must be removed after an examination and on the recommendation of the surgeon. Sutures are typically removed within five to seven days after placement. Absorbable sutures dissolve harmlessly in the body over time without intervention and become part of the body. This can take from ten days to eight weeks.

Nonabsorbable sutures are made of materials that are not metabolized by the body, such as silk, nylon, or polyester (Figure 46.39). The choice of suture material depends on the location of the injury or cut. Nonabsorbable sutures may or may not have coatings to enhance their performance characteristics. Currently, stainless steel wires and staples are also used as a nonabsorbable choice. They are commonly used in orthopedic surgery and for sternal closure in cardiac surgery. These types of "sutures" may also be used after orthognathic surgery to "hold" the surgically split bone together in the desired position.

Absorbable sutures or "catgut" are prepared from the intestines of sheep or goats or occasionally from those of hogs, horses, mules, pigs, or donkeys. Oddly enough, cat intestines are not used for sutures; therefore, it is assumed that the word was originally *kitgut*, with *kit* meaning "fiddle" (hence, "fiddle string") and that the present form has arisen through confusion between *kit* and *cat*.

Another explanation of the origin of the *cat* in "catgut" is that it is an abbreviation for cattle, which originally denoted not only cows, but all types of livestock. Al-Zahrawi, an inventor during the ninth century, observed that the catgut he used in his lute's string dissolved after a monkey ate part of it. This led him to the invention of absorbable types of sutures. Today, absorbable suture materials can be made from animal intestines, but most sutures are made from synthetic polymer fibers. Adding synthetic fibers has added quality to the material by decreasing the cost, lowering the suture reaction, and guaranteeing nontoxicity. The synthetic fiber sutures are very easy to handle.

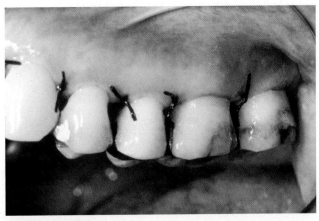

FIGURE 46.39
Silk sutures in the mouth.

Three kinds of catgut sutures are used:

1. *Plain gut:* untreated catgut
2. *Chrome gut:* treated and tanned with chromium salts to increase their persistence in the body
3. *Fast gut:* heat treated to allow more rapid absorption

Absorbable sutures are used in many of the internal tissues of the body. In most cases, three weeks is sufficient for the wound to close firmly. In rare cases, absorbable sutures can cause inflammation and be rejected by the body rather than absorbed. Various suture types are shown in Figure 46.40. A surgical suture packet is shown in Figure 46.41.

Recently, topical cyanoacrylate adhesives ("liquid stitches") have been introduced in combination with, or as an alternative to, sutures in wound closure. The adhesive is a liquid until it is exposed to water or water-containing substances or tissues, after which it hardens and forms a flexible film that bonds to the underlying surface. The tissue adhesive acts as a barrier to microbial penetration. Tissue adhesives may not be used near the eyes.

Over and over sutures (interrupted and continuous)

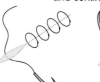

Subcuticular suture (interrupted and continuous)

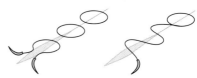

Horizontal mattress sutures (interrupted and continuous)

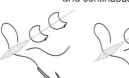

Vertical mattress sutures (interrupted and continuous)

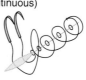

Lembert sutures (interrupted and continuous)

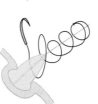

Cushing suture

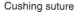
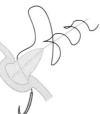

Everting suture

Lock - stitch suture

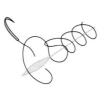

Halstod suture

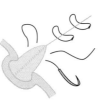

Connell suture

Purse-string suture

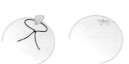

FIGURE 46.40
Types of sutures.

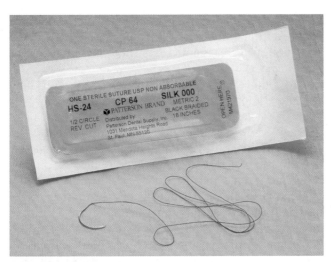

FIGURE 46.41
Surgical suture packet.

Another recent development in suture material is sutures coated with antimicrobial substances to reduce the chances of wound infection. These sutures have proven to be effective at keeping bacteria out of wounds.

Commonly used suture stitching techniques include the following:

* Simple interrupted stitch (or running)
* Mattress
* Horizontal mattress
* Vertical mattress
* Figure 8
* Continuous locking
* Subcuticular

Instruments for Sutures

Surgical needles come in various shapes, including straight, half-curved or ski, 1/4 circle, 3/8 circle, 1/2 circle, 5/8 circle, and compound curve (Figure 46.42). Needles may also be classified by their point geometry, such as tapered, cutting, reverse cutting, trocar point or tapercut, blunt points for sewing friable tissues, and side cutting or spatula points. Another kind of needle is atraumatic needles, which can be permanently swaged to the suture or can be designed to come off the suture with a sharp straight tug. These are also known as "pop-offs" and are commonly used for interrupted sutures, where each suture

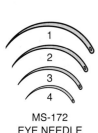

MS-172
EYE NEEDLE
3/8 Circle
Cutting Edge

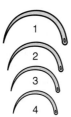

MS-176
EYE NEEDLE
1/2 Circle
Cutting Edge

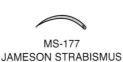

MS-177
JAMESON STRABISMUS
Cutting Edge

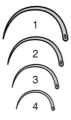

MS-176
EYE NEEDLE
1/2 Circle
Taper Point

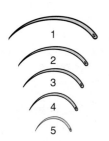

MS-155
LANE CLEFT PALATE
3/8 Circle
Cutting Edge

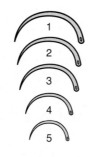

MS-156
LANE CLEFT PALATE
1/2 Circle
Cutting Edge

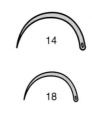

RC-14
RC-18
DENTAL
REVERSE CUTTING EDGE
1/2 Circle

FIGURE 46.42
Surgical needles.

is only passed once and then tied. Figure 46.43 shows the steps used to perform a simple suture knot.

How does a surgical assistant help with suture removals?

Suture Removal

Different parts of the body have different healing times; therefore, suture removal is done based on how much healing has been achieved to ensure that the wound is not going to open again or get infected. Commonly, facial wounds heal in 3 to 5 days, scalp wounds in 7 to 10 days, and joint wounds in about 14 days. A surgical dental assistant, based on the recommendation of the oral surgeon, provides postoperative instructions to the patient that include when the nonabsorbable sutures will be removed.

The suture removal procedure generally does not require anesthesia. The surgical assistant first cleans the debris accumulated on top of the suture knot by gently wiping it with an antiseptic, such as hydrogen oxide or chlorhexidine, to remove encrusted blood and loosened scar tissues. After the suture material can be seen clearly, the surgical assistant requests the oral surgeon to look at the sutured area to get approval that the healing is done and sutures can be removed. The surgical assistant may assist in suture removal or may be qualified to remove them independently as an expanded function. Sometimes, if the wound is large, not all the sutures will be removed at one time; instead, alternate sutures will be

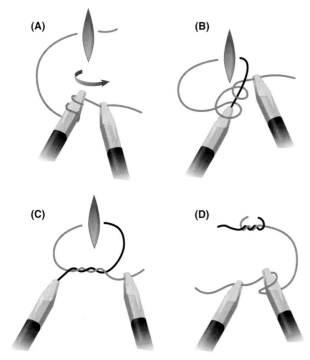

FIGURE 46.43
Suture knot steps.

removed as advised by the oral surgeon. Sutures are only removed from healed areas. If, while removing sutures, a small unhealed area is noticed, the oral surgeon should be informed.

To remove sutures, sterile forceps are used to hold the suture knot to make sure that the knot will not pass through the healing tissues, which can result in tearing of the new tissues. A surgical knife or suture scissors are used to cut the suture right underneath the knot and very close to the tissues, while the knot is pulled by the forceps. This is done to avoid passage of any outside suture material through the healing wound—exposure of the healing wound to outside suture material could result in an infection.

These relatively painless steps are continued until all sutures have been removed and lined up on a clean piece of gauze. The number of removed sutures is matched with the number of sutures the patient received as documented in the patient record. After suture removal, the healing wound is cleansed with an antiseptic. Suture adhesive may be applied if needed.

Postoperative Instructions for Sutures

Even after sutures have been removed, it is still important for the patient to be advised about the need to keep the wound area clean and free of debris. An antibiotic ointment may be prescribed to keep the wound disinfected or an antibacterial mouth rinse can be used for intraoral wounds. Patients should be advised to notify the dental office if a suture becomes loose or breaks off because the suture can always be resutured. The patient must notify the dental office if signs of infection are noticed including swelling, redness, bleeding, fever, or increased pain.

Instructions for Patient Care

Interpersonal communication is very important in building good patient and surgical team relations. The diagnosis and treatment options should always be presented clearly in lay terms to patients. Patients should be provided a list of instructions regarding their pre- and postoperative care. As an example, Tables 46-1 and 46-2, respectively, list some commonly prescribed preoperative and postoperative instructions for an extraction procedure.

Preoperative Instructions

Patients should understand that after a surgical procedure there may be some degree of discomfort or pain. Therefore, it is important for patients to take prescribed pain medication before and after the procedure as directed by the dentist. If the procedure is done under local anesthesia, then the patient may be advised to have some food with the medication. If the procedure is done under general anesthesia, the patient must take the med-

TABLE 46-1   Commonly Prescribed Preoperative Instructions for an Extraction Procedure

1. Take all premedications as prescribed.
2. Eat some food before arriving at the dental office for an extraction procedure. *Note:* If IV sedation is to be done, then the patient is advised not to eat for at least eight hours before the surgical procedure.
3. Bring a friend or a family member to escort you home after the procedure is done.

TABLE 46-2   Commonly Prescribed Postoperative Instructions After an Extraction Procedure

1. Do not disturb the healing area and avoid vigorous chewing, excessive spitting, or rinsing.
2. Use a pressure pack on the area of surgery by biting on the gauze pack placed by the dental staff.
3. If the bleeding persists for a long time, rinse with cold water and continue using pressure with a fresh gauze piece for another 30 minutes.
4. Moist tea bags wrapped with gauze may help control bleeding because tannic acid is a good hemostatic agent.
5. If active bleeding persists, notify the dental clinic.
6. Avoid overexertion because it may lead to postoperative bleeding and discomfort.
7. Keep the head elevated when lying down.
8. Take prescribed pain medication when pain is present.
9. Eat some food before taking most of the medications.
10. Avoid drinking any alcoholic beverages.
11. If the pain becomes severe, contact the dental office or urgent care center.
12. Drink lots of fluid, starting with clear fluids, such as water or broth, and then moving on slowly to teas, soups, and juices.
13. Dairy products should be avoided initially, and any hot liquid should be avoided until the bleeding has stopped.
14. Do not use a straw to drink beverages after intraoral surgery for several days because it may cause a blood clot to dislodge and may delay healing.
15. Eat healthy foods that are soft and require little or no chewing.
16. Take antibiotics as prescribed. (*Note:* Birth control pills may become ineffective when used with some antibiotics.)
17. Smoking must completely be avoided.
18. Notify the oral clinic if any abnormal signs are noticed.

ications but may not have anything else by mouth for at least eight hours preoperatively.

Why must a person not smoke after oral surgery?

Postoperative Instructions

Postoperatively, the patient should be advised not to disturb the healing area and to avoid vigorous chewing, excessive spitting, the use of a straw, or rinsing because these actions may delay initial healing, resulting in active bleeding or infection. If the patient was given anesthesia, then it is highly recommended that the patient be escorted home by a friend or relative.

The patient may be advised to use a pressure pack on the surgical area by biting on a gauze pack that has been placed by the dental staff. If bleeding persists, the patient can rinse with cold water and should continue using pressure with a fresh gauze piece for about 30 minutes. Moist tea bags wrapped with gauze may help with bleeding because tannic acid is a good hemostatic agent. If active bleeding persists, then the patient must notify the dental practice.

Oral surgery patients are typically advised to avoid overexertion because it may lead to postoperative bleeding and discomfort. The patient is also advised to keep his head elevated when he lies down. The patient should take prescribed pain medication when necessary. It is a good idea to instruct the patient to eat some food before taking medications because some medications can be disruptive to the gastrointestinal system. Patients should focus on eating healthy foods that are soft and require minimal chewing.

Patients should be advised to drink lots of fluids, starting with clear liquids such as water or a broth, and then slowly advance to teas, soda, soup, or juices. Dairy products should be avoided initially and hot liquids should be avoided until the bleeding has stopped. Patients should be told to avoid drinking any alcoholic or carbonated beverages. Alcohol can interfere with the effectiveness of some other drugs. Patients who have had an intraoral surgery procedure should be advised not to use straws in their beverages for several days. The use of straws can cause blood clots to dislodge and can delay healing.

Swelling or edema is a common occurrence with oral surgery. Swelling usually develops during the first 12 to 24 hours following surgery, often increasing on the second day. It should begin to subside by the third day. Patients should be advised that if swelling occurs it can be minimized by wearing an ice pack on the side of the face where the oral surgery was performed. The ice pack should be placed on the site for 30 to 45 minutes every hour while awake during the first 24 hours following the surgery. Anti-inflammatory medications such as Motrin or Advil may be suggested to help decrease swelling. Antibiotics may be prescribed to prevent any potential infection and the patient must take them as prescribed. Depending on the type of surgery, rinsing postoperatively with chlorhexidine mouth rinse may be advised. Note that birth control pills may become ineffective because of some antibiotics. Patients should continue taking any other prescribed medication, such as diabetes medication, as scheduled. Smoking must be avoided completely because it slows the healing process and contributes to the development of dry sockets. The patient must notify the oral clinic if any abnormal signs are noticed. If severe pain is present after 24 hours and is not being helped with prescribed analgesic, then the patient must contact the dental office or go to an urgent care center.

Postsurgical Complications

Patients should be informed about all possible post-surgery complications. Informed consent forms that outline possible complications in detail should be signed prior to surgery.

Dry socket (**alveolitis**) is the most common problem people experience following dental surgery extraction. Alveolitis is the result of premature loss of a blood clot in the empty tooth socket, resulting in bone exposure with lodged food and debris creating an offensive odor. This condition affects approximately one out of every five patients.

Dry socket occurs with greater frequency in people who smoke or are taking birth control pills or in individuals who are not following through on postoperative instructions. A clinical study trial of 267 women on birth control pills showed they were more susceptible to postoperative pain and dry socket.

Dry socket typically occurs in the lower jaw on the third to fifth day. The patient may first notice the pain starting in the ear and radiating down toward the chin. It frequently begins in the middle of the night and the pain can be extremely severe. Treatment involves placing a medicated dressing in the "empty" tooth socket, after removing all debris and flushing the area with warm water and antiseptic solution. This helps decrease the

Patient Education

The dental assistant can play a major role in addressing fears that oral surgery patients may experience. Utilizing effective interpersonal communication skills and the knowledge gained through education and/or experience, the surgical dental assistant can provide detailed preoperative and postoperative instructions that often help to relieve patient concerns.

Stress reduction is an important aspect of dental treatment. One way to determine whether or not a patient is very anxious about receiving dental treatment is to administer a standard questionnaire. Use of technology is a good tool for explaining to patients about the diagnosis and treatment plan. The Caesy system is a video-based patient education system that can be played either on multiple computers using its own proprietary "enterprise" system, or on individual DVD player/DVD computer units. It includes lots of 3-D animations of all the dental procedures which are commonly done in a dental office. It is a good tool for patient education as the patient can watch the procedure that is planned rather than just have the procedure verbally explained by the dentist or other dental team members.

pain and protects the socket from accumulating food particles. The pain from dry socket typically lasts for about 24 to 48 hours. The medicated dressing typically needs to be changed every day or two for five to seven days. The surgical assistant can change dressings and irrigate the socket if approved by the oral surgeon. A supplemental pain medication can be prescribed and an irrigation device is given to the patient to help keep food particles from lodging in the extraction site following removal of the dressing.

How is postsurgical edema managed?

SUMMARY

Oral surgery is a specialty of dentistry that involves the diagnosis and treatment of diseases, injuries, and defects of the hard and soft tissues of the oral and maxillofacial region. An oral surgeon is a specialist who treats the anatomic area of the mouth, jaws, face, and their associated structures.

The dental surgical assistant performs many specialized tasks requiring both interpersonal and advanced technical skills: (1) pre- and postsurgical patient assessment and monitoring, (2) use of specialized surgical instruments, (3) assisting with surgical procedures, (4) performing surgical asepsis and scrub, (5) assisting with pain control techniques, and (6) delivery of pre- and postsurgical instructions.

Dental surgical procedures can be completed in a private dental office or an operating room in a hospital. Surgical instruments are designed to apply adequate pressure in specific areas to loosen, retract, and remove bone tissue or teeth. Surgical asepsis is the procedure done to reduce or eliminate contaminants, such as bacteria, viruses, fungi, and parasites, from entering the operative field. Surgical asepsis includes disinfection of the clinical area, before and after the surgical procedure, the wearing of surgical attire, cleaning and sterilization of instruments, surgical hand washing, and donning of surgical (sterile) gloves.

Routine extractions are often performed in an oral surgeon's office. Sutures are the materials used to hold

SUMMARY (continued)

skin, internal organs, blood vessels, and all other tissues of the human body together after they have been severed by injury or surgery. Sutures are basically used to repair tissues and facilitate healing and keep the wound closed by stopping potential infection. Different parts of the body have different healing times; therefore, suture removal is done based on how much healing has been achieved to ensure that the wound is not going to open again or get infected. Depending on each state's dental practice act, the surgical assistant can assist in removal of sutures or can actually do the procedure. Before a patient's surgery is scheduled, the patient is provided with preoperative and postoperative instructions in a manner he can understand. The patient is informed in detail about all possible postsurgical complications, and the patient must sign the informed consent form that details the complications in writing. The most common postsurgical complication in dentistry is dry socket, or alveolitis, which results from the dislodging of a blood clot and lodging of food and debris and superimposed infection.

Professionalism

Some people are fearful of dental treatment—so fearful, in fact, that they avoid seeking it. These patients may feel physically ill when they come to a dental office. Many others, although they seek care, are very anxious about the prospect of dental treatment. These feelings have little regard for a patient's health status. Often, however, feelings of dread, fear, or anxiousness complicate a systemic condition. For instance, a fearful patient with a history of angina pectoris may have a heart attack or chest pain during a dental procedure.

The relationship between surgical team and patient is often a powerful one in the sense that the provider has the power to agitate or calm the patient by words and deeds. Eye contact, positive body language, use of words, tone of voice, and facial expressions are tools for maintaining a good patient–provider relationship by building the patient's confidence in the quality of treatment provided. If the practitioner appears to be inattentive or insensitive to the patient's needs, anxiety will increase. The worst would be if the practitioner appears to be patronizing, arrogant, or hostile, which would further increase the anxiety and can lead to serious future misunderstandings.

KEY TERMS

- **Alveolitis:** A postextraction complication resulting in inflammation of the alveolar process; also known as dry socket. p. 744
- **Ankyloglossia:** Shortness of the tongue's frenum; literally, "tongue tied." p. 737
- **Crepitus:** A clinical sign characterized by a peculiar crackling, crinkly, or grating feeling or sound under the skin or around the joints, for example, in the temporomandibular junction. p. 718

- **Diastema:** A gap between two teeth. p. 737
- **Exodontia:** The extraction of a tooth. p. 736
- **Luxate:** To put out of joint or out of place. p. 720
- **Malady:** A disease or disorder. p. 738
- **Malignant:** Tumor that is life threatening, such as a squamous cell carcinoma or basal cell carcinoma. p. 738

CHECK YOUR UNDERSTANDING

1. Oral and maxillofacial surgery can be indicated for a variety of reasons except
   a. alveolectomy.
   b. impaction removal.
   c. biopsy.
   d. removal of infected pulp from root canal.

2. The surgical assistant performs many specialized tasks except for
   a. pre- and postsurgical patient assessment and monitoring.
   b. surgical asepsis.

   c. excision biopsy.
   d. delivery of pre- and postsurgical instructions.

3. Which of the following is a special type of forceps designed with pointed beaks to fit into the furcation of the molar roots?
   a. #150
   b. #23K
   c. tissue
   d. 171L

CHECK YOUR UNDERSTANDING (continued)

4. These instruments look much like scissors with locking joints and serrated beaks.
   a. elevators
   b. forceps
   c. hemostats
   d. chisels

5. This is a hand instrument with a spoon-shaped face that is inserted in the socket or surgical site to remove infectious material, lesions, and/or debris.
   a. elevator
   b. curette
   c. root pick
   d. rongeur

6. A cystic sac containing teeth is a
   a. bone cyst.
   b. radicular cyst.
   c. dentigerous cyst.
   d. ranula.

7. Which of the following is used to control immediate bleeding after a dental surgical procedure?
   a. ice pack
   b. heat pack
   c. pressure pack
   d. wax in a gauze piece

8. Nonabsorbable sutures must be removed after an examination by and on the recommendation of the oral surgeon in what time period?
   a. 1 to 2 days
   b. 5 to 7 days
   c. 10 to 15 days
   d. 20 to 30 days

9. Patients should avoid drinking any alcoholic beverages before and after an oral surgical procedure because
   a. alcohol is expensive.
   b. alcohol can interfere with the effectiveness of some other drugs.
   c. alcohol can produce infection.
   d. alcohol can cause a scar issue.

10. Approximately one out of five postsurgical complications is
   a. bone fractures.
   b. profuse bleeding.
   c. dry socket.
   d. edema.

INTERNET ACTIVITIES

- Watch several animations regarding dental health at www.ada.org/public/media/videos/minute/index.asp#conditions
- To learn more about impacted teeth and surgical extraction, visit www.animated-teeth.com/wisdom_teeth/t1_wisdom_tooth.htm
- To play some cool games on surgical asepsis, visit www.studystack.com/matching-36541
- Watch a video on different kinds of sutures at http://cal.vet.upenn.edu/projects/surgery/index.htm

WEB REFERENCES

- American Association of Oral and Maxillofacial Surgeons www.aaoms.org/
- American Board of Oral & Maxillofacial Surgery www.aboms.org/General_Information/about_aboms.htm
- Caesy Education Systems www.caesy.com
- Centers for Disease Control www.cdc.gov/niosh/98-113.html
- Oral & Maxillofacial Surgery Questions Page www.calweb.com/~goldman/
- Oral & Maxillofacial Surgery Foundation www.omsfoundation.org/

47

Pediatric Dentistry

Learning Objectives

After reading this chapter, the student should be able to:

- Describe the roles of the pediatric team.
- Describe the pediatric office.
- Discuss the pediatric patient and his or her needs.
- Explain the diagnosis and treatment planning process.
- Discuss types of behavior management techniques.
- Describe common preventive procedures for children.
- Identify the difference between restorative, endodontic, and prosthodontic procedures.
- Describe common dental trauma emergencies.
- Identify signs of child abuse and neglect.

Preparing for Certification Exams

- Size and fit stainless steel crowns.
- Apply topical fluoride.

Key Terms

Alveolus	Open bay
Autonomy	Papoose board
Avulsed tooth	Pulpectomy
Coronal	Pulpotomy
Decalcification	Space maintainers
Exfoliate	T-bands
Nitrous oxide	Traumatic intrusion
Nonvital tooth	Vital tooth

Chapter Outline

- The Pediatric Team
- Pediatric Dental Office
- The Pediatric Patient
  - —Childhood Stages
- Patients with Special Needs
  - —Physical Conditions
  - —Mentally Challenged
  - —Mental Disorders
- Diagnosis and Treatment Planning
  - —Behavior Management Techniques
- Preventive Dentistry Procedures
  - —Coronal Polishing
  - —Fluoride Treatments
  - —Placement of Pit and Fissure Sealants
  - —Mouth Guards
  - —Interceptive Orthodontics
- Restorative Procedures and Equipment
- Endodontic Procedures
- Prosthodontic Procedures
- Dental Trauma
- Reporting Child Abuse and Neglect

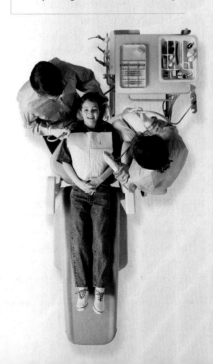

Pediatric dentistry is the specialty that treats children from birth through the teenage years. The main purpose of the pediatric practice is prevention. Applying preventive dentistry techniques and educating both patients and parents about oral health help to reduce dental decay, periodontal disease, and malocclusion. The health of a child and his or her teeth during the developmental stages is critical to the overall health of the child's permanent teeth. A child who learns good oral habits at an early age, including habits that lead to good nutrition, is likely to carry these habits over into adulthood. (See Chapter 16 for more information on oral nutrition.) A child's treatment needs are somewhat similar to those of an adult patient, which includes restoring and maintaining primary and permanent teeth. Due to the smaller size of primary teeth, special techniques must be used with pediatric patients.

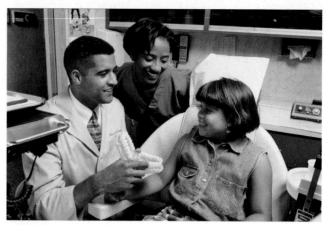

FIGURE 47.1
The pediatric dental team.

The Pediatric Team

The pediatric team is composed of a variety of individuals including the pediatric dentist, the dental hygienist, and the dental assistant (Figure 47.1). The pediatric dentist is trained as a specialist in the care of children's teeth. This specialty requires an additional two to three years of education beyond general dentistry. The pediatric dentist focuses on the physical, mental, emotional, and behavioral concerns of children and compromised adults.

Dental assistants and hygienists who work in pediatric dental offices must enjoy working with young people. Having patience and compassion is important to the success of dental treatment for children. Patients who build a relationship of trust with the assistant are more likely to be well-behaved patients and less likely to develop fears of going to the dental office. Dental team members can gain a patient's trust by being honest about treatment procedures and by taking the time to explain how equipment operates. In most states, dental assistants work independently with children and must be confident about managing children while they are receiving treatment. The assistant should be friendly and dedicated to reducing pediatric patient anxieties.

Pediatric Dental Office

The pediatric dental office should be colorful, fun, and friendly. The reception area typically contains games, children's books, and other items for entertaining children as they wait. Small chairs and tables are often placed in a dental office reception area to help make the patient feel comfortable and welcome. Some office waiting areas may offer items such as a fish tank and TV. Plants are typically discouraged in dental offices due to possible allergies that patients and their parents may have.

Inside the pediatric office, the environment is open and not restrained. Most pediatric practices have **open bay** operatories in which the dental chairs are placed in one large room with no structural walls between the chairs. Seeing other children being treated usually makes children feel more comfortable. This office design also helps to discourage misbehaving children because they usually will not act out in front of their peers. On some occasions, a private treatment area may be required to

---

Dental Assistant | PROFESSIONAL TIP

Familiarity with the special needs of the pediatric patient is important in all areas of dentistry. Some general practices treat children if no special precautions need to be taken. It is important that all dental assistants be trained in providing care to this special population.

Preparing for Externship

When preparing for an externship in a pediatric practice, it is important for you to feel comfortable and enjoy the presence of children. You may be asked to wear colorful scrubs. Remember to keep an open mind to learn new skills from your hands-on experiences.

treat children with behavior that is disruptive to other patients.

To assist in making the pediatric dental office fun and inviting, pediatric dental team members often wear fun and vibrant colored clothing. Other ways a pediatric office may create a more child-focused environment is through the use of colorful paint and wallpaper. Cartoon themes may be utilized to assist children in feeling more relaxed (Figure 47.2).

What responsibility does the dental assistant have in maintaining the appearance of the dental office?

The Pediatric Patient

Although some people believe that the pediatric dentist only takes care of young children, this is not true. The pediatric dentist typically sees children ranging in age from infancy up to age 18. Just like adult patients, children have fears, interests, and unique personalities that must be addressed by the dental team. Communicating with children according to their mental, emotional, and chronological maturity is extremely important. As a dental assistant it is important to be familiar with the stages of childhood and how these stages can influence how the pediatric patient will respond to dental care.

Childhood Stages
Infancy through Age 2

The child in this developmental stage is learning the skills needed to become independent. Motor skills develop rapidly during the first 3 to 8 months of a child's life. These skills include rolling over at 6 months, typically crawling between 8 and 10 months, and sitting alone at about 8 months. By the age of 2 the child has begun to walk independently and even begun to run and climb stairs.

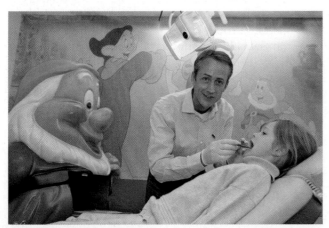

FIGURE 47.2
Pediatric treatment area.

Life Span Considerations
Always review a patient's medical and dental history for any physical conditions that could limit successful treatment. Children have short attention spans and need treatment to be as quick and efficient as possible. With the variety of ages, communicating with each child or compromised adult at their level of understanding is important.

The toddler stage, which begins at 12 to 18 months of age, is when the child begins to do some activities alone, and the struggle for **autonomy** begins to develop. The fight to become more independent is translated into the child's use of the word "no." Verbal skills are typically seen between the ages of 8 and 10 months when words such as "mama" or "dada" are spoken.

Children at this childhood stage begin to recognize familiar faces, but are still fearful of the unknown. They experience separation anxiety when their parents are not present. For this reason, it is important to ensure that parents are present during any child's treatment. Children at this stage respond well to play. If the dental assistant takes the time to establish rapport with 1- and 2-year-olds, then children's anxiety can be greatly diminished.

From about age 18 months to 2 years, children can start following simple directions from the dentist but have a very short attention span. Involvement of the parent helps to ensure that the child follows instructions for successful treatment. Children during this stage have difficulty sitting still for any period of time. Sometimes it may be important for a parent to hold the child during treatment in order to accomplish a procedure.

Ages 3 through 6

Children in this age group are considered to be in the preschool stage. Fine motor skills such as skipping, tying one's shoelaces, and throwing a ball overhand begin to develop. During this stage the child's growth rate begins to slow down and his psychosocial and cognitive development speeds up. The ability to interact with others increases as does the child's vocabulary.

Children at this age are often very curious and want to understand what is occurring. This often can be seen through the repetitive use of the question "Why?" Providing a mirror to the child to watch a simple dental cleaning can help to both relieve the child's anxieties and make the child feel as if she is assisting in the procedure (Figure 47.3). Praise and encouragement motivate children at this age. Through the utilization of praise and encouragement, children at this age will typically follow simple directions. Their attention span is a little longer than that of toddlers and they aim to please both parents and the dental team.

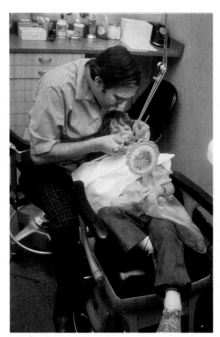

FIGURE 47.3
The pediatric patient.

Ages 7 through 9

During the school-age stage, development of socialization is important. Peer pressure begins to affect children's behavior. Their world expands greatly during this time due to the experiences acquired. Participation in school activities involving others helps children begin to learn how to accept rules and boundaries and overcome fears by gaining knowledge.

During this stage children's bodies are beginning to mature. Motor control continues to develop and fewer activities are dependent on parent participation. Cognitively, during these years children begin to develop in areas such as learning to tell time and to know the difference between current and past events. Relationships between objects can also be understood. Children at this stage can choose between right and wrong. As a dental assistant it is important for children at this stage to be praised for appropriate behavior.

Ages 10 through 12

The preadolescent stage is from the ages of 10 to 12 years. During this stage children experience rapid physical growth that includes the beginning of puberty for both boys and girls. During this stage children often feel physically awkward and unsure of their bodies. Children in the preadolescent stage are defining themselves and learning how to develop peer support groups.

Cognitively, preadolescent children can think logically but self-centered thinking is common. Children during this stage often have a false sense of immunity where they believe the concept of "it can't happen to me." It is important for the dental team to address these beliefs in

> ### Cultural Considerations
> The pediatric practice provides service to children from all cultural backgrounds. Try to become more familiar with different cultures. One cultural difference that may cause problems in dentistry because of the closeness of dental work is that of the distance between people that a particular culture prefers. The dental team can enhance knowledge of diversity by attending diversity classes or by reviewing information on the Internet about a specific culture. If there is a language barrier, ensure comprehension has occurred before beginning a dental procedure. Understanding and respecting cultural differences will enhance the dental experience for all patients.

order to assist the child in understanding how oral health issues can affect current and future dental needs.

Ages 13 through 20

The adolescent stage is the last stage of childhood and begins with the continuation of issues related to puberty that began near the end of the preadolescent stage. In this final stage of development, children are greatly concerned with appearance, usually wanting to gain knowledge about teeth and oral hygiene. As with the preadolescent stage, adolescents continue to have the "it can't happen to me" mentality. Children in adolescence also begin to question how things are done and begin to develop their own set of values and beliefs. Freedom of expression is significant to individuals in this stage.

For the dental team it is important to adolescent patients that they be treated like adults. Dental team members who belittle or speak down to the adolescent patient will have trouble gaining rapport.

Patients with Special Needs

The needs of a patient will assist in determining how and where the patient can be treated. Sometimes special needs cases cannot be completed in the dental office, and a hospital operating room has to be used. Children and some compromised adults with special needs include those

- with physical conditions,
- who have mental retardation (mild to severe), and
- with various mental disorders such as autism, Down syndrome, and cerebral palsy.

Physical Conditions

Several physical conditions might require special dental care. Categories of physical conditions that may affect the dental care of children include:

- Severe physical deformities such as those experienced by burn victims

- Cancer
- Extreme physical handicaps

Children with severe physical deformities may need to be seen in a hospital operating room. This is sometimes done in order to provide the child and the dental team as much comfort and safety as possible.

Mentally Challenged

A mental disability often begins in childhood and extends throughout life. The term *mentally disabled* refers to a child's undeveloped intelligence level, which can range from mild to severe. Mild disability describes children with IQs in the range of 50 to 70. These children generally develop social skills and can be treated in the dental office. Note, however, that comprehension levels can be affected, and dental team members must exhibit patience when working with a child who is mentally challenged.

Moderate mental disability describes children with IQs in the range of 35 to 55. These children usually can walk and talk and benefit from a special education program. They do become productive members of society, but may need special care for dental treatment. Severe mental disability describes children with IQs in the range of 20 to 40. These children usually do not communicate and may also have some type of physical disability. They will need special care for dental treatment and complete supervision as adults.

Mental Disorders

Patients with Down syndrome have an extra chromosome and exhibit mental and physical impairments (Figure 47.4). The physical characteristics of Down syndrome patients are peg-shaped teeth and almond-shaped eyes. The eruption schedule in patients with Down syndrome is commonly delayed, and they often have periodontal disease due to lack of good oral hygiene habits. Completing dental treatment depends on the mental capacity of the patient.

Cerebral palsy is a mental disorder of the central nervous system. This disorder affects the brain and motor skills of the patient and could cause seizures. Medications can be used to help relax the patient; sometimes the patient will need to be treated in the hospital for safety reasons.

Diagnosis and Treatment Planning

A pediatric examination is no different than that for an adult. A parent or legal guardian must be present with the child to complete a medical and dental history form. This form provides information regarding the child's past experiences and information on any existing allergies or medical conditions.

A child's first dental appointment should be between 12 months and 2 years of age. After the first visit the child should return twice a year for recall visits. The earlier the child is seen by a dentist, the sooner unhealthy habits can be corrected. During this appointment the dentist discusses the oral habits of the child. The main concerns of a dentist include thumb or finger sucking, bottle-feeding, pacifiers, and eating habits. Early correction of unhealthy habits can prevent some future problems with permanent teeth.

During the first examination both an intraoral and extraoral exam is performed. Charting of the teeth is also completed to evaluate the number and condition of the teeth (Figure 47.5). If decay is present at the first visit, radiographs may be taken depending on the age and cooperation of the child.

Behavior Management Techniques

It is always important to be honest with the pediatric dental patient. If a procedure is going to be a little uncomfortable, tell the patient in a way that can be understood in order to help him know what to expect. In children, fear is the main component of behavior problems. These fears are either subjective or objective. Subjective fears are developed from suggestions from other people. Objective fears are from the child's own experiences. A child's behavior can be managed in several ways:

- Using the distraction technique that refocuses the child's attention from the procedure to another source. Some pediatric offices have music or movies for children to enjoy, which can help take the child's mind off the occurring treatment.
- Use of mild sedation that includes giving the child premedication before treatment. This would be from a

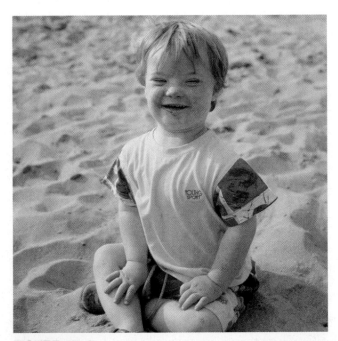

FIGURE 47.4
Child with Down syndrome.

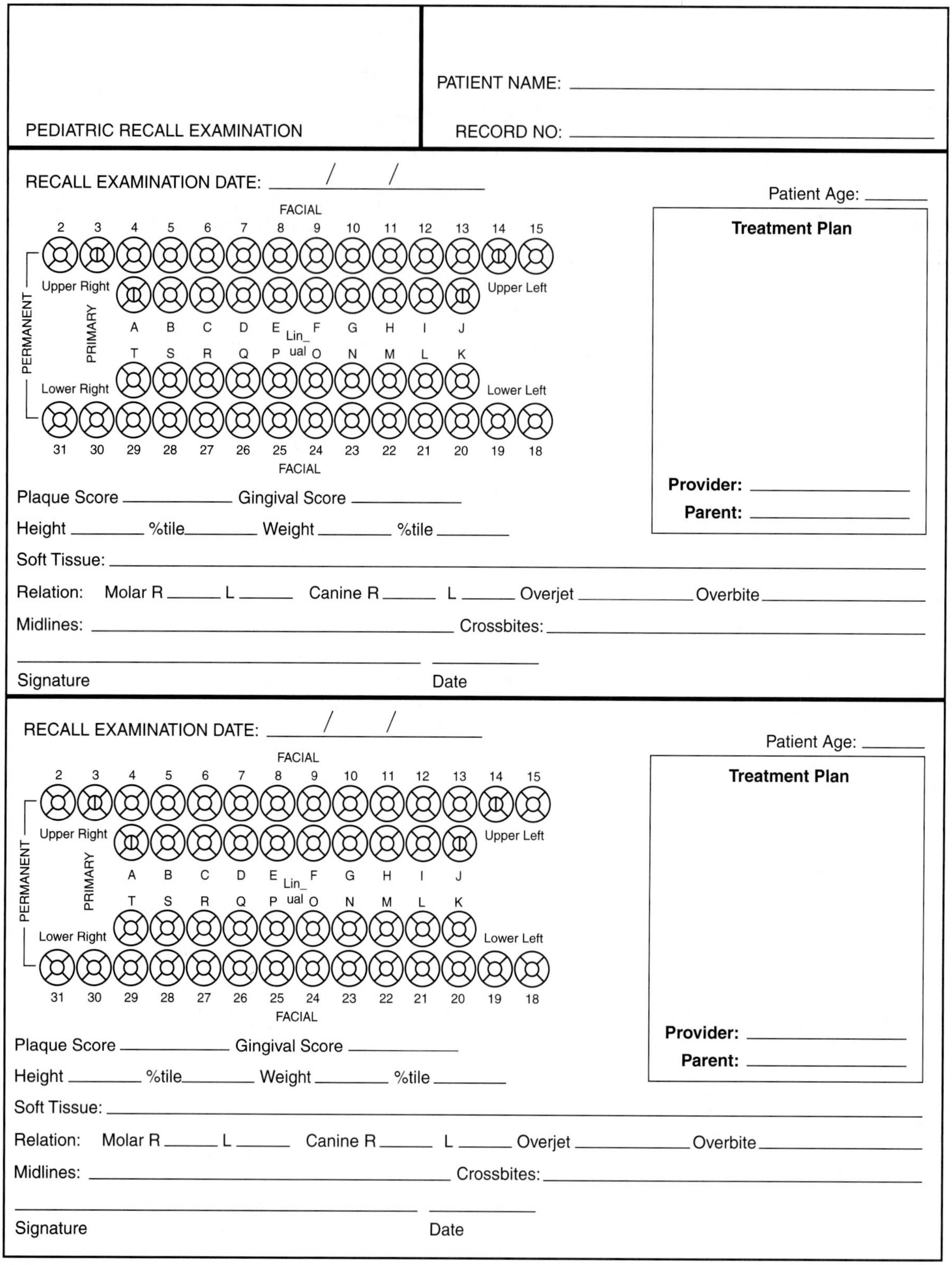

PEDIATRIC RECALL EXAMINATION

PATIENT NAME: ____________

RECORD NO: ____________

RECALL EXAMINATION DATE: ___/___/___

Patient Age: ______

FACIAL

2 3 4 5 6 7 8 9 10 11 12 13 14 15

PERMANENT — Upper Right — Upper Left

PRIMARY

A B C D E F G H I J

Lingual

T S R Q P O N M L K

Lower Right — Lower Left

31 30 29 28 27 26 25 24 23 22 21 20 19 18

FACIAL

Treatment Plan

Provider: ____________

Parent: ____________

Plaque Score ________ Gingival Score ________

Height ______ %tile______ Weight ______ %tile ______

Soft Tissue: ____________

Relation: Molar R ______ L ______ Canine R ______ L ______ Overjet ________ Overbite ________

Midlines: ____________ Crossbites: ____________

Signature ____________ Date ______

RECALL EXAMINATION DATE: ___/___/___

Patient Age: ______

FACIAL

2 3 4 5 6 7 8 9 10 11 12 13 14 15

PERMANENT — Upper Right — Upper Left

PRIMARY

A B C D E F G H I J

Lingual

T S R Q P O N M L K

Lower Right — Lower Left

31 30 29 28 27 26 25 24 23 22 21 20 19 18

FACIAL

Treatment Plan

Provider: ____________

Parent: ____________

Plaque Score ________ Gingival Score ________

Height ______ %tile______ Weight ______ %tile ______

Soft Tissue: ____________

Relation: Molar R ______ L ______ Canine R ______ L ______ Overjet ________ Overbite ________

Midlines: ____________ Crossbites: ____________

Signature ____________ Date ______

FIGURE 47.5
Pediatric chart.

prescription that the parent would administer to the child prior to arriving at the office. Common mild sedation may include a small dose of Valium. **Nitrous oxide** is another type of sedation used in the dental office before local anesthesia is given. These both help to relax the child before treatment begins.

- Modeling is effective because most children want to be the example of good behavior. This method consists of pointing out a well-behaved child to a misbehaving child.
- Gentle restraints are primarily used for safety in the office to keep children from hurting themselves or the

dental team. This is completed with the use of a **papoose board** that gently restrains the child's arms and legs (Figure 47.6). As with all methods, parental cooperation and consent is important to obtain prior to the use of any type of restraint.

- The "show and tell" technique helps to reduce anxiety by showing and explaining to the child what is going to be used *before* it is used (Figure 47.7).
- Voice control is a way to show the patient who is in charge. Note, however, that using an authoritative voice will only be effective if the child has respect for the members of the dental team.
- General anesthesia is an extreme method of behavior management that should be used only if the child is completely uncooperative and no other method has been successful. General anesthesia is generally used in a hospital setting.

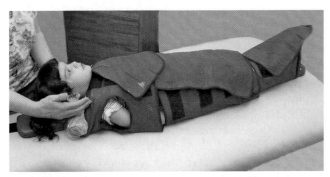

FIGURE 47.6
Papoose board.
Image courtesy Instructional Materials for the Dental Team, Lex., KY

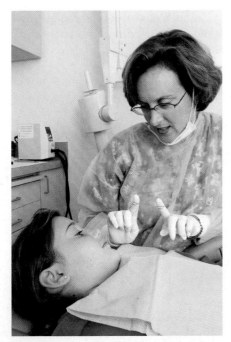

FIGURE 47.7
"Show and tell" behavior management technique.

Patient Education

Naomi is a 3-year-old girl who has been seen in Dr. Butler's office for the past year and is about to receive her first prophylaxis. As the dental assistant seats the child and begins to lean the chair back, Naomi begins to cry and ask for her mother. In this scenario you understand that the fear being expressed by this child came from not knowing what was about to happen to her. Always inform the patient before any procedure is performed. The show and tell technique can be used to reduce anxiety in children.

These methods should provide the dental team with various ways to manage different types of behaviors. Note that when utilizing behavior management techniques, it is critical for the dental team to acquire a parent or legal guardian's permission. This should be achieved verbally and in writing.

What are two behavior management techniques that can be utilized on a pediatric patient who is visiting the dental office for the first time?

Preventive Dentistry Procedures

Prevention is the key in pediatric dentistry. Correct brushing and flossing help to reduce plaque on the teeth that if not removed will turn into calculus buildup. Most children under age 10 do not have the dexterity to correctly clean all tooth surfaces. Parents play an active role in ensuring that the child's oral hygiene is addressed. Parents must be instructed and trained on both the importance of and steps for daily brushing and flossing of their children's teeth. Flossing the primary dentition, even though the teeth are not permanent, creates good habits. Once the permanent teeth do begin to erupt, children can be instructed on how to begin flossing for themselves.

As with adult dental patients, the pediatric patient may require dental care in addition to cleanings. Procedures done on the pediatric patient can include:

- Coronal polishing
- Fluoride treatments
- Placement of pit and fissure sealants
- Providing mouth guards
- Interceptive orthodontics

Coronal Polishing

Coronal polishing is a procedure completed in the dental office to remove stain and debris. The dentist, hygienist, or in some states the dental assistant uses a slow-speed handpiece with a prophy angle and polishing paste to clean the teeth. This preventive technique is completed twice annually to reduce calculus buildup and eliminate plaque accumulation. These biannual checkups help the dental team, the parents, and the child to work together to maintain good oral hygiene habits at home. (See Chapter 48 for more information about coronal polishing.)

Fluoride Treatments

Fluoride helps strengthen enamel and reduce dental decay. A child's age determines how much fluoride the child should receive. Systemic fluoride must be ingested every day during the tooth development stage for strong healthy teeth. Systemic fluoride is present in the body from various resources including foods with fluoride and water that has been fluorinated. When systemic fluoride is ingested, it circulates throughout the body and affects the developing teeth.

Fluoride has been added to most city-regulated water systems. If fluoride has not been incorporated into a city's water system, fluoride supplements should be prescribed by the dentist and given to the child on a daily basis. In addition, fluoride is applied topically twice a year after the coronal polishing procedure.

Fluoride is dispensed as a foam or gel that is placed into fluoride trays (Figure 47.8 and Procedure 47-1). Fluoride can also be dispensed as a rinse. (See Chapter 15 for more information about fluoride treatments.)

Placement of Pit and Fissure Sealants

Sealants are contained in a tooth-colored plastic covering that is placed on the occlusal surface to reduce dental decay in children. Sealants are mainly placed on newly erupted posterior permanent teeth due to the deep pits and fissures in the tooth structure. Sealants protect only the occlusal surface, so oral hygiene techniques must still be closely followed. The complete sealant procedure is

easy to accomplish on the child and no injection is required, making this preventive technique one that is favored by children and their parents. The placement of sealants has greatly reduced dental decay in children. (See Chapter 49 for more information about dental sealants.)

Mouth Guards

Children and teenagers who play sports must protect their teeth with mouth guards (Figure 47.9). Mouth guards help to prevent premature tooth loss or damage while engaging in a sport. They can be easily made in a dental office with a simple alginate impression for a custom fit. Mouth guards can also be purchased in a sporting goods store. Store-bought guards, however, do not provide as much protection or comfort as custom-fit mouth guards. Depending on the parents' preference, either type will provide at least some protection to the teeth.

Interceptive Orthodontics

Correcting oral habits and maintaining space for the eruption of the permanent teeth are common solutions for reducing or eliminating the eventual need for orthodontics. The two most common procedures performed to implement these solutions are the correction of oral habits and placement of space maintainers.

Thumb sucking and tongue thrusting are common oral habits that can be easily corrected. The correction of the thumb-sucking habit, however, is a very controversial subject. Some parents feel that the thumb is a comfort to the child, not realizing the adverse effect this habit has on the teeth. Prolonged thumb sucking causes the anterior teeth to protrude outward. The crib appliance is an example of a corrective appliance that can be placed in the patient's mouth to correct the thumb-sucking habit. Both the child and the parents are counseled to further help in the persuasion process of correcting the habit.

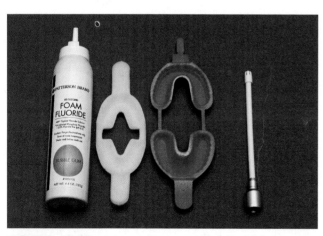

FIGURE 47.8
Fluoride trays.

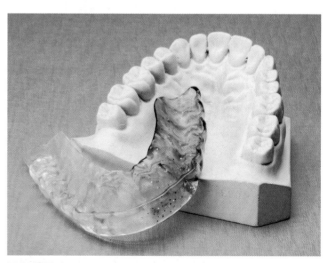

FIGURE 47.9
Mouth guard.

Procedure 47-1 Applying Fluoride for the Pediatric Patient

Dental assistants should be sure to check with their state dental practice laws to determine what tasks they are allowed to perform.

Equipment and Supplies
- Mirror, explorer, cotton pliers
- High-volume evacuator (HVE), saliva ejector, and air/water syringe
- 2 × 2 gauze sponges
- Fluoride solution (gel, foam, or rinse)
- Fluoride trays (correct size)
- Clock or watch

Procedure Steps
1. Fluoride should be applied after a coronal polish for best results.
2. Ensure the patient has no allergic reaction to fluoride (review health history).
3. Instruct patient not to swallow fluoride.
4. Place napkin and shield glasses on the patient.
5. Select correct tray size making sure all teeth are covered.
6. Place fluoride into tray about one-third full.
7. Dry patient's teeth with air or gauze sponge and instruct patient to hold the mouth open while the tray is inserted.
8. Place tray onto teeth and place saliva ejector between the maxillary and mandibular trays to remove excess fluoride.
9. Have patient close the mouth gently around the trays and saliva ejector.

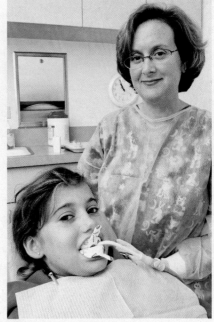
The placement of a fluoride tray.

10. Check the clock or watch for desired time according to the manufacturer's instructions.
11. When time has elapsed, remove the saliva ejector and trays from the patient's mouth.
12. Quickly remove excess fluoride from the mouth with the saliva ejector.
13. Instruct the patient not to eat, drink, or rinse for 30 minutes.
14. Document in the chart the type of fluoride used.

Tongue thrusting happens when the child's tongue pushes up against the anterior teeth during swallowing. This oral habit causes an open bite and can be corrected with therapy or an appliance.

One of the main purposes of the primary teeth is to hold the space for the permanent teeth. When primary teeth are lost prematurely due to a large amount of decay or an injury and the space is left open, the remaining primary teeth move and shift, causing severe crowding. **Space maintainers** are used to hold open the space where a primary tooth has been lost (Figure 47.10). Space maintainers are fixed or removable appliances specially designed for children. Fixed appliances are most commonly used

on children because they are cemented into place to eliminate the risk of losing the appliance.

Restorative Procedures and Equipment

Dental decay is the main reason tooth structure needs to be restored in children. Restoring primary teeth in children is very similar to restoring the teeth of adult patients. Many of the same materials and instruments are utilized. Adjusting the techniques and materials to the size of the patient is the main difference. For example, the

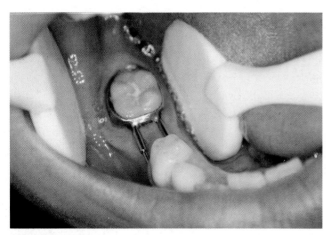

FIGURE 47.10
Space maintainer.
Image courtesy Instructional Materials for the Dental Team, Lex., KY

high-speed dental handpiece, burs, dental dam material, and dental dam clamp are all smaller in size to accommodate a child's mouth.

The restorative materials are amalgam, composite, and glass ionomers. The most commonly used material is amalgam for the posterior region although over time this may change due to some states beginning to require dentists to refrain from amalgam due to mercury involvement. Because children **exfoliate** their primary teeth, amalgam is the most cost-effective choice. For aesthetics (appearance) composite or glass ionomers are used mainly in the anterior area, but can also be used in the posterior if requested.

Matrix bands are used to replace missing walls on cavity preparations. In pediatrics, because of the smaller tooth size, custom matrices are more commonly used. One type is called **T-bands** (Figure 47.11), which are used on Class II restorations. T-bands are used without retainers and are made of brass strips. Spot-welded matrix bands are used on children. These are used without

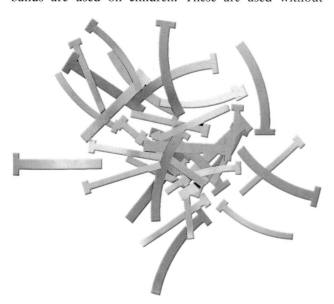

FIGURE 47.11
T-bands.
Courtesy Pulpdent Corporation

retainers and are custom fit with the use of a welding machine. Dental dams are used on children to help keep debris from falling back into the child's throat, to increase visibility, and to control the tongue during treatment. The smaller size 5 × 5 dental dam is commonly used on children.

Endodontic Procedures

Deep decay or injuries that involve the pulp of the tooth may require special treatment. Depending on the vitality of the tooth, the dentist can choose among three treatments: pulpotomy, pulpectomy, or extraction. The degree of infection determines the procedure needed.

In a **vital tooth**, a **pulpotomy** can be completed in which part of the tooth will remain vital or alive. When inflammation and infection are confined to the coronal portion of the pulp, a pulpotomy is recommended. A pulpotomy is the procedure for the pulp that has been exposed to infection only in the pulp chamber of a tooth. During a pulpotomy the pulp is removed from the **coronal** portion, leaving the pulp in the canals, which keeps the tooth vital (Procedure 47-2).

Near-pulp exposure is the condition in which the pulp has not yet been exposed, but the infection is close to it. Treatment includes removing the decay and placing a base of medication in an attempt to heal the pulp and to produce secondary dentin.

A **nonvital tooth** is one in which the pulp tissue is diseased or dead. A **pulpectomy** is the treatment used for a nonvital tooth when an infection has exposed the entire pulp in the crown and the root of the tooth (coronal and radicular) and must be completely removed.

In some cases the pulpotomy and pulpectomy procedures may fail. In such cases an extraction would be indicated.

Prosthodontic Procedures

Pediatric prosthodontic procedures are very simple compared to prosthodontic procedures in adults. For children, complete crown coverage is accomplished with stainless steel crowns. Stainless steel crowns are indicated for extreme decay, fractures, **decalcification**, and succeeding pulpectomy and pulpotomy procedures.

Crowns are used on both primary and permanent teeth and can be purchased in a set or separate with a variety of sizes from which to choose. Before a crown is placed, it must be contoured by the dentist. The dentist uses contouring pliers, scissors, and burs of choice to prepare the crown for placement. After preparation of the crown, it is permanently cemented into the mouth (Procedure 47-3).

Stainless steel is used on children because of its durability. Crowns are strong enough to last in the mouth until primary teeth are replaced with permanent ones. The use of stainless steel crowns on permanent teeth is for

Procedure 47-2 Assisting with a Pulpotomy on a Pediatric Patient

Dental assistants should be sure to check with their state dental practice laws to determine what tasks they are allowed to perform.

Equipment and Supplies

- Dental dam setup
- Cotton pellets, medication (formocresol)
- Anesthetic
- Cement (IRM or ZOE)
- Composite, amalgam, or stainless steel crown setup
- Burs (dentist's preference)

Procedure Steps

1. Place topical and dispense anesthetic.

2. Put on dental dam.

3. With a high-speed handpiece, access the pulp chamber through the occlusal surface of the tooth.

4. Remove the coronal portion of the pulp with the spoon excavator.

5. Dip cotton pellet into formocresol bottle, blot off excess with 2 × 2 gauze, and place inside pulp cavity for 5 minutes.

6. Remove cotton. Rinse and dry pulp cavity.

7. Prepare cement to a thick base consistency and put a layer over remaining pulp.

8. Place the restorative material (temporary or permanent) or stainless steel crown.

9. Remove the dental dam and check occlusion with articulating paper. Tip the patient's chin toward the floor to alleviate swallowing of the fluoride.

10. Freshen patient's mouth (rinse and dry).

11. Provide postoperative instructions to the patient and his/her parent or guardian.

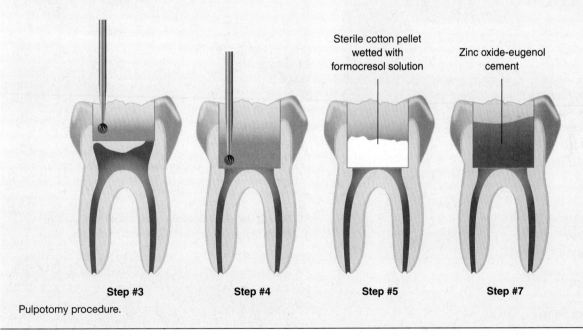

Sterile cotton pellet wetted with formocresol solution

Zinc oxide-eugenol cement

Step #3   Step #4   Step #5   Step #7

Pulpotomy procedure.

temporary purposes only. When the child becomes an adult, the crown must be replaced with a gold or porcelain crown. In rare cases dentures and partials can be constructed for children.

Dental Trauma

Accidents in children and adolescents are inevitable no matter how much precaution is taken. Dental injuries are a common sight in the pediatric practice. Dental injuries must be treated because the developing permanent teeth may be affected by an injury. The majority of injuries happen during the toddler years of life, but no child is exempt from a dental injury. The most common emergencies include fractures, traumatic intrusion, avulsed teeth, and displaced teeth.

Fractures (Figure 47.12), usually of the anterior teeth, are a common sight in pediatric practices. The

Procedure 47-3 Assisting with Placement of Stainless Steel Crowns on a Pediatric Patient

Dental assistants should be sure to check with their state dental practice laws to determine what tasks they are allowed to perform.

Equipment and Supplies

- Explorer, mirror, cotton pliers, spoon excavator, crown and bridge scissors, spatula, contouring pliers, articulating paper holder
- High- and slow-speed handpieces
- Diamond burs, green stones, polishing wheels
- Various sizes of stainless steel crowns
- 2 × 2 gauze sponges
- Cotton rolls
- Paper pad and cement
- Floss
- High-volume evacuator (HVE), saliva ejector
- Articulating paper

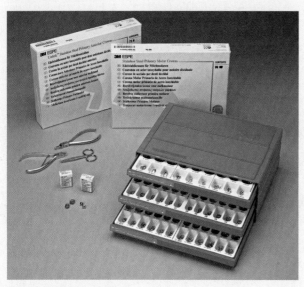

Stainless steel crown kit.
Courtesy 3M ESPE

Procedure Steps

1. Place topical in the *muccobuccal* fold. The dentist will dispense anesthetic near tooth to be restored.

2. Remove decay and reduce elevation and perimeter structure of the tooth with diamond burs.

3. Select correct size stainless steel crown for prepared tooth and place on tooth to ensure fit.

4. Use the crown and bridge scissors to adjust the height of the crown, making contact with the mesial and distal surfaces. Try adjusted crown on tooth to ensure fit.

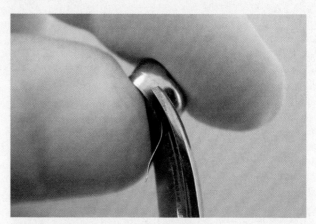

Stainless steel crown selected and trimmed.
Image courtesy Instructional Materials for the Dental Team, Lex., KY

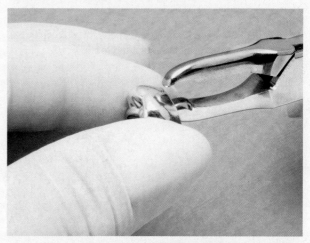

Crown contoured with contouring pliers and margins crimped with crimping tool.

5. Smooth jagged edges made by the scissors with a green stone and adjust shape with contouring pliers.

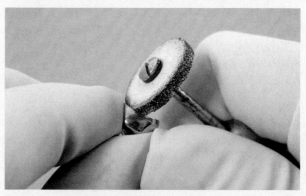

Crown margins smoothed with green stone.
Image courtesy Instructional Materials for the Dental Team, Lex., KY

continued on next page

Procedure 47-3 *continued from previous page*

6. Polish smooth with polishing wheels.

7. Seat crown on the tooth. Check bite with the articulating paper.

8. Mix permanent cement and place it inside the crown. Pass the crown to the dentist, who seats it in position. Ask the patient to bite down on a cotton roll.

9. Once the cement is dry, remove excess cement around the gingival margin with an explorer. Remove interproximal cement with floss by snapping between contacts, gliding the floss back and forth in the embrasure area to dislodge excess cement, and pulling the floss out toward the buccal side instead of back out through the contact.

10. Provide a final rinse to remove any small pieces of cement and refresh the patient's mouth.

11. Provide postoperative instructions to the patient and his/her parent or guardian.

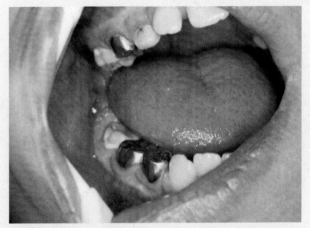
Crown placed on tooth.
Image courtesy Instructional Materials for the Dental Team, Lex., KY

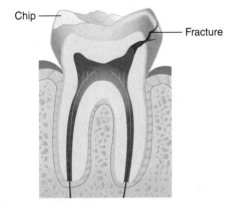
FIGURE 47.12
Tooth with a fracture and a chip.

dentist examines the teeth and documents the injury, and then performs tests on the tooth or teeth to determine vitality. Radiographs are taken to further assess the injury, and treatment will vary depending on the condition of the tooth. Fractures cause pulpal exposure and require immediate attention. At the emergency appointment, the pulp can be treated if needed but commonly the dentist will give the tooth a few months to heal before any further treatment is done. Once the tooth has completely healed, a permanent restoration is placed.

Traumatic intrusion occurs when the teeth are forced back into the **alveolus** with only part of the crown visible. In primary teeth this could cause infection or injury to the developing permanent tooth. This is the most severe type of injury because the alveolar socket is fractured and the periodontal ligament crushed, which could result in a ruptured blood vessel.

If the intrusion is 3 mm or less there is a good chance the tooth will re-erupt. If the intrusion is more than 6 mm, there is a greater chance of pulpal necrosis (death of pulp). In 96% of traumatic intrusion cases, pulpal necrosis occurs and eventually a pulpectomy is required. Allowing the tooth or teeth to re-erupt back into the mouth is the treatment of choice.

An **avulsed** tooth occurs when an entire tooth is forcibly knocked out of the dental socket. Immediate replanting of the tooth by a parent or guardian increases the tooth's long-term prognosis. If it is not replanted immediately, the tooth should be placed in a solution called Hank's balanced salt solution. This solution is the preferred solution because its chemical content is designed to keep the periodontal ligament alive. If this solution is not available, the tooth can be placed in milk, water, or a saline solution to keep it moist.

The avulsed tooth should never be scrubbed clean or washed. A gentle rinsing is sufficient. If the tooth is scrubbed, the periodontal ligaments may be disturbed or even removed, which reduces the ability of the tooth to reattach to the tooth socket.

The patient will need to see a dentist within 45 minutes if the replanting process is to succeed. After replanting the tooth, it will need to be splinted and may require a pulpectomy after healing. (See Chapter 44 for more information regarding endodontic procedures.) Replanting is not always successful, depending on the condition of the periodontal ligament. This treatment is completed only for permanent teeth. Primary teeth are not replanted because damage to the developing permanent teeth and the ligaments could occur. Therefore, if a primary tooth is avulsed, the treatment is to allow the socket to heal and to place a space maintainer where the tooth was. Once the eruption of the permanent tooth has occurred, the tooth's condition is evaluated and the need for further treatment is determined.

A displaced tooth occurs when a tooth is pushed from its original position. This causes severe periodontal ligament damage, and the tooth or teeth must be closely observed for vitality. The dentist will reposition the tooth and place a splint to hold it in position until complete healing has taken place, which occurs in about four to six weeks. After the tooth has healed, it is tested for vitality and treated accordingly. Avulsed and displaced tooth injuries are commonly found in the anterior area of the mouth and are typically caused by some type of fall the patient has experienced.

Reporting Child Abuse and Neglect

The subject of child abuse and neglect is a sensitive but important one. The dental team must be alert to protect children from abuse and neglect. Types of abuse include sexual, physical, emotional, and mental. Abused children may have injuries that will stand out to the dental team. Signs or signals to watch for are bruises or burns on the child's body and scars in the mouth or broken teeth. Neglect is a little harder to detect, but some signs may be visible to dental personnel. Children who have extensive decay, lack of hygiene, and who are not dressed appropriately for the weather may be exhibiting signs of neglect.

If any signs of abuse or neglect are suspected, the dental office policy regarding the reporting of child abuse or neglect should be followed. In a dental office typically the dentist must make the report to the state social services office or the police because he or she is the owner of the practice. Reports can also be anonymously submitted to the appropriate officials.

Once the suspicion has been reported to the authorities, a complete investigation is completed. Due to the severe consequences of abuse and neglect, the dental team should look for patterns of abuse or neglect over a period of time. If a dental assistant is suspicious of possible abuse or neglect, the information should be documented in the patient's chart and the information should be shared confidentially with the dentist. Remember that children play and can easily fall and injure themselves. A false accusation could traumatize an entire family.

What steps should the dental team take if a 3-year-old child is seen in the dental office with possible cigarette burns on the arms and cuts on the face?

SUMMARY

In this chapter we have discussed dental treatment for children, including prevention procedures and restoring and maintaining both primary and permanent teeth. The dental team must have a caring and compassionate attitude toward children and their needs. The dental assistant must show confidence to gain authority over the child and be the educator for both the patient and parents. Providing appropriate care to the pediatric dental patient is critical to having healthy teeth as an adult. The dental assistant can assist in ensuring that the pediatric patient has a positive experience at the dental office. This positive experience will translate into improved dental hygiene as a child and later as an adult.

Professionalism

Dentistry is a professional field and should always be treated as one. Professionalism begins with your appearance and attitude. Remember to leave your personal concerns outside of the office, and show respect to the doctor by referring to him or her by the doctor's last name only such as "Dr. Stackhouse." Show cooperation with coworkers by being a team player, and handle concerns professionally by following the chain of command.

KEY TERMS

- **Alveolus:** The socket of a tooth.   p. 759
- **Autonomy:** Independent functioning.   p. 749
- **Avulsed tooth:** A tooth forcibly separated from its socket.   p. 759
- **Coronal:** The portion of the tooth that can be seen clinically.   p. 756
- **Decalcification:** The removal of calcium salts from bone or teeth.   p. 756
- **Exfoliate:** The process of shedding the primary set of teeth.   p. 756
- **Nitrous oxide:** An inhaled flammable anesthetic and analgesic gas.   p. 752
- **Nonvital tooth:** Tooth in which the pulp tissue is diseased or dead.   p. 756
- **Open bay:** A room arrangement in which the dental chairs are placed in one large room with no structural walls between the chairs.   p. 748

- **Papoose board:** A restraint used for the safety of children.   p. 753
- **Pulpectomy:** Complete removal of all pulp tissues.   p. 756
- **Pulpotomy:** Removal of pulp tissue in the crown portion only.   p. 756
- **Space maintainers:** Appliance placed in the dental arch to prevent adjacent teeth from moving into space left by a missing tooth.   p. 755
- **T-bands:** A retainer free matrix made of brass; commonly used on primary teeth.   p. 756
- **Traumatic intrusion:** Tooth forcibly driven into the alveolus with only a part of the crown visible.   p. 759
- **Vital tooth:** Alive or healthy pulp tissue.   p. 756

CHECK YOUR UNDERSTANDING

1. Which specialty practice provides dental care for children and compromised adults?
   a. general dentistry
   b. endodontics
   c. pediatric dentistry
   d. orthodontics

2. What type of office design is a large open room with several chairs?
   a. reading room
   b. open bay
   c. quiet room
   d. study room

3. At what age should a child first visit the dentist?
   a. 12 months to 2 years
   b. 3 years to 6 years
   c. 2 years to 5 years
   d. 8 years to 12 years

4. What is a child's objective fear based on?
   a. child's own experience
   b. attitudes from others
   c. suggestions from others
   d. none of the above

5. Which behavior management technique names an instrument and demonstrates its usage?
   a. voice control
   b. subjective
   c. show and tell
   d. nonverbal

6. What should children who are involved in contact sports be custom fitted for?
   a. mouth guard
   b. space maintainer
   c. stainless steel crown
   d. all of the above

7. Which oral habit are crib appliances used to correct?
   a. tongue thrusting
   b. nail biting
   c. thumb sucking
   d. bruxism

8. Name the procedure that completely removes the pulp of a primary tooth.
   a. pulpotomy
   b. pulpectomy
   c. direct pulp capping
   d. apexogenesis

9. When a tooth is forcibly driven into the alveolus with only a part of the crown visible this is called what?
   a. traumatic intrusion
   b. displaced tooth
   c. avulsed tooth
   d. fracture

10. To whom should dentists report signs of child abuse?
    a. police
    b. social services
    c. both a and b
    d. none of the above

◉ INTERNET ACTIVITIES

- To gain further knowledge regarding pediatrics within the general practice, visit the Academy of General Dentistry's site at www.agd.org

- To learn more about the health of children's teeth, visit Kid's Health for Parents at http://kidshealth.org

◉ WEB REFERENCES

- American Academy of Pediatric Dentistry   www.aapd.org
- WebMD   www.webmd.com

48

Coronal Polishing

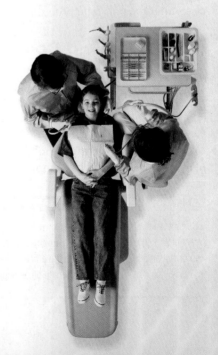

Learning Objectives

After reading this chapter, the student should be able to:

- Discuss the indications and contraindications for coronal polishing.
- Define selective polishing.
- Discuss polishing abrasives for aesthetic restorations.
- List and explain dental stains.
- Describe types of abrasives and uses for each.
- Explain dental handpieces and their attachments for coronal polishing.
- List the sequence of steps for coronal polishing.
- Explain the importance of flossing after polishing.
- Discuss the evaluation process after polishing.

Preparing for Certification Exams

- Receive and prepare patients for treatment, including seating, positioning the chair, and placing the napkin.
- Perform coronal polishing procedures.
- Identify features of rotary instruments.

Key Terms

Clinical crown

Endogenous stains

Exogenous stains

Extrinsic stain

Fulcrum

Intrinsic stains

Prophylaxis

Subgingival

Supragingival

Chapter Outline

- Coronal Polishing
  - Indications and Contraindications for Coronal Polishing
  - Selective Polishing
  - Polishing Aesthetic Restorations
- Dental Stains
- Coronal Polishing Materials and Equipment
  - Abrasives
  - Prophylaxis Angle and Handpiece
- Coronal Polishing Steps
  - Sequence of Polishing
  - Flossing After Polishing
  - Evaluation of Polishing

Coronal polishing is a proce-

dure that involves the removal of plaque and stain buildup on the crown surfaces of teeth. Coronal polishing is mainly utilized for cosmetic reasons, but can also be used as a tool to improve overall oral hygiene. This procedure involves using a slow-speed handpiece, a prophy angle with a rubber cup or brush, a basic setup (mirror, explorer, and cotton pliers), scalers, a disclosing agent, and a polishing agent. To efficiently assist the dentist or dental hygienist in the coronal polishing treatment, the dental assistant must be familiar with the procedure, the equipment, and the materials used.

Coronal Polishing

Coronal polishing is only one part of the **prophylaxis** procedure. A dental prophylaxis includes the complete removal of plaque, debris, and stains from the teeth. The complete prophylaxis procedure can only be performed by a hygienist or dentist. In some states a registered, certified, or expanded functions dental assistant can perform a coronal polish.

Coronal polishing includes removing **extrinsic stains** and soft deposits from the **clinical crown**. To make these stains more visible to the naked eye, disclosing agents can be used. Disclosing agents are made of a vegetable dye that stains the plaque present in the mouth red. This helps to educate patients about how to improve their brushing techniques, and it helps the operator ensure that all teeth are clean after the polishing procedure has been completed.

Indications and Contraindications for Coronal Polishing

There are several reasons, or indications, for why a patient may need a coronal polish. There are also contraindications that indicate when a patient should not be given this treatment.

Indications for coronal polishing include removal of plaque and stain so that a smooth surface results, there-

Cultural Considerations

Oral hygiene habits vary in different cultures. When caring for patients from other cultures, you need to be sensitive to the different beliefs you may come across. Teach all patients the importance of being proactive instead of reactive in their hygiene habits.

fore reducing plaque accumulation. Coronal polishing is also performed to prepare the teeth for placement of orthodontic bands, brackets, and enamel sealants. Fluoridated polishing paste is not recommended for these purposes. Coronal polishing can help to encourage patients to maintain good oral hygiene habits.

Many conditions could contraindicate a coronal polish. Contraindications for coronal polishing include the following:

- There is not enough stain present on the patient's teeth.
- The patient has a high risk of decay and has thin or malformed enamel.
- The patient's teeth are sensitive. In such a case, polishing is avoided because the polishing paste can cause the teeth to be more sensitive.
- The patient has had various types of restorations. Coronal polishing can leave scratches on gold, composite, acrylic, and porcelain restorations.

Selective Polishing

To evaluate a patient to determine if polishing is necessary, the dentist, hygienist, or dental assistant evaluates each tooth for stains ranging from mild to severe. Polishing that does not have to be done on all the teeth but rather on a few that are visibly stained is called selective polishing. Selective polishing is a procedure in which teeth are chosen for polishing according to the visibility of stain that is present.

Teeth that have no stain present are not polished to reduce unnecessary reduction of the fluoride-rich layer of enamel. Studies have shown that due to the abrasiveness of the polishing pastes used in dentistry a thin layer of enamel is lost each time a coronal polish is completed. Using the technique of selective polishing helps reduce stain buildup on stained teeth without losing enamel on unstained teeth.

After the stained teeth have been polished with a fine abrasive agent or brushed with a toothbrush and toothpaste, the remaining teeth are then polished with an extra fine abrasive to complete the coronal polishing procedure.

Polishing Aesthetic Restorations

When polishing aesthetic restorations, special care must be taken because of the delicate materials used to restore the teeth. Porcelain and composite restorations can be easily scratched by abrasive polishing agents. The restorations must first be identified as porcelain. Today, with the modern technology used in dentistry, many aesthetic restorations appear similar to natural tooth structure, which makes it difficult for the operator to identify natural teeth from restorations.

Prior to performing a polish on aesthetic restorations, it is important to examine the patient's mouth to chart where restorations are present. Once restorations have been located, they should first be polished with a mild abrasive agent or a special paste made for aesthetic restorations. Once this initial step has been completed, the remaining teeth can be polished.

Dental Stains

Dental deposits can be classified as any deposit or stain on the tooth structure and are considered either hard or soft. Stains can be located above the gingival tissues (**supragingival**) or below the gingival tissues (**subgingival**). Soft deposits consist of food debris or plaque and can be removed by coronal polishing. Hard deposits such as calculus, commonly referred to as *tartar*, need to be removed from the tooth structure by scaling both below and above the gingival tissue.

Dental stains are primarily an aesthetic concern. Most individuals are concerned with the appearance of their smile. A big smile can indicate confidence in one's appearance. Those who feel uncomfortable smiling may be experiencing this discomfort due to the appearance of their teeth.

Stains form as a result of several different causes. Some stains can be removed, whereas others cannot. Dental stains fall into two categories, either **endogenous stains** or **exogenous stains**. Knowing the difference between these two categories helps the dental assistant correctly inform patients about the treatments available to them. Endogenous stains are caused from disturbances during tooth development such as excessive amounts of fluoride (fluorosis) (Figure 48.1), medications given to a pregnant mother, or medications given during the devel-

opment of teeth. For example, if a child who is developing teeth is given the antibiotic tetracycline, the child's teeth could sustain a stain. This stain would not be able to be removed with coronal polishing (Figure 48.2).

Exogenous stains are caused by environmental sources. These types of stains can be further divided into two additional categories: **intrinsic stains** and extrinsic stains. The type of stain determines if the stain can be removed or not. Intrinsic stains are formed within the tooth structure and the stain becomes a part of the tooth structure. A nonvital tooth stain is a type of intrinsic stain. This stain occurs when the pulp is damaged. Extrinsic stains develop from outside sources such as food, drinks, or poor oral hygiene. Examples of extrinsic stains include brown, yellow, green, black, tobacco, orange, and chlorhexidine stains. Intrinsic stains cannot be removed with coronal polishing or scaling. Table 48-1 summarizes the types of intrinsic and extrinsic stains.

Brown and yellow stains are both associated with patients who have poor oral hygiene. These stains are commonly affiliated with an accumulation of plaque buildup that, if not removed, turns into calculus. Brown and yellow stains usually appear on the buccal and lingual surfaces of maxillary and mandibular teeth.

Green stains are found more often in children than adults and are often caused by poor oral hygiene. Green stains are located at the cervical third of the anterior teeth and are removable with scaling and polishing. Care must

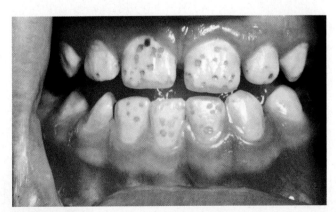

FIGURE 48.1
Severe fluorosis.

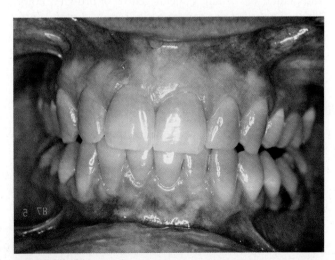

FIGURE 48.2
Tetracycline stain.

TABLE 48-1 Intrinsic and Extrinsic Stains

Intrinsic Stains	Description
Dental fluorosis	Brown and white spots of discoloration caused by ingestion of excessive fluoride during tooth development
Tetracycline	Gray to green stain caused by use of the antibiotic tetracycline during pregnancy while the teeth of the fetus are developing
Extrinsic Stains	
Brown	Can appear yellow to brown; caused by poor oral hygiene
Tobacco	Black to dark brown stain caused by the contents of the tobacco product
Green	Appears green and is caused by bacteria buildup from poor oral hygiene

be taken with removal of green stains due to the possible presence of decalcified enamel under the stain.

Black stains are normally found in female patients with good oral hygiene and are caused by natural sources. They appear at the gingival margin and are sometimes more difficult to remove.

Tobacco stains are the result of the tar combustion that occurs during cigarette smoking. This type of stain imbeds into the pits and fissures of the enamel, leaving a brown or black stain. The severity of the stain depends on the patient's oral hygiene habits.

Orange stains are usually seen on the lingual and facial surfaces of anterior teeth close to the gingival margin. These stains are thought to be caused by chromogenic bacteria that are often related to use of antibiotics.

Chlorhexidine stains are caused from the extended use of mouth rinses and toothpaste containing chlorhexidine. This stain can adhere to the tongue, restorations, and plaque and usually appears yellow or brown in color. These types of stains can be easily removed with toothbrushing or coronal polishing once the chlorhexidine usage has ended.

Patient Education

Many patients are concerned with the appearance of their teeth. For this reason, most patients are usually willing to listen to any tips given on how to keep their teeth white and healthy and reduce stain buildup. Extrinsic stains are easier to control than intrinsic stains by changing the patient's diet or oral habits. Intrinsic stains may need additional cosmetic dental care. Equipping patients with this information may help them to reduce stain buildup resulting in a whiter smile.

Coronal Polishing Materials and Equipment

To perform a coronal polish, various types of supplies are needed. The equipment needed to perform a coronal polishing procedure includes a slow-speed handpiece, a prophy angle, prophy brushes, a polishing cup, and abrasive materials (Figure 48.3).

Abrasives

Abrasives are materials that are used to remove dental stain and debris from the teeth. They are available in powders and pastes that are premixed or can be mixed in the office with water or mouthwash to form a paste. The paste must be moist when used to reduce the amount of friction generated by the handpiece on the tooth structure.

The pastes range in abrasiveness from extra fine to extra coarse. The paste with the least amount of abrasiveness that will effectively remove the stain should be selected. Because abrasives remove small amounts of enamel and could damage the gingival tissues, the finer abrasive agents should be tried first. Using finer abrasives more frequently than coarser abrasives will reduce enamel loss.

The types of abrasives that are commonly used are chalk, zirconium silicate, superfine silex, fine pumice, and silex. Chalk and zirconium are mild abrasives that do not abrade the tooth structure. Silicate and superfine silex are medium abrasives that remove light to medium stains. Silex is the most abrasive agent and is used to remove heavy stains.

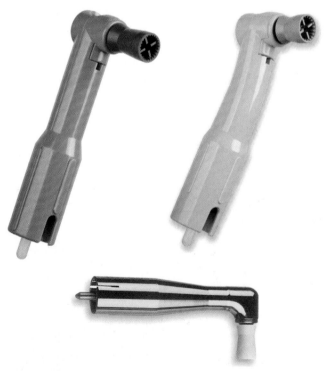

FIGURE 48.3
Disposable prophy angles with polishing cups.
Courtesy Young Dental

The use of an abrasive agent is only part of the stain removal process. The rate of abrasion impacts the ability to remove stains. The rate of abrasion is the force that is placed on the prophy cup through the handpiece. The pressure placed on the foot control (rheostat) determines the rotation speed of the cup.

Why should a dental assistant choose a mild abrasive for removing light stain buildup from a patient's teeth?

Prophylaxis Angle and Handpiece

One piece of equipment necessary to perform a coronal polish is the prophy angle. The prophy angle, which attaches to the slow-speed handpiece, can be either reusable or disposable. A reusable prophy angle must be sterilized and lubricated after each use; therefore, a disposable angle is more commonly used. The disposable prophy angle comes with the cup or brush already attached for convenience.

The polishing cup and prophy brush are both used during coronal polishing. The polishing cup attaches to the prophy angle (see Figure 48.3). The polishing cup is made of either natural soft flexible rubber or a synthetic material. Synthetic cups are used as an alternative for patients with latex allergies. The polishing cup is used prior to the use of the prophy brush. The prophy brush is used to clean the occlusal surfaces of posterior teeth.

When attaching the prophy angle to the handpiece, it is important to ensure that it is connected correctly. Once the attachment is secure, the handpiece is held in a modified pen grasp (Figure 48.4). The modified pen grasp can be described as holding the handpiece in a position similar to that used when writing. The fingers should be close to the prophy angle attachment with the remaining body of the handpiece resting on the hand between the thumb and forefinger.

After proper positioning has been accomplished, the operator must establish a **fulcrum** or finger-stabilizing point. A fulcrum provides stability for the operator and safety for the patient. The dental assistant uses two different types of fulcrums: intraoral and extraoral. The fulcrum will change depending on the tooth being polished.

When both position and stability have been established, the procedure is performed effectively and efficiently. When operating the handpiece, speed and technique are important. The slow-speed electric handpiece is controlled by a rheostat and rotates at a maximum of 20,000 revolutions per second, which produces heat that could cause pulp damage. Therefore, this procedure is technique sensitive. Finding the correct speed and pressure takes some practice. When the correct speed has been achieved, the sound emitted is a smooth even tone with no whine or whistle being heard.

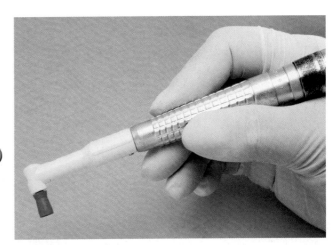

FIGURE 48.4
Modified pen grasp.

With steady even pressure on the polishing cup, the cup flares to reach into the gingival margin (Figure 48.5). An on/off motion is used to keep the cup moving on the tooth structure. This stroke overlaps to ensure complete tooth coverage (Figure 48.6). Only two to six seconds should be spent on each tooth, utilizing a substantial amount of paste to reduce friction. For instance, a full prophy cup of paste is only enough to clean two or three teeth.

Why is correct positioning and speed so important when using the prophy angle and handpiece?

Coronal Polishing Steps

Before beginning a coronal polishing procedure, both the patient and operator must be positioned correctly. Proper positioning helps to prevent injury and also operator and

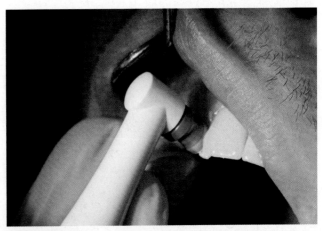

FIGURE 48.5
Example of rubber cup placement.
Image courtesy Instructional Materials for the Dental Team, Lex., KY

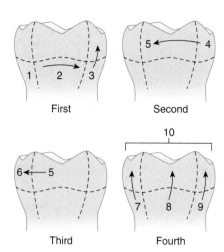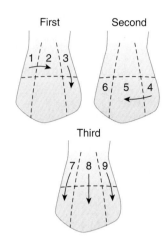

FIGURE 48.6
Polishing strokes for posterior and anterior teeth.

patient fatigue. The patient should be positioned according to the arch being cleaned. When the mandibular arch is being cleaned, the lower jaw is positioned parallel to the floor (Figure 48.7). The dental chair is adjusted to a 90-degree angle so that the operator is looking down on the arch. The headrest can be adjusted for the patient's comfort. To clean the maxillary arch, the patient's position is supine (completely lying flat) and the chin is slightly tilted upward (Figure 48.8). The operator's position depends on whether the operator is right- or left-handed. Figure 48.9 shows a right-handed operator seated in the correct position.

Sequence of Polishing

When completing a coronal polishing procedure, a system should be established to ensure no areas of the mouth are missed (Procedure 48-1). Development of the system can be left up to the operator. One suggestion is to begin in the upper right quadrant starting on

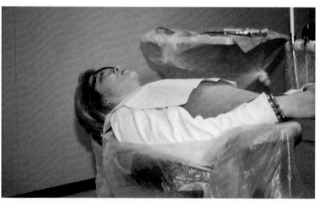

FIGURE 48.8
Patient's head positioned for polishing the maxillary arch.
Image courtesy Instructional Materials for the Dental Team, Lex., KY

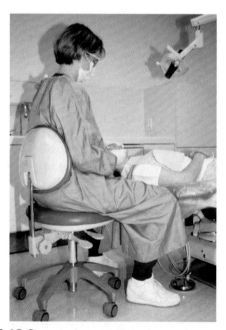

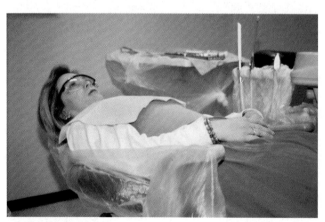

FIGURE 48.7
Patient's head positioned for polishing the mandibular arch.
Image courtesy Instructional Materials for the Dental Team, Lex., KY

FIGURE 48.9
A right-handed operator seated in the correct position.
Image courtesy Instructional Materials for the Dental Team, Lex., KY

Procedure 48-1 Performing a Coronal Polish

Equipment and Supplies

- Mirror, explorer, cotton pliers
- Saliva ejector, air/water tip
- Disclosing agent (liquid or tablet)
- Polishing paste (fine or extra fine)
- Dental floss
- Bridge threader
- 2 × 2 gauze squares
- Cotton tip applicator
- Prophy angle (disposable or sterile)
- Prophy brush (disposable or sterile)
- Slow-speed handpiece
- Patient hand mirror
- Patient toothbrush
- Red or blue pencil and dental tooth chart

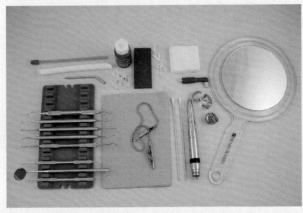

Coronal polishing supplies.
Image courtesy Instructional Materials for the Dental Team, Lex., KY

Procedure Steps

1. Review the patient's medical and dental history.

2. Greet and seat the patient. Place a napkin and eyewear on the patient and explain the procedure to the patient.

3. Check the patient's oral cavity for appliances and abnormal lumps or lesions (remove appliances).

4. Use a cotton tip applicator to place disclosing agent on the facial, buccal, lingual, and occlusal surfaces.

5. Once all tooth structures have been covered with the disclosing agent, rinse the patient's mouth.

6. Use a hand mirror to show the patient where plaque is present.

7. Identify on the dental tooth chart with red pencil the surfaces the patient has been missing when brushing. Provide the tooth chart to the patient when polishing is finished to review and correct missed areas.

8. Take the toothbrush and have the patient hold the hand mirror while you show the patient how to correctly clean all tooth surfaces.

9. Pick up the prophy angle and fill the prophy cup with polishing paste; spread the paste across up to three teeth to polish.

10. The operator can begin in the right maxillary quadrant on the posterior teeth or wherever the operator chooses as long as no areas are missed. Establish a fulcrum on the incisors or close to the area on which the operator is working. Use a mouth mirror for retraction.

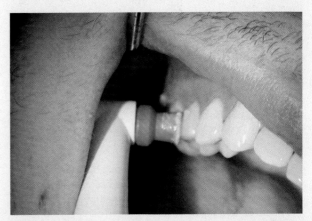

Polishing position on the maxillary right anterior facial surface.
Image courtesy Instructional Materials for the Dental Team, Lex., KY

11. Moving from the right maxillary posterior toward the anterior facial surface, retract the lip with a finger and establish a fulcrum on the teeth next to the tooth being polished.

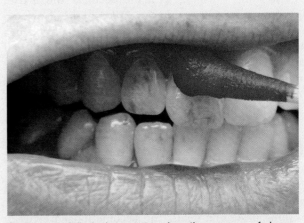

Application of disclosing agent to show the presence of plaque.
Image courtesy Instructional Materials for the Dental Team, Lex., KY

continued on next page

Procedure 48-1 *continued from previous page*

12. When the midline is reached, switch over onto the lingual surface of the maxillary right central moving toward the posterior area, using the mirror for indirect vision and making the fulcrum on the buccal surfaces of the maxillary.

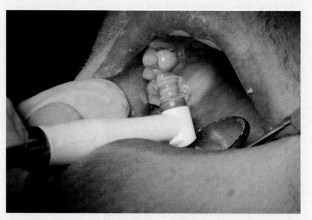

Polishing position on the maxillary right anterior lingual surface.
Image courtesy Instructional Materials for the Dental Team, Lex., KY

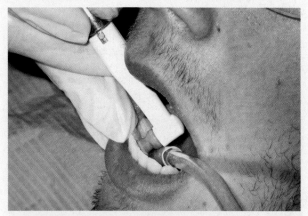

Polishing position on the maxillary right posterior buccal surface.
Image courtesy Instructional Materials for the Dental Team, Lex., KY

13. After polishing the last lingual surface of the most posterior tooth present, move onto the occlusal surface and polish the pits and fissures of the teeth moving from posterior to anterior. (A prophy brush can be used to clean this surface.)

14. When the midline is reached, rinse the patient's mouth two or three times and repeat steps until all quadrants have been polished.

15. When the teeth have been polished and rinsed, floss the interproximal surfaces of all teeth.

16. After completing the polishing procedure, dismiss the patient with a new toothbrush, floss, completed tooth chart, and any remaining instructions. (Fluoride treatment may be provided but only to children or patients with sensitive teeth.)

the buccal surface of the posterior teeth moving toward the anterior teeth, then making a loop over to the lingual surface of the anterior teeth moving toward the posterior, and finishing with the occlusal and incisal edges from posterior to anterior. Once all three surfaces have been polished, the patient should be provided a few rinses. Then the system should be repeated until all teeth have been polished. The operator should use the same sequence for every patient every time a polishing is done so as not to miss any areas, even if a patient is missing teeth in certain areas.

Flossing After Polishing

Flossing puts the finishing touches on the coronal polishing procedure. When all teeth have been polished and rinsed, floss is used to clean the interproximal spaces. Polishing paste and debris can become lodged between

the teeth and should be removed with floss. The floss must be rotated so that a clean piece is placed into each contact point. When the floss is being placed between the teeth, a gentle sliding motion must be used to prevent injury to the gingival tissue.

Evaluation of Polishing

When the coronal polishing procedure has been completed, the teeth should be evaluated for cleanliness. All tooth surfaces should be checked utilizing a mirror. If the teeth are clean, they will reflect light. Have the patient feel the teeth with his or her tongue. The teeth should feel smooth. If any surfaces have been missed, repolishing should occur before the patient is dismissed. When initially learning to perform the coronal polishing procedure, the operator can also use a disclosing agent in order to evaluate the polishing that has been performed.

Professionalism

As a new assistant to the field of dentistry, always keep an open mind with regard to styles and techniques that can be learned from other professionals. Listen to how your colleagues educate and interact with patients, and create a unique technique of your own.

Preparing for Externship

Based on the state in which you reside, dental assistants may be allowed to perform the coronal polishing procedure. It is important for the dental assistant to be confident when performing the procedure. Prior to performing the procedure, ask any questions you may have. If any questions arise during the procedure, take them directly to the dentist. Familiarize yourself with the office equipment and know where supplies are kept.

SUMMARY

The coronal polishing procedure can be completed by an expanded functions dental assistant in some states; therefore, having a complete understanding of the procedure and purpose is important. Some states require that dental assistants obtain additional training to do coronal polishing. Recognizing dental stains and aesthetic restorations determines type of polishing technique and materials the dental assistant should use. Ensuring that correct patient and operator positions are used will help the effectiveness of the polishing procedure.

KEY TERMS

- **Clinical crown:** The part of a tooth that is visible in the oral cavity.   p. 764
- **Endogenous stains:** Stains formed from within the tooth structure.   p. 765
- **Exogenous stains:** Stains formed from sources outside of the tooth.   p. 765
- **Extrinsic stain:** Stains on external surfaces of the teeth that can be removed with polishing.   p. 764
- **Fulcrum:** Finger stabilizing point.   p. 767
- **Intrinsic stains:** Stains formed from within the tooth structure that cannot be removed with polishing. p. 765
- **Prophylaxis:** Complete removal of all stain, debris, and calculus.   p. 764
- **Subgingival:** Below the gingival tissues.   p. 765
- **Supragingival:** Above the gingival tissues.   p. 765

CHECK YOUR UNDERSTANDING

1. Which of the following is not an example of an intrinsic stain?
   a. metallic stain
   b. tobacco stain
   c. dental fluorosis
   d. tetracycline stain

2. What are the indications for a coronal polish?
   a. tooth absorbs stain better
   b. gingival tissue damage
   c. teeth stay healthier
   d. motivates patient for better oral hygiene

3. _____ stains are on the outside of the tooth and can be removed by polishing and scaling.
   a. Intrinsic
   b. Extrinsic
   c. Nonvital tooth stain
   d. None of the above

4. Which surfaces is the prophy brush effective in cleaning?
   a. facial surfaces
   b. lingual surfaces
   c. occlusal surfaces with deep pits and fissures
   d. interproximal surfaces

5. What special precautions should be taken during the polishing of an aesthetic restoration?
   a. No special precautions are needed.
   b. Use a mild abrasive polishing paste with a rubber cup.
   c. Use a coarse abrasive polishing paste with a rubber cup.
   d. Do not polish aesthetic restorations.

CHECK YOUR UNDERSTANDING (continued)

6. A/an _____ provides stability for the operator and safety for the patient.
   a. fulcrum
   b. armrest
   c. handpiece angle
   d. handrest

7. The process of polishing the coronal surfaces and removing stains is called what?
   a. prophylaxis
   b. coronal polish
   c. sealant polishing
   d. both a and b

8. The process of carefully choosing which teeth to polish is called what?
   a. coronal polishing
   b. sequence of polishing
   c. selective polishing
   d. prophylaxis

9. What could happen if the speed of the prophy cup is too high?
   a. Teeth could be damaged.
   b. Gingival tissue could be damaged.
   c. Both a and b.
   d. None of the above.

10. Approximately how many seconds should it take to clean each tooth?
   a. 1 to 3 seconds
   b. 2 to 6 seconds
   c. 10 seconds
   d. 60 seconds

● INTERNET ACTIVITY

● To learn more about state regulations for coronal polishing, go to www.danb.org

● WEB REFERENCES

● American Dental Hygienists' Association www.adha.org/profissues/prophylaxis.htm
● Encyclopedia of Nursing and Allied Health http://health.enotes.com/nursing-encyclopedia/tooth-polishing
● South Dakota Department of Health www.state.sd.us/doh/dentistry/6-13-03minutes.htm
● Pub Med www.ncbi.nlm.nih.gov/entrez/query.fcgi?cmd=Retrieve&db=PubMed&list_uids=5258574&dopt=Abstract
● Vermont Board of Dental Examiners vtprofessionals.org

49

Dental Sealants

Learning Objectives

After reading this chapter, the student should be able to:

• Discuss the purpose and placement of pit and fissure sealants.

• Explain indications and contraindications for sealants.

• List the types of materials used for sealants and their storage.

• Describe the sequence of steps for performing a sealant procedure.

Preparing for Certification Exams

• Apply or assist in the application of pit and fissure sealants.

Key Terms

Acrylate

Chemically cured

Dental sealant

Filled resins

Light cured

Polymerization

Retention

Unfilled resins

Chapter Outline

• Dental Caries and Sealants

• Indications for Sealants

• Contraindications for Sealants

• Types of Sealant Materials

• Storage and Use of Sealants

• Precautions for Dental Personnel and Patients

• Factors in Sealant Retention

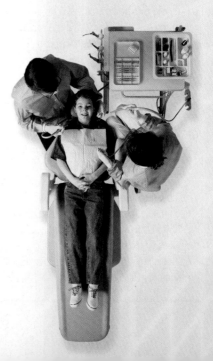

If proper dental hygiene is not utilized, sugar and bacteria can easily reside in the deep pits and grooves found in the anatomy of the posterior teeth (Figure 49.1). Sealants are used as a coating over those deep pits and grooves. A **dental sealant** is a hard clear, opaque, or tinted resin that is placed on the pits and fissures of the occlusal surfaces of caries-free teeth (Figure 49.2). The sealant helps make the tooth smooth and easier to keep clean and helps reduce tooth decay.

Sealants are more cost effective than restorations. Although sealants do not last as long as restorations, if properly cared for they can last up to seven years. The placement of sealants can usually be completed by dental assistants; regulations vary from state to state, however, so the dental practice act for the applicable state should be checked before performing the procedure.

Dental Caries and Sealants

Can a tooth with bacteria or a small carious lesion be sealed? It was once believed that if this were done, decay would develop under the sealant. Recent studies have proven that this typically does not occur. The bacterium that causes cavities can usually not survive under a sealant because it needs the sugars that are ingested daily to grow. Sealants are nearly 100% effective in protecting teeth from cavities. If decay does develop and progress under the sealant, restoration would be indicated.

Dental Assistant **PROFESSIONAL TIP**

Ms. Johnson is a single mother with three children. She is on a tight budget and her son has deep pits and fissures in his 6-year molars. Dr. Smith has recommended sealants be placed on all four of Elisha's molars. Ms. Johnson does not understand why he needs sealants if he does not have any cavities. How could Ms. Johnson be convinced to complete the treatment? The dental assistant would want to inform Ms. Johnson that by covering Elisha's molars with a sealant, cavities would be prevented on the chewing surfaces of those teeth. Sealants are also more cost effective than any type of restorative treatment available.

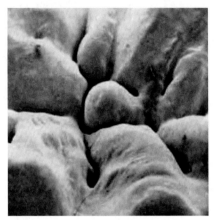

FIGURE 49.1
Microscopic view of occlusal pits and fissures.

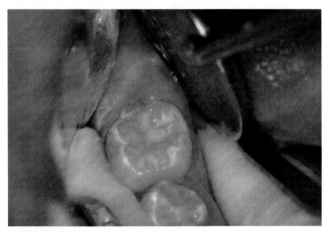

FIGURE 49.2
Molar with sealant in place.
Image courtesy Instructional Materials for the Dental Team, Lex., KY

Indications for Sealants

Dental sealants are primarily used for children, but all patients can benefit from their use. Sealants are used as a preventive tool to reduce dental caries during the high-decay periods experienced by young children and teenagers. Adults can benefit from sealants in some cases. If an adult has a small cavity that does not penetrate into the dentin, the decay can be removed and a sealant utilized instead of a restoration. Indications for enamel sealants include:

- Patients with a high volume of cavities on the occlusal surfaces
- Newly erupted molars

Life Span Considerations

Sealant application focuses mostly on children during the cavity-prone years, but many adults can benefit from sealant placement as well. If a cavity is small and has not penetrated into the dentin, the decay can be removed and a sealant can be used as an alternative to a restoration.

- Pits and fissures of primary and permanent teeth
- As a preventive procedure

Around age 3, Moriah received eight stainless steel crowns on all of her primary molars due to extensive decay. Now at age 7, the dentist has recommended sealants for Moriah's newly erupted 6-year molars. Why was this recommendation made?

Contraindications for Sealants

The use of sealants is not appropriate in some cases. Contraindications for enamel sealants include:

- Teeth with shallow grooves, because sugar and bacteria cannot easily hide in the shallow grooves
- Teeth that have been caries free for more than four years

Types of Sealant Materials

Sealant materials are available in many varieties (Figure 49.3). Knowledge of the types and differences allow the dental assistant to select the best product for each patient. Sealant colors are available in clear, opaque, or tinted. Some start out with a color tint, and then turn clear once they have set. Patients usually prefer the clear sealants for aesthetic reasons. Dental personnel, however, may prefer the opaque sealants because the opaque colors make the sealants visible to the dental team during future dental appointments. This helps the dental personnel to check the condition of the sealants to ensure they are still in place.

The type of sealant material used determines the **polymerization** process. Sealant materials are either **light cured** or **chemically cured** (self-cured). The light-cured process involves a one-component material that is set by a curing light. This process is preferred because the material can be manipulated as long as the operator wishes and will not harden until the curing light is placed on it. Chemically cured materials are two-paste materials: a base and catalyst. When the two materials are mixed, the setting process begins. This is known as autopolymeriza-

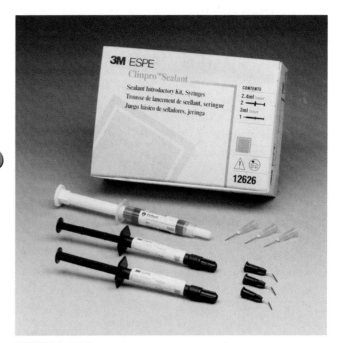

FIGURE 49.3
Sealant material.
Courtesy 3M ESPE

Patient Education

Sealants are used as a preventive procedure. Some patients have questions about why sealants are needed. Dental assistants need to explain the importance of the procedure, show the cost effectiveness of sealants, and answer any questions. Some of these questions may pertain to how long the sealant will last or whether a child can still acquire a cavity on the sealed tooth. Being able to effectively answer these types of questions ensures that the patient receives the preventive procedure needed.

Cultural Considerations

Many cultures do not believe in being proactive about dental treatment. Convincing some patients of the importance of a sealant may be a challenge. Being patient when dealing with patient questions and using visuals to explain the procedure will be helpful in ensuring patient understanding.

tion because the material begins to set as soon as the materials are mixed together. Complete setting time for chemically cured materials is indicated in the manufacturer's instructions.

Sealant materials are composed of dental composites or glass ionomers. Composites are preferred because they do not chip and wear away as fast as glass ionomers. The occlusal wear ability of the sealant is contributed by the filler. Sealants are available in either **filled resins** or **unfilled resins**. Filled sealants reduce the occlusal wear rate. Many dentists feel that because sealants are placed in the pits and fissures of the occlusal surface, the occlusal rate is insignificant. The important consideration to remember about filled sealants is that the sealant may need to be adjusted with a bur after placement. An unfilled sealant will wear naturally as the patient chews (Procedure 49-1).

Some sealant materials have the added benefit of fluoride release under the enamel sealant. Fluoride

Procedure 49-1 Applying Dental Sealants

Equipment and Supplies

- Mirror, explorer, cotton pliers
- Saliva ejector
- High-volume evacuator tip
- Air/water tip
- Slow-speed handpiece
- Light-curing unit
- White Arkansas stone (finishing bur)
- Pumice
- Dappen dish
- Prophy angle (disposable or sterile)
- Cotton rolls and/or dry angles
- Etchant
- Sealant material
- Articulating paper
- Fluoride gel or foam

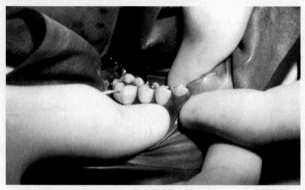
Placement of a dental dam.

3. The dentist checks the tooth to ensure no decay is present.

4. Moisten pumice with water to create a slurry consistency. Always make sure that the cleaning agent does not have any fluoride in it, because that would not allow the sealant to bond completely to the enamel rods.

5. Clean the occlusal surface with pumice and rinse thoroughly.

6. Place a cotton roll on the lingual and buccal surfaces. Dry the tooth completely with the air tip. Prior to using the air tip, be sure to clean out the air line by testing it on the patient's napkin or your glove.

7. Place acid etchant into the pits and grooves of the occlusal surface. Leave on for 30 to 45 seconds or according to the manufacturer's instructions.

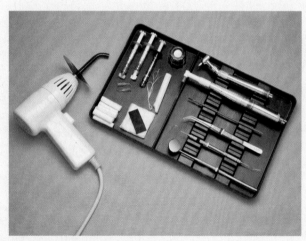
Sealant equipment and supplies.

Procedure Steps

1. Review the patient's medical and dental history.

2. Greet and seat the patient. Place a napkin and eyewear on the patient and tell her about the procedure. Instruct the patient on the importance of keeping the mouth open during the procedure to maintain a dry field (or place a dental dam).

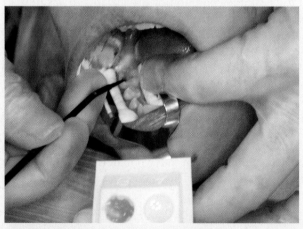
Etch application.
Image courtesy Instructional Materials for the Dental Team, Lex., KY

8. Completely rinse the tooth for a full 60 seconds.

9. Carefully replace cotton rolls as needed to ensure that no moisture gets on the etched surface.

continued on next page

Procedure 49-1 *continued from previous page*

10. Ensure teeth are completely dry, then dab the sealant on the occlusal surface covering all pits and fissures. Make sure the sealant is evenly placed across the surface. Light cure for 60 seconds.

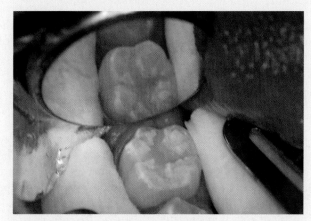

Sealant application.
Image courtesy Instructional Materials for the Dental Team, Lex., KY

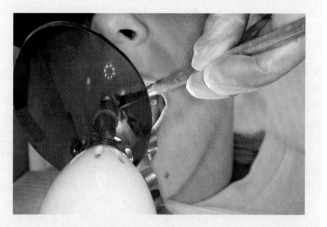

11. Check the sealant surface with the explorer for hardness.

12. Remove cotton rolls.

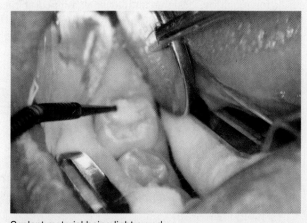

Sealant material being light cured.
Image courtesy Instructional Materials for the Dental Team, Lex., KY

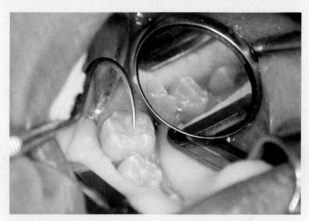

Placed sealant.
Image courtesy Instructional Materials for the Dental Team, Lex., KY

13. Check the occlusion with the articulating paper.

14. The dentist will make adjustments if necessary.

15. Fluoride may be applied to help remineralize the enamel.

16. Freshen the patient's mouth.

17. Give the patient postoperative instructions.

---

release in sealants helps to strengthen the enamel to help reduce future decay if the sealant is worn away over time.

Storage and Use of Sealants

When using any sealant product, it is always important to read and follow the manufacturer's instructions. Here are some general guidelines to follow:

- Replace caps after use.
- Do not expose to light or air.
- Check shelf life before use. Most sealants last for about 24 to 36 months.
- Some sealants can be stored in the refrigerator to extend the shelf life.

Precautions for Dental Personnel and Patients

Safety is always the main concern for both patients and the dental staff. Prior to performing any procedures on patients, it is always important to check the patient's heath history for any allergies.

When placing a sealant a phosphoric acid is used. For this reason, both the patient and the dental team should wear protective eyewear during sealant procedures. A dental dam may be used for additional protection. There are two types of etchant material: liquid and gel. The type used is based on the operator's preference.

When rinsing the patient's mouth, a controlled flow of water should be used with no air or spritz. This prevents the tissues from being burned with etch. If the etch contacts the skin or eyes, water should be used immediately to flush the area. For any further medical attention, the patient should be referred to the patient's personal physician.

Sealant materials contain **acrylate** or BIS-GMA, which could cause skin irritations; therefore, the dental assistant should always wear gloves when handling sealant materials. In some cases the acrylate can penetrate through the gloves. If this occurs the dental assistant should immediately remove the gloves and wash his or her hands immediately prior to regloving.

When using the ultraviolet curing light, special amber safety glasses should be worn by both the patient

Professionalism

As you grow in your new career, enjoy the interaction you will encounter with each patient. Remember, to serve another is a gift. Always carry yourself as a professional. The patients are watching how you interact with the entire dental staff. If a concern arises, follow the chain of command.

and the operator. Use of the ultraviolet curing light without protective eyewear can cause damage to the cornea of the eye over time.

Factors in Sealant Retention

The **retention** of the sealant depends on the effectiveness of its placement. Sometimes a small amount of decay may need to be removed before sealant is placed. The main factors that cause sealant failure are inadequate etching and moisture control. Etching opens up the enamel rods of the tooth. Saliva or moisture then closes up these rods, causing the sealant not to adhere to the tooth structure.

After placement of the sealant, an explorer is used to check for retention. Sealants should be examined at each recall visit to make sure they are not chipping away. If sealants are placed correctly, they can last up to seven years.

SUMMARY

Sealants are a preventive treatment to reduce dental decay. Although children primarily benefit from sealants, they can be utilized on adults. There are various types of sealant materials, and the dental assistant must be knowledgeable about the types and differences. Care should be given to the protection of both the patient and the dental team when using sealant materials and equipment. An effectively placed sealant will benefit the patient for many years.

Preparing for Externship

Depending on your state regulations, you may be asked to place a sealant alone. Ensure you understand the entire procedure completely before beginning and have the dentist check the finished product.

KEY TERMS

- **Acrylate:** A salt of acrylic acid. p. 778
- **Chemically cured:** Material that is set by the chemical process of mixing a base and catalyst together. p. 775
- **Dental sealant:** A hard clear, opaque, or tinted resin that is placed on the pits and fissures of the occlusal surfaces of caries-free teeth. p. 774
- **Filled resins:** Sealant material that contains filler particles. p. 775
- **Light cured:** Material that is set by a curing light. p. 775
- **Polymerization:** Process of setting a dental sealant. p. 775
- **Retention:** Ability of a dental sealant to adhere to the tooth structure. p. 778
- **Unfilled resins:** Sealant material that does not contain filler particles. p. 775

CHECK YOUR UNDERSTANDING

1. In preparation for sealant application, the teeth are polished with
   a. prophy paste.
   b. pumice.
   c. fluoride.
   d. etchant.

2. Sealants are indicated for
   a. caries-free posterior teeth.
   b. teeth with deep pits and fissures.
   c. primary and permanent teeth.
   d. all of the above.

3. What is the acid etchant responsible for in the sealant placement procedure?
   a. opening the enamel rods
   b. polishing the tooth structure
   c. both a and b
   d. none of the above

4. During sealant placement, what is the most important factor?
   a. isolation
   b. moisture control
   c. both a and b
   d. none of the above

5. Unfilled resin sealants are preferred because
   a. they must be adjusted with a bur after placement.
   b. they wear in naturally (no adjustments are needed).
   c. they reduce occlusal wear.
   d. all of the above.

6. Which sealant material undergoes autopolymerization?
   a. polymerization
   b. light cured
   c. chemically cured
   d. both b and c

7. When fluoride is added to a sealant material, what is the benefit?
   a. strengthens the enamel
   b. weakens the enamel
   c. prevents all future decay
   d. all of the above

8. Why are clear sealants *not* preferred by dental assistants?
   a. easily seen
   b. difficult to see at recall visits
   c. blend in with enamel color
   d. there is no preference

9. What are the contraindications for sealants?
   a. cavity-free teeth for more than four years
   b. teeth with occlusal decay
   c. teeth with shallow grooves
   d. teeth with occlusal restorations
   e. all of the above

10. What special precautions should be taken when using a curing light?
    a. No special precautions need to be taken.
    b. An amber shield should be used.
    c. Personal protective equipment should be worn.
    d. A lead apron should be worn.

INTERNET ACTIVITY

- Go to www.animated-teeth.com/tooth_sealants/t1_sealing_teeth.htm to learn more about dental sealants.

WEB REFERENCES

- Better Health Channel www.betterhealth.vic.gov.au/bhcv2/bhcarticles.nsf/pages/Dental_sealants?open
- Centers for Disease Control www.cdc.gov/Oralhealth/factsheets/sealants-faq.htm
- Dental Sealants www.usc.edu/hsc/dental/rest/OPER521a/
- Locate a Doc www.locateadoc.com/articles.cfm/888
- Science News Online www.sciencenews.org/pages/sn_arc97/11_22_97/fob1.htm

Orthodontics

Outline of Chapter

- The Orthodontist
- The Orthodontic Assistant
- The Orthodontic Office
- Understanding Occlusion
  —Etiology of Malocclusion
- The Alignment of Teeth and Arches
  —Benefits of Orthodontic Treatment
- Orthodontic Records and Treatment Planning
  —Medical and Dental History
  —Physical Growth Evaluation
  —Diagnostic Records
- Case Presentation
  —Financial Arrangements
- Specialized Instruments
- Orthodontic Treatment
  —Fixed Appliances
  —Separators
  —Orthodontic Bands
  —Bonded Brackets
- Auxiliary Attachments
  —Arch Wires
  —Elastomeric Ties or Ligature Wires
  —Power Products
- Headgear
- Adjustment Visits
- Oral Hygiene and Dietary Instructions
- Completed Treatment
  —Retention
  —Retention Appliances
- Treatment Options

Learning Objectives

After reading this chapter, the student should be able to:

- Identify the classes of malocclusion.
- List the types of orthodontic records used for treatment planning.
- Explain interceptive orthodontics and implementation.
- Describe the phases of orthodontic treatment.
- List the steps in the technique of placing elastic separators.
- Describe the function of an arch wire.
- Explain the use and function of headgear.
- Discuss the importance of retainer appliances and follow-up treatment.

Preparing for Certification Exams

- Receive and prepare patients for treatment, including seating, positioning chair, and placing napkin.
- Fabricate diagnostic models.
- Take intra- and extraoral photographs.
- Place and remove wire separators.
- Place and remove steel separating springs.
- Place and remove elastic ring separators.
- Preselect and fit orthodontic bands.
- Assist in the preparation, placement, and cementation of orthodontic bands.
- Remove excess cement from orthodontic bands.
- Assist in the preparation and direct bonding of orthodontic brackets.
- Place and remove arch wires.
- Place and remove ligature ties.
- Place and remove elastomeric ties.

Key Terms

Arch wire

Auxiliary attachment

Corrective (interceptive) orthodontics

Dentofacial

Distoclusion

Fetal molding

Ligature wire

Mesioclusion

Retainer

Orthodontics is a specialty of

dentistry that diagnoses, prevents, and treats dental and facial irregularities of growing and mature **dentofacial** (dentition and facial) structures. The term *ortho* means straight and *odont* means tooth.

The ages of orthodontic patients vary, with interceptive orthodontic treatments starting on patients as young as 7 years, or younger if needed. Interceptive orthodontic treatment allows the orthodontist to intercede or correct problems as they are developing. This is achieved in several ways, such as by removing the primary teeth or inserting a fixed or removable appliance that expands the jaw.

The Orthodontist

An orthodontist is a dental specialist who has completed college and four years of dental school and then completes an additional two- to three-year training program specializing in tooth movement (orthodontics) and guidance of facial development (dentofacial orthopedics). Orthodontists are uniquely educated experts in dentistry who straighten teeth and align jaws.

The Orthodontic Assistant

The orthodontic assistant is an individual in dentistry who has more autonomy than a general dental assistant. The orthodontic assistant participates in many functions within the office. Each state, through its dental practice act laws, governs the functions the orthodontic assistant is allowed to perform. Responsibilities can include assisting the orthodontist with treatment, educating the patient in oral and overall health, taking diagnostic impressions, taking radiographs and bite registrations, providing pre- and postoperative instructions to patients,

Dental Assistant PROFESSIONAL TIP

As a valuable member of the dental team, the orthodontic chairside assistant should have the most current knowledge of the latest materials and techniques. Orthodontic procedures require skill and patience. As a professional it is important to always stay current with new methods and equipment. Be sure to stay up to date in your field by taking continuing education classes and reading articles from professional dental journals.

Professionalism

As a valued member of the dental team it is important for the orthodontic assistant to present him- or herself in a professional manner. Being well groomed, punctual, and well spoken is only a start. The orthodontic assistant's attitude toward peers in the office should be helpful and cooperative. Disharmony among coworkers may make the patient feel uneasy and is unacceptable in the workplace.

and performing sterilization procedures. In some states, depending on the dental practice laws, dental assistants may also place arch wires, adjust headgear, place separators, fabricate vacuum machine–formed retainers, and fit orthodontic bands around molars.

The Orthodontic Office

The design of an orthodontic office is typically based on the "open bay" principle (Figure 50.1). As with pediatric dentistry, this design is used to accommodate and treat many patients at a time. Because very little equipment is required in orthodontic procedures, the open area can contain numerous patient chairs.

The patient care aspect of the office is typically divided into three areas: (1) an area to keep records confidential, (2) an area to take radiographs, and (3) an area to provide patient care for all stages of treatment. Orthodontic offices may also include a laboratory. This area is used for pouring impressions, trimming diagnostic models, and fabricating fixed and removable appliances.

Understanding Occlusion

The term *occlusion* simply means "contacts between teeth" and refers to the relationship between the maxillary and mandibular teeth when the upper and lower jaws are in the fully closed position. Normal occlusion occurs when there is ideal contact between the mandibular and

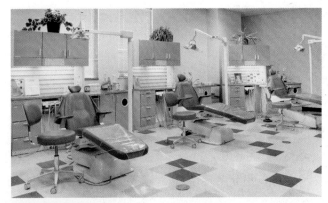

FIGURE 50.1
An open bay design.

maxillary arches. Any intra- or extra-arch deviations are considered a malocclusion.

The malocclusion classification system, known as the Angle classification system, was developed by Dr. Edward H. Angle (1855–1930) and is used today to describe how teeth and arch deviations are classified. Angle defines normal occlusion as an ideal mesiodistal relationship between the jaws and the dental arches. Therefore, a Class I occlusion (neutroclusion) is present when the mesiobuccal cusp of the maxillary first permanent molar occludes with the mesiobuccal groove of the mandibular first molar. In a Class I malocclusion the molar relationship is normal (or in neutroclusion), but deviations such as teeth being crowded in one or more areas within the arch are present.

A Class II malocclusion or **distoclusion** occurs when the mandibular teeth are distal to the maxillary teeth. The mesiobuccal cusp of the upper first molar occludes (by more than the width of a premolar) mesial to the mesiobuccal groove of the mandibular first molar. The maxillary incisors are in labioversion. The mandibular arch is in a distal relationship to the maxillary arch or said to be in distoclusion. This can be due to a deficiency of the lower jaw or an excess of the upper jaw. There are two types of Class II occlusions called divisions:

- **Class II, Division I**—The mandibular teeth are behind the upper jaw with a protrusion of the upper incisors.
- **Class II, Division II**—The mandibular teeth are behind the upper teeth, with the central incisors tipped labially.

The mandible and teeth are in mesial relationship to the maxillary teeth in a Class III malocclusion and are said to be in **mesioclusion.** The mesiobuccal cusp of the maxillary first molar occludes in the space between the distal cusp of the lower permanent first molar and the mesial cusp or the lower permanent second molar. Patients presenting with Class III malocclusion usually have a strong or protrusive chin, which can be due to either horizontal mandibular excess or horizontal maxillary deficiency. This is commonly referred to as an underbite. Figure 50.2 illustrates the three classes of malocclusion.

Etiology of Malocclusion

The three categories within the etiology of malocclusion are genetic, systemic (environmental), and local (habits). Genetic factors are responsible for deviations within the dentition and jaw sizes, just as our height and body frame are related to our genetics. Some dental heredity factors include:

- **Supernumerary teeth**—teeth in addition to the regular number of teeth
- **Ectopic eruption**—abnormal eruption of a permanent tooth out of normal alignment; causes abnormal resorption of a primary tooth

- **Irregular sizes**—irregularities in jaw sizes and teeth-to-jaw relationships
- **Congenitally missing teeth**—genetically missing teeth

Systemic factors include injuries at birth. These types of injuries fall under two major categories: fetal molding and trauma during birth. **Fetal molding** occurs when a limb of a fetus is pressed against another part of the body, such as an arm pressed against the mandible. This pressure can lead to distortion of the rapidly growing mandible. Trauma during birth may occur during the use of forceps in delivery. Injury to the developing teeth, jaw, and facial structures may occur. Dental trauma can lead to the development of malocclusion in a number of ways:

1. Damage to permanent tooth buds when an injury to primary teeth has occurred
2. Movement of a tooth or teeth as a result of the premature loss of a primary tooth
3. Direct injury to permanent teeth

Local habits that can create malocclusion include issues such as sucking habits of children involving the thumb, finger(s), or pacifier that can have an adverse effect on jaw and tooth development. Should these habits cause a malalignment within the permanent dentition, the malalignment can be treated with interceptive orthodontic appliances or behavioral changes.

When teeth do not occlude properly, undo stress and strain are placed on the surrounding muscle attachments, tissue, and bone. Problems with malalignment include digestive problems brought on by poorly chewed food and problems with temporomandibular joint (TMJ) pain due to the clenching and grinding of teeth. Whatever the reason for the malocclusion, misaligned teeth and/or jaws can compromise oral health and function.

Why is it important to see children at a young age for an orthodontic evaluation?

The Alignment of Teeth and Arches

During the initial orthodontic appointment, the occlusion is evaluated and noted along with deviations or misalignments with the dental arches. Here are some common problems:

- **Crowding**—Crowding of one or several teeth is the most common cause of malocclusion.
- **Overjet**—This severe protrusion of the maxillary anterior teeth causes a horizontal space between the mandibular facial surfaces of the lingual aspect of the maxillary anterior teeth (Figure 50.3).
- **Overbite**—This extreme vertical overlap of the maxillary teeth can be so severe that the mandibular anterior cannot be seen at all (see Figure 50.3).

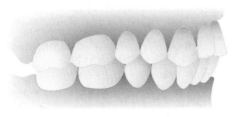
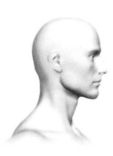

Class I

Mesognathic
profile

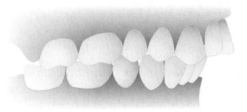

**Class II
Division 1**

Retrognathic
profile

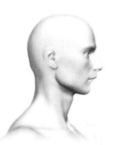

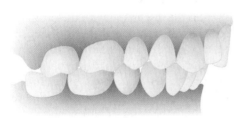
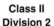

**Class II
Division 2**

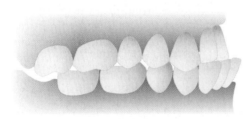

**Class III
Mesial occlusion**

Prognathic
profile

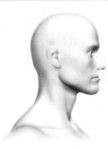

FIGURE 50.2
Class I, Class II, and Class III occlusions.

- **Cross bite**—A tooth or teeth that are in cross bite means that one or more maxillary teeth are lingual to the occluding mandibular tooth or teeth when in occlusion. This can mean there is a discrepancy in jaw size.

Most people have some malpositioning of teeth, and throughout the aging process the teeth continue to move ever so slightly. Orthodontic treatment is available at any age to correct, enhance, and improve malpositioned teeth. This type of treatment can eliminate not only the dental issue, but can help improve a patient's overall quality of life.

Benefits of Orthodontic Treatment

Besides boosting self-confidence and self-esteem through an improved appearance, orthodontic treatment brings the teeth, lips, and face into proportion. In this way, orthodontic treatment can benefit social and career success, as well as improve a person's general attitude toward life.

The pediatric patient can benefit through **corrective (interceptive) orthodontics**. This can be accomplished by placing a specialized fixed or removable appliance to

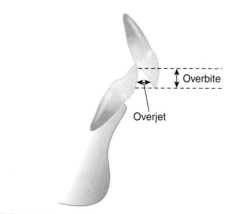

FIGURE 50.3
Overjet and overbite.

assist with jaw development or maintain space when a deciduous tooth is prematurely lost.

The adult patient can benefit from the utilization of orthodontic stability during periodontal treatment or simply tooth uprighting (the processes of vertical tooth positioning) and space maintaining for tooth replacement. The orthodontist works collaboratively with the adult patient's periodontist, general dentist, and/or prosthodontist for dental and jaw corrections.

Corrective orthodontics includes conditions that require correcting malrelationships and malformations of teeth and facial bones. Corrective orthodontics involves the orthodontist placing on the teeth bonded brackets or fixed orthodontic brackets that provide continual force that stimulates and redirects functional forces within the dentofacial structure. Corrective orthodontics includes:

- Fixed appliances (braces).
- Removable appliances for correction or maintenance of orthodontic treatment.
- Orthognathic surgery to correct jaw size discrepancies. This type of surgery is done only when the orthodontic problem is too severe to be corrected by other means.

What are some psychological effects that misaligned teeth can have on an individual?

Orthodontic Records and Treatment Planning

The initial visit to the orthodontist consists of an extensive examination of the face, jaws, and teeth, looking for symmetry between them. In the preliminary examination, a dental record is completed and documentation of the patient's oral habits or abnormal functions is noted.

The Angle classification of occlusion is determined on both sides of the patient's mouth and charted.

During the initial visit, a medical and dental history is taken and any questions or concerns the patient may have are answered. If the patient is a child, the parents are involved in the discussion with the orthodontist regarding expectations of treatment, aspects of care, and duration of treatment time. The expectations of the younger patient often differ from those of their parents with regard to dietary and drink restrictions in relation to orthodontic treatment. It is important that the dental team communicate with both the younger patient and the parent to ensure understanding of the treatment plan and the aftercare.

Sometimes the orthodontist may choose to delay treatment until further dental development has occurred. If treatment is delayed, the patient is placed on a recall appointment list to monitor growth. If treatment is recommended to begin, a second appointment is scheduled for completing the patient's diagnostic record.

How can the orthodontic team encourage patient motivation for the duration of orthodontic treatment?

Medical and Dental History

During the initial visit, a complete medical history is taken to evaluate the general health of the patient. It is important to take a good medical history to avert potential problems. Some conditions and medications can affect a patient's response to treatment. Although orthodontic therapy tends to be relatively bloodless, it is possible to cause bleeding by incidental injury to the soft tissues. For illnesses, such as endocrine problems, rheumatic fever, and prolonged bleeding, the patient should get a medical clearance and recommendations from a physician.

The dental history provides information concerning earlier dental treatments, for example, to treat caries incidences or deal with missing teeth. The outcome of orthodontic treatment might be affected by whether the patient has received routine dental care or only emergency dental care. For instance, the type of dental care the patient has sought in the past can be indicative of how motivated, dedicated, and enthusiastic the patient will be during orthodontic care.

Physical Growth Evaluation

The evaluation of physical growth by the orthodontist is critical in developing a successful treatment plan. The orthodontist must consider the differences between a patient's chronological and skeletal ages, because these factors affect the timing and method of treatment.

A lack of growth hormone causes a lag in the growth of bones, which is clearly apparent in a child's height. Growth hormone deficiency commonly causes a delay in the growth of a child's teeth and facial bones. More commonly, children with a growth hormone deficiency keep their deciduous teeth two to five years longer than average. It is not unusual to see 10- and 12-year-olds with primary teeth causing problems with eruption of the secondary dentition. These children are also more likely to be missing adult teeth, which may require orthodontic treatment or tooth replacement to correct.

Diagnostic Records

After the clinical evaluation is completed, the orthodontist will require diagnostic records. These records assist in the preparation of a patient's individualized treatment plan. Diagnostic records document such features as tooth angulations, dental crowding, and the presence of unerupted teeth.

Extraoral and intraoral photographs (digital or nondigital) and diagnostic impressions are taken as part of the initial diagnostic record. Photographs capture the

Cultural Considerations
Understanding the patient's needs is of the upmost importance. The orthodontic assistant must become more aware of cultural considerations related to the diversity of patients. Understanding the ethnocultural backgrounds of the dental patient will enable the assistant to be better at communication skills, patient motivation, and cooperation.

color, shape, texture, and characteristics of intraoral and extraoral structures. They are also helpful in case presentation and case documentation.

Three standard types of extraoral photographs are taken to evaluate the symmetry and balance of the face (Figure 50.4):

- A frontal view with lips in a relaxed position
- A frontal view with lips in a smile
- A profile view of the patient's right side with lips relaxed

Intraoral photographs consist of the following (Figure 50.5):

- Full frontal view (teeth in occlusion)
- Bilateral view (teeth in occlusion) back to the first molar
- Maxillary occlusal view, including palate and all occlusal surfaces

Two types of radiographs are also taken as part of the initial diagnostic record: cephalometric and panoramic radiographs. The cephalometric radiograph (Figure 50.6) is an x-ray that provides the orthodontist with a lateral view of the patient's head, teeth, and jaws. The cephalometric film offers valuable information about growth patterns to determine the course of treatment. An analysis of the cephalometric film helps the orthodontist determine

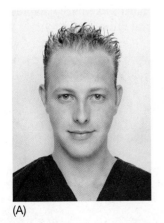 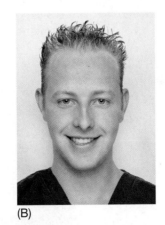 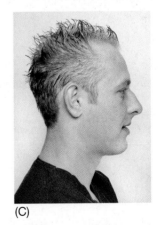

(A) (B) (C)

FIGURE 50.4
Standard extraoral photos: (a) frontal view with lips in relaxed position, (b) frontal view with lips in a smile, and (c) profile view of the patient's right side with lips relaxed.

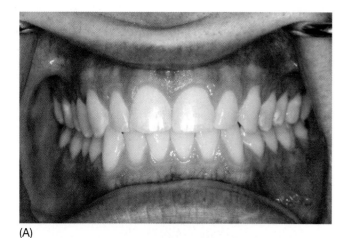

(A)

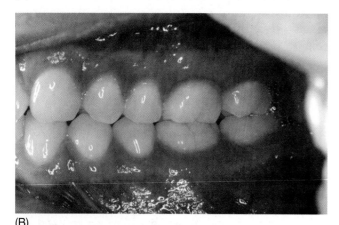

(B)

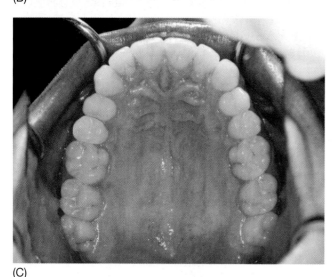

(C)

FIGURE 50.5
Intraoral photographs: (a) frontal view of an anterior bite, (b) side view of a right buccal bite relationship, and (c) occlusal view of maxillary teeth.
Images courtesy Instructional Materials for the Dental Team, Lex., KY

the current shape of the face, how the face has grown, and the expected growth. The orthodontic assistant will perform a cephalometric tracing to determine the relationship of certain landmarks. When the measurements are

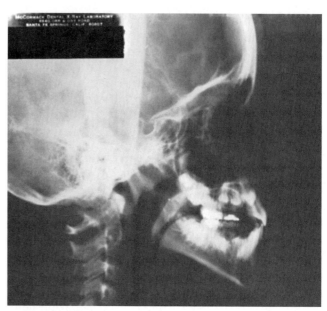

FIGURE 50.6
Cephalometric radiograph.

obtained, it is used for diagnosis, treatment planning, and/or assessment of treatment effects.

Panoramic radiographs (Figure 50.7) offer a comprehensive view of the maxillary and mandibular jaws, tooth development, roots of teeth, nerve positions, jaw structures, supernumerary teeth, joints including the temporomandibular joint, and missing or misplaced teeth.

In the last 10 years, digital radiology has become a common method of clinical evaluation in orthodontics. With the development of cost-effective intraoral and extraoral digital technology and an increase in dental practices becoming computerized, dental digital imaging has become an excellent alternative to conventional film imaging. An advantage of using digital images in orthodontics is that the cephalometric analysis can be easily accessed at the chairside computer for case presentation. Other advantages of digital radiology include the reduction of radiation and ease of storage. (Storage is done on a typical computer hard drive.) See Chapter 32 for more information on digital radiography.

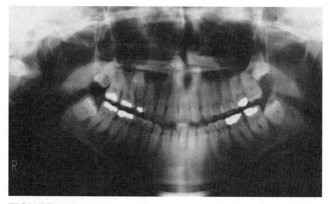

FIGURE 50.7
Panoramic radiograph for orthodontic treatment.

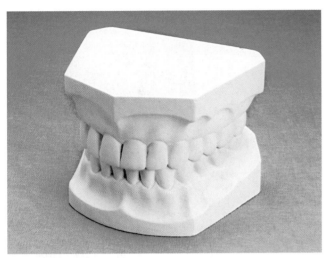

FIGURE 50.8
Diagnostic study model.

Diagnostic models are an essential part of record taking. They are used for diagnosis, case presentation, and patient identification. The orthodontic assistant generally fabricates the study models from accurate alginate impressions taken at the diagnostic records appointment. Study models are an accurate, positive replication of the patient's mouth, muscle attachments, and hard palate. These models are made with orthodontic plaster. The finished model is trimmed, polished, and symmetrically correct (Figure 50.8).

Case Presentation

Once the initial appointments have occurred, the orthodontist studies the information that was gathered and prepares a treatment plan for the patient. The treatment plan contains information on what is to be accomplished, the cost, and the approximate time treatment will take. A one-hour consultation appointment is scheduled for the patient, or guardian if the patient is under 18 years of age. The presentation includes the initial photographs, radiographs, cephalometric tracings, diagnostic models, and other adjunctive aids the orthodontist deems appropriate. The orthodontist or treatment coordinator presents the case, the approximate length of the treatment period, and the financial information to the patient/guardian. If treatment is accepted, a consent form is signed at that time and consecutive appointments are scheduled to begin treatment.

Financial Arrangements

Orthodontists commonly offer three types of financial arrangements: paying in full at the start of treatment, monthly payment plans, or semi annual payments. All financial plans consist of a formal, legally binding contract that states what percentage of the treatment is to be paid at the first appointment and what the fixed monthly payments are thereafter. Insurance coverage is considered at this time. Generally the subscriber of the insurance plan is responsible for submitting claims for reimbursement. On occasion, the orthodontic office submits the claims. (For more information on insurance procedures, see Chapter 55.)

Specialized Instruments

Orthodontic instruments primarily involve different types of pliers and band pushers. These are used to apply or remove bands and braces that correct and reshape the teeth and jaw structure. Here are some commonly used orthodontic dental instruments:

- **Orthodontic scaler** (Figure 50.9)—Utilized in bracket placement, removal of elastomeric rings, and removal of excess bonding or cement around bands or brackets.
- **Ligature director** (Figure 50.10)—Tucks twisted **ligature wire** ends into interproximal spaces.
- **Band (driver) pusher** (Figure 50.11)—Used to seat and position the band on the tooth. Can be used to contour the occlusal aspect of the band around the tooth. The working end has a round serrated tip to prevent slippage.
- **Bite stick**—Assists in band seating with the aid of the patient's biting force. The handle and tip are one piece made from autoclave material. The triangular steel working area is placed occlusal on the band (buccal/lingual) so the patient can bite onto the plastic stick. The biting force drives the band into position.
- **Bracket forceps (placement tweezers)**—Used to carry and place the bonded bracket on the tooth. Designed with a long-tipped, reverse action and serrated beaks to secure the bracket in place.

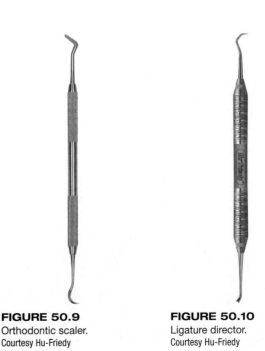

FIGURE 50.9
Orthodontic scaler.
Courtesy Hu-Friedy

FIGURE 50.10
Ligature director.
Courtesy Hu-Friedy

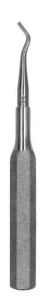

FIGURE 50.11
Band pusher.
Courtesy Hu-Friedy

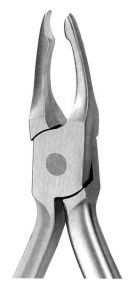

FIGURE 50.13
Crown and band contouring pliers.
Courtesy Hu-Friedy

Many different kinds of pliers are used in orthodontic treatments:

- **Bird-beak pliers (No. 139)** (Figure 50.12)—Used for seating separating springs and bending arch wire. The opposing beaks are conical and pyramidal. They are available in a variety of lengths.
- **Band contouring pliers** (Figure 50.13)—Used to recontour and adapt the O-band around the tooth. Beaks are tapered with a slight bow. One beak tip is concave and one is convex, allowing them to fit together for contouring orthodontic bands.
- **Weingart utility pliers** (Figure 50.14)—Used to hold orthodontic arch wire when placing or removing the

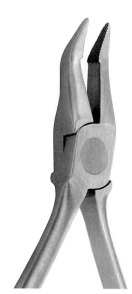

FIGURE 50.14
Weingart utility pliers.
Courtesy Hu-Friedy

wire from the mouth. The two opposing beaks have serrated tips that can be pointed, straight, or curved.
- **Tweed loop-forming pliers** (Figure 50.15)—Have one round and one concave opposing parallel beak. The beaks are used to form the omega loop and various other loops into an arch wire.
- **Posterior band remover pliers** (Figure 50.16)—Have two stainless steel beaks that are used to remove posterior bands. One beak is cylindrical with a replaceable nylon tip; the other is curved with a carbide insert. The cylindrical beak is placed onto the occlusal surface with the curved beak placed on the gingival surface of the band.

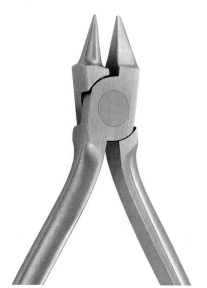

FIGURE 50.12
Bird-beak pliers with conical and pyramidal beaks.
Courtesy Hu-Friedy

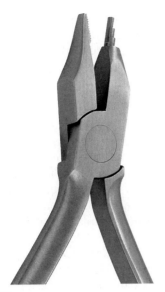

FIGURE 50.15
Tweed loop-forming pliers.
Courtesy Hu-Friedy

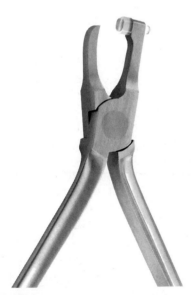

FIGURE 50.16
Posterior band remover pliers.
Courtesy Hu-Friedy

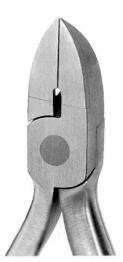

FIGURE 50.17
Pin and ligature cutter.
Courtesy Hu-Friedy

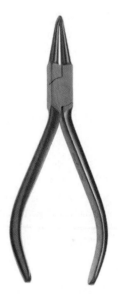

FIGURE 50.18
Howe utility pliers.
Courtesy Miltex Inc.

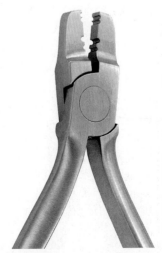

FIGURE 50.19
Lingual arch-forming pliers.
Courtesy Hu-Friedy

- **Pin and ligature cutter (ligature wire cutter)** (Figure 50.17)—Used to cut thin ligature wire. The beaks are tapered with carbide inserts that can be replaced or sharpened when worn.
- **Howe (110) utility pliers** (Figure 50.18)—Used for placing bands, tying ligature wire, and holding and adjusting the arch wire during placement and removal. Beaks are round and tapered with serrated pad tips.
- **Arch-forming pliers** (Figure 50.19)—Used to create form and contours in arch wires. The pliers have a concave, cylindrical beak that may be grooved or smooth.
- **Coon ligature-tying pliers** (Figure 50.20)—Used for tying wire ligature ties around brackets, bands, and arch

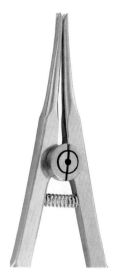

FIGURE 50.20
Coon ligature-tying pliers.
Courtesy Hu-Friedy

wires. The beaks are finely serrated and narrow to allow ease in ligature tying.

- **Distal end cutting pliers (Figure 50.21)**—Cut and hold (via a magnetic insert) the distal ends of arch wires that protrude distally from the buccal tube.

Orthodontic Treatment

Orthodontic treatment is more than just aligning teeth. The practice of orthodontics modifies and corrects facial growth using different appliances by placing force, torque, and pressure over a period of time. Some appliances are used to primarily move teeth (orthodontic), whereas others are used "orthopedically" to modify facial growth. Some appliances supply both orthodontic and orthopedic treatment effects. They come in several types: fixed, removable, and a combination of both. Orthodontic treatment can begin after the case presentation, providing all decayed teeth have been restored and a dental cleaning completed.

Fixed Appliances

Fixed appliances, or "braces" as they are commonly called (Figure 50.22), exert more pressure than removable appliances and can achieve more complex movements. They consist of small brackets that are bonded to the facial surface of the incisors and premolars, molar bands, arch wire, and auxiliaries that move the teeth in six different directions: mesial, distal, lingual, facial, apical, and occlusal.

An example of a fixed appliance is the attachments to bands and brackets that have a specialized function. The attached tubes and hooks make it possible to attach wires or elastics to the tooth allowing increased pressure in tooth movement. **Arch wires** are single wires that fit into the slots of brackets and tubes of bands. The bending of the wire and the resulting pressure cause the tooth or teeth to move in a desired direction.

Special Fixed Appliances

Special fixed appliances are used prior to, during, or after regular orthodontic bracket treatment. These appliances are cemented in place and have a specific function during a phase or phases of treatment. Types include lingual arch wires, space maintainers, palatal expansion appliances, and habit correction appliances.

The lingual arch wire appliance (Figure 50.23) conforms to the lingual aspect of the mandibular dental arch and is attached to molar bands that are cemented around the first molars. The lingual arch wire is used to promote or prevent tooth movement until permanent eruption takes place.

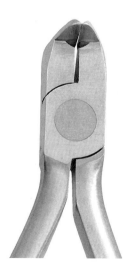

FIGURE 50.21
Distal end cutter.
Courtesy Hu-Friedy

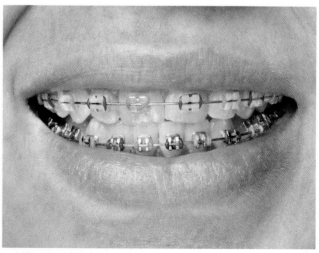

FIGURE 50.22
Intraoral frontal full set of braces.

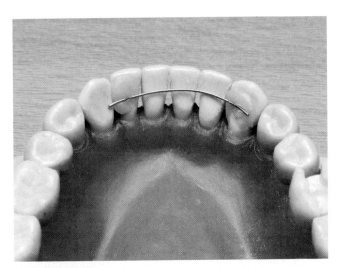

FIGURE 50.23
A lingual arch wire.

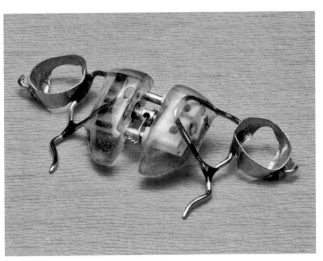

FIGURE 50.25
A palatal arch expander.

A space maintainer (Figure 50.24) is a fixed appliance worn to prevent adjacent teeth from moving into the space left by an unerupted or prematurely lost tooth. It consists of a band and wire loop soldered together. The wire loops provides space into which the permanent tooth can erupt. Space maintainers come in several varieties that adapt to patients' needs.

A palatal or upper jaw expansion appliance is placed to widen a narrow upper jaw and correct a cross bite. It is used to spread the midpalatal suture to create space where new bone cells are generated and mesh together, providing the teeth more room to erupt in a natural position.

The expander is made up of an acrylic palatal portion attached to a stainless steel framework that is soldered onto molar bands that are cemented around the molars, allowing for stability of the appliance (Figure 50.25). Inside the acrylic portion, a screw-like device is placed. By using a special key the patient turns the screw at precise intervals, which puts pressure onto the palate opening the midpalate suture for expansion. The timely use of an arch expander effectively minimizes or eliminates the need for braces when the patient gets older.

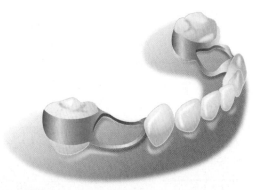

FIGURE 50.24
Two space maintainers in place holding the spaces open until the teeth erupt.

Steps in a Typical Orthodontic Treatment

A typical orthodontic treatment sequence is as follows:

1. Application of separators
2. Placement and cementation of posterior bands
3. Placement and bonding of brackets
4. Insertion of arch wire and application of ligature ties or elastomeric ties
5. Interval adjustment checks
6. Band and bracket removal
7. Placement of fixed or removable retention devices

Separators

For patient comfort and ease of placement of bands, separators are placed interproximally prior to fitting and cementing bands (Procedure 50-1 and Procedure 50-2). The use of a separator provides space and opens the contact points so they properly fit the molar bands. For the separators to achieve their purpose, they should stay in place for one week for tooth movement to occur. It is very important that separators stay in place; therefore, home care instructions must include that the patient check daily to verify the presence of the separator. Should a separator fall out, immediate replacement is necessary (Procedure 50-3). Separators come in several types: wire, steel springs, and elastomeric (elastic) separators.

Orthodontic Bands

An orthodontic band is a stainless steel circular metal strip that is adapted to fit closely around a tooth. Bands may have various components welded or soldered to them for use during treatment. They come in a variety of sizes, are anatomically correct, and are divided into maxillary and mandibular right and left. The occlusal edge is contoured or rolled, and the gingival edge is straight and

Procedure 50-1 Placing and Removing Brass Wire Separators

Equipment and Supplies Needed

- Basic setup: mouth mirror, explorer, cotton pliers
- Soft 20-mm brass wire
- Hemostat
- Ligature wire cutter
- Orthodontic scaler or condenser

Procedure Steps for Placing Brass Wire Separators

1. Bend brass wire into a C-shape or hook shape leaving a tail.

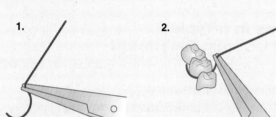

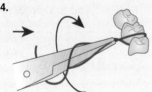

2. Use a hemostat to hold the brass wire. Insert the hook into the lingual interproximal space (usually between the second premolar and first and second molars).

3. Grab the tail of the brass wire and fold it over the contact by bringing it over to the facial.

4. Bring the ends of the wire together and twist using the hemostat. Make sure that the wire is not too tight or too loose.

5. Cut the wire using a ligature cutter. Fold the wire and tuck into the embrasure area using the orthodontic scaler or condenser.

Procedure Steps for Removing Brass Wire Separators

1. Using the ligature wire cutter, carefully lift the brass wire to the occlusal surface and cut the wire.

2. Use the hemostat to carefully remove both sections of the wire on the facial side.

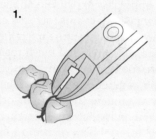

smooth making a well-formed adaptation around the molar.

Orthodontic bands may have buttons, cleats, or tubes attached for auxiliary power movement. When selecting an appropriate band for fitting, the dental assistant should perform a visual inspection at chairside to determine size, shape, and fit. An alternative to this method of selection is to adapt the bands to the patient's diagnostic cast prior to the appointment. This method may save some time at banding appointments.

How would you explain to a patient how orthodontic bands are fitted?

Procedure 50-2 Placing and Removing Steel Separating Springs

Equipment and Supplies Needed

- Basic setup: mouth mirror, explorer, cotton pliers
- Steel separating springs
- Bird-beak (No. 139) pliers
- Orthodontic scaler

Procedure Steps for Placing Steel Separating Springs

1. Grasp the spring at the base of the shorter leg using the bird-beak pliers.

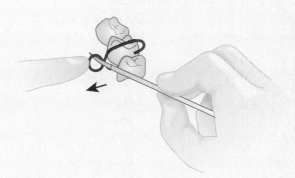

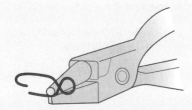

2. Place the bent end or curve hook end into the lingual embrasure. Pull the spring open to allow the shorter leg of the spring to slip beneath the contact from the lingual side to the facial side.

3. Carefully slip the spring into place with the helix or coiled side on the facial.

2. Place the orthodontic scaler into the coil or helix and lift upward until there is space between the upper arm and the occlusal aspect of the marginal ridge.

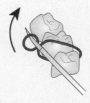

Procedure Steps for Removing Steel Separating Springs

1. Operator should place one finger of one hand over the spring to prevent it from coming off and injuring the patient.

3. While supporting the separator on the helix with the index finger, remove the upper arm of the spring and pull it toward the facial surface of the embrasure.

Fitting of Molar Bands

The maxillary and mandibular bands are initially seated on the tooth by finger pressure on the mesial and distal surfaces. After the initial placement a band pusher is used on the mesiobuccal and distolingual edges to seat the band. The band is placed close to the height of contour (marginal ridge). Then a bite stick (band seater) is placed on the buccal margins of the band, utilizing the patient's heavy biting force to drive the bands down for complete band seating (Figure 50.26).

Cementation of Orthodontic Bands

In selecting orthodontic band cement, strength should be considered as well as the use of a time-release fluoride proponent to aid in preventing decay under the band. Examples of cements include glass ionomers, polycarboxylate,

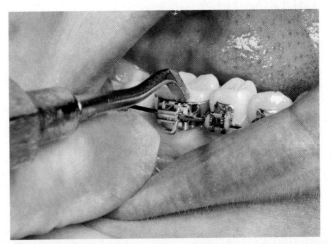

FIGURE 50.26
A band pusher being used to seat the band interproximally.

Procedure 50-3 Placing and Removing Elastomeric Ring Separators

Equipment and Supplies Needed

- Basic setup: mouth mirror, explorer, cotton pliers
- Elastomeric separators
- Dental floss
- Separating pliers
- Orthodontic scaler
- Patient protective eyewear

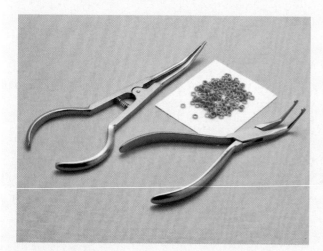

Procedure Steps for Placing Elastomeric Ring Separators

1. Place the elastic separator over the beaks of the separating pliers, making sure to squeeze the pliers to ensure the separator is secure.

2. Stretch and squeeze the ring separator, allowing one side of the separator to be inserted between the con-

tact areas. This can be done by using a back-and-forth motion, similar to flossing.

3. Release the tension of the pliers and disengage from the separator. Repeat this process on all teeth that will be receiving metal bands.

Procedure Steps for Removing Elastomeric Ring Separators

1. Using an orthodontic scaler, slip one end into the ring of the elastic separator.

2. Hold one finger of the hand over the separator so that it does not snap and hurt the patient.

3. Carefully pull the elastic separator using slight pressure to release it from the contact area.

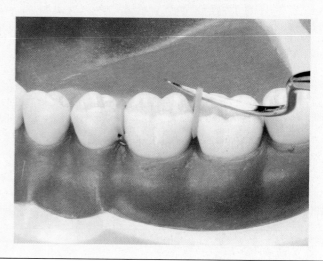

---

and zinc phosphate. However, zinc phosphate (the "gold standard") is being replaced with glass ionomer fluoride-releasing cement.

Generally, orthodontic band cement should be thick and have a long setting time to allow for adaptation and seating problems. For setting time, it is important to closely follow manufacturer's directions (Procedure 50-4). (For more information on dental cements see Chapter 35.)

Bonded Brackets

The bonded edgewise bracket is the most common type of attachment for fixed appliances (Procedure 50-5). The bracket is attached to a mesh, stainless steel backing pad that

is bonded to the enamel of the tooth. Brackets are bonded onto the facial surface of all anterior teeth. The bracket is designed with four tie wings so that an arch wire can be placed into the horizontal slot and the bracket can be ligated (held in place). Also available since 1979 are lingual brackets. Lingual brackets are designed to be aesthetically pleasing primarily for the adult patient. However, the comfort adjustment is often not well tolerated.

Orthodontic brackets have become more favorable because of the aesthetic and home care advantages. They are smaller, have a lower profile, and are easy to keep clean so the patient has better control over her oral health. Brackets may be made of stainless steel, ceramic, or acrylic and bonded directly to the teeth. They are

Procedure 50-4 Assisting in the Fitting and Cementation of Orthodontic Bands

Equipment and Supplies Needed

- Basic setup: mouth mirror, explorer, cotton pliers
- Cotton rolls or gauze squares
- Preselected orthodontic bands
- Chilled glass slab or paper pad
- Cement spatula (stainless steel)
- Band pusher
- Band seater
- Bite stick
- Scaler
- Band remover
- ChapStick, toothpaste, or utility wax

Preparation

1. Once the separators have been removed, polish the teeth with a rubber cup.

2. Rinse patient's mouth and air dry teeth. Cotton rolls are placed lingual and buccal to isolate the molars and keep the area dry.

3. Preselected bands are placed on a small square of masking tape with the occlusal surface down on tape and with the gingival margin placed upright.

4. Buccal tubes and any attachments are wiped with ChapStick, toothpaste, or utility wax to prevent cement from getting into them.

Procedure Steps for Mixing and Placing Cement

1. Once the orthodontist is ready to put the bands on, the assistant will mix the cement on the glass slab or mixing pad, carefully following the manufacturer's directions. The mixture should be thoroughly homogenous.

2. Load the first band by holding it by the margin of the masking tape, making sure that the gingival surface is upright.

3. While placing the spatula with cement over the margin, allow the cement to flow into the circumference of the band.

4. Transfer the band to the orthodontist, who will invert the band over the tooth. (*Note:* There are various ways that the orthodontist may want to transfer the bands; however, the transfer should be as smooth as possible. The bands must always be positioned so that they are handed to the orthodontist in the correct sequential order.)

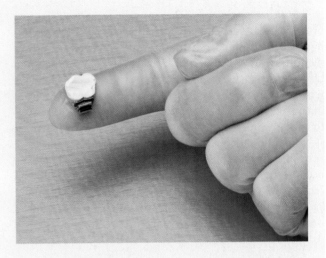

5. Transfer the band seater, bite stick, or any other instrument that the orthodontist might request until the band is properly seated. The patient is instructed to bite down gently, forcing the band down onto the middle third of the crown.

6. At this point, excess cement is forced out from under the gingival and occlusal margins of the bands and allowed to dry.

Procedure Steps for Removing Excess Cement

1. After the cement has reached the final stage of setting, remove the excess with an orthodontic scaler or explorer.

2. Thoroughly rinse any cement from the patient's mouth.

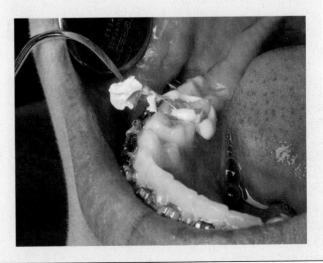

available in silver, gold, or natural tooth color (Figure 50.27). Ceramic and acrylic brackets are more popular because they are aesthetically pleasing and are not as noticeable as the stainless steel. The brackets are bonded using a composite resin similar to that used to restore anterior teeth.

Another style of bracket called a "self-ligating bracket," was developed in the 1970s. These brackets have been reengineered to simplify brackets and treatment systems. Self-ligating brackets have a "door" and hinge system where the door covers the slot of the arch wire when placed. The "door" takes the place of an auxiliary tie. Some of the advantages of using this system are that they cause less friction within the arch wire guide slot, enabling the teeth to slide and move faster; they are aesthetically pleasing; they promote efficient oral hygiene because they do not use auxiliary ties; and less time is required to make arch wire changes at each appointment. Self-ligating orthodontic companies include Orec's Speed Braces, Ormco's Damon System, GAC's In-Ovation, and Adenta's Evolution.

Auxiliary Attachments

Auxiliary attachments are essential to the contemporary edgewise appliance. They may be attached to molar bands or single brackets. They can be purchased presoldered onto the bracket or molar band, or the orthodon-

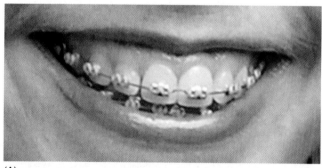
(A)

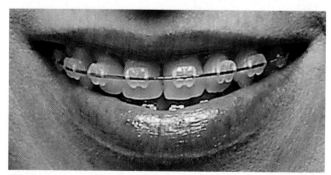
(B)

FIGURE 50.27
(a) Stainless steel "gold"-colored brackets and (b) tooth-colored brackets.
Courtesy American Association of Orthodontics

tist can weld them onto the band in the office. Some auxiliary attachments are headgear tubes. These are round tubes that are placed on the buccal surface of the maxillary first molar bands and are used to insert the end of the inner bow of the facebow appliance.

Attachments include edgewise tubes that are rectangular and placed on the facial aspect of molar bands and labial hooks located on the facial surfaces of the first and second molar bands for both arches. Their function is to hold the intra-arch elastics. Buttons or brackets located on the lingual portion of the bands serve to stabilize the arch and to act as reinforcement and as an anchor for tooth movement.

Arch Wires

The arch wire directs the teeth into the desired position. Arch wires are placed into the horizontal slots of the brackets and tubes in the molar bands. They are held in this position by a ligature or elastomeric tie. The arch wire produces a force that guides the movement of the teeth.

Many shapes and materials are used in the design of arch wires because each type of arch wire has a specific function that is unique to a particular movement. The orthodontic arch wire is the key to the outcome of orthodontic treatment.

Types of Arch Wires

During orthodontic treatment a variety of arch wires may be used. In the initial stages of tooth movement, a nickel titanium wire is used. This type of material is flexible, and resists permanent deformation, and adapts well to very crooked or crowded teeth with gentle force.

Stainless steel wire is stiffer and stronger than most types of arch wire. It is used to apply more force and stability to control tooth movement. It holds a permanent bend and withstands greater force, hence, it is known as the "working arch wire."

Beta titanium (TMA) is chosen when several bands are in place instead of brackets. This is an important wire that offers a combination of strength, flexibility, and memory.

Optiflex wire is a newer type of wire made from a composite material topped with a coating of optical glass fibers. This wire is aesthetically pleasing and is generally used in the initial stages of tooth alignment.

Shapes of Arch Wires

Arch wires are available in two shapes, round and rectangular (square). Round wires are used in the beginning stages of orthodontic treatment to exert gentle force. Their function is to level the arch and align teeth in an upright position. Round arch wires can be used to open a bite and slide teeth to close spaces. Rectangular or square arch wires are used in the final stages of treatment.

Procedure 50-5 Assisting in the Direct Bonding of Orthodontic Brackets

Dental assistants should be sure to check with their state dental practice laws to determine what tasks they are allowed to perform.

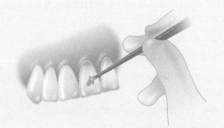

Equipment and Supplies Needed

- Basic setup: mouth mirror, explorer, cotton pliers
- Brackets
- Cotton rolls or lip retractors
- Pumice
- Slow-speed handpiece with prophy angle and rubber cup
- Bonding setup (acid etching and bonding agent)
- Orthodontic scaler

Preparation

1. First clean the teeth by using a prophy cup with pumice. (*Note:* A prophy paste without fluoride is acceptable. The use of fluoride will interfere with the bonding process.)

2. Rinse and dry the teeth. Place cotton rolls for isolation, and position lip retractors.

3. Dab the acid etchant solution onto the facial surface of the tooth that is to receive bonding. This solution remains on the tooth for a specific time according to the manufacturer's direction.

4. Dry the tooth, noticing the chalky appearance caused by the etching material.

Procedure Steps for Bonding the Brackets

1. The orthodontist applies a liquid sealant (usually the monomer of the bonding agent) to the prepared tooth surface.

2. The assistant places a small quantity of bonding material on the back of the specified bracket.

3. The assistant uses bracket placement forceps to transfer the bracket to the orthodontist.

4. The orthodontist places the bracket on approximately the middle third of the tooth.

5. Remove excess bonding agent with the scaler.

6. Bond the brackets to the teeth with a curing light.

7. Remove the cotton rolls and lip retractors from the mouth.

They function to position the crown and upright or align the root of the tooth in the maxillary and mandibular relationship and provide overall stability.

Elastomeric Ties or Ligature Wires

After the arch wire has been selected, measured, and placed into the slots of the brackets, it must be tied or ligated to keep it in place (Procedure 50-6). Elastomeric ties are made of plastic or rubber-like material and are stretched around the bracket to hold the arch wire in place. Figure 50.28 shows an elastomeric tie being removed.

The use of elastomeric ties results in less time being required for an arch wire change. Changing them is a quick job and patients enjoy selecting a color(s) to wear.

Ligature ties are thin wires that are twisted around the bracket to hold the arch wire in place. Generally ligature ties

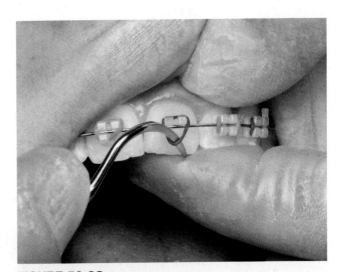

FIGURE 50.28
Removing elastomeric ties.

Procedure 50-6 Placing the Arch Wire and Ligature Ties

Dental assistants should be sure to check with their state dental practice laws to determine what tasks they are allowed to perform.

Equipment and Supplies Needed

- Basic setup: mouth mirror, explorer, cotton pliers
- Gauze and cotton rolls
- High-volume evacuator and/or saliva ejector
- Arch wire selected to fit
- Weingart pliers
- Bird-beak pliers
- Ligature wire and/or elastics
- Ligature cutting pliers
- Ligature tying pliers
- Distal end cutting pliers

Procedure Steps for Placing the Arch Wire

1. Insert the prefitted arch wire onto the brackets and into the buccal arch wire slot of the molar bands.

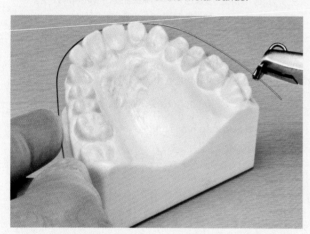

2. Securely fit the wire into the horizontal slots in the middle of the brackets. Tie the brackets with elastomeric ties or ligature wire.

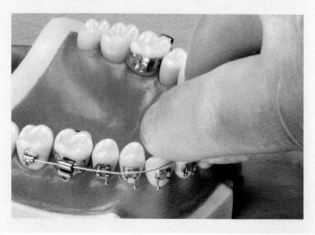

3. The elastomeric ties are placed over the brackets using a hemostat or ligature tying pliers. The ring ties are spread and placed on the gingival side of the bracket. They are then pulled down over the arch wire and wrapped around the occlusal side of the bracket.

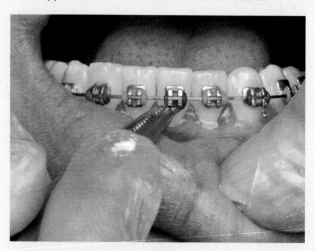

Procedure Steps for Placing Ligature Wire Ties

1. While holding the ligature wire between the thumb and index finger, wrap the wire around the occlusal and gingival wings of the bracket, going in a distal to mesial direction. Twist the ends of the wire together, using a hemostat or ligature tying pliers.

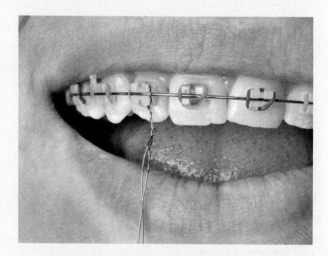

2. Using the pliers or hemostat, twist the ends of the ties for several rotations. Do not twist the wire too tight causing it to break.

continued on next page

Procedure 50-6 *continued from previous page*

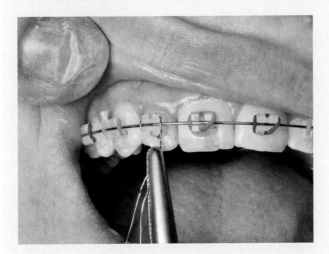

3. Repeat the process until the entire arch wire is tied.

4. The twisted ends of the ligature ties, or "pigtails" as they are often called, are cut with ligature wire cutting pliers to about 3 to 4 mm.

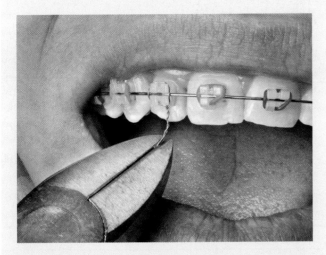

5. The pigtail is bent to allow it to be placed into the embrasure with a condenser.

6. After cutting and tucking the wire into the embrasure, run your finger over the area to check for sharp ends.

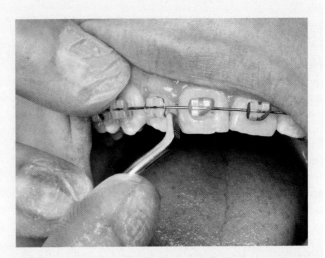

7. Check the distal ends of the arch wire, making sure you bend any leftover wire toward the tooth leaving only 1 mm of the wire extending out.

are 0.01-gauge stainless steel that may be tied in two ways. The ligature ties can either be tied around one tooth or several teeth, forming a figure 8. Either application usually begins at the most posterior tooth and works to the midline. Some ligature ties have hooks that have been soldered to them. These hooks are known as Kobayashi hooks. These hooks are ligated onto a bracket as needed to attach elastics.

Power Products

Several accessory products that are made of elastics are available. These products provide the ability for tooth movement during treatment. Elastic chain ties are contin-uous O's that form a chain. The power chain is used to apply gentle continual force on the teeth to close spaces or correct rotated teeth.

Elastics or rubber bands are used with the coopera-tion of the patient. They are placed from one tooth to another in the same arch or from one tooth to another in an opposing arch. The purpose of elastics is to close space between teeth and correct occlusal relationships between dental arches. The orthodontist determines the place-ment to create a specific direction of movement, and the dental assistant provides home care instructions to the patient. The success of using rubber bands relies greatly on patient cooperation.

The patient is instructed to use elastics to correct a Class II malocclusion. However, at the adjustment appointments it is obvious that he is not cooperating with elastic wear. What can be done to motivate cooperation with the patient?

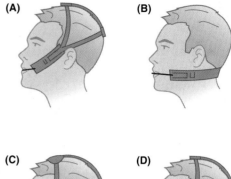

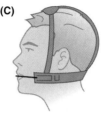
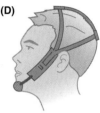

Headgear

Headgear is an orthodontic appliance that actively guides the growth and development of the jaw. It aids in correcting anteroposterior discrepancies. Ideally, the headgear is used to treat a Class II, Division I, malocclusion (increased overjet) along with fixed braces. Table 50-1 lists some common habits that affect the development of the jaw.

The headgear is attached to the molar bands and is anchored from the back of the head or neck. Its purpose is to stop the upper jaw from growing, hence, preventing or correcting an overjet. For the headgear to be effective, it is usually worn for a specific number of hours each day, with the majority of the time being during the sleeping hours.

The headgear consists of a padded strap that rests behind the patient's head and hooks onto the outside of the facebow (Figure 50.29). The inner portion of the facebow attaches into the buccal tube of the maxillary first molar. The facebow is used to stabilize or move the maxillary first molar distally and to create room in one arch. The outer portion of the facebow attaches to the special traction device (neck pad). The traction device applies extraoral force to achieve the desired results that the treatment indicates.

FIGURE 50.29
(a) High-pull headgear: a traction device that fits around the top of the patient's head and hooks into the maxillary molar buccal tubes. (b) Cervical traction: a traction device that fits around the patient's neck. The exerted force is parallel to the occlusal plane. (c) Combination headgear: used for both high-pull and cervical traction. Exerts its force along the occlusal plane and upward. (d) Chin cap: uses a combination of high-pull headgear and a chin cup that fits on the mandible to control the growth of the mandible in patients with Class III malocclusion.

Adjustment Visits

For orthodontic treatments to be successful, it is important for patients to attend their adjustment visits. These appointments are scheduled at specific intervals during treatment. At this appointment the arch wires are changed, loose bands are recemented, and broken brackets are replaced. It is essential that fixed appliances remain attached to the teeth during treatment. Should a bracket or band become loose, the tooth has a greater tendency to move out of alignment.

TABLE 50-1 Habits Affecting the Development of the Jaw

Habit Affecting Jaw Development	Effect
Anterior tongue thrust	The tongue rests on the lingual surfaces of the maxillary teeth, causing pressure to the teeth so that they move forward.
Lateral tongue thrust	The pressure of the tongue causes the bite to close, which may prevent the permanent teeth from erupting.
Tongue thrust	The tongue presses against the anterior teeth while swallowing. This pressure causes the anterior teeth to move forward.
Thumb and finger sucking	After the age of 5, continual sucking of fingers or thumb will cause the facial structure to be affected. Usually, the maxillary arch, palate, and anterior teeth are affected.
Bruxism	The involuntary grinding or clenching of teeth in movements other than chewing occurs, resulting in unnatural wear of enamel and pressure on the periodontal ligaments.
Mouth breathing	Continual mouth breathing can cause a change in the dentofacial structure. This can result in narrowing of the maxilla, leading to a pinched facial appearance.

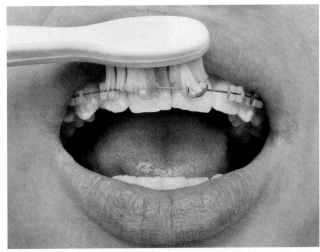

(A)

Adjustment visits are especially important for checking progress and evaluating oral hygiene. The orthodontic assistant (under direct supervision of the orthodontist) first checks the patient for any loose appliances, checks the patient's oral hygiene, and prepares the necessary setup for the treatment scheduled for that day. At this appointment, if an arch wire change is scheduled, the dental assistant removes the elastomeric ties and arch wire and addresses any oral hygiene concerns with the patient.

Oral Hygiene and Dietary Instructions

The orthodontic assistant provides oral hygiene instructions to the patient who is wearing brackets. Orthodontic bands and brackets offer an ideal environment to which food and debris can adhere. If the patient's hygiene is not of good quality, caries may become an issue. The assistant demonstrates how to brush the debris off of the braces by manipulating the brush around all four sides of the brackets and under the arch wire, and then demonstrates how to brush the teeth and tongue (Figure 50.30). The assistant should motivate and educate the patient on oral hygiene throughout treatment. Along with good brushing techniques, the patient must be taught how to

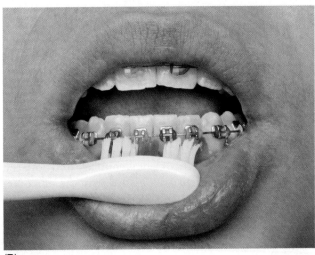

(B)
FIGURE 50.30
Brushing (a) the maxillary arch fixed appliances (braces) and (b) the mandibular brackets prior to brushing the teeth.

floss when fixed appliances are in place. The use of a "floss threader" will make flossing manageable (Figure 50.31). Other adjunctive oral hygiene aids include an end-tufted brush, a proxy brush, a rubber tip stimulator, and a water jet (e.g., Waterpik).

Some fruits and vegetables, such as apples and carrots, may be more difficult to eat during orthodontic treatment, but should not be avoided. The patient should be instructed on the importance of cutting up apples and carrots into small bite-sized pieces and then placing these items toward the back of the mouth to chew. The assistant should make recommendations to the patient on how to select and eat proper foods and what food items need to be avoided. Certain food items should be avoided because they can damage or break the bands, brackets, or arch wires. Table 50-2 lists some common types of food that should be avoided while undergoing orthodontic treatment.

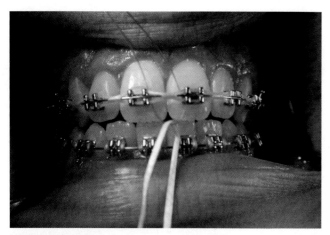

FIGURE 50.31
Floss being threaded under the arch wire with a floss threader.
Image courtesy Instructional Materials for the Dental Team, Lex., KY

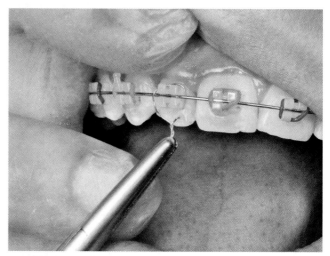

FIGURE 50.32
Removing the ligature wire.

Understanding growth, age, and tooth development assists in the orthodontic diagnosis. How does the growth of an individual play an important role in that diagnosis?

Completed Treatment

When the orthodontic treatment is complete and both the orthodontist and patient are satisfied with the outcome, the braces are removed and the retention phase begins (Figure 50.32) (Procedure 50-7). The removal appointment requires more time than an adjustment appointment. The instruments used are bracket removal pliers and band removal pliers. They are used along with a special technique that will not harm the enamel of the tooth:

- Band removal is accomplished by breaking the seal of the cement and lifting the bands off with a band remover.

- Bonded brackets are removed by causing a fracture in the bonding material, while being careful not to damage the enamel.
- Any residual cement or bonding material may be removed by using a scaling instrument or ultrasonic scaler.

Retention

The last phase of treatment is the retention phase, which may be the most important phase of the entire orthodontic process. In the retention phase, the active orthodontic treatment is over and retention or a holding pattern begins. During the active movement of treatment, the teeth moved slowly through the bone as osteoblast (new bone growth, spongy bone) was generated. Holding the teeth in the corrected position allows time for calcification to take place. If the retainer is not worn as instructed, the teeth drift out of ideal position.

TABLE 50-2 Orthodontics and Eating Habits

Foods to Avoid During Orthodontic Treatment	Outcome	Examples of Foods
Foods that contain sugar	High sugar content foods or drinks attack tooth enamel, causing decay around bands and brackets.	Cakes, candy, cookies, pies, coated cereal, soda, sports and fruit drinks containing sugar
Foods that are sticky	Loosen bands, bend arch wires, and break ligature ties.	Gummy bears, caramel, caramel corn, taffy, licorice, Starbursts, Sugar Daddies, chewing gum, chewy fruit snacks
Hard foods	Loosen bands and break bonded brackets off of the tooth. May also break and bend arch wires.	Chewing ice, popcorn, peanut brittle, jawbreakers, hard taco chips and taco shells, pretzels, hard candy, frozen candy bars
Husk foods	Often can lodge in between bands and brackets and beneath arch wires. Can cause irritation to gums.	Popcorn, peanuts, corn on the cob, meat on the bone

Procedure 50-7 Assisting at a Completion Appointment

Dental assistants should be sure to check with their state dental practice laws to determine what tasks they are allowed to perform.

Equipment and Supplies Needed

- Basic setup: mouth mirror, cotton pliers, explorer
- Gauze and cotton rolls
- Scaler
- Ligature wire cutting pliers
- Bracket and bonding material removal pliers
- Posterior band remover
- Ultrasonic scaler (optional)
- Prophy angle, prophy paste with fluoride
- Alginate impression material (preselected tray)

Procedure Step for Removing Elastic Bands

1. The elastic ties or bands are lifted and removed with a scaler. The elastic bands are then rolled over the bracket wings.

Procedure Steps for Removing Ligature Wire Ties

1. Using a ligature cutter, place the beaks of the cutter where the ligature wire is exposed. Cut the wire, making sure that you have hold of the wire.

2. Remove the wire from the wings of the bracket. Repeat this procedure on each bracket until all are removed.

3. The entire arch wire can now be removed by using a pair of Weingart pliers. Remove the arch wire by first pulling it out of the buccal tube on one end. Then, holding it securely, remove it from the opposite end.

Procedure Step for Removing Brackets

1. Remove the brackets using bracket-removing pliers. The lower beak of the pliers with the sharp edge is

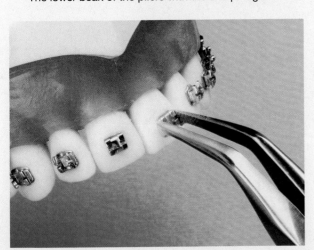

placed on the gingival edge of the bracket; the upper beak with the softer nylon tip is placed on the occlusal edge of the bracket. The pliers are then squeezed together, causing the sharp end of the pliers to break the bond and remove some of the cement.

Procedure Steps for Removing Bands

1. To remove the posterior bands, a pair of band-removing pliers is used. The cushioned end is placed on the buccal cusp of the tooth. The end with the blade is placed against the gingival edge of the band. The pliers are squeezed and the band is gently lifted toward the occlusal surface.

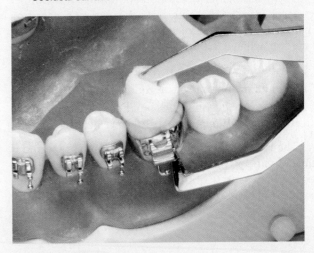

2. This same process is repeated on the lingual surfaces until the cement bond releases the band.

3. After all brackets and bands have been removed, the teeth are scaled with a hand or ultrasonic scaler to remove excess cement and bonding material.

4. Polish with a rubber cup and take completion photographs (intra- and extraoral).

5. After the teeth have been scaled and polished and there are no signs of cement or bonding material present, an alginate impression is taken on both arches for fabrication of retainers.

6. The patient is given an appointment for placement of the retainers. This may be later that day or in a week depending on the orthodontist's schedule. At this time, the patient is given instructions for wearing the retainer.

Note: The patient will also be seen periodically to make any adjustments to the retainer. Retention usually lasts for about two years.

To ensure long-term results, the retention phase is important for the following reasons:

* To allow for reorganization of gingival and periodontal tissues
* To support the teeth that are unstable so that the tongue and pressure of the cheeks do not cause a relapse
* To control growth changes

Retention Appliances

Various types of retention appliances are used. The specific type of **retainer** is selected by the orthodontist to adapt to the patient's individual treatment needs. Examples of retainers are positioner, Hawley, lingual bar, and invisible (clear) retainers.

The positioner is a custom-made appliance of rubber or elastic acrylic that fits over the patient's dentition when orthodontic treatment is complete. The positioner is used to achieve the following results:

* To maintain the teeth in their desired positions
* To stimulate and massage the gingivae
* To allow the alveolus to rebuild support around the teeth prior to the patient wearing a removable retainer

The Hawley retainer is the most common type and is made of self-polymerizing acrylic (rigid), with a wire bow on the facial aspects of the anterior teeth and wire clasps that hold around the molars for stability (Figure 50.33).

On the maxillary retainer the acrylic portion covers the palate. On the mandibular the acrylic is lingual of the anterior teeth to the floor of the mouth. In both retainers the wire should fit lightly between the contacts of the canines and premolars.

The lingual retainer is bonded directly to the lingual surface of the mandibular teeth from canine to canine. The metal bar is placed at the cingulum of the anterior teeth. This light steel wire is bent to provide lower incisor position during late growth. The patient is instructed to use a floss threader to clear around the area of the wire.

The invisible (clear) retainer is a clear acrylic (rigid) appliance that fits over the dentition only. The patient is instructed to wear the retainer full time until otherwise instructed by the orthodontist. The orthodontic assistant provides home care instructions on the care and maintenance of each appliance.

Postoperative treatment is continued for one year after a patient's braces are removed. Why are follow-up appointments required?

Treatment Options

With the onset of technology a recent alternative treatment option for fixed braces has become available. This technology is the application of Invisalign. Invisalign is a new orthodontic treatment system that works to

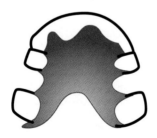
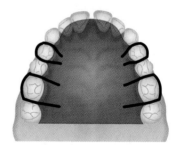
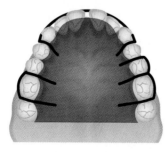
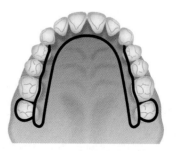

FIGURE 50.33
Hawley retainer appliances.

straighten teeth through the use of a series of clear plastic acrylic aligners. Invisalign eliminates traditional fixed brackets, bands, and wires. This concept does not work on all malocclusions. Along with a dentist's diagnosis, treatment plan, and great advances in 3-D computer technology, correction of malocclusions can occur.

Invisalign aligners are easy to remove and more comfortable than normal braces. The aligners are made of a material similar to that used to make whitening or fluoride trays, but are fabricated in a thinner, more precise and rigid material. A series of aligners is worn for about two weeks, 22 hours a day, removing only to eat, brush, and floss. When the teeth have moved to an interim desired position with one aligner, a new aligner is worn that moves the teeth to a new interim position. Aligners

continue to be changed until the teeth are in the final desired position.

To treat patients using the Invisalign appliance, a dentist must go through a certified program offered by the Invisalign manufacturer Align Technology. The dental assistant may also take a similar course that allows him or her to take polyvinyl silicone (PVS) impressions and bite registrations, x-rays, and intraoral and extraoral photographs. Invisalign offers modules on case presentation, management, and practice building for patient education.

What are some concerns that patients have prior to receiving orthodontic treatment?

SUMMARY

The orthodontic assistant is versatile, pleasant, knowledgeable, and skilled. There are many duties in the orthodontic office that are the responsibility of the assistant. The assistant may work with the dentist or function independently under the direction of the dentist. The functions vary as determined by each state's dental practice act.

The more credentials the assistant holds the more valuable he or she is to the practice. The orthodontic

assistant may elect to take a national examination (boards) for orthodontics offered by the Dental Assisting National Board and hold the certificate of orthodontic assistant. This entitles the assistant to take the expanded functions license exam for his or her particular state. Dental assistants must always be sure to check with their state requirements to determine what credentials are necessary to perform various functions.

KEY TERMS

- **Arch wire:** A contoured metal wire that provides force by guiding the movement of teeth during orthodontic treatment. p. 790
- **Auxiliary attachment:** Specialized attachment located on brackets and bands that is used to hold arch wires and elastics in place. p. 796
- **Corrective (interceptive) orthodontics:** Orthodontic treatment that creates space in the mouth, or reduces a patient's poor oral habits, prior to or instead of full orthodontic procedures. p. 783
- **Dentofacial:** Term used to describe structures of the teeth, jaws, and surrounding facial bones. p. 781
- **Distoclusion:** A Class II malocclusion in which the mesiobuccal cusp of the maxillary first molar occludes mesial to the mesiobuccal groove of the

mandibular first molar by more than the width of a premolar. p. 782
- **Fetal molding:** Condition that occurs when an arm or leg of a fetus presses against another forming bone, causing distortion of a rapidly growing area. p. 782
- **Ligature wire:** A light wire used to hold an orthodontic arch wire into a bracket. p. 787
- **Mesioclusion:** Term used to describe a Class III occlusion, in which the mesiobuccal cusp of the maxillary first molar is distal to the mesiobuccal groove of the mandibular first molar. p. 782
- **Retainer:** An orthodontic appliance used after orthodontic treatment to maintain teeth in their desired position. p. 804

CHECK YOUR UNDERSTANDING

1. Orthodontics is a specialty of dentistry in which a dentist must go to school several more years beyond that required for a regular dental degree. How many additional years must an orthodontist remain in school to receive a degree?

a. one year
b. two to three years
c. four years
d. five years

CHECK YOUR UNDERSTANDING (continued)

2. At what age should a person be referred for an orthodontic examination?
   a. 7 years
   b. 13 years
   c. 50 years
   d. all of the above

3. There is no vertical overlap of the teeth in an
   a. open bite.
   b. overbite.
   c. overjet.
   d. both a and b.

4. An Angle Class II malocclusion is also called a
   a. mesioclusion.
   b. neutroclusion.
   c. linguoclusion.
   d. distoclusion.

5. Damage to a tooth bud during development may be a/an _____ cause of malocclusion.
   a. developmental
   b. environmental
   c. genetic
   d. hereditary

6. In normal occlusion, which embrasure does the cusp of the maxillary canine occupy?
   a. between the mandibular central and lateral incisors
   b. between the mandibular canine and first premolar
   c. between the mandibular first and second premolars
   d. between the mandibular lateral incisor and canine

7. What food product(s) should you avoid while undergoing orthodontic treatment?
   a. vegetables
   b. chips, candy, and gum
   c. fruit
   d. milk

8. On the maxillary first molar bands, what is the buccal tube used for?
   a. arch wire
   b. elastics
   c. headgear
   d. torque springs

9. Which of the following is *not* a main method used to separate posterior teeth for the placement of bands?
   a. soft brass wire twisted tightly around the contacts
   b. steel springs placed around the contact point
   c. a metal disk wedged between the contact points
   d. elastomeric separators placed around the contact points

10. Excessive lip protrusion is most often caused by a
   a. Class I malocclusion.
   b. Class II malocclusion.
   c. Class III malocclusion.
   d. both a and b.

INTERNET ACTIVITIES

- Go to www.ada.org/public/media/videos/minute/index.asp to watch a short video on the field of orthodontics.
- Go to www.invisalign.com/generalapp/us/en/for/index.jsp to answer the following questions:
   a. What is Invisalign?
   b. How is this particular type of procedure done?
   c. Describe how the dentist or orthodontist becomes a certified Invisalign participant.
- Go to www.danb.org to obtain information about the Dental Assistant National Board Examination.
- Go to www.danb.org/main/statespecificinfo.asp for state specific dental practice act licensure requirements.

WEB REFERENCES

- American Association of Orthodontists www.braces.org
- American Dental Association www.ada.org/public/braces.faq.asp
- American Dental Association www.ada.org/public/media/videos/minute/index.asp
- Dental Assistant National Board www.danb.org
- Invisalign www.invisalign.com/general/app/us/en/for/index.asp

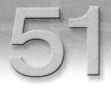

Assisting in Emergency Care

Learning Objectives

After reading this chapter, the student should be able to:

- Explain techniques to prevent medical emergencies in the dental office.
- List the emergency preparedness responsibilities of each dental team member.
- Discuss telephone protocol for emergency situations.
- Define the ABCD's of life support.
- Describe basic emergency kit items.
- Explain the use of the automated external defibrillator.
- Identify signs, symptoms, and treatments of emergencies, including syncope.
- Understand how to document an emergency situation.

Preparing for Certification Exams

- Recognize signs and symptoms related to specific medical conditions/emergencies likely to occur in the dental office.
- Respond to and assist in the management of chairside emergencies.
- Maintain emergency kit, prepare and post listing of emergency support personnel.
- Recognize signs and symptoms related to dental conditions.

Key Terms

Asthma

Angina pectoris

Automated external defibrillator (AED)

Cerebrovascular accident (CVA)

Edema

Epilepsy

Grand mal seizure

Hyperglycemia

Hyperventilation

Hypoglycemia

Myocardial infarction

Petit mal seizure

Postural hypotension

Syncope

Chapter Outline

- Preventing Medical Emergencies
- Emergency Preparedness
  - Responsibilities of Each Team Member
- Recognizing an Emergency
- Protocol for Emergency Situations
  - Cardiopulmonary Resuscitation
- Emergency Equipment and Supplies
  - Oxygen
- Emergency Responses
  - Shock Recognition and Treatment
  - Drug and Materials Sensitivity Related Emergencies
  - Cardiac Emergencies
  - Respiratory Emergencies
  - Other Emergencies
- Dental Emergencies
- Documentation of an Emergency

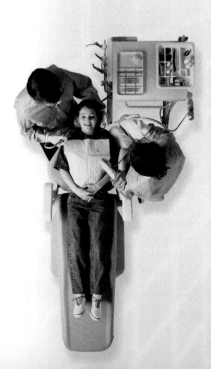

The dental team must be prepared not only to provide dental care to patients, but to offer emergency care in the unfortunate event that an emergency arises. Life-threatening emergencies can and do happen in dental offices. It can happen to anyone at any time. It is important for the dental assistant to be able to recognize specific emergency events and know what emergency care standards and equipment should be used to respond to emergencies. No one expects a life-threatening event to occur in the dental office, but if and when it does occur, it is important for each member of the dental team to be prepared and knowledgeable about how to respond appropriately.

Preventing Medical Emergencies

Many office emergencies can be prevented by being aware of the information provided by the patient in the form of a dental and medical health history. It is also important for the dental assistant to know how to obtain vital signs and to be able to interpret the results (Figure 51.1). (See Chapter 23 for more information about obtaining vital signs.)

Vital signs are helpful in determining a patient's current health status. With the basic information obtained from taking vitals, the dental team can be alerted to health issues that a patient may be having and possibly prevent a serious emergency from occurring.

A patient may be apprehensive and stressed because of the dental treatment. It is important for the dental assistant to recognize these signs and assist in creating an environment that calms the patient. The most important thing the dental assistant can do is be sensitive to the needs of each patient. The next important step is to be prepared.

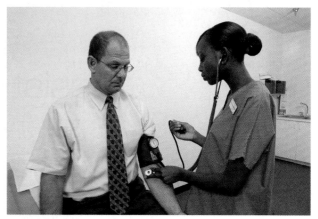

FIGURE 51.1
Assistant taking vital signs.

Life Span Considerations

People are living longer these days, so more elderly patients are being seen in the dentist's office. These individuals may have multiple health issues. The dental assistant should read each patient's health history completely, including information about any allergies and medications taken, and be prepared in the event of an emergency.

Emergency Preparedness

Regardless of the steps taken to prevent emergencies, not all of them can be prevented. If an emergency should happen, the dental team members must be prepared. This includes having an emergency plan in place, all of the necessary equipment and medications handy, and a list of clearly posted emergency phone numbers.

The dental assistant and the dentist must provide ongoing observation to ensure they respond to any emergency effectively. Ongoing observation involves paying attention to patients during dental treatment. Look to see if the patient's skin color changes, if the mood or anxiety level changes, and if the patient's breathing is normal or labored. Observance of vital signs is important to ensure that the members of the dental team can address any emergency situation.

The dental team members must remain calm in order to perform their assigned duties during an emergency. Dental health care personnel should also maintain a current certification for health care provider cardiopulmonary resuscitation (CPR) and/or advanced cardiac care. A basic first aid course that teaches how to control bleeding and treatment of burns and fractures will help the staff assist in other emergencies that may occur in the office. The dental team should be knowledgeable regarding the various responsibilities that each member of the dental team has in the event of an emergency in the office.

Dental Assistant PROFESSIONAL TIP

Dental assistants should attend continuing education classes in emergency care in order to ensure that their skills are current. The dentist and the rest of the staff will appreciate the dental assistant who has taken the initiative and shown the motivation to maintain the skills needed in an emergency.

Responsibilities of Each Team Member

Each person in the dental office must be aware of his or her responsibilities and functions in the event of a medical emergency. The combined effort of everyone leads to more efficient life-saving steps. The dental assistant is charged with multiple responsibilities:

- Notify the dentist of the emergency. The dentist has overall responsibility in every situation in the dental office.
- Alert other members of the dental team and request assistance when necessary.
- Administer basic life support (BLS) if necessary. This includes opening the airway, providing chest compressions, and obtaining the automated external defibrillator (AED), if available. The AED is not required in all states.
- Retrieve the emergency kit and oxygen.
- Assist the dentist in preparing emergency drugs and equipment.
- Monitor vital signs.

Most dental offices have instituted code words or phrases to indicate that an emergency is occurring in the office. By using these words, the dental assistant can notify the dental team of an emergency, yet avoid causing panic among the other patients. For example, three buzzes on the intercom may be used, or a page for "Dr. Red" may indicate to the staff that an emergency has occurred.

Each staff member in the dental office has responsibilities during an emergency. Even the front desk personnel or receptionist has key responsibilities in effectively responding to an emergency:

- Maintain updated emergency numbers that are easily accessible to everyone in the office (Figure 51.2). Ideally, numbers should be kept close to the telephone.
- Notify emergency personnel and when necessary provide explicit directions to the office. A script posted near the telephone can help the assistant provide important information to emergency personnel. This type of script is particularly useful if the assistant is nervous or upset.
- Direct emergency personnel to the office. This may require going outside and holding doors open for emergency equipment.
- Keep patients who are waiting to be seen calm, and reschedule patients if necessary.

If the dental office has more than one dental assistant, the responsibilities for responding to an emergency can be divided. For instance, one of the dental assistants can maintain the patient's airway, breathing, and circulation, place the patient in a comfortable position, and assess the patient's vital signs. The second dental assistant

EMERGENCY PHONE NUMBERS

Police Department: 303-339-8150

Fire Department: 911

Poison Control: 303-793-1127

Sky Ridge Hospital: 720-225-1000

FIGURE 51.2
Sample list of emergency phone numbers.

or hygienist is then free to retrieve the emergency kit and oxygen, prepare medications for the dentist, and search for information in an emergency reference book as needed.

The duties of a dentist during an emergency involve directing all team members, facilitating necessary treatment, and administering emergency medications. Additional personnel should assist wherever needed. All personnel in the office must be trained in all responsibilities and functions.

When a call has to be placed to report an emergency in the office, specific information should be provided to the 911 operator. Typically, the information needed includes:

- Nature of the emergency
- Name and age of victim (if possible)
- Exact location with address and phone number
- Name of the individual placing the call

During this call, it is important to provide as much information as possible to the operator and to stay on the line as long as required by the dispatcher.

What is the best way to prevent an emergency in the dental office?

Practice Drills

Conducting practice drills for handling an office emergency helps to ensure that all dental team members are clear about each person's specific role and function. Practice drills should be done routinely. Specific emergencies should be simulated so each staff member can practice performing his or her role. Regular practice will prepare the dental team to act in a calm and efficient manner during a real emergency. Practice and training should be annotated in employee records. This information may be valuable in the event of any legal actions.

What is the difference between a sign and a symptom?

Recognizing an Emergency

It is important to recognize any signs and symptoms exhibited by the patient and ensure that they are documented in the dental health record. A *sign* is what is observed about the patient, such as a change in breathing and skin color. A *symptom* is what the patient says she is experiencing or feeling. For example, the patient may say "My arm hurts" or "My skin is hot or itchy" or "I'm having trouble breathing." It is important to listen to the patient, but it is also important to observe the patient. A sign is more important than a symptom because it is observed by the dental team member.

Observation of the patient's pupils can provide valuable information about his medical condition:

- Normal pupils are each the same size. It is normal for pupils to constrict when exposed to light and dilate when exposed to dark.
- If the pupils are unequal, the patient could be experiencing stroke or brain damage from trauma.
- Failure of the pupils to constrict from light indicates a possible drug overdose.

The duties of the dental assistant are to recognize signs and symptoms and to provide support during the emergency. The dental assistant does not diagnose. This is the responsibility of the dentist.

Protocol for Emergency Situations

It is important that dental assistants have up-to-date credentials in CPR and training in obstructed airway management and obtaining vital signs. Reacting to an emergency should be an automatic response from the dental team. Knowing the links in the American Heart Association's chain of survival help to increase survival rates:

1. **Early access**—Activate EMS by calling 911.
2. **Early CPR**—Begin ventilations and chest compressions.
3. **Early defibrillation**—Use the AED.
4. **Early advanced care**—Emergency medical services (EMS) personnel provide basic life support, defibrillation, and may administer intravenous medications.

Cardiopulmonary Resuscitation

The following CPR information is strictly an overview of the process. To acquire a certification, individuals can contact the American Heart Association (AHA), the American Red Cross, or the National Safety Council. Typically, CPR training is offered to students as part of their dental assistant training or is required to be completed before entering into an accredited dental assisting program.

If an individual is having a heart attack, the greatest risk to the person occurs within the first two hours after onset of symptoms. An individual who receives CPR at the time a cardiac arrest occurs has a greater chance of survival than one who does not. For this reason it is important that all members of society, especially health care professionals, become trained in CPR. CPR is an emergency procedure in which a person's chest is compressed and ventilation is given following a certain protocol in an attempt to force air into the lungs (Figure 51.3). CPR provides artificial breathing and a heartbeat to the victim until advanced medical help arrives.

The advantage of CPR is that it provides immediate treatment for respiratory and cardiac arrest without the need for extra equipment. Respiratory arrest can result from drowning, stroke, choking, or any other injuries that lead to airway obstruction. Most people continue to have a pulse for several minutes after breathing ceases. Cardiac arrest is when circulation (heartbeat) and respiration (breathing) cease, and vital organs are deprived of oxygenated blood. Time is critical when administering CPR because brain damage can occur within four to six minutes after an arrest.

CPR is categorized into different steps. These steps are known as the ABCD's of CPR. The *A* stands for airway, the *B* for breathing, the *C* for circulation, and the *D* for early defibrillation. Procedure 51-1 addresses the first three of these four steps. The fourth step, defibrillation, is covered in Procedure 51-2.

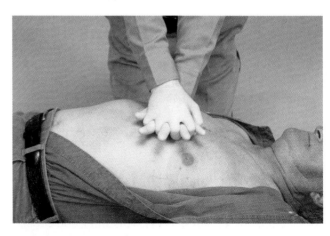

FIGURE 51.3
CPR compressions.

Procedure 51-1 Performing the ABCs of CPR

Equipment and Supplies

None

Procedure Steps

1. *Determine unresponsiveness:* Tap the patient's shoulder and shout: "Are you okay, are you okay?" Speak loudly and clearly.

2. *Activate EMS/obtain the AED:* Direct someone to call 911 and get the AED. (For an adult victim, phone first; for a child phone after one minute of CPR.) If you witness a child going unconscious, activate EMS, then begin CPR if necessary.

3. *Open the airway:* Use the head-tilt/chin-lift maneuver. Place one hand on the forehead, the other under the chin. The mouth should not be completely closed.

4. *Check for breathing:* Look, listen, and feel for breathing. Look for the chest to rise, listen for breathing sounds, and feel for air on your cheek. Continue for 5 seconds, but no more than 10 seconds.

5. *Provide two full breaths (each breath should take one second):* Put mouth over patient's mouth and pinch the nostrils. Use a pocket mask if available. If the chest does not rise, reposition the airway and try again. If the patient has a loose denture, remove it. If the denture fits, leave it in, because it will help with the mouth-to-mouth seal.

6. *Check the pulse:* Place two to three fingers on windpipe (Adam's apple) and slide fingers into the groove on the side of the neck nearest you. Check the carotid artery for 5 to 10 seconds along with signs of circulation/movement.

7. *If no pulse, begin chest compressions:* Deliver 30 chest compressions in less than 23 seconds. Using the heel of one hand with the other hand clasped on top, place the hands on the lower half of the sternum. Push hard and fast. Allow the chest to return to normal between compressions.

8. Continue the compression-to-ventilation ratio of 30:2 until the emergency crew arrives. After three cycles; check the pulse and reassess.

9. Document the emergency information and procedures in patient's dental health record.

The compression-to-ventilation ratio is 30:2 for all victims of any age, except for newborn babies. The current AHA guidelines state that an increased emphasis on chest compressions and early defibrillation increases the patient's chance of survival.

Some damage can occur when performing CPR such as injuries to the sternum, ribs, and other organs. Injuries are more likely to occur if incorrect procedures are used when administering CPR. To ensure that proper procedures and CPR techniques are followed, dental personnel should maintain a current CPR certification.

Automated External Defibrillator

Most cardiac arrest victims experience an abnormal heart rhythm called ventricular fibrillation. This abnormal rhythm must be stopped in order for a normal rhythm to resume. To do this, a defibrillator is recommended. Many dental offices are now equipped with an **automated external defibrillator (AED)**, which is an advanced computer that assesses the patient's condition and cardiac rhythms (Figure 51.4). It indicates when a shock is needed, and automatically defibrillates the patient if necessary.

Early defibrillation is often called the critical link in the chain of survival because it is the only way to successfully treat most sudden cardiac arrests. When cardiac arrest occurs, the heart starts to beat irregularly and blood is pumped inefficiently to the heart. If a normal

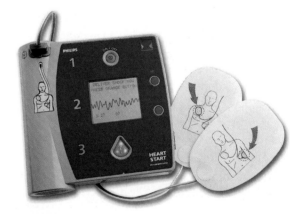

FIGURE 51.4
Automated external defibrillator.

heart rhythm is not restored in minutes, a person can die. In fact, for every minute without defibrillation the odds of survival drop 7% to 10%. A sudden cardiac arrest victim who is not defibrillated within 8 to 10 minutes usually has no chance of survival.

Why is an AED important to have in a dental office? What is the ratio of ventilations to compressions when performing CPR?

Procedure 51-2 Operating the Automated External Defibrillator

Equipment and Supplies
• Automatic external defibrillator

Procedure Steps

1. If there is no pulse, follow the ABC's of CPR (see Procedure 51-1).

2. Place electrodes on the patient's chest. (Follow AED instructions on machine.)

3. Press *Analyze* on the AED.

4. Announce "Everyone stand clear" while the machine analyzes the patient's heart rhythms.

5. If the AED unit indicates a shock is needed, make sure everyone is standing clear.

6. Give the shocks indicated by the unit.

7. Check the patient's pulse.

8. If a pulse is present, assess vital signs and keep patient comfortable until emergency medical services arrive.

9. If no pulse is present, press *Analyze* again and repeat the shock procedure if indicated.
   Safety note: Ensure that no bystanders or rescuers are touching the victim while the shock is being administered.

10. Document the emergency procedures in the patient's dental health record.

Emergency Equipment and Supplies

All dental offices should maintain at least the basic recommended emergency equipment and drugs. The American Dental Association suggests the following items be included in a dental office's emergency kit:

• Epinephrine injections (preloaded syringes)
• Antihistamine (Benadryl) that counteracts the effects of histamine and relieves allergies
• Anticonvulsant (Valium) in injection form for seizures
• Analgesic (Demerol) in injection form, which reduces the sensory function to the brain and relieves pain or anxiety
• Vasopressor for high blood pressure
• Antihypoglycemic, such as sugar packets or frosting, to be administered sublingually

• Nitroglycerin for chest pain; spray, sublingual tablets, or transdermal patches work well
• Bronchodilator (albuterol) inhaler to relax the bronchi in the event of an asthma attack
• Ammonia inhalant (a respiratory stimulant) for patients who faint
• Oxygen
• Automated external defibrillator

Other medications may be included depending on the dentist's training. Dentists must be trained and knowledgeable about indications, contraindications, and dosages of the medications in the emergency kits. Figure 51.5 shows an example of an emergency kit.

Professionalism

In preparing to work in the dental office for the first time, it is important for the dental assistant to have current CPR and first aid training. During orientation to the office, the dental assistant should become familiar with the protocol to be followed in the event of an emergency. Participating in routine drills conducted by the office will help to ensure that protocols are understood and learned correctly. Continue to act professional during all situations in the office. During an emergency, it may be easy to feel panicky but it is important to remain calm and keep the patient's needs paramount.

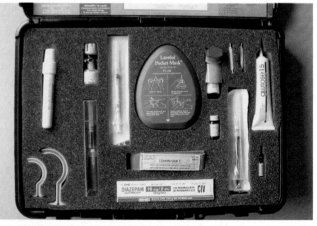

FIGURE 51.5
Emergency kit items.
Image courtesy Instructional Materials for the Dental Team, Lex., KY

Routine maintenance of equipment and supplies should be accomplished as well as weekly inspection of drugs for current expiration dates. The oxygen tanks should also be inspected along with the quality of the oxygen masks, intravenous (IV) lines, and blood pressure equipment to ensure that all are in working condition with no rips or tears.

Some larger dental offices maintain a "crash cart." This cart contains a defibrillator, oxygen, emergency medications, IV lines, oxygen masks, and CPR masks. Dental offices with a crash cart typically provide routine training on the use of the cart for emergencies. The emergency drugs, especially controlled substances, must be locked in a cabinet or crash cart. A log should be kept up to date, documenting when any substance was delivered or used, and any depleted supplies should be replaced as soon as possible.

Oxygen

Oxygen (O_2) is used to resuscitate patients who may be unconscious and is often used in emergencies (Figure 51.6). Oxygen cylinders come in different sizes. It is a good idea

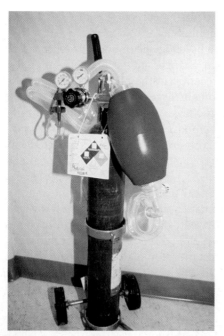

FIGURE 51.6
Oxygen equipment.
Image courtesy Instructional Materials for the Dental Team, Lex., KY

to maintain more than one cylinder for use in emergencies. In some larger clinics, oxygen containers are installed on the walls of each treatment room, making oxygen easily accessible if needed. An oxygen cylinder/tank is always colored green to distinguish it from other gases. Oxygen tanks are provided to dental offices by companies that specialize in providing medical equipment. The steps used to administer oxygen are shown in Figure 51.7.

Prior to administering oxygen a regulator must be attached to the oxygen tank. The regulator allows the pressure to be released at a specific rate. The flow of oxygen can be adjusted by a flow meter that controls the amount of oxygen.

Many attachments are available for administering oxygen. For sedated patients, a nasal cannula can be placed in the nostrils. For emergencies, an oxygen mask should be used. The mask should seal around the face so the oxygen does not leak out, depriving the patient of some of the intended oxygen. Another device that may be used with the oxygen mask is the Ambu-bag. An Ambu-bag is a valve-mask resuscitator used to provide artificial ventilation (breathing) to individuals who have difficulty breathing or who have stopped breathing completely. This can be used to resuscitate a patient with or without oxygen. The use of the Ambu-bag can increase a patient's respirations until normal breathing resumes.

Oxygen is a safe gas to administer; however, a few precautions should be followed such as not using oxygen around any open flame because oxygen is very flammable. Grease or oil of any kind will make oxygen explode. The dental assistant should ensure that no oil is on one's hands when operating an oxygen tank. The dental assistant should know how to administer oxygen in the event of an emergency. (See Procedure 51-3.)

How often should the drugs in an emergency kit be inspected? At what flow rate is oxygen administered?

Emergency Responses

Most emergencies in the dental office occur during high-stress, high-anxiety procedures such as surgical extractions or during the administration of anesthesia. The following are some physical changes that may be seen in a patient undergoing an emergency:

- Unconsciousness (unresponsive to stimuli)
- Altered consciousness (awake, but acting out of character or different than normal)
- Respiratory problems (difficulty breathing)
- Convulsions (uncontrollable muscle spasms)
- Chest pain

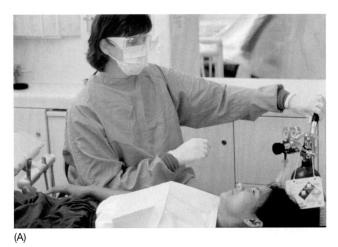

(A)

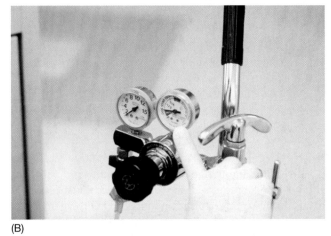

(B)

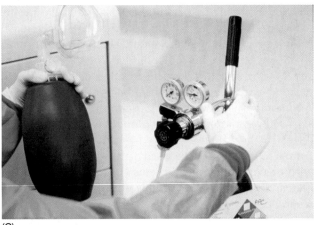

(C)

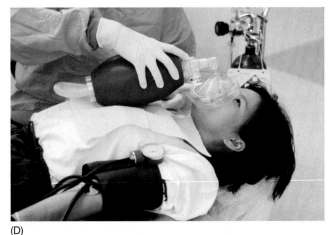

(D)

FIGURE 51.7
Steps in the administration of oxygen.
Images courtesy Instructional Materials for the Dental Team, Lex., KY

Shock Recognition and Treatment

When patients experience conditions that alter the intake of oxygen, the body may react by shutting down its systems. Shock changes the normal flow of blood through the vascular system. There are different types of shock in dentistry. Syncope is a result of shock.

Fainting/Syncope

High anxiety or stress and other underlying health problems can cause a patient to faint. This fainting, or **syncope**, is caused by an unbalanced distribution of blood to the brain and the rest of the body. Syncope is the most common medical emergency in the dental office and, if not corrected, can lead to death.

Syncope has been categorized as psychogenic and nonpsychogenic. Psychogenic factors include fear, pain, and anxiety. These factors can occur in the dental chair due to the sight of the needle or even in the reception areas. The waiting time can cause a patient's anxiety level to rise. Nonpsychogenic factors include physical causes, such as hunger or poor health. It is always a good idea to remind patients to eat breakfast or lunch prior to their dental appointment.

Once a psychogenic or nonpsychogenic factor is present, certain changes in the body occur. These changes trigger a reaction in the body that dilates the blood vessels, resulting in large amounts of blood being pumped to the arms and legs. With the patient sitting or lying in the chair, the blood cannot circulate throughout the body. This means there is a lack of oxygenated blood to the brain; without sufficient oxygen, the patient becomes unconscious.

The dental team may observe the signs of syncope when the patient begins to feel dizzy or light-headed, begins to sweat, or the patient's skin becomes pale. To restore oxygenated blood back to the patient's brain, the dental assistant should place the patient in the supine position. In this position the patient's legs, heart, and brain are at the same approximate level for equal distribution of blood flow. When a patient is placed in the supine position, the patient usually regains consciousness quickly. The subsupine position or Trendelenburg position, in which the patient's head is down on an inclined plane (i.e., lower than the feet), is a position used to help

Procedure 51-3 Administering Oxygen

Equipment and Supplies

- Oxygen cylinder
- Oxygen mask or nasal cannula
- Ambu-bag

Procedure Steps

1. Position the patient in the supine or subsupine position. The supine position is when the patient is lying down with his head, chest, and knees at the same level. The subsupine position is when the patient's head is lower than his heart and feet. This position is often used in emergencies.

2. Reassure the patient and explain the treatment being performed.

3. Ensure the green oxygen cylinder contains oxygen by opening the main valve at the top until gas starts to come out. Then close the valve immediately.

4. Attach the regulator by aligning the pin with the cylinder holes.

5. Open the valve two full turns. Check the pressure gauge to ensure that it reads 2,000 pounds per square inch (psi).

6. Attach the tubing from the mask or nasal cannula.

7. Position the mask over the patient's face. Ensure the mask forms a tight seal.

8. Attach the Ambu-bag if needed.

9. Start the flow of oxygen with the regulator control. The gauge should be set to flow at two to six liters per minute.

10. Observe the patient's color and response to the oxygen.

11. Document the emergency procedures in the patient's dental health record.

---

patients regain consciousness and is used in treating shock (Figure 51.8). If the patient has a head injury, however, this position is not used.

Ammonia inhalants are often used to try to revive a patient who has fainted. The ammonia causes muscle contractions, which cause more blood flow to the brain. If the patient fails to regain consciousness, the patient should be kept in the supine position with legs elevated and 100% oxygen being administered. EMS (911) should be activated. When syncope occurs, all dental treatment is postponed.

Postural Hypotension

Postural hypotension, also known as orthostatic hypotension, is the second-leading cause of syncope in dental offices. It is caused by insufficient blood flow to the brain, resulting from a change in position. Some basic signs and symptoms include low blood pressure and an altered state of consciousness or loss of consciousness. The time of unconsciousness is brief, only lasting a few seconds.

Many factors are known to be possible causes of postural hypotension. The most common is when a patient has been lying in a dental chair for a long period and then immediately stands up after the treatment. At this point, the patient may begin to exhibit the signs of syncope. It is important to immediately place the patient in the supine position in the dental chair. If the patient is pregnant and feels light-headed and faint, this is usually a result of pressure on the uterus and abdominal veins.

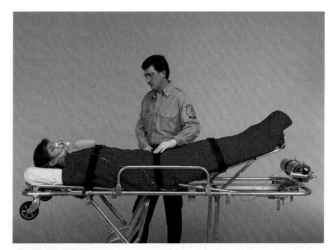

FIGURE 51.8
Patient placed in the Trendelenburg position on a gurney by an EMT.

Place the pregnant patient on her left side or put her in an upright sitting position to relieve the pressure on the blood vessels. To prevent postural hypotension, have the patient remain seated for a few minutes after treatment.

Allergic Reactions

A majority of the population is allergic to something. Sometimes the reaction is a minor rash; sometimes it can turn into a fatal anaphylactic reaction (a severe allergic reaction). The substance that enters the body and produces a hypersensitivity reaction is called an allergen. Most humans develop a natural acquired immunity to allergens; however, some individuals become overly sensitive to the allergen.

One of the best prevention methods for an allergic reaction is to know the patient's health history. The dental team should take note of any allergies or sensitivities, especially allergies to medications and dental materials. However, patients may still have a reaction to dental materials that they did not know they were allergic to. Different types of allergic reactions require various actions to be taken. For example, dermatitis, or a skin reaction, can occur and includes symptoms such as swelling (edema), redness (erythema), hives (urticaria), and blisters. The treatment is to remove the irritant. Sometimes the dentist will administer an antihistamine to reduce the swelling.

Anaphylactic Shock

A severe allergic reaction is called anaphylactic reaction or shock. This can happen to individuals who are extremely sensitive to allergens. It could occur when local anesthetic is being administered. The particular allergen enters the bloodstream, after which the person's blood pressure drops and the airway constricts, causing breathing problems. The person's tongue and throat swell, and

the individual may experience stomach pains. Other signs and symptoms may include itching or burning sensations, extreme swelling of tissues of the body, chest pain or tightness, or a rapid drop in blood pressure. These signs and symptoms are quick to occur.

The dental assistant should retrieve the emergency kit and oxygen immediately and place the patient in the supine position. If necessary, the dentist will administer an epinephrine injection in order to save the person's life. Oxygen relieves the patient's distress and is administered in conjunction with the epinephrine. Monitoring the patient's vital signs is critical and administration of CPR may be required as well as activating EMS.

Drug and Materials Sensitivity Related Emergencies

Drug emergencies happen as a result of adverse reactions to certain drugs or medications. Toxic reactions usually result from an excessive amount of a particular drug such as a local anesthetic. Too much local anesthetic injected into the body can be absorbed into the bloodstream, causing shaking, anxiety, uneasiness, and heart palpitations. This is a mild form of overdose, and the treatments involve placing the patient in the supine position, administering oxygen so that the anesthetic will redistribute in the blood, and maintaining an open airway. With much larger doses, life-threatening conditions can develop such as seizures. Treatment requires oxygen and notifying the EMS. The dental team may also need to perform basic life-saving steps.

Prevention is the key to avoiding a drug overdose. The patient should be questioned prior to treatment about allergies or hypersensitivities, such as latex allergies. The assistant and dentist should always double check the health history and question the patient regarding any latex allergy listed. If the patient has a latex allergy, ensure that nonlatex gloves and materials are used during treatment.

The dentist is giving a local anesthetic; the patient complains of her throat swelling, trouble breathing, and stomach pains. What emergency could she be experiencing and how should the dental assistant respond?

Cardiac Emergencies

The three most common cardiovascular emergencies likely to occur in the dental office include angina pectoris, myocardial infarction, and cardiac arrest. Due to the possibility of cardiac emergencies occurring in the dental office, it is important that all dental health care workers be certified in cardiopulmonary resuscitation.

Cultural Considerations

In any emergency, it is important to question patients about their symptoms and always reassure them. More than 30 million Americans speak Spanish as either their first or second language, making the United States the fifth largest Spanish-speaking population in the world. If the dental staff is not bilingual, it is helpful to know a few general emergency procedure phrases to assist the Spanish-speaking patient population. The following are some phrases that may be useful in the dental practice:

- Are you feeling well?: *No se esta sintiendo bien?*
- Are you feeling dizzy?: *Se siente mareado?*
- Remain calm, we're here to help: *Mantengase calmando, estamos aqui para usted.*

The following words help describe how the patient may feel:
- Cold: *frio*
- Disoriented: *desorientado*
- Hot: *caliente*
- Nauseated: *nauseado*

Other words and phrases that may be helpful for the assistant and the patient include:
- Open your mouth, please: *Abre la voca, por favor.*
- Bite: *muerdo*
- Don't move (for instance during a panoramic x-ray): *No se mueva.*
- Sit in the chair, please: *Sientese en la silla, por favor.*
- Spit: *escupir*
- Health history: *historia*
- Heart problems: *problemas del corazon*
- High blood pressure: *alta pression*
- Rheumatic fever: *fievre rhumatica*
- Epilepsy: *epilepsia*
- Allergic to medicine: *allergico a medicina*
- Taking any medicine?: *Tomando alguna medicina?*
- Pain: *dolor*
- Swelling: *inchado*

Angina Pectoris

A common heart disease that causes chest pain is called arteriosclerosis, or hardening of the arteries. The arteries become thick and hard, which causes narrowing of the walls of the arteries. The severity of the narrowing may cause patients to experience chest pains. This pain is called **angina pectoris**, which is the Latin term for "strangling of the chest." The pain occurs because the heart experiences oxygen deficiencies.

Angina is classified as either stable or unstable. A person who has stable angina may experience pain because of physical or emotional stress. Stable angina is usually controlled with medication. Unstable angina pain occurs even if the patient is at rest and medication such as nitroglycerin may not alleviate the pain. If the pain occurs in the dental chair, the dentist will check the health history and ask certain questions of the patient such as "What type of pain is it?" "Where is the discomfort?" "Did the nitroglycerin relieve the pain?" Armed with answers to these questions, the dentist can determine if the patient needs further emergency care.

The most common symptom of angina is pain in the center of the chest. During this time the patient should sit very still in order to alleviate the pain. The patient's skin may feel cold and clammy, and the patient's pulse and blood pressure rate may be high. The pain from angina usually lasts around three to eight minutes. The pain is usually relieved by a drug called nitroglycerin that is administered sublingually (under the tongue). Nitroglycerin can be administered in pill or spray form. It dilates the blood vessels so that the blood can flow throughout the body. If the patient has a history of angina pectoris, the patient will typically carry this drug with him. It is also maintained in the dental office emergency kit. The patient should be given oxygen, since the heart is not getting sufficient oxygenated blood during an angina pectoris episode. If the pain is not relieved by the nitroglycerin, the patient may be experiencing a heart attack. Keep the patient comfortable (sitting up or lying down) and activate the EMS.

Acute Myocardial Infarction

Acute myocardial infarction occurs when a portion of the myocardium (heart muscle) dies from lack of oxygen, usually caused by narrowing or blockage of the arteries (atherosclerosis). If the patient is experiencing an acute **myocardial infarction** (heart attack), typically the patient will initially deny it stating that it is probably indigestion. The signs are cold, clammy skin and heavy pressure or pain in the chest, shoulder, arms, back, and jaws. The patient will also experience shortness of breath, weakness, and anxiety. The pain associated with a heart attack usually happens while the patient is at rest. This pain can occur hours or even days prior to the actual heart attack. The pain can vary in intensity from extreme to almost nonexistent. The patient will eventually become unconscious.

When a patient is experiencing a heart attack the EMS should be activated immediately by calling 911. All dental treatment must be stopped, and nitroglycerin administered. Oxygen should be provided and the patient kept as comfortable as possible. In addition to receiving oxygen, it is recommended that a person experiencing a heart attack be given an aspirin to chew to help dissolve a blood clot that may have formed or to help with the flow of blood. Watch for signs of cardiac arrest, which is loss of circulation and breathing, and provide CPR if necessary. It is extremely important for the dental team to remain calm in this situation and assist the patient as directed by the dentist in charge.

Cardiac Arrest

Cardiac arrest is the sudden stopping of the heart and breathing. This can occur without warning, even in people with no suspected heart problems. It is referred to as sudden death. This sudden death can be caused by any of the following:

- Myocardial infarction
- Airway obstruction
- Drug overdose
- Seizures

The symptoms are sudden loss of consciousness, slow or absent respiration, and absence of blood pressure and pulse. The patient may show signs of profuse sweating and complete dilation of pupils. The treatment includes immediate CPR, defibrillation, and activating the EMS. Brain damage occurs within four to six minutes without oxygen.

Congestive Heart Failure

Congestive heart failure is a disorder in which the heart does not contract enough to provide adequate blood flow. The blood backs up and fluid accumulates in the lungs. The symptoms the patient may experience are fatigue, weakness, coughing, and respiratory distress. A person with heart failure may also have swelling of the hands and ankles. The patient will not be able to tolerate the supine position and may appear gray or cyanotic (bluish) in color. If these signs and symptoms occur, call for help immediately. Place the patient in the upright position and administer oxygen. Monitor vital signs until the EMS arrives.

What treatment is used for angina pectoris? What is the difference between myocardial infarction and cardiac arrest?

Respiratory Emergencies

When any patient experiences breathing problems, all dental treatment should be stopped and the cause of the breathing problem should be determined immediately. A patient deprived of oxygen for several minutes could experience serious damage to her body. The following respiratory emergencies may occur in the dental office.

Hyperventilation

Patients who have high anxiety from fear of treatment may start to breathe rapidly and shallowly and experience chest pain and a rapid heart rate. The patient may

also experience light-headedness and dizziness due to the lack of carbon dioxide. The patient may also experience muscle pain and tingling in the extremities. This is called **hyperventilation** or overbreathing.

When a patient is overbreathing, chemical changes happen in the body. Carbon dioxide levels in the blood decrease; the lower level of carbon dioxide reduces blood flow to the brain, which results in the dizziness, confusion, and agitation. Overbreathing also causes calcium levels to drop in the blood, which can result in muscle spasms or twitches.

When a patient is hyperventilating, it is important to attempt to keep the patient calm and instruct the patient to slow his breathing. Ensure that the patient is sitting upright. This helps alleviate fear and helps the patient to slow his breathing. The most effective treatment for hyperventilation is having the patient breathe into a paper bag or cupped hands (Figure 51.9). The rebreathing of the carbon dioxide helps alleviate the symptoms of hyperventilation. Once the dentist has determined that carbon dioxide levels have leveled off, oxygen may be administered.

The dental team can help prevent hyperventilation by attempting to keep the patient calm and discussing the patient's fears. If the dentist knows in advance of the patient's anxiety, he or she can administer an oral sedative to calm the patient prior to treatment.

Asthma

Asthma is a disorder of the respiratory tract, including the trachea, bronchi, and bronchioles. (See Chapter 4 for more information on the respiratory system.) It is reported most often in children and young adults. There

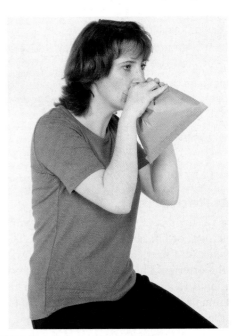

FIGURE 51.9
Treatment for hyperventilation.
Gary Ombler © Dorling Kindersley

are different categories of asthma. Extrinsic asthma is usually triggered by an allergen. Most people who have this type of asthma are already predisposed to allergies. Extrinsic asthma usually responds to medications and can be outgrown. Another type of asthma is called intrinsic asthma or infectious asthma. It is often seen in people over 30 years of age and is triggered by a type of bronchial infection.

An asthma attack can occur suddenly and without warning. When an individual is experiencing an episode of asthma, a wheezing sound is present; the bronchioles become narrow and there is an overproduction of mucus. The patient may have trouble inhaling and exhaling, he may begin to cough and sweat, and become very nervous. Patients who have a history of asthma typically carry their own inhalers (Figure 51.10); however, the emergency kit should be stocked with one as well.

Anxiety can trigger asthma attacks. It is important for the dental team to make every effort to prevent an asthma attack. For example, keep patient waiting times to a minimum, explain procedures to the patient, and use less-threatening terminology such as *handpiece* instead of *drill*.

If a patient experiences an asthma attack during treatment, stop all dental treatment and remove materials and instruments immediately. Position the patient in the upright position so that the patient can breathe easier. Have the patient use her bronchodilator. This should relax the bronchioles so the patient can breathe easier. Administer oxygen if available. Activate the EMS if the inhaler does not work. The dentist may decide to administer a shot of epinephrine from the emergency kit.

Obstructed Airway

Early recognition of airway obstruction is the key to a successful outcome. The dental office is one of the more common settings where airway obstructions can occur. When the patient is reclined back in the dental chair, the potential of a patient aspirating an object is high. These objects are slippery with saliva or blood, making it easy for them to slip from the dentist's hands or off of a handpiece.

Some of the causes of airway obstruction in the dental office can be prevented with a few easy techniques. For example, extracted teeth can be prevented from falling into the back of the throat by using a throat pack made of gauze. The dental assistant can prevent amalgam from blocking the airway by using a dental dam or high-velocity evacuation. Impression material can also block a patient's airway. To avoid this, ensure the patient is seated in the upright position while an impression is being taken. When trying on crowns, the assistant can place gauze across the back of the patient's throat as a screen. When trying the fit of a bridge or a dental dam clamp, a ligature, made of dental floss tied around the object, can be used to pull the object out if it falls down the back of the throat.

Foreign bodies may cause either partial or complete airway obstruction. With partial airway obstruction, the victim may have reduced exchange. With adequate air exchange, the victim can still cough and breathe. Poor air exchange can transition quickly to inadequate air exchange, which requires immediate action by the dental team. With complete obstruction, the victim is unable to speak, breathe, or cough and may clutch at her throat with her hands (the universal distress signal for choking). The Heimlich maneuver, which consists of subdiaphragmatic abdominal thrusts, is recommended for relieving airway obstruction (Figure 51.11 and Procedure 51-4).

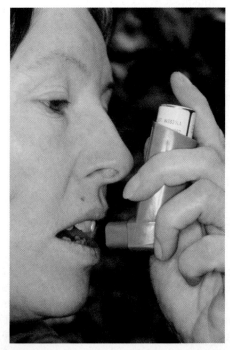

FIGURE 51.10
Asthma inhaler.

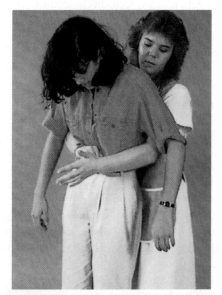

FIGURE 51.11
The Heimlich maneuver is one element of obstructed airway management.

Procedure 51-4 Managing an Obstructed Airway

Equipment and Supplies

None needed.

Procedure Steps

1. Determine whether the patient is choking by asking "Are you choking?" "May I help you?" (The patient may have her hands on her throat, which is the universal signal for choking.)

2. Position yourself behind the patient, place one of your legs between the patient's (for stability), and wrap your arms around her abdomen (see Figure 51.11). Let the patient know that you are there to help so she does not panic.

3. Place the thumb side of your hand between the navel and the xiphoid process (the notch at the end of the

lower part of the sternum). Grasp hands together. (For pregnant or obese people, wrap your arms around the chest, just under the armpits.)

4. Give quick inward, upward thrusts until the obstruction is expelled or the patient becomes unconscious.

5. If the patient becomes unconscious, lower her to the floor, check the airway, straddle her, and provide chest thrusts (similar to CPR chest compressions).

6. If the obstruction is relieved, but the patient is not breathing or does not have a pulse, call 911 and begin CPR.

7. Document the emergency procedures in the patient's dental health record.

Respiratory Arrest

When respiratory arrest occurs, the patient's breathing stops. However, the patient may still have a pulse for a short time. Artificial ventilation must be started immediately to maintain oxygen flow through the body. This artificial ventilation provides approximately 16% oxygen. If a pulse is not present, then begin chest compressions.

What is the universal distress signal for choking? How is an asthma attack treated?

Other Emergencies

Many emergencies can occur in the dental office, including cardiac and respiratory conditions and stroke. The dental health team should be prepared for the following emergencies.

Cerebrovascular Accident

Cerebrovascular accident (CVA) is commonly known as a stroke. CVAs are classified into three categories: cerebral embolism, cerebral hemorrhage, and cerebral thrombosis. An embolism occurs when a clot wanders from another part of the body and lodges itself in a cerebral artery, cutting off blood flow. A hemorrhage occurs when an artery ruptures and the head is filled with blood. This blood causes swelling and pressure on the brain. Cerebral thrombosis occurs when a clot actually forms in a cerebral artery, which results in lack of blood flow to the brain.

Strokes can happen to people of all ages; however, they more often occur in the elderly. In order for people to understand the severity of this condition, it is often referred to as a "brain attack," parallel to the term "heart

attack." Individuals experiencing a CVA must receive immediate care. Most CVA victims have predisposing factors such as arteriosclerosis, heart disease, and high blood pressure. Prevention is aided by the recognition and modification of the patient's risk factors. Risk factors include smoking, high blood pressure, heart disease, previous strokes, and heredity. Some of the signs and symptoms of a stroke are:

- Headache
- Slurred speech
- Unconsciousness/altered consciousness
- Paralysis on one side of the body
- Confusion or problems understanding
- Seizures

If these signs are present, the EMS should be activated, dental treatment stopped, vital signs monitored, and oxygen administered. Be prepared to administer CPR if necessary. Once the EMT arrives, he/she may determine that 81 mg of aspirin should be administered. This treatment has been shown to be effective in some people who have had strokes.

Epilepsy

Epilepsy is a chronic brain disorder characterized by recurrent seizures. The cause is mostly unknown; however, an accident that damages the brain can result in epilepsy. Heredity can also play a role in someone having epilepsy. Seizures may be mild to severe, ranging from loss of awareness to uncontrollable muscle spasms. The types of seizures are identified by the types of actions they produce. **Grand mal seizures** (also call tonic/clonic) are the most common and are characterized by loss of consciousness and uncontrollable muscle contractions/spasms. This type of seizure happens in different phases:

- **Prodromal**—The person may experience personality changes or an aura. Auras are actually small seizures. They are brief, localized, electrical brain discharges that often precede a more serious seizure. Auras can warn a person with epilepsy that a bigger seizure is on the way, giving the individual a chance to prepare by making a phone call or finding a safe place to lie down. A smell, sound, or light may trigger it. The person may have a frightened feeling or a euphoric feeling.
- **Convulsive**—The patient loses consciousness; the body becomes stiff and rigid, and then violently jerks.
- **Postictal**—This final phase consists of the patient slowly regaining consciousness. Confusion may occur and the person may go into a deep sleep.

A **petite mal seizure** (also called an absence seizure) is a seizure in which the patient exhibits a blank stare or a twitch or may blink rapidly. The patient is usually unaware of her surroundings for a short time. Another type of seizure is called a partial seizure. This involves a specific region of the brain. The victim may experience jerking movements on only part of his body. The person also may be in a trance-like state and tend to wander around.

If a patient is having a seizure it is important to ensure that the patient does not harm herself. The first thing to do if a seizure occurs is to remove all dental objects from the patient's mouth. Move all equipment away from the patient to avoid injury. Remove the patient's glasses and loosen her clothing. Keep dentures in the patient's mouth unless the dentures are causing an airway obstruction. Always keep hands out of the patient's mouth during a seizure to avoid injury to patient as well as the operator. Do not ever restrain the patient. During the restraining process, injury to the dental team member or to the patient could occur.

Keep the patient safe during the seizure. If possible, at the beginning of the seizure, gently place the person on his side to prevent possible aspiration of vomit. Once the seizure is over, place the patient in the recovery position (on his side) if he is not already in that position, reassure the patient, and allow the patient to fully recover. If the patient is injured during the seizure, stops breathing, or goes from one seizure to the next, then activate the EMS immediately.

Prevention is not always guaranteed; however, it is helpful to ensure that the patient's health history has been checked and that if a history of seizures does exist the patient is adhering to medication treatments. Sometimes seizures are triggered by stress. It is important to eliminate some of the stress and keep your patient as comfortable as possible.

Diabetes Mellitus

The term *diabetes mellitus* is sometimes referred to as "sweet urine," because people of ancient times observed that patients with diabetes urinated frequently and their urine tasted sweet. The term *diabetic* is translated as "running through a siphon," referring to those individuals who urinated frequently. *Mellitus* refers to honey because of the amount of sugar in the urine.

Diabetes is described as a metabolic disorder in which the pancreas produces insufficient amounts of insulin or no insulin at all. This means that the body is unable to adequately or effectively metabolize carbohydrates. Insulin is produced by the pancreas and when combined with the glucose from the food eaten provides fuel and energy for the body's metabolism to function properly.

Diabetes is classified as type 1 and type 2 diabetes. Type 1 diabetes is often referred to as juvenile diabetes or insulin-dependent diabetes mellitus (IDDM) and affects primarily children, although it has been known to affect older people as well. This type of diabetes is insulin dependent, which means that the person must give herself insulin injections. If the person does not take her insulin, she may lapse into a coma. Type 2 diabetes makes up the majority of diabetic cases. It is usually called adult-onset diabetes or non–insulin-dependent diabetes mellitus (NIDDM). It is normally diagnosed in obese, middle-aged patients and can be seen in obese children. It usually can be controlled with diet and medications that lower blood sugar.

Hyperglycemia and hypoglycemia may be complications of diabetes. They occur when there is too much or too little sugar in the body. These conditions can develop into emergencies. **Hyperglycemia** is too much sugar (glucose) in the blood and happens when there is a lack of insulin. The person may always be thirsty and urinate frequently. The patient's breath may have a sweet, fruity odor referred to as acetone breath. The patient's blood pressure will drop and his pulse will beat rapidly. The individual may also experience nausea, vomiting, fatigue, and abdominal pains. If left untreated, it can result in a diabetic coma, called diabetic acidosis. People who suffer from hyperglycemia require insulin injections. These individuals can test their urine and blood for glucose levels, to help prevent complications. If an emergency occurs, the EMS must be activated.

Hypoglycemia is known as insulin shock. This occurs due to too little sugar (glucose) in the body. This condition can occur in patients who do not have diabetes. Patients who skip meals and are anxious about a dental treatment could experience low blood sugar. Alcoholics suffer from low blood sugar because of a lack of stored glycogen (the main form of carbohydrate storage; converts to glucose for energy) in the liver. Glucose is fuel for the brain, so insufficient amounts can cause brain damage. A person with hypoglycemia may experience cold sweats, trembling, weakness, irritability, and confusion. The treatment includes getting the patient some type of sugar source such as frosting or sugar sublingually or a sugar drink.

Always ensure that patient histories have been reviewed for the presence of diabetes. Patients with diabetes should be asked if they have eaten or taken their medications prior to treatment. A thorough medical history should be taken for all patients diagnosed with diabetes.

Patients with diabetes are a challenge for the dental team. There is always the possibility that the patient will experience a diabetic coma or insulin shock while in the dental chair. Scheduling appointments shortly after meals is best for the patient. If the patient is experiencing other problems related to the diabetes such as high blood pressure or heart disease, dental treatment should be altered or postponed to avoid an emergency situation. People with diabetes also experience problems healing and are susceptible to infection. For this reason, the dental team needs to be especially careful not to cause tissue trauma. Always review the health history and be prepared to provide emergency treatment.

Table 51-1 provides an overview of the various types of emergencies that may be seen in a dental office.

What is the difference between hypoglycemia and hyperglycemia? Which type of seizure is characterized by a blank stare? **?**

Dental Emergencies

Some emergencies occur because of the dental treatment, not because of the health of the patient. A few of the dental emergencies that may occur are soft tissue injury, hemorrhage, and alveolitis. Whatever the emergency is, the assistant and the rest of the dental health care team should be calm and prepared to assist. Documentation should occur with all emergencies.

Soft Tissue Injuries

An anesthetic needle could break if the patient moves around too much. The assistant's job is to keep the patient calm. The removal of the needle may require a referral to a dentist with surgical experience. The incident must be recorded in the patient's dental health record in case legal action is later taken.

Soft tissue injuries also occur because the mouth is slippery due to the presence of blood and saliva. A wound or laceration can occur from any instrument. Soft tissue injuries in the dental office such as jabbing or suctioning of the tissue can be prevented with the use of proper techniques by the assistant. Patients may come in with soft tissue trauma due to sports injuries or a fall. The dental team should keep the patient calm and reassured while treating these injuries.

TABLE 51-1 Overview of Emergency Conditions and Procedures

Condition	Symptoms/Causes	Treatment
Syncope (fainting)	Light-headedness, cold sweat, skin becomes pale, loss of consciousness; caused by anxiety and unbalanced distribution of blood to the brain	Place patient in supine or subsupine position. The use of an ammonia inhalant will cause the patient to wake up.
Postural hypotension	Dizziness, fainting; lack of blood flow to the brain due to lying in dental chair for long periods, then quickly rising	Have patient sit back down in dental chair. Place her in a supine position if she faints.
Angina pectoris	Chest pain	Give patient his own nitroglycerin or provide from emergency kit.
Myocardial infarction	Chest pain that feels like "crushing pressure," pain radiating to jaw, arm, and back	Call 911, keep patient comfortable, monitor vital signs. Begin CPR if breathing and circulation stop.
Stroke	Paralysis on one side, slurred speech, double vision	Call 911, keep patient comfortable, monitor vital signs.
Hyperventilation	Rapid, shallow breathing; causes dizziness and chest pain due to lack of CO_2; caused by extreme anxiety	Keep patient calm. Have her breathe into a paper bag or her cupped hands.
Asthma	Respiratory difficulties, wheezing; triggered by an allergen or stress	Administer patient's inhaler or ask patient to self-medicate with inhaler if he is able to.
Allergic reaction	Rash, itching, hives; caused by an allergen	Administer Benadryl. For severe reaction (anaphylactic) administer epinephrine and call 911.
Seizure	Convulsions, involuntary muscle spasms, or blank stare	Keep patient safe, move nearby items and equipment away from patient. Monitor patient until seizure ends. Call 911 if patient becomes unconscious.
Hyperglycemia	Extreme thirst, frequent urination, nausea, vomiting; caused by too much sugar	Call 911. Hospital staff will administer insulin as needed.
Hypoglycemia	Cold sweats, trembling, irritability, confusion; caused by not enough sugar, too much insulin	Administer a sugar source, such as frosting, sublingually

Postextraction Hemorrhage

Hemorrhage can happen any time from a few hours to a few days after a tooth extraction. The bleeding from the extraction site may be light or heavy; however, any form of hemorrhage is serious. The symptoms of a postextraction hemorrhage may include bleeding that will not stop, large amounts of blood in the mouth, and physical weakness due to blood loss. To help stop the bleeding, place a moist gauze pack over the extraction site and instruct the patient to bite down firmly. The dentist may need to remove the gauze and place an absorbable gelatin sponge called Gelfoam, treated with a hemostatic agent called Surgicel. A hemostatic is something that reduces blood flow and helps form a clot.

Alveolitis

This condition is also known as dry socket. It occurs when a blood clot does not form after an extraction or when the clot is dislodged by smoking, using a straw, or spitting. The nerve endings in the bone are exposed to the air since there is no blood clot. This emergency is very uncomfortable for the patient. The dental team's goal is to keep the patient as comfortable as possible and provide treatment to alleviate the pain and possible infection.

The treatment involves placing eugenol gauze packing in the socket. The gauze is in the form of long strips that are treated with eugenol. Eugenol is a sedative medication made from cloves. The gauze is gently packed into the socket after the socket is gently irrigated of debris. This reduces the pain almost immediately by soothing the nerve endings and prevents food from getting lodged in the socket. The patient is then scheduled to return in one to two days for reevaluation and repacking of the socket if needed.

Patients may arrive with dental emergencies that require immediate attention. Maintain the emergency protocol that would be used if it were a medical emergency. The dental team should be prepared for any dental or medical emergency.

Documentation of an Emergency

Detailed documentation is crucial in the dental office, especially when an emergency occurs. As soon as possible after an emergency occurs, the dentist should document what happened from the beginning of the emergency. The dental chart should include the patient's signs and symptoms, the emergency care techniques and medications used by the dental health team, the patient's responses if any, and the emergency protocol the dental team followed.

The dentist must document whether the dental team responded appropriately or not. The dentist is ultimately responsible for the actions of employees. The dentist typically documents extensive details of the event, including

the patient's condition at the time the patient departs the dental office. The patient is then referred to her general physician for follow-up, and the emergency is annotated in the dental health record.

It is important to remember that prior to dental treatment, the dentist should question the patient extensively about his health history and annotate any changes in the patient's dental health record. An informed consent should also be used in addition to documenting the dental health record. The informed consent explains the procedure's risks and benefits. The patient's signature must be present on the informed consent in order for the procedure to take place. This information is crucial because it may be needed in a court of law at a later date.

Once the dental health record is complete with details and the patient has been transported to a hospital, the dental team should conduct a postemergency assessment. This is an evaluation of the team's performance, the equipment, and the situation in general. The assessment should consist of the following:

The Emergency Situation

- When was the emergency detected?
- Did the health history indicate a possible problem?
- What preventive measures were taken, if any?
- Were treatment recommendations followed?
- What could have been done differently?

The Performance of the Team

- How did the staff respond?
- Did everyone work in their assigned roles efficiently, or with panic and confusion?
- Did any team members have trouble?
- Do the team roles/assignments need to be modified?

Equipment and Supplies

- Was the emergency kit and oxygen in the correct location?
- Was the equipment functional?
- Were any drugs expired?
- Was CPR performed following the accepted standards?

The dentist and dental staff should review the answers to the assessment in order to improve their process if an emergency arises again. This helps the dental team in providing legal and appropriate patient care.

Most states have a Good Samaritan Act or laws that provide legal protection to those who provide emergency treatment. The dental team has an obligation to provide some kind of help or treatment. To encourage laypeople and dental health workers to help those in need, an example law might be worded as follows: Act in good faith and provide care that isn't negligent or reckless and act as a prudent person would within your own scope of training. When making the decision to help a victim, the provider must not abandon the victim.

SUMMARY

Preparedness is the key to managing medical emergencies in the dental environment. Emergencies can occur at any time and without warning, so it is important for the dental office to ensure that members of the dental team remain current in CPR certification, routine emergency drills are practiced, up-to-date emergency kits are maintained, and emergency numbers and the protocol for handling emergencies are familiar and available to all staff members. Medical emergencies are not always common in the dental office, but being prepared will help save lives.

KEY TERMS

- **Asthma:** Disorder of the respiratory tract. p. 818
- **Angina pectoris:** Chest pain. p. 817
- **Automated external defibrillator (AED):** A computer that assesses the patient's cardiac rhythm and automatically delivers defibrillation (electric shock). p. 811
- **Cerebrovascular accident (CVA):** Stroke; caused by insufficient blood flow to arteries in the brain. p. 820
- **Edema:** Swelling. p. 816
- **Epilepsy:** Chronic brain disorder characterized by recurrent seizures. p. 820
- **Grand mal seizure:** Uncontrollable, violent muscle contractions/spasms and loss of consciousness; also known as tonic/clonic seizures. p. 820
- **Hyperglycemia:** Too much sugar (glucose), not enough insulin in the blood. p. 821
- **Hyperventilation:** Light-headedness and dizziness caused by the rapid breathing leading to reduction in oxygen. p. 818
- **Hypoglycemia:** When the body has too little sugar and too much insulin; also known as insulin shock. p. 821
- **Myocardial infarction:** Heart attack or death of a heart muscle. p. 817
- **Petit mal seizure:** Short-term seizure characterized by a blank stare or eye twitch; also known as absence seizures. p. 821
- **Postural hypotension:** Insufficient blood flow to the brain as a result of a position change. p. 815
- **Syncope:** Loss of consciousness or fainting. p. 814

CHECK YOUR UNDERSTANDING

1. A seizure in which a person experiences loss of consciousness and involuntary muscle contractions is called a/an
   a. petit mal seizure (absence seizure).
   b. partial seizure.
   c. grand mal seizure (tonic/clonic).
   d. epilepsy.

2. Which type of diabetes mellitus is most severe?
   a. type 1
   b. type 2
   c. type 3
   d. type 4

3. Which of the following is not correct when calling 911 during an emergency?
   a. Give exact location with address and phone number.
   b. Give nature of emergency.
   c. Do not give patient's name due to privacy.
   d. Give your name.

4. An automated defibrillator is used
   a. in place of CPR.
   b. to shock the heart back into its normal rhythm.
   c. to read cardiac rhythms.
   d. both b and c.

5. Which of the following items should be in a dental office's emergency kit?
   a. epinephrine injection
   b. nitroglycerin
   c. inhaler
   d. all of the above

6. What color are oxygen tank cylinders?
   a. red
   b. blue
   c. yellow
   d. green

7. In what position would you place a patient who is suffering from syncope?
   a. supine
   b. subsupine
   c. upright
   d. both a and b

CHECK YOUR UNDERSTANDING (continued)

8. What is the treatment of choice for hyperventilation?
   a. epinephrine injection
   b. paper bag
   c. chest compressions
   d. inhaler

9. What condition is caused by too much insulin and too little sugar in the blood?
   a. hypoglycemia
   b. hyperglycemia
   c. epilepsy
   d. syncope

10. Where do you document an emergency and the emergency treatment provided?
    a. medical record
    b. you do not need to document them
    c. the dental health record
    d. the appointment book

INTERNET ACTIVITY

• Conduct research on the web to discover more information about the uses of an AED. A suggested website is www.redcross.org/services/hss/courses/aed

This is an AED information site from the American Red Cross.

WEB REFERENCES

• American Heart Association www.americanheart.org
• American Red Cross www.redcross.org
• National Safety Council www.nsc.org
• Spanish Health Terminology www.123teachme.com/learn_spanish/past_medical_history

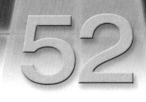

52

Communication Techniques

Chapter Outline

Learning Objectives

After reading this chapter, the student should be able to:

- Discuss the importance of good communication among members of the dental team.
- Explain the elements of effective verbal and nonverbal communication.
- Discuss Maslow's hierarchy of needs.
- Describe the channels of communication in the dental office.
- Define the different types of conflict.
- Explain the importance of understanding cultural diversity.
- Demonstrate appropriate telephone etiquette.
- Describe the parts of a letter.

Preparing for Certification Exams

- Understand the use and principles of communication.
- Use effective written communication techniques in preparing correspondence, reports, electronic mail, and other documents.
- Answer the telephone and conduct all phone conversations in a professional manner.
- Screen incoming calls and gather data.

Key Terms

Cultural diversity	Receiver
Downward channel communication	Salutation
Horizontal channel communication	Sender
Informal channel communication	Subjective fears
Nonverbal communication	Upward channel communication
Objective fears	Verbal communication

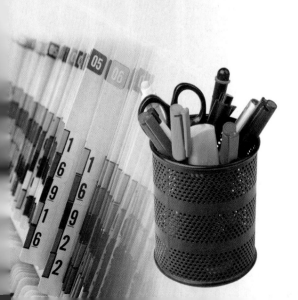

Communication is an important aspect of patient care. It is a two-way process in which information is shared among parties. It is accomplished through many modes such as written and spoken, behaviors and actions. To be a successful dental assistant, it is important to understand the delicate process of communicating with patients and coworkers and the cultural differences that may make communication difficult. Development of both effective verbal and nonverbal communications skills will ensure successful communication among members of the dental team and with dental patients.

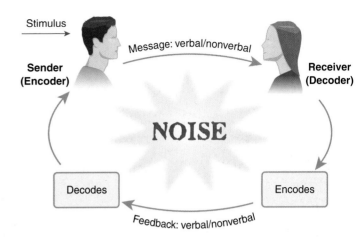

FIGURE 52.1
The communication process.

The Communication Process

Patients often arrive at the dental office with preconceived ideas about whether a certain treatment will be a good or bad experience. These ideas come from previous dental experiences or information from other sources. The dental assistant is an important member of the dental team who can assist in establishing the tone for the patient's dental visit.

Patients evaluate their dental experience based on the way they are treated on the telephone, how they are treated when they interact with front office personnel, and how they perceive they are being treated in the treatment room. Therefore, the way the members of a dental team communicate can affect the patient in either a positive or negative manner. Understanding the process of communication can help the dental assistant be more responsive to patient needs and in turn help to make the dental experience less frightening. The communication process includes the following elements (Figure 52.1):

1. **Sender**—the individual who is giving information to another person
2. **Message**—the idea that is translated into a message

3. **Mode/channel**—the mode by which the message is communicated, for instance, verbally or nonverbally, spoken or in writing, or via facial expressions—and intentional or not
4. **Receiver**—the recipient of the intended message
5. **Feedback**—the feedback provided by the receiver of the message.

The only way that communication can be truly effective is when the message is clearly sent so that the receiver understands the intended message.

Verbal Communication

The dental team can relieve patient fears through the simple act of proper and appropriate communication. Verbal communication consists of words used to transmit a message. **Verbal communication** can be spoken or written. Effective communication requires consideration of the words used. Words can have different meanings to different people. It is always helpful if a basic foundation of language exists between the dental team and the patients. Using technical jargon with patients may confuse them or lead them to believe something different than what is intended (Figure 52.2). When communicating with patients it is important to think before speaking. Table 52-1 describes some ineffective words that could confuse or scare patients and some effective replacements for those words.

The tone of one's voice is a significant factor in affecting how a patient may perceive the dental office experience. A dental assistant who uses a tone that conveys a friendly, confident, and professional attitude is likely to have patients who feel welcomed and confident in the dental team's abilities. Patients want to know not only that they are important to the dental practice, but they want to have a sense of confidence in the professionals who are performing the dental treatments. Sometimes the dental patient is apprehensive and unsure of what to

What Patients May Visualize with Negative Terms

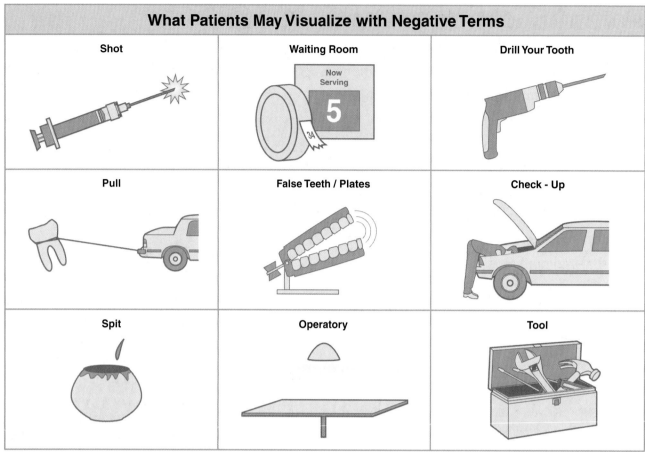

Shot	Waiting Room	Drill Your Tooth
Pull	False Teeth / Plates	Check - Up
Spit	Operatory	Tool

FIGURE 52.2
Images that patients may visualize when negative dental terms are used.

TABLE 52-1 Ineffective and Effective Dental Terms

Ineffective Words	Effective Words
Pain	Discomfort
Shot	Injection
Spit	Empty your mouth
Drill tooth	Prepare tooth
Acid etch	Condition
Waiting room	Reception area
False teeth	Dentures
Pull	Remove
Bill	Statement
Tool	Instrument
Operatory	Dental treatment room
Checkup	Examination
Price	Fee
Cancellation	Change in schedule

expect from the dental visit. Words that convey an appreciation of the patient's feelings help patients feel heard and understood. Encouraging words can be used to help patients begin to feel more positive about the dental experience.

Greeting a patient with a smile is important and can help diminish dread that the patient may be experiencing about the dental visit. Even if the day has been hectic, the dental team must treat each patient with as much enthusiasm as the first patient greeted earlier in the day. A positive attitude helps to make the patient feel comfortable and eases negative attitudes that can cause tension and stress.

Understanding Human Needs

To communicate effectively with patients, the dental team needs to concentrate on statements that are positive for the patient. At times the dental team begins conversations with patients by focusing on technical needs such as treating cracked teeth, decay, periodontal disease, or stained teeth. These are all valid needs; however, this type of discussion does not allow the patient to see the benefits of the treatment. People do not want to know technically why they should do something; rather they want to know how the treatment will relieve the present pain or benefit their overall oral health.

Many people go to the dentist to maintain their teeth for the rest of their lives. Others go to take care of a problem while it is still small so that they do not have to face perceived pain or expense that would come later if the problem were not addressed. Still others, possibly due to anxiety issues or financial concerns, wait until they experience pain before contacting the dentist for treatment. Discovering what motivates a patient to accept treatment is the key to communicating treatment options to patients. Positive statements are most important during case presentation for elective services. For example, when discussing the placement of veneers, the dental team member could describe the procedure as:

> Chips and permanent staining in the front teeth can detract from the rest of your facial features. Veneers

placed over your front teeth can correct these imperfections and help you achieve a beautiful smile. Veneers are thin, custom-made shells crafted of tooth-colored materials. Veneers give people a healthy, natural-looking smile with little or no discomfort.

Each patient has some basic needs that must be met. If these basic needs are not met, the patient is uninterested in fulfilling other needs. To understand patients, the dental assistant needs to understand a few general concepts related to basic human needs. A psychologist named Abraham Maslow (1908–1970) studied people in society and discovered many levels of needs (Table 52-2). The lower the needs in the hierarchy, the more fundamental these needs are and the more a person will tend to ignore the higher needs in order to pay attention to the lower needs. For example, when we are ill, we care little for what others think about us: all we want is to get better. The survival needs for food, shelter, and safety are usually fulfilled for most of us. We eat regular meals and have our house or apartment for shelter and safety. If these needs are not met, however, then we tend to do whatever it takes to fulfill those needs before we try to fulfill the need of acceptance or self-esteem. Appreciating and understanding the needs of patients is critical for successful communication.

Psychological needs are very real to patients. Patients come into the dental practice with subjective and objective

TABLE 52-2 Maslow's Hierarchy of Needs

The Five Needs
- **Physiological needs:** Deal with the maintenance of the human body. If we are sick, then nothing else matters until we recover.
- **Safety needs:** About putting a roof over our heads and keeping us from harm.
- **Belonging needs:** Has to do with the belief that if we are helpful and kind to others, they will want us as friends.
- **Esteem needs:** Reflect our need to attain a higher position within a group. If people respect us, we have greater power.
- **Self-actualization needs:** The desire to "become what we are capable of becoming," which would be our greatest achievement.

Three More Needs
Maslow later added three more needs by splitting two of the above five needs. Between esteem and self-actualization needs he added:
- Need to know and understand, which explains the cognitive need of the academic.
- Need for aesthetic beauty, which is the emotional need of the artist.

Self-actualization was divided into:
- **Self-actualization:** realizing one's own potential.
- **Transcendence:** helping others to achieve their potential.

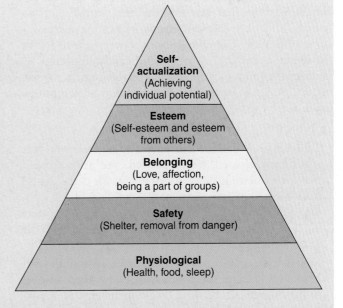

fears. **Subjective fears** are those fears that come from stories told by friends and families that can depict a negative side to dental treatment. **Objective fears** come from experiences and traumatic memories that the patient may have regarding past dental treatment. As a result of these types of fears, some patients are dental phobic. These patients are extremely terrified of dental treatment and must be treated with respect and patience. To meet the special needs of dental-phobic patients, the dental team must take extra steps to provide a positive atmosphere that is sincere and respectful.

All patients want to feel respected. It is important that the dental team be aware of the patient's time. If the office is running behind, the patient should be informed as soon as possible and given the choice to reschedule or wait. Always remain approachable for questions and concerns and resolve complaints as they arise.

Nonverbal Communication

Words are not the only element of good communication. Nonverbal communication relays messages as well. **Nonverbal communication** consists of communicating through body language and facial expressions. Facial expressions show different emotions such as feelings of happiness, sadness, excitement, confusion, and pain. Nonverbal communication that passes from the dental team to patients and vice versa can greatly impact the success of communication. Communication between members of the dental team can also be significantly impacted by nonverbal communication cues. For this reason a basic understanding of nonverbal cues is important. Emotions expressed by the dental patient in the form of nonverbal cues include:

* **Tenseness**—A patient in the reception area who has legs tightly crossed, hands clasped, and arms crossed may be exhibiting signs of being tense. It is the dental team's job to help the patient feel comfortable by talking to him and asking him about his weekend or offering him a magazine to read. (This may get his mind off of the treatment.)
* **Embarrassment**—A patient may cover her mouth with her hands because she is embarrassed by the condition of her mouth. As the dental team member, it is important to treat the patient with respect and kindness and not make an issue regarding the patient's possible feelings of embarrassment.

* **Anger**—The angry patient displays his emotion by acting defensive, with arms and legs tightly crossed. This may happen when patients perceive they are getting bad customer service or treatment. They may feel ignored by dental personnel or maybe feel as if they have been made to wait too long. It is the job of the dental team to recognize these signs and attempt to find out what the problem is. To prevent these situations, the dental reception personnel should always greet patients with a smile and a salutation as soon as patients enter the office. If the dental assistant is at the desk talking with a coworker when a patient walks in, the conversation should cease and attention should be directed toward the patient.

The dental health care team also sends out nonverbal cues that can affect the way the patient feels about the entire appointment experience:

* **Smiles**—Smiles send the message to patients that they are welcome and that the dental team is glad to see them. It helps patients feel more comfortable and less nervous, which in turn should result in return customers.
* **Attitude**—The dental team should consistently exhibit nonverbal cues that emanate enthusiasm and a genuine caring attitude rather than stress or frustration. Positive attitudes are contagious.

Listening Skills

Studies reveal that about 90% of all spoken words are never heard. Listening is one of the most difficult communication skills to obtain. To be a good listener, one must concentrate completely on the patient. Being a good listener requires specific skills and behaviors. For example, a common problem of listening is that of selective listening. A selective listener is an individual who only hears what he wants to hear. Eye contact is crucial while listening; it helps the listener focus more on what the sender of the message is saying.

When a patient is speaking it is important to not reply until the patient has finished her message. Do not concentrate on a reply until the patient is through speaking. Many times we try to formulate a reply or think about other things while we are trying to listen—and that does not work. We need to focus on the conversation we are currently having. Avoid getting impatient or being in a hurry to obtain information. It may be beneficial to get away from the outside distractions that make it difficult to focus on the message. Those distractions include others speaking, phones ringing, music, and other background noises.

The dental team should always actively listen when dealing with patients and coworkers (Figure 52.3). Active listening occurs when the receiver encodes the message and responds during a two-way communication. It may help to repeat back to the patient what the patient stated to ensure you have a complete understanding of his concerns. The dental health team should consistently work on developing and improving good active listening skills.

What type of communication is body language? What percentage of words do we actually hear? What is a more effective word for "drilling" a tooth? **?**

Communicating with Members of the Dental Team

Successful communication with those with whom we work is critical for success. Teamwork is the key to good relationships and a successful, efficient, well-run dental practice. The following are some tips to consider when working with the dental team:

- Work together and be receptive to other ideas.
- Avoid taking advantage of coworkers.

- Stay professional and avoid becoming emotional.
- Utilize open communication channels to allow for quicker conflict resolution.

Channels of Communication

Information can be communicated through various channels. In an organization, channels of communication include downward, horizontal, upward, and informal channels.

Downward channel communication is used to communicate information from the top of the organization down. Issues such as the organization's mission, vision, and goals are communicated through the downward channel. **Horizontal channel communication** occurs between peers (Figure 52.4). Information that is communicated using the horizontal channel includes goal setting and sharing day-to-day information to assist in ensuring that the goals of the office and the needs of the patients are being met. **Upward channel communication** reflects the flow of information from a lower level employee to an upper level employee in an organization (Figure 52.5). This type of communication includes feedback, requests for help, problem solving, and conflict resolution.

Informal channel communication is sometimes known as gossip or the "grapevine." Some organizations believe that the informal communication channel should be eliminated as much as possible. Although the informal channel can be problematic, managers can learn to use the informal channel as a means to discover how employees are thinking and feeling about various issues occurring in the office.

Because eliminating the informal channel is nearly impossible, it is wiser for managers to monitor the grapevine and to only intervene if this channel begins to be destructive to productivity and to the relationships of those within the organization. If employees are using the informal channel frequently, that may be an indication

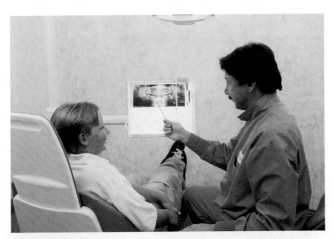

FIGURE 52.3
The dental assistant is in a listening position that shows interest in the patient.

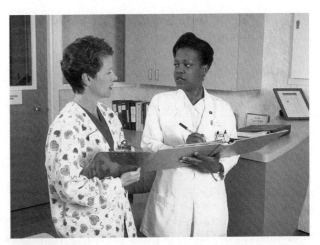

FIGURE 52.4
Horizontal communication.

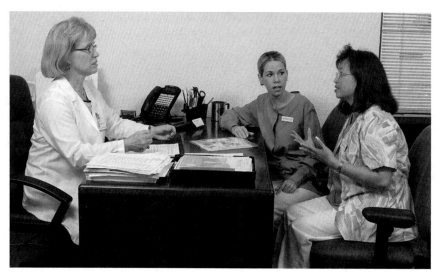

FIGURE 52.5
Upward communication.

that the other channels of communication in the organization are not working effectively. Informal communication channels can start rumors that can undermine an organization's effectiveness.

Barriers to Communication

Various barriers affect the success of communication. One of these barriers can be the working environment. An organization can either promote communication or inadvertently set up barriers that can cause stress in the dental team. This stress can often be observed or felt by patients, which further prevents effective communication from occurring. The following is a list of barriers that can create stress in the dental team and can cause a breakdown in communication:

- **Work overload/lack of sufficient staff**—An office that consistently sees a high volume of patients can cause stress on the dental team. This is particularly true if not enough staff members are available to handle the load. Heavy workloads can also be caused by high absenteeism rates of other staff members, accommodation of emergency patients, and increased administrative duties brought on by heavy phone traffic and poor scheduling of office staff.
- **Lack of understanding regarding roles and responsibilities**—A significant barrier to effective communication is when a lack of communication exists regarding the roles and responsibilities of each staff member in the dental office. Unclear roles can lead to miscommunication.
- **Change**—Most people react to change negatively. If change is communicated properly, office staff members are likely to react more positively. If change is not communicated, it can cause negative attitudes, which can be a barrier to effective communication. New techniques and policy changes should always be communi-

cated to the staff. The advantages and disadvantages of the change should be discussed along with ideas from the staff.

To minimize these types of communication barriers, management must play a significant role. It is up to management to address issues of overworked employees, training of staff regarding roles and responsibilities, and communicating change. All members of the dental team are important to ensuring that good communication continues to occur. Working together as a team can minimize barriers and possible conflicts in the workplace (Figure 52.6).

Cross-training, or learning each other's duties and tasks, is a great tool for use in respecting and understanding each other's jobs. It also helps the dental assistant become more productive in the organization.

Conflict

Conflict does at times occur in the workplace. Rest assured, though, that not all conflict is bad. How conflict

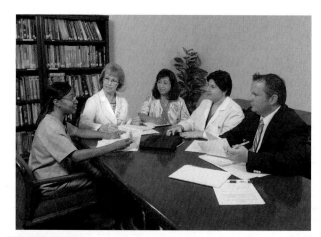

FIGURE 52.6
Dental team communicating.

is used can either be a hindrance or benefit to the situation. Conflict can be constructive if:

- the conflict results in the dental team members improving their decision-making skills.
- solutions to problems are identified.
- employees become more creative in their problem-solving methods because of the conflict.
- team and individual performances are improved due to the conflict that has occurred.
- the resolution of the conflict prevents lingering resentment.

Conflict can be destructive if it:

- causes stress and job burnout.
- minimizes communication.
- produces an atmosphere of mistrust.
- affects the quality of patient care.

Conflict and problem-solving tips include the following:

- Take responsibility for managing the problem or conflict. It is normal to avoid conflict, but it will not go away until it is dealt with.
- Uncover and discuss the real problem. For example, the conflict or complaint may appear to be the work assignment schedule; however, after talking with the conflicting people, it may be discovered that a personality clash exists. Once the problem is identified, steps to resolve it are easier.
- Set standards or goals to help resolve the conflict. The conflicting parties should have "buy-in" in order for conflict resolution to occur.
- Avoid arguments or emotional outbursts. When discussions are calm, resolution is quicker.

Conflict is not always easy to identify or resolve. Using the preceding tips is a start toward managing conflict in a professional manner. The management of conflicts is classified into different categories. The following categories describe the different styles of handling conflict:

- **Forcing or dominating style**—In this style, power, formal authority, and threats are used to handle the conflict. This method is used when quick action is needed or when implementing an unpopular decision.
- **Collaborating style**—In this style, an attempt is made to satisfy both conflicting parties. A win–win situation results when both parties put the needs of others or the organization ahead of themselves. This method is needed when decisions are important and require input from all involved.
- **Accommodating or obliging style**—This method accommodates one party's opinion by implementing their suggestions. It promotes harmony and stability. This is used when one party is unsure about his or her assessment of a situation.
- **Avoiding style**—This method takes a neutral position during conflict and is the best style to use when trivial issues are in conflict and if a "cooling-off" period is needed.
- **Compromising style**—This style tries to satisfy all of the needs of those involved in the conflict. It is used when a consensus cannot be reached to solve the problem.

Effective conflict management improves the organization and allows people to do their jobs better. It fosters creative thinking in the dental office and allows people to learn from mistakes. Conflict is inevitable in any organization. If it is handled correctly, however, it can improve morale and productivity. Team meetings should be held every day or at the least once a week for all dental team members to express new ideas or confront any problem in the office.

What type of communication channel does "gossip" fall under? How can conflict become positive?

Cultural Diversity

Cultural diversity addresses racial, ethnic, and religious differences. Dental patients come from various backgrounds. As a dental assistant, it is important to treat each patient with respect and avoid stereotyping individuals based on their cultural background and traditions. Sometimes patients want to discuss their cultural background or religious beliefs with dental team members. To better serve the dental patient, it is best to be open to discussing a patient's culture if the patient so chooses. Learning to listen and learn from patients is an important lesson that dental assistants should embrace. Demonstrating acceptance and a nonjudgmental attitude to all patients and avoiding the enforcement of one's own beliefs on patients is critical for successful relationships.

Patients and dental health care workers may have very different interpretations and ideas regarding dental treatments. These ideas and interpretations are influenced by cultural values, beliefs, and expectations about dental care. The following is a list of some basic cultural values and beliefs:

- The importance of the extended family, emphasized in Asian culture, often results in the extended family being highly involved in the dental care and decision making.
- Diet choices may be based on beliefs about what is healthy. Beliefs regarding diet could result in a refusal to eat certain foods that are being recommended to the patient to address nutritional issues.
- Beliefs about health and illness strongly influence behavior. Patients may be reluctant to obtain dental treatment or may refuse basic dental care due to their beliefs.

- Cultural beliefs may dictate what is appropriate to reveal or discuss. Some people may be raised to not whine or emotionally express pain. This may make it difficult for the dental team to initially determine problems.
- Race, ethnicity, and socioeconomic status can influence patients' decisions regarding dental treatment. Patients in poverty may lack the funds to follow the dentist's recommendations. These individuals may be uninsured and may refuse treatment that they consider unnecessary. Providers should try to understand the stress associated with poverty.
- Western values stress the importance of being direct and sharing one's opinion. Asian values stress politeness in verbal discussions. Asian cultures often use indirect means of expression, relying, for example, more on the nonverbal context for information than on the verbal context. Avoidance of self-disclosure and of public displays of emotion is characteristic. By being aware of these cultural differences, the dental assistant may want to begin by asking the Asian patient more general questions and then shifting to more specific ones.
- In the Western culture, it is common for health care providers to tell patients about treatments and diagnoses. In some cultures, patients may prefer not to know, because they fear that the very words may harm them.

Although cultural differences do exist, it is important to always remain mindful of not stereotyping any group of individuals. Always listen without judging and provide the best care possible for each and every patient. It may be helpful to have office forms available in the different languages of the patients who frequent the office. Tables 52-3 through 52-6 show basic terms in some common languages that may be encountered in the dental office.

Phone Skills

The telephone is usually the first contact the patient has with the dental office. Through conversations with the dental team over the phone, patients formulate their impressions of the professionalism and efficiency of the office. These impressions are formed by the tone of voice

TABLE 52-3 Basic Dental Terms in Spanish

English	Spanish
Mouth	La boca
Tooth	El diente
Pain	El dolor
Open	Abierto/a
Bite	La mordedura
Decay	La descomposicion
Filling	La empastadura
X-ray	La radiografia

TABLE 52-4 Basic Dental Terms in Russian

English	Russian
Mouth	рот(rot)
Tooth	зуб(zub)
Pain	боль(bol')
Open	открыть(ot-**krit'**)
Bite	кусатв(ku-**sat'**)
Decay	кариес(**ka**-ri-es)
Filling	пломба(**plom**-ba)
X-ray	рентген(rent-**gen**)

TABLE 52-5 Basic Dental Terms in French

English	French
Mouth	La bouche
Tooth	Le dent
Pain	La douleur
Open	Ouvrez
Bite	Mordez
Decay	Le carier
Filling	Le plombage
X-ray	X-ray

TABLE 52-6 Basic Dental Terms in German

English	German
Mouth	Der Mund
Tooth	Der Zahn
Pain	Der Schmerz
Open	Geoffnet (to have opened) Offfenen (to open)
Bite	Beißen
Decay	Die Karies Die Zahn Karies
Filling	Die Füllung
X-ray	Röntgenstrahlen

Cultural Considerations

Understanding different cultures can help you communicate better with dental patients. Make it a point to learn a little about various cultures; by doing so you will avoid insulting others.

used by the dental assistant and the overall treatment the patient receives during the phone conversation.

The dental assistant should develop a positive speaking image with particular attention paid to tone, volume, speed, and pitch. Every call needs to be answered in a pleasant and professional manner. The tone of your voice is greatly affected by a smile. When answering the phone it is important to smile. This is true even if your day has been difficult. The volume of your voice should be natural with use of good pronunciation. Attention should be given to slowing your speech for understanding and adjusting your pitch in order to emphasize important points.

Answering the Phone

Most dental offices have a standard greeting that all employees should use when answering the phone (Figure 52.7). A typical greeting would be "Good morning (or afternoon), Dr. Lafayette's office, Sue speaking. May I help you?" It is important to always identify the office and the name of the individual who is answering the phone. Never answer the phone by saying "Hold please" without getting a reply from the patient. The call could be an emergency. Other good telephone manners include these:

1. Answer the phone within three rings. The caller on the other end may be a prospective patient in need of immediate assistance. If the person has to wait, she may hang up and call another office hoping for a better response.

2. Do not answer the phone while eating or chewing gum. It is difficult for the caller on the other end to understand what is being said if the assistant is eating or chewing gum. It also does not reflect a professional image of the dental office.

3. Speak clearly, but not too fast, to ensure understanding of what is being communicated.

4. Do not use slang. The use of slang may give your caller the wrong idea about your office. He may feel that the office is unprofessional. Slang also leads to miscommunications.

5. Give your full attention to the caller. When assisting a patient at the desk and the phone rings, politely let her know that you must answer the phone and that you will return to her momentarily. Assist the caller, giving the person your full attention. If the call is going to take longer than expected, ask to place the caller on hold and then finish helping the patient at the desk.

6. Thank the caller and hang up last. To ensure the caller is finished speaking, let the caller hang up first to assure him that he has your complete attention.

Placing a Patient on Hold

At times a caller may need to be placed on hold. Prior to doing so, ask the caller "May I put you on hold for a moment?" Then wait for the caller to respond. If the caller agrees, place the individual on hold for no more than 30 seconds. If the caller states that being put on hold is not an option, it is important to be courteous and assist the individual at that time. The dental assistant may offer to call the patient back if she cannot be assisted at that time—this is not an ideal response, but may be necessary sometimes.

Some offices have an "on-hold" message that callers can listen to while waiting to speak with someone. Some on-hold messages have music or messages that explain the different services offered by the dental office. Be sure that the music and messages are appropriate and represent a professional image of the office.

Screening Calls

Patients who call into the office often want to speak directly to the dentist; however, this is not always possible. The dentist may be treating another patient and interruptions are not only inconsiderate to the patient in the chair, but may compromise infection control and decrease productivity. Politely inform the patient that the dentist is with a patient, and ask to take a message. Of course, there are always exceptions, such as family emergencies and calls from other dentists. Most offices have their own telephone policies on how to handle phone calls.

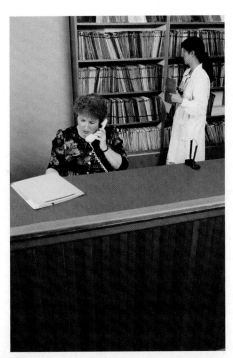

FIGURE 52.7
Assistant answering the telephone.

Taking Messages

When messages must be taken, it is important to correctly write down the information required for a callback. This information includes the caller's full name, phone number, the message, and the best times to return the call. Often preprinted message forms are used in dental offices to assist the receiver in obtaining the necessary information from the caller (Figure 52.8).

Once the caller has provided the information for the message, the information should be repeated back to the caller to ensure that the information has been correctly annotated. The dental assistant should not promise the caller a particular time when the callback will be made. If, however, the caller is promised a particular time for a callback, then it is critical to ensure that this occurs.

Once a message has been taken it should be given to the recipient as soon as possible. Patient messages that go to the dentist may require the dentist to have the patient's chart. If this is the case, be sure to attach the chart to the message prior to giving the message to the dentist.

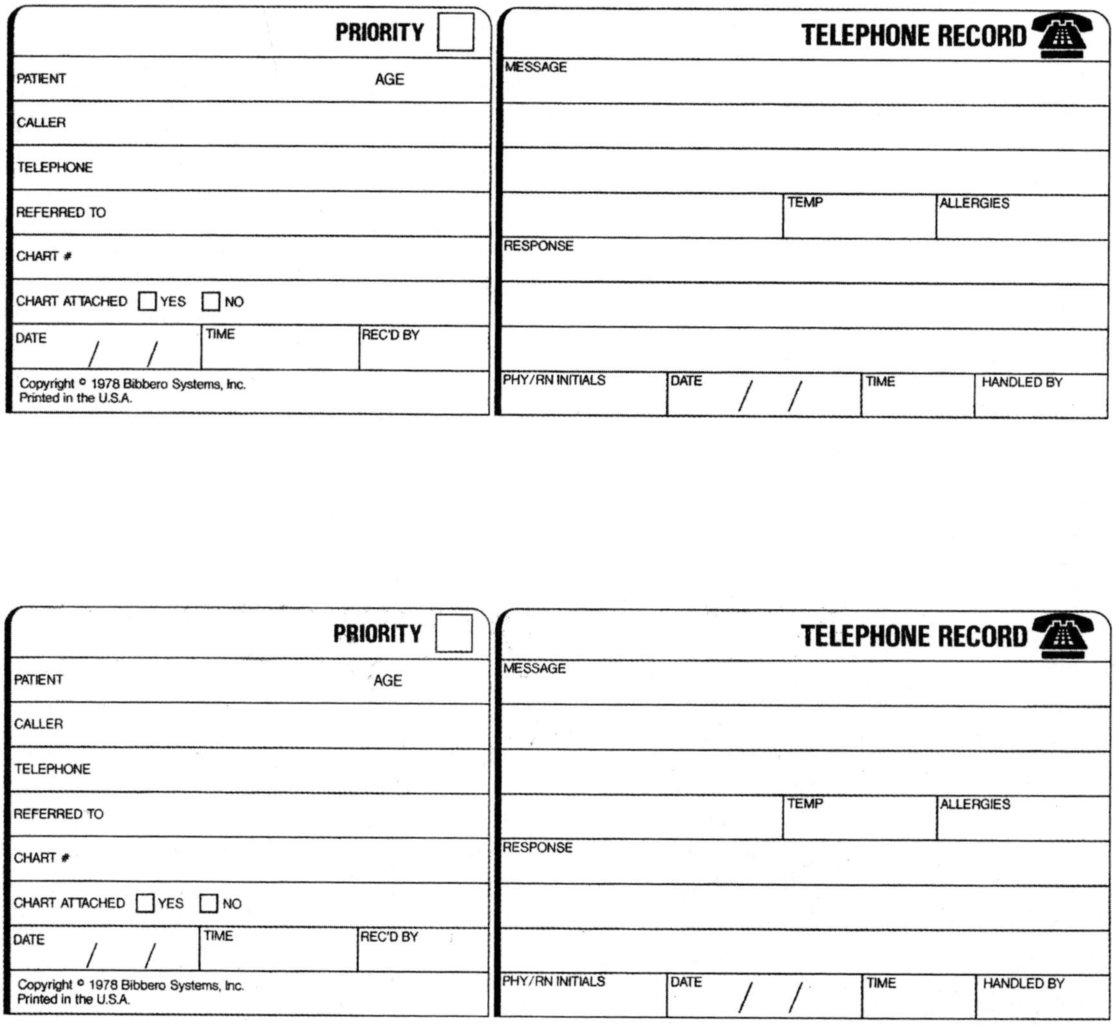
PRIORITY ☐
PATIENT AGE
CALLER
TELEPHONE
REFERRED TO
CHART #
CHART ATTACHED ☐ YES ☐ NO
DATE / / | TIME | REC'D BY

TELEPHONE RECORD
MESSAGE
TEMP | ALLERGIES
RESPONSE
PHY/RN INITIALS | DATE / / | TIME | HANDLED BY

PRIORITY ☐
PATIENT AGE
CALLER
TELEPHONE
REFERRED TO
CHART #
CHART ATTACHED ☐ YES ☐ NO
DATE / / | TIME | REC'D BY
Copyright © 1978 Bibbero Systems, Inc.
Printed in the U.S.A.
TELEPHONE RECORD
MESSAGE
TEMP | ALLERGIES
RESPONSE
PHY/RN INITIALS | DATE / / | TIME | HANDLED BY

FIGURE 52.8
Preprinted tear off Dental message pads.

Personal Phone Calls

Receiving or placing personal calls during working hours should be avoided. If a personal call must be made, it should be done during the employee's break and in a private area where patients will not overhear.

Answering Services

Receiving calls after business hours is often done through an answering service or the use of an answering machine. The answering service or machine relays an appropriate message to the patient that informs the patient about office hours and who to contact in case of an emergency. Messages should always be retrieved from the answering service or message center as soon as the office is open.

Answering services are typically not used when employees are in the office. These services are used for calls received after hours or if the dentist is out of town. The service allows the caller to speak to someone or leave a message. The service then contacts the on-call dentist or assistant, who will in turn contact the patient.

Another option that many offices use is the voicemail services offered by local telephone companies. Calls or messages can be retrieved by office personnel by calling an access number and entering a specific code number.

Office Equipment

Having the right equipment to conduct business is important for the efficiency of the dental office. Office equipment typically found in a dental office includes telephones, computers, a fax machine, a photocopier, and a printer.

Specific equipment for office telephones may include headsets. Telephone headsets for office use include an earphone and microphone that rests on the assistant's head and allows freedom of movement. The advantage of using a headset is that the assistant's hands are left free to retrieve materials that may be required to successfully conduct business on the phone.

Pagers and cell phones are other useful phone tools used by dentists to remain in touch with the office (Figure 52.9). Many dentists take calls during evening and weekend hours. Through the use of a pager or cell phone, the dentist on call can remain in touch with patients who may need attention during closed office hours.

A facsimile (fax) machine is a great communication tool for the dental office (Figure 52.10). It provides a quick way to convey information to insurance companies, dentists, and other health care providers. It is also a great tool to use when ordering supplies or equipment. The fax machine can save the office time in conveying information.

A fax machine is connected to a phone line and electronically sends and receives messages. At times confidential information must be sent immediately, and a fax machine is useful for doing that. A cover sheet with the

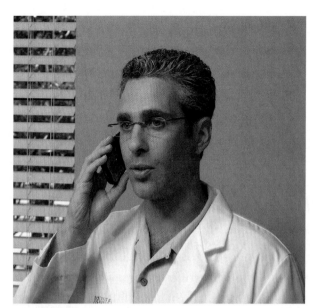

FIGURE 52.9
A dental professional staying in communication by use of a cell phone.

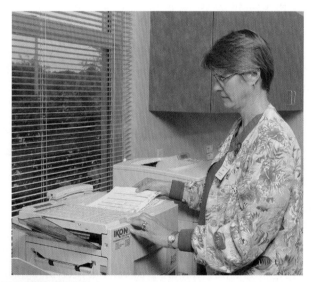

FIGURE 52.10
Using a fax machine.

intended recipient's name and the word "Confidential" is faxed first, then the confidential information. It is also a good practice when sending confidential information to call the recipient and have the person stand by to receive the intended information. Keeping the fax machine out of patient view will also help to maintain confidentiality. Following the Health Insurance Portability and Accountability Act (HIPAA) regulations and guidelines is crucial in maintaining patient privacy.

How should the dental assistant answer the phone? Is it appropriate to place a caller on hold? Why or why not?

Legal and Ethical Issue

Keep in mind that all communication with patients, verbal or written, is confidential. The Health Insurance Portability and Accountability Act has increased awareness of patient privacy. Ensure that you are familiar with the requirements you must follow as a dental assistant when it comes to ensuring confidentiality.

Written Communication

Dental offices use written communication to perform a multitude of tasks, such as creating business letters, newsletters, and employee manuals. Although advancements in computer software programs have made the creation of certain written materials easier, it is still important for the dental assistant to have basic skills in written communications.

To be a good communicator requires the efficient and effective use of both the written and spoken word. The first thing to know in order to accomplish written communication tasks required in the dental office is how to use the equipment. The computer is one of the most useful tools in the office. It allows the dental assistant to complete business letters, type office manuals and office newsletters, send and receive e-mail, schedule patients, and complete insurance forms. When first employed at a dental office, it is important to be oriented to the various office equipment and software programs used by the office. Training on the equipment can help to ensure efficiency.

Letters

One of the most important forms of communication between dentists, patients, and colleagues is correspondence through letters and memos. Letters can help to clarify information and are a useful and necessary form of communication in the dental office. Various types of written communication are used in dental offices. Letters sent out by the practice include letters to welcome patients to the practice, thank-you letters for referrals, letters of appreciation, and collection letters. Whenever correspondence is sent out from the office, it is important to ensure that the letter represents the image and professionalism of the office.

Attention should also be given to ensure confidentiality of patient information. HIPAA regulations have impacted the dental profession in terms of maintaining patient confidentiality. HIPAA established safeguards for dental and health care transactions that are transmitted electronically. Under HIPAA the dental office privacy standard must cover the following:

- **Protected health information**—Any information that can identify an individual, such as Social Security num-

ber, phone number, birth date, and name, must always be protected and out of sight of others.
- **Individual's rights**—Patients have the right to get copies of or otherwise access their dental information. Patients should be informed of the privacy policy in the office.
- **Use and disclosure**—This policy states that patient information cannot be disclosed without permission.

Continuous training for the dental health team is important to ensure everyone is doing what is required under HIPAA. Each person in the office must understand that he or she is responsible for protecting patient privacy. The American Dental Association is a good source of information regarding HIPAA policies in the dental office.

Parts of a Letter

When preparing a letter it is important to ensure that the professional image of the office is portrayed. The appearance of a letter makes a statement about the efficiency and professionalism of the office. The layout of a business letter is divided into several parts: the letterhead or heading, date, inside address, salutation, body, and the closing (Table 52-7):

- The letterhead or heading is usually preprinted with the name of the dentist, office address, and phone number. If the heading is not preprinted, it is typically placed about two inches from the top of the page and is centered.
- The date is typed two lines below the last line of the heading.
- The inside address is the information for mailing the letter and is typed four lines below the date. The letter address should match the envelope address and include the name of the person and his or her title on the first line, the company name on the second line, and then the city, state, and zip code on the last line. The two-letter state abbreviation in capital letters should be used. Leave two spaces after the state abbreviation before entering the zip code.
- The **salutation** is a formal greeting to the reader. This should begin two lines below the letter address, and should be even with the left margin. The word "Dear" is an appropriate salutation.
- The body consists of the actual message and begins two lines below the salutation. Typically paragraphs are single spaced with double spacing between each separate paragraph.
- The closing should be two lines below the last line of the body of the letter. Some common closings are "Sincerely," "Sincerely Yours," or "Respectfully."

Types of Letters

When writing letters, the assistant may choose a template and style from a word processing program. These

TABLE 52-7 Business Letter Basics

Heading: Twelve to 20 hard returns from top of page (if not using letterhead)

Date: Two hard returns below the last line of the heading or letterhead

Inside Address (Recipient's Address): Four to 12 hard returns below the dateline

Salutation or Greeting: Two hard returns below the last line of the inside address

Example: Dear Dr. Michaels:

Body: Two hard returns below the salutation (single spaced within paragraphs; double spaced between paragraphs)

Example: I am referring Jan Jones, age 11, to you for an orthodontic evaluation. Mrs. Jones will be contacting your office for an appointment. Jan seems to have a Class II, Division 1, malocclusion with crowding on the mandibular.

Enclosed are radiographs (panoramic, cephalometric, and FMXR) taken on November 12, 2008.

I look forward to your assistance.

Closing: Two hard returns below the last line of the body

Example: Respectfully,

Signature: Four hard returns below the closing; a handwritten signature should be used

Reference initials of typist and author: Two hard returns below title in the signature line

Example: LT:jg

Enclosure notation: Two hard returns below the reference initials

Example: Enclosure: Radiographs × 2

Copy notation: Two hard returns below all other notations

Example: cc: Dr. Harriet Myers

---

templates and styles can be modified to meet the needs and preferences of the office. There are a few basic styles from which to choose: the block style, the modified block style, and the simplified style (Figure 52.11).

In the block format, all sections begin at the left margin. The modified block format is the same as the block format, except the paragraphs are indented. The simplified letter is an efficient block style with the following exceptions: no salutation or complementary closing, the word "Subject" in the subject line is omitted, and lists are indented five spaces.

Characteristics of a Letter

An effective letter is one that is direct and contains a clearly stated message. When writing a letter, it is important to avoid using technical terms that might confuse or disinterest the recipient. Attention should be paid to ensure that the tone of the letter is both pleasant and professional. Use of words such as "please" and "thank-you" will keep the tone of the letter courteous and polite. Professionalism can be conveyed in a letter through the use of good grammar, complete sentences, and accurate spelling. Punctuation is another important aspect to a good letter or any written communication. The following is a list of some basic grammar techniques:

- Every sentence starts with a capital letter.
- Each sentence must have a subject and a verb. (The subject is what or whom the sentence is about. The verb

expresses an action or events or state of mind about the subject.)
- Commas are used to separate three or more words or phrases in a series.
- Commas are used between city and state names.
- Contractions, such as "don't" or "can't," are not used in formal business letters.
- Quotation marks are used to set off exact quotes from other sources.
- Numbers from one to nine are spelled out, and numerals are used for numbers 10 and above.

The use of active verbs most of the time will enhance letter-writing techniques. If the verb describes something that the subject is doing, the verb is active. If the verb describes something that is being done to the subject, the verb is passive.

Active: I recommend that the patient's molar be removed.

Passive: It was recommended by me for the patient to have the molar removed.

Avoid wordy sentences by eliminating unnecessary words. Put the meaning of the sentence in the subject and verb.

Wordy: Please refer to the fee that is enclosed.

Concise: Please refer to the enclosed fee.

Ensure that the sentence length and structure are varied. Use a combination of short and long sentences. Also

FIGURE 52.11
Example of the block style letter.

use parallel structure; this structure puts words and phrases in the same logical form.

Parallel: The position offers education, training, and money.

Nonparallel: The position is educational, offers you to be trained and money.

Finally, use positive as opposed to negative words and tones. Your message will have more of an impact if it is on the positive side. For example:

Negative: "You failed to show for your last appointment."

Positive: "We missed you at your appointment on 1 July."

Here are some good steps to follow when preparing a business letter:

1. **Gather information**—Be sure you have the correct, complete address for the recipient and all necessary information. For instance, if you are preparing a referral letter, be sure to include the nature of the problem that led to the referral. If the letter is an inquiry about a product, have the product name and number available.

Office Name
Street, City, State, Zip Code
Phone #, Fax phone #, Email

Month, day, year
(Line up date with signature block)

Mrs. Mary Smith
5522 E. Waters Street
Lake City, Iowa 44432

Dear Mrs. Smith:

(Indent each paragraph) After review of your radiographs and examination from August 1st, 2007, it is necessary to refer you to Dr. Glen Green for extraction of the lower left second bicuspid.

I will send Dr. Green the radiographs, along with detailed documentation of your examination.

Please call Dr. Green's office at 515-234-7777 and make an appointment as soon as possible. I am sure you will be pleased with the service he will provide for you. If you have further questions, please contact my office.

Respectfully,

First, MI, Last, DDS

Cc: (courtesy copy – optional)

(continued)

FIGURE 52.11 (continued)
Example of the modified block style letter.

2. **Create an outline**—Outlines help the writer stay organized.

3. **Develop a draft of the letter**—The draft, like the outline, allows the writer to review the letter to ensure the sequence is logical and make changes before sending it to the recipient.

4. **Review and revise the letter**—Always send out professional work. The letter represents the dental office. Be sure the letter professionally and clearly conveys the message.

5. **Proofread the letter**—Proofreading ensures the accuracy and completeness of the message being conveyed. Letters full of punctuation and spelling errors are not professional.

6. **Distribute the letter**—Letters are distributed nowadays via regular mail or e-mail.

7. **Store the document**—Typically the document is stored on the business office computer and saved to the daily backup system.

What types of letters are created and sent by a typical dental office?

```
┌─────────────────────────────────────────────────────────────┐
│                        Office Name                             │
│                Street, City, State, Zip Code                   │
│                 Phone #, Fax phone #, Email                    │
│                                                                │
│                                                                │
│   Month, day, year                                             │
│                                                                │
│                                                                │
│   Mrs. Mary Smith                                              │
│   5522 E. Waters Street                                        │
│   Lake City, Iowa  44432                                       │
│                                                                │
│                                                                │
│   NEW OFFICE MANAGER – JANE JONES, CDA (Subject line is all    │
│   captial letters) (No Salutation)                             │
│                                                                │
│   It is my pleasur eto inform you that Jane Jones is the new   │
│   Office Manager at our dental office.                         │
│                                                                │
│   She is a graduate of the Community University with over 10   │
│   years of dental assisting and office experience. She will be │
│   joining the practice as of August 1st, 2007.                 │
│                                                                │
│   Jane will be working primarily in the insurance section of   │
│   the office. We are looking forward to working with her. We   │
│   appreciate your patience and understanding while this        │
│   transition occurs.                                           │
│                                                                │
│                                                                │
│   FIRST NAME, MI, LAST NAME, DDS (All capital letters)         │
│                                                                │
└─────────────────────────────────────────────────────────────┘
```

FIGURE 52.11 (continued)
Example of the simplified style letter.

Electronic Mail

Correspondence is often sent electronically via e-mail. E-mail is usually intended to provide brief messages to coworkers or those outside the organization. It is important to remember that e-mail is not always secure and that HIPAA requires that patient information be protected. For this reason, confidential documentation or documentation with personal health information in it should not be sent via e-mail.

Even though e-mail is a quick message system, care should be given to proper punctuation and format. E-mails should follow proper etiquette rules such as using "please" and "thank-you." When communicating with coworkers or colleagues, the e-mail should still have a formal format. Always capitalize the appropriate words and check the document for correct spelling and punctuation. Capitalization of all words in an e-mail is poor e-mail etiquette because it can be interpreted as yelling. Keep in mind that personal e-mails sent from work should be kept to a minimum. Most offices have policies in place regarding personal e-mails. Sending inappropriate e-mails is never allowed.

Dental Office Procedure Manual

The dental office procedure manual is a resource that is used by all members of the dental team. This manual provides information on organizational goals and structure, personnel information, business office procedures, and clinical procedures. The manual should be developed and updated as needed by the entire dental team. (See Chapter 53 for more information regarding the dental office procedure manual.)

SUMMARY

Through the use of effective communication skills, the dental assistant can assist in helping the patient feel as comfortable as possible during a dental procedure. A dental assistant should obtain the skills necessary for listening and understanding verbal and nonverbal communication.

Consideration of each patient's background and culture can assist the dental assistant in communicating effectively with patients. In addition to effectively communicating with patients, it is important for the dental assistant to communicate well with coworkers. Proper communication with coworkers reduces stress and burnout and enhances the entire environment for staff and patients.

KEY TERMS

- **Cultural diversity:** Addresses racial and ethnic differences. p. 833
- **Downward channel communication:** Channel of communication that originates from an upper level employee of an organization and travels down to a lower level employee. p. 831
- **Horizontal channel communication:** Channel of communication that is used between members of an organization at the same level. p. 831
- **Informal channel communication:** Gossip; also known as the "grapevine." p. 831
- **Nonverbal communication:** Communicating through body language and facial expressions. p. 830
- **Objective fears:** Experiences and traumatic memories from prior treatments that may not have been positive. p. 830

- **Receiver:** The recipient of the intended message. 827
- **Salutation:** Formal greeting to a reader. p. 838
- **Sender:** The individual who is communicating a message to another person (the receiver). p. 827
- **Subjective fears:** Fears that come from stories told by friends and families. p. 830
- **Upward channel communication:** Channel of communication that originates from a lower level employee in an organization and travels to an upper level employee. p. 831
- **Verbal communication:** Consists of words used to transmit a message; can be spoken or written. p. 827

CHECK YOUR UNDERSTANDING

1. What type of communication makes use of body language?
   a. verbal
   b. nonverbal
   c. listening
   d. written

2. When should the telephone be answered?
   a. after one ring
   b. after three rings
   c. after four rings
   d. when you can get to it

3. Which piece of office equipment allows you to transmit hardcopy written messages?
   a. telephone
   b. pager
   c. voicemail
   d. facsimile machine

4. The salutation part of a letter is
   a. the introductory greeting.
   b. the actual message of the letter.
   c. the closing of the letter.
   d. the office address and phone number.

5. Dental practices send letters for which of the following reasons?
   a. to welcome patients to the practice
   b. to make a referral
   c. to collect a payment
   d. all of the above

6. Which type of communication channel includes goal setting?
   a. horizontal
   b. informal
   c. upward
   d. downward

7. The dateline of a letter is usually how many spaces below the heading?
   a. one
   b. two
   c. three
   d. four

CHECK YOUR UNDERSTANDING (continued)

8. Which of the following is an appropriate salutation?
   a. "Hi"
   b. "Hello"
   c. "Dear"
   d. none of the above

9. Which of the following elements are included when annotating a telephone message?
   a. caller's name
   b. caller's phone number

   c. what the call is in reference to
   d. all of the above

10. How does constructive conflict benefit the dental office?
    a. It affects quality of patient care.
    b. It causes unhealthy stress.
    c. It leads to new solutions to problems.
    d. It reduces job performance.

INTERNET ACTIVITY

- Research proper telephone techniques by visiting the following website: http://ec.hku.hk/epc/telephoning. Write a dialogue that you may use when answering the telephone at your dental office. With a partner, present it to the class.

WEB REFERENCES

- The Owl at Purdue http://owl.english.purdue.edu/handouts/pw/p_basicbusletter.html
- The Institute for Management Excellence www.itstime.com/aug97.htm
- American Dental Association www.ada.org/prof/resources/topics/hipaa/index.asp
- United States Department of Health and Human Services www.hhs.gov/ocr/hipaa

53

Practice Management Procedures

Learning Objectives

After reading this chapter, the student should be able to:

- Describe the purpose of operating manuals.
- Discuss future trends in records management in the dental office.
- Explain the importance of good record keeping.
- List the types of filing systems available.
- List three types of appointment scheduling techniques.
- Discuss the advantages and disadvantages of preventive recall programs.
- Compare and contrast the options for inventory management.
- Discuss the most common practices for maintenance and repair of equipment and supplies.

Preparing for Certification Exams

- Perform routine maintenance of dental equipment.

Key Terms

Calibration	Modified wave scheduling
Credit slip	Operating procedure manual
Double booking	Reorder point
Ergonomics	Shelf life
Lead time	Wave scheduling

Chapter Outline

- Operating Procedure Manual
  —Procedure Formats
- Computer Applications in the Dental Office
  —Hardware and Software
  —Computer Safety
  —The Future of Computers in the Dental Office
- Record Keeping
  —Clinical Records
  —Guidelines to Record Keeping
- Filing and Storing of Patient Records
  —Storing Files
  —Rules for Filing
  —Methods of Filing
- Appointment Scheduling
  —The Appointment Book
  —Using the Appointment Book
  —Scheduling Systems
- Preventive Recall Programs
- Inventory Management
  —Equipment
  —Supplies
  —Inventory Systems
- Equipment Repairs

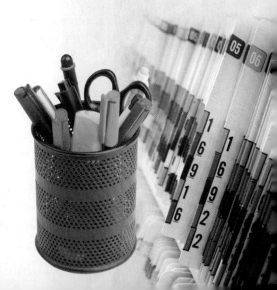

The success of a dental practice relies on sound practice management procedures. Certain business practices, such as utilizing computer applications, maintaining records, filing materials, and establishing an inventory system, are common to most businesses. Dental practices refine and tailor these practices to suit the needs of the particular practice. Business practices specific to the dental office include establishment of a scheduling system to address the needs of the practice, maintenance and care of dental equipment, and utilizing particular software computer applications appropriate for the practice.

Operating Procedure Manual

Operating procedure manuals are generally notebooks or three-ring binders that contain written directions for completing particular functions or tasks. Three-ring binders work well because pages can be easily removed, rearranged, or replaced. Procedures are a collection of methods that must be followed in order to achieve consistent performance of the task or work at hand. Hence, the purpose of the procedure manual is to ensure that tasks are performed uniformly and to allow for quality management and control. Procedures are commonly associated with repetitive or simplified work tasks. For instance, procedures in the dental office range from methods of autoclaving equipment to recording paychecks in the daily ledger.

Procedures should be written in a format that is easy to read and follow. Managers typically develop and write procedures. All written procedures must be coordinated with other departments and policymakers. This should be done to ensure that department procedures and policies are not in conflict with each other, and that procedures and policies are in sync with the overall objectives of the organization. Policies provide a guide for any actions to be taken.

The procedure manual also contains information regarding office communications, employment policies, Health Insurance Portability and Accountability Act (HIPAA) policy and regulations, Occupational Safety and Health Administration (OSHA) guidelines, and infection control policies and clinical procedures.

Procedure Formats

Procedures are written in different types of formats. Scores of software programs with varying formatting options are available for creating policy and procedure manuals. In the narrative type of format, procedures are written in paragraph form and usually consist of groups of statements that may contain special notes or explanations in subparagraphs, parentheses, or footnotes. Explanations for each procedure are written using complete and full sentences. The abbreviated narrative format is a combination of sentences and a listing of key terms and concepts. The playscript format, a well-known method used to write procedures, is used whenever necessary for relegating the responsibility to specific positions. Most procedure manuals are categorized and coded according to department, work type, or person who performs the procedure. The choice of format is usually that of the owner or chief administrator of the practice.

In addition to a suitable format, the procedure manual should be user friendly; that is, easy to locate, easy to handle, and easy to read. The idea is that the manual should be consulted and updated frequently so that all employees understand what is expected of them. If the rulebook is clear, concise, and current, it should be easier to follow.

The physical characteristics of the procedure manual are important too. For example, a loose-leaf system is preferred in some situations. The loose-leaf system provides the ability to easily replace obsolete information.

The procedure manual of the future is obviously electronic. The advantage of an electronic procedure manual is that it provides a format that is convenient to access and makes replacing obsolete information with up-to-date information very easy. Having procedures online also makes the manual more readily available to staff members. The deciding factor for most practices is the affordability of electronic resources.

Although the choice of format can be important, more important is the fact that the dental practice has an established and up-to-date operating procedure manual. The use of a complete and integrated procedure manual results in a more successful, efficient, and effective dental practice. Remember: less stress in the office increases morale and productivity.

Dental Assistant **PROFESSIONAL TIP**

Never leave a filing cabinet drawer open after you have finished with the filing. It is a safety hazard. Another employee could be walking along and not notice the drawer. The person could walk into the cabinet and easily be injured. It is a good practice to always clean up the office space in which you have been working. Cleanliness promotes safety, efficiency, and organization.

How can a policy manual help in getting everyone on the same page?

Computer Applications in the Dental Office

In today's business world most businesses and practices are somehow engaged in electronic data keeping and manipulation. Offices have computer technology, although it may not always be the latest and greatest version. Computers all have certain features. These features consist of both hardware and software components.

Hardware and Software

Hardware is the machinery necessary to process data. It consists of the physical tower, which contains the CPU or central processing unit; the monitor; the keyboard; the mouse; and all wires that run into and away from these components (Figure 53.1). The software is the part of the computer system that manages the data and is not visible. Examples of software include programs such as Microsoft Word or Excel.

Most of the time the office manager determines which hardware and software will be used and when they will be updated. The hardware needs to be updated less frequently than the software; however, each needs to be updated routinely. Hardware is typically updated when its capacity is diminished and the unit can no longer support the necessary software. Sometimes hardware just requires service as any electronic device would; for example, circuit boards may fail or cords could fray. Once a practice has turned a profit or has a cash surplus, it is a good idea to invest in upgrading the office computers, both the hardware and the software. Technology changes rapidly and allows for improved systems. These improvements ultimately can lead to improved customer service and increased profits.

Software is usually the part of the computer that is dealt with most often by the dental assistant. The dental assistant uses the computer for recording all types of information including but not limited to financial records, dental charting, and x-rays. The primary functions of the computer in the dental office are to manage the data. Every office should purchase programs with the specific needs of the office in mind. Word processing programs, spreadsheet programs, and programs that offer graphic art functions are typically found in a dental office. These programs can perform most of the basic tasks of a dental office. Numerous companies manufacture dental office software, including Dentrix, Eagle Soft, Denta Soft, and Easy Dent.

Word processing software is used for tasks such as writing letters to patients or referrals to other dentists and doctors and other general correspondence. Word processing functions that include the capacity to print labels are an asset to tasks related to marketing. The majority of businesses use a Windows operating system or a larger system that incorporates the Windows systems. Several packaged applications can be purchased that include word processing, spreadsheet, and database management programs. Spreadsheet programs are like worksheet programs with the added feature of having a calculator built into the program. Many of the word processing and spreadsheet programs have graphics features, which allow for the manipulation of data into such visuals as pie charts, graphs, and bar graphs. Some database management programs have graphic arts features. Database management is provided in the Windows format of Access. Access is a program that allows information to be retrieved in a variety of groupings. Larger database management needs can be met with larger systems. Many dental practices buy a specific data management program such as Dentisoft, Dentimax, or Dentrix. These programs are similar in the way they manipulate the data input. The difference may be in how the data are arranged and the various programs available in the data management program. For instance, some programs include financial management components and appointment scheduling features (Figure 53.2)

The safety and integrity of the data are of major concern to a dental practice. It is absolutely essential for the system to be backed up on a daily basis. This ensures that nothing is lost in the event of a computer failure. Viruses

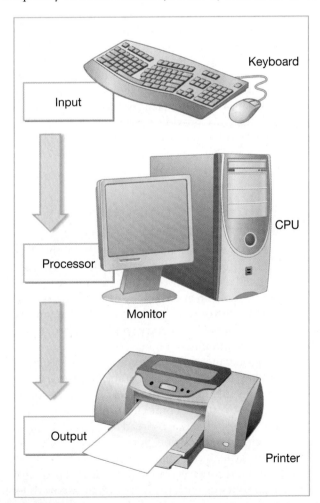

FIGURE 53.1
Computer hardware components.

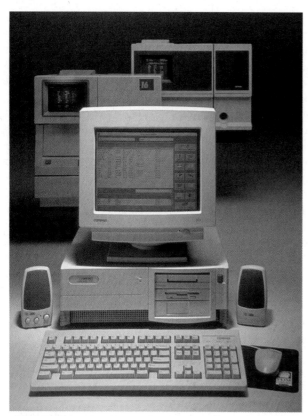

FIGURE 53.2
Patient data management system.

and other internal problems can be a threat to the security of a computer. Firewalls and antivirus software are available for a nominal fee and should be used.

Computer Safety

Computer safety is an issue facing more office workers than ever before. There are two main concerns when it comes to computer safety: the safety of the user and the safety of the data. With the increase in the use of computers, companies have seen an increase in injuries related to computer use. For instance, carpal tunnel syndrome, a condition affecting an individual's wrists, has been on the rise. This is due in part to the lack of attention given to ensuring that computer users are ergonomically aware.

Ergonomics is the body mechanics that are considered when humans use equipment and tools. The user must arrange the computer to protect the user's eyes, back, and wrists. When an individual is using a computer, the lighting can be very hard on the eyes. This is due to the glare both from the screen and the ceiling lights. Screen glare protectors can be purchased and applied to the monitor. It is also suggested that the user look away from the computer screen periodically to give the eyes a rest.

The seating position of the user in relation to the computer makes a difference in terms of the back and wrists. A person should sit with the monitor positioned just below eye level and in front of the user (Figure 53.3).

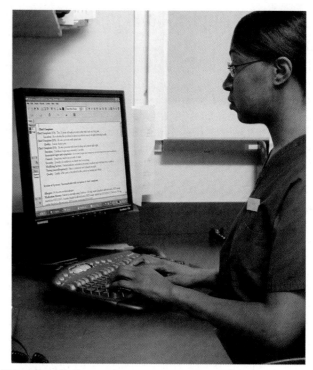

FIGURE 53.3
The computer user seated in an ergonomically correct position.

The back should be straight with support provided from the chair for the natural curves in the spine. The arms should be bent at about a 90-degree angle without using the armrests, and the keyboard should be close so that the user does not have to reach for the keys. Feet should be on the floor to provide maximum support. Other items for ergonomically correct positioning are available for purchase such as seat cushions, special wrist braces, and ergonomically designed keyboards.

The Future of Computers in the Dental Office

Computers in business are here to stay. How the dental office will be affected by computers in the years to come, however, is still unknown. Software of the future promises more graphics with an increased use of icons incorporated into a touch screen or run by voice control. These formats mean that less manual data entry will be required, leading to fewer errors and miscommunications.

Another advancement in computers that is currently taking hold in health care is that of the electronic record. Although some health care and dental facilities still use paper records, the future of the electronic record seems to be certain. Many offices are already considered "paperless" with electronic charting, appointments, billing, and radiology. Through the use of the electronic health record, patient records are more available and accessible. With the continuous push for more organizations to join the age of electronic records, further enhancements to electronic security will continue to be developed.

Why wouldn't a dental office want to go to paperless records?

Record Keeping

Record keeping is a high priority in the dental office. Not only do laws such as HIPAA require record keeping, but record keeping is essential in providing quality care to patients. The dental record goes by many names including the patient record or the dental chart. The chart contains examination records, radiographs, lab results, prescriptions, diagnoses, referrals, consent forms, and any correspondence. The chart does not contain financial information except for the name, address, and incidental information required by the insurance company. All charts should be filled out completely, accurately, and legibly.

The doctor owns the chart, and the patient owns the information. Patients have the right to view what is in the record and can request a copy of the file. Other parties may express an interest in the file as well. For example, insurance companies often want parts of the file to check on disbursements or to follow up in the matter of a complaint. If a patient pursues legal advice regarding an issue related to the dental practice, the attorney may request the patient's dental records. Sometimes, dental records are used for other legal matters such as identification in forensics. It is for these reasons that the chart should be kept in good shape, and all persons who handle the chart should be well trained and versed in the legal aspects of documentation.

Clinical Records

The clinical record includes a variety of forms excluding any financial information. The registration form (Figure 53.4) is one of the first forms a patient fills out along with the health questionnaire. The registration form and health questionnaire may be a combined form or may be separate. A pediatric patient should have the forms filled out by a parent or a legal guardian.

PATIENT REGISTRATION FORM
(Please Print)

Date: _____

Patient's Name: _____
       First   Middle   Last

DOB: ____/____/____
    Month Day Year

Address: _____
    Street   City State Zip

Phone: ____/____-_____
   (Area code)

Patient's SS#: ____-____-____ Driver's License #: _____ Occupation: _____

Method of payment (circle): cash check credit card insurance co-payment

Primary Insurance Co.: _____ Policy/Group #: _____

Medicare #: _____ Medicaid #: _____

Person Responsible For Payment: _____ Relationship _____
    First   Middle   Last

Address: _____ Phone: ____/____-_____
    Street   City State Zip   (Area code)

Employer Name: _____ Dept: _____
    First   Middle   Last

Address: _____ Phone: ____/____-_____
    Street   City State Zip   (Area code)

Spouse or Nearest Relative: _____ Relationship _____
    First   Middle   Last

Address: _____ Phone: ____/____-_____
    Street   City State Zip   (Area code)

How were you referred to this office? _____

_____

Statement of Financial Responsibility: I, _____ do hereby agree to pay all medical charges incurred by the above listed patient. I further understand that these charges are my responsibility, regardless of insurance coverage.

Responsible Person's Signature: _____

FIGURE 53.4
Patient registration form.

Legal and Ethical Issue

When working with charts and any other legal documents, make sure you document accurately, correctly, and completely. Be sure to present the information in the most objective way possible. If a patient has a behavior that is belligerent or rude, document the actual actions of the person, not your interpretation of the behavior. Describe the behavior without any commentary. For example, you might record that the patient was shouting obscenities and you can quote the actual words used. Do not record that you feel it was unnecessary behavior or that the patient was acting like a child. The latter phrases imply a judgment on your part, and it is best to document objectively and without emotion.

When a patient's information changes, it is important for the patient to fill out an update form. The update form provides the patient an opportunity to note any changes in her personal information, dental condition, finances, or anything else the patient wants the dental practice to know.

The clinical examination form (Figure 53.5) and the progress note can also be found in the dental chart. Typically, a new clinical exam form and progress note are created for each patient visit. The patient chart is also where laboratory requisitions are kept. States usually mandate that laboratory requisition forms and laboratory logs must be kept as a cross-reference. Other forms that are kept with the clinical record are the treatment plan form (Figure 53.6) and the signed informed consent form (Figure 53.7).

Guidelines to Record Keeping

To be sure that patient records are complete, certain guidelines should be followed by the dental team. Information that the dentist should document in patient records includes objective findings and other patient information such as medications prescribed, anesthesia administered, and conversations with the patient regarding treatment plans and recommendations.

General guidelines to documenting information in the patient chart include the following:

- Use black ink.
- Date every entry using the complete date: MM/DD/YYYY.
- Write legibly.
- Sign all entries.
- Never use correction fluid to correct an error in the chart. Inaccuracies and mistakes should be identified and corrected by striking one line through the error and making a notation per office policy to denote the reason for the correction. The notation is initialed and dated

if the mistake happened on the same day. If the mistake happened on a different date, another entry must be made that reveals the mistake and makes the correction, dated for the actual date of the later entry.

- Record all patient reactions in an objective manner.
- Track cancelled, missed, and rescheduled appointments. (This can be important for legal reasons.)
- Keep all statements factual and objective.
- Maintain confidentiality.
- Never alter a patient's record.

Filing and Storing of Patient Records

The equipment necessary for maintaining and storing paper files is very basic. Folders and filing cabinets are the most obvious equipment to use for storage. The folder itself can be either a folder style so that all of the documents fit inside a three-sided pouch, or the folder can be a two-sided, book-style folder that offers a few different sections and a more sturdy binding. To place forms in the patient record, forms are typically punched with holes at the top so that all forms lie flat, one on top of the next. Many dental offices use a color-coded system to mark the outside of the folders with the first few letters of the patient's last name (Figure 53.8). Sometimes the folders are marked with the year because this helps the assistant spot the current patient files more readily.

Other markings on the outside of the folder include any allergies the patient may have and sometimes the name of the insurance is listed. The name of the patient is usually typed onto a label with the Social Security number and birth date.

Patient files must be kept confidential and for an indefinite time frame. No clinical chart or financial records should be visible on the desk or in the operatory for other patients walking by to view. When not in use, all charts should be face down for confidentiality purposes and to abide by HIPAA regulations. Consent forms for releasing files must be signed by the patient. HIPAA prohibits information pertaining to an individual's health status from being displayed on the outside of a chart; however, a specific color-coding system can be utilized.

Storing Files

Patient files are kept in filing cabinets and other filing storage devices. Various types of filing cabinets are used, such as the vertical, open-shelf lateral (Figure 53.9), and movable types. The vertical file cabinet is the traditional standing kind with two to five drawers. These cabinets are cumbersome, require excessive storage space, and are heavy, especially the four- to five-drawer fireproofed cabinets. They also present a problem to the growing practice because they can fill up rather quickly.

DIAGNOSIS: MISSING TEETH and EXISTING PROBLEMS

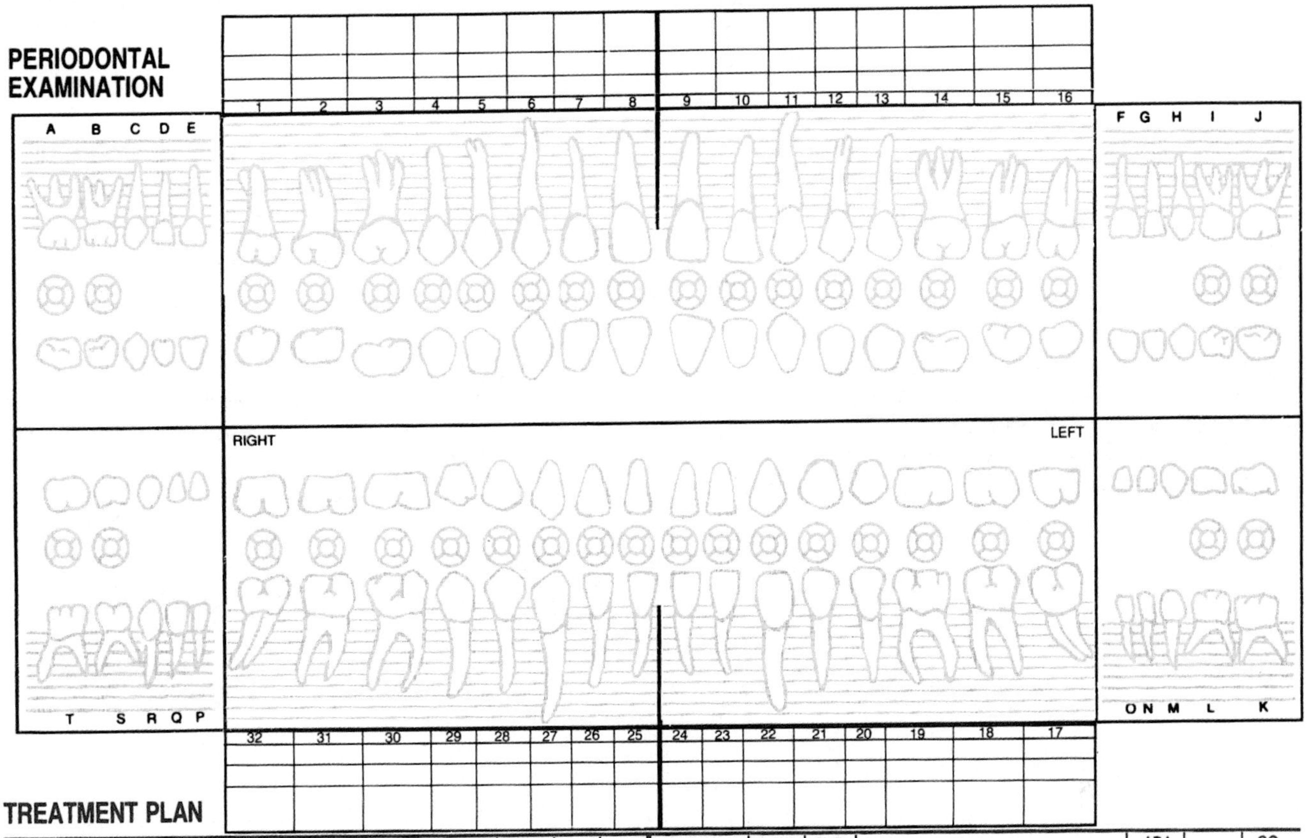

PERIODONTAL EXAMINATION

A B C D E

1 2 3 4 5 6 7 8 9 10 11 12 13 14 15 16

F G H I J

RIGHT

LEFT

T S R Q P

O N M L K

32 31 30 29 28 27 26 25 24 23 22 21 20 19 18 17

TREATMENT PLAN

DATE DIAGNOSED	TOOTH #	SUR-FACE	DESCRIPTION OF SERVICE	ADA CODE	FEE	CO-PAY	DATE DIAGNOSED	TOOTH #	SUR-FACE	DESCRIPTION OF SERVICE	ADA CODE	FEE	CO-PAY
			EXAMINATION										
			X-RAY: PANORAMIC: FMX: BWX:										
			DIAGNOSTIC MODELS										
			PROPHYLAXIS (CLEANING)										
			QUADRANTS SCALING & CURETTAGE										
			NITROUS-OXIDE GAS										

FIGURE 53.5

Clinical dental examination form.

Courtesy of Dr. Angela Osborn

| | Date: 08/21/2007 | **Angela Osborn** | | | | | Page: 01 |

Angela Osborn
9218 Kimmer Dr. Suite 106
Lone Tree, CO 80124
(303) 799-9993

All Treatment Plans for John J Doe
12121 S. Beautiful Smile St
Lone Tree, CO 80124
(303) 333-3333

Plan#	Code	Description	Tooth	Surface	Date Prop.	Date Comp.	Fee	PatAmt	InsEst
T1	D2950	Core Buildup, Including Any Pins	30		08/21/2007		298.00	149.00	149.00
T1	D2740	Crown-Porcelain/Ceramic Substrate	30		08/21/2007		1081.00	540.50	540.50
T1	D2950	Core Buildup, Including Any Pins	31		08/21/2007		298.00	149.00	149.00
T1	D2740	Crown-Porcelain/Ceramic Substrate	31		08/21/2007		1081.00	540.50	540.50
T1	D2393	Resin-based composite - three surfaces, posterior	2	MOL	08/21/2007		289.00	57.80	231.20
							3047.00	1436.80	1610.20

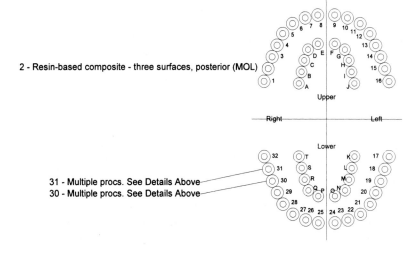

2 - Resin-based composite - three surfaces, posterior (MOL)

Upper

Right   Left

Lower

31 - Multiple procs. See Details Above
30 - Multiple procs. See Details Above

Primary Plan:

Stellar Marketing/Delta Dental Co	Maximum Benefits:	**1500.00**	Benefits YTD:	**0.00**
Subscriber: **John J Doe**	Deductible:	**50.00**	Current Plan:	**1610.20**
	Ded. Met?	**No**	Remaining:	**0.00**

I recognize this is an estimate only and is only valid for 3 months from date of proposal. The insurance coverage may vary from this estimated treatment calculation. I recognize that this is an estimate only and fully understand that I am ultimately responsible for payment in full for all treatment rendered.

Signature: _John Doe_   Date: _8-21 2007_

FIGURE 53.6
Treatment plan form.
Courtesy of Dr. Angela Osborn

The open-shelf lateral filing system is a tall series of shelves that have entry through a panel that slides down over the charts to keep them covered. These types of filing cabinets usually have four to five sections. All panels can be closed and locked for security purposes.

The vertical open-shelf system allows for expansion of the number of files and is more convenient to use than the other two types of cabinets. The files in a vertical open-shelf system are in full view and supports are placed within the cabinet to hold the files upright. The vertical open-shelf filing system is recommended for offices with plenty of storage space.

If space is limited and the practice is very large, then movable filing cabinets may be the ideal choice. They are a bit more expensive, but they are practical and simple to use. Movable filing cabinets are like the open-shelf lateral

ANGELA OSBORN DDS

9218 KIMMER DRIVE
SUITE 106
LONE TREE, CO 80124
PHONE 303.799.9993
FAX 303.799.9998

GENERAL CONSENT

Thank you for choosing our office for your dental care. We will work with you to help you achieve excellent oral health. While recognizing the benefits of a pleasing smile and teeth that function well, you should be aware that dental treatment, like treatment of any other part of the body, has some inherent risks. These are seldom great enough to offset the benefits of treatment, but should be considered when making treatment decisions.

Benefits of dental treatment can include: relief of pain, the ability to chew properly, and the confidence and social interaction that a pleasing smile can bring. Nonetheless, there are some common risks associated with virtually any dental procedure, including:

1. **Drug or chemical reaction.** Dental materials and medications may trigger allergic or sensitivity reactions.
2. **Long-term numbness (paresthesia).** Local anesthetic, or its administration, while almost always adequate to allow comfortable care, can result in transient or, in rare instances, permanent muscle numbness.
3. **Muscle or joint tenderness.** Holding one's mouth open can result in muscle or jaw joint tenderness, or in a predisposed patient, precipitate a TMJ disorder.
4. **Sensitivity in teeth or gums, infection, or bleeding.**
5. **Swallowing or inhaling small objects.**

While we follow procedural guidelines which most often lead to a clinical success, just like in any other pursuit in health care, not everything turns out the way it is planned. We will do our best to assure that it does. Please feel free to ask questions in regard to all dental procedures that are recommended to you.

I have read and understand the statement on this page:

John Doe   _8-21-07_
Patient's NAME please print   Date

John Doe   _8-21-07_
Patient's signature   Date

_____   _____
Parent's signature (if minor patient)   Date

FIGURE 53.7
Informed consent form.
Courtesy of Dr. Angela Osborn

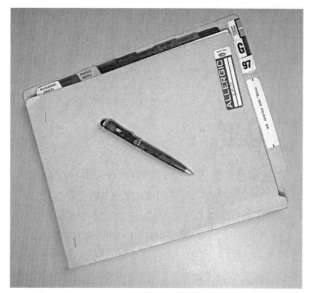

FIGURE 53.8
A color-coded record.

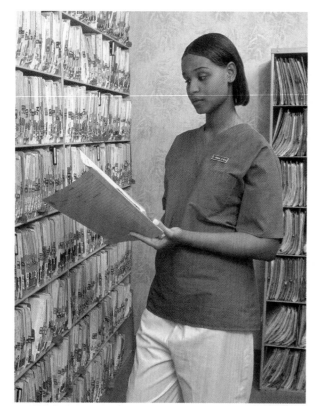

FIGURE 53.9
Vertical filing cabinets.

units except they are on rollers and can be moved by pushing them. Some of them are electronic and are moved by pushing a button.

Rules for Filing

Once the files are placed within the system, they are generally filed in an alphabetical format. Filing is the act of preserving and protecting the files and arranging them so that they can be retrieved quickly. Specific guidelines for filing include labeling folders clearly and correctly, maintaining enough space for additional papers in the file and for additional files to be placed on the shelves, and marking the shelves with the appropriate labels to identify the correct placement of the file.

Most offices use *out guides* when filing. These guides indicate where a file has been removed. The out guide is removed once the file is replaced. A form inside the out guide should include the date removed, to whom the file was released, and the purpose for the file's release.

The steps for filing include conditioning, releasing, indexing and coding, sorting, and finally storing and filing. Conditioning has four steps:

1. Remove all hardware including staples and paper clips from the folder.
2. Staple related papers together.
3. Items that are smaller than a page should be mounted on a standard sized piece of paper so that the file is neat and more manageable.
4. Mend any damaged records or pages by using reinforcements or transparent adhesive tape to press over ripped pages.

Releasing is the process of making a mark on the papers that are ready to be filed. The mark can be a stamp or the initials of the filing employee or dentist. For instance, after reading a lab or x-ray report, the dentist may initial or place a check mark on the document to indicate that it is ready to be filed. The mark is usually made on the upper left-hand corner of the document.

Indexing and coding of the files make up the next step. This step involves determining where the paper will be filed and indicating that decision on the paper. This indication can be a simple type of mark placed on the item to be filed.

The most critical step is sorting, which is to put the papers in the proper order for filing. It is recommended that large dental offices purchase a sorter from an office supply store to assist with the sorting function. A sorter is a flat piece of plastic that has progressively shorter pieces of plastic attached to the top. The separating pieces of plastic are marked with the letters of the alphabet so that the papers that go with the corresponding letters are sorted before actually going into the filing storage system.

The last filing step is to file and store the documents. Items should be placed one on top of the other face up in the chart and with the most recent document on top. It is also important for each document to be placed within the proper section of the file itself. Correspondence from other doctors, insurance companies, and patients is often kept in the last section of the file. X-ray reports and other lab reports usually have their own designated section within a chart.

Methods of Filing

Filing methods are categorized into three types: alphabetical, numeric, and subject. The alphabetical type is the most commonly used in the dental office. In very large practices or clinics, numeric systems are used, especially if Social Security numbers or computer-generated numbers are used to identify patients. Topical materials, business records, and correspondence are good reasons for using the subject method of filing.

Alphabetical Filing

Alphabetical filing is the oldest, most common system used to order information. Telephone books, dictionaries, and encyclopedias are good examples of alphabetical indexing. The rules for alphabetical filing are as follows:

- File by last name first, then first name, and then middle initial last. Begin by looking at two names that start with the same letter. Look at the second letter of the name and choose the closest letter to *A* to be the first file and the other to be second.

- Nothing comes before something. If the names are the same until the letters run out, the name with fewer letters comes before the one with more letters. For example, between *Adams* and *Adamson*, *Adams* is filed first alphabetically because all letters are the same until you have nothing to compare in the name *Adams* to the "o" in *Adamson*.

- Initials precede a name. For example, J. Smith comes before Jack Smith.

- Consider hyphenated names as one word.

- Disregard the apostrophe in alphabetizing. For example: Star's Cleaners still comes before Start Cleaning even though the apostrophe is in the same position as the "t."

- With names that are foreign or indistinguishable, file in the order in which it was written. For example, *Tu Lac Duc* is not a name where the first name is obvious so you would file it as it is written: T... U... .

- Consider the prefix of a name to be the first letter and think of the name as one word. For instance, *De Haviland* would be filed under the D's not the H's.

- Do not confuse *Mac* and *Mc*. File the names alphabetically as they appear without making an individual section just for them. (As always, however, check office policy because some offices file *Mc* and *Mac* separately.)

- Titles and terms of seniority should not be used for alphabetizing except as a last resort. For instance, if you have a file for Dr. Avery, but no first name, the file would be listed under "Avery, D."

- Titles without complete names are the first indexing unit. For instance, Dr. Avery without a first name listed will be filed as Avery, D.

- Disregard articles such as *A*, *An*, and *The* when filing.

    The alphabetical system has a few drawbacks. The correct spelling must be known for proper filing. As the number of files increases for a particular letter, more space is required to file that letter. So if a traditional filing cabinet is used, all of the drawers may have to be rearranged periodically to make the proper room. Locating the files can be a problem with the increased size of an alphabetical system. Use of color-coded labels can help minimize the problems with locating files.

Numeric Filing Systems

Numeric filing systems are recommended for extremely large practices with more than 5,000 charts. This type of system is an indirect filing system, unlike the alphabetical system, meaning that the numbers must be cross-referenced with a name. Many people object to this type of system because of the additional listing or the list of names that goes with the numbers, but it does have advantages. The files can be expanded by simply placing the new files at the back of the stack of files allowing for unlimited expansion. Confidentiality is more easily achieved in a numeric system because the name is not on the front of the chart. Color coding can be used in the numeric system as well because certain groupings of numbers can be given a corresponding color, which allows for a more easily visible group of files.

    The key for good filing practices, regardless of the filing method used, is for all members of the office staff to hold the placement of files and the rules of filing in high esteem. If even one member of the staff misfiles or is inconsistent about placing documents in the wrong sections of the chart, customer service and office efficiency can be drastically reduced.

Appointment Scheduling

Scheduling is a large part of any successful dental practice. Patients are brought in one at a time, and each patient has different needs and time requirements. Patients have their own agenda when it comes to scheduling, and certain procedures require more time than others. In some cases the doctor may perform the procedure required only in the morning hours and not in the afternoon or vice versa.

    Today most appointment scheduling in dental practices is done via computer, although some offices use dual systems in which appointments are recorded both electronically and manually. However, using dual systems increases the margin for error. The computer software systems used for appointment scheduling typically allow for pagination and columnation (Figure 53.10). The patient data are immediately accessed via the database, which supports the scheduling features of the software, and the insurance information is tied or toggled to the patient's appointment information.

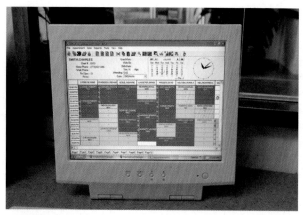

FIGURE 53.10
An example of a computerized scheduling format.

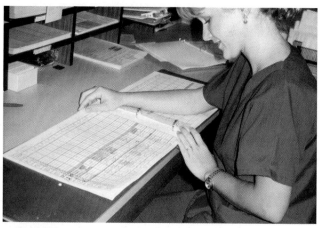

FIGURE 53.11
Using the appointment book.
Image courtesy Instructional Materials for the Dental Team, Lex., KY

Cultural Considerations

A recent practice that is becoming more common is that of Americans going to a foreign country for dental work. This is due primarily to the lower costs incurred with dental work done overseas. Patients should use caution when exchanging lesser fees for similar dental care in another country. Other countries' standards for cleanliness and aseptic techniques may vary. Americans take disinfection and sanitization for granted and expect the same care in another country. Because the standards may vary, a person could encounter unsafe conditions, which could ultimately be detrimental in their dental care and final results.

The Appointment Book

Recording appointments manually requires the use of an appointment book (Figure 53.11). Appointment books are available in all shapes and sizes. The layout of the book can range from one page per day to a week at a glance. Universal features of appointment books include columns for each dentist or for separate procedures and units or increments of time, usually in 10- or 15-minute intervals, referred to as units. Most appointment books are spiral bound or bound in a loose-leaf fashion and printed with common headings such as month, date, and day. Most of the holidays and religious observance days are printed directly on the page in advance and the sections for the weekend are usually smaller and off to the sides of the page.

Using the Appointment Book

If a manual appointment book is to be used, the book must first be prepared by marking off the times and days on which patient appointments will not be taken. Typically, this is done by the manager at the beginning of a new year before the appointment book becomes active.

The office manager goes through the appointment book and marks off any regular notations as well as any special events. Lunch hours, peculiar office closings, planned vacations, and meetings are some of the blocked off segments the manager addresses.

When using an appointment book, entries are typically recorded in pencil. This is done so that changes can be made easily in the event of cancellations or rescheduled appointments. Appointments to be booked require certain routine amounts of information. The patient's name, of course, is of the utmost priority. Sometimes the names of patients are similar and some are even pronounced exactly the same way. To minimize confusion, offices often cross-reference patient names by using the patient's Social Security number or date of birth. The home and business phone numbers are often recorded in the appointment slot in case the scheduler has a cancellation or if there is an office emergency that requires the dentist's attention. Some offices record a phone number in order to contact the patient as a reminder on the day before the appointment.

The treatment to be performed is recorded in the appointment book as well as the approximate length of the appointment. If the patient is a child, the age may be recorded in the appointment book. Sometimes special codes are used to describe certain statuses such as new patient or certain lab results and medications that may be prescribed in advance of the appointment.

Scheduling Systems

Efficient scheduling of appointments allows for the maximum number of patients to be seen in the least chaotic fashion. Most scheduling systems are designed around the needs of the patient, the preferences of the dentists, and the availability of facilities. Patient needs vary according to individual characteristics such as socioeconomic background, personal fears, or age. Distinguishing factors between patients often have to do with individual dental needs such as which procedure is being performed and how much of the dentist's time is required.

Some appointment scheduling systems are designed to address the dentist's personal preferences. These preferences include issues such as the dentist seeing certain types of patients in the morning versus the afternoon, the desire for a few minutes between patients for charting, and time at the end of the day for dictation. Some dentists like to spend more time with each individual patient, whereas other dentists prefer to have a steady stream of patients who are all seen very quickly.

Appointments are sometimes scheduled based on the availability of facilities or the operatory. For example, certain equipment stations are reserved for specific procedures such as cleanings and oral surgery.

Certain strategies are used to address these particular considerations: wave scheduling, modified wave scheduling, and double booking. All of the strategies deal with increments of time. The hours of the day are divided into specific units of time with the matrix preset to have lunch hours blocked out, breaks marked out, and a starting and ending point for when patients are to be seen. The length of the time blocks vary from office to office, but is usually 10 or 15 minutes.

One strategy that is recommended to help keep the office flowing smoothly is to leave two open appointment slots available on each day. This is known as a time buffer and can help in handling situations such as walk-in appointments, emergencies, and/or appointments that take longer than planned.

Wave scheduling is a scheduling system in which each appointment is allotted an average amount of time, and each patient is given the number of appointment slots that would be required to finish a necessary procedure based on average time required for that particular procedure. For example, a 15-minute slot would be assigned to a patient who needs a recheck (i.e., a brief follow-up visit due to previous treatment). Two 15-minute slots might be given to a new patient who needs x-rays and a cleaning. Sometimes the recheck takes more than a 15-minute time frame, but the 30-minute appointment might take only 20 minutes. In this way, the time averages out to fit the schedule evenly if not exactly.

Modified wave scheduling is based on the same time increments as wave scheduling, but the patients are set up with two or more appointments at once and then only one patient is scheduled for the next appointment slot, leaving the last slot open to allow for catching up in the schedule. Using the modified wave schedule, patients are typically scheduled to come in at the top of the hour and then none are scheduled for the last half hour. All patients are scheduled at the top of the hour, but the dental team has the entire hour to accomplish the patient care for all appointments scheduled in that hour. For example, a root canal, a cleaning, and a filling are scheduled at 10 a.m. and no other appointment is scheduled until 11 a.m. The preparation for each procedure is done right away and as the dentist gets to the next patient, the time taken for each of the procedures varies and allows for some flexibility in scheduling.

Another method of scheduling is **double booking**. In this method, two patients are scheduled at the same time. Double booking is typically not encouraged, but can work if each appointment is of a short duration. Sometimes two patients will have an appointment at the same time, but as long as they have different procedures, it is feasible to do.

One last scheduling strategy is called cluster scheduling. In cluster scheduling, patients are scheduled in groups according to the procedure required. For example, all root canals might be scheduled during the morning hours, and routine cleanings may be set aside for the afternoon hours. This strategy is used often in situations where equipment or space is scarce.

What additional scheduling strategies do you think might be effective for a dental office to consider?

Preventive Recall Programs

Dental offices rely heavily on having patients return for preventive care. The American Dental Association recommends that a person visit the dentist regularly to promote maximum oral care. Most insurance companies cover the costs of two cleanings or oral prophylaxis per year. Other reasons for recalling patients include denture checks, orthodontic progress checks, periodic evaluations, or endodontic treatments. With an effective recall program, the patient receives a notification to follow up with another appointment for service. The patient benefits by having better oral health, and the dental office benefits by having repeat customers.

The recall programs currently being used are much like appointment books. They were historically kept on paper, but are now most often kept using a computer

Life Span Considerations

People of all ages have a need for a dentist, even those who are edentulous (without teeth). Those who are without teeth are either the very young or the elderly population. The very young will not usually see a dentist until teeth start erupting. But the elderly population needs a different kind of attention—cleanings, extractions, and possibly dentures. Whatever services are required, elderly people generally like to have their appointments scheduled for early in the day. Be aware of your patients' needs and address their personal appointment preferences as needed.

software function. The computerized appointment calendar almost always contains several additional functions that may allow for mailing lists to be prepared and immediate access to insurance information and other patient data. It is much more effective to work with a computerized appointment schedule.

Dental office software is usually based on the old-fashioned method of using a tickler system. Tickler systems have been used for many years as a reminder system. Manual tickler systems consist of information being placed on index cards and then the cards are placed between dividers labeled by month. If a patient has an appointment in April and needs to return in six months, the scheduler makes a card to file in the September section so that the patient can be called or written to remind him to schedule an appointment for October. At the end of each month, the dental assistant pulls the cards and contacts those patients by either phone or mail.

Another common recall practice is to use the appointment book as a recall system. This system is known as the advanced appointment system and allows the office to keep track of future follow-up appointments. This system requires that the dental assistant look at future appointments to determine whom to contact for recall appointments.

Preventive recall programs are simpler to establish and easier to use if a dental practice is utilizing a computerized appointment book. Regardless of the type of recall program though, the theory is to keep the customer apprised of the appointments necessary to maintain proper oral hygiene (Figure 53.12).

Can you think of any other opportunities that would benefit from the use of a recall appointment system?

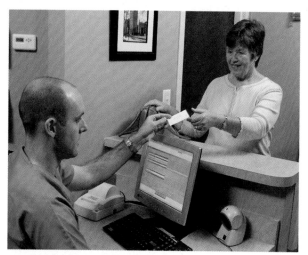

FIGURE 53.12
The patient is given an appointment card to remind her of the appointment made in advance.

Inventory Management

The term *inventory* suggests the creation of a complete list of all equipment and supplies that a dental practice has on hand. It is good practice for a business to take inventory of all of its equipment and supplies at least annually. It is a simplified process if a computerized system is in place, but even without electronic data processing, taking inventory is a good principle of business to practice.

Equipment

Equipment is divided into two categories: capital and expendable purchases. Capital purchases are normally those items that cost at least $500 and include things such as furniture, dental and surgical instruments, sterilizers, autoclaves, and radiological equipment. Some laboratory equipment, business machines, and major pieces of art are also considered capital expenses. Most of the items in this category have long lives and will not require immediate replacement. All items listed in an inventory should have the value of the item recorded.

Expendable items are less costly than capital items and include smaller instruments, syringes, and thermometers. All of these items should be listed in an inventory. The last thing that goes on the inventory is the usable supplies and medications on hand. An inventory of this nature would be instrumental when creating a new inventory for the following year. Comparison of the current inventory with the past one provides an invaluable tool for managing office supplies, preparing for tax purposes, and dealing with loss if a burglary or natural disaster occurs.

Supplies

Supplies are those items that are expendable and must be ordered and replaced fairly frequently. Several factors must be taken into account when determining which inventory supply system is to be used for tracking and reordering supplies to fill the dental practice's needs. Some items have a sensitive **shelf life**, which is the amount of time a product can be stored before the product is no longer usable.

Item, unit, and bulk prices must also be taken into account when ordering supplies. Some items are better purchased as a single item, but other items warrant a better deal if bought as a unit or in bulk. The best deals are usually obtained through bulk purchasing. For example, consider the purchase of dental floss. The item price would be the cost of one spool. The unit price would be the cost if the dental floss were packaged together as a unit, say, 12 spools to a package. The bulk price would be the cost if several 12-count packages were purchased. A price break is also sometimes offered for items that are purchased frequently.

Lead time should be a consideration when ordering supplies because this is the interval of time between when the order is placed and when it is received. The rate of use should be considered when determining the type of inventory system to put in place. Another consideration is the **reorder point,** the point that determines when a supply will be reordered based on lead time and the supply's rate of use.

Inventory Systems

Several inventory systems are available but they all have the same goals: to keep track of the supplies and to make sure they are available when needed. It is usually the duty of a designated employee to make sure inventory is managed. As stated previously, computer systems are invaluable, but there are other things that can assist as well. The tag system uses a reorder tag that is placed somewhere within the stock of that item. Once the tag appears, it is a sign that the item needs to be replenished. Information can be listed on the tag to facilitate reordering, such as line and item numbers and place of purchase. A sample inventory order form is shown in Figure 53.13.

Sometimes dental supply companies offer the service of placing the tags among the supplies. This action improves customer service and helps ensure that the products will be purchased again from that supply company. A more sophisticated system that is beginning to be used more frequently is a bar code system. The dental assistant can scan the bar codes on the product and transmit the data to the dental supplier. The supplier can then keep track of the inventory and provide more product when necessary. This system is the most efficient for the dental assistant.

When an order has been received, the packing slip must be evaluated to ensure that all items have been received and that they are as ordered. The packing slip indicates everything that is in the package. Sometimes items may have been back ordered and the packing slip will indicate this. The packing slip does not usually include information regarding the price or billing information. Damages to any of the products should be noted upon opening the packages. Those items should be returned for replacement or reimbursement. If an item is to be returned for any reason, a **credit slip** can be used. A credit slip alerts the dental office that it will not be billed for the returned items.

If an item was not included in a package, it may have been unavailable or placed on back order. Sometimes the item must be purchased from another warehouse. A back order slip or the packing slip will indicate when an item was not shipped.

Once the shipment has been unloaded and the contents checked, the dental assistant must put the items away in the proper storage area. Most stock should be rotated so that the older items are used before the newer items. Some of the supplies require special storage considerations such as refrigeration or away from light. The dental assistant should read the manufacturer's guidelines for proper storage recommendations and expiration dates.

Equipment Repairs

Most equipment comes with recommendations for maintenance and upkeep. Certain machines require **calibration,** which involves setting a machine to provide accurate measurements. Maintenance of equipment is

ORDER ITEM NAME: **ON ORDER**

ORDER QUANTITY: ____________ REORDER POINT: ____________

ORDER	QTY	REC'D	COST	PREPAID	ON ACCT	ORDER	QTY	REC'D	COST	PREPAID	ON ACCT

INVENTORY COUNT:

	JAN	FEB	MAR	APR	MAY	JUN	JUL	AUG	SEP	OCT	NOV	DEC
20 ___												
20 ___												

ORDER SOURCE: UNIT PRICE:

The King Company

222 East Maple Avenue

Anytown, IL 60000

FIGURE 53.13
A sample inventory order form.

performed routinely, either daily or periodically. Daily maintenance can range from simply wiping down the surfaces of the equipment to having to calibrate equipment each day.

Dental chairs should be disinfected after each patient, unless barriers have been used, and any dirt buildup in the seams of the chairs should be taken care of as soon as it is seen. Attention should be paid to always use the correct cleaning product for each type of equipment and to ensure that the cleaning is done according to the manufacturer's specifications. The chair base should be evaluated for cleanliness or any buildup of oil and debris. The sinks also require careful attention and cleaning. The sinks must be free of blood, plaster, amalgam, and other debris. The towel and soap dispensers should be wiped daily and filled as needed.

Other routine maintenance is performed at either weekly or monthly intervals. These tasks include cleaning the autoclave, changing solutions in the x-ray processing machine, changing light bulbs in the overhead lamps, and changing certain parts on the handpieces. It is good practice to include replacement parts in the office inventory and have the numbers of those parts available for use as needed, based on utilization patterns. Sometimes periodic care requires calling in an expert for the machinery or for the parts in question. For example, electrical wiring or hoses that run to the sink and the evacuator may need periodic attention from an expert.

Whenever a machine or piece of equipment fails, it is smart to do a quick assessment and look for the obvious problems. Sometimes the machine merely needs to be

Professionalism

When supplies that have been ordered arrive at the office, the most professional way to handle them is to do an immediate inventory of all items in the package. Each group of items should be counted and checked against the packing slip. If there is a shortage or any other kind of problem, the supply company should be contacted and notified of the discrepancy.

plugged into an electrical outlet. Always be on the lookout for frayed cords. If you find a frayed cord, do not use the appliance or device and do not wrap the cord with electrical tape. Rather, report the problem to the office manager who should disable and discard the item. Many of today's electrical appliances are computer operated and can be restored by rebooting the device.

Do not be afraid to call in the proper resources, such as the individuals who pick up biohazardous waste or the professionals who replace radiological chemicals, for some maintenance needs. In such situations, the dental assistant should call in professionals rather than try to perform the task him- or herself. On occasion, the item that is in need of repair may actually be in need of replacement. Those decisions are usually up to the dentist and/or office manager. A dental assistant may be asked to research the necessary item and report the best option for obtaining replacement equipment.

SUMMARY

The office management techniques used in a dental practice (other than the financial accounting systems) are critical for providing effective dental services to patients. The operating procedure manual is key to synchronizing the performance of each member of the dental team. The operating manual can be a living document, especially if it is consistently incorporated into the daily activities of the dental office.

Different types of software are available to the dental office for creating and updating the operating procedure manual and for other office needs such as records management, appointment scheduling, and patient care. Record keeping includes taking care of the reports and other paperwork within an individual patient file. Each file is stored in a filing system that is as large as necessary to accommodate the number of files that are being stored. Appointment scheduling can be performed according to the preferences of the dentist, the limitations of the equipment and office space, or patient need. HIPAA regulations are to be observed in every aspect of office management because it is

important to protect the privacy of patients and portability of their records.

Inventory management, including the upkeep of equipment, is usually organized according to a computerized system for tracking equipment and supplies used and how quickly they should be replaced. Supplies are different than capital expenses, which are usually large or expensive items such as real estate, x-ray or other heavy equipment, or furniture.

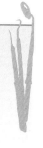

Preparing for Externship

During an externship, it is important for the dental assistant to ask questions and ensure good supervision of his or her actions is provided. Entering accurate information in a patient's chart is a must. If there is any doubt as to what should be entered the extern should ask for assistance.

KEY TERMS

- **Calibration:** The process of setting a machine to provide accurate measurements.   p. 859
- **Credit slip:** Slip of paper that alerts a dental office that it will not be billed for returned items.   p. 859
- **Double booking:** The scheduling of two patients for appointments at the same time.   p. 857
- **Ergonomics:** The body mechanics that are considered when a human uses equipment and tools.   p. 848
- **Lead time:** The interval of time between when an order is placed and when it is received.   p. 859
- **Modified wave scheduling:** A schedule based on the same appointment time increments as a wave schedule, but the patients are set up with two or more appointments at once and then only one patient is scheduled for the next appointment slot.   p. 857

- **Operating procedure manual:** Office manual that contains written directions for completing particular functions or tasks.   p. 846
- **Reorder point:** The point that determines when a supply will be reordered based on lead time and the supply's rate of use.   p. 859
- **Shelf life:** The time a product can be stored before it is no longer usable.   p. 858
- **Wave scheduling:** A scheduling system in which each appointment is allotted an average amount of time, and each patient is given the number of appointment slots that would be required to finish a necessary procedure based on average time required for that particular procedure.   p. 857

CHECK YOUR UNDERSTANDING

1. Two patients scheduled for 15-minute increments at the beginning of the hour is an example of which type of appointment scheduling?
   a. double booking
   b. wave scheduling
   c. modified wave scheduling
   d. none of the above

2. Which of the following are guides for actions to be taken?
   a. software
   b. certificate of deposit
   c. procedures
   d. policies

3. The mouse, wires, and central processing unit on a computer are considered to be what?
   a. hardware
   b. software
   c. spyware
   d. firewall

4. Which of the following is the term for a software program that is like a worksheet with a calculator built in?
   a. database
   b. word processing
   c. spreadsheet
   d. PowerPoint

5. What is the proper ergonomic angle of the arms at rest without using the armrest of a chair?
   a. 15 degrees
   b. 30 degrees
   c. 45 degrees
   d. 90 degrees

6. Which of the following information is not required for setting an appointment?
   a. patient's name
   b. patient's children's names
   c. patient's phone number
   d. patient's complaint

7. Which of the following is the name for a scheduling type that groups appointments according to procedure?
   a. wave scheduling
   b. modified wave scheduling
   c. cluster scheduling
   d. none of the above

8. Which of the following is true?
   a. Never alter a patient's record.
   b. Correction fluid may be used to correct mistakes in a chart.
   c. Appointment cancellations do not need to be tracked.
   d. None of the above.

9. Which is a type of filing cabinets?
   a. traditional vertical
   b. vertical open-shelf
   c. moving
   d. all of the above

10. Conditioning is a part of which process?
    a. ordering supplies
    b. filing
    c. reconciling the bank statement
    d. preparing the patient

INTERNET ACTIVITIES

- Go to www.sac.edu/students/support_services/ samanual/sarsrcs/sarmrk.html. Read about the responsibilities and qualities of an individual in charge of records.
- Go to www.watsonent.com/dent.htm and thoroughly read through the website. Once you feel you have gathered basic knowledge about the information provided there, pick five pieces of equipment and answer the following questions in complete sentences:

a. What is the piece of equipment called?
b. What is it used for?
c. Why is it important?
d. What would typically break or malfunction on the piece of equipment?
e. How and/or where can these tools be repaired?

WEB REFERENCES

- Ace Dental www.ace-dental.com/
- Burkhart www.burkhartdental.com/index
- Buy on Line Now www.buyonlinenow.com/hon-shelf-files.asp?source=aw
- Dental Assisting National Board www.danb.org/PDFs/Phase4.pdf
- Dental Resources www.dental-resources.com
- Dentimax www.dentimax.com/documentation/activitiesmenu.htm
- Investopedia www.investopedia.com/terms/i/inventory.asp
- Medical and Dental Standard Operating Procedures Library www.physicianswebsites.com/standard-procedures.htm
- Michigan Tech www.admin.mtu.edu/admin/procman/ch10/ch10p1.htm
- Nature.com www.nature.com/bdj/journal/v197/n11/full/4811866a.html

54

Financial Management

Learning Objectives

After reading this chapter, the student should be able to:

- Describe methods of patient payment for treatment.
- Explain the procedure and rationale for conducting a credit check.
- Explain the difference between manual and computerized accounting systems.
- Describe the purpose of a walk-out statement.
- Describe procedures for collection of past due accounts.
- Differentiate between fixed and variable overhead expenses.
- Describe standard taxes withheld from employee paychecks.

Preparing for Certification Exams

- Explain fees charged to a patient and financial arrangements.
- Collect fees and issue receipts or walk-out statements.
- Make and maintain financial arrangements with patients.
- Maintain patient account records.
- Follow up on delinquent accounts.
- Prepare checks for signature and maintain cash disbursement records.
- Balance the checkbook and reconcile bank statements.
- Maintain summaries of income and expenses.

Chapter Outline

- Accounting
  - Percentages
  - Decimals
- Preventive Account Management
  - Collecting Financial Data and Information
  - Fees and Financial Arrangements
- Accounts Receivable
  - Types of Accounts Receivable
  - Managing Accounts Receivable
- Collections
  - Collection Letters
  - Collection Calls
- Accounts Payable Management
  - Types of Expenses
  - Budgeting
- Writing Checks
  - Reconciling Bank Statements
- Payroll
  - Employee Information
  - Calculating Payroll
  - Form W-2: Wage and Tax Statement

Key Terms

Accounts payable

Accounts receivable

Aging account

Bonding insurance

Deposit slip

Expenditures

Fixed expenses

Gross salary

Net salary

Overhead

Pegboard system

Variable expenses

Walk-out statement

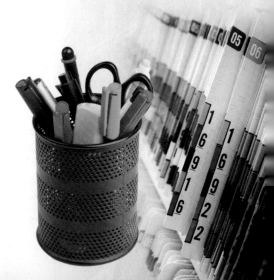

Dentistry is not only a health profession but also a business.

Maintaining a financial system for the dental practice to ensure sound business practices is the responsibility of the entire dental team. Responsible maintenance requires the ability to use basic accounting procedures and understand the dental practice's policies on fees and payments. Accounts receivable is the calculation of all money owed to the practice. Accounts payable is all money owed by the dental practice. The responsibilities of the dental assistant may entail collection procedures and payroll duties. Learning these skills makes the dental assistant a valuable and crucial asset to the organization and success of the dental office.

Accounting

Accounting involves the verifying and classifying of all transactions of accounts receivable and accounts payable. Usually a calculator or computer is used to add and subtract business computations. However, relying only on those devices without having a basic understanding of math computations can result in loss of cash flow due to mathematical errors. The following sections describe basic math procedures used for routine bookkeeping.

Percentages

When working with accounts receivable, percentages are often used. For instance, when working with insurance, percentages of deductibles must be determined. A computerized system will automatically calculate percentages, but if the office is using a manual system, then the dental assistant must fully understand the process of percentages in order to calculate the amounts correctly.

When changing a percent to a fraction, drop the percent sign, place the number over 100, and reduce the fraction:

$$5\% = 5/100 = 1/20$$

The fraction 5/100 was reduced to 1/20 by finding the lowest common denominator. For example: 5/100 divided by 5/5 equals 1/20.

If the numerator or top number is a decimal, multiply both top and bottom number (numerator and denominator, respectively) by the power of 10 to get rid of the decimal, as shown in the following example:

$$7.5\% = 7.5/100 = 75/1000 = 3/40$$

The top and bottom number were multiplied by 10 to get rid of the decimal. The answer is 75/1000. This number must be reduced so it was divided by 25, which is the lowest common denominator.

To change a percent into a decimal, move the decimal point two places to the left and remove the percent sign:

$$20\% = 0.20$$

$$3\% = 0.03$$

To find the percent of a number, convert the percentage to a decimal using the preceding example and multiply the specified number by the decimal. For example, to calculate 70% of $550:

$$
\begin{array}{r}
\$550 \\
\times .70 \\
\hline
\$385
\end{array}
$$

Decimals

When adding decimals, align all of the decimal points prior to doing the addition and subtraction. Add each column, beginning on the right and moving toward the left. For example:

$$
\begin{array}{r}
0.2 \\
48.25 \\
51.243 \\
+934.001 \\
\hline
1033.694
\end{array}
$$

When subtracting decimals, use the same procedure as above, however add zeros to have the same amount of numbers and aligned decimals. For example:

Instead of: 4.259   use: 4.259

              −2.14   −2.140

              Answer: 2.119

When multiplying decimals, multiply the equation as a normal multiplication problem. Count the number of digits to the right of the decimal point, then place the decimal point in the answer with the correct number of digits to the right of the decimal. For example:

$$\begin{array}{r} 500.25 \\ \times .30 \\ \hline 150.075 \end{array}$$

Although the dental assistant's traditional role is to assist the dentist during patient care, the dental assistant may be given the responsibility of managing the finances of the dental practice in the role of business assistant. Individuals assigned to managing accounts for the dental practice must keep all of their skills, including math, sharp and up to date.

Preventive Account Management

Several techniques are used to manage and control the money owed to the dental practice and money paid out by the dental practice. A sound financial policy is needed to manage accounts within any business. Today's dental practices face many financial challenges including providing improved quality care at reasonable costs to patients and addressing the financial needs of employees.

Many patients choose a dentist based on the financial payment plans offered by the practice. This challenges the dental practice to be flexible in addressing patient financial needs and may mean that customized payment plans will need to be established for individual patients. Preventive account management consists of collecting financial data and information, making financial arrangements with patients, and collecting on patient accounts.

Collecting Financial Data and Information

A patient's financial information is obtained when the patient completes the patient registration form prior to his appointment (Figure 54.1). This document lists who

PATIENT REGISTRATION FORM
(Please Print)

Date: ______________

Patient's Name: ______________________________ DOB: ____/____/____
First Middle Last — Month Day Year

Address: ______________________________ Phone: ____/____-______
Street City State Zip — (Area code)

Patient's SS#: ____-____-____ Driver's License #: __________ Occupation: __________

Method of payment (circle): cash check credit card insurance co-payment

Primary Insurance Co.: ______________ Policy/Group #: ______________

Medicare #: ______________ Medicaid #: ______________

Person Responsible For Payment: ______________________________ ______________
First Middle Last — Relationship

Address: ______________________________ Phone: ____/____-______
Street City State Zip — (Area code)

Employer Name: ______________________________ Dept: __________
First Middle Last

Address: ______________________________ Phone: ____/____-______
Street City State Zip — (Area code)

Spouse or Nearest Relative: ______________________________ ______________
First Middle Last — Relationship

Address: ______________________________ Phone: ____/____-______
Street City State Zip — (Area code)

How were you referred to this office? ______________________________

____

Statement of Financial Responsibility: I, ______________________________
do hereby agree to pay all medical charges incurred by the above listed patient. I further understand that these charges are my responsibility, regardless of insurance coverage.

Responsible Person's Signature: ______________________________

FIGURE 54.1
Patient registration form used to obtain financial information.

is responsible for the account financially, any insurance information, and employment information of the responsible party.

Credit reports also provide a way to gather information. The report lists creditors, amounts owed, and payment history. The dental practice can obtain these reports through a credit reporting agency. These reports can be used to determine a patient's typical payment patterns. If poor payment patterns exist, then the dental practice can refuse to make certain financial arrangements and require payment in full from the patient at time of service. Patient permission is required before reports are requested from credit reporting agencies.

Fees and Financial Arrangements

Once the dentist completes the patient examination or consultation, the treatment plan is developed. The dentist or the business assistant then determines an estimated fee for the future treatment. A fee schedule is used to define the charges for each service rendered. Fees are generally referred to as usual, reasonable, or customary. The term *usual fee* refers to the typical charge for a specific treatment. The term *reasonable fee* refers to a range of costs depending on the difficulty of the case. The *customary fee* is the average fee that dentists in the geographic area charge. Fees cannot be altered based on whether or not the patient has insurance, although cash discounts are frequently utilized.

The treatment plan and fee are documented and a copy given to the patient. The other copy is filed in the office records. The business assistant may be responsible for discussing the fees and financial arrangements with the patient. When discussing payment arrangements and fees, the conversation should be confidential and handled in a quiet, private place away from distractions and other patients. Payment or financial arrangements should be made prior to treatment, except in emergencies.

Consideration should be given to the dentist's stated fees, but also to the patient's ability to pay.

Once a payment plan that is equitable to the dental practice and the patient has been established, a contract and a budget plan are prepared. A billing statement is usually sent to the patient on a monthly basis. A billing statement is a monthly account of business transactions. It contains the following information:

- Date of the transactions
- Name of patient
- List of fees for each transaction
- Current account balances

The statement should include a return envelope in which the patient can mail his payment.

Accounts Receivable

Accounts receivable is the amount of money that is owed to the dental practice from patients for services rendered. Managing accounts receivable is referred to as bookkeeping and involves all transactions related to fee collection. The business assistant is responsible for handling other people's money. The business assistant is also responsible for securing the money, recording transactions properly, and keeping financial information confidential. Because of this high level of responsibility, this staff member may be bonded. This requires the dental practice to buy **bonding insurance**, which protects any monetary losses due to employee theft. Employees can be prosecuted for any type of theft.

Professionalism

Scenario: A patient displays her outrage in the reception area when the dental assistant presents the fee for a future dental extraction. She rants, raves, and starts to yell and curse, which gets the attention of the patients in the reception area and the treatment areas. The business assistant is clearly upset, but knows she must maintain her professionalism and somehow calm the patient. How should the assistant go about this? What could have been done to prevent the patient's public outburst?

Answer: The business assistant can help keep the patient and herself calm by not arguing or yelling back to the patient and asking the patient to discuss it in a more private setting.

The business assistant should have taken the patient to a private room and discussed the fee away from other patients.

Legal and Ethical Issue

Scenario: A patient's account of $300 is 60 days past due. The business assistant has sent out two billing statements, but no payment has been received. The dentist wants you to place a phone call to the patient reminding her about the overdue fee. You get busy during the day and forget to call the patient, so you call her at 6:30 A.M. the next morning. The patient is not very happy to receive a phone call that early in the morning and hangs up. You immediately call back and threaten a lawsuit if the payment is not made. Was the collections call handled properly? Why or why not?

Answer: The collection procedure was not handled properly because first the phone call was made too early in the morning. Second, dental team members are not to threaten patients/customers. They are simply to turn the case over to a collection agency.

Types of Accounts Receivable

The most common systems of bookkeeping used in dental practices are the pegboard system and a computerized bookkeeping system. Many dental practices use a computerized system instead of the manual pegboard system because a computerized system can perform more tasks such as charting and insurance coding. Computerized bookkeeping is also very useful for collection and correlations of statistical data related to treatments, efficiency, and cost breakdowns.

Pegboard System

The **pegboard system** is a manual handwritten system that consists of day sheets, charge slips, ledger cards, and receipt forms. This system of accounting is a "write it once" system, meaning that through the use of carbonized forms, information is recorded once, but used for multiple purposes. A pegboard is used to align all of the forms so that information entered is recorded simultaneously on various forms. Day sheets are used to record daily transactions for every patient. A new day sheet is used for each day of business. The day sheet typically consists of five sections, as indicated in Figure 54.2:

- **Section 1**—Patient transactions such as charges, credits, and current account balances are annotated.
- **Section 2**—Deposits for the day are annotated and transferred from Section 1. This includes cash and check payments.
- **Section 3**—A business analysis summary for each patient transaction is annotated.
- **Section 4**—All daily transactions are totaled and balanced in this section.
- **Section 5**—This section shows the total cumulative accounts receivable balance. This is the amount that is owed to the practice from all patients.

When the last day sheet of the month is completed, the accounts are totaled. Then patient ledger cards are totaled and compared to the accounts receivable day sheets. The totals should be exact. If there is a mistake, it must be found. The information on the patient ledger card is used to bill each patient.

Computerized System

A computerized bookkeeping system can be used for total patient management. In fact most offices use a

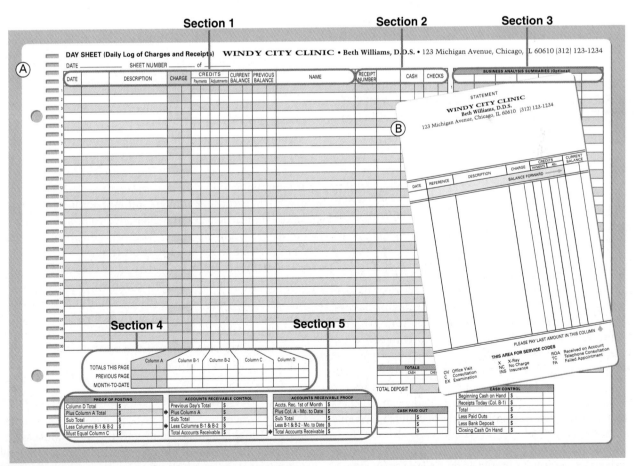

FIGURE 54.2
Sample pegboard day sheet with sections indicated. B is an illustration of a blank patient ledger card that would be used when completing the day sheet.

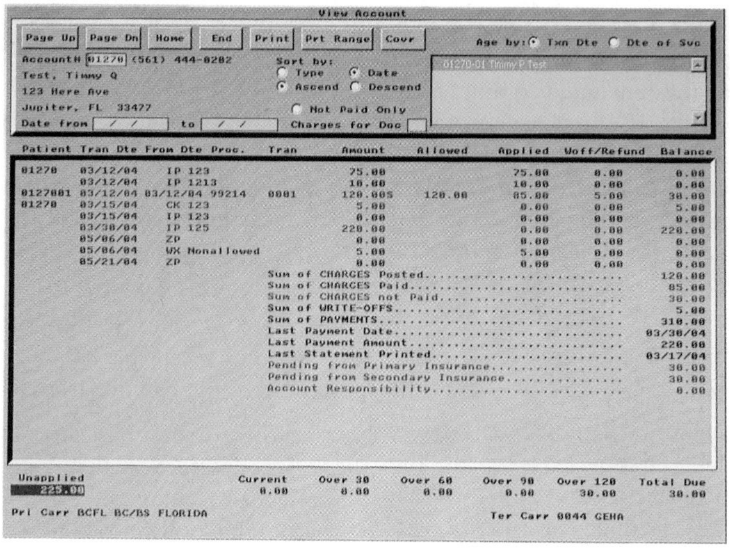

FIGURE 54.3
Computerized accounts receivable.

computerized patient management system. Systems such as Dentrix and EagleSoft provide dental offices with features for digital imaging; charting; taking notes, a health history, personal information; recording accounting and supply information; and of course payment and fee features. For example, when new patient data is entered into the system, numerous forms can be created such as a patient statement of fees and insurance claim forms. Through the use of computerized bookkeeping systems, accounts can automatically be calculated and financial reports easily created (Figure 54.3). Patient billing statements are generated monthly from the computer database. The statements inform patients of their financial status with the dental office.

The data is stored on a computer hard drive and backed up daily. The backup disks are stored in a safe place outside of the office in the event of fire or theft. Other advantages of a computerized bookkeeping system include its efficiency in patient billing and ease with which mistakes can be fixed.

Managing Accounts Receivable

Regardless of the system the office uses, the dental assistant will need to understand basic accounting principles. The bookkeeping process begins when the patient's appointment has ended. The charge slip is filled out by the dentist prior to the patient leaving the treatment room. The charge slip is handed to the business assistant at the front desk. The charge slip indicates the patient's current balance and treatment provided. The business assistant posts the information to the accounts receivable system for the patient.

Some offices have computers in each treatment room and the information is entered at the time of treatment. A daily journal or day sheet is used to document every patient appointment and every transaction. This is accom-

plished using the pegboard system or the computerized database system just discussed. The charge slip may be printed in duplicate to be used for accounts receivable, financial records, and as a receipt or walk-out statement for the patient. A **walk-out statement** shows the amount the patient paid, similar to a receipt, but also shows the patient's current balance if any is owed. The walk-out statement includes the patient's name, the date, and the type of service provided (Figure 54.4). Some offices give patients a postage paid envelope to encourage patients to mail payments as soon as possible.

Monthly Statements

A monthly statement is a request for payment from a patient. It is usually mailed to the patient with the account balance listed. The statement requests the amount be paid in full or, if previous arrangements were made, then the installment amount indicated must be paid. Finance charges may be added to accounts that are not paid within 30 days. The decision to add finance charges is made by the dental practice.

Statements are usually mailed at the same time each month. If the patient load is large, then the statements are mailed at different times of the month. For example, patients with last names beginning with A through M could be mailed statements during the first part of the month, and the remainder of the patients would then be billed at the middle of the month.

Receiving and Recording Payments

Every payment received must be entered immediately into the bookkeeping system and the daily journal. If a check is received, it should be endorsed with a restrictive endorsement to prevent anyone other than the dental practice from cashing it. Some dental practices provide the option for patients to pay with cash, check, or credit

STATEMENT OF ACCOUNT

Angela Osborn
9218 Kimmer Dr. Suite 106
Lone Tree, CO 80124
(303) 799-9993

Page:	1
Date:	08/21/2007
Acct. Nbr:	

Amount Due: **0.00**
Make Remittance Payable to:
Angela Osborn
Amount Enclosed: _____

John Doe
12121 S. Beautiful Smile St.
Lone Tree, CO 80124

Credit Card Number: _____
3 or 4 Digit Security Code: _____
Expiration Date: ____/____/_____

Signature: _____

Date	Name	Code	Description	Charges	Payments	Est. Ins. Portion	Est. Patient Portion
08/21/07	John J		Previous Balance				
08/21/07	John J	D2950	Core Buildup, Including Any Pins(Tooth # 30)	298.00			298.00
08/21/07	John J	D2740	Crown-Porcelain/Ceramic Substrate(Tooth # 30)	1,081.00			1,081.00
08/21/07	John J	D2950	Core Buildup, Including Any Pins(Tooth # 31)	298.00			298.00
08/21/07	John J	D2740	Crown-Porcelain/Ceramic Substrate(Tooth # 31)	1,081.00			1,081.00
08/21/07	John J	00001	Check		-2,758.00		

Account Aging	Current	Over 30	Over 60	Over 90	Total Balance		
	0.00	0.00	0.00	0.00	0.00		

Previous Balance	0.00
Current Payments	-2,758.00
Current Charges	2,758.00
New Balance	0.00

Angela Osborn * 9218 Kimmer Dr. Suite 106 * Lone Tree, CO 80124 * (303) 799-9993

FIGURE 54.4
Computerized walk-out statement.
Courtesy of Dr. Angela Osborn

card. Not many patients pay for dental treatment with cash; however, for the few that do, it is crucial to have change on hand. Some dental practices offer a discount for cash payments because patients who pay with cash save the practice time and money related to the costs of billing insurance companies or using credit. A computer-generated or handwritten receipt is given to the patient at the time of payment.

Checks are a means of ordering the bank to pay cash from the bank customer's account. The types of checks the business assistant may receive are certified checks, personal checks, money orders, and traveler's checks. A certified check is a guarantee that funds are available to cover the amount of the check. A personal check comes from an individual's account. When a personal check is written, there is no guarantee that funds are available. For this reason some offices will not take personal checks. A money order is used by people who usually do not maintain personal checking accounts. It is purchased for an exact amount and shows the name of the purchaser and who is to receive the money. Traveler's checks are designed for use by people who are away from home; however, a dental office may receive them. Traveler's checks are purchased through a bank and come in different denominations such as $10, $20, $50, and $100. When traveler's checks are purchased, they are signed by the purchaser. When used as payment, they are countersigned in the presence of the person who accepts payment.

If a dental practice accepts credit cards, a sign is typically posted at the front desk indicating which types of credit cards are accepted. When a practice accepts credit cards, the practice pays a fee for processing the cards, but that may be offset by the one big advantage of credit cards, which is that the payment is guaranteed.

Daily Posting of Payments

At the end of each day, the business assistant compares the day sheet or daily journal to the appointment book to ensure that each patient's information has been entered. Using the pegboard system or the computerized system, the assistant totals all figures. The total receipts should match the amount in the "cash" drawer. These two totals must balance. If the balances do not match, the error must be found.

Some hints to finding errors include re-adding columns and checking to see if the amounts may have been placed in the wrong columns. Corrections are made by drawing a line through the incorrect information, making a new entry, and initialing that change just like in a chart. Correction tape or fluid should never be used to cover an error.

Bank Deposits

The money received by a dental practice should be deposited on a daily basis into the practice's checking account. A **deposit slip** is an itemized copy of the money taken to the bank to be credited to the dental practice account (Figure 54.5). When a computerized system is

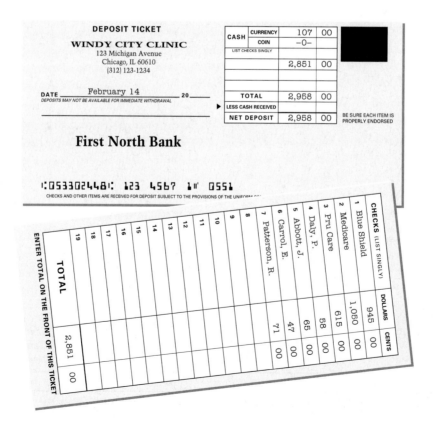

FIGURE 54.5
Deposit slip.

used, the computer generates a bank deposit slip from the funds entered into the accounts receivable program.

The deposit slip is printed with the practice name, address, and account number. The assistant ensures that the information is legible. All cash is listed together under the "Currency" row and checks are listed separately. The deposit slip is completed or printed in duplicate, and the copy is maintained in the dental practice records. Once the deposit is made, the amount should be entered into the check register of the dental practice.

Financial Reports

When managing finances for the dental practice, the business assistant must generate financial reports for the dentist and accountants to review any profits or losses and to ensure that there are no errors with regard to the financial health of the practice.

Audit reports track the daily transactions and verify that all transactions were posted correctly. This report is twofold: it identifies errors for correction and protects the employer from embezzlement. Embezzlement is the practice of stealing from an employer. The audit must be accomplished daily. The following steps outline how to complete the audit report:

1. Account for all charge slips.
2. Add the total charges. The charges should match the production total on the day sheet.
3. Match deposit slips and direct deposits with the amount of money collected.
4. Identify the types of payments (mail, insurance, credit card, check, cash).
5. Attach the day sheet, routing slips, daily schedule, and a copy of a deposit slip.

Financial reports determine the finances of the dental practice. A profit and loss statement is used to show if the dental practice is making or losing money. This information is used to report income and payroll taxes.

Accounts receivable reports categorize the amount owed to the dental practice from patients and insurance companies (Figure 54.6). The accounts receivable report is used when the administrative assistant must begin the collection process. See Procedure 54-1 for the steps in managing basic financial transactions.

What is the importance of the daily posting of payments?

ACCOUNTS RECEIVABLE BY RESPONSIBLE PARTY

Responsible Party		Current	30 Days	60 Days	90 Days	Contract	Total A/R	- Est. Ins.	= Due Now
8	Abbott, Joanna	$840.42	$0.00	$0.00	$0.00	$251.96	$1,092.38	$350.00	$742.38
3446	Abbott, Chris	$1,972.52	$0.00	$0.00	$0.00	$0.00	$1,972.52	$585.70	$1,386.82
3431	Abbott, Jeff	$2,169.13	$0.00	$0.00	$29.00	$0.00	$2,198.13	$844.00	$1,354.13
3434	Abernathy, Bill	$198.00	$0.00	$0.00	$19.12	$0.00	$217.12	$0.00	$217.12
3021	Abrams, Jill	$0.00	$0.00	$0.00	$85.00	$0.00	$85.00	$0.00	$85.00
3675	Adams, Joe	$0.00	$0.00	$0.00	$109.50	$0.00	$109.50	$0.00	$109.50
9	Adams, Kevin	$0.00	$0.00	$0.00	$53.60	$0.00	$53.60	$0.00	$53.60
2889	Ahuja, Andrew	$0.00	$0.00	$0.00	$68.60	$0.00	$68.60	$0.00	$68.60
1453	Albin, Matt	$0.00	$0.00	$0.00	$443.00	$0.00	$443.00	$0.00	$443.00
1120	Alexander, Sarah	$0.00	$0.00	$0.00	$80.00	$0.00	$80.00	$0.00	$80.00
15	Allen, William	$0.00	$0.00	$0.00	$150.00	$0.00	$150.00	$0.00	$150.00
2539	Allen, Mike	$100.00	$0.00	$0.00	$0.00	$0.00	$100.80	($0.00)	$100.80
2393	Allen, Cara	$0.00	$0.00	$0.00	$15.00	$0.00	$15.00	$0.00	$15.00
20	Allsop, Sue	$0.00	$0.00	$0.00	$59.00	$0.00	$59.00	$0.00	$59.00
23	Ambuehl, Mary	$0.00	$0.00	$0.00	$78.00	$0.00	$78.00	$0.00	$78.00
25	Ambuehl, Maya	$0.00	$0.00	$0.00	$80.12	$0.00	$80.12	$0.00	$80.12
26	Ames, Todd	$190.04	$0.00	$0.00	$0.00	$0.00	$190.04	$0.00	$190.04
30	Amsbary, Tina	$0.00	$0.00	$0.00	$12.60	$0.00	$12.60	$0.00	$12.60
31	Anderson, Mike	$0.00	$0.00	$0.00	$14.50	$0.00	$14.50	$0.00	$14.50
3488	Ankney, Bill	$0.00	$0.00	$0.00	$63.00	$0.00	$63.00	$0.00	$63.00
39	Ard, Ann	$0.00	$0.00	$0.00	$56.80	$0.00	$56.80	$0.00	$56.80

FIGURE 54.6
Accounts receivable report.

Procedure 54-1 Managing Basic Financial Transactions

Materials and Supplies Needed

- Dental charts for the day
- Daily appointment schedule
- Insurance information
- Day sheet
- Pen/pencil
- Computer if forms are computerized

Procedure Steps

1. On the day prior to the patient's appointment, the business assistant should:
   - Pull and review the patient's chart.
   - Confirm the appointment.

2. On the day of the appointment, the business assistant should:
   - Check the schedule.
   - Review dental charts.
   - When patient arrives, update financial and insurance information.
   - When treatment is complete, post transactions and schedule next appointment.

3. At the end of the day, the business assistant should:
   - Complete posting of daily transactions.
   - Process any mail payments.
   - Balance the day sheet and produce reports.
   - Complete an audit report.
   - Complete insurance processing.

Collections

It is essential to monitor the accounts receivable report to ensure collection of money owed to the practice is accomplished in a timely manner. The accounts receivable report contains information on each patient and the length of time that has passed between a charge being invoiced and the receipt of a payment for the charge. This is called an **aging account**. Periods of 30 days, 60 days, and 90 days are used to indicate the length of time money has been owed.

After reviewing the aging account, the business assistant may have to remind a patient that a payment is due. The collection process consists of reminders and strategies to try to collect payments that are due. The first reminder is a friendly reminder, a short letter generated by the computer after the first missed billing period. When using a manual system, several phrases that encourage payment can be placed on labels and attached to the billing statement. Computer programs can typically be set to include an appropriate message to the receiver. The following is an example of collection reminders:

- Prompt payment for your regular dental exams is appreciated.
- Don't delay. Your payment of $80.00 was due last month.
- Remember that you agreed to pay for your dental x-rays 30 days after your appointment.
- If you are having problems paying the balance of $125.00, please contact us.

If the friendly reminder does not work, and the balance remains unpaid after two billing periods, a tele-phone reminder is necessary. It is important to follow collection procedures that are regulated by the Fair Debt Collection Practices Act. This act requires that debt collectors treat people fairly by prohibiting certain methods of debt collections such as:

- Subjecting patients (debtors) to harassment or abusive treatment
- Calling debtors at inconvenient places or times such as at work or before the hours of 9:00 A.M. or after 8:00 P.M.
- Sharing debtor information with anyone except the debtor

Collection Letters

Offices that use computerized bookkeeping are typically set to produce automatic reminder notices regarding past due accounts for the office manager to use for daily reports. The computer system may also generate a reminder letter to be sent to the patient. When composing a collection letter it is important to personalize the letter for the patient's situation. The implication should always be made that the patient has good intentions. The letter should be brief, contain accurate data about the account, be firm regarding the necessity of payment, and politely include a "thank-you" in the closing of the letter. An overdue notice should never be sent on a postcard where the message is visible to others. Usually three types of collection letters are sent to patients for past due accounts: the first "friendly reminder" collection letter, an urgent collection letter, and the final collection letter (Figure 54.7). If attempts to collect fees using letters do not get results, then a collection telephone call is required.

<<Patient_First_Name>> <<Patient_Last_Name>>
<<Address_Line1>>
<<Address_Line2>>
<<City>>, <<State>> <<Zip>>

<<Date>>

Dear <<Patient_Title>> <<Patient_Last_Name>>,

We understand most of our patients are very busy people, and we are certain this is why we have not received payment on your account.

Since we have called this to your attention, please send us a check today.

Sincerely,

Walter H. Wiggins, D.D.S.

(A)

<<Patient_First_Name>> <<Patient_Last_Name>>
<<Address_Line1>>
<<Address_Line2>>
<<City>>, <<State>> <<Zip>>

<<Date>>

Dear <<Patient_Title>> <<Patient_Last_Name>>,

My financial secretary has advised me that your account has become seriously delinquent. I am sure that when you were in for your dental care you did not intend that your account be handled in this manner.

Unfortunately, and especially in these times, I am unable to continue to carry any accounts in a delinquent status.

Upon receipt of this note will you please call Mary Swilling, my financial secretary to make some arrangements. You will find that she is willing to cooperate with any realistic payment arrangement.

Sincerely,

Walter H. Wiggins, D.D.S.

(B)

(continued)

FIGURE 54.7
Examples of collection letters: (a) first collection letter, (b) urgent collection letter, and (c) final collection letter.

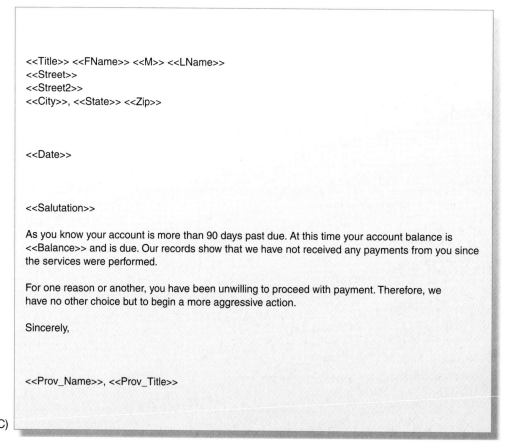

```
<<Title>> <<FName>> <<M>> <<LName>>
<<Street>>
<<Street2>>
<<City>>, <<State>> <<Zip>>


<<Date>>



<<Salutation>>

As you know your account is more than 90 days past due. At this time your account balance is
<<Balance>> and is due. Our records show that we have not received any payments from you since
the services were performed.

For one reason or another, you have been unwilling to proceed with payment. Therefore, we
have no other choice but to begin a more aggressive action.

Sincerely,



<<Prov_Name>>, <<Prov_Title>>
```

(C)

FIGURE 54.7 (continued)
Examples of collection letters: (a) first collection letter, (b) urgent collection letter, and (c) final collection letter.

Collection Calls

It can be difficult to telephone patients about past due accounts, but it must be accomplished with firmness and politeness. The call should never be demeaning. Although the office manager typically makes the collection phone calls, the dental assistant may at times be given this responsibility.

When making collection phone calls, it is important, prior to the call, to ensure that all of the necessary infor-

mation for the call is available. At the beginning of the call, the dental team member should confirm that the receiver of the call is the responsible party for the bill in question. Once this fact has been confirmed, try to obtain a commitment such as a date when the patient is going to pay the due amount. The caller should not apologize for the call—the call was necessary due to the payment being late. After the call, a follow-up confirmation letter should be sent. This letter confirms what was agreed on during the call. Collection calls should always be done in a private area out of listening range from other patients.

If attempts to collect payments do not work, then it may be necessary to obtain the services of an outside collection agency. A disadvantage of using a collection agency is that a percentage of the amount collected is kept by the agency as its service fee.

Why was the Fair Debt Collection Practice Act created?

Accounts Payable Management

Accounts payable is money owed by the dental practice. Usually the office manager ensures that accounts are paid

Life Span Considerations

The dental practice may have many elderly patients who are not comfortable with their personal information being stored on a computer or with computer-generated forms and letters. This may be because they are not computer literate. As the business assistant, you should take the time to explain to the patient about the computer security used in the office and how confidential information is secured. Also, prior to sending out computerized form letters or appointment reminders, spend a few extra minutes personalizing them—those few minutes will make a difference in how the patient feels about the dental practice.

in a timely manner and handled efficiently and ethically. Accounts payable tasks consist of writing checks, including payroll checks, verifying charges, and reconciling the checking account. To maintain accounts payable, the office manager must be efficient and organized. Many offices use a computerized system of accounts payable; however, the organizational steps that follow also apply if a manual system is used:

- Establish dates each month when checks will be generated or written. Pay attention to the due dates on invoices and the payroll date set by the dental practice. Ensure checks or automatic payments are sent 10 days prior to the due date to allow for adequate check processing times.
- Create a filing system of unpaid bills and due dates. When a bill arrives, check the due date and file it according to the system.
- Compare the invoices with the billing statement to ensure the charges are correct prior to sending the payment. If there are discrepancies, the office manager is responsible for correcting the error.
- Prepare the checks using a computerized system, a manual system, or automatic online payments.
- Annotate the date paid on the statement or invoice stub and include the check or transaction number. File in an appropriate file.

Types of Expenses

Many operating expenses are required when running a business. These expenses are referred to as **overhead**. Overhead includes things such as rent or mortgage, property taxes, payroll, consultants, legal and accounting services, supplies, utilities, housekeeping, and insurance. Overhead also includes laundry of uniforms, continuing education and professional association fees, and licensing. These overhead expenses usually fall into two categories: fixed and variable.

Fixed expenses are those that remain the same from month to month. Usually these are the rent or mortgage payments, payroll, and utilities. Salaries are not always fixed, however. Some employees work on an as-needed basis or as independent contractors; this is an example of a variable expense. **Variable expenses** change from month to month and include expenses such as dental supplies, laboratory fees, new equipment purchases, and repair fees.

Budgeting

The dental practice must have a financial plan or budget in order to meet the practice's account obligations. The budget is used to establish practice goals and to achieve a profit. The money spent to operate the practice is known as **expenditures**. Expenditures must be balanced with revenue, which is the amount of money received by the practice. A spreadsheet can be used to develop a budget and help calculate any changes in the budget for future goals. Gross income is the total of all professional income received. This pay, minus the payment of all practice expenditures, is the net income for the dental practice.

Organizing Expenditure Records

The bills for the dental practice should always be paid promptly. Major expenses should be paid by check or credit card. Petty cash is used to pay minor expenses. Petty cash is a set amount of money kept on hand for expenses that are paid immediately with cash. For example, when postage is needed, money can be taken out of the petty cash fund to pay for it. A voucher (Figure 54.8) should be filled out for all payments from the petty cash fund and the receipt for the item(s) purchased attached to it.

The business assistant should also document invoices, receipts, and cancelled checks and maintain them in a file. All unpaid bills are placed in an accounts payable folder that is separated into different categories such as rent, professional fees, salaries, supplies, utilities, and maintenance.

What is an example of variable overhead expenses? What is petty cash used for in the dental office?

Writing Checks

An account payable can be paid in many different ways, including with a check or electronically. Checks authorize a banking institute to transfer funds from one account to another account (Figure 54.9). Checks can electronically authorize the transfer of funds from accounts through the use of computer access. Procedure 54-2 explains the check writing steps that should be followed each time a check is written.

All transactions must be recorded in the checkbook register. The checkbook register is a record of deposits to

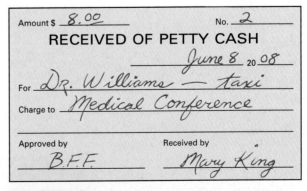

FIGURE 54.8
Petty cash voucher used for all payments from petty cash fund.

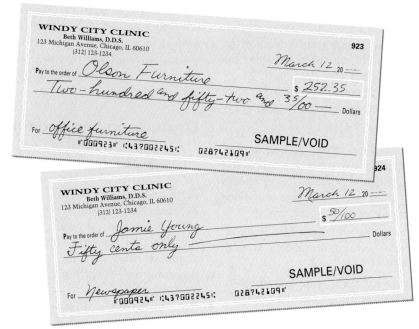

FIGURE 54.9
Correctly written checks.

and checks written by the practice. The documented information should include the date the check was written, the check number, the name of the payee (i.e., the intended recipient), and the amount and purpose of the check.

Reconciling Bank Statements

Most banks will send a bank statement to the dental practice every month. The bank statement shows the balance of the account at the beginning of the month, any deposits into the account, charges against the account, and the balance at the end of the month (Figure 54.10). To maintain accurate records, the business assistant should reconcile the bank statement as soon as it is received. The following steps describe how to reconcile the bank statement:

1. Arrange the checks in order by the check number.
2. Compare and verify the amount of each canceled check with the amounts listed on the bank statement. Check off all canceled checks and deposits in the checkbook register.
3. List the outstanding checks (the checks not yet returned to the bank). Include the check number and the amount. (This information comes from the checkbook register.)
4. Total the amount of the outstanding debits which include checks and debit charges. Then subtract the

Procedure 54-2 Writing Checks

Materials and Supplies Needed

- Pen
- Typewriter/computer
- Checks or printable check paper
- Checkbook ledger

Procedure Steps

1. Always use ink because it can not be altered. The ink can come from a pen, typewriter, or computer. Checks are printed on special paper that helps avoid the possibility of the check being altered or counterfeited.

2. Write accurately and neatly.

3. Enter the name of the person or company receiving the check in the *Payee* section. Write the complete company name as it appears on the statement. Titles such as Dr., Mr., or Mrs. are not used when writing a check.

4. Annotate the amount of the check in alpha and numeric form, for instance, "$233.24" and "Two hundred thirty-three and 24/100 dollars."

5. After the check has been written, have it signed by an authorized person (usually the dentist or office manager).

STATEMENT OF ACCOUNT

FIRST NORTH
BANK OF CHIGAGO
123 East Pearson, Chicago, IL 60611
(312) 321-1000

144808

WINDY CITY CLINIC	PAGE 1 OF 1
BETH WILLIAMS, D.D.S.	STATEMENT PERIOD
123 MICHIGAN AVENUE	FROM 08/01/05
CHICAGO, IL 60610	THRU 08/31/05
	CUST # 300-30-3000

---------------- ADVANTAGE CHECKING ACCOUNT ----------------

ACCOUNT NBR DD	12345	BEGINNING BALANCE	$2,646.63
AVG COLL BAL	$4,732.52	DEPOSITS/CREDITS	$8,000.00
MINIMUM BAL	$2,502.88	INTEREST PAID	$.00
TAX ID NUMBER	300-30-3000	CHECKS/DEBITS	$7,871.32 –
		SERVICE CHARGES	$5.00 –
		ENDING BALANCE	$2,770.31
		# DEPOSITS/CREDITS	1
		#CHECKS/DEBITS	11

DATE	DESCRIPTION		AMOUNT	BALANCE
				$2,646.63
08/01	BEGINNING BALANCE			2,621.68
08/01	CK#	872	24.95–	2,618.68
08/06	CK#	879	3.00–	2,543.68
08/08	CK#	883	75.00–	2,527.88
08/14	CK#	885	15.80–	2,502.88
08/15	CK#	886	25.00–	10,502.88
08/19	DEPOSIT		8,000.00	10,470.88
08/26	CK#	887	32.00–	7,970.88
08/26	CK#	888	2,500.00–	7,900.88
08/28	CK#	890	70.00–	7,775.31
08/28	CK#	889	125.57–	2,775.31
08/28	CK#	884	5,000.00–	2,770.31
08/31	MONTHLY MAINTENANCE FEE		5.00–	$2,770.31
08/31	ENDING BALANCE			

CHECK REGISTER

CHECK#	DATE	AMOUNT	CHECK#	DATE	AMOUNT
872	08/01	24.95	886	08/15	25.00
879*	08/06	3.00	887	08/26	32.00
883*	08/08	75.00	888	08/26	2,500.00
884	08/28	5,000.00	889	08/28	125.57
885	08/14	15.80	890	08/28	70.00

* INDICATES NON-CONSECUTIVE CHECK NUMBER(S)

FIGURE 54.10
Example of a bank statement.

amount of the outstanding checks and debit charges from the account balance on the bank statement.

5. Add any deposits that have been made but have not yet appeared on the statement, to the account balance.

6. After adding and subtracting the outstanding debits and credits, the resulting adjusted bank statement balance should match the balance in the checkbook register. If it does not, you will need to review all of the steps until the error is found.

Why should a check be printed or written in ink? What is the purpose of reconciling the bank statement?

Payroll

The administrative assistant or the office manager is assigned with creating and maintaining payroll records,

calculating payroll, producing payroll reports, and depositing taxes (Figure 54.11). Tax information can be obtained from the Internal Revenue Service's (IRS's) Publication 15, Circular E, *Employer's Tax Guide*. Publication 15 provides information about how to determine employee earnings, including tax withholdings, important dates to remember, and payroll documentation. Table 54-1 outlines the information provided in this publication.

The basic process of paying employees is as follows:

- The employer tracks hours worked by employees.
- The office manager calculates gross earnings.
- Deductions are calculated to get net pay.
- Paychecks are prepared.

Each employee must have a separate employee record, and the IRS requires that all payroll records be kept for at least four years. That is why it is important to keep accurate and efficient records. For tax reasons, employers must apply for an employer identification number using IRS Form SS-4. This is a nine-digit number

NAME	Joyce Walker		SOCIAL SECURITY NO.	123-12-1234
ADDRESS	22 W. Elm Avenue, Apt 3C		DATE OF EMPLOYMENT	6-30-05
	Goram City, MI 55555		TELEPHONE	(010)123-4567
EXEMPTIONS	1	HOURLY RATE	$10.00	

HOURS		GROSS SALARY	DEDUCTIONS					NET SALARY	DATE	CHECK NO.
REG.	O.T.		FWT	SWT	FICA					
80		800 –	72 –	14 –	61⁶⁰			652⁴⁰	7/14	276
80		800 –	72 –	14 –	61⁶⁰			652⁴⁰	7/28	414
72		720 –	64⁸⁰	12⁶⁰	55⁴⁵			587¹⁵	8/11	565
80	4	860 –	77⁴⁰	15⁰⁵	66²⁰			701³⁵	8/25	697
QUARTERLY TOTAL										
YEAR TO DATE										

FIGURE 54.11
An individual's payroll account.

TABLE 54-1 Contents of IRS Publication 15, Employer's Tax Guide

1. Employer Identification Number (EIN)
2. Who Are Employees
3. Family Employees
4. Employee's Social Security Number (SSAN)
5. Wages and Other Compensation
6. Tips
7. Supplemental Wages
8. Payroll Period
9. Withholding from Employees' Wages
10. Advance Earned Income Credit Payment
11. Depositing Taxes
12. Filing Form 941 or Form 944
13. Reporting Adjustments on Form 941 or Form 944
14. Federal Unemployment Tax
15. Special Rules for Various Types of Services and Payments
16. How to Use the Income Tax Withholding and Advance Earned Income Credit Payment Tables

assigned to sole proprietors or corporations and it is used for filing and reporting payroll information.

It is important to ensure that payroll records are kept confidential. They should be kept in a locked area, and unauthorized employees must not have access to this area.

Employee Information

All employees are required to file a federal income tax return by April 15 of every year. The amount of money withheld is approximately the annual tax the employee actually owes. The amount to withhold information comes from the *Employer's Tax Guide*. Every employee is required to complete Form W-4, Employee's Withholding Allowance Certificate (Figure 54.12). This form is used to determine the status of each employee and, hence, income tax deductions from wages.

All employees must have a copy of their Social Security card for the employer to use when reporting wages earned to the IRS. If an employee does not have a Social Security card or the card has a different last name (due to marriage or divorce), the employee is instructed to contact the Social Security Administration Office or go online at www.ssa.gov.

Form W-4 (2007)

Purpose. Complete Form W-4 so that your employer can withhold the correct federal income tax from your pay. Because your tax situation may change, you may want to refigure your withholding each year.

Exemption from withholding. If you are exempt, complete **only** lines 1, 2, 3, 4, and 7 and sign the form to validate it. Your exemption for 2007 expires February 16, 2008. See Pub. 505, Tax Withholding and Estimated Tax.

Note. You cannot claim exemption from withholding if (a) your income exceeds $850 and includes more than $300 of unearned income (for example, interest and dividends) and (b) another person can claim you as a dependent on their tax return.

Basic instructions. If you are not exempt, complete the **Personal Allowances Worksheet** below. The worksheets on page 2 adjust your withholding allowances based on itemized deductions, certain credits, adjustments to income, or two-earner/multiple job situations. Complete all worksheets that apply. However, you may claim fewer (or zero) allowances.

Head of household. Generally, you may claim head of household filing status on your tax return only if you are unmarried and pay more than 50% of the costs of keeping up a home for yourself and your dependent(s) or other qualifying individuals.

Tax credits. You can take projected tax credits into account in figuring your allowable number of withholding allowances. Credits for child or dependent care expenses and the child tax credit may be claimed using the **Personal Allowances Worksheet** below. See Pub. 919, How Do I Adjust My Tax Withholding, for information on converting your other credits into withholding allowances.

Nonwage income. If you have a large amount of nonwage income, such as interest or dividends, consider making estimated tax payments using Form 1040-ES, Estimated Tax

for Individuals. Otherwise, you may owe additional tax. If you have pension or annuity income, see Pub. 919 to find out if you should adjust your withholding on Form W-4 or W-4P.

Two earners/Multiple jobs. If you have a working spouse or more than one job, figure the total number of allowances you are entitled to claim on all jobs using worksheets from only one Form W-4. Your withholding usually will be most accurate when all allowances are claimed on the Form W-4 for the highest paying job and zero allowances are claimed on the others.

Nonresident alien. If you are a nonresident alien, see the Instructions for Form 8233 before completing this Form W-4.

Check your withholding. After your Form W-4 takes effect, use Pub. 919 to see how the dollar amount you are having withheld compares to your projected total tax for 2007. See Pub. 919, especially if your earnings exceed $130,000 (Single) or $180,000 (Married).

Personal Allowances Worksheet (Keep for your records.)

A Enter 1 " for **yourself** if no one else can claim you as a dependent . . . . **A** _____

B Enter "1" if:
- You are single and have only one job; or
- You are married, have only one job, and your spouse does not work; or
- Your wages from a second job or your spouse's wages (or the total of both) are $1,000 or less.

B _____

C Enter "1" for your **spouse**. But, you may choose to enter "-0-" if you are married and have either a working spouse or more than one job. (Entering "-0-" may help you avoid having too little tax withheld.) . . . . **C** _____

D Enter number of **dependents** (other than your spouse or yourself) you will claim on your tax return . . . . . . **D** _____

E Enter "1" if you will file as **head of household** on your tax return (see conditions under **Head of household** above) . **E** _____

F Enter "1" if you have at least $1,500 of **child or dependent care expenses** for which you plan to claim a credit . . **F** _____
(**Note.** Do **not** include child support payments. See Pub. 503, Child and Dependent Care Expenses, for details.)

G **Child Tax Credit** (including additional child tax credit). See Pub 972, Child Tax Credit, for more information.
- If your total income will be less than $57,000 ($85,000 if married), enter "2" for each eligible child.
- If your total income will be between $57,000 and $84,000 ($85,000 and $119,000 if married), enter "1" for each eligible child plus "1" **additional** if you have 4 or more eligible children. **G** _____

H Add lines A through G and enter total here. (**Note.** This may be different from the number of exemptions you claim on your tax return.) ▶ **H** _____

For accuracy, complete all worksheets that apply.
- If you plan to **itemize or claim adjustments to income** and want to reduce your withholding, see the **Deductions and Adjustments Worksheet** on page 2.
- If you have **more than one job** or are **married and you and your spouse both work** and the combined earnings from all jobs exceed $40,000 ($25,000 if married) see the **Two-Earners/Multiple Jobs Worksheet** on page 2 to avoid having too little tax withheld.
- If **neither** of the above situations applies, **stop here** and enter the number from line H on line 5 of Form W-4 below.

- **Cut here and give Form W-4 to your employer. Keep the top part for your records.** - - - - - - - - - - - - - - - - - - -

Form **W-4** Department of the Treasury Internal Revenue Service	**Employee's Withholding Allowance Certificate** ▶ Whether you are entitled to claim a certain number of allowances or exemption from withholding is subject to review by the IRS. Your employer may be required to send a copy of this form to the IRS.	OMB No. 1545-0074 2007

1 Type or print your first name and middle initial.	Last name	**2** Your social security number

Home address (number and street or rural route)	**3** ☐ Single ☐ Married ☐ Married, but withhold at higher Single rate. **Note.** If married, but legally separated, or spouse is a nonresident alien, check the "Single" box.
City or town, state, and ZIP code	**4** If your last name differs from that shown on your social security card, check here. You must call 1-800-772-1213 for a replacement card. ▶ ☐

5	Total number of allowances you are claiming (from line **H** above **or** from the applicable worksheet on page 2)	**5**
6	Additional amount, if any, you want withheld from each paycheck	**6** $
7	I claim exemption from withholding for 2007, and I certify that I meet **both** of the following conditions for exemption.	

- Last year I had a right to a refund of **all** federal income tax withheld because I had **no** tax liability **and**
- This year I expect a refund of **all** federal income tax withheld because I expect to have **no** tax liability.

If you meet both conditions, write "Exempt" here . . . . ▶ **7**

Under penalties of perjury, I declare that I have examined this certificate and to the best of my knowledge and belief, it is true, correct, and complete.

Employee's signature
 (Form is not valid unless you sign it.) ▶ _____ **Date** ▶ _____

8 Employer's name and address (Employer: Complete lines 8 and 10 only if sending to the IRS.)	**9** Office code (optional)	**10** Employer identification number (EIN)

For Privacy Act and Paperwork Reduction Act Notice, see page 2.	Cat. No. 10220Q	Form **W-4** (2007)

FIGURE 54.12

IRS Form W-4, Employee's Withholding Allowance Certificate.

(continued)

Deductions and Adjustments Worksheet

Note. Use this worksheet *only* if you plan to itemize deductions, claim certain credits, or claim adjustments to income on your 2007 tax return.

1   Enter an estimate of your 2007 itemized deductions. These include qualifying home mortgage interest, charitable contributions, state and local taxes, medical expenses in excess of 7.5% of your income, and miscellaneous deductions. (For 2007, you may have to reduce your itemized deductions if your income is over $156,400 ($78,200 if married filing separately). See *Worksheet 2* in Pub. 919 for details.) . . **1** $ _____

2   Enter: { $10,700 if married filing jointly or qualifying widow(er)
$7,850 if head of household
$5,350 if single or married filing separately }   . . . . **2** $ _____

3   **Subtract** line 2 from line 1. If zero or less, enter "-0-" . . . . **3** $ _____

4   Enter an estimate of your 2007 adjustments to income, including alimony, deductible IRA contributions, and student loan interest   **4** $ _____

5   **Add**   lines 3 and 4 and enter the total. (Include any amount for credits from *Worksheet 8* in Pub. 919) . **5** $ _____

6   Enter an estimate of your 2007 nonwage income (such as dividends or interest) . . . . **6** $ _____

7   **Subtract** line 6 from line 5. If zero or less, enter "-0-" . . . . **7** $ _____

8   **Divide** the amount on line 7 by $3,400 and enter the result here. Drop any fraction . . . . **8** _____

9   Enter the number from the **Personal Allowances Worksheet,** line H, page 1 . . . . **9** _____

10 **Add** lines 8 and 9 and enter the total here. If you plan to use the **Two-Earners/Multiple Jobs Worksheet,** also enter this total on line 1 below. Otherwise, **stop here** and enter this total on Form W-4, line 5, page 1   **10** _____

Two-Earners/Multiple Jobs Worksheet (See *Two earners/multiple jobs* on page 1.)

Note. Use this worksheet *only* if the instructions under line H on page 1 direct you here.

1   Enter the number from line H, page 1 (or from line 10 above if you used the **Deductions and Adjustments Worksheet**)   **1** _____

2   Find the number in **Table 1** below that applies to the **LOWEST** paying job and enter it here. **However,** if you are married filing jointly and wages from the highest paying job are $50,000 or less, do not enter more than "3."   **2** _____

3   If line 1 is **more than or equal to** line 2, subtract line 2 from line 1. Enter the result here (if zero, enter "-0-") and on Form W-4, line 5, page 1. **Do not** use the rest of this worksheet . . . . **3** _____

Note. If line 1 is *less than* line 2, enter "-0-" on Form W-4, line 5, page 1. Complete lines 4–9 below to calculate the additional withholding amount necessary to avoid a year-end tax bill.

4   Enter the number from line 2 of this worksheet . . . . **4** _____

5   Enter the number from line 1 of this worksheet . . . . **5** _____

6   **Subtract** line 5 from line 4 . . . . **6** _____

7   Find the amount in **Table 2** below that applies to the **HIGHEST** paying job and enter it here . . . . **7** $ _____

8   **Multiply** line 7 by line 6 and enter the result here. This is the additional annual withholding needed . . **8** $ _____

9   Divide line 8 by the number of pay periods remaining in 2007. For example, divide by 26 if you are paid every two weeks and you complete this form in December 2006. Enter the result here and on Form W-4, line 6, page 1. This is the additional amount to be withheld from each paycheck . . . . **9** $ _____

Table 1				Table 2			
Married Filing Jointly		**All Others**		**Married Filing Jointly**		**All Others**	
If wages from **LOWEST** paying job are—	Enter on line 2 above	If wages from **LOWEST** paying job are—	Enter on line 2 above	If wages from **HIGHEST** paying job are—	Enter on line 7 above	If wages from **HIGHEST** paying job are—	Enter on line 7 above
$0 - $4,500	0	$0 - $6,000	0	$0 - $65,000	$510	$0 - $35,000	$510
4,501 - 9,000	1	6,001 - 12,000	1	65,001 - 120,000	850	35,001 - 80,000	850
9,001 - 18,000	2	12,001 - 19,000	2	120,001 - 170,000	950	80,001 - 150,000	950
18,001 - 22,000	3	19,001 - 26,000	3	170,001 - 300,000	1,120	150,001 - 340,000	1,120
22,001 - 26,000	4	26,001 - 35,000	4	300,001 and over	1,190	340,001 and over	1,190
26,001 - 32,000	5	35,001 - 50,000	5				
32,001 - 38,000	6	50,001 - 65,000	6				
38,001 - 46,000	7	65,001 - 80,000	7				
46,001 - 55,000	8	80,001 - 90,000	8				
55,001 - 60,000	9	90,001 - 120,000	9				
60,001 - 65,000	10	120,001 and over	10				
65,001 - 75,000	11						
75,001 - 95,000	12						
95,001 - 105,000	13						
105,001 - 120,000	14						
120,001 and over	15						

FIGURE 54.12 (continued)
IRS Form W-4, Employee's Withholding Allowance Certificate.

Cultural Considerations

Scenario: A dental office hires a Spanish-speaking dental assistant to help with the patients who do not speak English. The new assistant speaks and reads very little English. What can the business assistant do to help the new employee fill out the IRS's W-4 tax form?

Answer: Publication 15, the *Employer's Tax Guide*, will allow the assistant to obtain the form in Spanish to help the new employee.

Calculating Payroll

To calculate payroll, all deductions must be subtracted from the gross salary to determine the employee's net salary. **Gross salary** is the amount of pay before any deductions have been taken out. **Net salary** is the amount of pay after deductions have been taken out. It is also called take-home pay.

The federal tax deductions include withholding taxes, Social Security taxes (FICA), Medicare taxes, and federal unemployment taxes (FUTA). Individual states may also collect taxes in addition to the federal deductions. Other deductions may include contributions to a retirement plan, health insurance, life insurance, and a savings program.

The employer must also pay quarterly payroll taxes to the government. The *Employer's Tax Guide* provides current information about employment tax rates.

Calculating Net Pay

Once an employer and an employee agree on a wage, the net pay can be determined. The following is an example of how an employee's net pay is determined:

1. The employee's hourly wage is $18 per hour.
2. For a 40-hour workweek, the gross salary is $720: 40 hours × $18 per hour = $720.
3. Then deductions are made from the gross salary: For 2008 the tax rate for Social Security is 6.2% and the tax rate for Medicare is 1.45%. These rates are combined and multiplied by the gross wages: 7.65% or .0765 × $720 = $55.08 is the amount to be deducted for FICA and Medicare taxes.
4. The amount of income tax withholding depends on the number of exemptions the employee has indicated on Form W-4. This amount is determined from a table in the *Employer's Tax Guide*. For this example, $86 in taxes have been withheld.
5. State and local taxes must be deducted. State and local taxes vary depending on the state. For this example, $50 has been deducted for state and local taxes.

6. Other deductions such as health care insurance for $50 a month may need to be deducted.

Utilizing the information in steps 1 through 6, the net, or take-home, pay would be calculated as follows:

Gross salary:	$720.00
Minus deductions:	
FICA $55.08	
Withholding tax $86	
State and local tax $50	
Health insurance deduction $50	
Total deductions:	−241.08
Net pay	$478.92

Form W-2: Wage and Tax Statement

Every year employees receive a copy of Form W-2, Wage and Tax Statement, from the employer (Figure 54.13). This is required to be mailed no later than January 31. The employee uses this information when filing personal income tax returns. One copy is for the federal tax return, one copy is for the state tax return, and one copy is for the employee's personal records. A copy is retained by the employer and a copy is sent to the IRS.

The following information is provided on Form W-2:

- Employer's name, address, and federal identification number
- Employee's name, address, and Social Security number
- Amount of federal income tax withheld
- Total wages paid to the employee
- Total FICA withheld
- Any state or local taxes withheld

What document must the business assistant become very familiar with when calculating payroll?

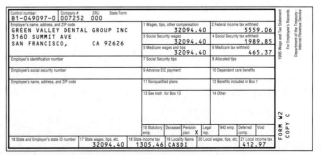

FIGURE 54.13
IRS Form W-2, Wage and Tax Statement.

SUMMARY

The financial management aspect of a dental practice can be a very challenging yet rewarding job. As a dental assistant, your responsibilities may go beyond patient care. Depending on the size and needs of the office, the dental assistant may be asked to participate in managing the finances of the practice. In this role, the individual must demonstrate knowledge in managing accounts receivable and accounts payable. Processing the office payroll may be another task required of this individual. The dental assistant who develops the skills needed to achieve these tasks will be a crucial member of the dental team. Being able to perform more than one job or responsibility may make you more employable.

Preparing for Externship

There are a lot of procedures to learn as a dental assistant. To become a well-rounded assistant, you should continue with your education, not only the clinical aspect of it, but the administrative as well. Go to www.danb.org and review the requirements for certification as a certified dental practice management administrator (CDPMA).

KEY TERMS

- **Accounts payable:** Amount of money owed by the dental practice. p. 874
- **Accounts receivable:** Amount of money that is owed to the dental practice from patients for services rendered. p. 866
- **Aging account:** The accounts receivable report that contains information on each patient and the length of time that has passed between a charge being invoiced and the receipt of a payment for the charge. p. 872
- **Bonding insurance:** Insurance that protects the practice against any monetary losses due to employee theft. p. 866
- **Deposit slip:** An itemized copy of the money taken to a bank to be credited to the dental practice account. p. 870
- **Expenditures:** Amount of money spent to operate the dental practice. p. 875

- **Fixed expenses:** Those expenses that remain the same from month to month. p. 875
- **Gross salary:** The amount of pay before any deductions have been taken out. p. 881
- **Net salary:** The amount of pay after deductions have been taken out; also called take-home pay. p. 881
- **Overhead:** The cost of running a business. p. 875
- **Pegboard system:** A manual, handwritten bookkeeping system; sometimes called the "write it once" system. p. 867
- **Variable expenses:** Those expenses that change from month to month. p. 875
- **Walk-out statement:** A receipt that shows the amount the patient paid and also the current balance if money is owed to the practice. p. 868

CHECK YOUR UNDERSTANDING

1. The walk-out statement provides all of the following information except
   a. the type of treatment provided.
   b. the patient's name and the date.
   c. the patient's birth date.
   d. the amount paid and the balance of the account.

2. What is another name for the pegboard bookkeeping system?
   a. computerized system
   b. "write it once" system
   c. accounts payable
   d. none of the above

3. An example of a variable expense is the cost of
   a. full-time salaries.
   b. mortgage or rent.
   c. supplies.
   d. utilities.

4. Which tax form does the employee complete when he or she is hired?
   a. Form W-2, Wage and Tax Statement
   b. Form W-4, Employee's Withholding Allowance Certificate
   c. Circular E
   d. accounts payable

CHECK YOUR UNDERSTANDING (continued)

5. The system for distributing money owed by the practice is
   a. accounts receivable.
   b. collections.
   c. embezzlement.
   d. accounts payable.

6. The employer identification number
   a. replaces the Social Security number of the dentist.
   b. must be applied for through the IRS.
   c. is used for filing and reporting payroll information.
   d. both b and c.

7. Which of the following is **not** a purpose of the Fair Debt Collection Practice Act?
   a. to provide fair treatment when collecting debts
   b. to share debtor information with other organizations
   c. to prohibit harassment while making collection calls
   d. to prohibit calling at inconvenient times

8. 60% of $475 is
   a. $2.85
   b. $28.5
   c. $285
   d. none of the above

9. How long must employees' payroll records be kept by the employer?
   a. 4 months
   b. 4 years
   c. 40 years
   d. none of the above

10. Which of the following information is included on Form W-2, Wage and Tax Statement?
    a. employer's identification number
    b. federal income tax withheld
    c. both a and b
    d. none of the above

● INTERNET ACTIVITY

• Access the IRS's *Employer's Tax Guide* at www.irs.gov/publications/p15/index.html and use it to determine the amount withheld for a dental assistant earning $600 per week, who claims two exemptions.

Answer:
$56.26.

● WEB REFERENCES

• Bridges to Algebra and Geometry www.learningincontext.com/Bridges/chapt07.htm
• Dental Economics www.dentaleconomics.com
• Dental Resources www.dental-resources.com
• Get Smarter.org www.getsmarter.org

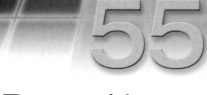

55

Dental Insurance

Learning Objectives

After reading this chapter, the student should be able to:

- Understand the terminology used in the dental insurance field.

- Review the options available for dental insurance.

- Compare the different types of dental insurance plans.

- Recognize the importance of educating patients about their dental insurance assistance.

- Differentiate between primary and secondary carriers.

- Identify dental procedure codes.

- Review processing, tracking, and management of claims.

- Explain the Health Insurance Portability and Accountability Act (HIPAA) of 1996.

Preparing for Certification Exams

- Know the dental insurance structure.
- Understand utilization of dental terminology.
- Identify the different types of dental insurance claims.
- Explain dental procedure codes and their importance.
- Describe the management of dental insurance claims.

Key Terms

Allowable charges

Benefit

Copay

Deductible

Exclusive provider organization (EPO) plan

Explanation of benefits (EOB)

Managed care

National Provider Identifier (NPI)

Preferred provider organization (PPO) plan

Upcoding

Waiting period

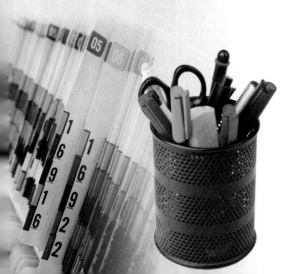

The dental insurance industry in the United States began as a by-product of the health insurance industry. Supposedly, the nation's first dental insurance plan was instituted in 1883 by the Denver and Rio Grande Western Railway's Hospital Association. The purpose of traditional dental insurance plans was, and still is, to encourage patients to seek preventive care and provide reimbursement to the insured for the cost of dental services.

In 1959, dental health maintenance organizations (HMOs) were formed and began to provide dental insurance. These types of plans were more popular and less expensive than traditional dental indemnity insurance. In addition to HMOs, preferred provider organizations (PPOs) began to be offered. Dental PPO insurance provides consumers with better service and fewer restrictions than dental HMO insurance. In the mid-1990s, discount dental plans became a large part of the dental insurance industry. Discount dental plans offered consumers access to affordable dental care at a reasonable price and with an emphasis on choice and service. Although dental insurance is available to any consumer who is willing to purchase the insurance, most individuals choose not to buy the coverage because of low or restrictive benefit coverage.

Dental Assistant PROFESSIONAL TIP

To perform your job well as a dental assistant, it is crucial that you understand dental insurance terminology. When presenting dental treatment plans to patients, the dental assistant may be asked what a specific term, such as "annual maximum benefit," means. Not every patient is knowledgeable about what his or her insurance plan entails. Patients are often busy and do not educate themselves about their dental insurance plans. The more information you can provide the patient, the better. Be prepared to answer quick and simple questions.

Professionalism

Learn from the doctors and other team members in the office. Support their decisions and utilize their knowledge to benefit the patient. Stay educated in the latest techniques and patient care. Always be professional and friendly in the presence of patients. Make sure you treat each patient with confidence and comfort.

Dental Insurance Terminology

Dental insurance terminology is a list of common terms and phrases related to dental insurance and the dental plan structure. These terms are utilized by dental insurance companies to communicate to dental offices and to the patient about the patient's insurance plan coverage. The more knowledge the dental assistant has about dental insurance, the more efficient and helpful the dental assistant can be in assisting the patient to understand insurance issues that may arise. When discussing a patient's insurance plan, a dental office team member must be able to explain the plan and its benefits to the patient or the individual who holds the insurance policy (the subscriber) such as a parent or spouse.

Situations arise daily within a dental office in which dental terminology needs to be used. For example, when a dentist is explaining a proposed treatment to a patient, he or she needs to use dental as well as laymen's terms that provide clarity about what is being said. This helps to ensure that the patient understands and accepts treatment options.

Use of dental terminology is also critical to the successful financial management of patient accounts. When reporting patient care to insurance companies, the dental team must use correct terminology in order to provide the insurance company with a clear picture of the patient's dental care. If the dental team does not understand and utilize specific terms when submitting a patient claim, the procedure may not be reported correctly to the insurance company, resulting in denial of payment.

In addition to medical terms, other terms common to the reimbursement process must be learned. For instance a term commonly used is **deductible**, meaning the amount of money the patient/subscriber must pay before the insurance plan will start to pay on any treatment. Many patients lack knowledge related to their own insurance plans. Although it is ultimately the subscriber's responsibility to understand his/her insurance plan and to accept the financial responsibility associated with it, it is in the best interest of the dental practice to ensure that insurance terminology and benefits are clearly explained so that patients understand how their insurance plan works. Both from a patient standpoint and from a business perspective, being able to discuss treatment options and dental insurance plans is important to a dental practice's continued success. Utilization of a form such as the patient ledger or statement of account can help in communicating the cost of treatment and the patient's financial responsibility (Figure 55.1). Clearly explaining a patient's treatment options and how payment of the treatment will be accepted can be a key factor in a patient accepting and receiving treatment.

How can a dental assistant help the doctor present treatment options along with the insurance estimate?

Dental Insurance Plans

Various types of insurance plans are available to dental patients. Some patients have dental insurance through their employers, whereas others purchase coverage through an independent insurance carrier.

Dental HMOs and DMOs

Dental HMOs and dental managed care organizations (DMOs) are similar to the traditional medical HMO in that consumers have a limited selection of dentists and the insurance plans are usually closed panel. **Managed care** refers to a cost containment system that directs the utilization of health benefits by (a) restricting the type, level, and frequency of treatment; (b) limiting access to care; and (c) controlling the level of reimbursement for services. The term *closed panel* refers to a type of managed care plan that contracts with dentists on an exclusive basis for services and does not allow the patient to see a dentist who is not contracted with the insurance company.

Typically, HMOs and DMOs offer the best deal in terms of limiting out-of-pocket costs for the subscriber of the insurance policy. Premium costs in these plans are also likely to be affordable. According to the National Association of Dental Plans, the average premium that an individual pays monthly to obtain dental HMO or DMO insurance is approximately $13 for single-person coverage.

Dental Preferred Provider Organizations

A **preferred provider organization (PPO) plan** is an insurance plan in which a purchaser of dental benefits receives services from certain dentists (i.e., preferred providers) who provide those services at specified rates that have been agreed on with the insurance company. A typical participating agreement gives the carrier, also known as the insurance company, the authority to set fees that the carrier will pay for charges rendered to the patient. Physicians who choose to be members of a PPO agree to accept the fee paid by the insurance company in addition to the deductible that is required of the patient.

If a patient goes to a dentist who is a preferred provider, the only amount the patient pays is the patient's

deductible and possibly a copay. A **copay** is a cost-sharing arrangement in which the insurance patient/subscriber pays a specified charge at the time of service, for example, $15 for an office visit. If the patient chooses to see a dentist of his choice who is not on the plan, the patient must understand that the insurance company will pay less and that the patient will pay more.

Why doesn't dental insurance cover all of the percentage of a fee given for dental treatment?

Dental Indemnity Plans

A dental indemnity plan is a traditional dental plan that lets subscribers receive a comprehensive range of dental services from the provider of their choice anywhere in the United States. The subscriber pays a percentage of charges for certain dental services and files a claim for reimbursement.

Exclusive Provider Organizations

Exclusive provider organization (EPO) plans are closed-panel plans that allow a particular group of insurance subscribers to receive dental care only from participating dentists (i.e., exclusive providers). EPO insurance plans are typically offered to groups of individuals through an insurance broker or the subscribers' employer. Under an EPO, if a patient decides to see a dentist who is not listed on the EPO panel, charges for services will not be covered by the plan. There are exceptions to this rule, particularly if the services received were due to an emergency or being out of the network area.

Because participating dentists are required to offer substantial fee reductions, many dentists elect not to participate in EPO-type plans. Under some benefits plans, participating dentists may be salaried employees of the EPO. An EPO contracts with a limited number of practitioners within a geographic area. Access to necessary specialized care can be restricted. The EPO also may limit the amount of services that a patient can receive in a given calendar year.

Alternative Plans

An example of an alternative plan is a discount plan that negotiates with various dentists for set discounts on certain procedures. The patient is responsible for paying for his/her services (minus the discount) at the time of treatment.

Unfortunately, many of these types of plans are unlicensed. Typically, when an employer and employee are selecting a dental insurance plan, it is important to look for companies that are licensed and meet state and federal guidelines.

Another alternative plan is a direct reimbursement plan. A direct reimbursement plan is a self-funded program

STATEMENT OF ACCOUNT

Angela Osborn
9218 Kimmer Dr. Suite 106
Lone Tree, CO 80124
(303) 799-9993

Page:	1
Date:	08/21/2007
Acct. Nbr:	

Amount Due: **0.00**
Make Remittance Payable to:
Angela Osborn
Amount Enclosed: _____

John Doe
12121 S. Beautiful Smile St
Lone Tree, CO 80124

Credit Card Number: _____
3 or 4 Digit Security Code: _____
Expiration Date: ____/____/_____
0
Signature: _____

Date	Name	Code	Description	Charges	Payments	Est. Ins. Portion	Est. Patient Portion
08/21/07	John J		Previous Balance				
08/21/07	John J	D2950	Core Buildup, Including Any Pins(Tooth # 30)	298.00			298.00
08/21/07	John J	D2740	Crown-Porcelain/Ceramic Substrate(Tooth # 30)	1,081.00			1,081.00
08/21/07	John J	D2950	Core Buildup, Including Any Pins(Tooth # 31)	298.00			298.00
08/21/07	John J	D2740	Crown-Porcelain/Ceramic Substrate(Tooth # 31)	1,081.00			1,081.00
08/21/07	John J	00001	Check		-2,758.00		

Account Aging	Current	Over 30	Over 60	Over 90	Total Balance		
	0.00	0.00	0.00	0.00	0.00		

Previous Balance	0.00
Current Payments	-2,758.00
Current Charges	2,758.00
New Balance	0.00

Angela Osborn * 9218 Kimmer Dr. Suite 106 * Lone Tree, CO 80124 * (303) 799-9993

FIGURE 55.1
Patient treatment estimate.
Courtesy of Dr. Angela Osborn

in which the employee is reimbursed by his/her employer. The plan is based on a percentage of dollars spent for dental care provided. The plan allows employees to seek treatment from the dentist of their choice. There is no insurance carrier involved.

Determining Eligibility

When a patient initiates contact with a dental office, it is important for a dental team member to verify the subscriber and family member's eligibility. In order for a patient to receive benefits for services rendered, the patient must be eligible. Eligibility requirements vary. For instance, when a subscriber begins new employment there is usually a 30- to 60-day **waiting period** before coverage becomes effective, that is, before the subscriber becomes "eligible" to receive benefits.

If a subscriber resigns from his/her job, is laid off, or retires, his/her coverage customarily terminates within 30 days from the notification of change of employment. However, the subscriber may have the option to continue coverage under the Consolidated Omnibus Budget Reconciliation Act (COBRA) of 1985. This entitles the subscriber to keep the same coverage; however, the subscriber is responsible for paying the entire premium, including any part previously paid for by the employer.

The guidelines and regulations for eligibility under other government programs, such as Medicaid and the Civilian Health and Medical Program of the Uniformed Services (CHAMPUS), vary greatly. Under Title IX of the federal Medicaid program, qualifying children up to age 20 living in households with incomes that are below federal poverty levels can be eligible for state-sponsored dental benefits. The federal government pays half of the fees for states that choose to sponsor adult dental Medicaid benefits. The dental benefits and dental plans associated with these benefits vary from state to state.

When working in an office that accepts patients enrolled in government programs, the dental assistant must be familiar with the specific forms of identification that indicate a patient is a subscriber to a government plan. This usually is an identification card or a proof-of-eligibility sticker. It is essential that the identification be verified each month because a patient's eligibility may change on a month-to-month basis.

Determining Benefits

If a patient's insurance plan is through the patient's employer, the employer who purchases the coverage as a benefit for the employee negotiates the benefits and limitations within the specific plan. The insurance carrier is responsible for covering only the negotiated treatment that is included in the plan. Each employee should be given access to a benefit booklet or Web address at which the specific benefits can be found. Before a patient pre-

Cultural Considerations

Dental assistants may find it challenging to discuss dental insurance with patients from other countries or cultures. Some cultures do not have dental insurance; others may not believe in Western dentistry. Therefore, they may not give their dental needs priority. It is important for you to be sensitive and help them understand their dental insurance while explaining the need for treatment.

sents to the dental office, it is important that the patient know what benefits his/her insurance plan provides. **Benefits** are the amount payable by a third party toward the cost of various covered dental services or the dental service or procedure covered by the plan.

When making an appointment with a patient, a dental team member typically retrieves information on the patient's insurance in order to help in determining what benefits the patient has. To retrieve more information on the patient's plan, the patient and/or dental assistant can do the following:

1. Call the insurance carrier and verbally obtain information about the benefits.
2. Call the insurance carrier and ask for a fax that details the benefits.
3. If available, go to the Web address provided and download, print, or save the benefits to a file for that individual patient's plan.

By learning about the patient's benefits prior to the initial appointment, the patient and the dental office can more accurately discuss any financial issues as related to possible treatments. This can ensure that the patient receives the amount of benefits to which he/she is entitled.

In addition to the type of insurance plan the patient has, other factors influence the amount of benefits that the patient is entitled to receive. The least expensive alternative (LEAT), also referred to as an alternative benefit, allows for reimbursement of the least expensive treatment. For example, when a patient presents to the dental office with numerous amalgam fillings that are old and have decay, the dentist may indicate the need for each to be replaced with a resin composite material. Rather than paying for resin composite fillings, the insurance carrier may offer the treatment alternative of paying an **allowable charge** (or maximum dollar amount) for amalgam fillings. The cost of an amalgam filling is less than that of a resin composite filling.

Another example would be when a dentist diagnoses the need to replace a patient's missing tooth with an implant, and the covered benefits do not include an implant, but they do cover the cost of a removable partial denture. Once the carrier pays the allowed charge (i.e., the lesser amount), the difference between the implant treatment fee and the alternative allowed charge paid by the carrier is the patient's responsibility.

How can a dental assistant be effective in educating patients about their insurance plans?

Coordination of Benefits

When a patient has two insurance companies (primary and secondary), the patient will receive payment from both carriers. The total payment received though may not be more than 100% of the total fees for dental treatment. For example, a patient is seen for services totaling $278. The primary carrier pays $205 on the claim for this service. Under coordination of benefits, the secondary carrier will only pay the difference between the total fee charged and the amount paid by the primary carrier. So, for this example, based on the individual insurance plan, the secondary carrier would only pay up to the remaining amount of $73.

Nonduplication of Benefits

When an insurance carrier has a nonduplication (also referred as "benefitless benefit" or carve-out) clause in its plan, a provision within the plan releases the carrier from responsibility for paying for services that are covered under the secondary insurance carrier's plan. Under these plans the reimbursement is limited to the higher amount allowed by the two insurance carriers rather than 100% of the fees charged. For example, if the fee charged is $278 and the primary insurance company only allows $205 for this service, and the secondary insurance company only allows $220 for this service, then the primary insurance company would pay the allowed $205. The secondary insurance company would only pay the difference between its allowed amount and the primary carrier's allowed amount, which is $15. This would equal the secondary carrier's primary allowed amount of $220. If the primary insurance company allowed a higher amount of the two carriers' allowed amounts, then the secondary carrier would pay nothing. The patient's responsibility would be to pay any remaining amount not covered by either insurance company.

Clarifying Primary and Secondary Carriers

When a patient has dual coverage, it is necessary to determine which carrier is the primary carrier and which is the secondary carrier. This is important because the primary carrier pays first, and then the secondary carrier pays an amount toward the remaining balance. When the patient is the insured, the patient's insurance carrier is always the primary carrier and the spouse's carrier is considered the secondary carrier.

When sending insurance claims, the primary claim is always sent first. Once the primary carrier sends payment, the secondary claim is then sent. The secondary claim is sent out with the **explanation of benefits (EOB)** form that was received from the primary carrier. An EOB contains information related to the claim and why the primary insurance company did or did not pay all or part of the claim. The copy of the EOB allows the secondary carrier to coordinate its response appropriately and send payment for the allowed benefits. Figure 55.2 provides an example of an EOB along with explanations of each box on the EOB.

The Birthday Rule

When determining which carrier is primary and which is secondary for dependent children or rider amendments, the birthday rule is implemented. The birthday rule is an insurance regulation utilized to determine coordination of benefits for dependent children based on the parents' dates of birth.

The birthday rule states that the primary carrier for the dependent is the insurance plan of the parent whose birth month and day is the earliest in the calendar year. The primary carrier for parents with the same birthday will be the plan that has covered the dependent for the longest period of time.

The birthday rule applies to parents who are not divorced. There are many factors to consider when parents are divorced or separated and when step-parents are involved. When filing claims that have both primary and secondary carriers, the primary claim is filed first. Once the primary carrier sends payment to the dentist with an attached explanation of how the bill will be paid, also known as the EOB, the claim can then be filed to the secondary carrier.

Understanding Limitations and Frequencies

Limitations are restrictive conditions stated in an individual or a group dental insurance plan. Certain procedures may simply not be covered as often as needed. A common example might be a plan that pays for a routine cleaning only twice a year, even though the patient requires a periodontal therapy type of cleaning every three months. Other plans may only cover dentures every five years. Limitations vary depending on the contract purchased.

HOW TO READ YOUR DENTAL EXPLANATION OF BENEFITS

You can access this form in the member section on our website at www.odscompanies.com.

1. The patient who had services performed.

2. This is the claim number for the services performed.

3. The provider who performed services.

4. The date the service was provided.

5. The type of service performed.

6. The code that describes the service performed.

7. This is the amount charged.

8. This is the amount (if any) that is being denied.

9. This shows any charges which have been applied to your plan's deductible. The deductible is subtracted from covered charges and is the responsibility of the patient.

10. This shows the amount you saved by using an ODS/Delta participating provider. You are not responsible for these provider discounts.

11. A covered charge is the amount allowed after disallowed charges, the deductible and provider discount are subtracted.

12. The co-pay is the difference between the covered charge and the amount paid. This amount is the patient's responsibility.

13. This shows the amount of benefit which has been paid by Oregon Dental Service.

14. The "Payee" identifies to whom Oregon Dental Service has made the benefit payment.

15. This shows the amount to be paid by the patient to the provider.

16. Explanations of codes in this column are listed at the bottom of the page under comments. *Additional explanation codes listed on reverse side.*

17. If there is a deductible, this section will identify the amount applied toward the annual deductible to-date and this section will also show the annual maximum met.

FOR SERVICES FROM TO (4.)	TYPE OF SERVICE (5.)	PROCEDURE CODE (6.)	TOTAL CHARGES (7.)	DISALLOWED CHARGES (8.)	DEDUCTIBLE (-) (9.)	PROVIDER DISCOUNT (10.)	REMAINING COVERED CHARGES (11.)	CO-PAY (12.)	TOTAL BENEFIT (13.)	PATIENT RESPONSIBILITY (15.)	COMMENTS (16.)
PATIENT: JUAN CLIENTE (1.)											
CLAIM: D55555521-00 (2.)			PROVIDER: SAM SANDER DMD (3.)								
0501 050105	EXAM: INITIAL	D0150	50.00	.00	.00	.00	50.00	.00	50.00	.00	
0501 050105	PROPHY: ADULT	D1110	60.00	.00	.00	.00	60.00	.00	60.00	.00	
0501 050105	XRAY : FM SERIES	D0274	40.00	.00	.00	.00	40.00	.00	40.00	.00	
	TOTALS		150.00	.00	.00	.00	150.00	.00	150.00	.00	
								PAYEE: SAM SANDER DMD (14.)			
PATIENT: JUAN CLIENTE											
CLAIM: D55555524-00			PROVIDER: SAM SANDER DMD								
0101 010106	AMAL: 2 SRF PERM	D2150	100.00	.00	25.00	25.00	50.00	10.00	40.00	35.00	R8
	TOTALS		100.00	.00	25.00	25.00	50.00	10.00	40.00	35.00	
								PAYEE: SAM SANDER DMD			
PATIENT: JOSE CLIENTE											
CLAIM: D55555526-00			PROVIDER: SAM SANDER DMD								
0101 010106	EXAM: INITIAL	D0150	50.00	.00	.00	.00	50.00	.00	50.00	.00	
0101 010106	PROPHY:ADULT	D1110	60.00	.00	.00	.00	60.00	.00	60.00	.00	
0101 010106	XRAY: 4 BITEWINGS	D0274	40.00	.00	.00	.00	40.00	.00	40.00	.00	
0101 010106	FLUORIDE: ADULT	D1204	20.00	.00	.00	.00	20.00	.00	20.00	.00	
	TOTALS		170.00	.00	.00	.00	170.00	.00	170.00	.00	
								PAYEE: SAM SANDER DMD			
PATIENT: MARIA CLIENTE											
CLAIM: D55555525-00			PROVIDER: SAM SANDER DMD								
0101 010106	AMAL: 2 SRF PERM	D2150	100.00	.00	25.00	25.00	50.00	10.00	40.00	35.00	R8
	TOTALS		100.00	.00	25.00	25.00	50.00	10.00	40.00	35.00	

COMMENTS:
*** PAYMENT FOR THESE SERVICES IS DETERMINED BASED ON THE SPECIFIC TERMS OF YOUR DENTAL PLAN OR DELTA'S AGREEMENTS WITH DELTA'S NETWORK DENTISTS.
R8   THE CHARGE EXCEEDS THE AMOUNT ALLOWED.

17.

JUAN CLIENTE	HAS MET $	.00 OF THE $ 25.00 PATIENT DEDUCTIBLE FOR THE 2005 BENEFIT YEAR.
	HAS MET $	150.00 OF THE $ 1,000.00 MAXIMUM FOR THE 2005 BENEFIT YEAR.
	HAS MET $	25.00 OF THE $ 25.00 PATIENT DEDUCTIBLE FOR THE 2006 BENEFIT YEAR.
	HAS MET $	40.00 OF THE $ 1,000.00 MAXIMUM FOR THE 2006 BENEFIT YEAR.
JOSE CLIENTE	HAS MET $	.00 OF THE $ 25.00 PATIENT DEDUCTIBLE FOR THE 2006 BENEFIT YEAR.
	HAS MET $	170.00 OF THE $ 1,000.00 MAXIMUM FOR THE 2006 BENEFIT YEAR.
MARIA CLIENTE	HAS MET $	25.00 OF THE $ 25.00 PATIENT DEDUCTIBLE FOR THE 2006 BENEFIT YEAR.
	HAS MET $	40.00 OF THE $ 1,000.00 MAXIMUM FOR THE 2006 BENEFIT YEAR.
THE FAMILY	HAS MET $	0.00 OF THE $ 75.00 FAMILY DEDUCTIBLE FOR THE 2005 BENEFIT YEAR.
	HAS MET $	50.00 OF THE $ 75.00 FAMILY DEDUCTIBLE FOR THE 2006 BENEFIT YEAR.

THIS IS NOT A BILLING. PLEASE SAVE THIS COPY FOR YOUR RECORDS.

Callout labels:
- Patient deductible for benefit year.
- Maximum met for the benefit year.
- Family deductible for the benefit year.
- This is not a billing. Please save this copy for your records.

If you have questions, please call our Dental Customer Service line between 7:30 a.m. and 5:30 p.m. Pacific Standard Time at 503-265-5680 (Portland area) or toll-free 1-877-277-7280.

DELTA DENTAL

THE **ODS** COMPANIES

FIGURE 55.2

Explanation of benefits (EOB) form with explanations for each area included on the form.
Courtesy of Oregon Dental Service (ODS). © 2007

Dental Explanation Codes and Comments

EXPLANATION CODES	COMMENTS
>4	MEMBER NO LONGER ELIGIBILE. PLEASE CHECK ID CARD.
D04	UNABLE TO DETERMINE BENEFITS. CLINICAL INFORMATION FROM PROVIDER WAS NOT RECEIVED TO SUBSTANTIATE NECESSITY.
D18	TOOTH COLORED (COMPOSITE) FILLINGS ON BACK TEETH ARE NOT A BENEFIT. ALLOWANCE HAS BEEN MADE FOR A SILVER (AMALGAM) FILLING.
D23	PORCELAIN CROWNS, IF POSTERIOR TO THE UPPER FIRST MOLAR AND LOWER SECOND BICUSPID, ARE OPTIONAL. BENEFIT IS FOR A FULL GOLD CROWN.
D29	PAYMENT IS PROVIDED FOR CAST RESTORATIONS, PORCELAIN CROWNS AND/OR A PROSTHETIC DEVICE ONCE IN A FIVE YEAR PERIOD.
D30	SPECIALIZED TECHNIQUES, PRECISION ATTACHMENTS, IMPLANTS AND COPINGS ARE NOT COVERED.
D40	AN ALTERNATIVE BENEFIT HAS BEEN PROVIDED BASED ON THE CONTRACT LIMITATION.
D62	PAYMENT IS NOT PROVIDED FOR ORTHODONTIC SERVICES, INCLUDING DIAGNOSIS AND TOOTH GUIDANCE APPLIANCES.
D76	IF PRIMARY INSURANCE DID NOT PAY THE AMOUNT AS SHOWN, PLEASE SUBMIT A COPY OF THEIR EXPLANATION OF BENEFITS FOR REVIEW AND/OR AN ADJUSTMENT.
D81	THE MAXIMUM BENEFIT ALLOWANCE UNDER THE NON-DUPLICATION PROVISION IS OUR NORMAL BENEFIT LESS THE AMOUNT PAYABLE UNDER THE PRIMARY PLAN.
D88	BASED ON CONSULTANT REVIEW, NECESSITY NOT ESTABLISHED. TREATMENT IS CONSIDERED PART OF THE RESTORATION.
D89	BASED ON CONSULTANT REVIEW, BENEFIT IS LIMITED.

EXPLANATION CODES	COMMENTS
D92	PORCELAIN/RESIN ONLAYS ON POSTERIOR TEETH ARE OPTIONAL. BENEFIT IS PROVIDED FOR METALLIC ONLAY.
L25	MAXIMUM BENEFIT HAS BEEN MET FOR THIS BENEFIT YEAR.
L35	ORTHODONTIC LIFETIME MAXIMUM HAS BEEN MET.
Q1	THIS CLAIM HAS PREVIOUSLY BEEN PROCESSED. PLEASE CHECK YOUR RECORDS.
R0	THIS SERVICE IS NOT COVERED.
R1	THE FEE CHARGED EXCEEDS THE MAXIMUM ALLOWANCE.
R5	THE MAXIMUM ALLOWED FOR SERVICES OF THIS TYPE HAS BEEN REACHED.
R6	THE CHARGE EXCEEDS THE DELTA AMOUNT ALLOWED.
R8	THE CHARGE EXCEEDS THE AMOUNT ALLOWED.
S5	TIMELY-FILING NOT MET. CLAIM SUBMITTED AFTER CONTRACT TIME LIMIT.
S6	DEPENDENT IS OVER MAXIMUM AGE.
W1	PROVIDER DISCOUNT HAS BEEN APPLIED.
W6	THE CHARGE EXCEEDS THE AMOUNT ALLOWED.
48B	INFORMATION REQUESTED FROM THE MEMBER ABOUT OTHER INSURANCE COVERAGE HAS NOT BEEN RECEIVED.
74	PLEASE SUBMIT A COPY OF THE PRIMARY CARRIER'S EXPLANATION OF BENEFITS. YOUR CLAIM WILL BE REVIEWED/ADJUSTED WHEN WE RECEIVE THIS INFORMATION.

If you can not find a specific explanation code listed above, or have further questions, please call the Dental Customer Service line at 503-265-5680 (Portland area) or toll-free 1-877-277-7280.

FIGURE 55.2 (continued)
Explanation of codes used in the comment section of the EOB.
Courtesy of Oregon Dental Service (ODS). © 2007

The contract may also exclude certain benefits or services, or it may limit the extent or conditions under which certain services are provided.

Frequencies are the number of times a type of treatment is allowed in a specified time frame. For example, sealants may have a frequency of once in a lifetime for permanent molars. Topical application of fluoride may only be allowed once in a 12-month period. Radiographs often have different frequencies for different types; for instance, the D0210 intraoral complete series (FMX) may only be allowed once every 36 months. (The "D" codes are discussed in the next section.) The D0274 bitewings (four films) can vary and be covered once or twice per 12-month period. It is important for both the patient and dental team to understand each limitation and frequency so that the patient can make an informed decision regarding treatment.

One important factor for a dentist and his or her staff to keep in mind when presenting treatment options to patients is to present the treatment options as the dentist diagnoses them. Some patients want to only have treatments performed that are paid for by their insurance company. For example, some insurance companies may not cover periodontal procedures or will enforce a frequency limitation on them. One procedure that usually has a frequency limitation is D4341 (periodontal scaling and root planing for four or more teeth per quadrant). The insurance company many limit this procedure to once every two years. A patient who is diagnosed to be periodontally involved may need to have the procedure performed once per year. It is the dentist and the staff members' responsibilities to explain the diagnosis and why treatment is in the best interest of the patient regardless of the insurance company's limitations. In this example, if the patient does not have the treatment performed as diagnosed by the dentist, the patient risks further complications with his/her oral health.

Dental Procedure Codes

Dental procedure codes are five-character alphanumeric codes that begin with the letter "D" and identify specific dental procedures. A dental procedure code cannot be changed or abbreviated by any licensee on any printed form or electronic transmission to a dentist, patient, or other recipient. To help ensure accurate recording and reporting of dental treatments, the American Dental Association (ADA) developed these codes, which are known as the Code on Dental Procedures and Nomenclature.

The ADA codes, known as CDT (Current Dental Terminology) codes, are listed in 12 categories of service, each with its own series of five-digit alphanumeric codes. The categories are listed by the type of service being performed; for example, the code for a preventive service such as a routine adult prophylaxis (D1110) is listed within the code series of D1000–D1999. It is important for the dental team to be knowledgeable about each of

these categories. By understanding each category, the dental office is able to submit the correct CDT code for treatment. The 12 categories and their code ranges are shown in Table 55-1.

The CDT codes are periodically reviewed and revised to reflect aggressive changes in dental procedures as they are recognized by dental professionals and those associated with the dental industry. On August 17, 2000, the CDT was named a Health Insurance Portability and Accountability Act (HIPAA) standard code set. This means that any claim submitted on a HIPAA standard electronic dental claim must use dental procedure codes from the version of the CDT in effect on the date of service.

The CDT codes are also used on dental claims submitted on paper, and the ADA maintains a paper claim form whose data content reflects the HIPAA standard electronic dental claim. The current version of the CDT code set has been in effect since January 1, 2007. It is available as the ADA publication titled *CDT 2007/2008*.

What are three different dental code categories?

Processing Claims

As alluded to in the preceding section, dental treatment claims can be filed either manually or electronically. Paper claim forms can be prepared and mailed to the carrier. These forms can be provided by the patient's specific insurance carrier, or the patient or dental office can go directly to the carrier's website (if available) and print the ADA claim form (Figure 55.3). The dental office's dental practice management computer software program may also have the capability to print the form.

Electronic Claim Submission

How an electronic claim form is submitted often depends on the dental practice management software system that the office is using. These systems typically have a specific vendor (clearinghouse) that the system uses for claims submission. Usually instructions for filing the claim electronically will be provided with the dental management software system.

Data that have been stored in the practice management software system are used to generate and submit claims. As a part of claims preparation, the practice management software system checks each claim to ensure the required information is included. The claims are then sent to the clearinghouse and from there on to each insurance carrier. The claims are transferred by use of modem, high-speed Internet, or cable connections. Check with the specific dental management software vendor for fees involved with sending claims electronically.

TABLE 55-1 The ADA's CDT Categories of Service and Five-Digit Alphanumeric Codes

Category of Service	Code Series	Description of Service
Diagnostic	D0100–D0999	Clinical oral evaluations, radiographs/diagnostic imaging, tests and examinations
Preventive	D1000–D1999	Dental prophylaxis, topical fluoride treatment (office procedure), space maintenance (passive appliances), nutritional counseling for control of a dental disease, tobacco counseling for the control and prevention of oral disease, oral hygiene instructions, sealants
Restorative	D2000–D2999	Amalgam restorations, resin-based composite restorations, gold foil restorations, inlay/onlay restorations, crowns (single restoration only), additional restorative services
Endodontics	D3000–D3999	Pulp capping, pulpotomies, endodontic therapy of primary and permanent teeth, endodontic retreatment, apexification/recalcification procedures, apicoectomy/periradicular services, other endodontic services
Periodontics	D4000–D4999	Surgical services (including usual postoperative care), nonsurgical periodontal services, other periodontal services
Prosthodontics, removable	D5000–D5899	Complete and partial dentures treatment including repairs and rebasing, interim prosthesis, other removable prosthetic services
Maxillofacial prosthetics	D5900–D5999	Facial moulage (sectional and complete) and treatment related to prostheses, including surgical stent and radiation carriers
Implant services	D6000–6199	Presurgical and surgical services, implant-supported prosthetics, other implant services
Prosthodontics (fixed)	D6200–6999	Fixed partial denture pontics, fixed partial denture retainers (inlays/onlays, fixed partial denture retainers) crowns (Other fixed partial denture services are found in codes D6920–D6999.)
Oral and maxillofacial surgery	D7000–D7999	Treatment and care related to extractions, alveoloplasty, vestibuloplasty, surgical treatment of lesions, treatment of fractures, repair of traumatic wounds including complicated suturing
Orthodontics	D8000–D8999	Orthodontic treatments and services
Adjunctive general services	D9000–D9999	Unclassified treatment, anesthesia, professional consultation, professional visits, drugs, miscellaneous services

Electronic vendors that are not structured within a practice management software system can also send claims electronically by contracting with a company that provides these services. These types of companies charge fees for filing the claims. It is best to research the different companies and the fees involved before deciding which type of electronic service to use.

A dental office may also wish to send electronic attachments such as periodontal charting, radiographs, narratives regarding a treatment date, or requests from a dental insurance carrier. To send these attachments electronically, the clearinghouse will utilize a third company that has the capability to send attachments. Sending claims electronically benefits the dental office by increasing the rate of claims submission and payment and reducing the paperwork load for the dental team.

Filling Out the ADA Claim Form

Regardless of whether a claim form is sent electronically or manually, in order for it to be processed and paid it is important to ensure that each form has the required infor-

mation. Each of the required information fields or "boxes" is numbered. On the ADA claim form, each of the boxes would be filled out as discussed in Table 55-2. A completed form would look like that shown in Figure 55.4.

Listed next are the general guidelines provided by the ADA regarding the completion of its claim form. The ADA claim form is designed so that the name and address of the third-party payer receiving the claim is visible in a standard #10 window envelope (see Box 3 in Figure 55.4). To place the form in an envelope, the "tick marks" printed in the margin provide reference as to how to properly fold the form.

1. In the upper right-hand corner of the form, a blank space is provided for the convenience of the payer or insurance company that can be used for the assignment of a claim or control number.

2. All boxes in the form must be completed unless it is noted on the form or in the instructions that completion is not required.

3. When a name and address field is required, the full name of an individual or a full business name, address, and zip code must be entered.

Dental Claim Form

HEADER INFORMATION

1. Type of Transaction (Mark all applicable boxes)

☐ Statement of Actual Services - OR - ☐ Request for Predetermination/Preauthorization

☐ EPSDT/Title XIX

2. Predetermination/Preauthorization Number

INSURANCE COMPANY/DENTAL BENEFIT PLAN INFORMATION

3. Company/Plan Name, Address, City, State, Zip Code

OTHER COVERAGE

4. Other Dental or Medical Coverage? ☐ No (Skip 5 - 11) ☐ Yes (Complete 5 - 11)

5. Name of Policyholder/Subscriber in #4 (Last, First, Middle Initial, Suffix)

6. Date of Birth (MM/DD/CCYY)	7. Gender ☐ M ☐ F	8. Policyholder/Subscriber ID (SSN# or ID#)

9. Plan/Group Number

10. Patient's Relationship to Person Named in #5 ☐ Self ☐ Spouse ☐ Dependent ☐ Other

11. Other Insurance Company/Dental Benefit Plan Name, Address, City, State, Zip Code

POLICYHOLDER/SUBSCRIBER INFORMATION (For Insurance Company Named in #3)

12. Policyholder/Subscriber Name (Last, First Middle Initial, Suffix, Address, City, State, Zip Code

13. Date of Birth (MM/DD/CCYY)	14. Gender ☐ M ☐ F	15. Policyholder/Subscriber ID(SSN# or ID#)

16. Plan/Group Number	17. Employer Name

PATIENT INFORMATION

18. Relationship to Policyholder/Subscriber in #12 Above ☐ Self ☐ Spouse ☐ Dependent Child ☐ Other

19. Student Status ☐ FTS ☐ PTS

20. Name (Last, First, Middle Initial, Suffix), Address, City, State, Zip Code

21. Date of Birth (MM/DD/CCYY)	22. Gender ☐ M ☐ F	23.Patient ID/Account# (Assigned by Dentist)

RECORD OF SERVICES PROVIDED

	24. Procedure Date (MM/DD/CCYY)	25.Area of Oral Cavity	26. Tooth System	27. Tooth Number(s) or Letter(s)	28. Tooth Surface	29. Procedure Code	30. Description	31. Fee
1								
2								
3								
4								
5								
6								
7								
8								
9								
10								

MISSING TEETH INFORMATION

34. (Place an 'X' on each missing tooth)

	Permanent																Primary										32. Other Fee(s)
	1	2	3	4	5	6	7	8	9	10	11	12	13	14	15	16	A	B	C	D	E	F	G	H	I	J	
	32	31	30	29	28	27	26	25	24	23	22	21	20	19	18	17	T	S	R	Q	P	O	N	M	L	K	33.Total Fee

35. Remarks

AUTHORIZATIONS

36. I have been informed of the treatment plan and associated fees. I agree to be responsible for all charges for dental services and materials not paid by my dental benefit plan, unless prohibited by law, or the treating dentist or dental practice has a contractual agreement with my plan prohibiting all or a portion of such charges. To the extent permitted by law, I consent to your use and disclosure of my protected health information to carry out payment activities in connection with this claim.

X _____

Patient/Guardian signature   Date

37. I hereby authorize and direct payment of the dental benefits otherwise payable to me, directly to the below named dentist or dental entity.

X _____

Subscriber signature   Date

ANCILLARY CLAIM/TREATMENT INFORMATION

38. Place of Treatment ☐ Provider's Office ☐ Hospital ☐ ECF ☐ Other

39. Number of Enclosures (00 to 99) Radiograph(s) Oral Image(s) Model(s)

40. Is Treatment for Orthodontics? ☐ No (Skip 41 - 42) ☐ Yes (Complete 41 - 42)

41. Date Appliance Placed (MM/DD/CCYY)

42. Months of Treatment Remaining

43. Replacement of Prosthesis? ☐ No ☐ Yes (Complete 44)

44. Date Prior Placement (MM/DD/CCYY)

45. Treatment Resulting from ☐ Occupational Illness/Injury ☐ Auto Accident ☐ Other Accident

46. Date of Accident (MM/DD/CCYY)

47. Auto Accident State

BILLING DENTIST OR DENTAL ENTITY (Leave blank if dentist or dental entity is not submitting claim on behalf of the patient or insured/subscriber)

48. Name, Address, City, State, Zip code

49. NPI	50. License Number	51. SSN or TIN

52. Phone Number	52A. Additional Provider ID

TREATING DENTIST AND TREATMENT LOCATION INFORMATION

53. I hereby certify that the procedures as indicated by date are in progress (for procedures that require multiple visits) or have been completed.

X _____

Date

54. NPI	55. License Number

56. Address, City, State, Zip Code	56A. Provider Specialty Code

57. Phone Number	58. Additional Provider ID

© 2006 American Dental Association, © MDC Systems & Services, Inc. / DentalMate, 2007

FIGURE 55.3

ADA claim form.

Courtesy of Dr. Angela Osborn

TABLE 55-2 Information Required on the ADA Claim Form

Header Information

Box 1	Type of Transaction: Statement of Actual Services, Request for Predetermination/Preauthorization, or EPSDT/Title XIX
Box 2	Predetermination/Preauthorization Number

Insurance Company/Dental Benefit Plan Information

Box 3	Primary insurance company (payer) information (Name, Address, City, State, Zip Code)
Box 4	Other Dental or Medical Coverage (This would be completed if the subscriber had a secondary insurance carrier.)
Box 5	Name of Policyholder/Subscriber in Box #4 (Last, First, Middle Initial, Suffix)
Box 6	Subscriber Date of Birth
Box 7	Subscriber Gender
Box 8	Subscriber Identifier (Social Security # or ID #)
Box 9	Plan/Group Number (number that identifies the employer with the insurance company)
Box 10	Patient's Relationship to Person Named in Box #5
Box 11	Other Insurance Company/Dental Benefit Plan Name, Address, City, State, Zip Code (This would be completed with the secondary carrier's information.)

Policyholder/Subscriber Information

Box 12	Policyholder/Subscriber Name (Last, First, Middle Initial, Suffix), Address, City, State, Zip Code
Box 13	Date of Birth (MM/DD/CCYY)
Box 14	Gender
Box 15	Policyholder Subscriber ID (SSN or ID#)
Box 16	Plan/Group Number
Box 17	Employer Name

Patient Information

Box 18	Relationship to Policyholder/Subscriber in #12 Above: Self, Spouse, Dependent Child, or Other
Box 19	Student Status: FTS (full time) or PTS (part time)
Box 20	Name (Last, First, Middle Initial, Suffix), Address, City, State, Zip Code
Box 21	Patient Date of Birth (MM/DD, CCYY)
Box 22	Patient Gender
Box 23	Patient ID/Account # (Assigned by Dentist)

Record of Services Provided

Box 24	Procedure Date (MM/DD/CCYY)
Box 25	Area of Oral Cavity (a two-digit numeric system used to report regions of the oral cavity to third-party payers)
Box 26	Tooth Systems [The ADA recognizes two major systems used for numbering teeth. The Universal/National System is used primarily in the United States, and the International Standards Organization System is used in most other countries. The Universal/National System for permanent (adult) dentition includes teeth numbers 1–32. Tooth number 1 is the patient's upper right third molar and follows around the upper arch to the upper left third molar. Tooth number 17 follows around the lower arch to the lower right third molar number 32. The Universal/National System order for primary (baby) dentition is the same as that of the permanent dentition; however, the primary teeth are designated by uppercase letters A through T, with A being the patient's upper right second primary molar and T being the lower right second primary molar.]
Box 27	Tooth Number(s) or Letter(s)
Box 28	Tooth Surface [the area (surface) of the tooth that applies for the specific procedure performed on the date of service listed]
Box 29	Procedure Code (the assigned CDT code for the performed procedure for the listed date of service)
Box 30	Description (a brief explanation of the procedure performed for the listed date of service)
Box 31	Fee (the fee assigned by the provider dentist)
Box 32	Other Fee(s)
Box 33	Total Fee (Add amounts from Boxes 31 and 32.)
Box 34	Missing Teeth Information (List any teeth missing for the patient on whom the procedure is being performed.)
Box 35	Remarks (Write specifics regarding the procedures performed for the listed date of service.)

(continued)

TABLE 55-2 Information Required on the ADA Claim Form *(continued)*

Authorizations

Box 36	Patient responsibility: The patient or guardian has to sign/give authorization that he or she will be responsible for payment of all charges associated with the procedures performed that are not covered by their dental benefit plan (insurance company). The patient and/or guardian consents (authorizes) for the use of protected health information to carry out payment activities in connection with the claim. Once the patient's signature is on file this can be used.
Box 37	Authorization of Payment: The subscriber authorizes direct payment of the dental benefits to be paid to the named dentist or dental entity.

Ancillary Claim/Treatment Information

Box 38	Place of Treatment: Provider's Office, Hospital, ECF (Extended Care Facility), or Other
Box 39	Number of Enclosures (00 to 99): Radiograph(s), Oral Images, and/or Model(s) (This is where the provider's office lists what is enclosed with the claim. Some procedures require radiographs, oral images, or models.)
Box 40	Is Treatment for Orthodontics? (If no, skip Boxes 41 and 42. If yes, complete Boxes 41 and 42.)
Box 41	Date Appliance Placed (MM/DD/YY)
Box 42	Months of Treatment Remaining
Box 43	Replacement of Prosthesis? (If prosthesis such as a crown or denture is being replaced, the insurance company has to know if it is a replacement.)
Box 44	Date of Prior Placement (MM/DD/YY) (If the prosthesis is being replaced, the insurance company has to have a record of the date the initial prosthesis was placed.)
Box 45	Treatment Resulting from: Occupational Illness/Injury, Auto Accident, or Other Accident
Box 46	Date of Accident (MM/DD/YY) (If prosthesis is being placed due to an accident, the insurance company has to have a record of the date of the accident.)
Box 47	Auto Accident State (If the prosthesis is being placed due to an auto accident, the state in which the accident took place must be listed.)

Billing Dentist or Dental Entity

Box 48	Billing Dentist or Dental Entity's Name, Address, City, State, Zip Code
Box 49	**National Provider Identifier (NPI)** Number (a standard unique identifier)
Box 50	License Number (dentist's state license number)
Box 51	SSN or TIN (billing dentist's Social Security number or federal tax identifier number)
Box 52	Phone Number (of billing dentist)
Box 52A	Additional Provider ID (These numbers are unique to a specific insurance company and the billing dentist.)

Treating Dentist and Treatment Location Information

Box 53	Signature: The treating dentist's signature is required in this box. The treating dentist may be different than the billing dentist. For example, when a dentist is an employee of a larger dental entity that is owned by another dentist, the dentist who actually performs the treatment is the treating dentist, and the dentist who owns the dental entity would be considered the billing dentist.
Box 54	NPI Number (of treating dentist)
Box 55	License Number (of treating dentist)
Box 56	Address, City, State, Zip Code (of treating dentist)
Box 56A	Provider Specialty Code (of treating dentist. A provider specialty code is assigned to each type of dental specialty, for example, oral surgeon, endodontist, orthodontist.)
Box 57	Phone Number (of treating dentist)
Box 58	Additional Provider ID (of treating dentist)

4. All dates must be written in a four-digit year format (20xx).
5. If the number of procedures reported exceeds the number of lines available on one claim form, the remaining procedures must be listed on a separate, fully completed form.

When a claim is being submitted to the secondary carrier, complete the form in its entirety and attach the primary carrier's EOB showing the amount paid by the primary carrier. The amount the primary carrier paid can be noted in the "Remarks" field (see Box 35 in Figure 55.4).

Dental Claim Form

HEADER INFORMATION

1. Type of Transaction (Mark all applicable boxes)

[✔] Statement of Actual Services - OR - [ ] Request for Predetermination/Preauthorization

[ ] EPSDT/Title XIX

2. Predetermination/Preauthorization Number

INSURANCE COMPANY/DENTAL BENEFIT PLAN INFORMATION

3. Company/Plan Name, Address, City, State, Zip Code

Delta Dental Co
P.O. Box 173803
Denver, CO 80217-3803

OTHER COVERAGE

4. Other Dental or Medical Coverage? [✔] No (Skip 5 - 11) [ ] Yes (Complete 5 - 11)

5. Name of Policyholder/Subscriber in #4 (Last, First, Middle Initial, Suffix)

6. Date of Birth (MM/DD/CCYY)	7. Gender	8. Policyholder/Subscriber ID (SSN# or ID#)
	[ ] M [ ] F	

9. Plan/Group Number

10. Patient's Relationship to Person Named in #5

[ ] Self [ ] Spouse [ ] Dependent [ ] Other

11. Other Insurance Company/Dental Benefit Plan Name, Address, City, State, Zip Code

POLICYHOLDER/SUBSCRIBER INFORMATION (For Insurance Company Named in #3)

12. Policyholder/Subscriber Name (Last, First Middle Initial, Suffix, Address, City, State, Zip Code

Doe, John J
12121 S. Beautiful St.
Lone Tree, CO 80124

13. Date of Birth (MM/DD/CCYY)	14. Gender	15. Policyholder/Subscriber ID (SSN# or ID#)
01/01/1968	[✔] M [ ] F	**332-33-3333**

16. Plan/Group Number	17. Employer Name
2222	**Stellar Marketing**

PATIENT INFORMATION

18. Relationship to Policyholder/Subscriber in #12 Above

[✔] Self [ ] Spouse [ ] Dependent Child [ ] Other

19. Student Status [ ] FTS [ ] PTS

20. Name (Last, First, Middle Initial, Suffix), Address, City, State, Zip Code

Doe, John J
12121 S. Beautiful St.
Lone Tree, CO 80124

21. Date of Birth (MM/DD/CCYY)	22. Gender	23. Patient ID/Account# (Assigned by Dentist)
01/01/1968	[✔] M [ ] F	**001755 0000006592**

RECORD OF SERVICES PROVIDED

	24. Procedure Date (MM/DD/CCYY)	25. Area of Oral Cavity	26. Tooth System	27. Tooth Number(s) or Letter(s)	28. Tooth Surface	29. Procedure Code	30. Description	31. Fee
1	08/21/2007	30	JP	30		D2950	Core Buildup, Including Any Pins	298.00
2	08/21/2007	30	JP	30		D2740	Crown-Porcelain/Ceramic Substrate	1081.00
3	08/21/2007	31	JP	31		D2950	Core Buildup, Including Any Pins	298.00
4	08/21/2007	31	JP	31		D2740	Crown-Porcelain/Ceramic Substrate	1081.00
5								
6								
7								
8								
9								
0								

MISSING TEETH INFORMATION

34. (Place an 'X' on each missing tooth)

Permanent																Primary									
1	2	3	4	5	6	7	8	9	10	11	12	13	14	15	16	A	B	C	D	E	F	G	H	I	J
32	31	30	29	28	27	26	25	24	23	22	21	20	19	18	17	T	S	R	Q	P	O	N	M	L	K

32. Other Fee(s)

33. Total Fee **2758.00**

35. Remarks

AUTHORIZATIONS

36. I have been informed of the treatment plan and associated fees. I agree to be responsible for all charges for dental services and materials not paid by my dental benefit plan, unless prohibited by law, or the treating dentist or dental practice has a contractual agreement with my plan prohibiting all or a portion of such charges. To the extent permitted by law, I consent to your use and disclosure of my protected health information to carry out payment activities in connection with this claim.

X **Signature On File**   **08/21/2007**
Patient/Guardian signature   Date

37. I hereby authorize and direct payment of the dental benefits otherwise payable to me, directly to the below named dentist or dental entity.

X **Signature On File**   **08/21/2007**
Subscriber signature   Date

BILLING DENTIST OR DENTAL ENTITY (Leave blank if dentist or dental entity is not submitting claim on behalf of the patient or insured/subscriber)

48. Name, Address, City, State, Zip code

Angela Osborn
9218 Kimmer Dr. Suite 106
Lone Tree, CO 80124

49. NPI	50. License Number	51. SSN or TIN
1578678637	7647	84-1580153

52. Phone Number	52A. Additional Provider ID
(303) 799-9993	

ANCILLARY CLAIM/TREATMENT INFORMATION

38. Place of Treatment

[✔] Provider's Office [ ] Hospital [ ] ECF [ ] Other

39. Number of Enclosures (00 to 99) Radiograph(s) Oral Image(s) Model(s)

40. Is Treatment for Orthodontics?

[✔] No (Skip 41 - 42) [ ] Yes (Complete 41 - 42)

41. Date Appliance Placed (MM/DD/CCYY)

42. Months of Treatment Remaining

43. Replacement of Prosthesis? [✔] No [ ] Yes (Complete 44)

44. Date Prior Placement (MM/DD/CCYY)

45. Treatment Resulting from

[ ] Occupational Illness/Injury [ ] Auto Accident [ ] Other Accident

46. Date of Accident (MM/DD/CCYY)

47. Auto Accident State

TREATING DENTIST AND TREATMENT LOCATION INFORMATION

53. I hereby certify that the procedures as indicated by date are in progress (for procedures that require multiple visits) or have been completed.

X *Angela Osborn*   **08/21/2007**
Signed (Angela Osborn)   Date

54. NPI	55. License Number
1578678637	7647

56. Address, City, State, Zip Code	56A. Provider Specialty Code
9218 Kimmer Dr. Suite 106 **Lone Tree, CO 80124-6733**	1223G0001X

57. Phone Number	58. Additional Provider ID
(303) 799-9993	

© 2006 American Dental Association, © MDC Systems & Services, Inc. / DentalMate, 2007

FIGURE 55.4
Completed ADA claim form.
Courtesy of Dr. Angela Osborn

Provider Identifiers

When submitting dental claims, a dental office or entity has specific numbers that are assigned to them. The Provider Specialty Code box refers to the type of dental professional who delivered the treatment (see Box 56A in Figure 55.4). Codes that can be used to describe the treating dentist can be found within the CDT book or on the Internet.

Clean Claims

In order for an insurance claim to be processed within the insurance companies' allowed time frame (generally 30 days), the claim has to be considered a "clean claim" by the insurance processing center. This means that all of the required fields on the claim form have been completed correctly. When a claim form is submitted correctly, payment can be made to the dentist and eliminates delayed payments and further work for the office staff.

Filling Out the Patient Registration Form

Dental claims contain confidential patient information. To submit a claim, the dental provider must have permission to release this confidential information. The provider obtains this permission via a "signature on file." The patient registration form (Figure 55.5) has signature boxes similar to those listed on the ADA claim form (see Boxes 36 and 37 in Figure 55.4). The patient is required to sign these boxes when completing the registration form. These signatures are required to be kept on file. When submitting claims electronically, there is no need to get the patient's permission for the release of the confidential information because the "signature on file" acts as a release. The person filling out the claim merely types "Signature on File" in the spaces provided in Boxes 36 and 37.

HIPAA and Electronic Transactions

HIPAA is a federal law that requires all health plans, health care clearinghouses, and any dentist who transmits health information in an electronic transaction to use a standard format and the ADA procedure codes.

Paper transactions sent by providers are not subject to this requirement.

Under HIPAA, the Department of Health and Human Services implemented transaction standards to protect the integrity of and advocate the standardization of electronic claims submissions. The goal of the program is to allow one standardized format for each specific transaction, with a standard set of codes. By doing this, electronic data transmissions are more efficient, which results in a cost savings for health care providers. For dentistry, the CDT codes are used to simplify transaction processing. Dental offices that do not file electronically must comply with the privacy rule and with the other aspects of administrative simplification that address security standards.

Management of Claims

The accurate maintaining of a dental office's accounts receivable is dependent on efficiently managing the insurance claims that are processed through the office. Most dental offices have a system in which they track claims. One of the more efficient ways of managing claims is to use a dental management software system. Various reports are typically available through most dental office

Legal and Ethical Issue

Most dental offices use their patients' personal information for a number of reasons, such as to call a patient's place of business or home to confirm scheduled appointments, to send electronic insurance claims via the Internet, and to relate various types of information to a dental laboratory. In order for an office to release this type of information, each patient must sign a HIPAA form. HIPAA helps ensure that all medical records, medical billing, and patient accounts meet certain consistent standards with regard to documentation, handling, and privacy. In addition, HIPAA requires that all patients be able to access their own medical records, correct errors or omissions, and be informed about how personal information is shared. Another provision involves notifying patients about an office's privacy procedures.

Statement of Financial Responsibility: I, _____ do hereby agree to pay all medical charges incurred by the above listed patient. I further understand that these charges are my responsibility, regardless of insurance coverage.

Responsible Person's Signature: _____

FIGURE 55.5
Signature area on patient registration form.

management software programs. These reports are essential in the monitoring of specifics such as:

- Claims that have been submitted for predetermination but have not been returned
- Claims that have been submitted for completed treatments, requesting payment, but have not been paid
- Claims that have been returned requesting further information from the carrier. These are considered to be pending

How do you determine benefits for a specific treatment plan prior to the date of service?

Insurance Fraud

Dental fraud is any crime in which an individual receives insurance money for filing a false claim, inflating a claim, or billing for services not rendered. Dental fraud takes many forms. Examples include:

- Billing for services not provided.
- Reporting a higher level of dental service than was actually performed. This is often called **upcoding**.
- Submitting a dental claim under one patient's name when services were actually provided to another person.
- Altering claim forms and dental records.
- Filing for noncovered services as if they were covered services.
- Changing the date of service on a claim form so it falls within a patient's benefit period.

- Routine waiving of a patient's copayment or deductible, if applicable.
- Performing services that are not suitable or necessary.

Fraud is sometimes called the "hidden crime" because many people do not even know it is occurring. Subscribers, sponsors, family members, and dentists are in a good position to detect and report possible fraud. The dentist's review of the claim form, prior to submission, and the subscriber's review of the dental insurance EOB form help to ensure that the information is accurate and truthful. Facts to confirm include the:

- type and number of services provided,
- date(s) of service,
- type of services reported, and
- amount collected from the patient as a deductible or copayment.

Most dental offices assign a staff member to ensure accurate and honest claims submission. It is important for the dental team to understand the consequences of submitting fraudulent claims.

Preparing for Externship

When starting your externship, someone from the dental office should give you a detailed tour of the insurance practices used in the office. Review what your duties are going to be and always ask questions. It is best to ask and be right. Do not let a patient leave with an answer you are unsure of. If you give a patient a wrong answer, you may create additional work for other team members and will appear unprofessional to the patient.

◉ SUMMARY

Dental insurance is designed to assist individuals by offsetting the costs of dental services. A dental office relies on its staff members to be comfortable with all aspects of providing dental services, which may include understanding dental insurance plans. The dental assistant can be a strong asset to the dental team if he or she is knowledgeable about dental insurance and its guidelines. When

the dental assistant is able to explain and educate the patient about dental insurance structures and benefits, the patient is better able to make decisions about proposed treatments. A dental assistant should follow the dental insurance policies set forth by the employer. Each dental office has its own set of polices and rules regarding dental insurance practices.

◉ KEY TERMS

- **Allowable charges:** The maximum dollar amount on which a benefit payment is based for each dental procedure. p. 888
- **Benefit:** The amount payable by a third party toward the cost of various covered dental services or the dental service or procedure covered by the plan. p. 888

- **Copay:** A cost-sharing arrangement in which the insurance patient/subscriber pays a specified charge at the time of service. p. 886
- **Deductible:** The amount of money the patient/subscriber must pay as part of the insurance plan. p. 885

KEY TERMS (continued)

- **Exclusive provider organization (EPO) plan:** Closed panel plan that allows a particular group of insurance subscribers to receive dental care only from participating dentists (i.e., exclusive providers).   p. 886

- **Explanation of benefits (EOB):** Document that details how a claim was processed and indicates the portion of the claim paid to the dentist and the portion of the claim, if any, the insurance subscriber needs to pay. An EOB is not a bill.   p. 889

- **Managed care:** Refers to a cost containment system that directs the utilization of health benefits by (a) restricting the type, level, and frequency of treatment; (b) limiting access to care; and (c) controlling the level of reimbursement for services.   p. 886

- **National Provider Identifier (NPI):** An identifier assigned by the federal government to all providers considered to be HIPAA-covered entities.   p. 896

- **Preferred provider organization (PPO) plan:** An insurance plan in which a purchaser of dental benefits receives services from certain dentists (i.e., preferred providers) who provide those services at specified rates that have been agreed on with the insurance company.   p. 886

- **Upcoding:** Reporting a higher level of dental service than was actually performed.   p. 899

- **Waiting period:** Period between employment or enrollment in a dental plan and the date when a covered person becomes eligible for benefits. Services subject to a waiting period could include any services related to placing crowns, bridges, or orthodontics. p. 888

CHECK YOUR UNDERSTANDING

1. What is the definition of a claim form?
   a. the amount payable by a third party toward the cost of treatment
   b. the measure of quality of care provided in a particular setting
   c. the form used to file for benefits under a dental benefit program; includes sections for the patient and the dentist to complete
   d. none of the above

2. How is the birthday rule established?
   a. by asking the insurance company how many children the subscriber has
   b. by determining which parent's birthday month and day (not year) falls earlier in the calendar year
   c. by sending the claim and letting the insurance company decide
   d. none of the above

3. Which of the following procedures is considered to fall under an insurance company's limitations and frequencies?
   a. radiographs
   b. application of fluoride
   c. sealants
   d. all of the above

4. If a subscriber is terminated from employment, what is the name of the continuation of insurance program?
   a. continued coverage act
   b. family reimbursement plan
   c. COBRA
   d. none of the above

5. What method of claim submission is not sent by mail?
   a. electronic
   b. fax
   c. phone
   d. none of the above

6. When was HIPAA created?
   a. 1888
   b. 1995
   c. 1996
   d. 2003

7. Which of the following would not be a standard source of claim submissions?
   a. by mail
   b. electronically
   c. by e-mail
   d. none of the above

8. What procedure category does a composite resin fall under?
   a. Diagnostic (D0100–D0999)
   b. Restorative (D2000–D2999)
   c. Prosthodontics, fixed (D6200–D6999)
   d. Oral Surgery (D7000–D7999)

9. What procedure category would an implant crown fall under?
   a. Diagnostic (D0100–D0999)
   b. Restorative (D2000–D2999)
   c. Adjunctive General Services (D9000–D9999)
   d. none of the above

CHECK YOUR UNDERSTANDING (continued)

10. What is the definition of a waiting period?
    a. period between employment or enrollment in a dental plan and the date when a covered person becomes eligible for benefits
    b. time when the dentist can see the patient for an appointment
    c. annual period in which employees can select from a choice of benefit programs
    d. none of the above

INTERNET ACTIVITIES

- To learn about the importance of using one's dental insurance before the end of the year go to http://dentistry.about.com/od/dentalcosts/tp/endofyear.htm. Note the importance of using the allowed yearly maximum.

- Go to www.deltadentalwa.com/pdfs/wdsuse.pdf and print the ADA claim form.

WEB REFERENCES

- American Dental Association www.ada.org
- Delta Dental of Colorado www.deltadentalco.com
- Humana Dental www.humanadental.com

56

Marketing Your Skills

Chapter Outline

- Professional Career Goals and Opportunities
  —Career Opportunities

- Locating Employment Opportunities
  —Newspaper Advertisements
  —School Placement Offices
  —Employment/Temporary Agencies
  —Internet Sources
  —Professional Organizations
  —Networking
  —Telephone Book

- The Résumé and Cover Letter
  —The Résumé
  —The Cover Letter

- The Interview and Follow-Up

- Employment Negotiations
  —Salary and Benefits
  —Letter of Agreement or Employee Contract

- Rights as an Employee
  —Americans with Disabilities Act
  —Family and Medical Leave Act

- Advancing Your Career
  —The Importance of Attitude and Healthy Living

Learning Objectives

After reading this chapter, the student should be able to:

- Identify the different career paths in the dental field.

- Explain the parts of a résumé.

- Develop a résumé and a cover letter.

- Explain how to prepare for an interview.

- Discuss employment negotiations for salary and benefits.

- Understand the rights of employees.

Preparing for Certification Exams

- Communicate effectively when interviewing for employment.
- Establish and maintain an up-to-date résumé and cover letter.
- Understand the Federal Equal Opportunity Employment Act.

Key Terms

Americans with Disabilities Act (ADA)

Cover letter

Family and Medical Leave Act (FMLA)

Federal equal opportunity and employment laws

Résumé

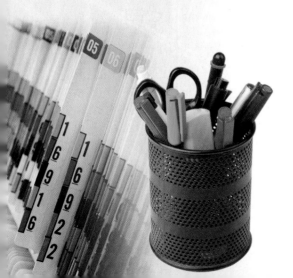

As you enter the field of dentistry as a new dental assistant, it is important to know how to locate jobs in the dental field and how to market your skills. This chapter discusses various career opportunities available to dental assistants, how to write a résumé that "speaks" success, and the proper demeanor to convey during a job interview. Rights as an employee and career advancement tips for the future are also presented.

Professional Career Goals and Opportunities

Before searching for career opportunities, you should first establish your goals. When determining your goals, it is important to look at both short-term and long-term goals. When setting goals, a few self-assessment questions should be answered:

- "Do I have the commitment it takes to work in the dental field?"
- "What are the challenges ahead?"

Answers to these questions can help you set your goals.

Another important area to assess is that of your skills. Some traits and characteristics are important for dental assistants to achieve. Taking the time to create a list of personal characteristics and traits and indicating where improvement must be achieved is an important activity. This activity will help you gain a more realistic view of what skills are currently held and what areas of weaknesses must be overcome. Desired traits and characteristics of a dental assistant include the ability to be:

- Prompt
- Motivated
- Self-starter
- Flexible
- Enthusiastic
- Compassionate
- Honest

Dental Assistant   PROFESSIONAL TIP

Educate patients about the profession of dentistry. The credentials of each member of the dental team should be proudly displayed in the dental office. Patients want to feel confident and comfortable with the professionals they have chosen to take care of their dental health.

Life Span Considerations

The future of dental assisting is growing at a rapid rate. As new skills are learned and experience gained, it is advantageous to document this information and continually update your résumé. Opportunities abound for good, highly qualified dental assistants.

- Humorous
- Good listener
- Technically skillful
- Dedicated/loyal
- Hard worker

Once the self-assessment is complete, it is time to set goals. Setting goals is typically easy—what is harder is accomplishing them. Many people fail at this because they fail to make a commitment to the goals they have set. When goals are defined they should be measurable, specific, and clear. An example would be "I will lose five pounds this month." An unclear goal statement may sound like this: "I will lose weight this week." The first statement is more specific and measurable. The second statement is vague, which means it may be harder to reach that particular goal.

Determining one's career philosophy is just as important as goal setting. During the job search, the dental assistant can spend time researching various organizations and the goals that each organization promotes. It is important to be sure that an organization's goals and philosophy fit well with the dental assistant's own goals and philosophy. The dental assistant should ask questions such as "Are my professional, social, and moral values compatible with this organization?" "How important are the office hours?" and "Is my moral philosophy compatible with the dental office's philosophy?"

Many dental assistants understandably take the first job that is offered to them without thinking about their own goals and philosophy. Instead, the dental assistant should examine his or her own professional career goals and then tie these goals into the many career opportunities available as a dental health care worker.

Career Opportunities

Dental assistants have a wide range of choices available to them now and in the future. Many of these opportunities open doors for future opportunities. The following subsections cover the many career opportunities available in the field of dental assisting.

Private Practice Offices

The dental assistant may seek employment with a solo dental office or group practice. The solo practice has only one dentist. The group practice may employ two or more dentists who offer many different services to their patients such as restorative and preventive procedures, endodontics, periodontics, prosthodontics, surgery, and orthodontics. Specialty offices focus on one area. Whichever practice is chosen, the dental assistant will be given many opportunities to work with the dentist and patients as well as to learn other duties.

Public Health Facilities

Public health dentistry involves working in clinics and schools that focus on preventing dental problems among the community. Dental assistants are employed in organizations that provide dental services at no cost to the patients. These programs are often funded by local and federal governments.

Hospital Dental Clinics

Dental assistants can work in hospitals in several different capacities. Some patients require general anesthesia to complete dental treatment. Either the dental assistant follows his or her dentist to the operating room or a dental assistant is hired directly by the hospital to work with the dentist. Working in hospital dentistry may require the assistant to assist in the treatment of patients who are confined to bed and providing preventive care.

Dental Schools

Dental schools hire assistants to assist individuals who are studying to be dentists. This type of setting provides the dental assistant with experience doing four-handed dentistry and assisting dentists with other patient care issues.

Educational Facilities

Community colleges, career schools, and technical schools hire experienced dental assistants to teach others to become dental assistants. This challenging, yet rewarding opportunity may require a bachelor's degree or higher. If you are interested in teaching, inquire at the particular school you would like to work at for further information. The requirements for teachers vary by state, and the American Dental Association (ADA) has specific requirements for teaching in an accredited program, including Dental Assisting National Board (DANB) certification. The ADA website (www.ada.org) contains more specifics for the dental assistant.

Consulting Industry

Experienced dental assistants may offer practice management concepts and skills to new or existing dental practices. They may have their own business or join a consulting firm. Topics covered by a consultant include ways to improve communication, productivity, and employee satisfaction. Practice management skills are necessary to take advantage of this opportunity.

Sales Industry

A person with the technical skills may also be able to sell dental products. Because the dental assistant can talk the dental language, he or she may be the best person for a dental product salesperson job. The experience gained through hands-on training, formal education, and experience will help sell products.

Insurance Industry

Insurance companies hire dental assistants to process dental claims. It helps to have a grasp of the Current Dental Terminology (CDT) codes when working in this capacity. If the dental assistant is seeking career expansion, working for an insurance company combines knowledge of dental procedures and terminology with the business aspect. This can lead to a rewarding and very different career as a dental assistant.

Forensics/Research Laboratories

Research laboratories in hospitals or medical centers look for experienced, knowledgeable dental assistants to work in research and possible forensic roles. The dental assistant is responsible for researching and documenting a variety of data. In the forensic field, the dental assistant's job is to assist the forensic dentist in charting and exposing radiographs on deceased individuals for the purpose of identification.

It is important for dental assistants to be aware of the many opportunities available to them. It is also critical to know how and where to find these opportunities.

What are some desirable traits of a dental assistant?

Locating Employment Opportunities

Jobs in dental assisting are increasing. According to the U.S. Department of Labor, compared to other occupations, dental assisting is projected to grow much faster through the year 2012. One of the reasons for this growth is that jobs in dental assisting will become available due to the expansion in the field of dentistry and the need to replace transferring assistants or retiring assistants.

Once dental assistants have determined which type of job they want to seek, it is important to learn about the many employment sources that can be used to find the right job position. As discussed in the following sections, places to seek out jobs include newspaper advertisements, school placement offices, employment or temporary agencies, Internet sources, professional organizations, word of mouth through networking, and the telephone book.

Newspaper Advertisements

The local newspaper is a good source of employment information. Dentists place advertisements in the classified section of the newspaper describing the positions they have available. Many newspapers post their classified ads sections online (Figure 56.1). To protect the privacy of the office, the dentist may list only a phone or fax number. The dental assistant should have a résumé and cover letter already prepared so that it is ready for faxing to prospective employers as jobs become available.

School Placement Offices

Dental offices often contact dental assisting schools when they are looking for new employees. Schools that offer dental assisting programs typically maintain a list of dentists that participate in the school's externship program and are interested in hiring new graduates. Students should make use of this valuable service. If attending a formal dental assisting school, this service is usually provided at no extra cost.

Employment/Temporary Agencies

Employment agencies are an ideal way to start a career for those individuals who want more experience prior to seeking a permanent position and for those who just want part-time employment. Once the résumé is complete, the dental assistant should send it to one of the local temporary agencies and then remain in touch with the agency on a consistent basis until placement is achieved. These agencies also help in finding full-time employment for the dental assistant.

Internet Sources

Many Web-based employment services are available. Most require posting of a résumé on their website. This may not be the best way to search for a job; however, it is an option that should not be ignored. One job site for dental health care workers called Dentalworkers.com assists with job searches. This site allows dental assistants to register, post a résumé, and search for job openings in their local area. Other online job search sites include Monster.com and Careerbuilders.com.

Professional Organizations

Dental assistant organizations and local dental societies often post employment opportunities. Membership is not always required to search for employment; however, membership is a good way to expand your career and network with people who are in the same field. Organizations that would be useful for the dental assistant to join include:

- American Dental Assistants Association (ADAA)
- Local dental assistant associations
- American Dental Association (ADA)
- Organization for Safety and Asepsis (OSAP)

Dental Assistant: Assoc. in Family Dentistry

Job ID	7703098
Company Name	Assoc. in Family Dentistry
Job Category	Healthcare
Location	Aurora, CO
Position Type	Full - Time, Employee
Salary	Unspecified
Experience	2 - 5 Years Experience
Desired Education Level	Associates
Date Posted	July 4, xxxx

DENTAL ASSISTANT

F/T, Busy office. Must be able to work incl. Eves & Sat hrs. Must be prof'l & positive. Salary commensurate with exp. Please Apply in person at: Assoc. in Family Dentistry, 15425 East Iliff Ave., Aurora, CO 80013; Fax Resume: 303-750-4637.

FIGURE 56.1
Sample job advertisement from a newspaper's online classified ads section.

Networking

Networking is meeting people and gaining job information through "word of mouth." A simple conversation at church or an event can provide the dental assistant with information on job availability. For example, your neighbor's dentist may have mentioned that she is expanding her office and is looking to hire extra assistants. That information is revealed to you through your neighbor. The result of this encounter may lead to an employment opportunity.

Telephone Book

The telephone book is another valuable resource for job opportunities. Obviously, this should not be the only method used to seek employment, but it does have some success. The prospective employee can search the telephone book for local dental offices in the area and fax, mail, or personally deliver his or her résumé to the offices. Sometimes dentists do not always advertise, so contacting them personally may lead the dental assistant to the perfect job.

The use of multiple sources when looking for a job results in maximum success. Some sources have higher success rates than others, so do not stick to just one method. Employment odds are increased if the dental assistant diversifies his or her options. It may take a little work, but it is well worth the effort. Before beginning the search, the dental assistant must have a résumé that will highlight skills and make him or her marketable.

What are some sources a dental assistant should use to search for employment?

The Résumé and Cover Letter

The term **résumé** refers to a summary of one's work experience and qualifications. A **cover letter** introduces the potential employee and provides a brief summary of why the individual is the right person for the job. Both of these documents should be printed on quality paper, usually white, off-white, or light gray.

These documents can be created using a word processing program. Several word processing programs provide résumé templates that allow you to create a professional, attractive résumé. The dental assistant may need to proofread and edit the résumé several times before it is ready to be sent to potential employers. Making a good first impression with potential employers is achieved by having a professional looking résumé.

The Résumé

Regardless of the style of your résumé, every résumé should include certain basic information. The following are some guidelines regarding the type of information that should be provided on a résumé:

- **Personal data**—Name, address, phone number, and e-mail address. Make the font for the name a little bigger than the rest of the information so it stands out to prospective employers. If an e-mail address is provided, ensure that it is a simple, appropriate address. Funny or inappropriate e-mail names do not impress future employers.
- **Career objective**—This lets the employer know about your current career goals. Consider this example: "To obtain a position as a clinical assistant in a general dentistry office, with a long-range goal of clinical coordinator." Another example would be "To gain a position as a clinical assistant in a team-oriented environment where I can utilize my skills and abilities."
- **Education**—List all colleges, universities, and vocational schools attended, with the date graduated or the number of hours earned. List the most recent school first. Be sure to list the skills obtained from dental assisting school.
- **Credentials or additional skills (optional)**—List certifications such as certified dental assistant (CDA), expanded duties, x-ray certification, CPR, and first aid.
- **Work experience**—List your work experience in chronological order. Include the place of employment, the dates employed, and the skills and jobs accomplished. A disadvantage to listing the dates of work experience is that it shows gaps in the work history or frequent job changes. If there are gaps in work history, the dental assistant can give reasons such as "homemaker," or "student." The dental assistant may include any volunteer work and acquired skills he or she may have accomplished during the gap in work history.
- **Affiliations and activities**—A list of special community activities, such as volunteer work, is important to list on your résumé. Honors received due to academics or other achievements also should be noted. Prospective employers value that information because it shows initiative and dedication. Other information that shows the dental assistant's value includes memberships in professional organizations such as the ADAA, American Medical Technologists, Toastmasters International, or other organizations that indicate you have had an ongoing interest in improving your skills.
- **References**—Note that references are not automatically provided with the résumé. They are placed on a separate sheet of paper and provided on request. References are lists of names and phone numbers of previous employers or acquaintances that can verify the dental assistant's abilities, skills, and character. Be prepared with the information in case the employer asks for it.

Keep these basic résumé tips in mind when preparing a résumé:

- Create several versions of your résumé so you can tailor each résumé to specific jobs as you apply for them.
- Use short, concise statements.

- List experience and capabilities clearly and accurately.
- Be accurate and honest.
- Keep your résumé to one page if possible.
- Use action verbs and "power" words to convey participation, involvement, and accomplishment (Table 56-1).

Figure 56.2 shows a sample résumé.

The Cover Letter

The cover letter is an introductory letter that communicates to the employer the dental assistant's potential and specific important attributes (Figure 56.3). A cover letter should always accompany the résumé unless the résumé is presented at the time of the interview. Cover letters exhibit certain similarities:

1. Introductory paragraph:
   a. Creates interest.
   b. States employment interest.
2. A paragraph that "sells":
   a. Highlights your strengths and abilities.
   b. Shows your value to the company.
3. Background summary paragraph that summarizes relevant experience.
4. Follow-up statement that provides a contact number and time that the assistant may be available.
5. Statement of appreciation such as "Thank you for your time and consideration" or "I look forward to discussing the possibility of working in your organization. Thank you."

The cover letter and the résumé make a personal statement about the dental assistant to the employer (see Procedure 56-1). A well-written letter and résumé suggest to the employer that the dental assistant takes pride in his or her work and is efficient and well organized.

What is the purpose of a cover letter?

The Interview and Follow-Up

The interview is a formal meeting that is designed to assess the qualifications of the dental assistant. Prior to the interview, there are many things to consider, includ-

Cultural Considerations

If the dental assistant is bilingual, that information should be in the résumé and in the cover letter. In today's diverse society, knowing another language may increase the chances of gaining employment and serving the community as a dental assistant.

TABLE 56-1 Action and Power Words That Can Be Used on a Résumé

Ability	Headed	Problem-solved
Accelerated	Hones	Produced
Accompanied	Honor	Programmed
Achieved	Humor	Proofread
Acquired	Imagination	Protected
Administered	Influenced	Questioned
Advised	Informed	Reasoned
Analyzed	Ingenuity	Recorded
Appreciate	Initiated	Recruited
Assisted	Innovated	Referred
Budgeted	Installed	Repaired
Built	Instituted	Represented
Capable	Instructed	Researched
Completed	Invented	Resolved
Composed	Judged	Restored
Confidence	Keynoted	Retrieved
Conscientious	Kept	Reviewed
Controlled	Listened	Set up
Decided	Led	Scheduled
Dependable	Learned	Showed
Determined	Maintained	Solved
Developed	Managed	Summarized
Distinctive	Mentored	Supervised
Diverse	Monitored	Supplied
Educated	Motivated	Studied
Enacted	Navigated	Superior
Encouraged	Negotiated	Taught
Energy	Observed	Tended
Enthusiasm	Obtained	Tested
Excellence	Operated	Trained
Exceptional	Ordered	Transcribed
Formulated	Organized	Typed
Finalized	Perceived	Understanding
Formed	Performed	Upgraded
Gathered	Persuaded	Utilized
Generated	Planned	Verified
Graduated	Predicted	Won
Guided	Prepared	Wrote
Handled	Presented	Zealous

ing researching the organization to which the dental assistant is applying. This can be done either by requesting information from the company or by researching the company on the Internet. Employers are impressed when applicants know about their company. Another reason to

NAME IN ALL CAPITAL LETTERS
Address in lower case
City, State, Zip
Telephone number
Email Address

Objective: Obtain a dental assistant position in a team-oriented general office where I can utilize the skills and have the opportunity for growth.

Education: (List all colleges, universities, and vocational schools, even if you didn't graduate. List the number of hours taken or the graduation date.)

Fall 2005   XXX Community College
AAS Degree, Dental Assisting
- Student Representative
- Graduated with honors
- DANB Infection Control Certified

Experience: (List work experience; company name, dates and relevant experience)

2005 to present   Linda Muse, DDS, MS   Colorado Springs, CO
- Assisted in four-handed dentistry
- Assisted in endodontics
- Responsible for infection control program
- Maintained dental health records
- Trained in expanded functions

2003 to 2005   Green's Apparel   Colorado Springs, CO
- Supervised employees
- Managed telephones
- Maintained accounts payable and receivable
- Organized work schedule

References: Available upon request

FIGURE 56.2
Sample résumé.

research the company is to find out if the company fits the philosophy of the assistant.

Preparation for the interview includes ensuring that appropriate clothing is available for the interview. Interview clothing is typical business attire such as a suit or nice pants or skirt with a dress shirt (Figure 56.4). Men should always wear ties, and women may wear hosiery if they choose. Loud colors should be avoided. Jeans, tank tops, flip-flops, or any flamboyant type of attire is not professional and must be avoided. Scrubs should not be

Your Address
City, State, Zip

Month, day, year

Office/Doctor's name
Address
City, State, Zip

Dear Dr. (last name):

I am writing in response to the advertisement in the May 15 edition of The Gazette for an infection control coordinator/chairside dental assistant.

Over the past year, I have gained much experience managing the infection control program in a general dentistry practice. I believe that I am the experienced, enthusiastic dental assistant that you are looking for. I am DANB certified in Infection Control and am currently awaiting the results of my Certified Dental Assistant examination.

Looking at my resume, you will see that I have the infection control experience that you are seeking. I am also proficient in the DENTRIX patient management software.

Please contact me for an interview to discuss the position. You may reach me at (719) 555-5155. I look forward to meeting you and your staff. I know I will be a valuable asset to your office.

Sincerely,

Your Name
Dental Assistant

Enclosure: Resume

FIGURE 56.3
Sample cover letter.

worn unless the interview is a working interview where the dental assistant will participate in clinical activities. This is sometimes done at a second interview.

Arriving on time to the interview is critical. Prior to the interview, the dental assistant should locate the office and obtain directions as needed. A practice run a few days prior to the interview may help to ensure that the location is easily found and that parking options are known. The time of the appointment and who will do the interviewing are pieces of information that should be obtained at the time the interview is set. Materials that should be taken to an interview include a portfolio that contains:

- Letters of recommendations
- References

Procedure 56-1 Preparing a Professional Résumé and Cover Letter

Materials Needed

- **Computer**
- **Résumé paper**
- **Printer**
- **Past employment information to include dates of employment**
- **Degrees and certificates**

Procedure Steps

1. Gather education and past employment information.

2. Type résumé following the sample format provided in Figure 56.2.

3. Use a 12-point font and a common, easy-to-read typeface.

4. Tailor the résumé to the specific job.

5. Avoid embellishing any information.

6. Proofread the résumé for any errors.

7. Have another individual proofread the résumé.

8. Ensure résumé is free of errors prior to printing.

9. Print on standard 8 1/2 × 11 inch white or ivory heavy paper.

10. Prepare cover letter specifically for the job position following the sample shown in Figure 56.3.

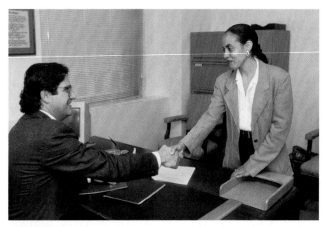

FIGURE 56.4
Professional interviewing attire.

- A copy of your résumé
- Copies of certifications
- College diplomas or transcripts
- Ink pen

To show radiographic skills, the dental assistant may also choose to place copies of a full mouth series of radiographs in the portfolio.

Some individuals are very comfortable with the interview process, whereas others need practice. For those who find interviewing difficult, practicing prior to the appointment is important. Practicing your interviewing skills with an instructor or other staff member at the college you are attending is a good option. Family members and friends can also participate in helping you become more comfortable with the interview process.

Professionalism

Maintain high personal standards at all times—prior to getting the job and after being hired. As a member of the health profession, it is important to be in good health and exhibit a professional appearance. Always have uniforms pressed, shoes clean, and in good condition. Performing beyond expectations will help with advancement in the company and, more importantly, make patients feel safe and comfortable. Membership in local, state, and national dental associations is also part of being a professional.

When practicing it is important to visualize the interview going well; this helps calm the nerves. Besides visualization, research helps. As stated earlier, researching the company sets the dental assistant apart from other applicants, but you must also research and be prepared to answer various types of interview questions. The number one question employers ask is "Why should I hire you for this position?" It is important to answer this question and all others with honesty and sincerity.

The following are questions an interviewer may ask, as well as some possible answers:

1. Tell me about yourself.

   Know your résumé details so you can state some of them.

2. Why do you want to work for this office?

   Research ahead of time to be ready for this question. Explain that you are impressed with, say, the company's policies, reputation, and potential growth.

3. Why should I hire you?

   A typical answer would be that you are qualified and your personal goals are compatible with those of the employer. Explain what strengths you can bring to the job.

4. What are your strengths?

   The interviewer really wants to know about your abilities to handle the job. Be honest but not arrogant, and proudly talk about your skills.

5. What are your weaknesses?

   You can turn this question to your advantage. If you work better knowing what's ahead of you all the time, then you can tell the employer that one of your weaknesses is that you need to work with a structured plan in order to prevent problems; this shows caring and organization.

6. Where do you want to be in five years?

   The employer is checking to see if you are going to stick around a while. Be careful answering this. You can tell them that you are seeking a team-oriented environment in which you can gain experience and growth.

7. Can you take radiographs?

   If you are experienced in taking radiographs, then say so. Show them a sample of your work. If you cannot take radiographs, do not mislead them— they may want you to do a working interview later at which you will be asked to take radiographs. It is always best to be honest.

8. Do you work better in a team or by yourself?

   Most of us can work in both capacities. Explain that you are a team player, but can also work well on your own.

9. Can you work a few late days or weekends?

   This question tells you that there may be some late days or weekend hours. One could ask how often this occurs and if it is on a rotating basis. Be honest and let the interviewer know if you can or cannot work the hours they are asking.

10. Why did you leave your last job?

    If you left on good terms, then you can reveal that information. If you did not leave on good terms then you might say you are seeking a change of career, seeking different, or more experience.

Questions about your personal life, such as "Are you married?," are illegal in the interview process. The dental assistant can choose how to handle those types of questions. Telling the interviewer that the question is illegal may be an option for you; however, that might anger the interviewer and ruin your chance of receiving the job. On the other hand, no one should be coerced into answering illegal questions. You must ask yourself if you really want to work in a place that ignores the law. After all, if they ignore the interviewing laws, you may wonder if they also ignore dental practice laws.

The interviewer will ask if the interviewee (the dental assistant) has any questions for the interviewer. The dental assistant should be prepared to ask questions or seek clarification about anything discussed in the interview. Questions should be relevant to the job. Salary questions can be asked and discussed during the first interview. Relevant questions asked by the potential employee include:

1. What are the job duties?
2. How will my progress be evaluated?
3. What promotional opportunities are available?
4. What are your expectations for this position?
5. What growth does the company project for the next five years?

This is also the time to seek clarification on anything not understood during the interview.

Once the interview is complete, thank the interviewer for his time and shake his hand. The dental assistant should inform the interviewer of his or her interest in the position. Some type of reference should also be made regarding a callback that the dental assistant hopes to get from the interviewer. Make sure a handwritten thank-you note is mailed to the interviewer immediately after the interview. This shows sincerity and interest in the position. An e-mail can be sent as a thank you, but some may consider this less personal.

When interviewing there are a few "do's and don'ts" to keep in mind: Don't chew gum or candy, don't crack your knuckles or any other body part, don't play with your hair or clothes, and don't answer your cell phone. In fact, your cell phone must be turned off during the interview. Some of the "do's" include being pleasant, smiling, answering questions honestly, and being respectful.

What do you do when asked about your personal information such as marital status?

Employment Negotiations

Keep in mind that negotiation of benefits and pay may occur during the first interview, although this conversation

Legal and Ethical Issue

Preparing and searching for employment requires a lot of work, but it will pay off. Be honest when writing a résumé. Do not embellish skills. If a particular skill cannot be done, then do not annotate it on the résumé. Employers want to hire honest, hard-working dental assistants.

is often saved for applicants who are called back for a second or third interview. Sometimes applicants may choose to ask questions about salary during the first interview if they require a specific salary. If the salary does not fall into a specific range, then the applicant and employer can avoid wasting time in a second interview.

For some people, negotiating the terms of employee benefits can be challenging. Before arriving at the interview, one should do some homework on how much pay and benefits are needed to make a living. This is done by preparing a monthly budget of household expenses, medical expenses, and vehicle expenses. In addition, researching the typical salary for dental assistants in the geographical area in which you are looking can help to ensure that you are not requesting a salary that is inappropriate. This can be accomplished by calling dental offices in the area to inquire as to the typical salary of dental assistants or one can go online to the U.S. Department of Labor, which provides data on the salary ranges for dental assistants nationally.

Salary and Benefits

A salary is the hourly wage and benefits paid to an employee for services. When an applicant is asked what salary is expected, it is important to inform the interviewer of a realistic amount. When projecting your salary, keep in mind the importance of a benefits package in conjunction with the salary. The benefits package should be discussed along with the salary, because when the benefits and salary are added it gives the dental assistant a better picture of the actual amount of pay for the work performed. Some of the specific benefits to ask about are:

- **Dental care for yourself and family**—Some offices provide free or reduced-cost dental care to their employees and dependents. This benefit is usually offered on a Saturday or other day the office is typically closed to regular patients.
- **Health insurance**—In today's society health care is very expensive so health insurance is an important benefit to discuss with future employers. Different packages are offered for single employees or employees with dependents.
- **Retirement plans**—Not every office offers retirement plans, but some will offer 401k savings plans. With this type of plan, the employer contributes a percentage of money and the employee contributes a percentage into a series of growth funds.
- **Uniform allowances**—Many dental offices want employees to wear specific colors and styles of uniforms and shoes. The employer may provide a uniform allowance to offset the cost of complying with these standards. The employer may also provide a cleaning allowance or provide in-house laundering in conformity with Occupational Safety and Health Administration standards.
- **Continuing education**—As a dental assistant it is important to continue your education through professional organizations such as the ADAA or by going to dental assisting expanded functions courses. Some dentists will pay continuing education registration fees or the annual dues for professional organizations.
- **Bonuses**—A bonus is an incentive employers use to keep employees motivated and productive. If the organization gives bonuses, the agreement contract will state under what conditions they are given.
- **Paid time off (PTO)**—Paid time off is an important benefit that employees need. At times it is offered after the probation period; other times it is offered after the first year of employment. The Fair Labor Standards Act does not require payment for time not worked, such as personal leave, vacations, sick leave, or federal or other holidays. These benefits are usually a matter of agreement between an employer and an employee.
- **Sick leave**—Although most people do not like to miss work, there are times when illnesses prevent people from working. During these times, it is good to know whether the employer provides sick leave. The agreement contract will state how many hours are offered and when the employee earns these sick leave hours. Federal law does not require employers to provide sick leave.

When discussing salary and benefits, it is also good to talk about employee evaluations, salary increases, and advancement opportunities within the organization.

Letter of Agreement or Employee Contract

A letter of agreement is prepared to ensure that certain topics of discussion are annotated prior to the official hiring (Figure 56.5). This document contains the job description, which specifically states the duties of the dental assistant in the office. The document contains the work schedule such as the days and hours the dental assistant is required to work, including the lunch hour and scheduled breaks. The document also includes the compensation agreed on including salary increases and bonuses. Work attire and if the employer provides a clothing allowance and/or laundering of scrubs is specified.

The employment agreement also states how long the new employee is on probation and terms under which the employee may be terminated. Probation or provisional employment is usually for a 90-day period. The purpose of the probationary period is for the employer to see if the employee is a good fit with the organization and can accomplish the assigned duties. It is also a chance for the assistant to see if the position is a good fit for him or her. Terms of termination such as how much notice an employee must provide prior to quitting are also spelled out in the letter of agreement.

What are three benefits to inquire about when you are hired?

EMPLOYMENT AGREEMENT
(Complete form in duplicate: one copy for the employer; one copy for the employee.)

EMPLOYEE'S NAME _Debbie Quigley, CDA_

Date _11/08/XX_   Full time/Part time _fulltime_

JOB TITLE _Chairside assistant to Dr. Hernandez_
See attached list for details of duties and responsibilities:

PRACTICE WORK SCHEDULE
(Your hours will be scheduled within these times.)

Usual days per week: S _____ M _✓_ T _✓_ W _½_ Th _✓_ F _✓_ S _½_

Usual working hours : _8:30_ to _5:30_ ; lunch _1 hr_ ; breaks _____ .

Work schedules are posted: _two weeks in advance. Assigned hours_ _may vary_

SALARY AND BENEFITS

Pay days: _every other friday_   Starting rate: _$ XX per hour_

Basis for increases: _review at 6 months, then annually_

Vacation days: _5_ ; Sick days: _5_ ; Personal time: _2_ .

Additional benefits: _group insurance is available_ _retirement plan after 3 years_

TERMINATION

For each new employee, the first _6_ weeks are a provisional period of employment. During this time, the new employee may leave or be dismissed without notice.

After this period, the employee is expected to give _2_ weeks notice.

If dismissed, the employee will receive _2_ weeks notice or the equivalent in severance pay.

In the event of fraud, theft, illegal drug use, or unprofessional conduct, the employee may be dismissed without notice or severance pay.

Debbie Quigley, CDA
Employee's signature

J. Hernandez, DDS
Employer's signature

FIGURE 56.5
Letter of agreement or contract.

Rights as an Employee

All employees for any organization have a right to fair treatment. According to **federal equal opportunity and employment laws**, employers cannot discriminate against an employee or applicant based on race, color, religion, sex, national origin, age, disability, marital status, or political affiliation.

It is important to research your rights as an employee. The Americans with Disabilities Act and Family and Medical Leave Act, discussed next, are just two valuable sources of information about employee rights.

Americans with Disabilities Act

Title 1 of the **Americans with Disabilities Act (ADA)** prohibits discrimination against existing employees and people with disabilities who are applying for employment. Under the ADA, employers are required to make certain reasonable accommodations to a job or work environment in order to help individuals with a disability perform their job duties. Required job tasks and the limitations of the employee determine the accommodations that must be provided. Accommodations may include specialized equipment, facility modifications, or adjustments to work schedules.

The law also applies to current employees who become disabled. The law requires that the employer make reasonable accommodations so that the employee can continue with the organization. Note that the ADA applies to companies that employ at least 15 people, so it may not apply to smaller dental practices.

Family and Medical Leave Act

The **Family and Medical Leave Act (FMLA)** provides certain employees with up to 12 weeks of unpaid, job-protected leave per year. It also requires that the individual's group health benefits be maintained during the leave. It allows employees to take reasonable unpaid leave for family and medical reasons. The FMLA applies to all public agencies, all public and private elementary and secondary schools, and companies with 50 or more employees. These employers must provide an eligible employee with up to 12 weeks of unpaid leave each year for any of the following reasons:

- The birth and care of the newborn child of an employee
- Placement with the employee of a child for adoption or foster care
- Care for an immediate family member (spouse, child, or parent) with a serious health condition
- To take a medical leave when the employee is unable to work because of a serious health condition

According to the U.S. Department of Labor, employees are eligible for leave if they have worked for their employer at least 12 months or, at least 1,250 hours during the past 12 months.

What is the purpose of the Family and Medical Leave Act?

Advancing Your Career

Dental assisting is a very rewarding career with great working conditions and hours. To continue to provide the best care possible to patients, the dental assistant may want to continue his or her education. Part of the dental assistant's responsibilities include complying with state and federal laws governing the practice of dentistry and acquiring and maintaining all credentials such as CPR. It is also important to stay challenged and knowledgeable about new techniques and materials. Some ways to advance your career as a dental assistant include the following:

- **Learn every aspect of the organization for which you work.** This includes both the clinical and administra-

Preparing for Externship

Write a practice cover letter and résumé that highlights your experience and your current skills. Have an instructor or classmate proofread it, and then use the information and questions in this chapter to conduct mock interviews. The more you practice interviewing, the more comfortable you will be in a real interview.

tive areas. This makes you a valuable employee who is flexible and able to take on other responsibilities when another worker is ill or on vacation. Learning all aspects of the job can also help with advancement in the organization.

- **Obtain national certifications.** This is not mandatory in every state but once obtained, it ensures the patients and the dentist of the assistant's knowledge and background in the field. It must be maintained by completing 12 continuing education units per year and paying an annual fee for the credentials. It also shows how serious the assistant is about his or her career and that he or she wants to stay updated on new techniques. National certification can be obtained through DANB. DANB studies show that certified assistants make, on average, $1.58 more an hour than noncertified assistants. More information about this can be found at www.danb.org.

- **Enroll in an expanded duty dental assistant course.** This additional education will enhance productivity in the dental office and possibly mean an increase in your salary and benefits package.

- **Join the American Dental Assistants Association professional achievement fellowship.** The ADAA offers the fellowship category to its members. There are two paths to this goal: clinical and business. Fellowship is available to those with documented educational achievements. This adds many hours of extra study and prestige to the profession.

The Importance of Attitude and Healthy Living

To achieve career success, the dental assistant must display some professional qualities and responsibilities. A positive attitude is the number one quality that employers desire from employees. If the dental assistant displays a positive attitude in everything he or she does, it will become contagious to coworkers and patients. A positive attitude allows for a better work environment. A positive attitude will help make patients feel more comfortable and willing to return for continued treatment.

Another important responsibility of the dental assistant is to maintain a healthy lifestyle. The assistant's outward appearance and health are a reflection of the organization. If the dental assistant is providing health care information to patients, then the dental assistant should display a healthy well-being. Achieving career objectives and advancing in this chosen career require a healthy lifestyle.

SUMMARY

Prior to taking a position in an organization, it is important to have a plan. When seeking employment, the dental assistant should look for the organization that best suits his or her skills. The dental assistant should know what aspect of dentistry interests him or her, and seek out certifications that will help obtain the perfect job. For help writing a résumé and finding employment, new dental assistant graduates can ask for help from the college's placement office or school instructors. Researching potential employers and preparing for interviews are critical steps to finding and obtaining employment.

KEY TERMS

- **Americans with Disabilities Act (ADA):** Prohibits discrimination against existing employees and people with disabilities who are applying for employment. p. 913
- **Cover letter:** Introduces the potential employee and provides a brief summary of why the individual is the right person for the job. p. 906
- **Family and Medical Leave Act (FMLA):** Allows employees to take reasonable unpaid leave for family and medical reasons. p. 914

- **Federal equal opportunity and employment laws:** Prevent an employer from discriminating against an employee or applicant based on race, color, religion, sex, national origin, age, handicapping condition, marital status, or political affiliation. p. 913
- **Résumé:** A summary of one's work experience and qualifications. p. 906

CHECK YOUR UNDERSTANDING

1. What kind of practice has two or more dentists?
   a. specialty
   b. general
   c. group
   d. sole

2. Which of the following is not appropriate dress for an interview?
   a. jeans
   b. dress pants
   c. skirt
   d. suit

3. The purpose of the cover letter is to
   a. highlight your skills.
   b. introduce yourself.
   c. explain your desire for the job.
   d. all of the above.

4. What is the purpose of the Americans with Disabilities Act?
   a. to keep employers from hiring individuals with disabilities
   b. to require the employer to make reasonable accommodations for individuals with disabilities
   c. to prohibit discrimination in hiring individuals with disabilities
   d. both b and c

5. Which of the following is not a trait of a dental assistant?
   a. honesty
   b. promptness
   c. aggressiveness
   d. compassion

6. Which of the following parts of a résumé lets the potential employer know about your career goal?
   a. the objective
   b. the thank-you letter
   c. credentials
   d. references

7. The Family and Medical Leave Act provides specific employees with up to how many weeks off in the event of illness or emergency?
   a. 6
   b. 10
   c. 12
   d. 14

8. Probation or provisional employment usually lasts how many days?
   a. 60
   b. 90
   c. 120
   d. 180

CHECK YOUR UNDERSTANDING (continued)

9. What should you do after an interview?
   a. Thank the interviewer and shake his or her hand.
   b. Ask the interviewer if he or she is going to hire you now.
   c. Immediately write and send a thank-you note.
   d. Both a and c.

10. Which of the following is a good way to advance your career as a dental assistant?
   a. Learn all aspects of the field.
   b. Enroll in an expanded functions course.
   c. Display a positive attitude.
   d. All of the above.

● INTERNET ACTIVITIES

- Identify possible opportunities by doing an Internet search on dental assistant employment.
- Search the Department of Labor website at www.doleta.gov and find the job opportunities and statistics pertaining to dental assisting, or go to www.careerone.com to find opportunities in your area.

● WEB REFERENCES

- Job search engines www.dentalworkers.com, www.dentaltown.com, www.careerone.com
- Dental Assisting National Board www.danb.org
- Occupational Information Network http://online.onetcenter.org
- Résumé information http://resume.monster.com/
- U.S. Department of Labor www.doleta.gov

Appendix

Dental and Other Professional Organizations in the United States

Academy of Dental Materials, Inc.
21 Grouse Terrace
Lake Oswego, OR 97035
Phone: 503-636-0861
Fax: 503-675-2738
Internet: www.academydentalmaterials.org

Academy of General Dentistry
211 East Chicago Avenue, Suite 900
Chicago, IL 60611-1999
Phone: 888-243-3368
Fax: 312-440-0559
Internet: www.agd.org

Academy of Prosthodontics
Internet: www.academyofprosthodontics.org

American Academy of Cosmetic Dentistry
5401 World Dairy Drive
Madison, WI 53718
Phone: 608-222-8583 or 800-543-9220
Fax: 608-222-9540
Internet: www.aacd.org

American Academy of Pediatric Dentistry
211 East Chicago Avenue, Suite 1700
Chicago, IL 60611-2637
Phone: 312-337-2169
Fax: 312-337-6329
Internet: www.aapd.org

American Academy of Periodontology
737 N. Michigan Avenue, Suite 800
Chicago, IL 60611-6660
Phone: 312-787-5518
Fax: 312-787-3670
Internet: www.perio.org

American Association of Oral and Maxillofacial Surgeons
9700 West Bryn Mawr Avenue
Rosemont, IL 60018-5701
Phone: 847-678-6200 or 800-822-6637
Internet: www.aaoms.org

American Association of Orthodontists
401 North Lindbergh Boulevard
St. Louis, MO 63141-7816
Phone: 314-993-1700
Fax: 314-997-1745
Internet: www.braces.org

American Association of Women Dentists
216 West Jackson Boulevard, Suite 625
Chicago, IL 60606
Phone: 800-920-2293
Fax: 312-750-1203
E-mail: info@aawd.org
Internet: www.aawd.org

American Board of Oral and Maxillofacial Surgery
625 North Michigan Avenue, Suite 1820
Chicago, IL 60611
Phone: 312-642-0070
Fax: 312-642-8584
Internet: www.aboms.org

American Cancer Society
Phone: 800-ACS-2345
Internet: www.cancer.org

American College of Prosthodontists
211 E. Chicago Avenue, Suite 1000
Chicago, IL 60611
Phone: 312-573-1260
Fax: 312-573-1257
Internet: www.prosthodontics.org

American Dental Assistants Association
35 East Wacker Drive, Suite 1730
Chicago, IL 60601-2211
Phone: 312-541-1550
Fax: 312-541-1496
Internet: www.dentalassistant.org

American Dental Association
211 East Chicago Avenue
Chicago, IL 60611-2678
Phone: 312-440-2500
Internet: www.ada.org

American Dental Education Association
1400 K Street, NW, Suite 1100
Washington, DC 20005
Phone: 202-289-7201
Fax: 202-289-7204
Internet: www.adea.org

American Dental Hygienists' Association
444 North Michigan Avenue, Suite 3400
Chicago, IL 60611
Phone: 312-440-8900
E-mail: mail@adha.net.
Internet: www.adha.org

American Heart Association
7272 Greenville Avenue
Dallas, TX 75231
Phone: 800-AHA-USA-1 or 800-242-8721
Internet: www.americanheart.org

American National Standards Institute
1819 L Street, NW, 6th floor
Washington, DC 20036
Phone: 202-293-8020
Fax: 202-293-9287
Internet: www.ansi.org

American Red Cross
2025 E Street, NW
Washington, DC 20006
Phone: 703-206-6000
Internet: www.redcross.org

American Society for Testing and Materials
100 Barr Harbor Drive
P.O. Box C700
West Conshohocken, PA, 19428-2959
Phone: 610-832-9500
Internet: www.astm.org

Aurum Ceramic Dental Laboratories LLP
Phone: 800-363-3989
Fax: 888-747-1233
Internet: www.aurumgroup.com

Bureau of Labor Statistics (BLS)
Postal Square Building
2 Massachusetts Avenue, NE
Washington, DC 20212-0001
Phone: 202-691-5200
Internet: www.bls.gov

CAESY Education Systems
1201 SE Tech Center Drive, Suite 110
Vancouver, WA 98683
Phone: 800-685-2599
E-mail: info@caesy.com
Internet: www.caesy.com

Centers for Disease Control and Prevention
1600 Clifton Road
Atlanta, GA 30333
Phone: 404-498-1515 or 800-311-3435
Internet: www.cdc.gov

Children's Dental Health Project
2001 L Street, NW, Suite 400
Washington, DC 20036
Phone: 202-833-8288
Fax: 202-318-0667
Internet: www.cdhp.org

Contemporary Dental Assisting
AEGIS Communications, LLC
104 Pheasant Run, Suite 105
Newtown, PA 18940
Phone: 215-504-1275
Internet: www.contemporarydentalassisting.com

Dental Assisting National Board
444 N. Michigan Avenue, Suite 900
Chicago, Illinois 60611
Phone: 1-800-FOR-DANB (312-642-3368)
Fax: 312-642-1475
Internet: www.danb.org

Department of Health and Human Services
200 Independence Avenue, SW
Washington, DC 20201
Internet: www.hhs.gov

Department of Labor (DOL)
Frances Perkins Building
200 Constitution Avenue, NW
Washington, DC 20210
Phone: 877-US-2JOBS
Internet: www.doleta.gov

Environmental Protection Agency (EPA)
Ariel Rios Building
1200 Pennsylvania Avenue, NW
Washington, DC 20460
Waste Hotline: 800-372-9473
Fax: 703-308-8686
E-mail: OSWWasteWise@epa.gov
Internet: www.epa.gov

Food and Drug Administration (FDA)
5600 Fishers Lane
Rockville, MD 20857
Phone: 888-INFO-FDA (888-463-6332)
Internet: www.fda.gov

Hispanic Dental Association
3085 Stevenson Drive, Suite 200
Springfield, IL 62703
Phone: 217-529-6517 or 800-852-7921
Fax: 217-529-9120
E-mail: HispanicDental@hdassoc.org
Internet: www.hdassoc.org

Humboldt-Del Norte Dental Society
P.O. Box 6368
Eureka, CA 95502
Internet: www.hdnds.org

Journal of Maxillofacial and Oral Surgery
6277 Sea Harbor Drive
Orlando, FL 32887-4800
Phone: 877-839-7126
Fax: 407-363-1354
E-mail: usjcs@elsevier.com
Internet: http://journals.elsevierhealth.com/periodicals/
yjoms

Journal of the American Dental Association
211 East Chicago Avenue
Chicago, IL 60611-2678
Phone: 312-440-2500
Internet: www.jada.ada.org

Medline Plus
8600 Rockville Pike
Bethesda, MD 20894
Internet: http://apps.nlm.nih.gov/medlineplus

Merck & Co., Inc.
One Merck Drive
P.O. Box 100
Whitehouse Station, NJ 08889-0100
Phone: 908-423-1000
Internet: www.merck.com

National Association of Dental Laboratories
325 John Knox Road, Suite L103
Tallahassee, FL 32303
Phone: 850-205-5626 or 800-950-1150
Fax: 850-222-0053
Internet: www.nadl.org

National Council on Radiation Protection and Measurements
7910 Woodmont Avenue, Suite 400
Bethesda, MD 20814-3095
Phone: 301-657-2652
Fax: 301-907-8768
Internet: www.ncrponline.org/

National Institute of Dental and Craniofacial Research
Phone: 301-402-7364
Fax: 301-480-4098
E-mail: nidcrinfo@mail.nih.gov
Internet: www.nidcr.nih.gov

Occupational Safety and Health Administration
200 Constitution Avenue, NW
Washington, DC 20210
Phone: 800-321-OSHA (800-321-6742)
Internet: www.osha.gov

Oral Cancer Foundation
3419 Via Lido, Suite 205
Newport Beach, CA 92663
Phone: 949-646-8000
Fax: 949-496-3331
E-mail: info@oralcancerfoundation.org
Internet: www.oralcancerfoundation.org

Oral Health America
410 N. Michigan Avenue, Suite 352
Chicago, IL 60611
Phone: 312-836-9900
Fax: 312-836-9986
E-mail: liz@oralhealthamerica.org
Internet: www.oralhealthamerica.org

Organization for Safety and Asepsis Procedures (OSAP)
P.O. Box 6297
Annapolis, MD 21401
Phone: 410-571-0003 or 800-298-OSAP (800-298-6727)
Fax: 410-571-0028
E-mail: office@osap.org
Internet: www.OSAP.org

Pan American Health Organization
525 23rd Street, NW
Washington, DC 20037
Phone: 202-974-3000
Internet: www.paho.org

Rihani International, Inc.
1647 Cranston Street
Cranston, RI 02920
Phone: 401-942-0670
Fax: 401-942-1360
E-mail: rihani@rihani.com
Internet: www.rihani.com

Academy of Fixed Prosthodontics Office of the Secretary
31 Emory Road
Winnipeg, Manitoba, R3T 3K9, Canada
Phone: 888-220-9386
Fax: 204-275-1285
E-mail: aafpsmith@mts.net
www.fixedprosthodontics.org

British Dental Association
64 Wimpole Street
London, W1G 8YS, United Kingdom
Phone: 020 7935 0875
Fax: 020 7487 5232
E-mail: enquiries@bda.org
www.BDA-dentistry.org.uk

Canadian Dental Assistants' Association
2255 St. Laurent Boulevard, Suite 203
Ottawa, ON K1G 4K3, Canada
Phone: 613-521-5495
Fax: 613-521-5572
E-mail: info@cdaa.ca
www.cdaa.ca

Canadian Dental Association
1815 Alta Vista Drive
Ottawa, Ontario, K1G 3Y6, Canada
Phone: 613- 523-1770
Fax: 613-523-7736
E-mail: info@cda-adc.ca
www.cda-adc.ca

FDI World Dental Federation
13 Chemin du Levant
l'Avant Centre, F-01210 Ferney-Voltaire, France
Phone: 33 4 50 40 50 50
Fax: 33 4 50 40 55 55
E-mail: info@fdiworldental.org
www.worlddental.org

First Dental Media Ltd
Rose House
223 Quinton Lane
Birmingham B32 2UD, United Kingdom
E-mail: info@firstdentalmedia.com
www.dental-videos.com

Global Health Council
1111 19th Street, NW, Suite 1120
Washington, DC 20036
Phone: 202-833-5900
Fax: 202-833-0075
www.globalhealth.org

Health Volunteers Overseas
1900 L Street, NW, Suite 310
Washington, DC 20036
Phone: 202-296-0928
www.hvousa.org

International Association for Dental Research
1619 Duke Street
Alexandria, VA 22314-3406
Phone: 703-548-0066
Fax: 703-548-1833
www.iadr.org

Ivoclar Vivadent
AG Bendererstrasse 2
9494 Schaan, Principality of Liechtenstein
Phone: 423 235 35 35
Fax: 423 235 33 60
E-mail: info@ivoclarvivadent.com
www.ivoclar.com

KerrHawe SA
Via Strecce 4
P.O. BOX 268 6934
Bioggio, Switzerland
Phone: 41 91 610 05 05
Fax: 41 91 610 05 14
www.kerrhawe.com

Mexican Dental Association (Asociación Dental Mexicana)
Ezequiel Montes No. 92 Col. Tabacalera Mexico, DF, 06030, Mexico
Phone: 011 52 55 3000 0350
Fax: 011 52 55 3000 0351
E-mail: admfederacion@prodigy.net.mx
www.adm.org.mx

Pierre Fauchard Academy
An International Honor Dental Association
Phone: 800-232-0099
www.fauchard.org/contact/contact.php

World Health Organization
Avenue Appia 20
CH-1211 Geneva 27, Switzerland
Phone: 41 22 791 2111
Fax: 41 22 791 3111
www.who.int/en

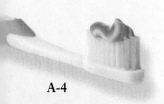

Abnormalities of Teeth
http://dentistry.umkc.edu/practition/assets/AbnormalitiesofTeeth.pdf

About Cosmetic Dentistry
www.aboutcosmeticdentistry.com

Academy of Dental Materials
www.academydentalmaterials.org

Academy of General Dentistry
www.agd.org

Academy of Prosthodontics
www.academyofprosthodontics.org

Ace Dental
www.ace-dental.com

ADAM
adam.about.com;

http://medicalimages.allrefer.com/large/scurvy-corkscrew-hairs.jpg

Advanced Endodontics of Houston
www.advanced-endodontics.com/surgical_therapy.html

Advanced Endodontics of Westchester, PLLC
www.westchesterendo.com/doct_microsurgery.html

American Academy of Cosmetic Dentistry
www.aacd.org

American Academy of Fixed Prosthodontics
www.fixedprosthodontics.org

American Academy of Pediatric Dentistry
www.aapd.org

    Dental Care for Special Child
    www.aapd.org/publications/brochures/specialcare.asp

American Academy of Periodontology
www.perio.org

American Association of Oral and Maxillofacial Surgeons
www.aaoms.org/oms.php

American Association of Orthodontists
www.braces.org

American Association of Women Dentists
www.aawd.org

American Board of Oral and Maxillofacial Surgery
www.aboms.org/General_Information/about_aboms.htm

American Cancer Society
www.cancer.org

American College of Prosthodontics
www.prosthodontics.org

American Dental Assistants Association
www.dentalassistant.org

    Ethics and Code of Conduct
    www.dentalassistant.org

American Dental Association
www.ada.org

    Anesthesia for the Dental Visit
    www.ada.org/prof/resources/pubs/jada/patient/patient_06.pdf

    Braces
    www.ada.org/public/braces.faq.asp

    Council on Scientific Affairs: The Use of Dental Anesthesia
    www.ada.org/public/topics/anesthesia_faq.asp

    Dentures
    www.ada.org/public/topics/dentures_faq.asp

    Education information
    www.ada.org/public/careers/team/index.asp

    Educational videos
    www.ada.org/public/media/videos/minute/index.asp

    HIPAA Information
    www.ada.org/prof/resources/topics/hipaa/index.asp

    Oral health topics
    www.ada.org/public/topics/cleaning.asp

    Radiographs, update and recommendations
    www.ada.org/prof/resources/pubs/jada/reports/report_
      radiography.pdf

American Dental Board of Anesthesiology
www.adba.org/index.html

American Dental Education Association
www.adea.org

American Dental Hygienists' Association
www.adha.org

    Prophylaxis
    www.adha.org/profissues/prophylaxis.htm

American Heart Association
www.americanheart.org

    Picture of Heart
    www.americanheart.org/downloadable/heart/1023826501754
      walletcard.pdf

American National Standards Institute
www.ansi.org

American Red Cross
www.redcross.org

American Society for Testing and Materials
www.astm.org

American Society of Dentist Anesthesiologists
www.asdahq.org

American Society of Regional Anesthesia and Pain Medicine
www.asra.com

Aurum Ceramic Dental Laboratories LLP
www.aurumgroup.com

Aurum Ceramic Product Collection
www.aurumgroup.com/usa/default.htm

Better Health Channel
www.betterhealth.vic.gov.au/bhcv2/bhcarticles.nsf/pages/Dental_
  sealants?

Biology—Anatomy of the Brain
www.biology.about.com/library/organs/brain/blcerebellum.htm

Brazilian Dental Journal
www.forp.usp.br/bdj/t0182.html

Bridges to Algebra and Geometry
www.learningincontext.com/Bridges/chapt07.htm

British Dental Association
www.BDA-dentistry.org.uk

British Dental Journal
www.nature.com/bdj/journal/v199/n8/full/4812913a.html

    Crowns and other extracoronal restorations: Impression
    materials and technique
    www.nature.com/bdj/journal/v192/n12/full/4801456a.html

Bureau of Labor Statistics Occupational Outlook Handbook
www.bls.gov/oco/ocos097.htm

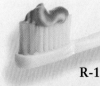

Burkhart
www.burkhartdental.com/index

Buy Online Now: Chart Cabinets
www.buyonlinenow.com/hon-shelf-files.asp?source=aw

Buyers Guide to Dental Products
www.dentalcompare.com

California Committee on Dental Auxiliaries licensing information
www.comda.ca.gov/licensing/index.html

Exam information
www.comda.ca.gov/exam_rdh.html

CAESY Education Systems
www.caesy.com

Cathode tube
library.thinkquest.org/19662/low/eng/cathoderays.html

Centers for Disease Control and Prevention
www.cdc.gov

Latex allergy information
www.cdc.gov/niosh/98-113.html

Infection control guidelines
www.cdc.gov/OralHealth/infectioncontrol/guidelines/
infection_control_guidelines.ppt or
www.cdc.gov/mmwr/preview/mmwrhtml/rr5217a1.htm

Sealants
www.cdc.gov/Oralhealth/factsheets/sealants-faq.htm

Children's Dental Health Project
www.cdhp.org

Clinical Practice: Introducing Digital Radiography in the Dental
Office: An Overview
www.cda-adc.ca/jcda/vol-71/issue-9/651.pdf

Colgate Professional
www.colgateprofessional.com

Colgate World of Care
www.colgate.com

Contemporary Dental Assisting
www.contemporarydentalassisting.com

Cranial nerves
mywebpages.comcast.net/wnor/cranialnerves.htm

Crest Oral B patient education
www.dentalcare.com/soap/patient/english/menu.htm

DataFace
http://face-and-emotion.com/dataface/anatomy/head_lateralview.jsp

Delta Dental of Colorado
www.deltadentalco.com

Dental Assistant National Board
www.danb.org

Dental Assisting Core Competencies Study
www.danb.org/PDFs/Phase4.pdf

Dental cements
www.dentalcements.com

Dental Compare: The Buyers Guide for Dental Professionals
www.dentalcompare.com

Dental Economics
www.dentaleconomics.com

Dental, Oral, and Craniofacial Data Resource Center: Periodontal
Diseases
http://drc.hhs.gov/report/pdfs/section3-diseases.pdf

The Dental Place
www.brushfloss.com/faq.htm

Dental Resources
www.dental-resources.com

Pulpectomies
dentalresource.org/topic58pulpotomypulpectomy.html

Dental Sedation Teachers Group: Conscious Sedation
www.dstg.co.uk/teaching/conc-sed/

Dental videos
www.dental-videos.com

DentiMax
www.dentimax.com/documentation/activitiesmenu.htm

DENTSPLY International
www.dentsply.com

Diabetes and Periodontal Disease
www.seniorhealth.about.com

Digital Dentist
www.thedigitaldentist.com

Diseases Info
phoenity.com/diseases/pellagra.html

DoctorSpiller.com
www.doctorspiller.com

DPRWorld.com
www.dprworld.com/

The Endo Experience
www.endoexperience.com/emergencydiagnosis.htm

Environmental Protection Agency
www.epa.gov

First Dental Media Ltd.
www.dental-videos.com

Flesh and Bones: Prevention of Periodontal Disease
www.fleshandbones.com/readingroom/pdf/864.pdf

Food and Drug Administration
www.fda.gov

Foundations in Continuing Dental Education
www.nurseslearning.com/courses/fice/fde0033/c11/index.htm

Free Education on the Internet
www.free-ed.net

Fundamentals of dental radiography
www.free-ed.net/free-ed/MedArts/DentalRad01.asp

Get Body Smart
www.getbodysmart.com/ap/skeletalsystem/skeleton/axial/skull/
quizzes/markings/sutures/animation.html

Get Smarter.org
www.getsmarter.org

GC America, Inc.
www.gcamerica.com

The Guardians.com
www.theguardians.com

Head Start Information and Publication Center
www.headstartinfo.org

Heraeus Kulzer
www.heraeus-kulzer-us.com

HIPAA Information
www.hipaaadvisory.com

Hispanic Dental Association
www.hdassoc.org

History of radiography
www.ndt-ed.org/EducationResources/CommunityCollege/
Radiography/Introduction/history.htm

HIV and Periodontal Disease
www.hivdent.org

Human Anatomy Online
www.innerbody.com/index.html

Humana Dental
www.humanadental.com

Humboldt-Del Norte Dental Society
www.hdnds.org

Hypothalamus Gland
www.heumann.org/body.of.knowledge/k1/hypothalamus.html

In Vitro Comparison of Peak Polymerization Temperatures of 5 Provisional Restoration Resins
www.cda-adc.ca/jcda/vol-67/issue-1/36.html

Indiana State Department of Health: Dental Radiography Study Guide
www.in.gov/isdh/regsvcs/radhealth/pdfs/dental_study_guide.pdf

Infection Control Today
www.infectioncontroltoday.com

Institute for Management Excellence
www.itstime.com/aug97.htm

Investopedia
www.investopedia.com/terms/i/inventory.asp

Invisalign
www.invisalign.com/general/app/us/en/for/index.asp

Ivoclar Vivadent
www.ivoclar.com

Job search engines
www.dentalworkers.com
www.dentaltown.com
www.careerone.com

Joseph S. Dovgan, DDS: Root canal retreatment
www.endodovgan.com/Endoinfo_NSRET.htm

Journal of Oral and Maxillofacial Surgery
journals.elsevierhealth.com/periodicals/yjoms

Journal of the American Dental Association
http://jada.ada.org

The Use of Dental Radiographs
http://jada.ada.org/cgi/content/full/137/9/1304

Why Switch to Digital Radiography
http://jada.ada.org/cgi/content/full/135/10/1437

Panoramic and Cephalometric Extraoral Dental Radiograph Systems
http://jada.ada.org/cgi/content/full/133/12/1696

Management of Endodontically Treated Teeth
http://jada.highwire.org/cgi/content/full/136/5/611

Kerr Hawe SA
www.kerrhawe.com

KODAK Dental Radiography Series: Successful Panoramic Radiography
www.kodakdental.com/documentation/film/N-406SuccPanRad.pdf

www.kodak.com/documentation/film/N-406PanRad.pdf

Locate a Doc
www.locateadoc.com/articles.cfm/888

Louisiana State University Health Sciences Center
www.medschool.lsuhsc.edu

Loyola University Medical Network
www.meddean.luc.edu/lumen/DeptWebs/microbio/med/gram/tech.htm

Gross anatomy
www.meddean.luc.edu/Lumen/MedEd/GrossAnatomy

Mayo Clinic
www.mayoclinic.com

Medical and Dental Standard Operating Procedures Library
www.physicianswebsites.com/standard-procedures.htm

Medline Plus
www.nlm.nih.gov/medlineplus/gumdisease.html

Merck & Co., Inc.
www.merck.com

Michigan Tech
www.admin.mtu.edu/admin/procman/ch10/ch10p1.htm

Muscular Dystrophy Association education information
www.mdausa.org/publications

National Association of Dental Laboratories
www.nadl.org

National Council on Radiation Protection and Measurements
www.ncrponline.org

National Institute of Allergy and Infectious Diseases
www.niaid.nih.gov

National Institute of Dental and Craniofacial Research
www.nidcr.nih.gov

National Institute of Neurological Disorders and Stroke
www.ninds.nih.gov

National Kidney Foundation, Inc.
www.kidney.org

National Museum of Dentistry
www.dentalmuseum.org

National Safety Council
www.nsc.org

Net Wellness: Consumer Health Information
www.netwellness.org/healthtopics/dentalseniors/tobaccocancerODA.cfm

Occupational Information Network
http://online.onetcenter.org

Occupational Safety and Health Administration (OSHA)
www.osha.gov

Anesthetic Gases: Guidelines for Workplace Exposures
www.osha.gov/dts/osta/anestheticgases

Odontocat: Prevention
odontocat.com/angles/prevplacaang.htm

Ohio State University College of Dentistry
www.dent.ohio-state.edu/anesthesiology/faculty.php

Open Wide: Oral Health Training for Health Professionals
www.mchoralhealth.org/OpenWide/mod1_4.htm,

www.mchoralhealth.org/OpenWide/mod1_3.htm

Oral and Maxillofacial Surgery Foundation
www.omsfoundation.org/

Oral and Maxillofacial Surgery Questions
www.calweb.com/~goldman/

Oral Cancer Foundation
www.oralcancerfoundation.org

Oral Health America
www.oralhealthamerica.org

Organization for Safety and Asepsis Procedures
www.osap.org

Otolaryngology Houston: Geographic Tongue
www.ghorayeb.com/TongueGeographic.html

The Owl at Purdue
http://owl.english.purdue.edu/handouts/pw/p_basicbusletter.html

Physicians' Desk Reference
www.pdrhealth.com

Pierre Fauchard Academy
www.fauchard.org

Premier Dental
www.premusa.com/dental/prosthetic.asp

Preventive Care for Child Development
www.craigentinny.co.uk/Children/tooth_development.htm

Procter and Gamble's Premier Portal for Dental Professionals
www.dentalcare.com

Pub Med
www.ncbi.nlm.nih.gov/entrez/query.fcgi?cmd=Retrieve&db=PubMed&list_uids=5258574&dopt=Abstract

Resume information
http://resume.monster.com

Rihani International, Inc.
www.rihani.com

RX List.com
www.rxlist.com

Science News Online
www.sciencenews.org/pages/sn_arc97/11_22_97/fob1.htm

Signet: The Best of Digital Dental X-Ray Panoramic Technology
www.dxis-net.com

South Dakota Department of Health
www.state.sd.us/doh/dentistry/6-13-03minutes.htm

Spanish Health Terminology
www.123teachme.com/learn_spanish/past_medical_history

Thyroid imaging
http://web.tiscali.it/thyroidimaging/pic_gozzonod3.htm

University of Arkansas Department of Neurobiology and
    Departmental Sciences
www.uams.edu/neuroscience_cellbiology

University of California at Los Angeles: Relief of Pain and Suffering
www.library.ucla.edu/biomed/his/painexhibit/panel1.htm

University of Illinois at Chicago, College of Dentistry,
    Department of Endodontics
www.uic.edu/depts/endo/apico.html

University of Iowa, Oral Pathology Image Database
www.uiowa.edu/~oprm/AtlasHome.html

University of Michigan Medical School
http://anatomy.med.umich.edu/nervous_system/infratem_tables.html

    Oral cavity studies
    www.med.umich.edu/lrc/coursepages/M1/anatomy/html/
        surface/head_neck/oral_cavity.html

University of Texas Medical Branch
www.utmb.edu

University of Virginia
www.healthsystem.virginia.edu/uvahealth/adult_oralhlth/
    implants.cfm

U.S. Department of Agriculture: MyPyramid.gov
www.mypyramid.gov

U.S. Department of Health and Human Services
www.hhs.gov/ocr/hipaa

U.S. Department of Labor
www.doleta.gov

Vermont Board of Dental Examiners
www.vtprofessionals.org/opr1/dentists/pubs/diduno.html

Virginia Commonwealth University, School of Dentistry
www.dentistry.vcu.edu

Web4Health
http://web4health.info/en/answers/ed-pictures.htm

WebMD
www.webmd.com/hw/dental/hw12228.asp

    Dentures
    www.webmd.com/oral-health/guide/dental-health-dentures

Wikipedia
http://en.wikipedia.org/wiki/Oral_and_maxillofacial_surgery

World Center for Implantology
www.enexus.com/dental-implant/doctor.htm

Xylitol.org
www.xylitol.org

abandonment: Withdrawing care from a patient without reasonable notice or without providing a referral for completion of dental treatment.

abrasion: The mechanical wearing away of tooth structure.

abscess: A collection of pus in a localized area.

abutment: A natural tooth or implant used to support or anchor a fixed or removable dental prosthesis.

accounts payable: Amount of money owed by the dental practice.

accounts receivable: Amount of money that is owed to the dental practice from patients for services rendered.

acid etchant: A bonding technique in which tooth structure is etched with phosphoric acid to create the rough surface necessary for mechanical and micromechanical bonding.

acquired immunodeficiency syndrome (AIDS): Disease that destroys the body's immune system.

acrylate: A salt of acrylic acid.

active immunity: Immunity that is artificially acquired from immunizations; sometimes called adaptive immunity.

adhere: To hold onto a surface.

aerobic bacteria: Bacteria that depend on oxygen to survive.

aesthetic dentistry: Operative dentistry to emulate natural beauty; cosmetic dentistry.

aesthetics: Refers to how a provisional restoration looks; also spelled *esthetics*.

aging account: The accounts receivable report that contains information on each patient and the length of time that has passed between a charge being invoiced and the receipt of a payment for the charge.

air/water syringe: Device that is utilized to emit air, water, and a combination of both in a spray; also known as a *three-way syringe*.

ala: The winged flare of the nostril.

ala–tragus line: Line that runs from the winged flare of the nostril (ala) to the opening of the ear (tragus).

ALARA concept: A radiation protection concept that states all exposures should be kept "as low as reasonably achievable."

allowable charges: The maximum dollar amount on which a benefit payment is based for each dental procedure.

alloy: A mixture of metals.

alveolar bone: The bone that supports the teeth of both the mandible and maxilla.

alveolar crest: The highest peak in the alveolar process.

alveolar process: The part of the mandible and maxilla that contains the tooth sockets.

alveolar socket: The opening within the alveolar bone that houses the roots of the teeth.

alveolitis: A postextraction complication resulting in inflammation of the alveolar process; also known as dry socket.

alveolus: The socket of a tooth.

alveoplasty: Surgical procedure performed to shape and contour alveolar ridges.

amalgam: A soft metal made of alloy mixed with mercury to restore form and function to teeth.

ameloblasts: Enamel-forming cells.

American Dental Assistants Association (ADAA): Professional organization that represents the profession of dental assisting.

American Dental Association (ADA): Professional organization that represents the profession of dentists in the United States.

American Medical Technologists (AMT): An organization of medical professionals that administer tests so dental assistants can become registered.

Americans with Disabilities Act (ADA): Prohibits discrimination against existing employees and people with disabilities who are applying for employment.

anaerobic bacteria: Bacteria that are destroyed by contact with oxygen.

analgesics: A diverse group of drugs used to relieve pain; also known as *painkillers*.

anatomic portion: The portion of a model that includes the teeth and oral structures.

anatomical crown: The portion of the tooth that is covered with enamel.

anesthetic: Medication that produces the temporary loss of feeling or sensation.

angina pectoris: Sudden and sharp chest pain.

ankyloglossia: Shortness of the tongue's frenum; literally, "tongue tied."

anode: The positive electrode in the x-ray tube/glass envelope.

anorexia: Common eating disorder for the male and female teen population. Involves daily starvation and excessive exercise to prevent weight gain.

anteroposterior plane: A forward–backward plane that is aligned with a specific landmark.

anterior: The front of the mouth or the front teeth.

anxiety: A physiological state characterized by cognitive, somatic, emotional, and behavioral components including fear, apprehension, or worry.

apex: Peaked tip at the end of each root.

aphthous ulcers: Painful ulcers appearing in the oral cavity as a circular lesion with a yellow center and a red outline or halo; sometimes referred to as a canker sore.

apical foramen: Opening in the apex of each root.

apicoectomy: The surgical removal of the apical portion of a tooth.

appendicular: Region of the body pertaining to the arms and legs.

apposition: The process in which tissue and tooth formation occur; fourth stage of tooth development.

arch wire: A contoured metal wire that provides force by guiding the movement of teeth during orthodontic treatment.

articulate: To join together.

articulation: The action of two or more bones meeting to form a junction (i.e., a joint).

articulator: A device used to reproduce the patient's jaw movements.

aseptic: Free from contamination by disease-producing microorganisms.

assistant's zone: Positioning zone that is based on the clock concept. For a right-handed operator, the dental assistant is positioned in the zone from 2 to 4 o'clock; for a left-handed operator, the dental assistant is positioned in the zone from 8 to 10 o'clock.

asthma: Disorder of the respiratory tract.

asymmetry: A lopsided unevenness or irregularity in facial features.

atom: The basic unit of all matter.

atria: Upper chambers of the heart.

attrition: The wearing away of the chewing surface of the teeth during their normal function; final stage of tooth development.

autoclave: Sterilizer that uses moist heat, under pressure.

automated external defibrillator (AED): A computer that assesses the patient's cardiac rhythm and automatically delivers defibrillation (electric shock).

automatic processor: Machine that automatically processes film through each stage of the developing process.

automatrix: Matrix system used to create a temporary wall to support the tooth restoration without using a retainer.

autonomy: Independent functioning.

auxiliary attachment: Specialized attachment located on brackets and bands that is used to hold arch wires and elastics in place.

avulsed tooth: A tooth forcibly separated from its socket.

axial wall: Internal surface of a cavity preparation positioned parallel to the long axis of the tooth.

axial: Portion of the body pertaining to the head, neck, and trunk.

bacteria: Small one-celled microorganisms.

basal cell carcinoma: Cancerous lesion that does not metastasize; most commonly found on areas of the skin that have been exposed to the sun. Occurs more often in individuals with fair skin tones.

basic setup: Instrument setup consisting of a mouth mirror, an explorer, and cotton pliers.

BCE: Before common era. Refers to the same dates as "BC" or "before Christ"; for example, 5000 BC = 5000 BCE.

beam alignment device: Device used to position the primary beam by aligning the position-indicating device.

benefit: The amount payable by a third party toward the cost of various covered dental services or the dental service or procedure covered by the plan.

bevel: The slanted cutting edge on the blade of a hand instrument that is used to place a distinct beveled angle at the enamel margins of a cavity preparation.

biofilm: A community of microorganisms that accumulates on surfaces inside moist environments such as dental unit waterlines, allowing bacteria, fungi, and viruses to multiply, which can increase a patient's susceptibility to transmissible diseases; previously called dental plaque.

biological indicators: Spore tests (vials or strips) that contain bacterial spores; used to determine if sterilization has occurred.

bisecting angle technique: Method of exposing radiographs in which the position-indicating device and x-ray beam are directed perpendicular (at 90 degrees) to an imaginary line that equally bisects a triangle created by the long axis of the tooth and the film.

bite registration: A record of how the patient's maxillary and mandibular arches occlude.

bitewing radiograph: Radiograph used primarily to examine the interproximal surfaces of the teeth.

bloodborne pathogens: Organisms transferred through blood or body fluids that cause infectious disease.

bonding: *Verb:* Adhering tooth-colored resin composite to a tooth surface to create a bond. *Noun:* Tooth-colored resin composite that is bonded, sculpted, hardened, and polished to tooth surfaces; usually used for aesthetic purposes.

bonding insurance: Insurance that protects the practice against any monetary losses due to employee theft.

border molding: Part of the final impression, where softened compound or wax is placed along the borders of the denture.

brachial: Pertaining to the arm.

bradycardia: A slow heart rate.

bridge threader: Used to thread dental floss to clean underneath a bridge or other dental appliance.

bruxism: Excessive grinding of the teeth.

buccal: Surface next to or toward the cheek of posterior teeth.

bulimia: Eating disorder in which overeating is followed by vomiting.

calcification: The process in which tissue becomes hardened due to calcium deposits; fifth stage of tooth development.

calculus: Hardened plaque, a mineralized deposit on teeth formed by saliva, debris, and minerals; also called tartar.

calibration: The process of setting a machine to provide accurate measurements.

cancellous bone: Lightweight, sponge-like bone located in the interior area of the bones; it is more porous than dense bone.

Candida albicans: An oral yeast infection presenting as a thick, white covering on oral mucosa; also called moniliasis.

candidiasis: Disease caused by the fungus *Candida albicans*; also called oral thrush.

carbohydrates: Sugars and starches used for energy.

carcinoma: Cancerous lesion of the epithelium (tissue that lines the mouth) that spreads into bone and connective tissues.

caries: An infectious disease that results in the localized destruction of the teeth.

cariogenic agent: Agent that causes caries.

cariology: The study of the caries process.

carotid: The pulse felt at the neck on either side of the trachea.

carpal tunnel syndrome (CTS): An injury associated with repetitive or continuous flexing and extending of the wrist.

cartilage: Tough nonvascular, flexible, connective tissue.

carvers: An instrument with sharp cutting edges used to shape tooth anatomy into restorations.

cassette: A protective film-holding container with two intensifying screens; used to hold extraoral film during exposure.

cast model: A gypsum replica of the mouth made from an impression of a patient's mouth.

cast post: Metal post created by a laboratory to be placed into an endodontically treated tooth to improve retention of a cast restoration.

cathode: The negative electrode in the x-ray tube/glass envelope.

cavitation: The formation of cavities or holes in tissue or teeth.

cavity: Breakdown in the anatomy of the teeth; usually caused by caries.

cavity wall: One of several walls of a cavity preparation.

CE: Common era. Refers to the same dates as "AD" or "anno Domini"; for example, AD 1996 = 1996 CE.

celluloid strip: Transparent polyester strip used to create a temporary wall to support the tooth restoration of an anterior tooth; often known as a Mylar strip.

cementoblasts: Cementum-forming cells.

Centers for Disease Control and Prevention (CDC): Federal agency that makes recommendations on health and safety issues.

centric occlusion: The position of the mandible when the teeth are biting fully together.

centric relationship: Jaws positioned in a way that will produce a centrally related occlusion.

cephalometric radiograph: Profile of the head and face showing both bone and soft tissue.

cerebrovascular accident (CVA): Stroke; caused by insufficient blood flow to arteries in the brain.

charting: The process of recording information about the patient's mouth and dentition.

chemically cured: Process of mixing two materials together to create a chemical reaction that makes a material harden (set).

chemically cured: Material that is set by the chemical process of mixing a base and catalyst together.

chief complaint: The symptom or group of symptoms that represents the patient's reason for seeking care.

civil law: Noncriminal legal action that a patient may pursue against a dentist that may result in a compensation lawsuit for pain, suffering, and loss of wages resulting from a dental treatment or dentist's actions.

clinical crown: The portion of the crown that is visible in the oral cavity.

colony-forming units (CFUs): Unit of measure for numbers of viable bacteria per milliliter.

Commission on Dental Accreditation: Evaluates and provides accreditation for programs for dentists, dental assistants, and dental hygienists in the United States.

commissures: The corners of the mouth.

compact bone: Hard and dense layer of bone.

complete denture: Dental prosthesis that replaces all missing teeth in a full arch or arches.

complete mouth rinse: A rinse that is generally performed once all oral procedures have been completed; sometimes during long dental procedures, when the patient's entire mouth needs refreshing, a complete rinse may be performed.

compliance: Adherence to official standards.

composite resin: Tooth-colored filling material made of silica or porcelain particles interlaced with liquid resin.

comprehensive oral exam: An extensive evaluation and recording of all extraoral, intraoral, and soft tissue findings.

cone cut: An error created when only part of an image is seen on a radiograph due to improper alignment of the position-indicating device with the film.

connectors: Elements of a partial denture that unite the working parts into one unit.

consultation room: Specified room or meeting area where diagnosis, financial information, treatment, and/or treatment planning, as well as extensive personal or health-related issues, are discussed concerning the patient.

contaminated waste: Regulated waste that is potentially infectious and/or sharp.

contour: The overall shape or form of the original tooth structure.

contra-angle: The angle at the head of the slow-speed handpiece to which burs attach.

contrast: Differences in densities on adjacent areas of a radiograph.

copay: A cost-sharing arrangement in which the insurance patient/subscriber pays a specified charge at the time of service.

core buildup: The restorative material that recreates the lost tooth structure of the anatomical crown (also known as just a *buildup*); part of the cast post that extends into the anatomical crown.

coronal: The portion of the tooth that can be seen clinically.

corrective (interceptive) orthodontics: Orthodontic treatment that creates space in the mouth, or reduces a patient's poor oral habits, prior to or instead of full orthodontic procedures.

cover letter: Introduces the potential employee and provides a brief summary of why the individual is the right person for the job.

credit slip: Slip of paper that alerts a dental office that it will not be billed for returned items.

crepitus: A clinical sign heard upon movement that is characterized by a peculiar crackling, crinkly, or grating feeling or sound under the skin or around the joints, for example, in the temporomandibular junction.

criminal law: Involves a state or government action against individuals who perform nonlegal procedures or violate laws. Such lawsuits can result in disciplinary action, fines, and/or imprisonment.

critical items: Items that penetrate soft tissue and directly contact bone, blood, and other body fluids.

crown: A restoration covering or replacing a major part of or the entire clinical crown of a tooth.

cultural diversity: Addresses racial and ethnic differences.

cumulative trauma disorder (CTD): An injury associated with ongoing stresses to the joints, muscles, nerve, and tendons.

curing: Chemical or physical process that improves the properties of a dental material, such as hardness and strength.

D.D.S.: Doctor of Dental Surgery.

debridement: Removal of debris, including necrotic nerve tissue, from a tooth root canal.

decalcification: The removal of calcium salts from bone or teeth.

deciduous: The first set of teeth in a human; also known as primary.

deductible: The amount of money the patient/subscriber must pay as part of the insurance plan.

demineralization: The loss of minerals from the body or teeth.

density: The overall blackness on a radiograph.

Dental Assisting National Board (DANB): Provides a nationally recognized test for front-office professionals or chairside assistants to become certified in their profession.

dental chair: The center for all clinical and treatment activity. The chair is designed for the patient's comfort and allows the operator and/or assistant to provide treatment to the patient in an efficient manner.

dental dam: Thin latex or latex-free barrier used to isolate a specific tooth or teeth during treatment.

dental film holder: A device used to stabilize the film in the patient's mouth.

dental handpiece: A mechanical device designed for use with rotary instruments.

dental jurisprudence: The governing laws in the science of dentistry.

dental lamina: Growth of the oral epithelium that will eventually form the teeth.

dental operatory/treatment room: Clinical or control area where dental treatment is performed.

dental papilla: Tissue from the mesoderm layer that will form dentin and pulp.

dental practice act: Legal restrictions set forth by each state legislative body that describe the statutes regarding performance guidelines for licensed and nonlicensed dental health care professionals.

dental sac: Capsule that contains the developing tooth; it will also form the cementum, periodontal ligament, and some alveolar bone.

dental sealant: A hard clear, opaque, or tinted resin that is placed on the pits and fissures of the occlusal surfaces of caries-free teeth.

dental team: Team consisting of various dental specialists such as periodontists, prosthodontists, and oral maxillofacial surgeons; also includes general dentists, dental hygienists, and dental assistants.

dental unit: Consists of handpieces, air/water syringes, saliva ejector, possibly an oral evacuator or ultrasonic scaler, along with numerous other options depending on operator's preferences.

dentin: Tissue that makes up the bulk of the tooth; it is covered by cementum on the root and enamel on the crown.

dentinal tubules: Microscopic canals running through dentin.

dentition: Tooth arrangement; in position.

dentofacial: Term used to describe structures of the teeth, jaws, and surrounding facial bones.

denture base: Referred to as the saddle, it holds the denture teeth and acrylic that covers the alveolar ridges.

deposit slip: An itemized copy of the money taken to a bank to be credited to the dental practice account.

desiccation: The removal of all moisture from an area; the process of drying out.

diastema: Space between two teeth; place where adjacent surfaces do not touch.

diastolic: The bottom number of a blood pressure reading; represents the amount of pressure during the relaxation phase of the heartbeat.

die: A precise replica of a prepared tooth created from an impression used by the dental laboratory to make the cast or milled restoration.

differentiation: Changes in the function of cells in the tooth bud and development of teeth occurs; third stage of tooth development.

disinfection: Process that prevents growth of disease-carrying microorganisms.

distal: Surface of tooth away from the midline.

distocclusion: A Class II malocclusion in which the mesiobuccal cusp of the maxillary first molar occludes mesial to the mesiobuccal groove of the mandibular first molar by more than the width of a premolar.

Doctor of Dental Medicine (D.M.D.): The degree a person receives on graduation from dental school; awarded to individuals who complete clinical hours of training in dentistry and successfully complete board examinations. This degree is the same as the D.D.S. degree. The degree awarded is determined by the university.

Doctor of Dental Surgery (D.D.S.): The degree a person receives on graduation from dental school; awarded to individuals who complete clinical hours of training in dentistry and successfully complete board examinations. This degree is the same as the D.M.D. degree. The degree awarded is determined by the university.

double booking: The scheduling of two patients for appointments at the same time.

downward channel communication: Channel of communication that originates from an upper level employee of an organization and travels down to a lower level employee.

droplet transmission: A disease that occurs from splash or splatter to the mucosa (mouth/eyes) or nonintact skin.

drug interaction: The effect a drug can have when taken with another drug.

dry angle: Triangular-shaped, absorbent wafer-like pad used for moisture control.

dry heat sterilizer: Sterilizer that uses heated, dry air to sterilize instruments.

dual-curing process: A process in which the material begins to harden through self-curing and then requires a final cure with a visible light unit.

due care: The actions any reasonable or prudent dental care professional would perform under similar circumstances.

duplicating film: Film used specifically for duplicating or copying existing radiographs.

duration: The lasting effect of an anesthetic agent.

edema: The presence of abnormally large amounts of fluid in the tissues; swelling.

edentulous: Without teeth.

electromagnetic radiation: The production of a wavelike energy through space and matter.

elongation: A vertical angulation error that occurs when there is insufficient vertical angulation of the position-indicating device to the film.

embrasure: The V-shaped space formed by the contour and position of adjacent teeth.

embryology: The study of how a human being develops through three stages before birth.

emphysema: A breathing condition characterized by the stretching out of the alveoli or the air sacs in the lungs.

emulsion: A coating on the film that gives it greater sensitivity to radiation.

enamel organ: Tissue arising from the ectoderm layer that will form the enamel.

endocardium: Thin lining inside the heart.

endodontics: The specialty that involves the treatment of the tooth pulp and periapical tissues.

endodontist: A dentist who specializes in the diagnoses and treatment of dental pulp diseases.

endogenous stains: Stains formed from within the tooth structure.

endosteal implant: Implant that is surgically placed in the bone. Four types are available: blade, cylinder, screw, and transitional (provisional).

engineering control: The use of a device that minimizes the risk of exposure to infectious material.

epiglottis: Elastic cartilage covered with mucous membrane that forms a part of the larynx; its function is to close off the larynx during swallowing.

epilepsy: Chronic brain disorder characterized by recurrent seizures.

epithelial: Tissue consisting of tightly packed cells that form a covering over external and internal body surfaces.

ergonomics: The study and adaptation of how people work, including the anatomic and physiological characteristics of people in the work environment.

erosion: Chemical wearing away of tooth structure.

eruption: The process of a tooth breaking through the gum tissue to grow into place in the mouth; sixth stage of tooth development.

erythema: Redness of the tissues, often due to inflammation.

ethical drug: Any drug that requires a prescription.

etiologic: Factors causing disease.

eugenol: A clear to pale yellow, oily aromatic liquid made from clove oil that is sometimes used in dentistry as an anti-inflammatory and antimicrobial. Contains soothing qualities and has a pleasant, spicy, clove-like taste.

event-related sterilization: Instrument packages that remain sterile unless an event causes contamination (i.e., wet or torn packages).

exclusive provider organization (EPO) plan: Closed panel plan that allows a particular group of insurance subscribers to receive dental care only from participating dentists (i.e., exclusive providers).

exfoliation: The normal process of losing, shedding, or falling out of primary teeth.

exodontia: The extraction of a tooth.

exogenous stains: Stains formed from sources outside of the tooth.

exothermic reaction: A chemical reaction that produces heat during the setting of a material.

expanded function: Advanced task that requires increased skill and training performed by a dental auxiliary when delegated by a dentist in accordance with the governing state dental practice act.

expanded functions dental assistant (EFDA): Dental assistant who can perform certain intraoral procedures delegated by the dentist after the dental assistant has been specially trained in the expanded functions per the applicable state dental act.

expenditures: Amount of money spent to operate the dental practice.

expiration: The exhaled portion of a respiration.

Explanation of Benefits (EOB): Document that details how a claim was processed and indicates the portion of the claim paid to the dentist and the portion of the claim, if any, the insurance subscriber needs to pay. An EOB is not a bill.

exposure control plan: A plan that explains exposure determination for employees to help minimize occupational exposure to bloodborne pathogens.

express contract: Verbal or written words that are agreed on in an established contract.

extirpation: Removal of infected pulp tissue within a tooth.

extraoral: Outside the mouth.

extraoral film: Film designed to be used outside of the mouth during x-ray exposure.

extraoral radiographs: X-rays taken outside of the mouth.

extrinsic stain: Stains on external surfaces of the teeth that can be removed with polishing.

exudate: A fluid-type substance that forms as a result of the inflammatory process; the fluid contains bacteria, leukocytes or white blood cells, dead cells, degenerated tissues, and tissue fluid.

fabricated: Made or constructed.

facebow: Part of an articulator that is used to record the relationship of the maxillary arch to the horizontal axis rotation of the mandible.

facial: Surface of tooth toward the face.

facultative bacteria: Bacteria that can live with or without oxygen.

Family and Medical Leave Act (FMLA): Allows employees to take reasonable unpaid leave for family and medical reasons.

fats: Nutrients used for body insulation and energy; also known as lipids.

federal equal opportunity and employment laws: Laws that prevent an employer from discriminating against an employee or applicant based on race, color, religion, sex, national origin, age, handicapping condition, marital status, or political affiliation.

fetal molding: Condition that occurs when an arm or leg of a fetus presses against another forming bone, causing distortion of a rapidly growing area.

fiber-optic system: A system used with a high-speed handpiece that uses fiber optics to illuminate the oral cavity.

filled resins: Sealant material that contains filler particles.

filler: Silica or porcelain particles that add strength to composite resins.

film: The term used to describe the film packet and its components prior to it being developed or processed.

film processing: A series of chemical steps that converts a film into a radiograph.

film speed: Establishes the amount of radiation and time needed to expose a film.

fissure: A deep furrow running along a developmental groove.

fixed expenses: Those expenses that remain the same from month to month.

fixed partial denture: A prosthetic replacement of one or more missing teeth cemented or attached to abutment teeth or implant abutments adjacent to the space.

flash sterilization: Procedure that uses a quick flash of heat to sterilize instruments.

fluoridation: The process of adding fluoride to the public water supply.

fluorosis: White or brown discolorations of tooth enamel with surface defects called mottling.

foramina: Openings in bone allowing for passage of nerve and blood vessels.

foreshortening: A vertical angulation error that occurs when there is excessive vertical angulation of the position-indicating device to the film.

fossa: An irregularly shaped depression on the surface of a tooth.

four-handed dentistry: Clinical procedures performed by the operator and an assistant in a structured dental environment.

framework: Metal skeleton of a removable partial to which remaining units are attached.

Frankfort plane: A horizontal line from the upper margin of the ear to the lower margin of the eye orbit.

frenectomy: Surgical removal of the frenum.

frenula: Folds of tissue connecting the cheeks and lips to the alveolar mucosa.

frequency: The number of wavelengths passing through a fixed point per given period of time.

fulcrum: The pivotal point or support used to stabilize and control a dental instrument. This "finger rest" point in the mouth is designed to rest and support the hand while using an instrument or handpiece in the patient's mouth; also helps prevent slipping while providing stabilization for the operator's hand during procedures.

furcation: The region of a multirooted tooth at which the roots divide.

furcation involvement: Loss of interradicular bone between multirooted teeth as a result of periodontal infection.

galvanic: Relating to an electric shock due to two different metals coming in contact.

generic: Drugs that are sold without a brand name and/or trademark.

gingivectomy: Surgical excision of the gingiva.

gingivitis: Inflammation of the gingiva.

gingivoplasty: Surgical reshaping of the gingival tissue.

glenoid fossa: A shallow depression within the temporal bone.

grand mal seizure: Uncontrollable, violent muscle contractions/spasms and loss of consciousness; also known as tonic/clonic seizures.

Green Vardiman Black: Referred to as the "grand old man of dentistry." Black was responsible for the standardization of cavity preparations.

gross or frank caries: Obvious severe destruction of the tooth by decay.

gross salary: The amount of pay before any deductions have been taken out.

gypsum: Material used to create diagnostic cast models of a patient's maxillary or mandibular arch.

halitosis: Bad breath.

handpieces: Instruments that aid the dentist in tooth preparation and the removal of dental decay.

Hazard Communication standard: Statement of OSHA regulations regarding how the employer must protect employee health if hazardous chemicals are used in the workplace.

hazardous waste: Chemical waste that is potentially harmful to humans or the environment because it is highly reactive, toxic, corrosive, contaminated, combustible, carcinogenic, or degraded.

Health Insurance Portability and Accountability Act (HIPAA): An act passed by Congress to address the security and privacy of health data.

hemostasis: The process by which the body controls bleeding.

hepatitis: A viral infection that affects the liver.

herpetic whitlow: Painful crusting ulcerations on the fingers or hands resulting from exposure to the herpes virus.

high-volume evacuator (HVE): Device used to remove saliva, blood, water, and debris from a patient's mouth.

HIPAA: See *Health Insurance Portability and Accountability Act (HIPAA).*

Hippocrates: the "father of medicine."

Hippocratic oath: An obligation to refrain from wrongdoing and to treat patients to the best of one's ability.

histology: The study of the composition and function of tissues.

holding solution: Solution in which instruments are placed prior to placing them in an ultrasonic cleaner.

homeostasis: The process of all body functions performing together to maintain harmony in the body.

homogenous: The characteristic of having a uniform structure or composition throughout.

horizontal angulation: Proper alignment of the position-indicating device in a side-to-side or back-and-forth direction.

horizontal channel communication: Channel of communication that is used between members of an organization at the same level.

human immunodeficiency virus (HIV): A virus that attacks a specific type of white blood cell that controls the body's immune response.

hydrophilic: A tendency toward compatibility with water or complete wetting ability.

hydrophobic: A tendency away from water, an aversion to it, and less wetting ability.

hyperglycemia: Too much sugar (glucose), not enough insulin in the blood.

hyperplasia: Excess folds of tissue that result from an ill-fitting denture.

hypertension: High blood pressure.

hyperthyroidism: Overactive thyroid function.

hyperventilation: Light-headedness and dizziness caused by rapid breathing that causes a reduction in oxygen intake.

hypoglycemia: When the body has too little sugar and too much insulin; also known as insulin shock.

hypothyroidism: Underactive thyroid function.

Ida Gray: The first African American woman to graduate with a dental degree.

imbibition: The process of absorbing water, causing swelling.

immunocompromised: Condition in which a person is at risk for a disease due to a weakened immune system.

implant: A titanium, screw-like device specially designed to be placed surgically within the mandibular or maxillary bone as a means of providing for a dental prosthesis.

implied contract: A contract that is implemented by the patient's actions, not verbally or written; also known as *implied consent.*

impression: A negative replica of a person's teeth and oral structures into which dental plaster or stone is placed in order to make an accurate copy or positive replica of the patient's dentition.

incipient caries: The initial formation of tooth decay.

incisal: The biting or cutting edge of anterior teeth.

induction: The time from injection to the time when complete anesthesia is achieved.

infectious waste: Regulated waste that has been in contact with blood or other body fluids.

infiltration: A type of local anesthesia in which the anesthetic solution is injected directly into the gingival and alveolar tissue sites to numb the nerve endings in the area.

informal channel communication: Gossip; also known as the "grapevine."

informed consent: The procedure of fully informing a patient about the choices the patient has regarding dental care.

informed refusal: Occurs when the patient refuses treatment after he or she has been fully educated regarding the consequences of not receiving the treatment.

initiation: The bud stage or start of tooth development; first stage of tooth development.

inlay: A gold, porcelain, or resin filling made to fit a prepared cavity cemented or bonded in place to restore a decayed or broken tooth.

innate immunity: The general protection that humans are born with; also known as natural immunity.

insertion: The movable end of a muscle.

inspiration: The inhaled portion of a respiration.

intensifying screen: A device used in a cassette that converts x-ray energy into light, which causes a decrease in the amount of time needed to expose the film.

interproximal: The space between adjacent contacts of teeth in the same arch.

intraoral: Inside the mouth.

intraoral film: Film designed to be used in the mouth during x-ray exposure.

intrinsic stains: Stains formed from within the tooth structure that cannot be removed with polishing.

ion: An electrically charged particle.

ionization: The process through which electrons are lost from the shell of an atom.

ionizing radiation: Radiation that is capable of producing ions by adding or removing electrons from the shell of an atom.

irreversible pulpitis: Condition in which inflamed tooth pulp is unable to respond to treatment and the patient's symptoms of pain continue.

isolation: Process of keeping the operative area or teeth separate and dry.

Josiah Foster Flagg: Man who invented the dental chair.

Kaposi's sarcoma: Malignant bluish-purple vascular tumor; an opportunistic neoplasm that may occur in people with HIV infection.

labial: Surface of tooth toward the lips.

lactobacilli: Bacteria that produce lactic acid from fermentable carbohydrates.

lamina dura: Compact bone that lines the socket of the alveolar process.

laminar flow: Occurs when water flows fastest in the middle and slower on the edges of tubing.

latent image: An invisible image that is in the emulsion of the film after exposure to radiation and prior to developing.

latent infection: An ongoing infection with recurrent symptoms.

lateral: From the side.

lathe: A rotary machine used during grinding, finishing, and polishing procedures.

lead time: The interval of time between when an order is placed and when it is received.

leakage radiation: Radiation that escapes or leaks out of the tube head.

leukoplakia: Usually a precipitating factor for cancer; appears as a white leathery patch that cannot be identified as any other white lesion.

ligature wire: A light wire used to hold an orthodontic arch wire into a bracket.

light cured: Process of using a high-intensity light to make a material harden (set).

light cured: Material that is set by a curing light.

limited area mouth rinse: A rinse performed during a clinical procedure when the dentist pauses during treatment.

line angle: Junction of two surfaces in a cavity preparation; cavity line angle.

linea alba: A long fold of tissue along the buccal mucosa next to where the teeth come together.

lingual: Surface of tooth next to the tongue.

lining mucosa: A thin delicate tissue that covers the inside of the cheeks, vestibule, soft palate, undersurface of the tongue, and floor of the mouth.

long axis of the tooth: An imaginary line passing vertically, or lengthwise, through the tooth that divides the tooth in half.

Lucy B. Hobbs: First woman to graduate from dental school.

luting: To bond or cement together.

luting agent: A viscous material placed into a dental prosthesis that attaches the prosthesis firmly to the tooth by means of a chemical reaction.

luxate: To put out of joint or out of place.

malady: A disease or disorder.

malignant: Tumor that is life threatening, such as a squamous cell carcinoma or basal cell carcinoma.

malleability: The property of being shaped or formed under pressure without breaking.

malpractice: Incorrect or negligent treatment by a professional.

managed care: Refers to a cost containment system that directs the utilization of health benefits by (a) restricting the type, level, and frequency of treatment; (b) limiting access to care; and (c) controlling the level of reimbursement for services.

mandible: The bone of the lower jaw.

margin: The junction where the provisional meets the tooth structure.

Maryland bridge: A type of fixed partial denture that does not require crowns, but may require a minimally invasive preparation to the lingual aspect of the adjacent teeth; also known as a *resin-bonded bridge.* The wings of the prosthesis are bonded to the lingual surfaces of adjacent natural teeth.

masseter: The principal muscle of mastication that closes the mouth.

mastication: The act of chewing.

masticatory mucosa: A dense thick mucosa that is designed to withstand the trauma of chewing; it covers the hard palate, tongue, and gum tissue.

Material Safety Data Sheet (MSDS): Written document that provides comprehensive information about a chemical and information about how to contact its manufacturer.

matrix: The binding substance that holds filler particles together, especially in a composite resin.

matrix band: Strip or band placed so as to serve as a retaining outer wall that supports the tooth restoration to recreate proper form and function.

matrix system: The device used to help the dentist restore anatomic contours and proximal contact to the proximal tooth.

maxilla: Two bones that form the upper jaw.

maxillary tuberosity: A rounded prominence of bone located posterior to the maxillary molars.

mechanical bruxism: Excessive grinding of the teeth.

mentalis: Muscle of the chin that protrudes the lower lip and wrinkles the skin.

mesial: Surface of tooth toward the midline.

mesioclusion: Term used to describe a Class III occlusion, in which the mesiobuccal cusp of the maxillary first molar is distal to the mesiobuccal groove of the mandibular first molar.

microbiology: The study of living organisms too small to be seen without a microscope.

midsagittal plane: A horizontal line perpendicular (at a right angle) to the floor. This line divides the body into two equal parts: right and left halves.

milled restoration: A precision-cut piece of ceramic that fits a die for a crown, inlay, or onlay.

milliampere (mA): A unit of measurement used to determine the amount of electrical current; 1 mA is equal to 1/1,000 of an ampere.

minerals: Found in the earth's crust and also used like vitamins for body functions.

mini implant: A threaded implant placed using minimally invasive microsurgery for long-term denture stabilization.

mixed dentition: Mixture of permanent and primary teeth present in the mouth at same time; exists until all primary teeth fall out.

model trimmer: A machine used to grind and contour gypsum cast models.

modified wave scheduling: A schedule based on the same appointment time increments as a wave schedule, but the patients are set up with two or more appointments at once and then only one patient is scheduled for the next appointment slot.

motion economy: Refers to the manner in which a person can conserve energy while performing a task.

mucoperiosteum: Membrane that is formed by the combination of the mucosal and periosteal surfaces.

multiple sclerosis: Progressive weakening of the muscles due to nerve damage.

muscular dystrophy: A group of diseases marked by progressive atrophy or a wasting away of the muscle tissue.

musculoskeletal disorders (MSDs): Painful disorders that affect the muscles and bones of the neck, the shoulders, and back. Carpal tunnel syndrome is an example of this type of disorder.

mutans streptococci: Bacteria with significant potential to cause dental caries.

myelin sheath: Protective, insulated covering that surrounds some nerves.

Mylar: A trademarked, thin polyester film.

myocardial infarction: Heart attack or death of a heart muscle.

myocardium: Middle layer (muscular wall) of the heart.

National Children's Dental Health Month: Initiated by the American Dental Association to observe children's dental health; occurs during the month of February each year.

National Provider Identifier (NPI): An identifier assigned by the federal government to all providers considered to be HIPAA-covered entities.

necrotic pulp: Nonvital pulp that is dead and gangrenous.

negligence: Failure to use a standard of care that a reasonable person would apply under related situations.

net salary: The amount of pay after deductions have been taken out; also called *take-home pay.*

nitrous oxide: An inhaled flammable anesthetic and analgesic gas.

noncritical items: Items that come in contact with intact skin only.

nonverbal communication: Communicating through body language and facial expressions.

nonvital tooth: Tooth in which the pulp tissue is diseased or dead.

nucleus: Control center portion of a cell that is responsible for growth, repair, and reproduction of cells.

nutrients: Obtained from food and used by the body for various daily functions.

obesity: Condition of a person who is 20% over the desired weight for height and build.

objective evaluation: Portion of dental examination that consists of any observations regarding the patient made by members of the dental team.

objective fears: Experiences and traumatic memories from prior treatments that may not have been positive; contrast with *subjective fears.*

obturate: To fill the root canals of a tooth.

obturator: Constructed prosthetic device designed to close a congenital or acquired opening in the palate.

occlusal: Chewing surface of the posterior (back) teeth located on the molars and bicuspids.

occlusal film: Intraoral film used to examine large areas of the upper or lower jaws.

odontoblasts: Dentin-forming cells.

odontogenesis: Tooth production; the origin and formation of the tooth.

onlay: A cast or milled restoration designed to cover the occlusal surface of at least one cusp of a posterior tooth; used to restore a decayed or broken tooth.

open bay: A room arrangement in which the dental chairs are placed in one large room with no structural walls between the chairs.

operating procedure manual: Office manual that contains written directions for completing particular functions or tasks.

operative dentistry: Common term for restorative or aesthetic dentistry that restores decayed or defective teeth to proper form and function.

operator's zone: The location the person performing the procedure operates within. Based on the clock concept, the right-handed operator is positioned at and performs in the zone from 7 to 12 o'clock; the left-handed operator does so in the zone from 12 to 5 o'clock.

opportunistic infection: An infection that is normally caused by a nonpathogenic organism in people with weakened immune systems.

oral and maxillofacial surgeon: A dentist who specializes in the treatment of the entire facial structure due to injury or disease.

oral evacuation: Process of removing excess fluids, saliva, blood, or debris from the oral cavity during operative dental procedures.

oral pathologist: A dentist who specializes in examining tissue samples to provide proper diagnosis and treatment of biopsy results.

organelle: Special component of a cell that performs a particular function for the cell.

origin: The fixed attachment of a muscle.

orthodontist: A dentist who corrects malocclusions by realignment of the teeth and/or joints.

osseointegration: A biological bonding process that fuses healthy bone to a metallic implant, usually titanium.

osteoblasts: Cells responsible for forming bone.

osteoclasts: Cells responsible for destroying bone.

osteonecrosis: Bone death resulting from poor blood supply to an area of bone.

other potentially infectious materials (OPIM): Items that have been in contact with fluids and tissues designated by the Centers for Disease Control and Prevention as possibly capable of spreading disease.

Otto Walkoff: German dentist credited with taking the first x-rays of teeth in 1896.

outline form: The shape of the area of a cavity preparation.

overbite: A vertical overlap of the maxillary teeth with the mandibular arch.

overdenture: Denture base that rests on the endodontically retained prepared teeth or on an implant instead of the tissue and bone.

overhead: The cost of running a business.

overjet: A horizontal overlap of the maxillary teeth with the mandibular arch.

overlapping: A horizontal angulation error that occurs when the x-ray beam is not at 90 degrees to the tooth and film, and images from two adjacent structures are superimposed on top of each other.

pain: Defined by the International Association for the Study of Pain as "an unpleasant sensory and emotional experience associated with actual or potential tissue damage, or described in terms of such damage."

palate: The roof of the mouth.

palladium (Pd): A soft, silver-white, tarnish-resistant, naturally occurring metal related to platinum; considered a precious metal.

palpation: Process of examining by applying the hands or fingers to the external surface of the body to detect evidence of disease or abnormalities.

panoramic radiograph: An extraoral film that shows a wide view of both upper and lower jaws on one radiograph.

papoose board: A restraint used for the safety of children.

paralleling technique: Method of exposing periapical radiographs in which the long axis of the tooth and the film are situated parallel with each other and the position-indicating device is directed at the center of the film and tooth at a 90-degree angle, or perpendicular, as directed by the locator ring.

parietal: Pertaining to the walls of a body cavity.

partial denture: Dental prosthesis that replaces one or more missing teeth in an arch or arches where at least one natural tooth remains.

passive immunity: Immunity from an outside source that lasts for a short time.

patent drugs: Drugs that can be obtained without a prescription; referred to as over-the-counter drugs.

pathogenic: Disease producing.

pathogens: Microorganisms that are capable of causing disease.

pedodontist: A dentist who specializes in dental treatment for children.

pegboard system: A manual, handwritten book-keeping system; sometimes called the "write it once" system.

pellicle: A thin layer of salivary proteins coating the surface of the teeth.

penicillin: The first antibiotic.

percussion: Gentle tapping on the crown of the tooth.

periapical abscess: Infection from within the tooth that spreads out through the apex and into the surrounding bone.

periapical radiograph: Radiograph that shows the desired teeth and the surrounding areas including the apices.

pericardium: Fibrous (double-walled) sac that surrounds the heart.

periodontal debridement: The removal of calculus, plaque, and its by-products from the coronal and root surfaces and tissue wall and pocket to promote healing.

periodontal pocket: A sulcus that has deepened beyond three millimeters due to some type of pathology.

periodontal probe: An instrument that is demarcated at specific units of measurement and is used to determine the depth of the periodontal sulcus or pocket.

periodontist: A dentist who specializes in the treatment of the surrounding structures that support the teeth due to injury or disease.

periodontitis: Inflammation of the periodontium that involves loss of supporting bone.

periodontium: Soft and bony supporting structure of tissues that surrounds the teeth.

periosteum: Tough, fibrous lining that covers the compact coronal bone.

permanent dentition: Second set or succedaneous teeth.

perpendicular: Intersecting at or forming a right angle, or a 90-degree angle, to the tooth and film packet, creating a corner (the opposite of parallel).

personal protective equipment (PPE): Protective clothing, masks, gloves, and eyewear used to protect health care workers from exposure to bloodborne and airborne pathogens.

petit mal seizure: Short-term seizure characterized by a blank stare or eye twitch; also known as *absence seizures*.

pharmacokinetics: The study of how drugs enter the body, circulate throughout, and exit the body.

pharmacology: The study of drugs.

pharynx: Passageway for air and food.

philtrum: A vertical groove between the nose and upper lip.

phobia: Exaggerated internal fears held by people.

photon: Small bundle of pure energy that has no mass or weight.

Pierre Fauchard: Known as the "father of modern dentistry."

pit: A small pinpoint depression on the surface of a tooth that is caused by the failure of the union of the developmental grooves.

plaque: A sticky, usually tooth-colored film on teeth that is formed by and harbors bacteria and their by-products; also known as a *biofilm*.

platinum (Pt): A silver-white precious metal that does not corrode in air.

polymerization: A chemical process that causes two materials to harden together, as in the setting of a dental sealant.

pontic: An artificial tooth on a fixed partial denture or bridge.

porcelain-fused-to-metal crown (PFM): An indirect restoration in which porcelain is fused to the external surfaces of a casting to imitate the appearance of natural tooth structure; usually provides full coverage.

position-indicating device (PID): A cylinder (or cone) affixed to the tube head that is used to align the x-ray with the film in the patient's mouth.

posterior: The back of the mouth.

postural hypotension: Insufficient blood flow to the brain as a result of a position change.

preceptorship: Studying and training for a field under the guidance of a professional already practicing in the field.

preferred provider organization (PPO) plan: An insurance plan in which a purchaser of dental benefits receives services from certain dentists (i.e., preferred providers) who provide those services at specified rates that have been agreed on with the insurance company.

primary dentin: Dentin formed prior to tooth eruption.

primary dentition: First set of 20 teeth; also called deciduous or baby teeth.

primary radiation: Initial radiation produced at the tungsten target that exits the tube head.

proliferation: Production of new parts; the bud and early cap stages of tooth development.

prophylaxis: Complete removal of all stain, debris, and calculus.

prostheses: Artificial replacements for teeth and other oral structures.

prosthodontist: A dental specialist whose practice is limited to the restoration of the natural teeth and/or the replacement of missing teeth with artificial substitutes.

proteins: Nutrients used for muscle tissue construction and repair; come from sources such as meat, eggs, and nuts.

provisional: A temporary crown or bridge that is made to cover and protect a prepared tooth or teeth while the permanent prosthesis is being fabricated.

proximal: Place where a tooth contacts its neighbor in the same arch.

public health dental official: Provides dental health care on county, state, and national levels by providing education and demonstration of proper oral hygiene instruction to elementary schools, high schools, businesses, and the general population/community.

pulmonary disorders: Problems that involve the lungs and the breathing process.

pulp: Tissue composed of blood and lymph vessels, nerve and connective tissues, and odontoblasts.

pulpal wall: The internal surface of a cavity preparation positioned perpendicular to the pulp of the tooth; the floor of the preparation.

pulpectomy: Complete removal of all pulp tissues.

pulpitis: Inflammation of the tooth pulp.

pulpotomy: Removal of pulp tissue in the crown portion only.

quadrant: One-fourth of the mouth.

radial: Pertaining to the bone of the forearm.

radiograph: A one-dimensional view of a three-dimensional subject; a film after it has been exposed to x-rays and developed to show images on a film; also known as *x-ray* or *film*.

radiolucent areas: Dark portions of a radiograph that represent soft tissues (for example, dental pulp) that allow x-rays to pass through; space and air are also radiolucent.

radiopaque areas: Light or white portions of a radiograph that represent areas of dense tissue that absorb x-rays, not allowing them to pass through; examples include enamel, dentin, bone, and various metal restorations.

rampant caries: Quickly developing decay apparent throughout the mouth.

receiver: The recipient of the intended message.

recession: Apical migration of the gingival margin leading to exposure of the cementoenamel junction.

reciprocity: Allows an individual to transfer licensure, with the same rights, from one state to another without having to retake licensure exams.

recommendation: Official public or private agency statement of the best way to comply with a regulation.

regulated waste: Infectious, sharp, or hazardous waste.

regulation: Official government agency rule that must be followed.

reline: Process to improve the internal fit of a dental prosthesis (full, partial, or overdenture) by resurfacing the tissue side of the prosthesis.

remineralization: The restoring of minerals to tooth structure.

reorder point: The point that determines when a supply will be reordered based on lead time and the supply's rate of use.

res gestae: Statements made at the time of an alleged negligent act that are admissible in court as evidence.

res ipsa loquitur: "The act speaks for itself" (Latin). The cause is obvious.

resorption: Process that causes portions of the alveolar ridge to shrink.

respondeat superior: "The master answers" (Latin). The employer is responsible for all employee actions.

restoration: Measures taken to return a defective tooth to proper form and function with the use of a dental material.

restorative dentistry: Area of dentistry that restores decayed or defective teeth to proper form and function; an area of operative dentistry.

rests: Element of a removable partial denture that makes contact with a tooth to provide vertical and horizontal support.

résumé: A summary of one's work experience and qualifications.

retainer: An orthodontic appliance used after orthodontic treatment to maintain teeth in their desired position.

retention: Ability of a dental sealant to adhere to the tooth structure.

retention form: The shape of a cavity preparation; designed to prevent displacement of the dental material.

reversible pulpitis: Condition in which inflamed tooth pulp is able to respond to treatment.

rheostat: Foot-controlled or pedal device that is used to operate and control the dental handpieces.

risk management: Actions implemented to minimize legal risks to the dental practice.

root planing: Procedure that removes cementum or surface dentin that may contain calculus, is rough, or is contaminated with toxins or microorganisms.

root surface caries: Decay found on the root surfaces of teeth.

saliva ejector: Device used to remove fluids such as small amounts of saliva or water from a patient's mouth; also known as a *low-volume evacuator.*

salutation: Formal greeting to a reader.

sarcoma: Malignant neoplasm beginning in supportive and connective tissue such as bones.

scaling: The removal of biofilm, calculus, and stains from the crowns and roots of teeth.

scatter radiation: A form of secondary radiation that occurs once the primary beam has interacted with matter and then is deflected off in a different direction.

secondary dentin: Dentin formed after tooth eruption that remains for the life of the tooth.

secondary radiation: Occurs when the primary beam comes in contact with and passes through any type of matter.

sectional matrix: Small kidney bean–shaped matrix that is held in place by a spring-loaded ring to create natural contacts and profile. The Palodent sectional matrix system is an example.

sedative: A material that has a soothing effect on the patient.

self-curing process: The hardening or setting process when two chemical materials are mixed.

semicritical items: Items that come in contact with tissues, but do not penetrate soft tissue or bone.

sender: The individual who is communicating a message to another person (the receiver).

shelf life: The time a product can be stored before it is no longer usable.

sialolith: A stone in a salivary duct.

slime layer: A matrix produced by some bacteria from their cell walls.

smear layer: A very thin layer of debris on newly prepared dentin.

sol: A viscous liquid whose particles become attached to each other, forming a loose mass.

space maintainers: Appliance placed in the dental arch to prevent adjacent teeth from moving into space left by a missing tooth.

sphygmomanometer: Instrument used to take blood pressure readings; also known as the blood pressure cuff.

spore: Layers of protective membranes formed by some bacteria.

squamous cell carcinoma: Malignant lesion that metastasizes (travels) into surrounding tissues or into the lymph nodes of the body.

standard: Official government agency statement of the regulations governing a specified issue.

standard precautions: A standard of care that protects health care workers from pathogens that are spread by blood and other potentially infectious material.

static zone: The area above or behind the reclined patient. Based on the clock concept, that would be from 12 to 2 o'clock for a right-handed operator and from 10 to 12 o'clock for a left-handed operator.

stent: A sterile, clear acrylic template positioned over the alveolar ridge that enables the location of the exact position of a dental implant; any material used to make a mold of an original contour.

sterilization: A process that kills all living microorganisms; the ability to destroy all living organisms and endospores.

stomodeum: A primitive mouth.

straight attachment: The nose cone connection for a slow-speed handpiece.

Streptococcus mutans: The primary bacteria found in dental plaque.

stroke (cerebrovascular accident): A bleeding lesion or a tear in the brain.

subgingival: Below the gingival tissues.

subjective evaluation: Portion of the dental examination that consists of the patient's observations about why the patient decided to visit the dentist.

subjective fears: Fears that come from stories told by friends and families; contrast with *objective fears.*

subperiosteal implant: Implant that is placed on top of alveolar bone with abutment posts or bars rising above the mucoperiosteum; used primarily when the alveolar bone has atrophied (wasted away), usually as a result of a failed or poorly fitting denture.

subsupine position: Position in which patient is reclined in the dental chair with the patient's head positioned lower than the feet. This position is also called the *Trendelenburg position.*

succedaneous teeth: Permanent teeth that replace primary teeth.

sulcus: Space between the tooth and the free gingiva.

supernumerary teeth: Extra teeth.

supine position: Position in which patient is reclined in the dental chair with the patient's nose and knees at the same level.

suppuration: The formation of pus; often in the gingival sulcus related to inflammation.

supragingival: Above the gingival tissues.

suture: An immovable line of union between two bones.

syncope: Loss of consciousness or fainting.

syneresis: The process of contracting and shrinking with time as a result of losing water.

systemic fluoride: Fluoride that is delivered to the tooth via the body's bloodstream.

systolic: The top number of a blood pressure reading; represents the force of the heart as it contracts.

tachycardia: A fast heart rate.

T-bands: A retainer free matrix made of brass; commonly used on primary teeth.

temporomandibular joint: The encapsulated synovial joint between the temporal bone of the skull and the condyle of the mandible.

tertiary dentin: A reparative dentin that forms in response to injury or irritation.

tetanus: Disease caused by bacteria often found in soil; the bacteria often enter the body via a wound in the skin.

time-related sterilization: Type of sterilization in which the shelf life of instruments is identified with an exact expiration date.

titanium: Type of metal that is most compatible with human tissues and bone.

Tofflemire retainer: Mechanism that holds the matrix band in position; also known as a *universal retainer.*

topical fluoride: Fluoride treatment that is applied to the surface of tooth enamel.

tori: Oral maxillary, mandibular, or palatal bone growths projecting outward from the surface.

tort: Intentional or unintentional act that causes harm.

trade name: Name given to a drug by the particular manufacturer that sells the drug.

tragus: The prominence of fleshy tissue located toward the middle opening of the ear.

transfer zone: The area through which materials and instruments are passed. This area is across the patient's chest. Based on the clock concept, for a right-handed operator this would be in the zone from 4 to 7 o'clock and for a left-handed operator in the zone from 5 to 8 o'clock.

transosteal implant: Implant that is inserted through the mandible from the inferior border.

traumatic intrusion: Tooth forcibly driven into the alveolus with only a part of the crown visible.

traumatic occlusion: An occlusion that does not properly articulate, causing additional pressure to a specific area of a tooth and causing the pulp to feel "bruised."

triturate: The mechanical combination of dental materials.

trituration: The mixing of alloy with mercury to form amalgam.

tuberculosis: A bacterial infection that affects the lungs.

tungsten target: Portion of the anode struck by electrons (focal spot).

ultrasonic cleaner: Cleaning system that loosens and removes debris by the use of sound waves in a liquid.

unfilled resins: Sealant material that does not contain filler particles.

unit dose concept: Prevents contamination of bulk supplies by dispensing only enough to complete the procedure.

universal precautions: Precautions used to protect patients and health care workers from coming into contact with contaminated body fluids.

universal retainer: Mechanism that holds the matrix band in position; also known as a *Tofflemire retainer*.

upcoding: Reporting a higher level of dental service than was actually performed.

upright position: Position in which patient is seated with the dental chair back at a 90-degree angle. This position is used for patient entry and release from the dental chair.

upward channel communication: Channel of communication that originates from a lower level employee in an organization and travels to an upper level employee.

uvula: A fold of mucous membrane attached to the back of the soft palate.

variable expenses: Those expenses that change from month to month.

vasoconstrictor: Type of drug that constricts blood vessels; used to prolong anesthetic action and to control bleeding.

veneer: Ultrathin layer of composite resin or porcelain bonded to the facial surface of teeth.

ventricle: Lower chamber of each half of the heart.

vermilion border: Transitional area between the skin of the face and mucous membrane of the lip.

vertical angulation: Proper alignment of the position-indicating device in an up-and-down direction.

vertical dimension: The space occupied by the height of the teeth in relaxed and normal occlusion.

viruses: The smallest microorganisms.

visceral: Pertaining to the internal organs or the covering of the internal organs.

viscosity: The property of a material that causes it to flow or not flow easily; the resistance of a material to flow.

vital tooth: Alive or healthy pulp tissue.

vitamins: Nutrients derived from natural sources such as plants; they are needed for healthy body functioning and prevention of diseases.

waiting period: Period between employment or enrollment in a dental plan and the date when a covered person becomes eligible for benefits. Services subject to a waiting period could include any services related to placing crowns, bridges, or orthodontics.

walk-out statement: A receipt that shows the amount the patient paid and also the current balance if money is owed to the practice.

washer/disinfector: Automatic cleaning system designed to clean and disinfect instruments using a high-temperature cycle.

wave scheduling: A scheduling system in which each appointment is allotted an average amount of time, and each patient is given the number of appointment slots that would be required to finish a necessary procedure based on average time required for that particular procedure.

wavelength: Distance between the crests or high point of the radiation waves.

wedge: Wood or plastic, usually triangular or anatomic apparatus placed in the embrasure space to secure the matrix to the tooth and provide the proper contour for restoring a Class II cavity.

wettability: The capacity of a material to flow over a surface and capture all irregularities.

whitening: Process of brightening stained, discolored teeth with in-office or at-home systems.

Wilhelm Conrad Roentgen: German physicist who discovered radiographs (x-rays) in 1895.

written consent: A written document signed by the patient that provides consent to receive treatment.

xerostomia: Dryness of the mouth caused by an abnormal reduction in salivary secretion.

x-radiation (x-ray): High-energy ionizing electromagnetic radiation.

zygomatic: Pertaining to the cheekbone.

zygote: The first stage in embryonic development.

Index

I-1

cultural diversity, 833–834, 834t, 843
dental office procedure manual, 842
dental team members, dealing with, 831–833, 831f, 832f, 843
Internet activity, 844
listening skills, 830–831, 831f
nonverbal communication, 830, 843
office equipment, 837, 837f
phone skills, 834–837, 835f, 836f
verbal communication, 827–830, 828f, 828t, 829t, 843
Web references, 844
written communication, 838–842, 839t, 840–842f, 843
Community dental health programs, 8–9, 8f
Compact bone tissue (cortical bone), 43, 43f, 69
Complete (full) dentures
components of, 663, 663f, 665
considerations and indications for, 662
explained, 658, 665
purpose of, 661–662
Complete mouth rinse, 398, 411
Complete proteins, 244
Complex cavities, 130
Compliance, explained, 272–273, 280
Complications, postsurgical, 744, 745
Composite resins
advantages and disadvantages, 256f, 526–527
cement, 551t, 556, 556f, 557, 557t, 559
coupling agent, 527
curing lights, 528
explained, 524, 535
fillers, 527, 535
finishing and polishing, 528, 530
forms of, 527, 528f
instruments for, 365, 365f
order of application, 539t
preparing, placing, curing, and finishing, procedure for, 529
resin matrix, 527, 535
tooth preparation, 527
Compound, dental, 594
Compound cavities, 130
Comprehensive examinations
comprehensive oral exams, 318, 326
medical conditions, discovering, 320
Compressive stress, 521, 521f
Computed tomography (CT), 515
Computer-controlled local anesthesia delivery system, 428–429
Computerized system of accounts receivable, 867–868, 868f
Computers in the dental office
appointment scheduling, 855, 856f
future of, 848
hardware and software, 847–848, 847f, 848f
record storage, 302
safety, 848, 848f, 861
Concrescence of teeth, 159
Condensation silicone impression materials, 570
Condensers, 363, 364f
Cone cut error, 488, 503
Confi-Dental, 543
Confidentiality
e-mail, 842
patient records, 306–309, 308f, 309f, 326
principle of, 26–27, 28
Conflict in the workplace, 832–833
Congenital conditions
developmental disorders, 157
missing teeth, 782

Congestive heart failure, 337
Connective tissue, 37, 38f
Connective tissue grafts, 710
Connectors for partial dentures, 660f, 660–661, 661f, 665
Consent, implied, 24
Consent, informed. See Informed consent
Consolidated Omnibus Budget Reconciliation Act (COBRA) of 1985, 888
Consultation appointments, 659
Consultation rooms, 293, 303
Consulting industry, career opportunities in, 904
Consumer-Patient Radiation Health and Safety Act, 467
Contaminated waste, 199, 276, 280
Contour, explained, 645, 654
Contra-angle attachments for handpieces, 369, 369f, 376
Contra-angle retainers, 615f, 616
Contracts, explained, 24, 28
Contrast on radiographs, 453
Control panels of dental x-ray units, 445, 447f
Controlled Substances Act, 417, 417t
Convalescent stage of infections, 178
Convulsive phase of seizures, 821
Coon ligature-tying pliers, 789–790, 790f
Coordination of benefits, 889
Copay, explained, 886, 899
Copper in amalgam, 523
Corded direct sensors, 515, 515f
Core buildup, 632–633, 641
Coronal (frontal) plane, 32, 34f, 35f
Coronal polishing, 763–772
aesthetic restorations, 764–765
dental assistant expanded function, 12
dental stains, 765–766, 765f, 766t, 771
evaluation of, 770
explained, 764, 771
indications and contraindications, 764
Internet activity, 772
materials and equipment, 766–768, 766f, 767f, 768f, 771
pediatric patients, 753–754
procedure for, 769–770
selective polishing, 764
sequence of, 768–770
steps in, 767–770, 768f
Web references, 772
Coronal portion of tooth, 756, 761
Coronary artery disease, 50
Corrective (interceptive) orthodontics, 783–784, 805
Corrosion control for instruments, 259
Cortical bone (compact bone tissue), 43, 43f, 69
Cotton pliers, 360–361, 361f
Cotton roll isolation, 398–400, 399f, 400f
Coulombs per kilogram (C/kg) unit of radiation measurement, 449
Council on Dental Education of the ADA, 718
Coupling agents for composite resins, 527
Cover letters
explained, 906, 915
preparing, procedure for, 910
sample of, 909f
tips for, 907
Coverage, provisional, for crowns, 636–637
CPR. See Cardiopulmonary resuscitation (CPR)
CRA (Clinical Research Associates) Foundation, 273–274, 274t

Cranial bones
ethmoid bone, 74f, 74t, 75, 76f
frontal bone, 74, 74f, 74t, 76f, 91
function of, 73
occipital bone, 74f, 74t, 75
parietal bone, 74, 74f, 74t, 76f, 91
sphenoid bone, 74–75, 74f, 74t, 76f
temporal bones, 74, 74f, 74t, 91
Cranial nerves
explained, 55, 55t
head and neck anatomy, 87–88, 88f, 89f
Cranial Nerves Web site, 92
Crash carts, 813
Credentialing for dental assistants, 14–15
Credit slips, 859, 859f, 861
Crepitus, 79, 91, 321, 326, 718, 745
Crest Oral B Patient Education Web site, 239
Creutzfeldt-Jakob (mad cow) disease, 200
Criminal law, 24, 28
Critical items, explained, 254, 254t, 269
Critical organs, radiation effects on, 449
Crohn's disease, 60t
Crookes, William, 444
Crookes-Hittorf cathode tubes, 444, 444f
Cross bite, 783
Cross-training in the dental office, 18
Crowding of teeth, 782
Crown and bridge scissors, 366, 366f
Crown lengthening surgery, 712–713, 712f
Crowns
assisting with, procedure for, 638
cementation appointment, 637
final impression and bit registration, 636
fixed prosthodontics, 630, 630f, 631f, 641
gingival retraction cords, placing and removing, 635–636
preparation, 632
procedure for, overview of, 632–637, 632f, 633f, 634f, 641
provisional coverage, 636–637
retention for, 632–633, 633f, 641
retraction, types of, 633–634, 634f
shade selection, 632, 632f
stainless steel, 756–757, 758–759
tissue management, 633–636, 634f
Cryer elevators, 721f
CT (computed tomography), 515
Cueria, Malvina, 7
Cultural Considerations
amalgam, lawful use of, 600
apprehensions, relieving, 344
beliefs and health care practices, 217
bilingual dental assistants, 739
children from other cultures, 750
cleft palate and lip occurrence rate, 106
communication with patients, 411
communication with patients of other cultures, 834
crown aesthetics, cultural definitions of, 631
demonstration for non-English speaking patients, 470
dental anxiety, 434
dental implants, language barriers regarding, 673
dental insurance, 888
dental restorations as cultural statements, 533
dental sealants, importance of, 775
dental tourism, 334
dental work in foreign countries, 856
diet and dental hygiene, 211
disease transmission, 178

Pearson Education, Inc.

YOU SHOULD CAREFULLY READ THE TERMS AND CONDITIONS BEFORE USING THE CD-ROM PACKAGE. USING THIS CD-ROM PACKAGE INDICATES YOUR ACCEPTANCE OF THESE TERMS AND CONDITIONS.

Pearson Education, Inc. provides this program and licenses its use. You assume responsibility for the selection of the program to achieve your intended results, and for the installation, use, and results obtained from the program. This license extends only to use of the program in the United States or countries in which the program is marketed by authorized distributors.

LICENSE GRANT

You hereby accept a nonexclusive, nontransferable, permanent license to install and use the program ON A SINGLE COMPUTER at any given time. You may copy the program solely for backup or archival purposes in support of your use of the program on the single computer. You may not modify, translate, disassemble, decompile, or reverse engineer the program, in whole or in part.

TERM

The License is effective until terminated. Pearson Education, Inc. reserves the right to terminate this License automatically if any provision of the License is violated. You may terminate the License at any time. To terminate this License, you must return the program, including documentation, along with a written warranty stating that all copies in your possession have been returned or destroyed.

LIMITED WARRANTY

THE PROGRAM IS PROVIDED "AS IS" WITHOUT WARRANTY OF ANY KIND, EITHER EXPRESSED OR IMPLIED, INCLUDING, BUT NOT LIMITED TO, THE IMPLIED WARRANTIES OR MERCHANTABILITY AND FITNESS FOR A PARTICULAR PURPOSE. THE ENTIRE RISK AS TO THE QUALITY AND PERFORMANCE OF THE PROGRAM IS WITH YOU. SHOULD THE PROGRAM PROVE DEFECTIVE, YOU (AND NOT PRENTICE-HALL, INC. OR ANY AUTHORIZED DEALER) ASSUME THE ENTIRE COST OF ALL NECESSARY SERVICING, REPAIR, OR CORRECTION. NO ORAL OR WRITTEN INFORMATION OR ADVICE GIVEN BY PRENTICE-HALL, INC., ITS DEALERS, DISTRIBUTORS, OR AGENTS SHALL CREATE A WARRANTY OR INCREASE THE SCOPE OF THIS WARRANTY.

SOME STATES DO NOT ALLOW THE EXCLUSION OF IMPLIED WARRANTIES, SO THE ABOVE EXCLUSION MAY NOT APPLY TO YOU. THIS WARRANTY GIVES YOU SPECIFIC LEGAL RIGHTS AND YOU MAY ALSO HAVE OTHER LEGAL RIGHTS THAT VARY FROM STATE TO STATE.

Pearson Education, Inc. does not warrant that the functions contained in the program will meet your requirements or that the operation of the program will be uninterrupted or error-free.

However, Pearson Education, Inc. warrants the diskette(s) or CD-ROM(s) on which the program is furnished to be free from defects in material and workmanship under normal use for a period of ninety (90) days from the date of delivery to you as evidenced by a copy of your receipt.

The program should not be relied on as the sole basis to solve a problem whose incorrect solution could result in injury to person or property. If the program is employed in such a manner, it is at the user's own risk and Pearson Education, Inc. explicitly disclaims all liability for such misuse.

LIMITATION OF REMEDIES

Pearson Education, Inc.'s entire liability and your exclusive remedy shall be:

1. the replacement of any diskette(s) or CD-ROM(s) not meeting Pearson Education, Inc.'s "LIMITED WARRANTY" and that is returned to Pearson Education, or

2. if Pearson Education is unable to deliver a replacement diskette(s) or CD-ROM(s) that is free of defects in materials or workmanship, you may terminate this agreement by returning the program.

IN NO EVENT WILL PRENTICE-HALL, INC. BE LIABLE TO YOU FOR ANY DAMAGES, INCLUDING ANY LOST PROFITS, LOST SAVINGS, OR OTHER INCIDENTAL OR CONSEQUENTIAL DAMAGES ARISING OUT OF THE USE OR INABILITY TO USE SUCH PROGRAM EVEN IF PRENTICE-HALL, INC. OR AN AUTHORIZED DISTRIBUTOR HAS BEEN ADVISED OF THE POSSIBILITY OF SUCH DAMAGES, OR FOR ANY CLAIM BY ANY OTHER PARTY.

SOME STATES DO NOT ALLOW FOR THE LIMITATION OR EXCLUSION OF LIABILITY FOR INCIDENTAL OR CONSEQUENTIAL DAMAGES, SO THE ABOVE LIMITATION OR EXCLUSION MAY NOT APPLY TO YOU.

GENERAL

You may not sublicense, assign, or transfer the license of the program. Any attempt to sublicense, assign or transfer any of the rights, duties, or obligations hereunder is void.

This Agreement will be governed by the laws of the State of New York.

Should you have any questions concerning this Agreement, you may contact Pearson Education, Inc. by writing to:

Director of New Media
Higher Education Division
Pearson Education, Inc.
One Lake Street
Upper Saddle River, NJ 07458

Should you have any questions concerning technical support, you may contact:

Product Support Department: Monday–Friday 8:00 A.M. –8:00 P.M. and Sunday 5:00 P.M.-12:00 A.M. (All times listed are Eastern). 1-800-677-6337

You can also get support by filling out the web form located at http://247.prenhall.com

YOU ACKNOWLEDGE THAT YOU HAVE READ THIS AGREEMENT, UNDERSTAND IT, AND AGREE TO BE BOUND BY ITS TERMS AND CONDITIONS. YOU FURTHER AGREE THAT IT IS THE COMPLETE AND EXCLUSIVE STATEMENT OF THE AGREEMENT BETWEEN US THAT SUPERSEDES ANY PROPOSAL OR PRIOR AGREEMENT, ORAL OR WRITTEN, AND ANY OTHER COMMUNICATIONS BETWEEN US RELATING TO THE SUBJECT MATTER OF THIS AGREEMENT.